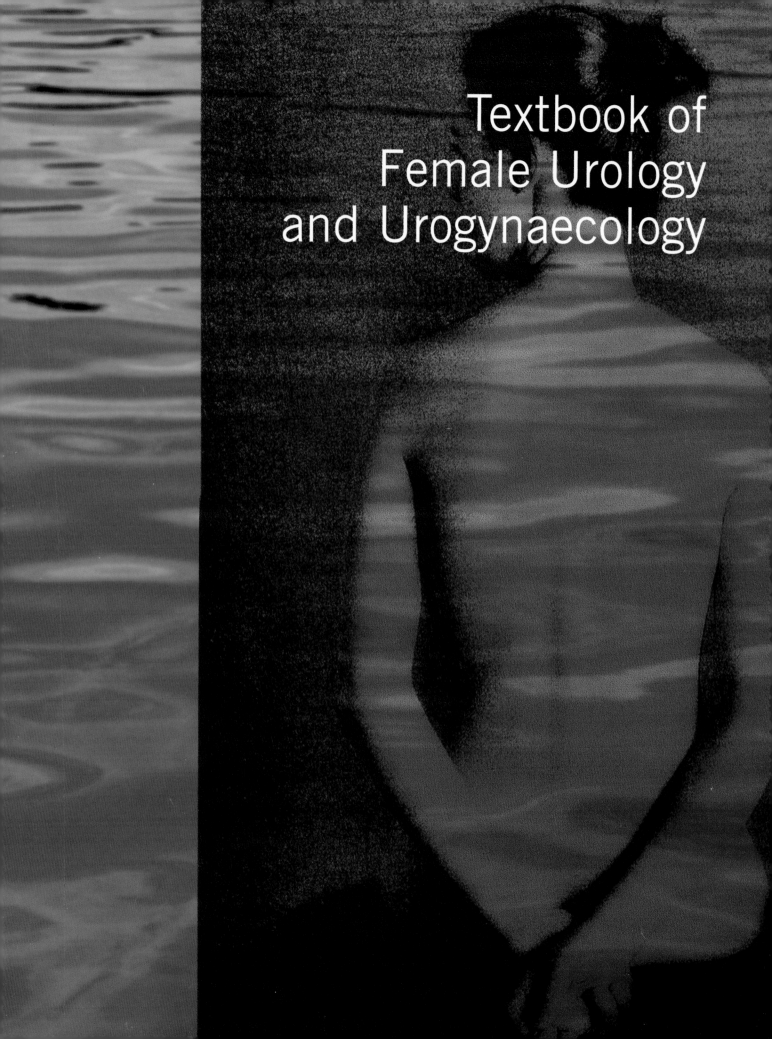

Textbook of
Female Urology
and Urogynaecology

Textbook of Female Urology and Urogynaecology

Edited by

Linda Cardozo MD FRCOG
Professor of Urogynaecology, King's College Hospital, London, UK

David Staskin MD
Director, Continence Center, Beth Israel Deaconess Medical Center
Assistant Professor of Surgery/Urology
Harvard Medical School, Boston, MA, USA

ISIS
MEDICAL
MEDIA

©2001 by Isis Medical Media Ltd, a member of the
Taylor & Francis group

First Published in the United Kingdom in 2001
by ISIS Medical Media, The Livery House,
7–9 Pratt Street, London NW1 0AE
Tel.: +44 (0) 20 74822202
Fax.: +44 (0) 20 72670159
E-mail: info.dunitz@tandf.co.uk
Website: http://www.dunitz.co.uk

Although every effort has been made to ensure that all owners of copyright material have been acknowledged in this publication,
we would be glad to acknowledge in subsequent reprints or editions any omissions brought to our attention.

The Authors have asserted their right under the Copyright, Designs and Patents Act 1988
to be identified as the Authors of this Work.

Although every effort has been made to ensure that drug doses and other information are presented accurately in this
publication, the ultimate responsibility rests with the prescribing physician. Neither the publishers nor the authors can be
held responsible for errors or for any consequences arising from the use of information contained herein.
For detailed prescribing information or instructions on the use of any product or procedure discussed herein,
please consult the prescribing information or instructional material issued by the manufacturer.

A CIP record for this book is available from the
British Library.

ISBN 1 901865 05 3

Distributed in the USA by
Fulfilment Center
Taylor & Francis
7625 Empire Drive
Florence, KY 41042, USA
Toll Free Tel.: +1 800 634 7064
E-mail: cserve@routledge_ny.com

Distributed in Canada by
Taylor & Francis
74 Rolark Drive
Scarborough, Ontario M1R 4G2, Canada
Toll Free Tel.: +1 877 226 2237
E-mail: tal_fran@istar.ca

Distributed in the rest of the world by
ITPS Limited
Cheriton House
North Way
Andover, Hampshire SP10 5BE, UK
Tel: +44 (0)1264 332424
E-mail: reception@itps.co.uk

Artwork by Adrian and Gudrun Cornford
Cover image courtesy of Science Photo Library (photographer, Cristina Pedrazzini)

Page layout and design by J&L Composition Ltd, Filey, North Yorkshire, UK
Image Reproduction by Expo Holdings Malaysia
Printed and bound by Imago China

Contents

**SECTION IV –
TREATMENT OF INCONTINENCE,
PROLAPSE AND RELATED CONDITIONS**

Contributors

Paul Abrams MD FRCS
Professor of Urology, Bristol Urological Institute, Southmead Hospital, Bristol, UK

Kate Anders
Urogynaecology Nurse Specialist, Urogynaecology Unit, King's College Hospital, Denmark Hill, London, UK

Karl-Erik Andersson MD PhD
Professor and Head, Department of Clinical Pharmacology, Lund University Hospital, Lund, Sweden

Rodney A. Appell MD FACS
Head, Section of Voiding Dysfunction and Female Urology, Department of Urology, The Cleveland Clinic Foundation, Cleveland, OH, USA

Christopher Benness MBBS MD FRCOG FRANZCOG CU
Urogynaecology Unit, Prince Alfred Hospital, Sydney, Australia

John Bidmead MBBS MRCOG
Research Fellow, Department of Urogynaecology, King's College Hospital, London, UK

Marc-Olivier Bitker
Professor of Urology, Hopital de la Pitié, Paris, France

Jerry G. Blaivas MD
Clinical Professor of Urology, Cornell Medical Center, UroCenter of New York, New York, NY, USA

Kari Bø PhD, PT, Exercise Scientist
Professor, Norwegian University of Sport and Physical Education, Oslo, Norway

Kelvin Boos MD BSc MRCOG MRCP
Department of Urogynaecology, King's College Hospital, Denmark Hill, London, UK

Alain P. Bourcier PT
Consultant Urodynamics, Department of Urology, Tenon Hospital; Director of Training Programme, Institut Français De Réadoptation Uro-Génitale, Paris, France

Linda Brubaker MD FACOG FACS
Professor and Director, Section of Urogynecology and Reconstructive Pelvic Surgery, Loyola University Medical Center, Maywood, IL, USA

Linda Cardozo MD FRCOG
Professor of Urogynaecology, Department of Urogynaecology, King's College Hospital, London, UK

David C. Chaikin MD
Clinical Assistant Professor, Department of Urology, Cornell Medical Center, New York, NY; Associate Attending Urologist, Morristown Memorial Hospital, Morristown, NJ, USA

Charlotte Chaliha MA MB Bchir MRCOG
Specialist Registrar, St George's Hospital, Urogynaecology Unit, Department of Obstetrics and Gynaecology, Cranmer Terrace, London, UK

Michael B. Chancellor MD
Director of Neurourology and Urinary Incontinence Programs, University of Pittsburgh School of Medicine, Pittsburgh, PA, USA

Christopher Chapple BSc MD FRCS (Urol)
Consultant Urological Surgeon, Department of Urology, Royal Hallamshire Hospital, Sheffield, UK

Rowan J. Connell
National Medical Laser Centre, Charles Bell House, London, UK

Geoffrey W. Cundiff MD FACOG
Associate Professor, Director of Division of Gynecological Specialties, Johns Hopkins Medicine, Baltimore, Maryland, USA

Alfred Cutner MD MRCOG
Consultant Gynaecologist, University College Hospital, London, UK

Helen Dallosso PhD
Research Fellow, Department of Epidemiology and Public Health, University of Leicester, Leicester, UK

John O. L. DeLancey MD
Norman F. Miller Professor of Gynecology and Associate Chair for Gynecology, Department of Obstetrics and Gynecology, University of Michigan Medical School, Ann Arbor, MI, USA

Ananias C. Diokno MD
Chief, Department of Urology, William Beaumont Hospital, Royal Oak, MI, USA

Roger R. Dmochowski MD FACS
Medical Director, North Texas Center for Urinary Control, Fort Worth, TX, USA

Richard W. Dover MRCPI MRCOG
Research Fellow, Royal Surrey County Hospital, Guildford, UK

Harold P. Drutz BA MD DRCS(C) FACOG FSOGC
Professor and Head, Section of Urogynecology, Department of Obstetrics and Gynecology, University of Toronto, Ontario, Canada

Keith Edmonds MB ChB FRCOG FRANZCOG
Consultant Gynaecologist, Queen Charlotte's and Chelsea Hospital, London, UK

J. Andrew Fantl MD
Women's Gynecologic Care, PC, Smithtown, NY, USA

Clare J. Fowler MBBS MSc FRCP
Reader and Consultant in Uro-Neurology, Department of Uro-Neurology, The National Hospital for Neurology and Neurosurgery, Queen Square, London, UK

Su Foxley
Continence Advisor, Optimum Health

Robert M. Freeman MD FRCOG
Consultant Obstetrician and Gynaecologist, Urogynaecology Unit, Directorate of Obstetrics and Gynaecology, Derriford Hospital, Plymouth, UK

Mimi L. Gallo RNC MSN CRNP
Adult Nurse Practitioner, Beth Israel Deaconess Medical Center, Boston, MA, USA

Roxane Gardner MD MPH
Instructor, Obstetrics, Gynecology and Reproductive Biology, Harvard Medical Center, Cambridge, MA, USA

Cheryle B. Gartley BSc
President and Founder, The Simon Foundation for Continence, Wilmette, IL, USA

H. Roger Hadley MD
Professor and Chairman, Division of Urology, Loma Linda University Medical Center, Loma Linda, CA, USA

Judy Haken
Continence Advisor, Optimum Health

Marie-Andrée Harvey MD
Research and Clinical Fellow, Division of Urogynecology, Department of Obstetrics and Gynecology, Brigham and Women's Hospital, Boston, MA, USA

Jean J. C. Hay-Smith MSc Dip Phys MNZCP
Lecturer, School of Physiotherapy, Division of Health Sciences, University of Otago, Dunedin, New Zealand

Bernard T. Haylen MD FRCOG FRANZCOG CU
Urogynaecologist, St Vincent's Hospital, Darlinghurst, Sydney, Australia

Sender Herschorn BSc MDCM FRCSC
Associate Professor Surgery/Urology, University of Toronto, Division of Urology, Sunnybrook and Women's Health Sciences Centre, Toronto, Ontario, Canada

Andrew Hextall MRCOG
Specialist Registrar in Urogynaecology, Department of Urogynaecology, King's College Hospital, Denmark Hill, London, UK

Paul Hilton MD FRCOG
Consultant Gynaecologist and Subspecialist in Urogynaecology, Directorate of Women's Services, Royal Victoria Infirmary, Queen Victoria Road, Newcastle upon Tyne, UK

Polly N. Hughes BSc MB ChB
Urogynaecology Research Fellow, Bristol Urological Institute and Department of Obstetrics and Gynaecology, Southmead Hospital, Bristol, UK

Gerry J. Jarvis MA FRCS FRCOG
Consultant Gynaecological Surgeon, St James's University Hospital, Leeds, UK

Janine K. Jensen MD
Assistant Professor, Department of Obstetrics and Gynecology, University of California at Irvine, Orange, CA, USA

Suk Young Jung MD PhD
Neurology and Female Urology Fellow, Division of Urologic Surgery, University of Pittsburgh School of Medicine, Pittsburgh, PA, USA

Mickey M. Karram MD
Associate Director, Department of Obstetrics and Gynecology, Good Samaritan Hospital, and Associate Professor of Obstetrics and Gynecology, University of Cincinnati, Cincinnati, OH, USA

Con Kelleher MD MRCOG
Consultant Obstetrician and Gynaecologist, Department of Obstetrics and Gynaecology, Guys and St Thomas' National Health Service Trust, London, UK

Margie A. Kahn MD
Director of Urogynecology, Assistant Professor, University of Texas Medical Branch, TX, USA

Vik Khullar BSc MRCOG
Subspecialty Trainee in Urogynaecology, Urogynaecology Unit, King's College Hospital, London, UK

Young H. Kim
Assistant Professor, Department of Surgery, Division of Urology, Brown University School of Medicine, Providence, RI, USA

Andrew J. Kirsch MD FAAP
Associate Clinical Professor of Urology, Director of Pediatric Urology Fellowship, Emory University School of Medicine, Children's Healthcare of Atlanta, Atlanta, GA, USA

Kathleen C. Kobashi MD
Fellow, Tower Urology Institute for Continence, Cedars-Sinai Medical Center, Los Angeles, CA, USA

Neeraj Kohli MD
Director, Division of Urogynecology and Reconstructive Pelvic Surgery, Mount Auburn Hospital/Beth Israel Hospital, Harvard Medical School, Boston, MA, USA

Devinder Kumar
Consultant Colorectal Surgeon, St George's Hospital, Cranmer Terrace, London, UK

Mark Lamah MB FRCS
Royal Surrey County Hospital, Egerton Road, Guildford, Surrey, UK

Jaqueline M. Lavin
Specialist Registrar in Obstetrics and Gynaecology, Saint Mary's Hospital for Women and Children, Whitworth Park, Manchester, UK

Gary E. Leach MD
Clinical Professor or Urology, University of Southern California and Director, Tower Urology Institute for Continence, Cedars-Sinai Medical Center, Los Angeles, CA, USA

Wendy W. Leng MD
Assistant Professor, Division of Urology, University of California San Francisco, CA, USA

Gunnar Lose MD DMSc
Chief Gynaecologist, Department of Obstetrics and Gynaecology, Glostrup County Hospital, University of Copenhagen, Glostrup, Denmark

Kevin R Loughlin MD
Professor of Surgery (Urology) Department of Urology, Brigham and Women's Hospital, Harvard Medical School, Boston, MA, USA

Adam Magos BSc MD FRCOG
Consultant Obstetrician and Gynaecologist, Minimally Invasive Therapy Unit and Endoscopy Training Centre, University Department of Obstetrics and Gynaecology, The Royal Free Hospital, Hampstead, London, UK

James Malone-Lee
Barlow Professor of Geriatric Medicine, Royal Free and University College London School of Medicine, London, UK

Jill Mantle BA FCSP Dip TP
Research physiotherapist, Department of Urogynaecology, King's College Hospital, Denmark Hill, London, UK

Anders Mattiasson
Co-ordinating Chairman of the Standardization Committee of the International Continence Society, Department of Urology, Lund University Hospital, Lund, Sweden

Catherine W. McGrother MB BS FFPHM
Senior Lecturer in Epidemiology, Faculty of Medicine, University of Leicester, Leicester, UK

Edward J. McGuire MD
Professor and Director, Division of Urology, University of Texas-Houston Medical School, Houston, TX, USA

Fiona K. Mensah MSc
Research Associate in Statistics, Department of Epidemiology and Public Health, University of Leicester, Leicester, UK

Richard J. Millard MB BS FRCS FRACS
Associate Professor and Head, Department of Urology, Prince of Wales Hospital, Randwick, Sydney, NSW, Australia

Tariq Miskry MB BS MRCOG
Clinical Research Fellow, Minimally Invasive Therapy Unit and Endoscopy Training Centre, University Department of Obstetrics and Gynaecology, The Royal Free Hospital, Hampstead, London, UK

Ash K. Monga
Consultant Gynaecologist, Princess Anne Hospital, Coxford Road, Southampton, UK

Jacek L. Mostwin MD DPhil
Professor of Urology, James Buchanan Brady Urological Institute, Johns Hopkins Medical Institutions, Baltimore, MD, USA

Diane K. Newman RNC MSN CRNP FAAN
Adult Nurse Practitioner, Director of Clinical Services, DKN Medical Associates, Philadelphia, PA, USA

Victor Nitti MD
Assistant Professor, Department of Urology, and Director of Neurourology and Female Urology, New York University School of Medicine, New York, NY, USA

Sarah I. Perry PhD
Research Associate, Department of Epidemiology and Public Health, University of Leicester, Leicester, UK

Eckhard Petri
Head and Professor of Gynaecology and Obstetrics, Schwerin Medical School, Schwerin, Germany

Damian Jin Chye Png MBBS FRCS MMed FAMS
Assistant Professor and Consultant Urologist, Division of Urology, Department of Surgery, National University of Singapore, Singapore

William Porter MD
Resident, Department of Obstetrics and Gynecology, University of Cincinnati, Cincinnati, OH, USA

Stephen Radley MB BS FRCS Ed. (Gynaecology) MRCOG
Senior Registrar in Obstetrics and Gynaecology andResearch Fellow in Urogynaecology, Royal Hallamshire Hospital, Urology Research, Sheffield, UK

David Rickards FRCR FFRDSA
Consultant Uroradiologist, University College Hospitals, London, UK

Andrea Rockall FRCR
Senior Registrar, Department of Radiologu, University College Hospitals, London, UK

Eric S. Rovner, MD
Assistant Professor of Urology, Division of Urology, Department of Surgery, Hospital of the University of Pennsylvania, PA, USA

H. Jane Rufford MBBS MRCOG
Research Fellow, Department of Urogynaecology, King's College Hospital, London, UK

Anita Saltmarche RN MHSc
President, HealthCare Associates, Clinical Associate, Faculty of Nursing, University of Toronto, Ontario, Canada

Stefano Salvatore
Divisione di Ginecologia Chirurgica, Ospedale Bassini, Cinisello Balsamo, University of Milan, Bicocca, Italy

Karen C. Sasso RN BSN MSN CCCN
Clinical Nurse Manager, Evanston Northwestern Healthcare, Evanston Hospital, Continence Center, Evanston, IL, USA

Jane A. Schulz MD FRCS(C)
*Assistant Professor, Department of Obstetrics and Gynecology, University of Alberta
Urogynecology Unit, Mount Sinai Hospital, Toronto, Ontario, Canada*

P. J. R. Shah FRCS
*Consultant Urologist to UCL Hospitals and Royal National Orthopaedic Hospital
Trust, London, UK*

Christine Shaw PhD
*Research Fellow, Department of Epidemiology and Public Health, University of
Leicester, Leicester, UK*

Mark C. Slack MBBCh MMed(UCT) FCOG(SA) MRCOG
*Consultant Gynaecologist, Division of Urogynaecology, Department of Obstetrics
and Gynaecology, Peterborough Hospitals NHS Trust, Peteborough, UK*

A. R. B. Smith
*Consultant Gynaecologist, Saint Mary's Hospital for Women and Children,
Manchester, UK*

Howard M. Snyder III MD FFAP FACS
*Professor of Urology, University of Pennsylvania School of Medicine, The Children's
Hospital of Philadelphia, Philadelphia, PA, USA*

Stuart L. Stanton FRCS FRCOG
*Professor of Pelvic Surgery and Urogynaecology, St George's University Hospital,
Urogynaecology Unit, Department of Obstetrics and Gynaecology, Cranmer Terrace,
London, UK*

David Staskin MD
*Director, Continence Center, Beth Israel Deaconess Medical Center and Assistant
Professor of Surgery/Urology, Harvard Medical School, Boston, MA, USA*

Abdul Sultan MD MRCOG
*Consultant Obstetrician and Gynaecologist, Mayday University Hospital, Thornton
Heath, Surrey, UK*

Christopher J.G. Sutton MA FRCOG
Consultant Gynaecologist, Waterden Road Clinic, Guildford, Surrey, UK

Steven E. Swift MD
*Associate Professor of Obstetrics and Gynaecology, Department of Obstetrics and
Gynaecology, Medical University of South Carolina, Charleston, SC, USA*

James P. Theofrastous MD
*Director of Urogynecology & Reconstructive Pelvic Surgery, Department of Obstetrics
and Gynecology, Mountain Area Health Education Center; Associate Clinical
Professor, UNC Chapel Hill School of Medicine, Asheville, NC, USA*

M. Chrystie Timmons MD
Director, Gerigyn, P.A., Chapel Hill, NC USA

Philip M. Toozs-Hobson MB BS MRCOG
*Consultant, Obstetrics and Gynaecology, Birmingham Women's Hospital,
Birmingham, UK*

Philip E.V. Van Kerrebroeck MD PhD Fellow EBU
Professor of Urology, Chairman of Department of Urology, University Hospital Maastricht, Maastricht, The Netherlands

Eboo Versi MA DPhil MB BChir MRCOG
Associate Professor of Obstetrics, Gynecology and Reproductive Biology, Chief, Division of Urogynecology, Department of Obstetrics and Gynecology, Brigham and Women's Hospital, Harvard Medical School, Boston, MA, USA

Mark E. Vierhout MD PhD
Consultant, Ikazia Hospital, Rotterdam, The Netherlands

David B. Vodušek MD PhD
Medical Director, Division of Neurology, University Medical Centre and Professor of Neurology, University of Ljubljana, Ljubljana, Slovenia

Adrian Wagg MB MRCP
Senior Lecturer in Geriatric Medicine, Royal Free and University College School of Medicine, University College Hospital, London, UK

K. Waldeck
Department of Clinical Pharmacology, Lund University Hospital, Lund, Sweden

Mark D. Walters MD
Head of the Section of General Gynecology and Urogynecology/Reconstructive Pelvic Surgery, Cleveland Clinic Foundation, Department of Gynaecology and Obstetrics, Cleveland, OH, USA

Anne M. Weber MD
Cleveland Clinic Foundation, Department of Obstetrics and Gynaecology, Cleveland, OH, USA

Alan J. Wein MD
Professor and Chief of Urology, Hospital of the University of Pennsylvania, Urology Division, Philadelphia, PA, USA

Jeffrey P. Weiss MD
Clinical Adjunct Assistant Professor/Urology, Cornell University, Weill School of Medicine, New York Presbyterian Hospital; USA

Don Wilson MD FRCS FRANZCOG CU
Professor of Obstetrics and Gynaecology, Dunedin School of Medicine, University of Otago, Dunedin, New Zealand

Brian G Wise
Consultant Urogynaecologist, William Harvey Hospital, Ashford, Kent, UK

Stephen A. Zderic MD
Assistant Professor, Pediatric Urology, Children's Hospital of Pennsylvania, Department of Urology, Philadelphia, PA, USA

Foreword

Urinary and faecal disorders, as well as pelvic organ prolapse, are frequent problems that are not life threatening but which have a significant impact on the quality of life of women of all ages. In tertiary referral centres, and increasingly in the community; in the UK, parts of Europe, and in the United States, a multidisciplinary team of physicians, surgeons, nurse and therapists work together in order to enhance the management of their patients. The American Board of Urology and the American College of Obstetrics and Gynecology recently announced their intention to create a joint postgraduate fellowship, representing the infancy of the developing field of pelvic surgery. This initial combination of female urology ('gynaeco-urology') and urogynaecology into a single programme recognizes the vital need for surgeons to master concepts and techniques from urology, gynaecology and colorectal surgery, in order to become the 'pelvic surgeons' of the future.

Our vision during the conception of this book was to assemble an international group of authors from various fields, in order to avoid the polarization of ideas which occurs in many textbooks as a natural product of the basic training and interests of the contributors. The authors includes urologists, gynaecologists, specialist nurses and physiotherapists who are considered experts in their fields. Our mission during the construction of the outline was to produce a comprehensive volume which would chronicle past contributions, document the present state of the art, and serve as a foundation for preparing the reader for future developments in the field.

The product is a text arranged in sections, enabling the reader to access areas of interest; the extensive bibliographies are intended to facilitate further study of the subject. The section on surgery has been formatted to serve as a text and atlas, and is intended to provide information pertaining to the decision-making process as well as the technical aspects of the surgical procedures.

Finally, we humbly recognize, as the text goes to press, that it is impossible to cover all aspects of female urology and urogynaecology comprehensively, and that the rapid pace of advances in the field makes it difficult to be completely up to date.

As editors, we are truly grateful to all those authors who have contributed. Researching and writing demands a considerable amount of time and effort, and we are grateful to the authors who sacrificed 'quality time' outside of their required hours of clinical and scientific work to make this project a reality. In addition we are grateful to the publishers, Isis Medical Media Ltd, for producing a book of high quality, which should enhance the minds, the practices and the bookshelves of those who own it.

Finally, we would like to thank our patients, who place their trust in us each and every day. We hope that this textbook contributes to the quality of their care and to the ability of those who will care for them in the future.

Linda Cardozo, David Staskin

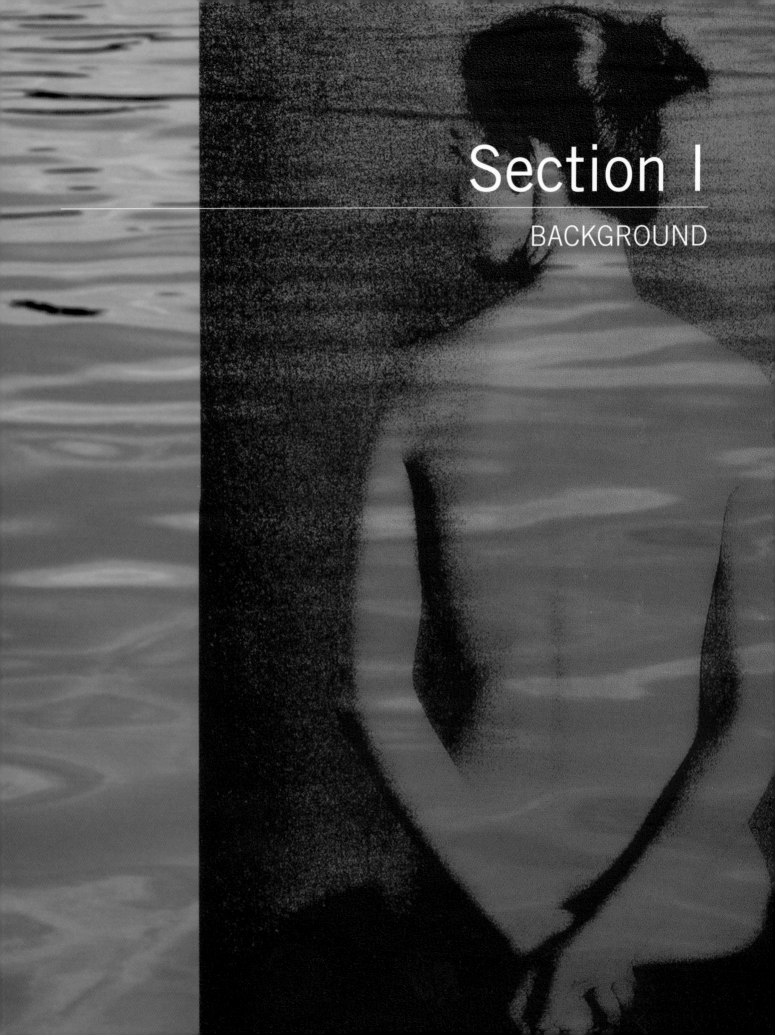

Section I

BACKGROUND

1

History of urogynaecology

H. P. Drutz, J. A. Schulz

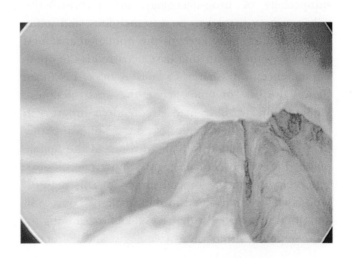

INTRODUCTION

As we move into a new millennium, accompanied by many new advances in the field of urogynaecology and reconstructive pelvic surgery, it is appropriate to take time to reflect on the events of the last century, and to make suggestions for future directions. With the significant increase in our post-menopausal female population there is a growing demand for improved quality of life and management of pelvic floor dysfunction. We no longer contemplate *whether* women will grow older but, rather, *how* they will grow older. The life expectancy for women has almost doubled through the 20th century. In 1923, Professor Sir Arthur Keith, in his Hunterian Lecture on 'Man's posture: its evolution and disorders'[1] stated

> every movement of the arms, cough or strain sets going a multitude of 'water hammers' within the abdominal and pelvic cavities. Every impulse sets the bladder knocking at the vaginal exit … it is the continual repetition of small forces, more frequently than the sudden application of a great effort which wear down the vaginal defence.

Although it has long been recognized that factors such as childbearing and chronic increases in intra-abdominal pressure contributed to pelvic floor prolapse, only recently has there been growing demand to manage all of the resulting problems. Urinary incontinence is now the most common reason for admission to long-term institutionalized centres in Canada and the United States. Billions of dollars are spent every year on nappy (diaper) and pad products, but this does nothing to correct the underlying problem of incontinence.

Reviewing the last century of progress in the new subspecialty of urogynaecology and reconstructive pelvic surgery proved to be a tremendous, and somewhat daunting, task. Perhaps the quotation that best summarizes the events that have occurred is the opening sentence from Charles Dickens' *A Tale of Two Cities*: 'It was the best of times, it was the worst of times'. Undoubtedly, we have made tremendous progress in this burgeoning new field; however, a political battle-field was perpetuated with the division of the female pelvic floor between urologists, urogynaecologists, gynaecologists and colorectal surgeons. This political feud is cleverly illustrated in the article of Louis Wall and John DeLancey with its well-known drawing of the competing urologist, gynaecologist and colorectal

surgeon.[2] This is one of the many challenges that must be overcome in providing overall women's healthcare as we move into the 21st century. A multidisciplinary approach to managing female pelvic floor dysfunction must be advocated to provide women with appropriate care in the areas of urinary and faecal incontinence, urogenital ageing, conservative management and reconstructive pelvic surgery.[3]

Voltaire, the French philosopher of the 'age of enlightenment', said 'these truths are not for all men nor for all times'. From this we must humbly accept the concept that the truths we believe in today regarding our management of women with pelvic floor disorders must be constantly reassessed and modified with scientific advancements and research. Similarly, the epigram by Alphonse Karr (1849), *plus ça change plus c'est la même chose* (the more things change, the more they stay the same) also reflects the changes during the past century, especially in the field of surgical intervention, where in many cases we have continued to reinvent the wheel. The significant events in this field over the last century are reviewed below.

PROGRESS IN THE 20TH CENTURY

Treatment

In 1892, Poussan proposed the concept of urethral advancement for the management of urinary incontinence.[4] He suggested 'introducing a bougie into the urethra, resecting the external meatus and portion of the urethra, and then after torsion of the canal to one hundred and eighty degrees, it is transplanted to a point just below the clitoris'. By the turn of the century, four main treatments for stress urinary incontinence were outlined:

1. injection of paraffin into the region of the urethra;
2. massage and electricity;
3. torsion of the urethra;
4. advancement of the external urethral meatus.

A century later, we are still trying to identify the best urethral bulking agent. Research with paraffin, Teflon (poly[tetrafluorothene]), silicone, collagen, autologous fat, carbon particles, and various copolymers has failed to identify an ideal medium.

In his landmark 1913 paper, Kelly outlined operations for managing urinary incontinence in women.[5] These included the following:

- puncture of the bladder and insertion of a catheter;
- closing the urethra and creating a vesico-abdominal fistula;
- closing the vagina and creating a rectovaginal fistula;
- compression of the urethra with an anterior colporrhaphy;
- periurethral injection of paraffin;
- advancement of the urethral meatus to the clitoris.

Kelly suggested that 'the torn or relaxed tissues of the vesical neck should be sutured together using two or three vertical mattress sutures of fine silk linen passed from side to side'. In his first publication, he described 16 patients as being well and four patients in whom the procedure was not successful, giving a success rate of 80%. However, further evaluation has revealed that the long-term success, using only these sutures to correct stress incontinence, falls to roughly 60%.[6] This decline may be related to gradual postoperative elongation of the smooth muscle in which the sutures were placed.[7] With coincident suburethral plication of the pubourethrovaginal ligaments of the urogenital diaphragm, the long-term results of a Kelly plication are significantly better.[8]

Sling procedures were pioneered in the early 1900s by three European physicians. Goebell first suggested transplantation of the pyramidalis muscle in 1910.[9] This was followed by Frankenheim who, in 1914, recommended using the pyramidalis or strips of rectus muscle as a suburethral sling by attaching the muscle to overlying fascia.[10] In 1917, Stoeckel suggested combining the techniques of Goebell and Frankenheim and adding plication of the vesical neck.[11] Throughout the 20th century, there have been many variations of sling procedures described in the literature. In 1907, Giordano suggested the use of gracilis muscle by wrapping it around the urethra.[12] Shortly thereafter, in 1911, Souier described the use of levator ani muscles by placing them between the vagina and urethra,[13] and, in 1923, Thompson recommended the use of strips of rectus muscle, surrounded by fascia, to be passed in front of the pubic bones and around the urethra.[14] The next key event in the development of surgery to the anterior compartment was the development of the bulbocavernosus muscle fat pad graft by Martius in 1929.[15] This has found wide use in fistula repairs and reconstruction of the anterior vaginal wall. In 1968, John Chasser Moir[16] introduced the concept of the gauze hammock operation as a modification of the original Aldridge[17] sling procedure described in 1942. Chasser Moir recognized that 'operations of this type do no more than support the bladder neck and urethrovesical junction and so prevent the undue descent of parts when the woman strains or coughs.'

Victor Bonney, in 1923, stated 'incontinence depends in some way upon a sudden and abnormal displacement of the urethra and urethrovesical junction immediately behind the symphysis'.[18] This was followed in 1924 by a description from B. P. Watson of 'the muscle sheet that normally supports the base and neck of the bladder' and his statement that 'so far as the incontinence of urine is concerned, the important sutures are those which overlap the fascia at the neck of the bladder and so restore it to its normal position'. In reviewing Watson's work with anterior colporrhaphy, he was able to obtain 'perfect control' in 65.7% of cases, 'improvement' in 21.9%, and 'no success' in 12.4%.[19] These figures are in keeping with others that have been reported for anterior colporrhaphy. Therefore, it was apparent that hypermobility of the bladder neck was an issue, and that the anterior colporrhaphy was not a satisfactory operation for stress incontinence.

The next landmark in genitourinary surgery occurred in 1949 with the publication of the paper of Marshall, Marchetti and Krantz on 'The correction of stress incontinence by simple vesicourethral suspension.' They suggested that this operation was 'particularly valuable for patients whose first procedure failed.' In their first 44 patients, they described 82% with excellent results, 7% with improvement and an 11% failure rate.[20] Shortly thereafter, in 1950, H. H. Fouracre Barns described the 'round ligament sling operation for stress incontinence'; this technique was popularized by Paul Hodgkinson.[21] In 1961, John Burch first described his modification of the Marshall–Marchetti–Krantz procedure; he proposed a retropubic colpourethropexy that took the anterolateral aspects of the vault of the vagina and attached them to Cooper's ligament.[22] Burch recognized the potential complications of this procedure if done alone, including the recurrence of creation of an enterocele or rectocele, the development of ventral/incisional hernias and even the possibility of a vesicovaginal fistula.

Diagnosis and investigation

As the number of procedures offered for the treatment of stress incontinence increased, there were also significant advances in the urogynaecological diagnostic procedures available. In 1882, Mosso and Pellacani described cystometry using a smoked drum and a water manometer.[23] An aneroid barometer for cystometric evaluation was developed by Lewis in 1939.[24] Jeffcoate and Roberts, in 1952, introduced the concept of radiographic changes in the posterior urethrovesical angle.[25] These changes were further modified in 1956, by Bailey in England, who described seven variations in the urethrovesical angle on radiographic studies.[26] Later modifications were performed by Tom Green in the United States in 1962, when he described Green types 1 and 2 incontinence.[27] Identification of the posterior urethrovesical angle by lateral bead chain cystography was introduced by Hodgkinson in 1953.[28]

By 1956, Von Garrelts had introduced the concept of uroflowmetry.[29] In 1964, Enhorning, Miller and Hinman combined cystometry with radiographic screening of the bladder;[30] this was followed a few years later in 1969 by Brown and Wickham's introduction of urethral pressure profilometry.[31] Another landmark occurred in 1971, when Patrick Bates, Sir Richard Turner-Warwick and Graham Whiteside introduced synchronous cine pressure–flow cystography, with pressure and flow studies.[32] This was the beginning of the field of videourodynamics. Equipment was further expanded with the introduction of the micro-tip transducer, in 1975 by Asmussen and Ulmsten, for measuring urethral closure pressure.[33]

Further investigational advances occurred in the latter part of the 20th century. These included the introduction of the Urilos monitor in 1974 by James, Flack, Caldwell and Smith.[34] This device allowed evaluation of dampness to determine whether the fluid lost was urine. In 1981, Sutherst, Brown and Shawer developed the pad-weighing test as an objective measure of the severity of urinary incontinence.[35]

In 1961, Enhorning suggested that 'surgical treatment for stress incontinence is probably mainly beneficial because it restores the neck of the bladder and

the upper part of the urethra to the influence of intra-abdominal pressure.'[36] This introduced the concept of pressure transmission ratios and the idea that successful operations for stress urinary incontinence worked by restoring the urethrovesical junction to an intra-abdominal position. In 1956, Jeffcoate added further interpretation of our investigative techniques when he attempted to caution gynaecologists, stating 'the absence of the posterior urethrovesical angle is merely a sign of incompetence of the internal sphincter. The presence of an angle is a function of the involuntary muscle at the urethrovesical junction, not of the muscle of the pelvic floor,'[37] and so the simplistic approach of static cystourethrograms began to be questioned. Green had suggested that if one saw a radiographic diagnosis of type 1 incontinence, this could readily be repaired with an anterior colporrhaphy; the type 2 stress incontinence required a retropubic urethropexy. A number of authors, including Drutz in 1978,[38] have confirmed the limited accuracy of static cystourethrograms.

By 1953, Paul Hodgkinson had recommended 'that if on anteroposterior straining radiograph, the urethrovesical junction is depressed 4 cm below the lower border of the symphysis, I believe the objective of the operation can be accomplished through anterior colporrhaphy.'[28] A decade later, Hodgkinson commented on the frequency of detrusor dyssynergia, with grade 1 defined as detrusor contraction in response to coughing and heel jouncing; grade 2 was spontaneous automatic detrusor contractility when recumbent. Hodgkinson recognized the importance of discovering this condition prior to performing any surgery for stress urinary incontinence.[39]

Success rates

As we approached the 1970s, we began to recognize that operative failures in the treatment of stress urinary incontinence mainly involve three areas,[40] as follows:

1. incorrect diagnosis and the fact that bladder instability (and not just simple stress incontinence) may have been the cause of the incontinence;
2. the wrong operation may have been chosen and some operations probably give better long-term results;
3. the concept of technical failure.

We recognized that the vaginal approach to primary stress incontinence probably gave only a 50–60% success rate, whereas the suprapubic approach achieved at least 80%. In 1973, J. E. Morgan discussed indications for primary retropubic urethropexy: these included minimal pelvic floor relaxation, chronic chest disease, occupations involving heavy lifting, patients heavily involved in athletics, and obesity.[41] In 1970, Hodgkinson stated that 'the most durable operation for stress incontinence is a retropubic urethropexy and the least durable is a vaginal repair.' Hodgkinson quoted a 92.1% success rate with his own 404 patients that had a retropubic urethropexy.[40] The other movement in the 1970s was of the urologists and gynaecologists toward endoscopic bladder-neck suspensions such as the Pereyra, Raz and Stamey suspensions; numerous variations including the Gittes and Cobb–Raagde were described in the literature. In the 1990s we have now realized that the long-term results of these needle suspension procedures are also not as good as those of the retropubic procedures.

THE WAY AHEAD

Now, as we approach the 21st century, we must consider what lies ahead. The main fields of responsibility as urogynaecologists and reconstructive pelvic surgeons include the following:

- education;
- surgery;
- uropharmacology;
- neurophysiology;
- behaviour modification;
- collagen;
- ultrasonography/magnetic resonance imaging (MRI).

Regarding education, we need to focus on education of our colleagues in obstetrics and gynaecology, family practice, geriatrics and community healthcare, as well as the public. The awareness must be increased that incontinence is not a normal effect of ageing: the many myths, including 'everyone gets it' and 'it can't be treated', must be dispelled. Urogenital ageing must be stressed as part of menopause management, and conservative management in the community should be promoted. The other aspect of education is the training of new sub-

specialists in the field of urogynaecology and reconstructive pelvic surgery. Board certification is now available in Australia and board recognition has been established in the United States. The International Urogynecology Association (IUGA) is now establishing international standards of training in conjunction with FIGO (International Federation of Gynecology and Obstetrics) and the WHO (World Health Organization).

Within the field of surgery for pelvic floor problems, we need to re-evaluate what we do. Over 200 operations have been described for stress incontinence. Randomized controlled trials, with adequate patient numbers and follow-up of at least 2 years, are required for the evaluation of new and existing procedures. The role of bulking agents is still controversial and the ideal medium has yet to be discovered. New pharmacological agents continue to be produced; well-designed, placebo-controlled trials are mandatory for their evaluation. Neurophysiology is another developing area: work is being done to determine if there are certain factors in labour that lead to irreversible changes to the pelvic floor. Another outstanding question is whether abnormalities in the electromyographic patterns predict success or failure of different treatments. We continue to develop new modes of conservative management, including behaviour modification and devices; further studies are needed to clarify the specific areas of use for these therapies.

The role of collagen in pelvic floor disorders is a fascinating area. We need both effective qualitative and quantitative assays to determine whether there are certain defects of collagen in patients with pelvic floor dysfunction. Also, we need to establish whether there are genetic markers that could be screened for to determine certain 'at-risk' patients. Perhaps there is a select group of patients that should be counselled to have delivery by caesarean section; this group may also require the use of synthetic materials for reconstruction of their pelvic floor. We need to look at the relationship of collagen to oestrogen and the general effects of urogenital ageing to see if they are independent factors.

We are in the midst of a revolution in imaging technology. The development of three-dimensional ultrasonography and progress with MRI have allowed a new approach to evaluating defects associated with stress urinary incontinence and pelvic floor disorders. Progress in the field of ultrasonography has been hampered by a lack of standardization of terminology; this was recognized by the German Association of Urogynecology, who attempted to make recommendations for standardization of methodology.[43] The fact that different methods are used (such as abdominal, perineal, introital, vaginal and rectal) has further impeded progress in this field. Recent papers have investigated the urethra and surrounding tissues with intra-urethral ultrasonography; their authors have proposed that sphincter measurements can be a prognostic factor in patients who underwent operations for stress urinary incontinence.[44] Beco stated that 'Doppler and colour studies will play an increasing role in the evaluation of urethrovesical disorders.'[45] With new developments in MRI, and especially dynamic MRI, these techniques will also play a growing part in investigation and research.

CONCLUSIONS

At the International Continence Society meeting in 1986, Sir Richard Turner-Warwick gave an address in which he defined the urogynaecologist as 'neither the general urologist nor the general obstetrician and gynaecologist, but someone who has special training and expertise in genitourinary problems in women.'[46] Today, we should expand this definition to include urogynaecology and reconstructive pelvic surgery. Such a physician implies a surgeon with specialized training in the conservative and surgical management of women with urinary and/or faecal incontinence, persistent genitourinary complaints and disorders of pelvic floor supports.

As Marcel Proust said, 'We must never be afraid to go too far, for the truth lies beyond.' We must humbly accept that the 'truths' that we identify today almost certainly will have to be changed in the future. However, if we work collaboratively to produce well-designed scientific research, we should be able to establish truths that stand the test of time in our ongoing quest to improve the quality of life for women with pelvic floor problems.

ACKNOWLEDGEMENT

This chapter is an adaptation of the Presidential Address from the 21st Annual International Urogynecology Association Meeting, 1996: Drutz HP. The first century of urogynecology and reconstructive pelvic surgery: where do we go from here? *Int Urogynecol J* 1996; 7: 348–353

REFERENCES

1. Keith A. Man's posture: its evolution and disorders. *Br Med J* 1923; II: 451–454

2. Wall LL, DeLancey JOL. The politics of prolapse: a revisionist approach to disorders of the pelvic floor in women. *Perspect Biol Med* 1991; 34: 486–496

3. Nager CW, Kumar D, Kahn M, Stanton SL. Management of pelvic floor dysfunction. *Lancet* 1997; 350: 1751

4. Poussan. *Arch Clin Bord* 1892. No. 1

5. Kelly HA. Incontinence of urine in women. *Urol Cutan Rev* 1913; 17: 291

6. Bergman A, Elia G. Three surgical procedures for genuine stress urinary incontinence: five year follow-up of a prospective randomized study. *Am J Obstet Gynecol* 1995; 173: 66

7. Wall LL, Norton PA, DeLancey JOL. *Practical Urogynecology*. Baltimore: Williams and Wilkins 1993; 153–190

8. Nichols DH, Randall CL. *Vaginal Surgery*. Baltimore: Williams and Wilkins 1996; 218–256

9. Goebell R. Zur operativen Besierigung der angeborenen Incontinentia vesical. *Z Gynäk Urol* 1910; 2: 187

10. Frankenheim P. Zentral Verhandl. d. Deutsch. *Geseusch Chir* 1914; 43: 149

11. Stoeckel W. Über die Verwändung der Musculi Pyramidales bei der opeutinen Behandlung der Incontinentia Urinae 1917; 41: 11

12. Giordano D. Twentieth Congress Franc de Chir 1907; 506

13. Souier JB. *Med Rec* 1911; 79: 868

14. Thompson R. *Br J Dis Child* 1923; 20: 116

15. Martius H. Sphincter und Harndöurenplastic aus dem Musculus Bulbocavernosus. *Chirurgie* 1929; 1: 769

16. Chasser Moir J. The gauze-hammock operation (a modified Aldridge sling procedure). *J Obstet Gynaecol Br Commonw* 1968; 75: 1–9

17. Aldridge AH. Transplantation of fascia for relief of urinary stress incontinence. *Am J Obstet Gynecol* 1942; 44: 398–411

18. Bonney V. On diurnal incontinence of urine in women. *J Obstet Gynaecol Br Emp* 1923; 30: 358–365

19. Watson BP. Imperfect urinary control following childbirth and its surgical treatment. *Br Med J* 1924; 11: 566

20. Marshall VF, Marchetti AA, Krantz KE. The correction of stress incontinence by simple vesicourethral suspension. *Surg Gynecol Obstet* 1949; 88: 509–518

21. Fouracre Barns HH. Round ligament sling operation for stress incontinence. *J Obstet Gynaecol Br Emp* 1950; 57: 404–407

22. Burch JC. Urethrovaginal fixation to Cooper's ligament for correction of stress incontinence, cystocele and prolapse. *Am J Obstet Gynecol* 1961; 81: 281–290

23. Mosso A, Pallacani P. Sur les fonctions de la vessie. *Arch Ital Biol* 1882; 1: 97

24. Lewis LG. New clinical recording cystometer. *J Urol* 1939; 41: 638–645

25. Jeffcoate TNA, Roberts H. Stress incontinence. *J Obstet Gynaecol Br Emp* 1952; 59: 865–720

26. Bailey KV. A clinical investigation into uterine prolapse with stress incontinence: treatment by modified Manchester colporrhaphy. Part II. *J Obstet Gynaecol Br Emp* 1956; 63: 663

27. Green TH Jr. Development of a plan for the diagnosis and treatment of urinary stress incontinence. *Am J Obstet Gynecol* 1962; 83: 632–648

28. Hodgkinson CP. Relationship of female urethra and bladder in urinary stress incontinence. *Am J Obstet Gynecol* 1953; 560–573

29. Von Garrelts B. Analysis of micturition: a new method of recording the voiding of the bladder. *Acta Chir Scand* 1956; 112: 326–340

30. Enhorning G, Miller E, Hinman F Jr. Urethral closure studied with cine roentgenography and simultaneous bladder–urethral pressure recording. *Surg Gynecol Obstet* 1964; 118: 507–516

31. Brown W, Wickham JEA. The urethral pressure profile. *Br J Urol* 1969; 41: 211–217

32. Bates CP, Whiteside CG, Turner-Warwick R. Synchronous cine/pressure/flow cystography: a method of routine urodynamic investigation. *Br J Radiol* 1971; 44: 44–50

33. Asmussen M, Ulmsten U. Simultaneous urethrocystometry and urethral pressure profile measurements with a new technique. *Acta Obstet Gynaecol* 1975; 54: 385–386

34. James ED, Flack F, Caldwell KP, Smith. Urine loss in incontinent patients: how often, how much? *Clin Med* 1974; 4: 13–17

35. Sutherst JL, Brown M, Shawer M. Assessing the severity of urinary incontinence in women by weighing perineal pads. *Lancet* 1981; 1: 1128–1130

36. Enhorning G. Simultaneous recording of intravesical and intraurethral pressure: a study of urethral closure pressures in normal and incontinent women. *Acta Chir Scand* 1961; 276 (Suppl): 1

37. Jeffcoate TNA. Bladder control in the female. *Proc R Soc Med* 1956; 49: 652–660

38. Drutz HP, Shapiro BJ, Mandel F. Do static cystourethrograms have a role in the investigation of female incontinence? *Am J Obstet Gynecol* 1978; 130: 516–520

39. Hodgkinson CP, Ayers MA, Drukker BH. Dyssynergic detrusor dysfunction in the apparently normal female. *Am J Obstet Gynecol* 1963; 87: 717–730

40. Hodgkinson CP. Stress urinary incontinence. *Am J Obstet Gynecol* 1970; 1: 1141–1168

41. Morgan JE. The suprapubic approach to primary stress incontinence. *Am J Obstet Gynecol* 1973; 49: 37–42

42. Khullar V, Salvatore S, Cardozo LD, Hill S, Kelleher CJ. Three dimensional ultrasound of the urethra and urethral sphincter: a new diagnostic technique. *Neurourol Urodyn* 1994; 13: 352–353

43. Shaer G, Koelbl H, Voigt R *et al*. Recommendations of the German Association of Urogynecology on functional sonography of the lower female urinary tract. *Int Urogynecol J* 1996; 7: 105–108

44. Hermans RK, Klein HM, Muller U *et al*. Intraurethral ultrasound in women with stress incontinence. *Br J Urol* 1994; 74: 315–318

45. Beco J. Personal communication, November 1996

46. Turner-Warwick R., International Continence Society Proceedings Boston, Mass., USA 1986

2

Epidemiology (USA)

A. C. Diokno

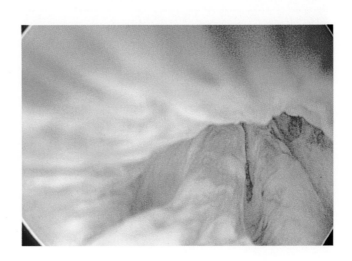

INTRODUCTION

Epidemiology is defined as the study of the relationships of various factors determining the frequency and distribution of diseases in a community.[1] However, one may consider the epidemiological study of urinary incontinence (UI) to be in its infancy. Epidemiological studies dealing with UI are sparse and methodologies are extremely varied. Furthermore, there is no consensus on the definition of UI among investigators dealing with this subject. As a consequence, there is conflicting information, especially in the prevalence rates. Another major issue in studying UI is the fact that incontinence itself is a condition with many varied types, occurring in many different segments of the population. Students of the epidemiology of UI must therefore account for all these variabilities when evaluating data from these studies.

PREVALENCE OF URINARY INCONTINENCE

The prevalence of UI is defined as the probability of being incontinent within the defined population group within a specified period of time Among women of all age groups, it is reasonable to state that the prevalence of UI increases with age and increasing debility: it is highest among groups of people who are older, debilitated and institutionalized.

One of the classic studies of UI prevalence was conducted by Thomas *et al.*[2] by postal survey to selected health districts in the London boroughs and neighbouring health districts in the late 1970s. In that survey,

incontinence was defined as involuntary excretion or leakage of urine in inappropriate places or at inappropriate times twice or more a month, regardless of the quantity of urine lost. Incontinence was further subdivided into regular UI for a loss twice or more per month, and occasional for less than twice per month. The response rate from this postal survey was excellent, at 89%. Table 2.1 shows the prevalence rates for regular and occasional incontinence in women aged 15 to more than 85 years. There appear to be three age tiers to the prevalence of regular incontinence in women: the first level is at 15–34 years, when the prevalence is lowest (4–5.5%); the second tier is at 35–74 years (prevalence 8.8–11.9%); the third is at 75 years and older (16%).

In a more focused epidemiological study on UI, Diokno and his group[3] performed face-to-face household interviews with respondents who were 60 years and older, living in their households in the community of Washtenaw County, Michigan in the mid 1980s. This epidemiological study funded by the National Institutes of Health (NIH) was entitled 'Medical, Epidemiologic and Social Aspects of Aging', now better known as the MESA project. In this project, incontinence was defined as urine loss of any volume beyond the respondent's control, with a minimum frequency of six times within the last 12 months. Any loss of less than six days but fitting any of the known mechanisms of urine loss – such as urge and/or stress loss – was also considered to be UI. A total of 1955 respondents participated, a participation rate of 65.1%. Table 2.2 shows that, in this community,

Table 2.1. *Prevalence of urinary incontinence (UI) in women*

Age group (years)	Regular UI (%)	Occasional UI (%)	Total UI (%)
15–24	4.0	11.9	15.9
25–34	5.5	20.0	25.5
35–44	10.2	20.7	30.9
45–54	11.8	21.9	32.9
55–64	11.9	18.6	30.5
65–74	8.8	14.6	22.4
75–84	16.0	13.6	29.6
> 85	16.2	16.2	32.4

Data adapted from ref. 2.

Table 2.2. *Prevalence of urinary incontinence in women aged 60 years and over*

Age	Continent*	Incontinent*	Total
60–64	193 (60.9)	124 (39.1)	317
65–69	192 (65.3)	102 (34.7)	294
70–74	111 (58.7)	78 (41.3)	189
75–79	105 (62.5)	63 (37.5)	168
80–84	64 (64.6)	35 (35.4)	99
85+	50 (64.1)	28 (35.9)	78
Total	715 (62.4)	430 (37.6)	1145

* Percentages in parentheses.
Data adapted from ref. 2.

the prevalence of UI in women aged 60 years or older was 37.6%. There was no significant difference in the rates between any age groups in this sample.

The prevalence of incontinence in this population was also assessed on the basis of other bladder symptoms of the female respondents. The prevalence of self-reported infection or irritation was 17.4%, whereas the prevalence of bladder-emptying symptoms was 9.1%. Urinary incontinence was significantly more prevalent among women with irritation infection (46.4%) and bladder-emptying symptoms (44.8%) than among women who were asymptomatic (34.5%) As expected, irritative voiding symptoms were more prevalent than were of bladder-emptying symptoms.

Another area that was explored was the prevalence of UI among respondents from white or ethnic minority groups. The MESA survey showed that the prevalence rate among white women was 39% in contrast to 23.8% among black women respondents. There was no significant difference in the prevalence rates between white and black male respondents (18.5 and 19.7%, respectively). The reason for the discrepancy in the rates in women is not clear from our data. There are also some suggestions at various forums that the prevalence of incontinence among Pacific Islanders may be less than the prevalence rates reported in Europe and North America. Certainly, these issues need clarification and steps are under way through funded NIH studies to examine the issue of ethnicity of UI.

Many prevalence studies have been published, some before but many after the two cited above. With regard to young women, Wolin[4] in 1969 published his survey of healthy student nurses 17–25 years of age and reported that 51% had experienced stress UI, with 16% experiencing major or regular urine loss. In the group of middle-aged women who were surveyed, Burgio et al.[5] reported a 30.7% prevalence of regular incontinence, which was defined as at least once a month, among healthy women between 42 and 50 years of age. Similarly, Elving et al.[6] reported that 26% of women aged 30–59 years had experienced UI at some time in adult life. They also reported 14% to have perceived UI at some time in adult life. Several published epidemiological studies confirm the high prevalence rate among the elderly population: Brocklehurst et al.[7] reported a 23% prevalence of UI among women aged 65 years or more; Milne et al.,[8] on the other hand, reported a 42% prevalence, which probably represents the higher bounds of the problem.

UI is much more prevalent among institutionalized women. Ouslander et al.,[9] in a survey of seven nursing homes, reported a UI prevalence rate of 50% among all patients surveyed. Hansen et al.[10] reported a 58.5% prevalence of UI in Danish nursing homes. In an acute-care hospital setting, the reported prevalence of UI reported by Sullivan and Lindsay[11] was 19%, whereas Willington[12] estimated that 30% of unselected elderly women admitted are incontinent of urine.

INCIDENCE AND REMISSION

Incidence is the probability of becoming incontinent during a defined period of time. Determining the incidence of a condition or disease is helpful in determining the onset of the condition as well as in understanding the risk factor of the condition. The MESA survey at Washtenaw County, Michigan established the incidence rate of UI in the United States.[13] The incidence rate among women who were continent during the initial baseline interview and became incontinent a year later was 22.4%; the incidence of UI during the third-year interview of respondents who were still continent during the second interview was 20%.

Campbell et al.[14] reported an incidence rate of incontinence among women aged 65 years and older in New Zealand to be about 10% in a 3-year period. Burgio et al.[5] reported a 3-year incidence rate among middle-aged healthy women to be 8%. Elving *et al.*,[6] in their survey of Danish women, showed a steady increase in the incidence of incontinence to the age of 59 years; unfortunately, they did not study women beyond that age to determine further the trend in incidence rate.

The MESA survey also analysed the remission rate for urinary incontinence. The remission rate – that is, women who were incontinent at the baseline (first) interview and became continent during the second interview a year later – was 11.2%. A similar rate (13.3%) of the incontinent respondents at the second interview reported being continent a year later at the third interview. Campbell *et al.*[14] reported a remission rate of 13% over a 4-year period among New Zealand women who had been incontinent.

TYPE AND SEVERITY OF URINARY INCONTINENCE

Prevalence and incidence of types of UI

In epidemiological studies, as in clinical investigations, the type of UI must be defined. In most surveys, stress and urge type are easily definable from well-established questionnaires. In general, incontinence is considered of be the stress type when the urine loss was experienced at the time of physical exertion (such as coughing, laughing, sneezing, etc.). Urge incontinence is defined as involuntary loss of urine preceded by a sudden urge to void. When the urine loss is associated with both stress and urge, it is considered to be of mixed type. Because of the difficulty in identifying the overflow type, when the urine loss is associated with neither the stress nor the urge type, the incontinence is labelled 'other'. However, when the survey respondents were taken one step further into urodynamic testing, the type of incontinence has been classified into the various urodynamic types according to the pathophysiological abnormality.

The MESA survey conducted by Diokno *et al.*[3] in Washtenaw County, Michigan reported the prevalence of the types of clinical incontinence encountered among their respondents. The most common type reported by these women aged 60 years and older was the mixed stress and urge type (55.5%), followed by the stress type (26.7%), then the urge (9.0%) and other (8.8%) types. Wells *et al.*[15] studied a series of 200 women 55–90 years of age who presented to a continence clinic: they reported a prevalence of 35% stress, 26% urge, 22% mixed urge/stress, and 19% other categories.

Herzog *et al.* reported, from the MESA survey, the natural history of both continent and incontinent respondents for 2 years.[13] Most continent women who developed UI developed a stress or mixed urge/stress type. Women with stress UI either remained so or developed a mixed type of urge and stress incontinence, whereas women with the mixed type did not change.

Prevalence and incidence of severity of UI

In epidemiological studies, severity has been categorized by the frequency of incontinent episodes, by the volume of urine loss or by the frequency of difficulty in controlling the flow of urine. The Diokno MESA study[3] reported the severity of UI among its 60-year-old respondents in terms of the number of days per year that urine loss was experienced and the volume of urine loss per day. As shown in Table 2.3, if severe or significant UI is considered to be the loss of at least 1 tablespoonful of urine per day, on at least 50 days a year (approximately once a week), then 25.8% of women respondents aged 60 years and older at the time of the MESA survey had severe incontinence.

The patterns of change in the severity of UI in the MESA survey were also analysed.[13] For the purpose of reporting the severity over time, the following definitions were established: respondents with mild incontinence were those who reported low frequency (1–9 days/year) and/or small volume (less than one half-teaspoon per day for less than 300 days/year); those with severe incontinence were those who reported high frequency (300 or more days/year) and/or large volume (more than a quarter cup per day on 50 or more days/year); those respondents with intermediate volume and/or frequency were considered to have moderate incontinence. On the basis of these severity levels, continent respondents who became incontinent were most likely to develop a mild form of incontinence. About half of those who were classified originally as mildly incontinent remained so and very few became severely incontinent. Among those who reported moderate incontinence, most remained moderately incontinent or changed to mildly incontinent, with very few advancing to severe incontinence. Among women who were severely incontinent at baseline, most remained severely incontinent.

Table 2.3. *Percentage of severe incontinence, as judged by volume and frequency of urine loss, in 60-year-old women*

Volume of urine lost in 24 hours	No. of days with urine loss				Total percentage*
	1–9	10–49	50–299	300–365	
Drops < $\frac{1}{2}$ tsp	16.1	11.6	5.6	3.0	36.3 (135)
$\frac{1}{2}$ tsp–< 1 tbsp	9.7	9.7	7.5	3.2	30.1 (112)
1 tbsp–< $\frac{1}{4}$ cup	4.6	4.6	5.4	3.2	17.8 (66)
$\frac{1}{4}$ cup or more	2.4	2.4	4.3	6.7	15.8 (59)
Total *	32.8 (122)	28.3 (105)	22.8 (85)	16.1 (60)	100.0 (372)

* Number of patients in parentheses.
Data adapted from ref. 3.

Prevalence of voiding frequency

The prevalence of voiding frequency is receiving greater attention as more and more studies are being conducted for conditions related to bladder dysfunction. For example, pharmacological interventions as well as behavioural techniques aimed at improving bladder function usually affect the frequency of voiding day and night. It is therefore imperative that a comparative standard is available on which to base any observations related to frequency of voiding prior to, during and after an intervention.

The MESA study has established the distribution of voiding frequency among the elderly (60 years and older) living in a community, who are likely to be the subjects of pharmacological and behavioural interventions aimed at controlling abnormal voiding.[3] It appears that the normal daily frequency of urination in this age group is no more than eight times, as 88% of all our asymptomatic respondents reported that range. To be more specific, 47.3% of asymptomatic women reported that they voided six to eight times, 34.8% voided four or five times, and 5.5% voiding one to three times daily.

In terms of nocturia – which was defined as the frequency of being awakened from sleep and getting up to void – 93% of asymptomatic women voided no more than twice at night. In contrast, 25% of women with irritative symptoms and 24% of women with difficulty in emptying the bladder voided three or more times each night. These data suggest that abnormal bladder function has a significant effect on the frequency of voiding.

PREVALENCE OF URODYNAMIC MEASURES AMONG CONTINENT AND INCONTINENT ELDERLY WOMEN

To establish the urodynamic characteristics of both continent and incontinent elderly women living in a community, a series of urodynamic tests were conducted on those MESA respondents who volunteered to undergo such tests.[16,17] This study provided information on the prevalence of the various parameters in the urodynamic tests that are of interest in the evaluation of incontinent patients but for which there are no well established data from control subjects. The MESA survey data established the sensitivity and specificity of the various urodynamic tests, from which it was concluded that such tests – including uroflow, cystometrography, static urethral profilometry and stress cystography – should be used, not to screen and diagnose UI but, rather, to confirm clinical manifestation. Urodynamic testing, by virtue of its ability to identify various mechanisms of UI, is believed to be helpful not only in determining the category of therapeutic approach but also in assessing outcomes of therapy.

The MESA survey studied a random sample of non-institutionalized ambulatory elderly women, both continent and incontinent; an initial clinical evaluation was followed by a series of urodynamic evaluations. A total of 258 self-reported continent and 198 self-reported incontinent women underwent the clinical evaluation comprising history taking, physical examination (including pelvic examination) and urinalysis. From these groups, 67 continent and 100 incontinent women underwent urodynamic testing including an initial non-instrumented uroflow test, followed by catheterized post-void volume measurement, followed by filling cystometry, static and dynamic urethral profilometry, provocative stress test and lateral stress resting and straining stress cystogram.

Uroflowmetry

The uroflow measures of peak flow rate (PFR) and average flow rate (AFR) were analysed according to the voided volume at increments of 100 ml. When volume was controlled, the mean PFR and AFR did not differ significantly between respondents who were continent and those who were incontinent. The flow rates did not differ between women with competent sphincters and those with urethral incompetency. The continuity of the urinary stream was not associated with continence status nor with the clinical type of incontinence (i.e. urge, stress, etc.)

Post-void residual volume

A post-void residual volume of 0–50 ml was found in 78.1% of continent and 86.5% of incontinent women; 9.7% and 8.4% had residuals of 51–100 ml; 2.4% and 1.6% had residuals of 101–150 ml, and 9.7% and 3.5% had residuals of 151 ml or more, respectively. There was no statistical difference between continent and incontinent women with regard to prevalence of a residual urine volume greater than 50 ml. These data give rise to questions regarding the post-void residual volume in relation to the diagnosis of overflow incontinence: the determining factor for overflow incontinence may be the same factor as for urge and/or stress incontinence, and the abnormal post-void residual volume may be coincidental or a contributory factor rather the primary reason for the incontinence.

Bladder capacity

Among the women volunteers, 79% of continent volunteers and 64% of incontinent volunteers had a bladder capacity of 300 ml or more; however, this difference in bladder volume between continent and incontinent subjects was not significant. The mean cystometric bladder capacities among 60–64-year-old continent and incontinent subjects were 381.8 and 442.7 ml, respectively; for 65–69-year-old subjects they were 421.6 and 370.0 ml, for those aged 70–74 years they were 410.3 and 414.2 ml; for those aged 75–79 years they were 350.3 and 426.8 ml, and for those aged 80 years old or more they were 318.3 and 408.3 ml, respectively. These results refute the notion that the bladder capacity of the elderly is smaller than normal, if we consider a bladder capacity of 300 ml or more to be normal.

Uninhibited detrusor contraction

The diagnosis of uninhibited detrusor contraction was based on the definition by the International Continence Society. The overall prevalence of uninhibited detrusor contraction in women was 7.9%; the prevalence of uninhibited detrusor contraction among continent respondents was 4.9%, whereas for incontinent subjects it was 12.2%. The difference between the two prevalence rates was not significant. However, comparison of the bladder capacity between female respondents showed that the capacity in women with uninhibited detrusor contraction was 364 ml, whereas in those without uninhibited contraction it was 404 ml; the difference was statistically significant at $p < 0.05$. This may explain the increased frequency, urgency and smaller voided volumes of patients with detrusor instability.

Static and dynamic urethral pressure profilometry (UPP)

The mean functional urethral length (FUL) did not change significantly as the age of the subjects increased, but the values of the maximum urethral pressure (MUP) and the maximum closure pressure (MCP) showed a significant progressive reduction as age increased ($p = 0.002$ and $p = 0.0003$, respectively). This progressive reduction of MUP and MCP reinforces the belief that elderly women are more predisposed to stress urine loss.

The parameters of UPP for supine subjects did not show any significant difference between continence and incontinence. However, for standing subjects, significant differences were observed between continent and incontinent groups with respect to MUP, which was significantly ($p = 0.0025$) lower in the incontinent compared with the continent group. Likewise, the MCP and the FUL were significantly reduced in standing but not in supine incontinent subjects when compared with the continent group.

The results of dynamic profilometry were reported as either positive (zero or positive reading), corresponding to incontinence, or negative (corresponding to continence). There was no significant difference between incontinent and continent subjects in the supine position, but there was between the groups in the standing position. Despite this significant difference, there was a great deal of overlap between the results for the continent and incontinent groups, invalidating a diagnosis based on this test alone.

Lateral stress cystography

Comparison between continent and incontinent subjects and between those with different types of incontinence, with regard to urethral axis, posterior urethrovesical angle (PUV) and distance of urethrovesical junction to the urogenital diaphragm (UGD), showed that incontinent respondents had a significantly ($p = 0.001$) wider PUV angle than did continent respondents; however, no significant difference was observed between stress and non-stress types of incontinence. There was no difference in the urethral axis and the position of the bladder neck in relation to the UGD between the groups according to continence status or clinical type of incontinence. There was a significantly greater mean PUV angle among incontinent subjects with an incompetent

sphincter than among continent subjects with a competent sphincter ($p = 0.004$); however, neither the measurements of the urethral axis nor the location of the UGD differed between these two groups.

Provocative stress test

A provocative cough stress test was found to be significantly correlated to continence and incontinence status and, more specifically, to the stress type of urine loss with or without urge loss ($p \leqslant 0.0005$). Table 2.4 depicts the results of the stress test, showing a 98.5% specificity. The result of the stress cystogram, when correlated with the stress test, showed a strong association ($p = 0.009$). A urethral axis of 30 degrees or more is more likely to give rise to a positive stress test than is an axis of less than 30 degrees. The stress test can be performed as part of the initial office evaluation and does not require special equipment: there is no morbidity, it is inexpensive and (more importantly) it has extremely high specificity; it should be a part of everyone's initial evaluation. However, a negative test in someone who is experiencing UI does not rule out its existence, as the sensitivity of the test often is only 40%.

MEDICAL CORRELATES OF URINARY INCONTINENCE

Health correlates

Several health conditions were noted in the MESA survey[18] to be significantly associated with UI in women.

Table 2.4. *Comparison of results of provocative stress test with self-reported severity of incontinence in elderly women*

Stress test result	Continence*	Incontinence* Mild	Moderate	Severe	Total
Absent	70 (98.6)	31 (86.1)	9 (52.9)	17 (54.8)	127
Present	1 (1.4)	5 (13.9)	8 (47.1)	14 (45.2)	28
Totals	71 (100)	36 (100)	17 (100)	31 (100)	155
Not determined[†]	4	0	0	3	

* Percentages in parentheses.
[†] Also, five with no severity of incontinence, two with stress absent, three with stress present.
Data adapted from ref. 17.

Surveys showed that physical mobility problems, specific neurological symptoms, lower urinary tract symptoms, bowel problems and history of genital surgery are more prevalent among those who are incontinent than among those who are continent. Other factors associated with female geriatric incontinence include a history of parent or sibling incontinence, incontinence either during pregnancy or *post partum*, vaginal infection and the use of female hormones.

Subjects with mobility problems were defined in the survey as users of wheelchairs or walking aids, those with diagnosed arthritis or those with a fall during the last year. In those incontinent women with mobility problems, the urge type of incontinence was significantly more prevalent than any other type.

With regard to urinary tract problems, incontinent respondents had significantly more urinary tract infections; pain, burning or stinging while urinating; hesitancy; urgency to void, and slow stream, than did the continent respondents. Similarly, the proportion of women who reported coughing and sneezing was often significantly higher among incontinent than continent respondents.

With regard to bowel problems, more women with UI reported faecal incontinence and constipation than did those who were continent. Women in the group with stress incontinence were the least likely of all those with UI to lose control over their bowels. These findings further underline the multifactorial issues confronting caregivers treating elderly incontinent women.

With regard to familial and personal history of incontinence among female respondents, more incontinent respondents reported an incontinent parent or sibling than did continent respondents. There was also a significantly higher response rate among incontinent respondents than continent respondents with regard to incontinence experienced during adolescence.

As far as pregnancy is concerned, there was no difference in the proportion of nulliparous women between continent and incontinent respondents. Among incontinent women, however, there were more nulliparous women in the group with urge incontinence than in the groups with stress or mixed types of incontinence. Those women who had been pregnant at least once were asked if they had been incontinent during any pregnancy and whether they had been incontinent shortly after any delivery: more incontinent than continent respondents reported that they had been incontinent during pregnancy or *post partum*.

Women who were incontinent reported a higher rate of female hormone use (10.4%) than did continent respondents (6.1%). It is not known whether the higher rate of hormone use among incontinent respondents is related to treatment of incontinence.

Use of diuretics

The MESA survey[19] identified 36.9% of female respondents to be current users of a diuretic medication, although no significant difference was found in the prevalence of incontinence between users and non-users of diuretics. However, in men, incontinence was significantly more prevalent among those diuretic users found to have uninhibited detrusor contractions on cystometry than in those users who did not have such contractions. This could not be assessed in women because the number of women in the group with uninhibited contractions was too small for analysis. Nevertheless, these findings suggest that care providers should be aware of the potential provocative effect of diuretics in a patient with pre-existing detrusor instability and that, if possible, diuretics should be avoided in this group of patients.

PATIENT STRATEGIES TO CONTROL URINE LOSS

The MESA survey also studied the various strategies by which women cope with their incontinence:[20] 69% of incontinent women were using one or more methods to control their urine loss. This degree of coping was significantly greater than that in their male counterparts, 55% of whom reported the use of one or more methods to contain their urine loss. For most (55%) incontinent women, absorbent products such as sanitary napkins, toilet tissue and absorbent garments were the most popular means. The second most common strategy (in 42%) was to locate a toilet upon arrival at an unfamiliar place. Voiding manipulation – such as scheduled urination, voiding before leaving home, and other conscious efforts to plan urination – was practised by 28% of female incontinent respondents. Alteration of the diet and fluid intake to control incontinence was reported by 16% of respondents, and 12% did pelvic muscle exercises; only 6% of women reported taking medication for their incontinence.

Jeter *et al.*[21] in 1990 reported the results of a postal survey sent to 36,500 members of the advocacy group HIP (Help for Incontinent People, Inc.), with a response rate of 33%. Results showed that most incontinent persons had tried alternative ways to manage their urine loss. Pelvic muscle exercises had been tried by only 14% of respondents and were in use by only 7.7% at the time of the study. With regard to medical consultation, 37% of respondents had consulted a urologist, 35% their family doctor and 17% their gynaecologist. Over 50% (range 52–61%) of respondents who consulted their physician reported that their condition did not improve; the degree of improvement (or lack of it) was not related to the severity of incontinence. These data were subsequently updated by another survey conducted by HIP (now known as NAFC [National Association For Continence, Spartanburg, SC, USA]). The report published in the spring issue of the NAFC journal *Quality Care* reported an increasing rate of dissatisfaction with the outcome of treatment:[22] in 1992 34.6% of the member respondents were dissatisfied with treatment they had undergone; in 1995, this rate increased to 62.1%. Nevertheless, in the same report in 1992 65.9% reported no change in their condition, in contrast to an improvement in the 1995 survey showing that the 'no change' response had fallen to 46.7%. Similarly, in 1992 only 24.6% considered that their condition had improved, whereas in 1995 the improvement rate increased to 41.4%.

CONCLUSIONS

UI is a highly prevalent condition that affects women of all ages, domicile or health status. In elderly women, the incidence and remission rates appear to be significant. UI is highly correlated with several medical conditions. Several urodynamic parameters help to explain the mechanism of incontinence whereas others raise questions on the validity of long-standing concepts of bladder function and dysfunction. Although some urodynamic tests have shown significant differences between continent and incontinent subjects, the values overlap, thus hindering meaningful interpretation.

Future studies must be aimed at unifying the definition of survey parameters in UI. As epidemiological studies of UI are at an early stage, many fields remain unexplored; these must be investigated, so that the insights provided by such epidemiological data can be used in the areas of causality and prevention.

REFERENCES

1. *Dorland's Illustrated Medical Dictionary* 26th edn. Philadelphia: WB Saunders, 1985; 451
2. Thomas TM, Plymat KR, Blannin J, Meade TW. Prevalence of urinary incontinence. *Br Med J* 1980; 281: 1243
3. Diokno AC, Brock BM, Brown MB, Herzog AR. Prevalence of urinary incontinence and other urologic symptoms in the noninstitutionalized elderly. *J Urol* 1986; 136: 1022–1025
4. Wolin LH. Stress incontinence in young, healthy nulliparous female subjects. *J Urol* 1969; 101: 545–549
5. Burgio KL, Matthews KA, Engel BT. Prevalence, incidence and correlates of urinary incontinence in healthy, middle-aged women. *J Urol* 1991; 146: 1255–1259
6. Elving LB, Foldspang A, Lam OW, Mommsen S. Descriptive epidemiology of urinary incontinence in 3100 women age 30–59. *Scand J Urol Nephrol Suppl* 1989; 125
7. Brocklehurst JC, Dillane JB, Griffiths L, Fry J. The prevalence and symptomatology of urinary infection in an aged population. *Gerontol Clin* 1968; 10: 242
8. Milne JS, Williamson J, Maule MM, Wallace ET. Urinary symptoms in older people. *Mod Geriatr* 1972; 2: 198
9. Ouslander JG, Kane RL, Abrass IB. Urinary incontinence in elderly nursing home patients. *J Am Med Assoc* 1984; 248: 1194
10. Hansen FR, Theissen KA, Krakauer R. Urinary symptoms in elderly women in nursing homes. *Ugeskr Laeger* 1990; 152: 3242–3244
11. Sullivan DH, Lindsay RW. Urinary incontinence in the geriatric population of an acute care hospital. *J Am Geriatr Soc* 1984; 32: 646
12. Willington FL. Significance of incompetence of personal sanitary habits. *Nurs Times* 1975; 71: 340
13. Herzog AR, Diokno AC, Brown MB, Brock BM. Two year incidences, remissions and change patterns of urinary incontinence in noninstitutionalized older adults. *J Gerontol* 1990; 45: 67–74
14. Campbell AJ, Reinken J, McCosh L. Incontinence in the elderly: prevalence and prognosis. *Age Ageing* 1985; 14: 65–80
15. Wells TJ, Brink CA, Diokno AC. Urinary incontinence in the elderly woman: clinical findings. *J Am Geriatr Soc* 1987; 35: 933–939

16. Diokno AC, Brown MB, Browk BM *et al.* Clinical and cystometric characteristics of continent and incontinent noninstitutionalized elderly. *J Urol* 1988; 140: 567–571

17. Diokno AC, Normalle DP, Brown MB, Herzog AR. Urodynamic tests for female geriatric urinary incontinence. *Urology* 1990; 36: 431–439

18. Diokno AC, Brock BM, Brown MB *et al.* Medical correlates of urinary incontinence in the elderly. *Urology* 1990; 36: 129–138

19. Diokno AC, Brown MB, Herzog AR. Relationship between use of diuretics and continence status in the elderly. *Urology* 1991; 38: 39–42

20. Herzog AR, Fultz NH, Normalle DP *et al.* Methods used to manage urinary incontinence by older adults in the community. *J Am Geriatr Soc* 1989; 37: 339–347

21. Jeter KF, Wagner DB. Incontinence in the American home. *J Am Geriatr Soc* 1990; 38: 379–383

22. *Quality Care.* 1996; 14: 2

3

Epidemiology (Europe)

C. W. McGrother, C. Shaw, S. I. Perry, H. M. Dallosso, F. K. Mensah

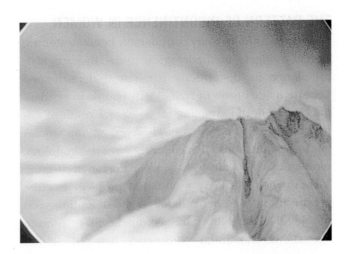

INTRODUCTION

Epidemiology is the study of disease in populations. It is primarily concerned with identifying clues to causation and estimating need as a basis for service provision. Accordingly, it considers associated environmental, lifestyle and co-morbidity factors and definitions of disease in terms of symptoms, severity, impact and natural history. Epidemiology is primarily an observational science that relies on understanding and controlling methodological imperfections to achieve a reasonable interpretation of available data. The main epidemiological indices are *prevalence* – the proportion of a population having a disease at a point in time – and *incidence* – the rate of occurrence of a disease in a population over a period of time.

Urinary incontinence is a symptom of lower urinary tract disorder, but it is only one among several significant urinary symptoms. Urinary incontinence is not a disease in the sense of being a discrete pathological entity; indeed, the symptom of incontinence is common to several different types of lower urinary tract disorders. Incontinence may also be conceptualized as an impairment (i.e. a functional abnormality), a disability (i.e. a restriction) or a handicap (i.e. a social disadvantage), depending on its severity and individual tolerance. Here again, other urinary symptoms, such as urgency, may contribute significantly to the overall disability arising from a lower urinary tract disorder. Thus, incontinence can serve as a *marker* rather than a *measure* of disease and need. Within these limitations, existing epidemiological studies provide useful insights into the pattern and extent of bladder disorder in the female population.

THE PATTERN OF INCONTINENCE IN WOMEN

Prevalence estimates vary considerably between studies, largely owing to methodological issues. In particular, prevalence in the elderly is often underestimated because of exclusion of frail elderly people in residential care from the sampling frame or as a result of disproportionate non-response. However, among studies on total populations selected for rigorous methodology, most estimates for any leakage are in the range 20–30%. Incontinence is clearly a common problem but the precise prevalence depends upon the definition used (Table 3.1). The pattern of incontinence in relation to age shows substantial consistency between studies

(Fig. 3.1). The prevalence peaks at around ages 45–55 years then dips between ages 55–70 years and increases again beyond age 70 years. The presence of a peak followed by a decline, in women, suggests that at least one of the underlying disorders represented may recover to some extent.

'Daily' leakage shows a lower prevalence but similar pattern to 'any' leakage, except for a disproportionately greater increase in prevalence in old age (Fig. 3.2). Severe forms of incontinence in women are therefore relatively common in old age, whereas mild forms of incontinence are most common in mid-life. Men show a lower but similar increase in prevalence in old age

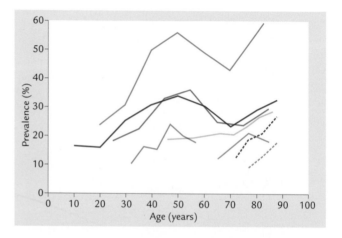

Figure 3.1. *Prevalence of urinary incontinence in women. (Data from refs. 1 —, 2 —, 3 ---, 4 —, 5 —, 6 —, 7 ---, and 8 —.)*

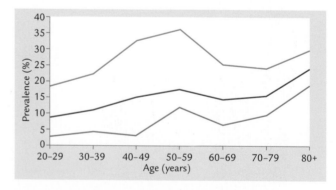

Figure 3.2. *Prevalence of severe incontinence in women, where severity is defined as multiplication of frequency by severity of incontinence, the values depicted being typical for the categories as defined: slight (— leakage of a few drops several times a month), moderate (— daily leakage of a few drops) and severe (— larger amounts at least once a week).*

Table 3.1. *Prevalence and definition of urinary incontinence in women in European studies*

Author/year/country	Base population	Response (%)	Definition	Prevalence (%)
Thomas[4] 1980 England*	GP register; age ≥ 15 years	89	Involuntary leakage of urine • occasional – less than twice a month • (regular – twice or more per month)	27 (9)
Yarnell[2] 1981 South Wales[†]	GP register (+ total population); age ≥ 18 years	96	Do you have any problems with 'waterworks' <u>and</u> • do you ever lose urine at any time? • (wetting weekly or more)	45 (12)
Sandvik[5] 1993 Norway*	Total population register; age ≥ 20 years	77	How often do you experience urine leakage? • drops or little × less than once a month • (drops × weekly or more × monthly)	29 (16)
O'Brien[9] 1991 England*	GP register; age ≥ 35 years	79	Two or more leaks in any one month	16
Elving[8] 1989 Denmark*	Total population register; age 30–59 years	85	Any urinary incontinence in a year	17
Hørding[10] 1986 Denmark[§]	Total population register; age 45 years	85	Loss of urine after strong desire to void or coughing, running etc.	22
Milsom[6] 1993 Sweden*	Total population register; age 46–88 years	75	Defined according to International Continence Society guidelines (question not specified)	21
Vetter[3] 1981 South Wales[†]	GP register; age ≥ 70 years	95	Do you ever wet yourself? • as little as a few drops once a week • (a few drops daily or more)	18 (7)
Tilvis[11] 1995 Finland[‡]	Total population register; ages 75, 80, 85 years	82	Subjects asked whether they suffer from incontinence	20
McGrother[7] 1986 England[†]	GP register (+ total population); age ≥ 75 years	94	Do you have difficulty in controlling your water? • occasional – twice a week or less • (frequent – more than twice a week)	12 (5)
Lagaay[12] 1992 Netherlands[†]	Total population register; age ≥ 85 years	94	Do you suffer from involuntary loss of urine?	28

Method of data collection: * postal questionnaire; [†] structured interview; [‡] combination; [§] unclear.

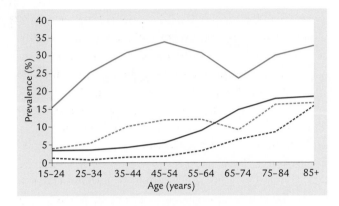

Figure 3.3. *Prevalence of urinary incontinence in men (—) and women (—): any leakage (solid) or monthly leakage (dashed).*

(Fig. 3.3); however, men show no peak at all in mid-life, which suggests that the self-limiting disorder is associated with the female sex.

STRESS AND URGE INCONTINENCE

In women, genuine stress incontinence (GSI) and detrusor instability (DI) are the two most commonly recognized clinical disorders of the lower urinary tract. Several studies have shown a relationship between these disorders and the symptoms of stress and urge incontinence. Studies that have relied on standardized questions have shown good validity:[13,14] for example, the sensitivity and specificity of pure stress was 78% and 84%, of pure urge 61% and 95%, and of combined stress and urge 68% and 79%, respectively, in these studies.

Although the symptoms of stress and urge incontinence may not be sufficiently accurate predictors to be clinically diagnostic for surgical interventions, they provide adequate markers with which to examine the different patterns of behaviour of the two leading bladder disorders. Overall, stress incontinence is the most prevalent type of incontinence reported by women. However, the proportion with urge incontinence increases with age to the point where stress and urge incontinence are almost equally common in old age (29% and 25%, respectively, in those aged 75 years or over; Fig. 3.4).

The symptom of stress incontinence may occur alone or in combination with urge incontinence. Among the few reliable studies available, that of Yarnell *et al.*[2] is

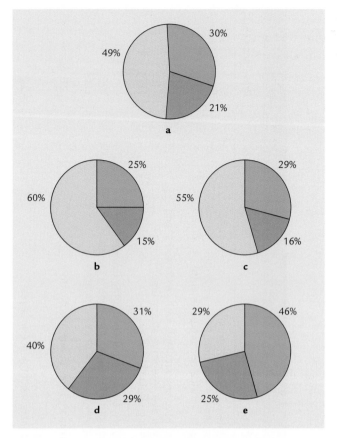

Figure 3.4. *Prevalence of stress incontinence ( ), urge incontinence ( ) and combined stress + urge incontinence ( ) in women by age group: (a) 25+ (b) 25–34; (c) 45–54; (d) 65–74; (e) 75+ years.*

fairly consistent with others in showing a rise in prevalence across the reproductive years with a mid-life peak and a subsequent decline (Fig. 3.5). The pattern is similar for stress incontinence alone and stress combined with urge incontinence, except that in combination there is also a progressive increase with age. This pattern suggests a connection between GSI and the reproductive and menopausal periods followed by 'recovery' in a proportion of cases before age-related factors become dominant. Recovery may occur naturally, in response to treatment or by adaptation (e.g. avoidance of provocation).

In keeping with other studies, urge incontinence (either alone or in combination with stress incontinence) shows a progressive increase with age, with no decline in mid-life (Fig. 3.6). Thus the overall pattern of incontinence is likely to be the result of the summation of the two main clinically recognized disorders, with GSI accounting for the mid-life peak in women and DI contributing primarily to the overall increase with age. The increase and overlap of both disorders in old age may explain the preponderance of severe incontinence at this stage. Little information is available on the population prevalence of other underlying conditions or types of incontinence, such as nocturnal enuresis.

THE EXTENT OF NEED

When deciding on treatment, it is important to consider not only the severity of symptoms but also the psychological and social impact. The impact of inconti-

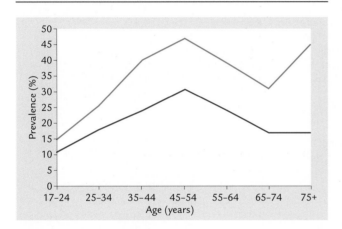

Figure 3.5. *Prevalence of stress incontinence: (—) pure stress; (—) pure stress + combined stress and urge.*

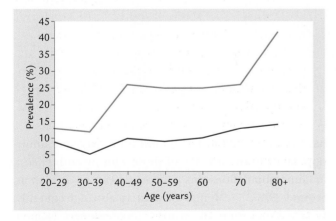

Figure 3.6. *Prevalence of urge incontinence: (—) pure urge; (—) pure urge + combined stress and urge.*

nence may be measured directly by asking questions about the bothersome, problematic or worrying nature of symptoms. The prevalence of bothersome incontinence has been reported mostly as being between 7 and 12% of the total population studied (Table 3.2).

There is a relationship, although not a strong one, between symptom severity and the perception of bother: 14% of women with mild incontinence have been found to be worried by their condition, compared with 24% with moderate and 29% with severe incontinence.[16] There is also evidence that this perception of bother is related to different types of incontinence: it has been reported that 8% of women with pure stress incontinence, 16% of women with pure urge incontinence and 29% of women with mixed incontinence identified their symptoms as causing problems.[2] Although there is evidently a correlation between symptom severity and direct measures of 'bother', it is apparent that relatively few women, even those experiencing severe symptoms, consider such symptoms to be a problem. Overall, the direct approach suggests that only about one-third of women in the community who have urinary incontinence experience any impact on their lives.

The impact of incontinence may also be measured indirectly by assessing the restricting effect of symptoms on daily activities, social activities, relationships and emotions. Urinary incontinence can have a significant effect on an individual's life. The strategies that people adopt to manage the condition sometimes involve exhaustive, time-consuming rituals of frequent toileting, changing and washing garments, and avoidance of social contacts – which can ultimately render the individual socially isolated.[18] Often, however, people cope fairly successfully with the condition but at the cost of avoiding certain activities and arranging their environments to accommodate the problem: for example, they may visit only those places where they know the location of toilet facilities.[19]

Table 3.3 details several of the more methodologically rigorous epidemiological studies, which suggest that between 1 and 5% of the population suffer some restriction in their daily social activities as a result of urinary incontinence. Activities most commonly affected are shopping, visiting friends and sporting activities. Other studies report restrictions in sport and leisure activities (such as exercise, walking, dancing, going to the cinema, holidays, and visiting and

Table 3.2. *Prevalence of bothersome urinary incontinence in women*

Author/year	Age (years)	Aspect of bother measured	Population prevalence (%)
Harrison[15] (1994)	20+	Worry	8.5
Lagro-Janssen[16] (1990)	50–65	Worry	5.0
Sandvik[5] (1993)	20+	Problem	25.0
Yarnell[2] (1981)	18+	Problem	7.0
Samuelsson[17] (1997)	20–59	Embarrassment	12.4

Table 3.3. *Prevalence of restriction of activities due to urinary incontinence*

Author/year	Age (years)	Restriction in activities	Population prevalence (%)	Percentage of incontinent sample
Lam[22] (1992)	30–59	No. of activities: 1 or more	3.0	19.4
		2 or more	1.0	6.3
		Type of activity: social	3.0	17.4
		sport	2.0	15.7
		sexual	1.1	5.9
Lagro-Janssen[16] (1990)	50–65	Restricted in activities	3.0	24.6
Harrison[15] (1994)	20+	Shopping and walking	3.7	20.5
		Travelling long distances	5.3	29.5
		Keep fit	3.9	21.8
		Social life	2.6	14.1
Yarnell[2] (1981)	18+	Social life	1.1	2.8
		Social and domestic life	0.9	2.3
Brocklehurst[25] (1993)	30+	Using public transport	2.5	34.0
		Visiting friends	3.5	47.0
		Going out to work	2.4	33.0
		Going to supermarket	4.0	44.0
Rekers[19] (1992)	35–79	Must know where toilet is	1.3	7.6
		Sport	0.5	2.9
		Going to church	0.3	1.5
		Visiting relatives	0.3	1.5
		Going shopping	0.2	1.2
		Work	0.2	1.2
		Sexual activities	0.1	0.6

entertaining friends) and in activities of daily living (such as bending, lifting and shopping).[20,21] Travel becomes problematic, with initial avoidance of long journeys and, eventually, also of short journeys. Relationships may be affected, particularly sexual relationships, as incontinence can occur during coitus.[22] Disturbance of sexual relations due to incontinence has been reported in 1.1%[22] and 0.1%[19] of community populations (i.e. in 1–4% of those with incontinence); in clinic populations this proportion can be as high as around 40%.[21,23] Mental distress is also a frequently reported outcome of urinary incontinence: women with incontinence experience shame and embarrassment, loss of self-esteem, anxiety and depression.[24]

Table 3.4. *Extent of use of services by women with urinary incontinence*

Author/year	Age (years)	Percentage of incontinent sample who sought help
Lagro-Janssen[16] (1990)	50–65	32
Harrison[15] (1994)	20+	13
Yarnell[2] (1981)	18+	9
Brocklehurst[25] (1993)	30+	47
Samuelsson[17] (1997)	20–59	9
Seim[26] (1995)	20+	20
Rekers[19] (1992)	35–79	28

Restriction in social activities is correlated with severity of symptoms: the larger the volume or the more frequent the leakage, the greater the psychosocial effects. Of women with mild incontinence, 12% were reported to be restricted in social activities, whereas 31% of women with moderate or severe symptoms suffered restriction in activity.[16] It has also been suggested that restriction depends upon the type of incontinence, with urge or mixed incontinence having a greater impact than stress incontinence alone.[20] Overall, the indirect approach suggests that only about one-tenth of women in the community who have urinary incontinence experience a disabling (i.e. restricting) effect on their lives.

A further perspective on the extent of need is provided by the take-up of services. Reported consultation rates vary considerably, depending on the sample and the definition of incontinence, but it is often estimated that between one-fifth and one-third of women with incontinence have actually spoken to a doctor (Table 3.4). Consultation rates increase with increasing severity and impact of incontinence, but the association is not strong:[19] for example, 44% of women with incontinence at least once a week sought help compared with 22% with lesser incontinence. Even among women reporting worry about their symptoms, only one-third had spoken to a doctor and, among women reporting more severe restriction to their social life, only one-half had consulted a health professional.

A major reason for this discrepancy (i.e. women with a problem who fail to seek help) between the patient's perceptions of the problem and help-seeking behaviours are misconceptions of the aetiology and natural history of the condition. Many women view incontinence as the inevitable result of childbearing and older age, and consider it an inappropriate use of consulting time.[27] There is a general lack of awareness of the range of treatments, as others do not consult a doctor because they fear surgery;[27] those that are aware of treatments may have low expectations of their efficacy.[15] Unfortunately, these views are often reinforced by health professionals: for example, 17% of one sample of incontinent women had sought help, only to be told that 'urinary incontinence is a common phenomenon which increases with age, and nothing can be done'.[28] Age also plays a part, with younger people being more likely than older people to seek help.[19]

In summary, most studies suggest that 20–30% of women experience some leakage of urine, but only 7–12% perceive this to be problematic in some way, whereas 1–4% suffer actual restriction to their daily activities as a result of incontinence; 4–10% of women have spoken to a doctor at some stage about incontinence. Clearly, the extent of need depends on definition, and further clarification is required of the factors involved in determining need.

INCONTINENCE IN INSTITUTIONS

Urinary incontinence is much more prevalent among elderly women living in institutions than among those living at home[1,7,29] (Table 3.5). If anything, the difference in prevalence is underestimated: the threshold for defining incontinence in institutions tends to be higher, as it relies on observations from carers rather than self-reported incontinence. The higher prevalence is probably due to the selection of frail, dependent and incontinent individuals into residential care.[3,11,30,31] Prevalence estimates are likely to vary over time and between countries, depending on the configuration of residential care. In Great Britain, the evidence suggests that between 30 and 70% of patients in geriatric and psychogeriatric wards experience urinary

incontinence, compared with 30–60% of residents in nursing homes and 15–30% in residential homes.[12,32–36] A census of all people aged 64 years and over in long-term care in Leicestershire, England in 1991 showed that these differences were related to the level of dependency among residents (Table 3.6). Prevalences are likely to vary within settings, as admission and management policies change and as residents age.

Table 3.5. *Prevalence of urinary incontinence* among elderly women*

| Age group (years) | Place of residence | | | | All women | |
	Community (%)	(n)	Institutions (%)	(n)	(%)	(n)
75–79	8	31	–	4	9	35
80–84	14	34	–	1	13	35
85+	12	15	36	16	18	31
All ages (902)[†]	11	80	32	21	12	101

*Incontinence defined as difficulty in control.
[†] Total sample size
From ref. 7 with permission.

Table 3.6. *Prevalence of incontinence* in elderly people[†] in residential care*

| Type of home | Incontinence | | Dependent (%) |
	Urine (%)	Double (%)	
NHS geriatric	31	27	61
NHS psychogeriatric	28	37	47
NHS acute	21	9	35
Private nursing	30	33	70
Private residential	19	10	32
Local authority	21	14	26
Voluntary	6	4	17
Other	15	8	24
All places	23	18	39

*Incontinence defined as at least one incontinent episode weekly.
[†] Mean age, 83 years; proportion of women, 79%.
From ref. 36 with permission.

The Leicestershire study also illustrates that, in institutions, almost half of those with urinary incontinence also experience faecal incontinence. This is a far higher proportion than in the general population, where only 1% of women aged 65 years or more have been found to have faecal or double incontinence, compared with 12% with regular urinary incontinence.[4,37]

ASSOCIATED FACTORS

Most aetiological studies have been in mixed age groups in relation to undifferentiated incontinence and, probably for these reasons, show many inconsistencies. In young women, incontinence is mainly a symptom of GSI; in elderly women, almost half of all cases may be secondary to dementia and mobility problems and half to various bladder disorders, primarily DI.[38] These diseases have different aetiologies; associated factors will therefore vary, depending on the mix of cases and the age range of the sample in each study.

There is reasonable consistency between population studies over the main morbidities associated with incontinence in old age:[3,11,29,38,39] primarily, these include dementia, depression, anxiety and poor mobility (Table 3.7). An association with neurological disease was observed to occur in advanced old age in women. Somewhat weaker links were reported for cardiovascular disease (including stroke, diabetes and respiratory disease) but not with musculoskeletal disease. The strong association with dementia tends to colour attitudes towards treatment of incontinence in elderly people. It is worth noting that, among all people aged 75 years or more, only 20% of those with incontinence were reported to be cognitively impaired[38] (Table 3.8).

In younger women there have been few longitudinal studies on defined populations capable of eliminating bias and disentangling the cause-and-effect sequence. In one cohort study, following childbirth, factors associated with the development of stress incontinence were high birth weight, prolonged second stage of labour, use of forceps, and vaginal delivery;[40] maternal age was the dominant predictor of late-starting and persistent stress incontinence; those in social classes I and II and white (i.e. non-Asian) women appeared to be at increased risk.

Table 3.7. *Morbidity associated with incontinence in old age*

Morbidity	Prevalence in the population	
	With urinary incontinence (%)	Without incontinence (%)
Dementia*	15.0	2.4
Depression[†]	10.2	2.7
Anxiety[†]	17.6	5.3
Mobility*	68.0	37.0
Neurological[‡]	40.8	25.9
Genital[‡]	35.6	25.4
Urinary tract[‡]	63.4	48.7
Cardiovascular[‡]	60.6	52.7

*Age 75+ years men and women.[38]
[†] Age 70+ years men and women.[3]
[‡] Age 85 years women only.[29]

Table 3.8. *Prevalence of dementia, locomotor problems and incontinence in elderly people*

Morbidity	Prevalence (%)	n
Dementia, locomotor problems and incontinence	1.7	20
Dementia and incontinence	0.2	2
Dementia and locomotor problems	1.7	20
Dementia alone	0.4	5
Locomotor problems and incontinence	6.7	80
Locomotor problems alone	30.8	370
Incontinence alone	3.7	45
Continent	54.9	660
All persons	100	1202

From ref. 38 with permission.

NATURAL HISTORY OF INCONTINENCE

In order to calculate the incidence and remission rates of a condition it is necessary to conduct repeated prospective surveys on a large random sample of the population over a number of years. For this reason, there are very few prospective studies available and there have been no reports of incidence in Europe as yet.

Estimates of incidence rates can be calculated from data collected retrospectively. In one such study in Denmark, a postal questionnaire, completed by 2631 women aged 30–59, asked if they had ever experienced a period of urinary incontinence and, if so, when it had started.[8] The incidence of 'any incontinence' as an adult ranged from 0.54 to 1.4% per year, and for incontinence that was a social or hygienic problem the range was 0.32–0.78% per year, increasing with age. In another retrospective study in England, among those aged 75 years or more living at home, the incidence of incontinence (i.e. difficulty in controlling the urine) was estimated at 1% in the previous year.[7] If this is a true picture, the pattern of increase in new cases with age would indicate that incontinence is not merely the continuation of a childhood problem but arises for new reasons – and increasingly so with advancing age.

Retrospective studies are subject to problems with recall. Episodes of incontinence may be forgotten, or there may be difficulty in recalling the correct year of onset, especially in the distant past. These reports are therefore likely to underestimate the true incidence, especially among the elderly with memory defects.

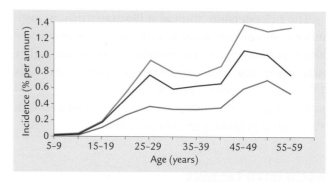

Figure 3.7. *Incidence of urinary incontinence in women by age: (—) all incontinence; (—) pure stress + combined stress and urge; (—) pure urge + combined urge and stress.*

However, the advantage of retrospective studies is that they readily provide a perspective of incidence over a lifetime. In this respect, the overall incidence of incontinence mirrors the pattern of prevalence in younger women (Fig. 3.7). The pattern of incidence of urge and stress incontinence, either alone or in combination, is also consistent with the pattern of prevalence in younger women. Among those men and women aged 75 and over, analysis of the duration of incontinence gives some indication of the relatively large increase in incidence in old age (Fig. 3.8).

Incontinence is subject to remission in a proportion of cases. One study estimated that 33% of those originally identified as reporting some incontinence were no longer incontinent 3–12 months later.[1] Undoubtedly, there are problems with the reliability of questions

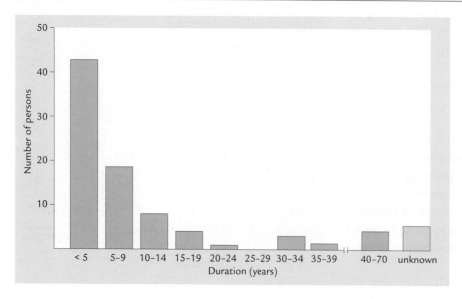

Figure 3.8. *Duration of urinary incontinence in elderly people.*

used to identify incontinence, but this and evidence elsewhere suggests that, in a proportion of cases, incontinence may be episodic and may remit, possibly naturally but also in response to treatment.

OTHER URINARY SYMPTOMS

There have been relatively few epidemiological studies of other important symptoms related to incontinence in women, namely frequency, urgency and nocturia. The prevalences of such symptoms reported in one Danish population are shown in Figure 3.9.[41] It is apparent that potentially significant symptoms are quite common (e.g. hourly frequency, with a 2–8% prevalence). However, there is little validated guidance on the pathological levels of such symptoms, making interpretation difficult.

In younger women, frequency shows a peak in prevalence around ages 30–39, which coincides with the peak childbearing ages. The pattern is similar for frequency and urgency, which suggests that there may be similarities in the underlying conditions for these symptoms. In contrast, nocturia shows a steady increase with age, suggesting a different underlying pathology, strongly related to ageing.

The true pattern of such symptoms in the total population, particularly in the elderly, is difficult to gauge because of substantial variation in response rates in different age groups, as shown by the Danish study. It is likely that the bias stems from a probable loss of cases among infirm or institutionalized elderly women, who often fail to respond to postal questionnaires. Studies that have focused on elderly women in particular generally show high prevalence rates for significant urinary symptoms (Table 3.9).

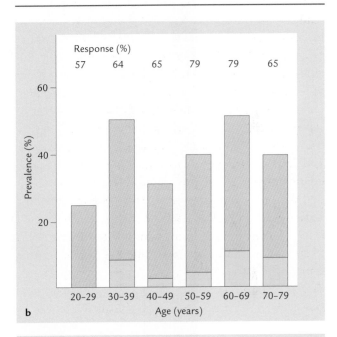

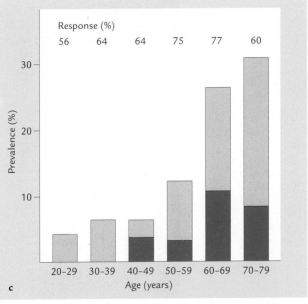

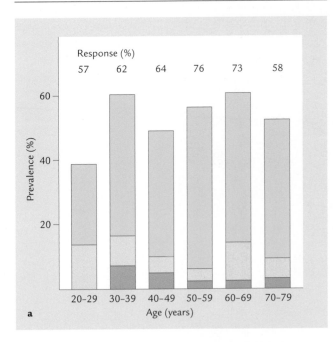

Figure 3.9. *Prevalence of urinary symptoms in women:*
(a) frequency (2–3-hourly; 1–2-hourly; hourly);
(b) urgency ('now and then'; every day);
(c) nocturia (twice; ■ ≥ 3 times).

Table 3.9. *Prevalence of other urinary symptoms in older women in European studies*

Study (year) /population	Frequency	Prevalence Age (years)	%	Urgency	Prevalence Age (years)	%	Nocturia	Prevalence Age (years)	%
Brocklehurst[42] (1971) / general practice list	Can you go for longer than 2 hours in the day time without having to pass urine?	All 65+	9	Do you have to go to pass urine in a hurry?	All 65+	32	Do you ever get up at night to pass urine (twice or more)?	65–70 71+ All 65+	14 35 28
Milne[43] (1972) / Edinburgh population	Has there been any change in how often you pass urine in a day?	62–69 70+ All 62+	16 30 23	Do you lose control of your bladder if unable to go to the lavatory as soon as you need to pass urine?	All 62+	20	Do you rise to pass urine at night (twice or more)?	62–69 70–79 80+ All 62+	18 31 41 26
Kok[39] (1992) / Community residents only	More than seven voids a day	60–84 85+ All 60+	11 13 11	Strong desire to void accompaniied by fear of leakage	60–84 85+ All 60+	7 21 11	More than twice a night	60–84 85+ All 60+	9 17 11

REFERENCES

1. Yarnell JWG, St Leger AS. The prevalence, severity and factors associated with urinary incontinence in a random sample of the elderly. *Age Ageing* 1979; 8: 81–85

2. Yarnell JWG, Voyle GJ, Richards CJ, Stephenson TP. The prevalence and severity of urinary incontinence in women. *J Epidemiol Community Health* 1981; 35: 71–74

3. Vetter NJ, Jones DA, Victor CR. Urinary incontinence in the elderly at home. *Lancet* 1981; ii: 1275–1277

4. Thomas TM, Plymat KR, Blannin J, Meade TW. Prevalence of urinary incontinence, *Br Med J* 1980; 281: 1243–1245

5. Sandvik H, Hunskaar S, Seim A *et al.* Validation of a severity index in female urinary incontinence and its implementation in an epidemiological survey. *J Epidemiol Community Health* 1993; 47: 497–499

6. Milsom I, Ekelund P, Molander U *et al.* The influence of age, parity, oral contraception, hysterectomy and menopause on the prevalence of urinary incontinence in women. *J Urol* 1993; 149: 1459–1462

7. McGrother CW, Castleden CM, Duffin H, Clarke M. Provision of services for incontinent elderly people at home. *J Epidemiol Community Health* 1986; 40: 134–138

8. Elving LB, Foldspang A, Lam GW, Mommsen S. Descriptive epidemiology of urinary incontinence in 3,100 women age 30–59. *Scand J Urol Nephrol Suppl* 1989; 125: 37–43

9. O'Brien J, Austin M, Parminder S, O'Boyle P. Urinary incontinence: prevalence, need for treatment and effectiveness of intervention by nurse. *Br Med J* 1991; 303: 1308–1312

10. Hørding U, Pedersen K, Sidenius K, Hedegaard L. Urinary incontinence in 45 year old women. *Scand J Urol Nephrol* 1986; 20: 183–186

11. Tilvis RS, Hakala S, Valvanne J, Erkinjuntti T. Urinary incontinence as a predictor of death and institutionalization in a general aged population. *Arch Gerontol Geriatr* 1995; 21: 307–315

12. Lagaay AM, Van Asperen IA, Hijmans W. The prevalence of morbidity in the oldest old, aged 85 and over: a population-based survey of Leiden, The Netherlands. *Arch Gerontol Geriatr* 1992; 15: 115–131

13. Lagro-Janssen ALM, Debruyne FMJ, Van Weel C. Value of the patient's case history in diagnosing urinary incontinence in general practice. *Br J Urol* 1991; 67: 569–572

14. Versi E, Cardozo L, Anand D, Cooper D. Symptoms analysis for the diagnosis of genuine stress incontinence. *Br J Obstet Gynaecol* 1991; 98: 815–819

15. Harrison GL, Memel DS. Urinary incontinence in women: its prevalence and its management in a health promotion clinic. *Br J Gen Pract* 1994; 44: 149–152

16. Lagro-Janssen TLM, Smits AJA, Van Weel C. Women with urinary incontinence: self-perceived worries and general practitioners' knowledge of problem. *Br J Gen Pract* 1990; 40: 331–334

17. Samuelsson E, Victor A, Tibblin G. A population study of urinary incontinence and nocturia among women aged 20–59 years. *Acta Obstet Gynaecol Scand* 1997; 76: 74–80

18. Mitteness LS. The management of urinary incontinence by community living elderly. *Gerontologist* 1987; 27: 185–193

19. Rekers H, Drogendijk AC, Valkenburg H, Riphagen F. Urinary incontinence in women from 35 to 79 years of age: prevalence and consequences, *J Obstet Gynecol Reprod Biol* 1992; 43: 229–234

20. Sandvik H, Kveine E, Hunskaar S. Female urinary incontinence: psychosocial impact, self care, and consultations. *Scand J Caring Sci* 1993; 7: 53–56

21. Norton PA, MacDonald LD, Sedgwick PM, Stanton SL. Distress and delay associated with urinary incontinence, frequency and urgency in women. *Br Med J* 1988; 297: 1187–1189

22. Lam GW, Foldspang A, Elving LB, Mommsen S. Social context, social abstention, and problem recognition correlated with adult female urinary incontinence. *Dan Med Bull* 1992; 39: 565–570

23. Sutherst JR. Sexual dysfunction and urinary incontinence. *Br J Obstet Gynaecol* 1979; 86: 387–388

24. Macaulay AJ, Stern RS, Stanton SL. Psychological aspects of 211 female patients attending a urodynamic unit. *J Psychosom Res* 1991; 35: 1–10

25. Brocklehurst JC. Urinary incontinence in the community – analysis of a MORI poll. *Br Med J* 1993; 306: 832–834

26. Seim A, Sandvik H, Hermstad R, Hunskaar S. Female urinary incontinence—consultation behaviour and patient experiences: an epidemiological survey in a Norwegian community. *Fam Pract* 1995; 12: 18–21

27. Jolleys JV. Reported prevalence of urinary incontinence in women in a general practice. *Br Med J* 1988; 296: 1300–1302

28. Simeonova Z, Bengtsson C. Prevalence of urinary incontinence among women at a Swedish Primary Health Care Centre. *Scand J Prim Health Care* 1990; 8: 203–206

29. Hellstrom L, Ekelund P, Milsom I, Mellstrom O. The prevalence of incontinence and use of incontinence aids in 85 year old men and women, *Age Ageing* 1990; 19: 383–389

30. Johanson JF, Irizarry F, Doughty A. Risk factors for fecal incontinence in a nursing home population. *J Clin Gastroenterol* 1997; 24: 156–160

31. The Royal College of Physicians. *Incontinence: Causes, Management and Provision of Services.* London: Royal College of Physicians of London; 1995

32. Clarke M, Hughes AO, Dodd KJ *et al.* The elderly in residential care: patterns of disability. *Health Trends* 1979; 11: 17–20

33. McLauchlan S, Wilkin D. Levels of provision and of dependency in residential homes for the elderly: implications for planning. *Health Trends* 1982; 14: 63–65

34. Capewell AE, Primrose WR, Macintyre C. Nursing dependency in registered nursing homes and long term care geriatric wards in Edinburgh. *Br Med J* 1986; 292: 1719–1721

35. Stott DJ, Dutton M, Williams BO, Macdonald J. Functional capacity and mental status of elderly people in long-term care in west Glasgow. *Health Bull* 1990; 48: 17–24

36. Peet SM, Castleden CM, McGrother CW. Prevalence of urinary and faecal incontinence in hospitals and residential and nursing homes for older people. *Br Med J* 1995; 311: 1063–1064

37. Thomas TM, Egan M, Walgrove A, Meade TW. The prevalence of faecal and double incontinence. *Community Med* 1984; 6: 216–220

38. McGrother CW, Jagger C, Clarke M, Castleden CM. Handicaps associated with incontinence: implications for management. *J Epidemiol Community Health* 1990; 44: 246–248

39. Kok ALM, Voorhurst FJ, Burger CW *et al.* Urinary and faecal incontinence in community-residing elderly women. *Age Ageing* 1992; 21: 211–215

40. MacArthur C, Lewis M, Knox G. *Health after Childbirth.* London: HMSO, 1991

41. Sommer P, Bower T, Nielsen KK *et al.* Voiding patterns and prevalence of incontinence in women. *Br J Urol* 1990; 66: 12–15

42. Brocklehurst JC. Dysuria in old age. *J Am Geriatr Soc* 1971; 19: 582–519

43. Milne JS, Williamson J, Maule MM, Wallace ET. Urinary symptoms in older people. *Mod Geriatr* 1972; 2: 198–212

4

Epidemiology (Australia)

R. J. Millard

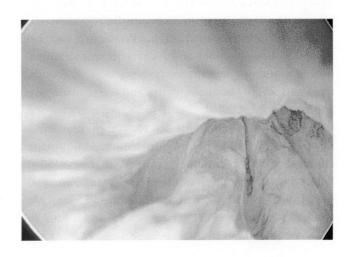

INTRODUCTION: THE SYDNEY SURVEY

In geographical terms, Australia is the driest continent on Earth; regrettably the same cannot be said of its inhabitants. The Australian population is multicultural, having been derived largely from waves of immigrants from Britain and the Mediterranean and Balkan countries for much of its 200 year post-colonization history, and from Asian and Central European countries more recently. Studies show that 5–6% of adult Australians have regular or severe urinary incontinence, a prevalence remarkably similar to that reported from other basically Caucasian populations.[1,2]

Data regarding prevalence in Australia have been available since a study in Sydney in 1983.[3] No systematic study of general prevalence has been conducted since that time. However, the longitudinal Women's Health Australia study, involving over 40 000 women,[4] has provided new data on prevalence in women[5] and may yield new data on the incidence of incontinence over the next 10–20 years as the cohorts age.

The problem with all surveys aimed at assessing the prevalence of incontinence is how to define urinary incontinence. Do we wish to know only how many people have regular and severe incontinence, assuming that we could define what we meant by even this term? Alternatively, is it relevant to know about all levels of urinary incontinence that occur in the community? Is whether the individual chooses to wear an incontinence pad or appliance a good indicator of significant incontinence?

To circumvent these issues, the 1983 Sydney survey attempted to ascertain the prevalence of all present and all past urinary incontinence and to stratify the type, severity and frequency of occurrence of the incontinence problems discovered in the study population. The study was designed to ascertain the prevalence of urinary incontinence in Australia. Prevalence was correlated with age, gender and socio-economic stratification. An attempt was made to define at-risk groups, types and severity of incontinence and use of protective appliances. A detailed, 38-question, self-report questionnaire was devised and tested for comprehensibility in small focus groups before distribution. A multistage cluster-sampling technique was used to target 3000 adults in 1000 homes, randomly selected from 100 postal districts. All 3000 were telephoned to increase compliance and to check data received, and a total of 1256 completed questionnaires were analysed.

Three hospitals (1666 beds) and 15 nursing homes (1631 beds) were also surveyed by questionnaires sent to staff, and the data from these establishments were analysed separately.

A total of 293 individuals admitted to some degree of present urinary incontinence or leakage by day, and 51 also had some loss of urine at night. In all, 301 persons (24%) – 13% of the male and 34% of the female respondents – had some degree of urinary loss. Eight people were incontinent only at night. The male-to-female ratio among those with urinary leakage was 1:2.7, with females accounting for 73% of sufferers. The frequency of urinary loss is shown in Table 4.1.

Leakage was more common in members of blue-collar families (27%) than in members of white-collar families (25%). Students and those in full-time employment tended to have half the prevalence of incontinence (13% and 16%, respectively) reported by the other groups (30–34%). Housewives had the highest prevalence of incontinence overall (40%).

The mean duration of all leakage problems was 8.8 years; 18% reported leakage for less than a year, whereas 23% had had problems for 15 or more years; 17% could not specify the duration of their problem.

The 293 positive respondents were asked to specify circumstances under which they experienced leakage (more than one answer was allowed) (Table 4.2).

All 293 individuals who reported some current degree of leakage were asked to quantify the severity of the urine loss (Table 4.3).

Severe incontinence was twice as common in blue-collar than in white-collar families, but minor degrees

Table 4.1. *Frequency of incontinence episodes*

Frequency	Percentage of respondents		
	Male	Female	Overall
Often wet	2	4	3
Once a day	2	4	3
Once a week	1	3	2
Once or twice a month	0	4	2
Rarely	8	18	13
Never wet	87	66	76

Table 4.2. *Circumstances in which respondents experienced leakage*

	Percentage of respondents	
	Males (n = 79)	Females (n = 214)
Coughing or sneezing	5	61
Straining or lifting	5	12
Urge	27	35
Giggle	9	30
No warning or provocation	1	7
Post-micturition dribble	59	8
With urinary infections	8	10
Other	8	9
Total*	122	172

* Respondents may have more than one type of incontinence

Table 4.3. *Quantification of severity of urinary loss in 293 respondents*

	Percentage of respondents		
Urinary loss	Male (n = 79)	Female (n = 214)	Overall
Always wet	0	2	2
Flooding	0	2	1
Moderate loss	8	5	5
Slight loss	25	41	37
Just a spot	66	49	54

Table 4.4. *Percentage frequency and severity of leakage in 293 respondents wet by day**

Type of incontinence	Frequency				
	Often	1/day	1/week	2/month	Rarely
Coughing	15	12	9	12	52
Strain	31	7	7	14	41
Urge	20	11	8	10	50
Giggle	15	13	7	8	56
No warning	38	19	6	6	31
Post-micturition	22	15	4	11	48
Other	12	15	4	19	50

	Severity				
	Always	Flood	Moderate	Slight	Drops
Coughing	1	2	2	46	48
Strain	7	3	10	38	41
Urge	1	3	7	35	52
No warning	19	6	6	38	19
Post-micturition	2	2	2	27	69
With UTI	–	–	7	37	56
Other	4	4	8	50	35

* A patient may have more than one type of incontinence. UTI, urinary tract infection.

of leakage were equally prevalent. The type of incontinence was correlated with severity and frequency of leakage episodes as shown in Table 4.4.

In most cases, incontinence occurred infrequently and was of minor severity. What stands out is the relatively more frequent nature of the leakage of the quiet dribbling incontinence type, which occurs without warning or provocation.

Nocturnal incontinence

Incontinence at night was reported by 51 (26 female and 25 male) individuals, a prevalence of 4% of the population over the age of 10 years. The frequency of nocturnal incontinence is shown in Table 4.5 correlated with sex and age group.

Treatment experience

Perhaps reflecting the minor nature of the problem for the majority of the positive respondents, 70% of the 301 with leakage had never sought any treatment. However, 31% of the women and 26% of the men had sought

Table 4.5. *Frequency of nocturnal incontinence, correlated to sex and age group*

Frequency	Overall percentage	No. and sex		Age group (years)				
		M	F	10–29	30–44	45–59	60–74	75+
Most nights	8	2	2	2	0	1	1	0
Once a month	4	2	0	1	0	1	0	0
Occasionally	16	5	3	6	1	1	0	0
Rarely	73	16	21	19	7	8	0	3
				28	8	11	1	3
	Percentage wet in age group			5.6	2.3	4.4	1	8

help from general practitioners (24%), from specialists (14%) or from other health professionals (1%). (Respondents may have sought help from more than one healthcare professional.) Those most likely to seek help were over 60 years of age, and either blue-collar or unemployed persons. This may be explained by the fact that it is the elderly and those from blue-collar families who have the highest prevalence of urinary leakage and also the more severe degrees of incontinence.

At the time of the study 93 people were having treatment for incontinence, representing 31% of the 301 with current leakage. This is similar to the treatment rate reported by Thomas *et al.*[1] The types of treatment being received were pharmaceutical agents in 33%, appliances in 8%, bladder/muscle training in 13%, and surgery in 24% of patients.

RELATIONSHIP BETWEEN INCONTINENCE AND AGE GROUP

The prevalence of incontinence and its relationship to age group and gender is shown in Figure 4.1 and in Table 4.6. The increased prevalence seen with increasing age is particularly prominent in men over 60 years of age. The normal female preponderance is lost in old age, with a consequent rise in overall prevalence. The high (40%+) prevalence rate in the over-60 age groups is similar to that found in other studies[6] and to the prevalence of incontinence found in nursing homes.[7] Those over 60 years of age reported more severe and more frequent episodes of incontinence than did younger people.

Even young women have a higher prevalence of incontinence than young men, and this trend is accentuated after 30 years of age, possibly as a result of

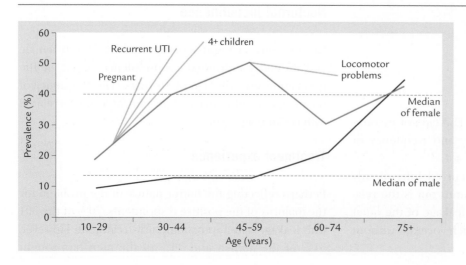

Figure 4.1. *Prevalence of incontinence according to age and sex (— female [n = 214]; — male [n = 79]).*

Table 4.6. *Prevalence of incontinence, and its relationship to age group and gender*

No. of individuals	Age group (years)					Overall
	10–29	30–44	45–59	60–74	75+	
Sample total	498	354	250	117	37	1256
Female	243	194	129	64	21	651
Wet*	47	75	64	19	9	214
	(19)	(39)	(50)	(30)	(43)	(33)
Male	255	160	121	53	16	605
Wet*	25	20	16	11	7	79
	(10)	(13)	(13)	(21)	(44)	(13)

* Percentages in parentheses.

pregnancy and childbirth. This was particularly apparent in the rates of stress urinary incontinence, which increased from 7% in the 10–29 year-old group to 26% in 30–44-year-old women and to 36% in the 45–60-year-old group. These data are similar to those obtained from the Australian Women's Health study.[5] The relationship between incontinence type and age group is shown in Table 4.7, which emphasizes the rising prevalence of urge incontinence in the elderly and the high rate of simple stress incontinence in middle age.

PRECIPITATING FACTORS

The 301 individuals who were 'wet day or night' were requested to identify the 'cause' of their leakage problem (Table 4.8). Hysterectomy was blamed for incontinence in 7% of the women, mostly by women from

Table 4.7. *Relationship between incontinence type and age group*

Incontinence	Percentage female	Percentage in age group (years)					Overall percentage
		10–29	30–44	45–59	60–74	75-plus	
Cough/sneeze	97	25	53	63	33	44	46
Strain/lift	86	7	13	12	7	–	10
Urge	78	31	29	28	50	56	33
Giggle	90	29	25	24	13	19	24
No warning	94	6	5	6	3	6	5
Post-micturition	37	26	24	18	23	6	22
With UTI	78	11	12	4	7	13	9
Other	77	14	10	5	7	6	9
No./group size		72/498	97/354	78/250	30/117	16/37	
Prevalence (%)		14	27	31	26	43	30
Percentage of responses/sufferers*		150	171	161	143	150	159

* A patient may have more than one type of incontinence. UTI, urinary tract infection.

blue-collar families or those off the workforce, compared with only 1% of the women from white-collar families. Incontinence associated with urinary tract infection was also twice as common in women from blue-collar families. The association between incontinence and hysterectomy and other pelvic surgery has been observed in other studies by Foldspang[8] and Parys.[9]

The relationship between incontinence and number of children is shown in Figure 4.2. The first child and pregnancy virtually doubled the prevalence of incontinence in women from 20% to about 40%. There was no change then until the fourth child, when the prevalence rose to 56%. The effect of parity has been noted from other studies.[1,2,6,10] Women from blue-collar families were more likely than others to blame childbirth for their incontinence.

A recent study of incontinence during pregnancy was reported by Chiarelli.[11] In a cross-sectional descriptive study using a five-item structured interview, 336 women were approached and 304 participated (90%): overall, 64% reported stress urinary incontinence during pregnancy; in the last month of pregnancy 57% reported stress incontinence (with or without urge incontinence) while 42% had urge incontinence (with or without stress incontinence). Among the 195 women experiencing incontinence, 25% lost only a few drops, 57% lost sufficient to dampen the underwear or pad and 18% reported severe loss. The leakage had started during the first trimester in 8%, in 18% in the second

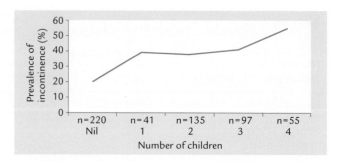

Figure 4.2. *Relationship between incontinence and number of children.*

trimester and in 47% in the last trimester of the most recent pregnancy whereas for 20% leakage had begun in a previous pregnancy, in 6% it began after the birth of a previous child and only 3% indicated that they had been incontinent before any of their pregnancies. For 49% leakage was not at all bothersome, 31% found it a little bothersome, 16% quite bothersome and 4% extremely bothersome.

Chi-square analysis showed four factors to be significantly associated with continence status – namely, previous delivery mode, parity, chronic cough and bouts of sneezing. Women who had previous vaginal deliveries were 2.5 times more likely to be incontinent than those who had no previous delivery or had only caesarean section. Those who reported previous forceps delivery were 10 times more likely to be incontinent than those with no prior delivery. Only 8% of the women had had their pelvic floor muscles tested during their pregnancy.[11]

RISK FACTORS INFLUENCING INCONTINENCE

An analysis of potential risk factors was undertaken. The groups found to be associated with higher rates of incontinence are shown in Table 4.9.

The association between incontinence and cystitis has been noted by Mommsen *et al.*,[12] who found a six-fold increase in experience of incontinence.

A more detailed analysis of risk factors in women has emerged from the Women's Health Australia project[5] (Table 4.10). This longitudinal study involved three cohorts of women – young (age 18–23 years), middle aged (age 45–50 years) and older (70–75 years) at the time of the baseline survey. The women were selected randomly[4] from the Australian Medicare database covering all women resident in Australia. During 1996, 14 761 young women, 14 070 middle-aged women and

Table 4.8. *Cause of leakage identified by 301 individuals who were 'wet day or night'*

Cause	Percentage of individuals	
	Male	Female
Urinary tract infection	5	13
Hysterectomy	–	7
Childbirth/pregnancy	–	31
Menopause	–	5
Prostatectomy	5	–
Other operation	4	2
Miscellaneous	13	32
No cause identified	69	32

Table 4.9. *Groups found to be associated with higher rates of incontinence*

Risk factor	Percentage incontinence in group	Percentage incontinence in remainder
Diabetes	36	24
CVA	25	24
Neurological disorder	29	24
Locomotor difficulty	45	24
Over 75 years of age	43	24
Recurrent UTI	55	24
Pregnancy	45	34
Four (or more) children	56	34

CVA, cerebrovascular accident; UTI, urinary tract infection.

12 893 older women completed baseline surveys (respectively, 48, 54 and 41% of those of each group invited to take part). The baseline questionnaire consisted of 252, 285 and 260 items, respectively, for each of the age cohorts. Participants were asked whether they had leaked urine in the last month 'never', 'rarely', 'sometimes' or 'often': responses other than 'never' were taken as indicating incontinence. The advantages of this study were its large sample size and the representative nature of the sample. The limitation was the use of a single non-validated question about leaking urine which fails to differentiate between different types of incontinence.

The prevalence of leaking urine in young women was 12.8% (95% confidence interval [CI] 12.2–13.3); in middle-aged women it was 36.15% (CI 35.2–37.0), and in older women 35.0% (CI 34.1–35.9).[5] These figures are similar to those reported by the earlier Australian prevalence study.

Table 4.10. *Adjusted odds ratios for variables associated with leakage of urine in women*

Variable	Odds ratio (95% confidence intervals)		
	Young (18–23 years)	Middle-aged (45–50 years)	Older (70–75 years)
Parity			
0	1.00		
1	2.82 (2.37–3.35)	1.58 (1.29–1.93)	0.88 (0.71–1.0)
2	2.59 (1.86–3.61)	1.66 (1.41–1.95)	1.14 (0.96–1.36)
3 or more	4.84 (2.54–9.20)	1.81 (1.54–2.12)	1.16 (0.98–1.36)
Constipation			
Never	1.00		
Rarely	2.13 (1.86–2.42)	2.46 (2.24–2.71)	2.67 (2.38–2.99)
Sometimes	2.86 (2.43–3.36)	2.16 (1.94–2.40)	2.05 (1.82–2.31)
Often	2.66 (2.07–3.40)	2.31 (1.84–3.35)	2.21 (1.87–2.61)
BMI			
Underweight < 19.9	1.00		
Ideal 20–24.99	1.08 (0.94–1.23)	1.31 1(1.10–1.55)	1.19 (1.00–1.40)
Overweight 25–29.99	1.34 (1.13–1.60)	1.47 (1.23–1.75)	1.39 (1.16–1.65)
Obese 30–40	2.09 (1.67–2.61)	2.05 (1.70–2.46)	1.82 (1.49–2.23)
Very obese > 40	1.82 (1.07–3.09)	2.49 (1.84–3.35)	3.29 (2.05–5.29)
Burning and stinging*			
Never	1.00		
Rare	2.94 (2.59–3.33)	2.17 (1.96–2.42)	2.45 (2.18–2.76)
Sometimes	4.19 (3.56–4.93)	2.71 (2.35–3.14)	2.99 (2.62–3.41)
Often	4.93 (3.60–6.74)	4.29 (2.85–6.45)	7.97 (5.71–11.12)

BMI, body mass index; * indicative of a history of urinary tract infection.
Data provided by P. Chiarelli; personal communication and ref. 5.

Parity was significantly associated with the prevalence of incontinence in young women but was less strongly correlated in the other age groups. There was a strong association between any degree of constipation and urinary leakage.

In middle-aged women, those with high body mass index (BMI > 25) and constipation were those most likely to experience leakage of urine. Hysterectomy alone had a lower odds ratio for leakage, whereas women who reported a prolapse repair either alone or with a hysterectomy were more likely to leak. Neither current use of hormone-replacement therapy nor duration of use were associated with leaking urine.

In the older cohort, the effect of parity was obscured. Pelvic surgery of any kind had a positive association with incontinence. Those with high BMI and those with a history suggestive of urinary tract infection (burning and stinging) were more likely to report incontinence.

At all ages, women who reported leaking urine had lower scores on the physical and mental component of the Swedish Short Form 36 (SF36) inventory, suggesting a lower quality of life for these women compared with continent women.

PAST EXPERIENCE OF INCONTINENCE IF NO PROBLEM AT PRESENT

The 955 respondents who denied any degree of urinary leakage at the present time were asked to report if they had ever experienced urinary leakage since they were 17 years of age. Replies showed that 16% of men and 30% of women had had previous experience of leakage: in 6% leakage had occurred occasionally and in 17% it had been experienced only rarely. The pattern of previous incontinence was similar to that found among those who admitted to present leakage.

CHILDHOOD INCONTINENCE AND RELATIVE RISK

Of the whole group of 1256 respondents, 21% (269) recalled having problems as a child with bedwetting. The occurrence of this problem was equal in males and females. In addition 9% (114 respondents, 67% female) recalled having had urinary leakage at school. Bedwetting was apparently more common in white-collar families (25% of whom were affected) than in blue-collar families (where only 20% recalled problems).

Childhood nocturnal enuresis was recalled by 269

individuals. As adults, 11% of these individuals still wet the bed while 32% had diurnal incontinence. Childhood bedwetters accounted for 57% of all those currently wet at night and 30% of all those wet by day (Table 4.11). Childhood bedwetters appeared to carry a five-fold increased risk of nocturnal incontinence in adult life compared with non-bedwetters. They were also at higher risk of developing some degree of urinary incontinence by day, with 1.7 times the prevalence rate of non-bedwetters. Of 114 respondents (9%) wet at school, 39% were wet by day at the time of the survey, accounting for 15% of all those now wet; 7% of the group now suffer from incontinence at night and account for 16% of all those now wet at night (Table 4.12). Individuals with incontinence in childhood at school carry a three-fold risk of night-time incontinence as an adult and twice the risk of diurnal incontinence than their fellows who had been dry at school.

The epidemiology of childhood enuresis in Australia has been independently studied by Hawkins[13] in 1962 and by Bower et al.[14] in 1996. The former took a sample of 1000 children in one general practice only and found a prevalence of nocturnal enuresis (of one or more nights per week at school age) of 18%; daytime incontinence was not evaluated. The 1996 study by Bower[14] used a self-administered questionnaire distributed to parents with children 5–12 years of age, at the eight largest polling stations of three electorates. Voting is compulsory in Australia and these electorates were selected to represent voters of high (9000), middle (7600) and lower (9000) socioeconomic classification. Of the 3111 parents approached, 2292 (74%) responded. The prevalence rate was 15% for nocturnal enuresis, 2% for isolated day wetting and 4% for combined day and night wetting; overall, 79% of children were dry, 18.9% had nocturnal enuresis and 5.5% had daytime incontinence. Whereas daytime wetting did not show a gender bias, 60% of children with enuresis were

Table 4.11. *Present incontinence among those recalling nocturnal enuresis as a child*

Current	Childhood bedwetter	Childhood non-bedwetter
Percentage wet at night now	11	2
Percentage wet by day now	32	19

Table 4.12. *Incontinence among those wet at school*

Current	Wet at school	Dry at school
Percentage wet at night now	7	2
Percentage wet by day now	39	19

Table 4.13. *Prevalence (%) of enuresis*

Type	Male (n = 277)	Female (n = 181)	Overall
Nocturnal enuresis	11.3	7.6	18.9
Daytime wetting	2.7	2.8	5.5
Total	14	10.4	

Frequency	Night	Day
Every day	2.4	0.6
2+/week	2.7	0.8
1/2 weeks	0.9	0.3
1/month	1.8	0.4
<1/month	11.1	3.4

Table 4.14. *Frequency of significant urinary incontinence in 10 men and 75 women*

Frequency of incontinence	Percentage	
	Male	Female
Often wet	50	25
Once a day	30	27
Once a week	20	25
Once or twice a month	–	23

male, regardless of whether the enuresis was primary or secondary (Table 4.13). The families of only 33.8% of enuretic children had sought professional help for the problem. Family strategies used were reward charts (16%), waking the child to void (30%), fluid restriction (43%) and waiting for maturity (51%). Non-enuretic children woke spontaneously to void at night in 80% of cases; by contrast, enuretic children woke only 49% of the time. There was a significant difference in the incidence of a positive family history between enuretic and dry children: among dry children, 55.5% had no family history, whereas only 30.6% of enuretics had no known family history. These figures corroborate the findings of the earlier general population study,[3] suggesting that 100 000 children wet the bed each night in Australia.

PREVALENCE OF SIGNIFICANT INCONTINENCE IN THE POPULATION

The results detailed above indicate that some urinary incontinence is experienced by many people. The problem has been identification of the rate of troublesome and significant leakage from most of the infrequently wet individuals. Using computer analysis, the entire sample was filtered to exclude all those with rare episodes of leakage and those who had 'just a spot' or slight loss of urine only, on infrequent occasions; patients who had leakage only with urinary infections were also excluded. The remainder were considered as having 'significant' urinary incontinence: of these 85 people 10 were men and 75 were women. The frequency with which they experienced incontinence is shown in Table 4.14.

Infrequent urinary incontinence was rare in those women over 65 years of age Whereas frequent leakage was unusual in patients under 35 years of age. The degree of wetness experienced is detailed in Table 4.15. Minor leakage volumes were rare over 65 years of age. Whereas those 'always wet' tended to be younger (< 64 years old), the elderly tended to have 'moderate loss' or 'flooding'. Of this group only 40% of both sexes had ever sought treatment: 30% of each sex had seen their general practitioner, and specialists had seen 30% of the men but only 17% of the women. This low percentage of people seeking treatment reflects the fact that about 40% of each sex needed to wear protective underwear; the remainder managed by hygienic measures alone.

The pattern of incontinence reported by those who were deemed to have significant incontinence is shown in Table 4.16.

Among the men with frequent incontinence, small-volume post-micturition loss was most commonly a complaint of younger men; older men suffered from urge incontinence (especially in the 75+ age group, in which this occurred in 20%). By contrast, females

Table 4.15. *Degree of wetness in respondents with significant urinary incontinence*

Degree of wetness	Percentage	
	Male	Female
Always wet	0	4
Flooding	0	4
Moderate loss	30	11
Slight loss	70	48
Just a spot	0	33

Table 4.16. *Pattern of incontinence reported by those deemed to have significant incontinence*

Incontinence type	Percentage	
	Male	Female
Coughing or sneezing	–	67
Straining or lifting	–	17
Urge	50	43
Giggle	10	27
No warning or provocation	10	12
Post-micturition dribbling	40	11
	110	177

* More than one response was allowed.

tended to have more than one cause of leakage, with stress incontinence predominant (particularly in middle-aged women). Urge incontinence in women appeared to be equally prevalent at all ages, but its severity grew with advancing years; flooding urinary loss was reported only by those over 50 years of age.

URINARY INCONTINENCE IN PEOPLE IN INSTITUTIONS

A parallel study was conducted to determine the prevalence of incontinence among those in institutional care: 15 nursing homes in the Sydney area were surveyed; one public hospital (824 beds) and two private hospitals (842 beds) were also investigated.

Incontinence in Nursing Homes

The staff of 15 of the larger nursing homes across the city were asked to fill out profiles of their patients' continence status (Table 4.17). Among the 1631 residents of these nursing homes 596 were incontinent, a prevalence rate of 37%. Most of those who were incontinent were over 70 years of age. The ratio of males to females was close to 1:1, but females outnumbered males in the homes by 2.6:1; as a result there were more wet women than men. Wet men tended to be slightly younger than wet women. The degree of incontinence reported in this group is shown in Table 4.18, correlated with mobility status. There was no significant difference between the degree of incontinence found in men and women in nursing homes. Residents who were chair-bound tended to have the highest rates of incontinence.

If the prevalence found in this survey (37%) is applied

Table 4.17. *Continence status of patients in 15 of the larger nursing homes in Sydney*

Degree of wetness	Percentage		
	Male	Female	Overall
Always wet	39	40	39
Flooding	15	13	13
Moderate loss	31	35	34
Slight loss	13	10	11
n	194	394	596

to the population of all nursing homes in Australia, an estimated 22 000 incontinent individuals might be expected to be found in these establishments.

Incontinence in hospitals

In order to assess the prevalence of incontinence, the staff of one large public hospital and two small private hospitals were asked to make a count of incontinence among their patients. In the public hospital 3.4% of the 824 patients had incontinence known to the nursing staff and 71% of these were over 71 years of age. This may be an underestimate in that many patients who were able to manage their own incontinence may not have been known to the ward nursing staff.

In the two small private hospitals the prevalence of

Table 4.18. *Degree of incontinence analysed by patient mobility*

Mobility	Percentage of patients incontinent				
	Always wet	Flooding	Moderate	Slight	Overall
Ambulant	10	11	20	44	18
Chair-bound	76	64	54	27	61
Bedridden	8	16	3	–	6
Mobile aided	6	9	23	27	15
n	234	80	200	66	596

incontinence was 13 and 22%, respectively. There was a high proportion of psychiatric patients, of whom 15% were incontinent; 40% of the geriatric patients in these hospitals were incontinent.

PREVALENCE OF INCONTINENCE IN AUSTRALIA

Among adult Australians, 24% of individuals admit to having some urinary loss and 6% of the population have significant or frequent urinary leakage. Of those who currently have no incontinence (76%), 23% have experienced some urinary leakage in their past adult life. Of those who currently suffer some form of leakage 73% are female, but women account for 88% of those with severe incontinence (M:F ratio = 1–7.5). The female predominance disappears over the age of 60. A summary of the prevalence of incontinence is shown in Table 4.19. If the figures for significant present incontinence are applied to the census figures, it can be estimated that as many as 960 000 adults in Australia may experience regular or severe incontinence; however, fewer than half of these ever seek professional help.

REFERENCES

1. Thomas TM, Plymat KR, Blannin J, Meade TW. Prevalence of urinary incontinence *Br Med J* 1980; 281: 1243–1245

2. Jolleys JV. Reported prevalence of urinary incontinence in women in general practice. *Br Med J* 1988; 296: 1300–1302

3. Millard RJ. The incidence of urinary incontinence in Australia. *Br J Urol* 1985; 57: 98–99

4. Brown WJ, Bryson L, Byles J *et al.* Women's Health Australia: Recruitment for a national longitudinal cohort study. *Women's Health* 1998; 28: 23–40

5. Chiarelli P, Brown W, McElduff P. Leaking urine – prevalence and associated factors in Australian women. *Neurourol Urodyn* 1999; 18; 567–577

6. Milsom I, Ekelund P, Molander U *et al.* The influence of age, parity, oral contraception, hysterectomy and menopause on the prevalence of urinary incontinence in women. *J Urol* 1993; 149: 1459–1462

7. Ouslander JG. Urinary incontinence in nursing homes *J Am Geriatr Soc* 1990; 38: 289–291

8. Foldspang A, Mommsen S, Elving L, Lam GW. Parity as a correlate of adult female urinary incontinence prevalence. *J Epidemiol Community Health* 1992; 46: 595–600

9. Parys B, Haylen B, Hutton J, Parsons K. The effects of simple hysterectomy on vesicourethral function. *Br J Urol* 1989; 64: 594–599

10. Mommsen S, Foldspang A, Elving L, Lam GW. Association between urinary incontinence in women and a previous history of surgery. *Br J Urol* 1993; 72: 30–37

Table 4.19. *Summary of prevalence of incontinence in Australia*

Incontinence	Percentage of individuals		
	Male	Female	Overall
Childhood enuresis	21	21	21
Past incontinence (in adult life)	16	30	23
All present incontinence	13	34	24
Ever incontinent as an adult	28	53	41
Significant incontinence now	2	11	6

11. Chiarelli P, Campbell E. Incontinence during pregnancy: prevalence and opportunities from continence promotion. *Aust N Z J Obstet Gynaecol* 1997; 37: 66–73

12. Mommsen S, Foldspang A, Elving L, Lam GW. Cystitis as correlate of female urinary incontinence. *Int Urogynaecol J Pelvic Floor Dysfunct* 1994; 5: 135–140

13. Hawkins DN. Enuresis: a survey. *Med J Austr* 1962; 23: 979–980

14. Bower WF, Moore KH, Shepherd RB, Adams RD. The epidemiology of childhood enuresis in Australia. *Br J Urol* 1996; 78: 602–606

5

Quality of life and urinary incontinence

C. Kelleher

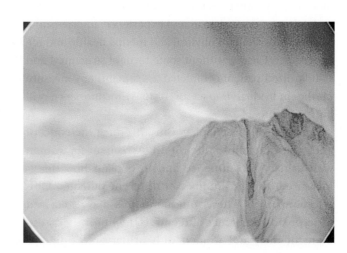

INTRODUCTION

Urinary incontinence is a common condition among women of all ages, and may significantly impair the lifestyle of those affected. It is usually as a result of the impact of incontinence on women's lives that help is sought from the medical profession, although this may occur only after many years of suffering.[1]

Urinary incontinence is a complex problem resulting from many different causes and for which many different approaches to treatment exist. It is also complex because of the different ways and varying severity with which it affects the lives of sufferers.

Typically, an assessment of the nature of urinary symptoms is made using standardized symptom questionnaires. An accurate diagnosis of the cause of urinary symptoms requires urodynamic assessment. On the basis of these investigations and an assessment of the severity of symptoms, appropriate treatment is instituted.

Assessing the impact of clinical problems, and the wishes of patients for treatment, is so fundamental to good clinical practice that it is usually assumed to have taken place in one form or another prior to clinical decision-making. It is partly for this reason, and because as clinicians we have traditionally measured the severity of our patients' symptoms for them, that patient-assessed subjective health measures have crept slowly into mainstream clinical and research practice.

Unfortunately, the complexities of urinary incontinence and other similar conditions render such simplistic and non-standardized assessments inaccurate. Urinary symptoms affect different women in different ways and have a variable influence on their physical, psychological, social, domestic and interpersonal lifestyles. These are modified by other factors – which include age, race and culture; personal goals and experience; interpersonal relationships; general physical and mental health; and life expectancy. Clearly, without some form of structured and standardized patient-completed assessment, any measure of the individual impact of urinary incontinence will be inaccurate.

The aim of this chapter is to introduce the concept and value of quality-of-life (QoL) assessment for women with urinary incontinence and to explain how this is measured, using a number of different validated QoL questionnaires. These questionnaires have received widespread acceptance and endorsement for the assessment of men and women with urinary incontinence and are now included in all clinical studies of continence care. Measurement of the QoL of incontinence sufferers is so important for the assessment and treatment of this condition that, in some studies, it is replacing the traditional urinary symptom and urodynamic outcome measures that have previously been used.

WHAT IS QUALITY OF LIFE?

There is no consensus definition of QoL, although it is linked to the World Health Organization (WHO) definition of health as being 'not merely the absence of disease, but complete physical, mental, and social well-being'.[2] It is a multidimensional concept, and has come to mean a combination of patient-assessed measures of health, including physical function, role function, social function, emotional or mental state, burden of symptoms and sense of well-being.[3]

HOW TO MEASURE QUALITY OF LIFE

QoL is usually measured with questionnaires completed by patients or their carers and, although many different questionnaires are now available, each conforms to the same basic structure. The questionnaires consist of a variable number of domains (or sections), usually one to seven, which gather information focused on particular aspects of health and QoL[4] (Table 5.1).

QUALITY-OF-LIFE QUESTIONNAIRES

Two major types of QoL questionnaire are available – namely, generic and disease specific. Irrespective of their type, all questionnaires have been previously validated and their reliability tested to ensure their psychometric value for the assessment of QoL[4] Questionnaires that have not been through this lengthy design process have

Table 5.1. *Dimensions of quality of life*
• Physical function, e.g. mobility, self care, exercise
• Emotional function, e.g. depression, anxiety, worry
• Social function, e.g. intimacy, social support, social contact, leisure activities
• Role performance, e.g. work, housework, shopping
• Pain
• Sleep/nausea
• Disease-specific symptoms

unproven value and should not be used in clinical studies where QoL is a stated outcome measure.

Generic questionnaires (e.g. the Nottingham Health Profile [NHP],[5] UK Short Form 36 [SF36] health status questionnaire,[6] Sickness Impact Profile [SIP],[7] Psychosocial Adjustment to Illness Scale [PASI][8]) are designed as general measures of QoL, applicable to a wide range of different populations and clinical conditions, and are not specific to a particular disease, treatment or age group. They allow comparisons to be made between different patient groups and between patients with and without medical complaints. Extensive previous research using these questionnaires has provided comparative and normative data which are of value in QoL studies. Normative values are obtained from large population surveys of people without medical complaints, and the results are usually available in the instruction manuals provided with properly validated questionnaires. Normative data are stratified by age, social class and sex.

An example of the use of such data for the comparison of women with urinary incontinence or with rheumatoid arthritis, and women without medical complaints, using the SF36 health status questionnaire[9] is shown in Figure 5.1. The data were obtained from a study in Sweden of 411 women with detrusor instability (DI), all of whom completed the SF36 questionnaire. As can be seen, women with urinary incontinence due to DI suffer greater impairment in vitality and social function, and greater emotional problems than women with rheumatoid arthritis or neither condition. Understanding the unique impact on patients' lives of different medical conditions ultimately improves the treatment we are able to offer.

Unfortunately, generic questionnaires necessitate non-specific questioning, and scoring systems applicable to widely varying states of health, and therefore lack sensitivity when applied to women with conditions, such as urinary incontinence, that are not life-threatening. This is particularly important in respect of the inability of such questionnaires to detect clinically important improvement in QoL when incorporated into clinical trials.

Disease-specific questionnaires aim to overcome this problem and are designed to assess, with greater complexity and accuracy, the impact of specific medical complaints. A number of different condition-specific

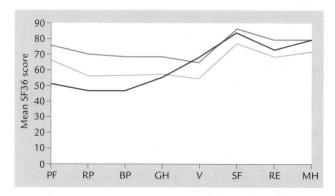

Figure 5.1. *An example of the use of the Short Form 36 (SF36) health status questionnaire to compare women with different medical conditions (overactive bladder; rheumatoid arthritis) and normal (i.e. fit, healthy) adults ( ). The domains of the SF36 shown are: PF, physical function; RP, role, physical; BP, bodily pain; GH, general health; V, vitality; SF, social function; RE, role, emotional; MH, mental health. A lower score indicates a poorer quality of life. (Data from ref. 9.)*

questionnaires have been designed for the assessment of urinary incontinent women. Only questionnaires of published validity and reliability are discussed in this chapter.

A sensible approach for clinical trials is the inclusion of both a disease-specific and a generic questionnaire that have previously been used successfully in similar studies.

APPLICATIONS OF QUALITY-OF-LIFE MEASURES IN UROGYNAECOLOGY

Perhaps the most obvious use for standardized health measurement profiles is as outcome measures in clinical trials. They are of particular value for the comparison of treatments with little apparent difference in objective clinical outcome, but where patient morbidity is reduced. An example would be the comparison of established and new surgical procedures for the correction of genuine stress incontinence (GSI), or different medications for the treatment of DI.

An additional value of QoL measures is their ability to determine the significance to patients of changes in objective clinical parameters, which (although they may achieve statistical significance) may be clinically irrelevant. An example could be a change in nocturia from six to five voids per night, which, while generating significant *p* values in clinical studies may confer little if any QoL improvement to the patient. Another example may be the assessment of a new surgical procedure for the treatment of GSI whereby GSI is cured but at the expense of voiding difficulties and detrusor instability.

In addition to these obvious clinical applications QoL assessment may prove to be important for health services research and the allocation of financial resources within an already overutilized and underfunded health service. Economic evaluations in continence care have concentrated on nursing-home populations and only few estimates of the overall costs to society are available.[10,11] Although costs are therefore difficult to calculate and are undoubtedly underestimated, research data in the USA have estimated the cost of continence care to be in excess of US$16 billion.[12] This can be expected to increase further with the current shift towards a larger elderly population.

QoL is an important outcome in economic evaluations of continence care and is the most obvious measure of effectiveness of treatment from the patient's point of view. It expresses an important economic benefit, and something one is willing to pay for either individually or collectively. In order for QoL instruments to be useful for cost-effectiveness analysis, a single composite questionnaire score is required. This involves the summation of data from all the individual domains of a QoL questionnaire to produce an overall score or index. Such calculations assume either that the individual domains are weighted with respect to their individual importance to the overall score or, as is more usually the case, that the individual domains contribute equally to the overall questionnaire result. The calculation of weighting is beyond the scope of this chapter.[4] Results of QoL questionnaires are not usually presented in the form of a single index, as this loses valuable information regarding the domains of QoL that are most affected by a clinical condition.

Once the healthcare expenditure required to produce a certain level of improvement in QoL is known, this can be used to compare the effects of expenditure in other areas of continence care or in other conditions. An example of this form of calculation would be the use of quality-adjusted life years (QALY), which is a measure incorporating both QoL and survival obtained by multiplying life years by a weight reflecting the QoL of that year.[13]

The level of willingness to pay for a reduction in incontinence problems is another form of cost–utility analysis and may be an indication of both the physical and psychological burden of patients with urinary incontinence. 'Willingness-to-pay' questionnaires ask women the amount they are willing to spend to achieve a specified improvement in their clinical condition. A study in Sweden has shown that the severity of symptoms of urge incontinence, expressed as frequency and leakages, is correlated with patients' QoL, as well as the amount that they are willing to pay for a given percentage reduction in their symptoms[13]. It is unclear whether this form of hypothetical analysis would be applicable in populations where healthcare is entirely free and the costs of delivering health are rarely considered by patients.

It has been shown that many women with urinary incontinence do not seek help for their problems, or delay obtaining medical advice.[1] Whether help is sought for urinary incontinence does not appear to depend on the duration or severity of incontinence or on patient education.[14] Although some women are insufficiently worried about their symptoms to want treatment,[15,16] this is not the normal situation, and embarrassment, poor information and a fear of admitting to urinary incontinence may play a major part in the reasons for delayed presentation. QoL questionnaires would therefore be useful in population surveys to determine the burden of incontinence and to calculate the service provision and expenditure required to provide appropriate continence care.

The ultimate aim for QoL assessment is the inclusion of short and meaningful questionnaires into routine clinical practice; unfortunately, as yet, no single questionnaire is either short enough or widely enough accepted to fulfil this role.

Some of the potential applications for QoL questionnaires are listed in Table 5.2.

PREDICTORS OF QUALITY-OF-LIFE IMPAIRMENT FOR INCONTINENT WOMEN

Urinary incontinence results in impairment in many aspects of the QoL of sufferers, yet it is impossible to predict, on the basis of urinary symptoms and urodynamic diagnosis alone, the degree of this impairment.[17]

Little is known about the effect of age on the subjective severity of urinary incontinence. Gjorp *et al.*[18] found that 72% of a sample of 79 elderly women with genitourinary symptoms felt them to be normal for

GSI + OVB
vs QOL

Table 5.2. *Applications of quality-of-life measures*

- Screening and monitoring for psychosocial problems in individual patient care
- Population surveys of perceived health problems
- Medical audit
- Outcome measures in health services or evaluation research
- Clinical trials
- Cost–utility analyses
- An adjunct to the clinical review

elderly people. In addition, Norton *et al.*[1] have shown that elderly women tend to present later for the assessment and treatment of urinary incontinence,[1] although there is insufficient evidence to support the assumption that their urinary symptoms are less troublesome.

It is possible that the earlier presentation of younger women reflects a greater knowledge about incontinence and its treatment, as neither symptom severity nor diagnosis affected presentation to the same degree. It is also possible that urinary incontinence may affect the young and old differently: for example, incontinence often results in sexual dysfunction[19–21] and exercise restriction, which may be more problematic for younger women.

Unfortunately, many assumptions are often made regarding the impact of urinary incontinence in the elderly, despite insufficient research. Our own studies have shown that QoL is often significantly improved by bladder-neck surgery in elderly women, yet age itself is a major factor upon which surgery may be denied to such patients.

Although it would be expected that the duration of symptoms and severity of leakage are major predictors of QoL impairment, symptom duration and severity of urinary incontinence *per se* do not appear to correlate well with QoL. At present it is unclear whether QoL deteriorates with a longer duration of urinary symptoms, as prospective studies are difficult to perform. This would, however, be particularly interesting to ascertain for women with DI, where it has been shown that those with a poorer QoL are less likely to respond to conventional treatments.[22] The reason for this may be that urinary symptoms are of greater severity and therefore less likely to improve,[23] although it would be important to determine if earlier intervention would prevent inevitable QoL deterioration and improve the chance of successful treatment. This would also

encourage the wider availability of community continence clinics and improve the initial management of urinary symptoms in primary care.

The urodynamic diagnosis appears to be a major factor predicting QoL impairment. It has been shown by a number of studies that women with DI have a greater QoL impairment than those with GSI.[24,25] Wyman *et al.*[26] attributed this to the fact that women with DI are less able to predict incontinent episodes and have more precipitating factors, more severe leakage and, therefore, less feeling of control over their bladder symptoms than those with GSI. In addition, interpersonal and sexual problems appear to be particularly common amongst urinary incontinent women, and are greater for women with DI than for those with GSI.[21,22]

Undoubtedly, targeting treatment towards women with greater QoL impairment and isolating particular problem areas in the management of urinary incontinence would be of great benefit to continence carers, and ultimately would improve the treatment of incontinent women.

RELATIONSHIP OF QUALITY-OF-LIFE WITH CLINICAL MEASURES

On the whole, few and weak relationships have been found between the presence of urinarysymptoms (including incontinence) and clinical measures such as urodynamics. Lower urinary tract symptoms are diagnostically disappointing and additional information from urodynamic evaluation is needed in order to make an accurate diagnosis and propose specific and effective therapies.[17,27,28]

Assessing the impact of urinary incontinence on the well-being of individuals can be accomplished using a symptom-impact evaluation, or QoL questionnaire. Symptom-impact questionnaires measure the degree to which a patient is bothered by the presence of a symptom, rather than measuring whether a symptom is present or absent. Such a system is used in various of the condition-specific QoL questionnaires designed for the assessment of urinary incontinent patients (see Table 5.3 on page 54).

Comparing symptom impact and symptom presence is an important concept. In one study by Jolleys *et al.*,[29] the prevalence of symptoms did not correlate with their 'degree of bothersomeness'. For example, although only 14% of patients had nocturia (more than one episode), 67% found it bothersome; in contrast, 78% of patients had terminal dribbling but only 19% found it bothersome. Individual patient's views of bothersomeness vary significantly, and are modified by many different factors. The objective degree of symptom severity, such as the number of pads worn or the amount of urine lost, is therefore less important than an individual's overall outlook on the problem.

If the impact of symptoms is to be used to compare individuals with different urinary problems, then a system of weighting the significance of the individual symptoms is essential in order to make any valid comparisons between different diagnostic groups. It would, for example, be difficult to compare the symptom impact for women with predominantly irritative bladder symptoms with that of women with predominantly stress symptoms when both are scored on the same scale. This is particularly important when questionnaires are used as outcome measures in clinical trials and the type of symptoms changes. In this context, the assessment of QoL or, rather, the impact of the presence of any symptoms on various aspects of the lifestyle of patients, allows for more meaningful and stable comparison both between patients, and for the same patient before and after treatment.

QUALITY OF LIFE STUDIES OF URINARY INCONTINENT WOMEN

A number of studies have attempted to measure the QoL of incontinent women. Such studies vary in their design, their methodology, the criteria used for the diagnosis of urinary incontinence and (where stated) the definition of QoL. The majority of studies have made no attempt to diagnose objectively the cause or presence of incontinence at all, despite the fact that urinary symptoms and objective urodynamic diagnoses correlate poorly.

Incontinence has, however, been shown to reduce social relationships and activities,[30–32] to impair emotional and psychological well-being[33] and to impair sexual relationships.[19–21] Some studies report that incontinence causes (at the very least) avoidance behaviour and careful planning to avoid or conceal incontinent episodes, and also causes considerable inconvenience.[34,35] In addition, embarrassment and diminished self-esteem are common reactions to incontinent episodes.[35,36]

GENERIC QUALITY-OF-LIFE ASSESSMENT

Few studies in the literature have used generic, validated, QoL instruments to assess women with urinary incontinence. Hunskaar and Vinsnes[24] used the SIP,[7] a validated 136-item questionnaire, to assess 70 women attending a self-referral centre for incontinent patients. Women were divided on the basis of age into two groups (middle-aged: 40–60 years; elderly: over 70 years), and on the basis of symptom questionnaires into stress and urge symptom subgroups. Women were asked to respond to SIP items only if they considered them attributable to their bladder symptoms. Mean scores on the SIP were low for both groups, but the study concluded that the impact of urinary incontinence on QoL was both age and symptom dependent. Younger women scored significantly higher on the SIP, as did women with urge symptoms. Sleep, rest, emotional behaviour, mobility, social interaction and recreational activities were most commonly affected.

The study unfortunately lacked objective urodynamic assessment; the sample sizes were small, and no account was taken of the women's ages in the comparison of QoL scores. Similarly, the practice of encouraging women to respond only to those questionnaire items that are attributable to their urinary symptoms may introduce inaccuracies in both the scoring and interpretationof QoL measures. This is particularly problematic in an elderly population, the members of which may be unsure of the cause of their QoL impairment, and unsure which problems are attributable to urinary incontinence and which to other causes.

Grimby *et al.*[25] examined the NHP scores from 120 elderly women (65–84 years old) with urinary incontinence compared with 313 76-year-old women without urinary symptoms. Their data were obtained from a large population study of 6000 women living in the city of Gothenburg, Sweden; the overall response rate to this parent study was 70.1%. Elderly women (over 70 years of age) with subjectively reported urinary incontinence were subdivided into those with urge incontinence (48 women; 40%), stress incontinence (34 women; 28.3%) or both (38 women; 31.7%) on the basis of a pad test, a urinary diary, a cough provocation test and a clinical history, but without the benefit of urodynamic investigations. The mean age of the incontinent group was 75.4 years and that of the continent control group 76 years.

Unfortunately, the total number of incontinent women in the parent study was not stated and the women included in this study were merely the first 120 women in whom incontinence could be demonstrated by either a pad or cough provocation test. No attempt was made to determine incontinence in the control group by similar tests, and continence was assumed on the basis of their lack of admission to this symptom. Ideally, for a true control group, cough provocation and pad tests should also have been performed on these women, and the number of women in the test and control groups should have been matched.

Using the NHP, Grimby *et al.* showed a significantly higher level of both emotional impairment and social isolation among the incontinent women.[25] They also showed a higher level of emotional disturbance among women with urge and mixed incontinence than among those with stress incontinence. Women with urge incontinence had significantly greater sleep disturbance than the control women.

Sand *et al.*[37] used the SF36 health status questionnaire to assess the efficacy of treatment for women with GSI entered into a prospective, randomized, double-blind, placebo-controlled trial comparing the use of an active pelvic floor stimulator with that of a sham device: 35 women used the active device and 17 the sham device, the latter acting as controls. A significant benefit of the active device was demonstrated by both objective measures (pad testing, urinary diary, vaginal muscle strength) and subjective measures (urinary symptom questionnaire, severity of urinary incontinence visual analogue scale), although no significant improvement was seen in SF36 scores. It is highly likely that this result was attributable to the small number of women entered into the study, and that results would have been different had a disease-specific measure been used.

Although generic QoL questionnaires may not be sufficiently sensitive to clinical improvement for inclusion in smaller clinical trials, they may be of value in the prediction of the success (and therefore the selection) of treatment for incontinent women. We have shown that, for women with DI, a poorer QoL measured using the PAIS[8] can predict women for whom treatment is less likely to succeed with anticholinergic therapy (Fig. 5.2). This may reflect a greater severity of DI in these women, whose urinary symptoms would be expected to be harder to cure. It is interesting to spec-

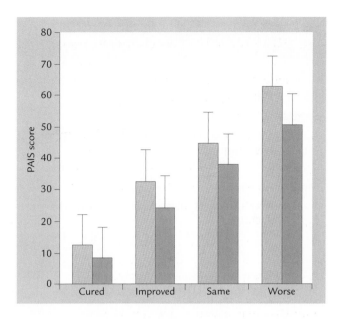

Figure 5.2. *Psychosocial Adjustment to Illness Scale (PAIS) scores for 171 women with detrusor instability before (■) and after (■) treatment (> 6 months) with anticholinergic therapy. A higher score indicates a poorer quality of life. (Data from ref. 46.)*

ulate that, if it were possible to commence treatment earlier in the natural history of this condition, when QoL impairment is potentially less, the treatment outcome would be more successful. Using the same questionnaire, we have shown that women with greater QoL impairment attributable to GSI are more likely to consider colposuspension a subjective success. This reflects the success of this type of surgery for women with severe GSI, but also may be of value in the selection and prioritization of those women who would be most likely to respond to surgery (Fig. 5.3).

DISEASE-SPECIFIC QUALITY-OF-LIFE ASSESSMENT OF URINARY INCONTINENCE

In recognition of the importance of QoL assessment of incontinence sufferers, and the lack of sensitivity of generic questionnaires, a number of different condition-specific QoL questionnaires have been developed, or are at various stages of development. Only those questionnares with proven validity and reliability testing are mentioned in this chapter. A few of the more advanced questionnaires have data regarding responsiveness in clinical studies. A list of selected condition-specific QoL questionnaires is shown in Table 5.3. Cont.

Table 5.3. *Recommended condition-specific quality-of-life questionnaires*

Symptom assessment and QoL impact

1. Kings Health Questionnaire[38]

Symptom assessment

1. Bristol Lower Urinary Tract Symptoms (BFLUTS)[39]
2. Urogenital Distress Inventory (UDI)[40]
3. Symptom Severity Index (SSI)[41]

QoL assessment

1. Incontinence Impact Questionnaire (IIQ) and IIQ-7 (short form)[26,40]
2. Quality of life in persons with urinary incontinence (I-QoL)[42]
3. SII[41]
4. York Incontinence Perceptions Scale (YIPS)[43]
5. Stress Incontinence Questionnaire (SIQ)[34]
6. Psychosocial Consequences Questionnaire[44]

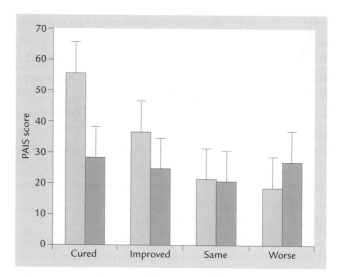

Figure 5.3. *Psychosocial Adjustment to Illness Scale (PAIS) scores for 112 women with genuine stress incontinemce before (▨) and after (■) colposuspension (> 6-month follow-up). A higher score indicates a poorer quality of life (QoL). Women with higher quality of life (QoL) scores prior to treatment were more likely to consider their surgery to have been successful. (Data from ref. 46.)*

Table 5.4. *Kings Health Questionnaire*

PART I
General health perception
1. How would you describe your health at present?

Incontinence Impact
2. How much do you think your bladder problem affects your life?

PART II
Role limitations
3a. To what extent does your bladder problem affect your household tasks (e.g. cleaning, shopping etc.)?
3b. Does your bladder problem affect your job, or your normal daily activities outside the home?

Physical limitations
4a. Does your bladder problem affect your physical activities (e.g. going for a walk, run, sport, gym etc.)?
4b. Does your bladder problem affect your ability to travel?

Social limitations
4c. Does your bladder problem restrict your social life?
4d. Does your bladder problem limit your ability to see/visit friends?

Personal relationships
5a. Does your bladder problem affect your relationship with your partner?
5b. Does your bladder problem affect your sex life?
5c. Does your bladder problem affect your family life?

Emotions
6a. Does your bladder problem make you feel depressed?
6b. Does your bladder problem make you feel anxious or nervous?
6c. Does your bladder problem make you feel bad about yourself?

Sleep/energy
7a. Does your bladder problem affect your sleep?
7b. Do you feel worn out or tired?

cont.

Table 5.4. *Kings Health Questionnaire (cont.)*

Severity measures
Do you do any of the following; if so how much?
8a   Wear pads to keep dry?
8b   Be careful how much fluid you drink?
8c   Change your underclothes when they get wet?
8d   Worry in case you smell?
8e   Get embarrassed because of your bladder problem?

PART III
We would like to know what your bladder problems are and how much they affect you. From the list below choose only those problems that you have at present. Leave out those that do not apply to you.

• *Frequency*	Going to the toilet very often
• *Nocturia*	Getting up at night to pass urine
• *Urgency*	A strong and difficult-to-control desire to pass urine
• *Urge incontinence*	Urinary leakage associated with a strong desire to pass urine
• *Stress incontinence*	Urinary leakage with physical activity, e.g. coughing, sneezing
• *Nocturnal enuresis*	Wetting the bed at night
• *Intercourse incontinence*	Urinary leakage with sexual intercourse
• *Frequent waterworks infections*	
• *Bladder pain*	
• *Difficulty passing urine*	
• *Other (Please specify)*	

Copies of each of these questionnaires can be obtained from their authors upon request. The content of the Kings Health questionnaire (KHQ) is summarized in Table 5.4 and the full version of the questionnaire and scoring system can be obtained from the authors.

Validation studies of the KHQ have shown that women with DI have greater QoL impairment attributable to their urinary symptoms than women with GSI, or than women with urinary symptoms but normal urodynamic investigation results (Figs 5.4, 5.5).[38] The KHQ has also been included in trials of the new antimuscarinic drug tolterodine for the treatment of DI. Clinical studies have demonstrated significant improvement in all domains other than personal relationships for women receiving tolterodine for the treatment of their DI (Fig. 5.6).[45] These data were obtained during a study of 411 women with DI included in a randomized controlled trial of tolterodine for the treatment of DI, and demonstrate the responsiveness of the KHQ to change in clinical trials. Further studies using the KHQ and other condition-specific questionnaires are currently in progress, evaluating both new and established surgical treatments of GSI. The KHQ has been translated into seven languages and is therefore now available for inclusion in multicentre, international trials.

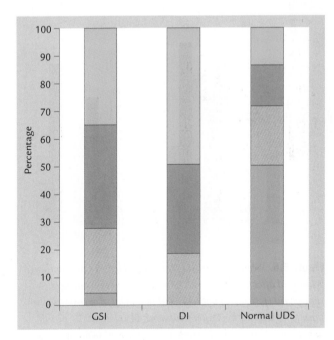

Figure 5.4. *Responses to the question 'How much do you think your bladder problem affects your life?' in Part I of the Kings Health Questionnaire for women with genuine stress incontinence (GSI), detrusor instability (DI) and normal urodynamic investigations (UDS):* ■ *not at all;* ▨ *a little;* ▨ *moderately;* ▨ *a lot. More women with DI are moderately or greatly affected by their bladder problems than women with GSI or normal UDS.*

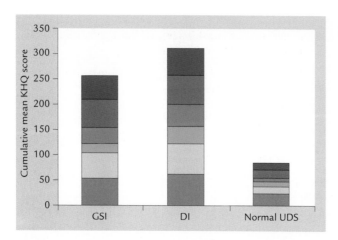

Figure 5.5. *Cumulative mean scores on Part II of the Kings Health Questionnaire for women with GSI, DI and normal UDS:* ■ *sleep;* ■ *emotions;* ■ *personal problems;* ■ *social limitations;* ■ *physical limitations;* ■ *role limitations. The cumulative scores for women with DI are greater than those for women with other diagnoses, indicating a greater QoL impairment.*

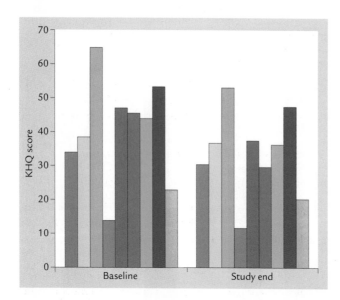

Figure 5.6. *Scores on Part II of the Kings Health Questionnaire before and after treatment with tolterodine, demonstrating a significant (p < 0.01) improvement in all QoL dimensions other than personal relations after treatment:* ■ *emotions;* ■ *health perception;* ■ *incontinence impact;* ■ *personal relations;* ■ *physical limitations;* ■ *role limitations;* ■ *severity measures;* ■ *sleep/energy;* ■ *social limitations. (Data from ref. 45.)*

CONCLUSION

This chapter offers an introduction to the concept of QoL assessment for the assessment of urinary inconti-

nent patients, to the types of questionnaire available and to their potential uses. Assessing the effects of urinary incontinence from the point of view of the patient is essential if we are to understand fully the impact of this condition and to offer effective treatment.

REFERENCES

1. Norton PA, MacDonald LD, Sedgwick PM, Stanton SL. Distress and delay associated with urinary incontinence, frequency and urgency in women. *Br Med J* 1998; 297: 1187–1189

2. World Health Organization. Definition of health from preamble to the constitution of the WHO basic documents, 28th edn. Geneva: WHO, 1978; 1

3. Coulter A. Measuring quality of life. In: Kinmonth AL, Jones R (eds) *Critical Reading in General Practice.* Oxford: Oxford University Press, 1993

4. Streiner DL, Norman GR. *Health Measurement Scales, a Practical Guide to their Development and Use.* Oxford: Oxford Medical Publications, 1993

5. Hunt SM, McEwen J, McKenna SP. Measuring health status. A new tool for clinicians and epidemiologists. *J R Coll Gen Pract* 1985; 35: 185–188

6. Jenkinson C, Coulter A, Wright L. Short Form 36 (SF-36) health survey questionnaire. Normative data for adults of working age. *Br Med J* 1993; 306: 1437–1440

7. Bergner M, Bobbitt R, Carter W, Gibson B. The sickness impact profile: development and final revision of a health status measure. *Med Care* 1981; 19: 787–805

8. Derogatis LR, Derogatis MF. *The Psychosocial Adjustment to Illness Scale (PAIS and PAIS SR) Administration, Scoring and Procedures Manual-II.* Towson, MD: Clinical Psychometric Research, Inc., 1990

9. Johannesson M, O'Connor RM, Kobelt-Nguyen G, Mattiasson A. Willingness to pay for reduced incontinence symptoms. *Br J Urol* 1997; 80: 557–562

10. Hu TW. The impact of urinary incontinence on healthcare costs. *J Am Geriatr Soc* 1990; 38: 292–295

11. Hu TW. The economic impact of urinary incontinence. *Clin Geriatr Med* 1996; 2: 673–687

12. Fantl JA, Newman DK, Colling J. *Urinary Incontinence in Adults: Acute and Chronic Management. Clinical practice guideline No. 2,* 1996 update. AHCPR Publication 96-0682. Washington DC: US Public Health service. Agency for Health Care Policy and Research, 1996

13. Kobelt G, Economic considerations and outcome measurement in urge incontinence. *Urology* 1997; 50 100–107

14. Burgio KL, Ives DO, Locher JL *et al.* Treatment seeking for urinary incontinence in older adults. *J Am Geriatr Soc* 1994; 42: 208–212

15. Memel DS, Harrison GL. Urinary incontinence in women: its prevalence and its management in a health promotion clinic. *Br J Gen Pract* 1994; 44: 149–152

16. Lagro-Janssen AL. Value of patient's case history in the diagnosis of urinary incontinence in general practice. *Br J Gen Pract* 1990; 40: 331–334

17. Jarvis GJ, Hall S, Stamp S *et al.* An assessment of urodynamic examination in incontinent women. *Br J Obstet Gynaecol* 1980; 87: 893–896

18. Gjo0rp T, Hendriksen C, Lund E, Stromgard E. Is growing old a disease? A study of the attitudes of elderly people to physical symptoms. *J Chron Dis* 1987; 40: 1095–1098

19. Sutherst JR. Sexual dysfunction and urinary incontinence. *Br J Obstet Gynaecol* 1979; 86: 387

20. Kelleher CJ, Cardozo LD. Sexual dysfunction and urinary incontinence. *J Sex Health* 1994; 3: 186–191

21. Hilton P. Urinary incontinence during sexual intercourse: a common but rarely volunteered symptom. *Br J Obstet Gynaecol* 1988; 95: 377–381

22. Moore KH, Hay DM, Imrie AH. Oxybutynin chloride (3 mg) in the treatment of women with idiopathic detrusor instability. *Br J Urol* 1990; 66: 479–485

23. Moore KH, Richmond DH, Sutherst JR, Manasse P. Is severe wetness associated with severe madness in detrusor instability? *Neurourol Urodyn* 1992; 11: 460–461

24. Hunskaar S, Vinsnes A. The quality of life in women with urinary incontinence as measured by the sickness impact profile. *J Am Geriatr Soc* 1991; 39: 378–382

25. Grimby A, Milstrom I, Molander U *et al.* The influence of urinary incontinence on the quality of life of women. *Age Ageing* 1993; 22: 82–89

26. Wyman JF, Harkins S, Choi S *et al.* Psychosocial impact of urinary incontinence in women. *Obstet Gynecol* 1987; 70: 378–380

27. Versi E, Cardozo L, Anand D, Cooper D. Symptoms analysis for the diagnosis of genuine stress incontinence. *Br J Obstet Gynaecol* 1991; 98: 815–819

28. Bergman A, Bader K. Reliability of the patient's history in the diagnosis of urinary incontinence. *Int J Gynaecol Obstet* 1990; 32: 255–259

29. Jolleys JV, Donovan JL, Nanchahal K *et al.* Urinary symptoms in the community: how bothersome are they? *Br J Urol* 1994; 74: 551–555

30. Iosif S, Hendriksson L, Ulmsten U. The frequency of disorders of the lower urinary tract, urinary incontinence in particular, as evaluated by a questionnaire survey in a gynaecological health control program. *Acta Obstet Gynaecol Scand* 1981; 60: 71–76

31. Breakwell SL, Noble Walker S. Differences in physical health, social interaction, and personal adjustment between continent and incontinent housebound aged women. *J Commun Health Nurs* 1988; 5: 19–31

32. Kutner NG, Schechtman KB, Ory MG *et al.* Older adults' perceptions of their health and functioning in relation to sleep disturbance, falling, and urinary incontinence. *J Am Geriatr Soc* 1994; 42: 757–762

33. Herzog AR, Fultz NH, Normolle DP *et al.* Methods used to manage urinary incontinence in older adults in the community. *J Am Geriatr Soc.* 1989; 37: 339–347

34. Nochajski TH, Burns PA, Pranikoff K, Dittmar SS. Dimensions of urine loss among older women with genuine stress incontinence. *Neurourol Urodyn* 1993; 12: 223–233

35. Lagro-Janssen AL, Smits A, van Weel C. Urinary incontinence in women and the effects on their lives. *Scand J Prim Health Care* 1992; 10: 211–216

36. Ouslander JG, Hepps K, Raz S, Su Hong L. Genitourinary dysfunction in a geriatric outpatient population. *J Am Geriatr Soc* 1986; 54: 507–514

37. Sand PK, Richardson DA, Staskin DR *et al.* Pelvic floor stimulation in the treatment of genuine stress incontinence: a multicentre placebo controlled trial. *Neurourol Urodyn* 1994; 13: 356–357

38. Kelleher CJ, Cardozo LD, Khullar V, Salvatore S. A new questionnaire to assess the quality of life of urinary incontinent women. *Br J Obstet Gynaecol* 1997; 104: 1374–1379

39. Jackson S. Donovan J, Brookes S *et al.* The Bristol Female Lower Urinary Tract Symptoms Questionnaire: development and psychometric testing. *Br J Urol* 1996; 7: 805–812

40. Shumaker SA, Wyman JF, Uerbersax JS *et al.* Health related quality of life measures for women with urinary incontinence. The Urogenital Distress Inventory and the Incontinence Impact Questionnaire. *Quality Life Res* 1994; 3: 291–306

41. Black N, Griffiths J, Pope C. Development of a symptom severity index and a symptom impact index for stress incontinence in women. *Neurourol Urodyn* 1996; 15: 630–640

42. Wagner TH, Patrick DL, Bavendam TG *et al.* Quality of life in persons with urinary incontinence, development of a new measure. *Urology* 1996; 47: 67–72

43. Lee PS, Reid DW, Saltmarche A, Linton L. Measuring the psychosocial impact of urinary incontinence. The York Perceptions Scale (YIPS). *J Am Geriatr Soc* 1995; 43: 1275–1278

44. Seim A, Hermstad R, Hunskaar S. Management in general practice significantly reduces psychosocial consequences of female urinary incontinence. *Quality Life Res* 1997; 6: 257–264

45. Kobelt G. Personal communication, 1998

46. Kelleher CJ. The Impact of Urinary Incontinence on the Quality of Life of Women. MD Thesis, University of London, 1995

6

Communication: the key to effective incontinence assessment, treatment and patient satisfaction

A. Saltmarche, C. Gartley

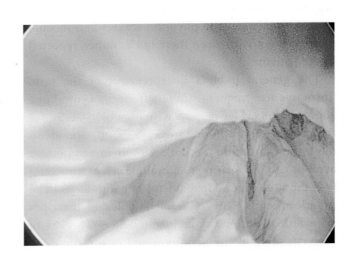

INTRODUCTION

Urinary incontinence is both physically bothersome and emotionally upsetting. Women affected by it often feel embarrassed, ashamed and alone because of the accompanying social stigma, which may cause them to hide their symptoms from their family, friends and healthcare professionals and, in some cases, even to deny the problem to themselves. Knowing the stigma attached to incontinence, and fearing a potential accident, the sufferer may live in constant dread of being ostracized if discovered. Nevertheless, the incontinent patient's emotional distress and anguish may not be evident to the healthcare professional at first glance.

This chapter focuses on the social and psychological aspects of incontinence in women. Of the estimated 14.5 million people in North America who experience incontinence, approximately 85% are women; however, millions still suffer in silence. What better reason is there, then, for gynaecologists and urologists to make this issue an important part of their clinical practice and research?

THE MEANING OF INCONTINENCE

Society dictates acceptable norms for our behaviour related to the timing and location of emptying our bladders. The International Continence Society defines incontinence as 'involuntary loss of urine which is objectively demonstrable and a social or hygienic problem'.[1] Although it is helpful for the healthcare community to have a widely accepted definition of incontinence, it may actually be a disservice to the individual who has the problem. If 'objectively demonstrable' means that incontinence exists only when 'induced' during assessment in the office or laboratory, what diagnosis can the physician make when incontinence is not actually seen there but is, rather, reported by the patient?

The general public's interpretation of the term 'incontinence' frequently differs from the clinical one above, and many lay persons have no understanding of the problem at all. In one survey, 45% of respondents did not recognize the word: 38% of them had no idea at all or gave an incorrect definition such as 'problems with the stomach and inability to cope with life'.[2] In an American study, 58% of women indicated that they knew little to nothing about incontinence.[3] This lack of understanding of the definition and of the condition itself may lead to confusion between the healthcare professional and the patient, who may not know or may deny that she is incontinent, although she may readily admit to 'loss of bladder control' or to 'leaking'.

CONSEQUENCES OF INCONTINENCE

The consequences of incontinence, which are numerous, vary throughout the population. Some women cope reasonably well by making small changes to their daily activities. Others feel the impact more, experiencing embarrassment, humiliation and fear – which in turn, diminishes their willingness to participate in relationships, sexual activities and social events.[4] The fact that urinary incontinence affects different women in different ways may explain why only approximately 50% of sufferers welcome the prospect of medical treatment.[5]

It has been noted that objective tests take no account of the patient's perception of the problem, and that a poor correlation exists between the subjective degree of bother that symptoms cause and objective measures of the degree of incontinence.[6,7] This is because many factors other than the severity of urinary leakage affect the perception of incontinence as a significant health problem: such factors include age, culture, social class, interpersonal relationships, social support, underlying aetiology, duration of symptoms, and other current illnesses.

UNDER-REPORTED AND UNDERTREATED

A great deal of evidence indicates that not only is incontinence under-reported but also that it is undertreated. This evidence was collected from the following medical sources: the Consensus Conference hosted by the National Institutes of Health in 1988; the Clinical Practice Guidelines developed in 1992 and updated in 1996; and the conference hosted in 1998 by the International Continence Society and the World Health Organization, in Monaco.

Many women may find the need to use a sanitary napkin quite normal, and view urinary leakage as an extension of their menstrual cycle, or of ageing or childbirth. Even though some women may consider incontinence normal, they may also be embarrassed and humiliated, or fear being stigmatized, and may therefore decide not to speak to a healthcare professional. Other women may not disclose the problem because of a belief that nothing can be done to cure or improve the leakage.

Many healthcare professionals themselves accept incontinence as inevitable or unresponsive to treatment because so little importance is placed on the topic in the medical curriculum and texts. Still a closet issue, incontinence receives scant attention from journalists and lacks militant consumer groups and lobbyists who could 'open the closet door' and push incontinence onto the political agenda, with the attendant funding for services and research.

THE CHALLENGE OF PHYSICIAN–PATIENT COMMUNICATION

Because incontinence is under-reported and under-treated it is clear that the physician–patient lines of communication need to be opened. Research indicates that women often fail to communicate clearly to their physician the symptoms of their incontinence and the impact of it on their lives. When they do broach the topic, their reference may be furtive, such as 'I have to go to the bathroom more often now', or ' I'm leaking during exercise class' (Saltmarche R, Cherrie P, Frydrych S. Unpublished data, 1998). In a busy clinical practice, the physician may not hear a patient's vague reference to her symptoms clearly enough to help her. If the complaint is heard, it may pale in comparison with other life-threatening conditions to which the physician must attend.

Many women do not take time out of their busy daily schedules even to reflect on how incontinence affects their lives, and may not actually be aware of the changes made to cope with the problem. Other women, feeling embarrassed, may not think their symptoms important enough to warrant their doctor's time. Still others may fear bad news and the options for treatment; these patients say nothing, when what they need most is to talk about an issue that causes distress and greatly diminishes their quality of life.[8]

Having spoken with thousands of individuals who experience incontinence, we believe that many women either do not feel that they are heard by their physicians or are not satisfied with the quality of communication. Nor, generally speaking, are they satisfied with treatment or outcomes. In an attempt to assist with the dialogue between patient and physician, a paper on *A Patient's Rights and Responsibilities* was developed.[9] Patients' rights and responsibilities were revised (Table 6.1) and rights and responsibilities for the physician were developed.

Table 6.2, which outlines the physician's rights and responsibilities, is not an attempt to assign responsibility, as much as it is an attempt to improve communication. Much work is still needed to ensure that women who experience incontinence and, the resulting shame and embarrassment will, first, come forward to seek medical intervention and, second, will receive the necessary care. It is hoped that outlining the expectations of both parties will reduce confusion or misunderstanding. The rights and responsibilities for patients and physicians demonstrate that they are both partners in the assessment, treatment and measurement of outcomes.

Research has found that more than 90% of physicians believe that serious medical problems could be avoided if patients were more willing to talk about

---

Table 6.1. *Incontinence: the patient's rights and responsibilities*

As a patient, you have a right to:

- the knowledge that incontinence can be cured, treated or effectively managed
- a quality of life not restricted by continence issues
- receive care from a healthcare professional who is interested and knowledgeable about incontinence, and comfortable discussing body functions
- participate in the patient/healthcare partnership
- written materials describing potential treatment options so you can actively participate in decision-making
- be aware of any potential negative outcomes of surgical, medical or management treatment for incontinence
- ask questions about the assessment, treatment options or potential outcomes
- refuse or delay a recommended treatment or decide when 'enough is enough'

As a patient, you have a responsibility to:

- provide complete and accurate information to your healthcare professional
- ask all questions to clarify your knowledge about your condition
- follow the treatment plan agreed upon
- notify your healthcare professional if you stop following the treatment plan
- seek out another healthcare professional if your incontinence is not being addressed to your satisfaction

Table 6.2. *Incontinence: the physician's rights and responsibilities*

As a physician, you have a right to:

- complete and accurate information from the patient
- a patient who is willing to actively participate in the physician/patient partnership
- be notified if the patient stops following the treatment plan

As a physician, you have a responsibility to:

- not accept incontinence as inevitable
- provide adequate assessment and treatment for incontinence
- provide verbal and written information for the patient so she understands the assessment, treatment options, including potential risks, benefits and probable outcomes
- refer the client to another healthcare professional if you or the patient deem it necessary

their problems. Studies have also revealed that time, education, fear and embarrassment are major obstacles to effective patient–physician communication. Furthermore, 67% of doctors say they are not able to spend enough time with their patients and that they consider this a 'somewhat serious' to 'very serious' problem in their practices.[8]

The physician's lack of time and fast work pace may generate a sense of urgency, giving the patient the impression that she is not heard, or that there is not sufficient time for her to tell her story or talk about her experience with incontinence. When the physician does make time to listen to the patient (and this may be the first time she is able to tell her story), the feedback is very complimentary. 'When my doctor was willing and open to discuss my leaking, it made me feel less ashamed and more comfortable. I was determined to faithfully do all of the recommendations', said one participant. 'I was thrilled to have my doctor explain my condition so that I understood it and the possible treatments available and the potential positive and negative sides of it', said another in the same study (Saltmarche R, Cherrie P, Frydrych S. Unpublished data, 1998).

THE ART OF ASKING QUESTIONS

As physicians and other healthcare professionals develop skills and expertise in assessments and diagnoses, they learn to direct their questioning, to address the presenting complaint or problem. Although this approach may provide the most effective and efficient method of obtaining the data, it does not always allow the patient the opportunity to express specific concerns. This may result in the woman being left with the feeling that she has not been heard – or, potentially, may be detrimental, relevant information not having being obtained.

As an introduction to discussing incontinence – a sensitive and embarrassing issue for many women – it may decrease the discomfort level of the patient to use open-ended questions to initiate the assessment process, such as 'What was life like before you starting experiencing loss of bladder control?' This question may assist patients to reflect and recognize how they have gradually changed their lives, in an attempt to decrease accidents or to reaching the lavatory in time.

Another such question might be 'Can you tell me how the loss of bladder control has affected your day-to-day activities?' Understanding the impact of the condition is important on a number of levels: it may demonstrate the patient's interpretation of significance; it may illustrate motivation to participate actively in the potential treatment options, and it may indicate willingness to undergo more invasive forms of treatment.

THE VOIDING DIARY AS A COMMUNICATION TOOL

The voiding diary may offer both the busy physician and the apprehensive patient an opportunity to achieve their goals of establishing open lines of communication, by jointly selecting the most appropriate treatment and evaluating outcomes. Requesting the patient to complete the voiding diary and asking her to consider the implications of incontinence for her daily life, not only provides the clinician and the patient with objective data but also requires the woman to reflect carefully on her condition and whether it has significantly changed her life. This exercise may decrease the amount of time required to solicit the necessary information as much as it may help the woman to describe her symptoms and their implications for her life. It may also provide a starting point for discussing mutual goals of treatment and measuring outcomes. (See also chapter 15.)

The voiding diary may offer another positive benefit in that, for most women who experience incontinence, it is not just the physical toll that the condition exacts but also the psychological trauma and the social barriers it creates. Individuals, although not actually incapacitated by incontinence, choose to abandon certain activities because they dread the prospect of leaking and being humiliated. Before a particular patient feels like resuming her 'old' life, she will need not only to control her symptoms but also to gain the confidence that she can do so consistently. Naturally, this process will take time, patience and emotional support. The diary will demonstrate real improvement over time, which may help the woman to regain her confidence and to obtain sufficient self-assurance to resume relinquished activities.

IMPROVING PATIENT SATISFACTION

As clinicians, we are educated and trained to 'solve' and 'fix' the health problems of the people who come to see us. Traditionally, to achieve this goal, we take the patient's history, make a diagnosis and select a solution(s) to fix the problem. Perhaps this well-intentioned approach leaves the patient feeling isolated and unheard – an object, not a person. If the patient feels excluded from the process, this does not encourage her to take responsibility for completing her treatment. Although the ultimate outcome is important for both parties, for the patient the two-way communication and the step-by-step process to achieve that outcome may he equally important, if not more so. We believe that the establishment of open, informative communication will lead to the development of a mutually beneficial partnership with the patient. In the long run, this kind of

relationship may decrease the overall time that the physician may need to spend with the patient, and may result in more successful outcomes and greater patient satisfaction.

REFERENCES

1. Andersen J, Abrams P, Blaivas JG, Stanton SL. The standardization of terminology of lower urinary tract function. *Scand J Urol Nephrol Suppl* 1988; 114: 5–9

2. Canadian Continence Foundation *Incontinence in Canada*. Commissioned healthcare survey by Angus Reid Group, 1998

3. Bladder Health Council Health Survey conducted by Yankelovich Partners. *Informer*. Chicago: Simon Foundation for Continence, 1995; spring–summer issue: 3.

4. Norton C. The effects of urinary incontinence in women. *Int Rehabil Med* 1988; 4: 9–14

5. O'Brien J, Austin M, Sethi P, O'Boyle P. Urinary incontinence: prevalence, need for treatment and effectiveness of intervention by nurse. *Br Med J* 1991: 303: 1308–1312

6. Wyman J, Harkins S, Choi S *et al.* Psychosocial impact of urinary incontinence in women. *Obstet Gynecol* 1987; 70: 378–380

7. Ryhammer AM, Djurhuus JC, Laurgerg S, Hermann AP. No relationship between self-reported urinary incontinence and pad test weight gain in healthy perimenopausal women. *Neurourol Urodyn* 1995; 14: 456–457

8. Koop CE. Take Time to Talk educational program. New York: Pharmacia & Upjohn, 1997.

9. Gartley C. Incontinence: a patient's rights and responsibilities. *Informer*. Chicago: Simon Foundation for Continence, 1995: spring–summer issue: 3.

7

The evolution of continence nurse specialists

M. L. Gallo, D. K. Newman, K. C. Sasso

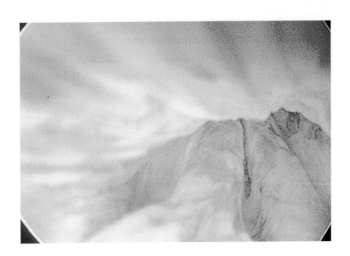

INTRODUCTION

Urinary incontinence (UI) is a devastating condition that affects approximately 13 million Americans, about 5% of the population.[1] Among Americans between the ages of 15 and 64 years, the prevalence of UI ranges from 1.5% to 5% in men and from 10% to 30% in women.[2,3] Of people over the age of 65 years, 20–35% are incontinent.[4] In the USA, society incurs a significant economic burden as a result of UI. In 1995, the direct cost of caring for incontinent persons over the age of 65 years in the community and nursing homes was estimated to be US\$26.3 billion annually in the USA.[5] This figure reflects the resources spent to treat UI and to mitigate its effects. These costs are predominately for palliative rather than rehabilitative services. Fewer than 10% of these patients will seek treatment. Many people who are incontinent will not even mention the problem to their healthcare provider; this may be related to feelings of embarrassment and shame or to a belief that the condition is hopeless and occurs naturally with ageing.[6]

The personal consequences of incontinence are numerous. Some patients may experience anxiety, depression, social isolation and low self-esteem related to their bladder problems. Often, UI causes the patient to stop working, travelling or participating in social events with friends and family. In addition, family members, particularly spouses, share the frustrations and limitations when the patient refuses to participate in situations outside the home for fear of being incontinent. In some situations, UI can predispose a patient to long-term care facilities. A study examining reasons for institutionalization found that 44% of family members reported that UI was a significant factor in placing a relative in long-term care.[7] Lastly, prolonged incontinence can result in medical complications such as skin irritation, infection and decubitus ulcers.

One of the greatest obstacles to effective management of incontinence is the perception that incontinence is inevitable and irreversible – a perception almost as common among healthcare providers as among patients.[8] As a result, many individuals turn to the use of products such as absorbent pads and supportive aids, without having this condition properly diagnosed or treated.[9] However, over the past 15 years, in many countries the nursing professional has come to the forefront as the primary healthcare provider for persons with UI. In countries such as Great Britain, Australia, Singapore and Germany, government-regulated health systems have supported the role of nurses in the field of UI. In the USA, advanced practice nurses (APNs), nurse practitioners (NPs) and clinical nurse specialists (CNSs), have become increasingly interested, knowledgeable and informed about the assessment, diagnosis and treatment of patients suffering with UI. Such nurses are developing a nursing subspecialty in the care of individuals with incontinence to meet the rising demands of this growing population. This chapter outlines the role of the nurse in various countries and the growth of the APN as a leader of incontinence nursing care in the USA.

A GLOBAL PERSPECTIVE OF THE CONTINENCE NURSE SPECIALIST

The scope and extent of nursing services for incontinence differ throughout the world. One model that has been comprehensively developed is in Great Britain, where 'continence nurse advisors' were developed. In 1977, Great Britain developed a national system for nurses to be trained to care for patients with UI.[10] The goal was for the nurse to be the reference point on the subject of incontinence, both urinary and faecal. Multiple branches of the government funded these nursing specialists and assigned them to a geographical location, usually a district health authority, and determined the scope of practice. Many of the original positions were created in conjunction with research-based urology clinics. Often, a nurse was hired to work on a research grant by assisting with urodynamic testing. From this limited position, many nurses became interested in caring for incontinent patients and sought information about conservative and surgical methods of patient care. However, because so little was published about the nursing role in the care of incontinent patients, many inquisitive nurses began conducting their own research and publishing their findings in nursing journals.

Initially, the growth of the continence nurse advisor was slow but, as manufacturing companies developed disposable products, many health authorities saw the need for an advisor to assist with their use. Initially, these nurses acted as 'pad and pant' nurses. The role evolved into that of a CNS. Through publications and experience, continence advisors and physicians throughout Great Britain have contributed greatly to the expansion of knowledge about the assessment and treatment of patients with UI. In addition, many physicians developed specialty continence assessment clinics, and promoted the role of the continence advisor as a major contributor in the British healthcare system. Currently, the continence nurse advisor has four main areas of responsibilities: (1) clinical, involving patient assessment, management and treatment; (2) administrative, including monitoring supplies, protocols and the budget for incontinence in their specific health district; (3) education for patients, consumers and other nurses; and (4) research. This specialty of incontinence nurses has evolved into a national professional organization – the Association for Continence Advice (ACA) – which includes both nurses and physical therapists who treat persons with incontinence. In 1998, the ACA held its Second International Conference on Urinary Incontinence in Edinburgh, drawing nurses from 15 countries.

Despite such advances by the continence nurse advisor, the adequacy of knowledge possessed by basic nurses and other health professionals within this area of care has been questioned by Great Britain's governing agencies, the Royal College of Nursing and the King's Fund. Reports of the King's Fund (1983) and the Royal College of Nursing (1982) speculated that health professionals lacked sufficient knowledge about incontinence, owing to inadequate education at either basic or post-basic levels. A study by Cheater in 1992 surveyed experienced and student nurses in one health district in England to establish the level of educational preparation and knowledge about continence management:[11] the results indicated that, despite considerable advances in the management of UI in recent years, many nurses, irrespective of experience, lacked sufficient knowledge about incontinence upon which informed nursing practice should be based. Therefore, more research needs to be conducted in Great Britain to assess the educational preparation and knowledge of all nurses involved in continence care.

NURSING SERVICES FOR INCONTINENCE IN THE USA

In comparison to Great Britain, the USA falls behind in the development of a specific role for nurses who specialize in the area of incontinence. The USA does not have a national health system and/or network of specialized continence nurse advisors. However, when the

history of nursing in the USA has been reviewed, the care of persons with elimination problems has been documented, since the time of Florence Nightingale, as integral to basic nursing care. Nightingale's 1859 *Notes on Nursing* noted the basics of elimination care when she wrote that 'chamber pots without a lid should be utterly abolished and they must be emptied frequently'.[12] In the 1800s, discussion of incontinence health was correlated with the problem as a childhood dilemma and mentioned the use of rubber urinals in adults. In the 1920s, general nursing textbooks included a section on care of the patient with incontinence or urology problems, with treatments mentioned consisting of hot packs, sitz-baths and avoidance of cold feet. At that time, nursing management of UI consisted mainly of how to care for and use catheters. As early as 1922, conservative and preventative measures such as pelvic muscle exercises were suggested in women after childbirth to improve pelvic support.[13] Not until the 1950s were additional non-surgical treatments of UI suggested, including such treatments as electrical stimulation, pessaries and silver nitrate applied to the urinary meatus. It was during this period that nursing textbooks began to devote several pages to incontinence, expanding management options to include skin care, management with a catheter, penile clamp, external catheters and incontinence pads.[14] Conservative management of incontinence was first seen as a role for nurses in 1960. During this time, nurses involved in long-term care attempted to improve both faecal and urinary incontinence; however, these programmes were met with resistance from both staff and patients, who accepted UI as a normal part of care.[15] In 1968, the first nursing model for incontinence care was expressed through the publication of a manual on bowel and bladder care.[16] This was also the time when nursing expanded incontinence care to include subspecialties such as rehabilitation patients – particularly those with spinal cord injury.

Part of the problem with UI care in the USA is that the nursing care is fragmented and is practised by several levels of nurses – from nursing assistants or aides to APNs. As the care is fragmented, so is nursing's approach to basic assessment, treatment and management strategies. As manufacturers have introduced more disposable products into the US retail market, nursing strategy for management of UI has centred around containment. Although UI prevalence rates for persons living in extended-care facilities and in their

homes are over 50%, prevention techniques and rehabilitative treatments are not routinely initiated by
nurses caring for these patients.[17,18] This is a growing
dilemma that will only worsen as the US population
ages. However, most in the medical and nursing community will agree that nurses play a central role in the
care of incontinent older adults. In the long-term care,
acute care and home care settings, the nurse may be the
only healthcare professional who detects and begins the
assessment and treatment of incontinence. In most
institutional healthcare settings, nurses not only provide direct patient care but are also responsible for the
philosophy, standard and policy of care while supervising the performance of other nursing staff members.
The duties and responsibilities of the nurse specialist
for incontinence care in the USA are similar to the role

outlined by more structured programmes in place in
other countries. The nurse has become the expert
incontinence clinician, educator, administrator and
researcher. However, no federal initiative has recommended formation of incontinence specialists. Therefore, a more formal structured movement in this
nursing subspecialty is not likely in the near future.

This is disturbing as the nurse has a key role in the
prevention of incontinence and the restoration of continence[19,20] (see Table 7.1). Where this is not a viable
goal, the nurse is instrumental in helping the patient,
the patient's family and caregivers (where relevant) to
cope effectively with the physical, psychological, social
and economic consequences of the problem. The nurse
needs to have a thorough knowledge of the various ways
in which normal bladder function may become

Table 7.1. *Identification of nurses, educational preparation and incontinence-related care*

Nurse	Education/licensure	Incontinence-related care
Nurse Assistant (NA) Nurse's Aide	Certification usually through technical school instruction	• Detects UI • Modifies diet • Toilets patient • Changes products, devices and pads • Inspects skin and applies product
Licensed Practical Nurse (LPN)	Practical Nursing education programme State Licensure	• Detects UI • Reviews bladder records • Assesses and implements diet modification • Toilets patient • Implements a scheduled toileting programme • Teaches bladder-retraining and urge-inhibition techniques • Implements appropriate use of products and devices • Inspects skin and applies product

Registered Nurse (RN)	Diploma in Nursing
	
	Associate Degree in Nursing
	
	Bachelor's Degree in Nursing or Outside Nursing
		• Identifies UI
		• Carries out basic assessment of UI, to include history, physical examination and baseline urological assessment
		• Educates and counsels patients/families and caregivers
		• Conducts nursing interventions, to include:
		  1. Scheduled toileting programmes
		  2. Bladder retraining
		  3. Behaviour modification
		  4. Implementation of the use of devices and products
		• Supervises non-professional staff
		• Implements bladder health promotion strategies

cont.

Table 7.1. *Identification of nurses, educational preparation and incontinence-related care (cont.)*

Nurse	Education/licensure	Incontinence-related care
Advanced Practice Nurse (APN)	Master of Science in Nursing Master of Science	• Identifies UI • Carries out basic assessment of UI, to include comprehensive history, mental, functional and environmental assessment
Nurse Practitioner (NP)	Certificate through the American Nurses Credentialing Center	• Carries out complete physical examination, to include assessment of genital prolapse with fitting of pessary

Clinical Nurse Specialist (CNS)	Meets individual State requirements for APN	• Carries out baseline urological assessment
		• Conducts complex urodynamic study with interpretation of data
		• Conducts additional studies such as laboratory tests
		• Identifies patients who need referral to other medical specialists
		• Educates and counsels patients/families and caregivers
		• Conducts nursing interventions, to include:
		  1. Scheduled toileting programmes
		  2. Bladder retraining
		  3. Behaviour modification
		  4. Pelvic muscle rehabilitation with biofeedback therapy and interpretation of data
		  5. Neuromuscular pelvic muscle stimulation
		  6. Implementation of the use of devices and products
		• Prescribes pharmacological intervention
		• Supervises non-professional staff
		• Implements bladder health promotion strategies

UI, urinary incontinence.
Adapted from ref. 21.

impaired and how illness, injury and psychosocial factors may adversely affect the bladder. Then, in response to these problems, nurses are able to carry out systematic assessments and appropriate and informed interventions. Continence nurse specialists can serve as clinical support for nurses who have incontinent patients, as catalysts for improved care and coordination of services, and as educators and researchers.[22] Since 1980, chapters on the nursing care of persons with incontinence have been included in most nursing textbooks, both general nursing texts and specialty books such as geriatrics, women's health, obstetrics and gynaecology, and urology. Several nurses have written textbooks specifically on UI;[23,24] in addition, nurses have been instrumental in publishing books specifically for consumers that deal with every aspect of UI.[25–27]

EDUCATION FOR THE CONTINENCE NURSE IN THE USA

Although many nurses have great expertise in caring for incontinent patients, there are no academic or clinical proficiency requirements in order to be considered a continence nurse specialist. However, in 1993, the Wound, Ostomy, and Continence Nurses Society (WOCN) developed the first certification programme for continence care nurses. To be eligible for this examination the nurse must:

• hold current licensure as a registered nurse,
• have a baccalaureate degree, and either
  1. complete either an enterostomal therapy nursing programme or a specialty nursing programme accredited by WOCN, and also complete at least

2000 hours (1 year's full-time experience in the specialty), or

2. complete 4000 hours (2 year's full time) in the continence specialty area.[28]

To date, the number of nurses certified through this process has not been significant, probably because of views of specific requirements. The norm is that most nurses in the USA obtain their knowledge and skill through self-motivated activities: these activities include reading medical and nursing journals, attending professional meetings, observing clinical findings of other healthcare professionals (urologists, urogynaecologists or gynaecologists) and joining professional organizations to discuss topics related to the care of incontinent patients. In 1998, Jacobs and colleagues[28] surveyed nurses attending a national conference on UI about their educational preparation related to this condition. Respondents reported that less than half (40%) received academic education including course work in accredited post-baccalaureate or graduate programmes related to UI. However, most nurses (76%) obtained instruction at professional conferences, continence clinics supervised by nurse practitioners or physicians, 'on-the-job' training, self-study and in-service programmes.

Specialty nursing associations addressing continence care are summarized in Table 7.2.

Despite the fact that nursing interventions for patients with UI are effective,[9, 29] most individuals in the USA do not report this condition to their healthcare provider. In most cases, once the UI has been reported, providers do not assess or treat accurately; this is not surprising, as most nurses do not receive basic training in this field. To help remedy this neglect, the US Department of Health and Human Services, Agency for Health Care Policy and Research (AHCPR) in 1996 recommended that 'first and foremost, information about UI be included in the curricula of undergraduate and graduate health professional schools'.[9] However, Colling[30] notes that more than half the faculty who teach geriatric content in nursing programmes lack any formal education specifically related to UI. In another study, Norton found that UI is rarely treated as a separate subject in schools of nursing.[31] Information about the evaluation and treatment of incontinence is more likely to be learned in fragments, or during on-the-job training when confronted with a patient with skin breakdown associated with UI. Morishita *et al.*[32] describe UI content that is reportedly taught in most nursing school curricula, but the didactic component is only

Table 7.2. *Specialty nursing associations addressing continence care in the USA*

Organization	Address	Telephone
American Nephrology Nurses Association	East Holly Ave. Box 56 Pitman, NJ 08071-0056	(609) 256-2320
Association of Rehabilitation Nurses	4700 W. Lake Ave. Glenview, IL 60025	(847) 375-4710
Association of Women's Health, Obstetric, & Neonatal Nurses	2000 L. Street, Suite 740, Washington, DC 20036	(202) 261-2400
National Alliance of Nurse Practitioners	325 Pennsylvania Ave. SE, Washington, DC	(202) 675-6350
National Conference of Gerontological Nurse Practitioners	P.O. Box 270101, Fort Collins, CO 80527-0101	(970) 493-7793
Society of Urologic Nurses & Associates	East Holly Ave. Box 56 Pitman, NJ 08071-0056	(609) 256-2335
Wound, Ostomy, & Continence Nurses Society	1550 S. Coast Hwy., Suite 201, Laguna Beach, CA 92651	(888) 224-9626

Reproduced from ref. 21 with permission.

2 hours in length and clinical experience is left to chance, offering little assurance that practice and feedback are obtained. In addition, formal curriculum content in undergraduate nursing programmes tends to be 'informed orientated' and structured to facilitate students' recall of information to pass state licensure examination. Educational competencies for continence care at the basic preparation level for beginning professional practice courses has been summarized by Jirovac *et al.*[21] (Table 7.3). Specific knowledge about UI, as well as the broader area of gerontological nursing, is not tested in undergraduate programmes, which makes adequate coverage of UI content in the curriculum unlikely.

In graduate nursing curricula, little is published about UI content in primary care or geriatric nursing programmes. Nevertheless, studies show that nurses prepared at the graduate level (CNSs and NPs) who demonstrate a desire and interest in this field have made a commitment to manage and treat patients with UI effectively. With appropriate education, nurses can manage UI effectively,[33] and may reduce the costs of caring for patients with incontinence.[34]

ADVANCED PRACTICE NURSES

A group of nurses in the USA – APNs – are coming to the forefront as primary providers for persons with UI. APNs are CNSs, NPs, nurse midwives, and nurse anaesthetists. They are registered professional nurses who have received a Master of Science degree in nursing. Educational competencies for continence care by the Master's-prepared APN have been described (Table 7.4). These healthcare professionals are knowledgeable about a wide range of medical health conditions and work closely with a physician collaborator to maximize patient outcomes in acute, primary, home, outpatient and long-term care settings. Despite great diversity among client populations, practice setting and specific function, all APNs have the same role as practitioner, consultant, educator, researcher, administrator and leader.[35]

NPs and CNSs commonly work in areas of patient care traditionally managed solely by physicians. In the USA, the NP and CNS roles are similar. A study in 1990 noted likeness in the core curriculum of all NP and CNS academic programmes, with differences in added courses for NPs in pharmacology, primary care, physical assessment, health promotion, nutrition and history taking.[36] The major cause of role differentiation between the NP and the CNS has been described in the practice setting, with the CNS working in acute care and the NP working in ambulatory or primary care. Because of similar role delineation, many authors have suggested that a merger of CNS and NP graduate nursing programmes would be cost-effective and would allow for greater job mobility.[37]

ADVANCEMENT OF ADVANCED PRACTICE NURSING SERVICES

The APN role is growing, owing to an increase in nursing graduate programmes, research that demonstrates the cost-effectiveness of APNs and the expansion of innovative practice and consultation models.[38,39] However, the most significant growth in the use of the APN to provide healthcare services has been in the changes in laws in 1989 and 1997 that allow these services to be reimbursed directly by the federal Medicare insurance programme. The 1997 law removed the restrictions on the type of settings and geographical areas in which Medicare pays for the professional services for the APN. Payment is a percentage (85%) of the physician fee schedule amount. Prior to 1998, the APN providing services to persons in their home or in private-practice settings could provide these services only through direct physician supervision, which meant that the physician was physically in the medical office or with the APN when making a home visit. The APN must continue to work in collaboration with a physician; this occurs when the APN works with a physician to deliver healthcare services within the scope of the practitioner's professional expertise as defined by individual state laws. However, in certain instances, such as in a hospital setting and in long-term settings, if payment is already being received as part of the overall facility costs for furnishing services, separate payment cannot be received for the APN services. The setting where the law is most applicable and can expand the APNs services is the private-practice setting. In the USA, the scope of an APN's service and practice differs depending on geographical location. Restrictions on scope of practice and prescriptive authority may differ in specific states.[40] The APN can invoice for services using ICD-9 and CPT codes. In the area of UI, reimbursement has been realized through the use of evaluation and management visit codes, biofeedback therapy, patient education and therapeutic activities procedure codes.

Table 7.3. *Educational competencies for continence care: basic preparation for beginning professional practice*

A professional nurse will be able to independently:

1. Obtain a focused health history to include:
   a. the presence of risk factors for urinary incontinence (UI) and medical conditions that may be contributing to UI and identifying patients at risk for the development of UI
   b. confirming the presence and effect of UI subjectively
   c. a detailed exploration of the symptoms of UI and associated factors including symptoms of leakage, frequency, urgency, and nocturia (failure to store); and retention and overflow (failure to empty)
   d. medication review including prescription and nonprescription drugs to identify those patients whose medications may negatively affect urine control
   e. bowel pattern to include frequency, consistency, and usage of any assistive products (e.g., dietary measures, prescription and nonprescription medications including suppositories and enemas)
   f. functional, environmental, social, and cognitive factors that may contribute to or result in UI

2. Obtain an intake and output record that includes:
   a. voiding records from patients that include time and onset of incontinent episodes, voiding pattern, 24-hour recording with diurnal and nocturnal frequency, amount voided, amount leaked, activity when leakage occurred, and presence of inadequate or excessive output
   b. intake record with 24-hour pattern of fluid intake that includes amount, frequency, and type of oral intake

3. Obtain diagnostic measures to detect evidence of urinary tract infection and other disorders contributing to incontinence that may include:
   a. urinalysis or the use of a chemically treated dipstick to detect hematuria, pyuria, bacteriuria, glycosuria, or proteinuria
   b. obtaining clean catch or catheterized urine specimen for culture and sensitivity
   c. obtaining catheterized urine specimen to detect amount of urine in bladder or post void residual (PVR) urine volume

4. Conduct a physical examination that includes:
   a. focused abdominal exam to estimate suprapubic fullness; to rule out palpable hard stool, and to evaluate bowel sounds
   b. examination of the genitals including skin integrity of perineum, appearance of urethral meatus, and presence of prolapse
   c. rectal exam including evaluation of sphincter tone, perineal sensation, and presence or absence of faecal impaction
   d. confirming the presence of UI objectively and evaluation of the force and character of urine stream during voiding with observation of actual toileting of client
   e. a functional assessment including mobility, self-care ability, cognitive ability (mental status exam), and communication patterns

5. Assess environment

6. Initiate nursing interventions that include:
   a. strategies that promote bladder health (fluid hydration, caffeine reduction, bowel programs, dietary strategies, weight reduction, smoking and alcohol reduction)
   b. educating and counseling patients and families (e.g., anatomy and physiology of genitourinary system, factors affecting continence, etiologic factors related to UI, treatment options available to patients who may benefit from scheduled voiding regimens without further testing)
   c. identifying patients who require further evaluation before therapeutic intervention; collaborating with physicians or advanced practice nurses regarding diagnosis, intervention plan, expected outcomes, and ongoing evaluation
   d. implementing scheduled toileting programs for functional incontinence and evaluating its effectiveness
   e. supervising nursing staff in the implementation of prompted voiding and scheduled toileting programs and evaluation of its effectiveness
   f. evaluating patients with indwelling catheter for voiding trial and initiation of bladder training
   g. teaching pelvic muscle exercises to patients at risk for developing stress incontinence
   h. implementing bladder training programs for early symptoms of stress or urgency
   i. implementing of scheduled toileting programs for patients at risk for developing functional incontinence before UI develops
   j. identifying patients who would benefit from assistive devices to maintain continence
   k. recommending appropriate containment devices and topical therapy for prevention and management of perineal skin breakdown

Reproduced from ref. 21 with permission.

Table 7.4. *Educational competencies for continence care: Master's preparation for advanced practice (e.g. CNS, NP, Nurse Midwife)*

In addition to competencies of a professional nurse, an advanced practice nurse will be able to:

1. Conduct a physical examination that includes:
   a. a general examination if indicated to detect conditions such as edema and other problems that may contribute to UI
   b. an abdominal exam to detect masses and evaluate bowel sounds
   c. a neurological exam
   d. a pelvic exam to evaluate pelvic muscle strength, perineal structure, perineal skin status (estrogenization of vaginal mucosa), signs of pelvic descent
   e. a rectal exam to evaluate presence or absence of reflexes, resting anal sphincter tone, anorectal sensation, sphincter function
   f. provocative stress testing
   g. with additional education may include urodynamic testing such as uroflowmetry, cystometry, simple cystometry, a filling cystometrogram, or a voiding cystometrogram and may also include videourodynamics and interpretation of urodynamic data

2. Evaluate assessment findings including:
   a. identifying patients in need of further laboratory tests
   b. identifying patients in need of medical referral

3. Identify patients who may benefit from behavioral intervention for their UI and prescribe and direct comprehensive continence program (may include prescriptions), may include:
   a. bladder training
   b. directing caregivers regarding specifics of a habit training program, prompted toileting, and other scheduled voiding regimens
   c. directing caregivers regarding specifics of a prompted toileting program
   d. teaching patients to perform pelvic muscle exercises. May include the use of vaginal cones, electrical stimulation and biofeedback
   e. individualizing a plan that incorporates drug management
   f. designing and implementing continence programs for patients with neurogenic bladders (clean intermittent cath, self catheterization)

4. Recommend topical therapy for management of perineal skin breakdown, dermatitis related to UI

5. Evaluate individual patient outcomes on an ongoing basis

6. Develop management program for chronic, long term incontinence to include the use of alternative measures and supportive devices

Reproduced from ref. 21 with permission.

ADVANCED PRACTICE NURSES AS PROVIDERS OF CONTINENCE CARE

As previously noted, the APN is active in the evaluation, diagnosis and treatment of patients with UI, as the APN is usually prepared educationally at the graduate nursing level. Although no educational programme includes continence care as part of the prescribed curriculum, the basic knowledge of health assessment and applied research is incorporated in graduate nursing education (see Table 7.1). With desire, patience and commitment to providing incontinence care, these nurses seek learning opportunities to meet their educational needs: they may receive on-the-job training from a practising physician (such as a urogynaecologist, urologist or gynaecologist) trained and interested in the care of women with urinary dysfunction; they may also learn from preceptorships available from these physicians and from attendance at instructional seminars or conferences on continence care. Regardless of the method used to obtain information about continence care, the APN is currently active in providing this much-needed service.

INCONTINENCE PRACTICE OF THE ADVANCED PRACTICE NURSE

The APN is a skilled professional who provides expertise in the assessment, diagnosis, treatment and/or management of UI. This entire scope of practice includes skill in history taking, physical examination, urodynamic and pelvic floor muscle evaluation, and in varied non-surgical treatment and management plans.

Patient history

The patient's medical, social, gynaecological and urological history is best obtained using a detailed history form that is completed by the patient and reviewed by the APN. A voiding diary covering 24–48 hours can assess the number of, and time interval between, micturition episodes, as well as fluid intake, urine volume and any incontinence episodes associated with an urge or physical activity. This allows the APN to guide patient history enquiry to determine the direction of the evaluation plan. Asking the patient to quantify UI by recounting the number of leaking episodes per week resulting from a cough/laugh/sneeze, or with an urge, and the duration of each symptom, will help determine the type of UI and the effect on the patient. A patient will be more likely to make a commitment to treatment if an individualized care plan is developed that will resolve or ameliorate the primary reason for seeking treatment of the UI.

A thorough review of a patient's pharmacological therapy may reveal potential side effects that contribute to UI (such as those from diuretics or α-blockers), or urinary retention (from tricyclic antidepressants, anticholinergics or α-adrenergics) or urgency/frequency symptoms in women not on oestrogen-replacement therapy. Dietary factors should also be investigated to see whether urinary symptomatology may be related to excessive caffeine, alcohol or fluid intake contributing to urgency/frequency symptoms or increased diuresis. Excessive fluid intake or a reverse diuresis detected on the voiding diary can also contribute to nocturia and/or nocturnal enuresis. The patient history responses will guide the APN in the physical assessment of the patient and, subsequently, to an accurate diagnosis and treatment or management plan.

Physical examination

The three major assessment components to the physical examination of the woman with UI are neurological, gynaecological and urodynamic.

The focus of the neurological examination is on the lower extremities and perineum. Assessment of the lower extremities for normal, symmetrical strength and for deep tendon reflexes is a way to assess the lumbosacral spinal cord. The testing of sharp and dull sensation around the thighs above the knee can determine whether the lower micturition centre is intact.[41] The sacral reflexes are examined by demonstrating a contraction of the levator ani muscles after stroking the labia majora overlying the bulbocavernosus muscles (bulbocavernosus reflex), or via a tap on the clitoris (clitoral reflex). The cough reflex causes contraction of the pelvic floor muscles, and stroking the skin next to the anus will elicit an 'anal wink' reflex. Any abnormality of these reflexes would suggest further investigation by a physician, preferably a neurologist.[42]

The gynaecological or pelvic examination entails inspection of the vulva and vagina for signs of oestrogen deficiency, skin irritation, inflammation or infection. Genital tract infection can lead to increased afferent sensation of the urethra, causing irritative voiding symptoms such as urgency, frequency and/or dysuria, which may confuse the diagnosis of urinary dysfunction.[41] The vagina is inspected for any abnormalities and, with the use of a Sims' speculum, the degree of any anterior, posterior or apical compartment defects (such as a cystocele, rectocele, enterocele or uterovaginal prolapse) may be assessed. Bimanual vaginal and digital rectal examinations are performed to rule out pelvic pathology; the latter also tests for anal sphincter tone and presence of stool. Pelvic muscle strength and endurance may be assessed during rectovaginal examination.

A simple Q-tip test can determine any urethral hypermobility contributing to stress incontinence: a straining angle of greater than 30 degrees, in our practice, is considered to be hypermobility of the bladder neck. Further urodynamic assessment of urethral closure-pressure profiles and leak-point pressures would further differentiate the diagnosis between genuine stress incontinence (GSI) with urethral hypermobility with or without intrinsic urethral sphincteric deficiency.

The urological component of the examination starts with measurement of post-void residual (PVR) urine. Practitioners' opinions vary on what amount is considered a normal PVR. According to the 1996 Clinical Practice Guidelines, a PVR of less than or equal to 50 ml, is considered to be within normal limits.[29] A PVR can be raised as a result of infection, functional obstruction, mechanical obstruction from pelvic organ prolapse, or neurological factors. A PVR obtained from straight catheterization of the bladder can be checked for infection or diabetes by a simple dipstick urinalysis and/or sent to the laboratory for culture and sensitivity tests to rule out bacteriuria contributing to the patient's urge incontinence.

A simple way to screen for stress incontinence is the urinary stress test. This is best accomplished with a patient who has a full bladder, is standing, is coughing and is performing a Valsalva manoeuvre, in order that urinary leakage can be observed. If urine continues to leak without increased intra-abdominal pressure, then detrusor instability (DI) can be considered in the working diagnosis and warrants further investigation. Patients with genital prolapse may need to have the prolapsed organ supported with a pessary, proctoswab or Sims' speculum in order that urine leakage can be observed.

Additional urodynamic tests may be part of the assessment performed by the APN. These would range from uroflowmetry and simple cystometrics, to complex multichannel urodynamic testing. If the patient's subjective complaints suggest urge or mixed incontinence and the patient does not wish for surgical intervention, the least expensive cystometrics can be performed to obtain a diagnosis of DI. If the patient complains of mixed incontinence and is considering surgical intervention to treat the incontinence, or if the diagnosis suggests urethral sphincteric deficiency or neurological voiding dysfunction, then quantitative multichannel urodynamic testing that includes urethral closure-pressure profiles and electromyography (EMG) studies should be considered. APNs not able to perform such tests should refer the patient to a continence centre.

TREATMENT OF UI

The APN can direct the treatment options specific to the patient's diagnosis of GSI, DI, mixed incontinence (GSI and DI), overflow or functional incontinence.

Treatment success depends on the patient's compliance with the treatment plan and their ability to follow the plan physically, emotionally and financially. The APN can provide many non-surgical treatment options to cure or ameliorate incontinence, as outlined below.

Pelvic floor muscle rehabilitation

Pelvic floor muscle rehabilitation is used in the treatment of GSI and DI. The patient performs pelvic muscle exercises (PMEs), known commonly as 'Kegel' exercises, on a daily basis until continence is restored or significantly improved. The goal is to increase strength, control and coordination of both slow- and fast-twitch muscle fibres. In the past few years, most incontinence specialists have been advocating a more aggressive programme that includes prescribing PMEs three times per day and performing the exercises in three positions (lying, standing and sitting). The patient is taught to hold the muscle contraction initially for 3 seconds with an equal time of relaxation. As muscle strength and control improve, the patient is instructed to lengthen the time of the contraction to 5, then 10 seconds. Patients perform 100–150 exercises over a period of 6–8 weeks.[43]

Very often, patients need assistance to perform these exercises correctly. The use of biofeedback therapy assists the patient in identifying and isolating the pelvic floor muscles with visual and auditory cues displayed on a monitor. EMG, pressure probes (vaginal or rectal) or perianal EMG surface electrodes are used to display the patient's pelvic floor muscular strength, duration, relaxation and isolation on a monitor viewed by the patient. EMG surface electrodes can be placed on the abdomen to monitor accessory muscle activity during the pelvic muscle contraction.

Pelvic floor electrical stimulation is used in conjunction with biofeedback therapy to help with pelvic muscle isolation or as a separate treatment for GSI or urge incontinence. Pelvic floor stimulation units are available for patient home use and are set at different frequencies – 50 Hz for GSI; 10 or 12.5 Hz for DI.

Weighted vaginal cones provide proprioreceptive biofeedback where the weight of the cone on the superior surface of the perineal muscles provides the woman with the sensation to contract her pelvic floor muscles to retain the cone in the vagina. The cones range in weight from 20 to 70 g. Vaginal-cone therapy can be used alone as a method to increase pelvic muscle strength or in conjunction with a PME programme.

Behavioural modification

Behavioural modifications include bladder retraining, urge inhibition, timed toileting, habit training, prompted voiding, fluid management and elimination of bladder irritants. Bladder retraining is primarily used with patients having DI but, as outlined in the 1996 Clinical Practice Guidelines, it can be used for mixed and stress incontinence.[9] The patient voids in regimented time intervals, with gradual increases in the time intervals between voids as the patient learns to inhibit the urge to void. The APN instructs the patient on bladder inhibition techniques such as performing pelvic muscle contractions, position change (i.e. if standing, change to sitting), deep breathing, and/or distraction, to help inhibit the sensation of urgency in order to delay voiding. The goal is to restore normal bladder function and voiding pattern.[44] The patient must be cognitively intact and motivated to comply with the treatment, for it may take 3–4 months to restore continence.

Timed voiding and habit training are forms of behaviour modification; however, unlike bladder retraining, these therapies control incontinence but do not normalize physiological bladder function. The goal is to keep the patient dry by regular toileting. With timed voiding, the patient's daytime voids are scheduled at fixed intervals, such as every 2 hours, or only on even hours, regardless of the patient's voiding pattern. In habit training, the patient voids in accordance with the times of incontinence indicated on the voiding record, in order to prevent incontinent episodes. For those patients cognitively impaired, prompted voiding is utilized: with this therapy, a caregiver prompts the patient to void at timed intervals, in order to keep the patient dry; the key is positive reinforcement for the patient, and caregiver consistency.[45] Patients with urinary symptoms of urgency and frequency should be receiving diet counselling to limit caffeine intake, as this is a known bladder irritant and diuretic.[46] Caffeine is found in cola beverages, coffee, tea, chocolate and certain non-prescription medications; its diuretic effect can increase bladder volume and contribute to both stress and urge incontinence.[47]

Some patients may take in excess fluid in order to keep the urinary pH elevated (to prevent acidic urine from causing urinary urgency and frequency); however, this may contribute to incontinence from excessive urine in the bladder. The APN would counsel these patients on the normal adult daily intake (1.5–2.0l) and inform them that overconsumption of fluids can only contribute to their incontinent episodes.[21] When nocturia or nocturnal enuresis is a problem, the APN would suggest that the patient should limit fluid intake after the evening meal.

Sometimes, a patient with a diagnosis of DI complains only of nocturnal enuresis and/or nocturia without incontinence during the day. Requesting a 48-hour voiding diary – which records urinary frequency, fluid intake and urine output – can help determine if the patient has reverse diuresis or daytime urinary frequency. If reverse diuresis is a concern, limiting fluids after the evening meal, or even taking a medication such as DDAVP (desmopressin acetate), will help to decrease nocturnal urine output and allow urine production to occur during the patient's waking hours.

Medication

Pharmacotherapy is used to treat both stress incontinence and DI. Prescription of medications and monitoring of effects are integral to an APNs practice; if the APN does not have prescriptive authority, then collaboration with a physician as part of a practice would allow the prescription of various medications. The classes of drug used to treat DI are anticholinergic agents, musculotropic relaxants (antispasmodics), tricyclic antidepressants and calcium-channel blockers.[46]

GSI is best treated with α-adrenergic to increase urethral sphincteric tone and decrease episodes of stress incontinence from increased outlet resistance. Patients with mixed incontinence can use a tricyclic antidepressant such as imipramine for the anticholinergic effect to control DI and increase urethral sphincteric tone from the α-adrenergic effect.[46]

MANAGEMENT OF URINARY INCONTINENCE

The history of nursing in the USA shows that early approaches to nursing care of incontinence centred around managing the problem through containment of the urine loss by using products and devices.

Therefore, the APN who specializes in this field must become the expert in the use of this 'equipment'.

Devices

In many cases, rehabilitative treatments in women are not appropriate and the use of certain intra-vaginal devices may be the best option for managing the UI. Pelvic organ support devices (pessaries) are being recommended to provide support to women with genital prolapse and to alleviate symptoms of urgency, frequency and UI. Another intravaginal support device has been used to treat stress UI by repositioning and supporting the bladder neck. These new products, specifically the incontinence ring and the bladder-neck support prosthesis have been used in patients to manage stress UI. These devices are most successful if there is little or no genital prolapse, so that the device remains within the vagina, supporting the bladder neck.

Occlusive urethral devices have been marketed for internal and external use to control urine loss from stress UI. An example of an internal urethral device is a disposable catheter-like product appropriately sized for women's urethral length. This device is inserted in the urethra and a retention air balloon is inflated to prevent urine loss during physical activity. A metal tab at the opposite end prevents the device migrating into the bladder. The device is inserted to prevent urine loss during increases in intra-abdominal pressure, and is worn until the urge to void is present as a result of normal bladder filling. A string is pulled which releases a valve and the device is removed so that the patient can urinate. The patient who opts for this device must be cognitively intact with good manual dexterity.

External occlusive devices adhere to the urethral meatus by means of a light adhesive and/or suction. These devices are useful in patients with mild stress incontinence and who have the manual dexterity to apply and remove the device.

Protective pads

Many sizes and styles of protective absorbent pads are currently available to manage UI. Patients choose the type of protective pads to suit the amount and type of urinary leakage. Patients with mild infrequent stress incontinence wear pads marketed for menstrual flow containment (panty liner, mini pad and maxi pad) or use toilet tissue or paper towels instead of a pad to save expense. For some of these women, wearing a vaginal tampon can provide support to the bladder neck and prevent mild stress incontinence. For worse incontinence, pads the size of a sanitary pad have a special gelling material to absorb the urine. Incontinence protective wear ranges from the incontinence pad to a full adult nappy (diaper) or briefs, available in various sizes and absorbencies.

Patients with irritation or skin breakdown from the wearing of pads can use cloth panties, which have removable washable inserts. Skin care must become an important part of the patient's daily routine, with application of barrier ointments to the perineal area to promote skin healing and prevent skin deterioration.

When assisting a patient in the choice of the appropriate protective product to manage incontinence, it is important to consider the physical, psychological and financial concerns of the patient. If immobility exists with excessive incontinence, a full adult diaper with protective pads for the bed may be the appropriate choice. Active women with moderate-to-severe incontinence might find the diaper functional but, psychologically, objectionable because of its similarity to a baby's nappy. Cost of the protective pads is another consideration and is why some patients would rather use toilet paper and change it with every void, than buy commercial products to manage incontinence. Incontinence pads and products have a role in the management of incontinence but should not be a substitute for seeking professional help to treat the condition of urinary incontinence.

Use of catheters

Some patients may require catheterization to empty their bladders, owing to temporary postoperative retention after a continence-restoring surgical procedure, or because of a neurological defect that impairs bladder emptying. The APN can teach patients clean intermittent self-catheterization (CISC) in either of these instances. Provided that patient is cognitively intact and has adequate manual dexterity, CISC is the best way to manage temporary or prolonged bladder emptying. The most important principle relating to the management, with CISC, of inadequate bladder emptying is frequent catheterization to avoid overdistention of the bladder.[21] Excessive bladder volumes can contribute to urine dribbling (overflow incontinence), to decreased bladder contractility and to infection. CISC is a simple task where the only equipment needed is a 12 or 14 F 6-inch straight catheter, cleaned with soap and rinsed well with tap water after use. The catheter is stored in a clean plastic bag and reused until it becomes too soft or brittle. Methods to teach patients CISC include both the use of a mirror and the 'blind' method: as these women learn both methods of CISC, usually the 'blind' method allows for more flexibility in lifestyle without the nuisance of carrying a mirror, using a catheter guide or finding a suitable place to position the mirror in order to perform the catheterization.

Patients with urinary retention and the need for prolonged catheterization, but who lack the mobility and good manual dexterity needed for CISC, may be helped with the use of some newer products to relieve urinary retention that are still under clinical investigation. Most of these products are catheter-like devices placed into the patient's urethra with a retention balloon at the bladder neck. Bladder drainage is attained by activating a valve to allow urine to drain. This is best used on cognitively intact patients who have enough manual dexterity to activate a valve and empty their bladder contents.

For cognitively and/or physically impaired patients, an indwelling Foley catheter can be used, provided that catheter care is maintained. Routine care involves daily meatal cleaning with soap and water. Routine catheter changes should be based on individual patient assessment. Routine irrigation of catheters is discouraged. Sometimes an indwelling catheter is used temporarily to help heal the perineal skin breakdown resulting from prolonged UI.

CONCLUSIONS

The APN is capable of providing assessment, diagnosis, and treatment and management options for patients in need of continence care. These services can be provided to the patient by an APN functioning in a fully equipped continence clinic with a collaborating physician or at the patient's bedside in a long-term care facility, although this is limited by the resources available at the bedside. The APN is an important resource to the patient in need of continence care and represents an educator, counsellor and practitioner. Although a national approach to incontinence nursing care has not been formulated in the USA, the APN has evolved into this nursing subspecialty and responsibilities are similar to those identified in countries where 'continence nurses' are organized. However, the care of persons with incontinence is a part of all levels of nursing care. Continence education of nurses in the USA continues to develop in both nursing school and training programmes; hence, this expansion of knowledge is leading to more positive outcomes for patients with incontinence.

REFERENCES

1. National Kidney and Urologic Diseases Advisory Board. *Barriers to Rehabilitation of Persons with End-stage Renal Disease or Chronic UI*. Workshop summary report Mar 7–9. Bethesda, MD: National Kidney and Urologic Diseases Advisory Board, 1994

2. Burgio KL, Matthews KA, Engel BT. Prevalence, incidence and correlates of UI in healthy, middle-aged women. *J Urol* 1991; 146: 1255–1259

3. Harrison GL, Memel DS. UI in women: its prevalence and its management in a health promotion clinic. *Br J Gen Pract* 1994; 44(381): 149–152

4. Mulcahy JJ. UI. *Urol Nurs* 1993; 12(3): 525–531

5. Wagner TH, Hu T. Economic costs of urinary incontinence. *Urology* 1998; 51: 355–361

6. Newman DK, Burns PA. Significance and impact of UI. *Nurse Pract Forum* 1994; 5(3): 130–133

7. Johnson MJ, Werner C. We have no choice: a study of familial guilt feelings surrounding nursing home care. *J Gerontol Nurs* 1982; 8: 641–645, 654

8. Doughty DB. Preface. In: Brewer D, Bryant R, Hampton B, Ooka M, Van Niel J (eds) *Urinary and Fecal Incontinence: Nursing Management*. St Louis, MO: Mosby Year Book, 1991; ix

9. Urinary Incontinence Guideline Panel. *Urinary Incontinence in Adults: Clinical Practice Guideline*. AHCPR Publication No. 92–0038. Rockville, MD: Agency for Health Care Policy and Research, Public Health Service, U.S. Department of Health and Human Services, March 1996

10. Roe B. *Clinical Nursing Practice: The Promotion and Management of Continence*. New York: Prentice Hall, 1992

11. Cheater FM. Nurses' educational preparation and knowledge concerning continence promotion. *J Adv Nurs* 1992; 17: 328–338

12. Wells T. Nursing research on urinary incontinence. *Urol Nurs* 1994; 14: 109–112

13. Young H, Davis DM, Johnson FP. *Young's Practice of Urology, Based on Study of 12,500 Cases*, Volume 1. Philadelphia: WB Saunders, 1926

14. Homer B, Henderson V. *Textbook of the Principles and Practice of Nursing*, 5th edn. New York: Macmillan, 1955

15. Saxon J. Techniques for bowel and bladder training. *Am J Nurs* 1962; 62: 69–71

16. Bergstrom D. *Care of Patients with Bowel and Bladder Problems: a Nursing Guide*. Minneapolis: American Rehabilitation Foundation, 1968

17. Ouslander JG, Palmer MH, Rovner BW *et al.* Urinary incontinence in nursing homes; remission and associated factors. *J Am Geriatr Soc* 1993; 41: 1083–1089

18. Noelker L. Incontinence in elderly cared for by family. *Gerontologist* 1987; 27: 194–200

19. Newman DK, Wallace J, Blackwood N, Spencer C. Promoting healthy bladder habits for seniors. *Ost Wound Manage* 1996; 42: 18–28

20. Sampselle CM, Burns PA, Dougherty MC *et al.* Continence for women: evidence-based practice. *J Obstet Gynecol Neonatal Nurs.* 1997; 26: 375–385

21. Jirovec MM, Wyman JF, Wells TJ. Addressing urinary incontinence with educational continence-care competencies. *Image* 1998; 30(4): 375–378

22. Smith DA, Newman, DK. The role of the continence nurse specialists. In: Jeter K, Faller N, Norton C (eds) *Nursing For Continence*. Philadelphia: WB Saunders, 1990; 267–272

23. Jeter K, Faller N, Norton C. *Nursing For Continence*. Philadelphia: WB Saunders, 1990

24. Palmer M. *Urinary Incontinence: Assessment and Promotion*. Maryland: Aspen Publications, 1996

25. Bruning N. *What You Can Do About Bladder Control*. New York: Dell Books, 1992

26. Burgio KL, Pearce KL, Lucco AJ. *Staying Dry, A Practical Guide to Bladder Control*. Baltimore: Johns Hopkins University Press, 1989

27. Newman DK. *The Urinary Incontinence Sourcebook*. Los Angeles, CA: Lowell House, 1997

28. Jacobs M, Wyman JF, Rowell P, Smith D. Continence nurses: a survey of who they are and what they do. *Urol Nurs* 1998; 18(1): 13–20

29. National Institutes of Health Consensus Development Panel. Conference on Urinary Incontinence in Adults. *J Am Med Assoc* 1989; 261: 2685–2690

30. Colling J. Educating nurses to care for the incontinent patient. *Nurs Clin North Am* 1988; 23: 279–289

31. Norton C. *Nursing for Continence*. Beaconsfield, England: Beaconsfield Publishers, 1986

32. Morishita L, Uman G, Pierson C. Education on adult urinary incontinence in nursing school curricula: can it be done in two hours? *Nurs Outlook* 1994; 42: 123–129

33. Pearson BD, Droessler D. Continence through nursing care. *Geriatr Nurse* 1988; 9: 347–349

34. MEDSTAT. Market Scan Report for UI Panel. DHHS Publication No. NCHS 86–121. Washington: US Department of Health and Human Services, 1986

35. Kerr KL, Renaud-Tessier A, Smellie-Decker M *et al.* Clinical privileging for advanced practice nurses. *Nurse Pract* 1996; 21: 94, 97–98

36. Newmant BJ. Health care dollars and regulation sense: the role of advanced practice nursing. *Yale J Regul* 1992; 9(2): 417–487

37. Joel LA. The CNS and NP roles: controversy and conflict. *Am J Nurs* 1995; 95(4): 7

38. Newman DK, Parente CA, Yuan JR. Implementing the Agency for Health Care Policy and Research Urinary Incontinence Guidelines in a home health agency. In: Harris MD (ed) *Handbook of Home Health Care Administration*, 2nd edn. Gaithersburg, MD: Aspen, 1997; 394–403

39. Newman DK, Palumbo MV. Planning an independent nursing practice for continence services. *Nurse Pract Forum* 1994; 5(3): 190–193

40. Newman DK. Program and practice management for the advanced practice nurse. In: Hamric AB, Spross JA, Hanson CM (eds) *Advanced Nursing Practice*. Philadelphia: W.B. Saunders, 1996; 545–568

41. Sand PK. Evaluation of the incontinent female. *Curr Probl Obstet Gynaecol Fertil* 1992; 15: 107–151

42. Sand PK, Ostergard DR. The lumbosacral neurologic examination. *Urodynamics and the Evaluation of Female Incontinence, a Practical Guide*. London: Springer-Verlag, 1997; 11–13

43. Messick GM, Powe CE. Applying behavioral research to incontinence. *Ost Wound Manage* 1997; 43(10): 40–42, 44–46, 48

44. McDowell BJ, Burgio KL, Candib D. Behavioral and pharmacological treatment of persistent urinary incontinence in the elderly. *J Am Acad Nurse Pract* 1990; 2: 17–23

45. Hesnan K. ET nurses expanding our practice, *Ost Wound Manage* 1992; 38: 12–19

46. Montella JM, Wordell CJ. Effect of drugs on the lower urinary tract. In: Ostergard DR, Bent A (eds) *Urogynaecology and Urodynamics Theory and Practice*, 4th edn. Baltimore: Williams and Wilkins, 1996; 271–280

47. Newman DK, Steidle C, Wallace DW. Urinary Incontinence: An Overview of the Diagnosis and Management. *Am J Managed Care* 1995; 1(1): 68–74

48. Newman DK. Urinary incontinence management in the USA: the role of the nurse. *Br J Nurs* 1996; 5: 79–88

49. Pierson CA. Pad testing, nursing interventions, and urine loss appliances. In: Ostergard DR, Bent A (eds) *Urogynaecology and Urodynamics Theory and Practice*, 4th edn. Baltimore: Williams and Wilkins, 1996; 251–269

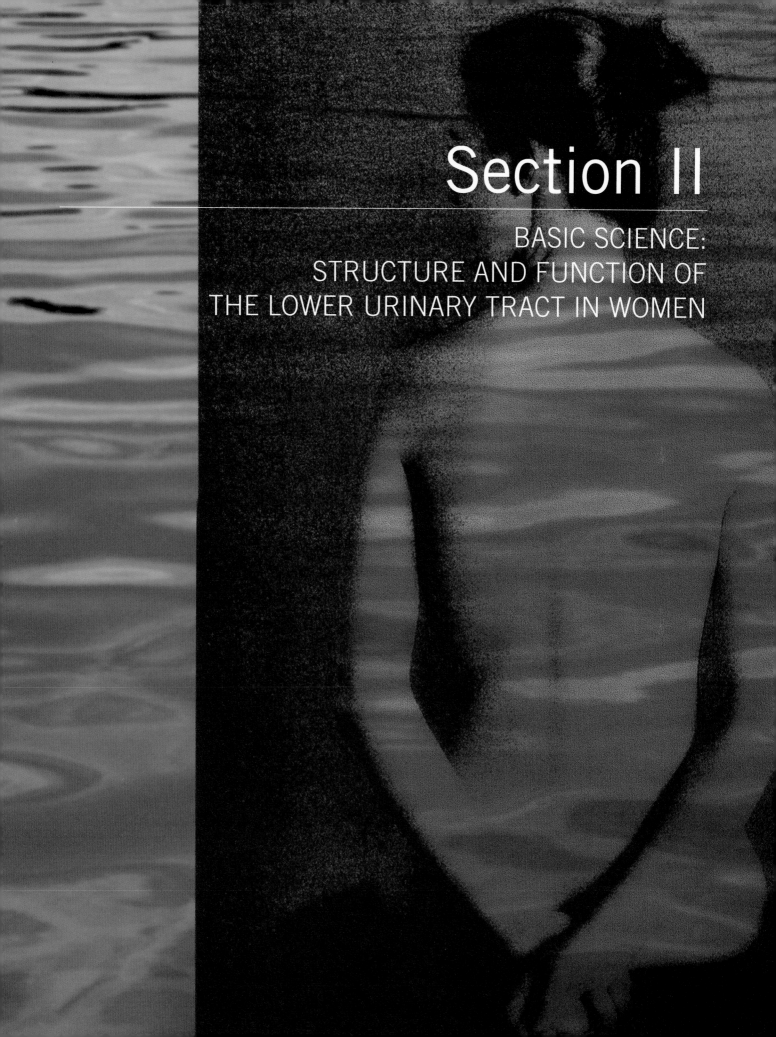

Section II

BASIC SCIENCE:
STRUCTURE AND FUNCTION OF
THE LOWER URINARY TRACT IN WOMEN

8

Classification of voiding dysfunction

D. R. Staskin

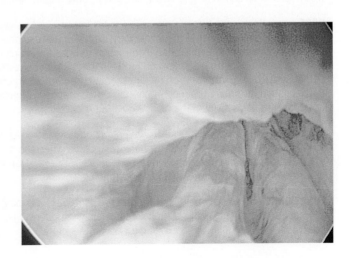

INTRODUCTION

The purpose of a classification system is communication. The value of grouping, correlating and interrelating facts and concepts into an organizational structure can be measured by the ability of the final product both to provide a logical framework for introducing new academic information into the existing knowledge and to act as a useful clinical tool for diagnosing and treating disease. Voiding dysfunction may be classified by clinically derived symptoms and signs and/or by objective findings – by structure (anatomy) and/or function (physiology) or by disease states and/or the lower urinary tract presentation. The decision to adopt a single classification system, or the attempt to devise a system inclusive of all of lower urinary tract function and dysfunction, is certainly ideal but is confounded by the problem of keeping the system simple while describing complex relationships.

CLASSIFICATION: COMBINING SYMPTOMS AND FUNCTION

The classification of voiding dysfunction exclusively by symptoms is descriptive and facile, but has been demonstrated to lack both sensitivity and specificity for the pathophysiology of the underlying condition. The classification of incontinence by symptoms with the definitions of 'genuine' function is presented in Table 8.1.

A functional approach to voiding divides the lower urinary tract into the areas of the 'bladder' and 'bladder outlet' during 'storage' and 'emptying' and classifies the activity as 'overactive', 'normal', or 'underactive'. The International Continence Society (ICS) has adopted this methodology, and it can be combined, for the purpose of illustration, with the 'symptomatic' classification (Table 8.2). The ICS classification defines the pathophysiology of voiding dysfunction based on the descriptive terminology of 'activity': an overactive bladder represents an unwanted increase in detrusor pressure during urinary storage; an underactive bladder describes the failure to generate a sufficient detrusor contraction during bladder emptying; an overactive outlet (obstruction during emptying) and an underactive outlet (decreased resistance during storage) describe abnormalities in bladder-neck and urethral dysfunction. The usefulness of this functional classification is that the pathophysiology may be confirmed with urodynamic findings. A classification of neurogenic voiding dysfunction, based on the level of the neurological lesion, can also be correlated with functional bladder activity and symptoms (Table 8.3).

Table 8.1. *Symptomatic classification with function*

STRESS – symptom – *the involuntary loss of urine with activity (cough, laugh, sneeze, lift, strain).*
Genuine stress incontinence (GSI) – *the involuntary loss of urine resulting from an increase in intra-abdominal pressure which overcomes the resistance of the bladder outlet in the absence of a true bladder contraction.* The decrease in bladder outlet or urethral resistance may result from poor anatomical support of the bladder neck (urethral hypermobility) or a loss of urethral function (intrinsic sphincter deficiency). **Clinical confusion**: the patient describes the symptom of urine loss with activity but the aetiology of leakage is actually an uninhibited bladder contraction; similarly, many patients will describe GSI as a sensation, which is confused with 'urge'; finally, stress and urge incontinence may coexist.

URGE – symptom – *the loss of urine with the feeling of urgency, voiding before the ability to toilet.*
Genuine urge incontinence – *the involuntary loss of urine resulting from an increase in bladder pressure secondary to a true bladder contraction.* An involuntary contraction may be the result of a suprasacral (spinal or intracranial) neurological lesion that results in uncontrolled reflex contractions (detrusor hyperreflexia) or may be idiopathic (detrusor instability). Patients may demonstrate other symptoms of 'motor urgency' (frequency, urgency, nocturia) without urinary loss. 'Sensory urgency' describes the sensation of urinary urgency without a true contraction. **Clinical confusion**: the patient has decreased sensation, and loses urine from motor activity of the bladder without the feeling of 'urge'.

OVERFLOW – *the involuntary loss of urine resulting from urinary retention.* The retention may result from inadequate bladder contractility or outlet obstruction. Urinary loss occurs when the bladder pressure overcomes the urethral resistance owing to bladder contractility, increases in intra-abdominal pressure or urethral relaxation. **Clinical confusion**: the symptoms that are described may be a mixture of stress and urge complaints.

FUNCTIONAL – *the involuntary loss of urine resulting from a deficit in the ability to perform toileting functions secondary to physical or mental limitations.* **Clinical confusion**: the underlying pathophysiology of stress, urge or overflow incontinence may coexist, as well as difficulty in eliciting an accurate history.

Table 8.2 *International Contnence Society classification**

Bladder	Outlet
Overactive (urge)	Overactive (retention)
Normoactive	Normoactive
Underactive (retention)	Underactive (stress incontinence)

*Symptoms in parentheses.

The interrelationship, both anatomically and neurophysiologically, between the bladder outlet and the pelvic floor, necessitates a system which recognizes the individual contributions and the combined effects of the urethral mechanisms and pelvic structures which compose the bladder outlet on bladder activity. Isolating the bladder outlet, urethra or sphincter mechanism from the levator complex does not allow the integration of important relationships between pelvic floor activity and the detrusor. For example, in classifying 'genuine stress incontinence' (GSI), knowledge of the ability to maintain anatomical support through constant and augmented levator tone, and of learning to identify, contract or coordinate the external sphincter–levator complex during increases in intra-abdominal pressure, is critical to the understanding of continence. An understanding of the pathophysiology of 'urge incontinence' requires that the relationship between resting pelvic floor tone and the active contraction of the pelvic floor on the detrusor is considered, although definitive reflex arcs in the human have not yet been identified. Pelvic floor activity may contribute to both the reflex inhibition of the detrusor and the more practical ability to block, mechanically, bladder motor activity until toileting is accomplished. The initiation of voiding requires pelvic floor relaxation. Obstructive voiding symptoms or urinary retention may result from the inhibition of detrusor contractility, through the complete inhibition of detrusor initiation or by 'pseudodyssynergia' of the voluntary sphincter during voiding. A functional approach that incorporates pelvic floor activity should be proposed, and in the future, refined (Table 8.4).

Table 8.3. *Neurogenic voiding dysfunction*

(a) Neurogenic classification*

Bladder/detrusor	Outlet/sphincter
Hyperreflexic (<u>overactive</u> – *urge*)	Uncoordinated (<u>overactive</u> – *obstruction)*
Normoreflexic	Coordinated
Areflexic (<u>underactive</u> – *retention*)	Denervated (<u>underactive</u> – *stress incontinence*)

(b) Expected behaviour of the bladder, internal sphincter and external sphincter based on location of the lesion

	Bladder	Internal sphincter	External sphincter
Infrasacral	Areflexic, underactive	Innervated	Denervated, underactive
Spinal	Hyperreflexic, overactive	Uncoordinated if T6 or above	Dyssynergic, overactive
Suprapontine	Hyperreflexic	Coordinated	Coordinated

*Underlining denotes <u>function</u>; italic type denotes *symptoms.*

Table 8.4. *Expanded functional classification of voiding dysfunction including pelvic floor activity*

I. OUTLET DYSFUNCTION: BLADDER OUTLET AND PELVIC FLOOR

A. UNDERACTIVE OUTLET (DECREASED URETHRAL RESISTANCE)
   Symptomatic: GSI

1. Anatomical support defects (GSI-A) (types I and II GSI):
   Pathophysiology: anatomical motion creates inequities in transmission pressures to bladder and outlet, overcoming urethral resistance, and/or and shear forces create unequal motion of anterior and posterior urethra
   (a) anatomical defects of fascia, muscles, ligaments and bony pelvis
   (b) functional support: muscular contraction – denervation or loss of identification, strength or coordination of levator musculature

2. ISD (GSI-ISD) (type III) (LUCP)
   Pathophysiology: deficiency of urethral closure mechanism secondary to decreased innervation, vascularization or trauma to mucosa, submucosa or smooth or skeletal musculature of urethra
   (a) proximal urethral sphincter: bladder neck and proximal urethra (GSI-ISD-p)
   (b) external sphincter: denervation or loss of voluntary or reflex control (GSI-ISD-d)
   (c) combined total proximal and external sphincter deficiency (GSI-ISD-t)

3. Combined GSI (GSI-A-ISD)
   Pathophysiology: a degree of both anatomical motion and sphincter dysfunction

4. Failure to inhibit the detrusor: decreased pelvic floor activity
   Pathophysiology: failure to contract pelvic floor releases detrusor reflex and decreases ability to inhibit active contraction
   (a) neurological: (infrasacral) denervation (areflexia of pelvic floor)
   (b) behavioural: failure to contract pelvic floor (lack of identification/strength/coordination)
   (c) mechanical: damage to pelvic floor structures with intact innervation

B. OVERACTIVE OUTLET (INCREASED URETHRAL RESISTANCE)
   Symptomatic: overflow incontinence/retention; frequency–urgency

1. Anatomical obstruction (physical blockage)
   Pathophysiology: increased outlet resistance secondary to compression or narrowing
   (a) iatrogenic: surgical (e.g. for urinary incontinence)
   (b) other: congenital, inflammatory, neoplastic, traumatic

2. Functional obstruction (failure of relaxation)
   Pathophysiology: increased outlet resistance secondary to failure of normal relaxation
   (a) neurogenic: detrusor sphincter dyssynergia (smooth or skeletal musculature)
   (b) behavioural: failure to relax pelvic floor musculature or external sphincter

3. Combined anatomical and functional obstruction

4. Inhibition of detrusor activity: increased pelvic floor activity
   Pathophysiology: failure to relax pelvic floor inhibits initiation of detrusor activity and inhibits ability to develop or continue a sustained detrusor contraction
   (a) neurological: (suprasacral) overactivity/hyperreflexia (dyssynergic pelvic floor activity)
   (b) behavioural: failure to relax pelvic floor (learned, acquired, maladaptive, psychogenic)
   (c) situational: 'voluntary' inhibition secondary to environment or pain

II. BLADDER DYSFUNCTION

A. OVERACTIVE BLADDER (INCREASED INTRAVESICAL PRESSURE)
   Symptomatic: urge incontinence (with or without sensation)

1. Uninhibited detrusor contractions: motor urgency
   Pathophysiology: increased intravesical pressure overcomes urethral resistance or causes sensation of urinary urgency
   (a) bladder instability:
       primary = idiopathic, subclinical neurological, or symptomatic phasic detrusor activity;
       secondary = obstruction, reflex urethral relaxation
   (b) detrusor hyperreflexia:
       suprapontine (intracranial) neurological lesion (with or without sphincter control);
       spinal (suprascral) neurological lesion (with or without sphincteric dyssynergia)

cont.

Table 8.4. *Expanded functional classification of voiding dysfunction including pelvic floor activity (cont.)*

2. Decreased compliance
    Pathophysiology: increased intravesical pressure secondary to decreased accommodation
    (a)   fibrosis: radiation, inflammation, immune response
    (b)   neurological: loss/reversal of accommodation reflex – conus medullaris or peripheral

3. Combined detrusor contractions and decreased compliance

4. Pelvic floor underactivity (see I.A.4 above)

B.   UNDERACTIVE BLADDER (DECREASED INTRAVESCIAL PRESSURE)
Symptomatic: overflow incontinence/retention

1. Peripheral denervation or neuropathy
    Pathophysiology: decreased contractility secondary to absent neural input
    (a)   congenital, inflammatory, neoplastic or trauma lesion to peripheral nerves
    (b)   diabetes or other metabolic cause

2. Detrusor myopathy
    Pathophysiology: decreased contractility secondary to smooth muscle damage
    (a)   fibrosis/collagen deposition
    (b)   inflammation/obstruction /overdistension

3. Pharmacological inhibition
    Pathophysiology: decreased contractility secondary to receptor blockade
    (a)   anticholinergics
    (b)   smooth muscle relaxants/spasmolytics/membrane stabilizers

4. Pelvic floor overactivity (see I.B.4 above)

III.   COMBINED OUTLET AND BLADDER DYSFUNCTION (I and II)

IV.   DISORDERS OF SENSATION

A.   DECREASED SENSATION

1. Decreased bladder sensation
    Pathophysiology: denervation, myopathy, behavioural, pharmacological
    (a)   decreased sense of fullness and normal urge response
    (b)   loss of sense of fullness/urge warning only with active contraction
    (c)   loss of sense of fullness/urge incontinence without appreciation of 'urge'
    (d)   urinary retention without appreciation of distension

2. Decreased bladder outlet and pelvic floor sensation
    Pathophysiology: denervation, myopathy, behavioural, pharmacological causing decreased ability to identify/contract/coordinate
    (a)   bladder overactivity (I. A. 4): failure to inhibit?
    (b)   bladder underactivity (II.B.4): failure to initiate?
    (c)   contributory to decreased bladder sensation? (IV.A.1.a–d)
    (d)   sexual dysfunction—anorgasmia

B.   INCREASED SENSATION

1. Increased sensation of the bladder/bladder outlet
    Pathophysiology: neuropathic, inflammatory, mucosal permeability defect, psychogenic
    (a)   frequency–urgency symptoms
    (b)   suprapubic and pelvic pain syndromes

2) Increased sensation of the pelvic floor/bladder outlet
    Pathophysiology: neuromuscular myalgia, neuropathic, inflammatory, psychogenic
    (a)   levator myalgia
    (b)   frequency–urgency and pelvic pain syndromes

3) Combined deficit

GSI, genuine stress incontinence; ISD, intrinsic sphincter deficiency; LUCP, low urethral closure pressure.

A FUNCTIONAL APPROACH: INCORPORATING PELVIC FLOOR ACTIVITY

The underactive outlet

The bladder outlet (sphincteric mechanism) is responsible for 'outlet resistance' during urinary storage. The bladder outlet remains closed at rest. Resistance to leakage is provided by the intrinsic closure pressure along the length of the urethra. The urethra can be divided into two functional areas: these are (a) the 'proximal' sphincteric mechanism – a product of mucosa, submucosa, smooth muscle and non-striated skeletal muscle incorporating the bladder neck and proximal urethra – and (b) the distal mechanism or 'external' sphincteric mechanism located in the middle of the 'anatomical urethra' and intimately related anatomically and physiologically to the levator ani complex. Anatomical support facilitates transmission of intra-abdominal pressure to both areas and is provided by both the anterior vaginal wall and its attachments to the pelvis, and by the constant tone (slow-twitch fibres). Active contraction (fast-twitch fibres) of the levator complex can increase this support, but is usually seen only after pelvic muscle training, and is not a 'normal' reflex.

GSI is the involuntary loss of urine *per urethram* – which occurs when intravesical pressure overcomes the urethral resistance owing to an increase in intra-abdominal pressure in the absence of a true bladder contraction. Urethral closure pressure is maintained by preserving or augmenting anatomical support and by increasing the intrinsic activity of the external sphincter complex. The preservation or enhancement of the anatomical backboard facilitates pressure transmission in the proximal and distal sphincteric mechanism, and preserves the anatomical relationships of the sphincteric components to maintain or increase closure pressure. Proper anatomical support provides an obvious mechanical advantage and, just as importantly, allows efficient action of the individual structures.

Type I or type II GSI is classified as 'poor anatomical support', associated with bladder-neck and urethral motion. However, an understanding of the contribution of pelvic floor activity and dysfunction allows one to appreciate that the aetiology of urinary leakage is probably multifactorial. Classically, an important event in maintaining continence is the preservation of intra-abdominal pressure transmission to the bladder neck and proximal urethra with respect to the bladder during stress manoeuvres. In addition, inhibiting the rotational motion of the urethra prevents a relative differential in the movement of the posterior urethra with relation to the anterior urethra, and the development of a shearing force between the anterior and posterior urethral walls which decreases urethral coaptation and compression. The most fixed point, and the area of maximal pressure transmission during increases in intra-abdominal pressure, is the external sphincter – levator complex in the mid-anatomical urethra. Transmission forces as well as active sphincteric contraction provide urethral resistance during stress manoeuvres.

The combination of defects at many levels of the sphincteric mechanism may combine to decrease urethral resistance. Type III GSI, intrinsic sphincter deficiency or low urethral closure pressure describe a deficiency in any of the intrinsic urethral functions detailed above, through atrophy, denervation, devascularization or scarring. The degree of pudendal nerve denervation during childbirth may contribute to deficiencies in anatomical support both by affecting levator support and by decreasing intrinsic sphincter function.

It is reasonable to assume that the complex aetiology of GSI is a mixture of anatomical support abnormalities and intrinsic sphincter abnormalities. The pathophysiology is related to the relative loss of mechanical (ligamentous) support of functioning (innervated) intrinsic (urethral) and extrinsic musculature (slow- and fast-twitch fibres of the levator complex). Therapy may be directed at correcting the defect, or compensating for the deficiency, by increasing the function of another component that contributes to urethral resistance.

The overactive bladder

The central and peripheral nervous systems mediate bladder (detrusor) control through complex voluntary pathways and reflex arcs. Central afferent control of the bladder smooth musculature is mediated by the reflex and voluntary contractions of the pelvic floor and sphincter musculature, which suppress bladder contractility and prevent urge incontinence. The relaxation of the urethral sphincter during voiding, and dyssynergic activity in spinal cord injury, have been documented. It is not known whether the specific anatomical areas of the urethra or pelvic floor (sphincter urethrae, compressor urethrae, urethrovaginal sphincter, bulbocavernosus, anal sphincter, levator complex) act in unison, individually, or at all in detrusor inhibition in normal subjects.

The underactive bladder and overactive outlet

During the initial phase of bladder emptying, the pelvic floor and external sphincter relax in order to decrease urethral resistance and facilitate low-pressure flow. In addition, this relaxation decreases the reflex inhibition of bladder contractility. Relaxation is followed by a detrusor contraction, which continues until voiding is completed. Failure to empty the bladder may be due to elevated outlet resistance or to impaired contractility of the bladder. The most commonly observed clinical aetiology of elevated outlet resistance is non-neurogenic (obstruction following incontinence surgery). Neurogenic outlet obstruction, commonly seen following injury to the suprasacral spinal cord, is due to a loss of coordination between the bladder and sphincter (detrusor sphincter dyssynergia). When emptying failure is secondary to bladder dysfunction, it may be a result of either detrusor smooth muscle pathology or insufficient neural stimulation of the detrusor. Insufficient neural stimulation may occur at the neuromuscular level (pharmacological), with nerve impairment (neuropathy), or with alterations in central control of micturition (conus medullaris, spinal column or brain). The impairment of detrusor contractility by the absence of pelvic floor relaxation is evident in spinal cord disease (failure to empty following adequate sphincterotomy in the spinal cord patient due to incomplete detrusor contractions) and parkinsonism (failure to empty secondary to pelvic floor bradykinesia).

Sensory disorders

Traditional classification systems have focused on motor rather than sensory activity. Disorders of bladder and bladder outlet sensation may result from central or peripheral denervation, from psychological causes, or from pharmacological agents such as pain medications. The role of decreased sensation in the function of the pelvic floor and the interaction between the pelvic floor and bladder with relation to the sensory pathway on the micturition reflexes await further investigation. The pudendal nerve is responsible for the innervation of pelvic floor structures as well as of the genital skin, urethral mucosa and anal canal. Proprioceptive information of the periurethral musculature and sensory innervation of the levator ani muscles are also mediated by the pudendal branches.

Increased sensation or pain attributed to the bladder is a major clinical challenge. The symptoms of urinary frequency, urgency and suprapubic pressure often result in diagnostic evaluations and therapy for bladder disorders, even in the absence of definitive findings of mucosal or smooth muscle abnormality. Pain that may originate from fascial, muscular or neurological aetiologies within the pelvic floor should be included in the differential diagnosis of the patient with urethral or bladder syndromes.

CONCLUSIONS

The effect of the pelvic floor–levator complex dysfunction on 'bladder symptoms' and normal voiding behaviour deserve increased attention. Currently, otherwise effective therapy may be ineffective when the lower urinary tract, in exclusion of the pelvic floor, is considered as the sole source of the problem.

9

Basic embryology

R. J. Connell, A. Cutner

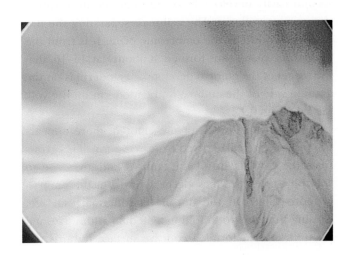

INTRODUCTION

From a single cell at conception, the embryonic phase consists of the first 8 weeks of life when all the tissues of the body differentiate and the structures form. The second phase of development is when these structures grow and mature; this is known as the fetal phase. By the end of week 8, the embryo has an identifiable human shape.[1,2]

This chapter briefly describes the initial differentiation of the tissue planes and then describes further development of the female lower urinary tract.

EARLY EMBRYONIC DEVELOPMENT

The fertilized ovum undergoes a series of mitotic divisions, known as cleavage: 40–50 hours after fertilization, the four-cell stage is reached. The dividing ball of cells is known as the morula, because of its resemblance to a mulberry (fruit of the genus *Morus*). Towards the end of the first week the morula contains 16 cells and enters the uterine cavity. Soon after this the morula becomes so large that, in order to maintain adequate nutrient supply, a cavity develops – the extra-embryonic coelom.[2,3] This cavitation neatly facilitates the formation of (a) the inner cell mass at one end of the morula and (b) the surrounding outer cell mass. The former develops into the tissues of the embryo and the latter into the tissues of the trophoblast. With further accumulation of fluid and growth, the morula becomes known as the blastocyst.

The single-layered endoderm forms on the surface of the inner cell mass, facing the blastocyst cavity; the remaining cells form the ectoderm. Cavitation within the ectodermal cell layer results in the amniotic cavity. A second cavity develops below the endoderm, forming the primary yolk sac. The cell mass separating the two cavities is known as the embryonic plate. It is from the embryonic plate, thus formed at about day 14–16, that the tissues of the embryo develop;[2,4,5] ectoderm is on the amnion side of the embryo and endoderm on the yolk sac side (Fig. 9.1).

With further growth of the embryo, there appears the primitive streak derived from ectoderm. This grows from the caudal end of the embryo and gives rise to the third layer, the mesoderm. Growth of the embryo is more rapid on the dorsal (endodermal) surface, causing the embryo to fold in a median and horizontal plane; hence, it forms a concave surface towards the

yolk sac. The yolk sac is invaginated by further lateral growth of the mesoderm, which meets medially (Fig. 9.2). The mesoderm itself then cavitates to form the coelomic cavity:[2,5] at the caudal end, fusion of the ectodermal and endodermal layers forms the cloacal membrane (Fig. 9.3); at the cephalic end of the embryo, the same fusion forms the buccopharyngeal membrane.[4]

From the cephalic end of the primitive streak, a further ectodermal development is the neural plate; with further growth, this develops into the neural groove. Neural folds develop on the lateral walls of the groove and, with further growth, the folds meet in the midline, forming the neural tube. The neural tube gives rise to

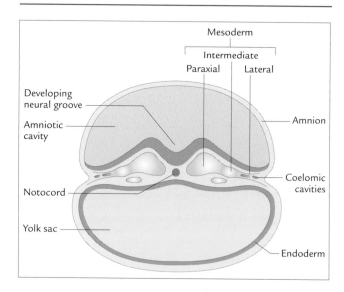

Figure 9.1. *Cross-section of a 17-day-old embryo.*

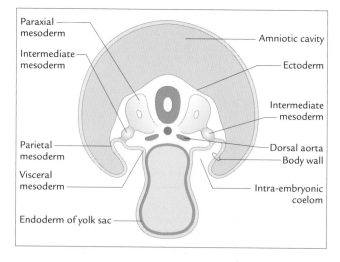

Figure 9.2. *Transverse section of a 25-day-old embryo.*

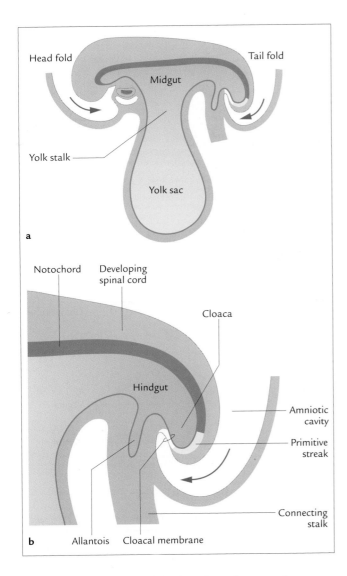

Figure 9.3. *Formation of the cloacal membrane at the caudal end of a 4-week-old embryo: (a) lateral view illustrating the folding of the embryo; (b) detail of the caudal end of the embryo showing the formation of the cloacal membrane, and the position of other structures.*

the central nervous system. Ectoderm also forms the mucous membrane of the lower anal canal and urogenital tract.[4,5]

Mesoderm differentiates to form blocks of cells (somites) in 43 pairs. These form the future bones, cartilage and ligaments; skeletal muscle; dermis and subcutaneous tissues of the skin; the blood vessels; heart and blood cells; and the lymph vessels and tissue.[5,6]

DEVELOPMENT OF THE FEMALE URINARY SYSTEM

Early bladder development

The endoderm folds with the growth of the embryo in such a way that the yolk sac becomes invaginated. The invaginated yolk sac forms the gut; it communicates with the extra-embryonic yolk sac by way of the vitellointestinal duct, which later forms part of the umbilical cord. Continued folding results in the approximation of the cloacal membrane and the proctodeum. The cloacal membrane breaks down to form the anal and genital orifices. At the head end, the buccopharyngeal membrane and the foregut meet in a similar way, the membrane breaking down to form the mouth.[6,7]

A diverticulum (termed the allantois) develops from the hindgut; it appears on about day 16.[6] At the junction of the two is the future site of development of the bladder, which later becomes a fibrous cord – the urachus (the median umbilical ligament in adults). That part of the hindgut connected to the allantois is the cloaca. By 6 weeks a wedge of mesenchymal tissue – the urorectal septum – divides the cloaca; this division results in the formation of an anterior part (the primitive bladder) and a posterior part (the anorectal canal) (Fig. 9.4).[8–10]

The endoderm forms the future epithelial lining of the entire alimentary tract and the cells of the bladder (excluding the trigone), parts of the urethra and the lining of the vagina.

The upper urinary tract

The upper urinary tract comprises the kidneys and ureters.

Kidneys and ureters

Three sets of kidneys develop in humans. These structures are analogous to the excretory units of primitive fish and amphibians, and higher animals.[10]

Pronephros

At around the start of week 4, in the cervical region, the mesoderm forms segmental tubular cell masses, known as the nephrotomes,[11] which are certainly non-functional in humans.[12] By the end of that week this

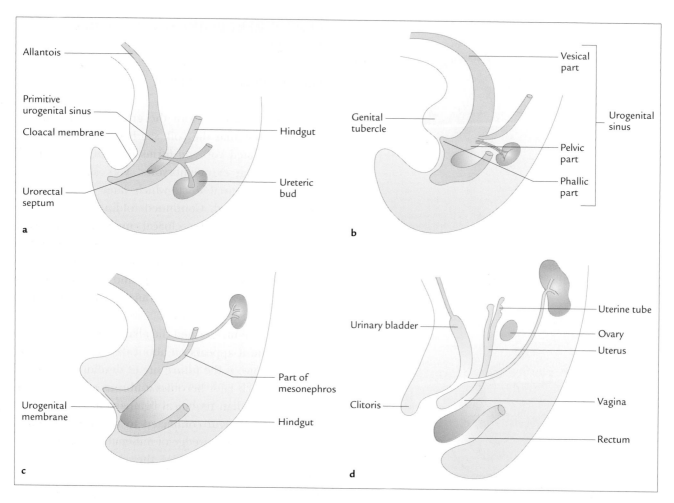

Figure 9.4. *Longitudinal section of a fetus showing division of the cloaca at (a) 5 weeks, (b) 8 weeks, (c) 10 weeks and (d) 12 weeks.*

pronephros has degenerated but most of the pronephric ducts are utilized by the mesonephros.

Mesonephros

With regression of the pronephros, mesoderm in the region of the 8th somite develops into tubules.[13] It differentiates into the mesonephric ducts and the nephron units,[13] which soon develop communications and lengthen. Laterally the tubules become the collecting (mesonephric) duct. As the duct lengthens, more nephron units develop. The mesonephric duct extends caudally to the anterior part of the cloaca (the primitive bladder) on each side.[8–10,13] The mesonephric ducts divide the primitive bladder into two parts – the upper vesicourethral canal and the lower urogenital sinus. The upper part of the vesicourethral canal dilates, forming the bladder; the caudal part forms the proximal urethra. The urogenital sinus forms the distal urethra.

Metanephros

The metanephros appears in week 5;[13] it develops from the mesonephric mesoderm and gives rise to the permanent kidney. It becomes functional by week 6. Outgrowths of the mesonephric ducts near the insertion into the cloaca give rise to the ureteric buds;[12–14] these grow cranially into the mesoderm of the intermediate cell mass, which forms the metanephrogenic cap. The inferior part of the ureteric bud dilates to form the ureter; the superior part dilates to form the renal pelvis.[13]

The metanephric kidney starts its existence as a caudal structure. With growth of the body it eventually attains a more cranial position in the abdomen. This ascent is associated with a changing blood supply (Fig. 9.5).[13]

Glomerular filtration starts at about week 9, increasing markedly after birth.[10,14,15]

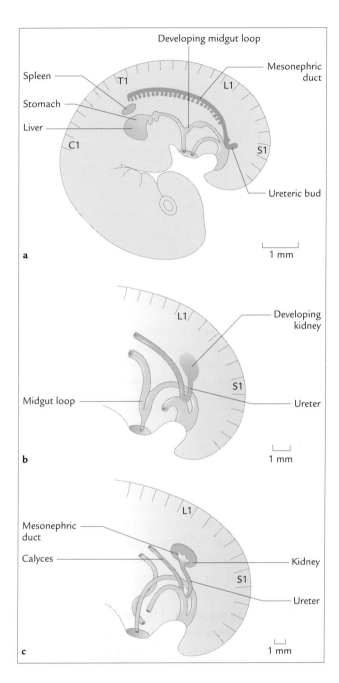

a

Spleen

Stomach

Liver

C1

T1

Developing midgut loop

L1

Mesonephric duct

S1

Ureteric bud

1 mm

b

Midgut loop

L1

Developing kidney

S1

Ureter

1 mm

c

Mesonephric duct

Calyces

L1

Kidney

S1

Ureter

1 mm

Figure 9.5. *Relative shift of position of the kidneys with time: (a) 5 weeks, (b) 6 weeks and (c) 7 weeks after fertilization.*

The lower urinary tract

The lower urinary tract consists of the bladder and urethra.

Bladder and urethra

Partitioning of the cloaca by the urorectal septum by week 8 results in the anorectal canal and the urogenital sinus.[8–12,16] The urogenital sinus is divided into three parts – the upper, the pelvic and the phallic. The large upper part forms the bladder, and is continuous with the allantois, connecting the apex of the bladder to the umbilicus.[17] The allantois forms the urachus, which is the median umbilical ligament in the adult. The next part of the urogenital sinus is the narrow pelvic part forming the urethra; the last part is the phallic part.

The caudal ends of the mesonephric ducts enter the lower part of the immature bladder separately. The bladder gradually grows and absorbs the caudal part of the mesonephric duct. With continued growth of the bladder, the ducts eventually open through the lateral angles of the bladder. More caudal to the bladder, the mesonephric ducts come to lie progressively closer together, and eventually fuse to form the urethra (Fig. 9.6). The part of the bladder bounded by, and derived from, the mesonephric ducts becomes the future trigone, which can be defined by week 6 (Fig. 9.6). The lower urinary system is made up of an epithelial lining, connective tissue, smooth muscle and striated muscle.

Epithelium

The cells of the urinary tract epithelium are of a common origin, yet differentiate at an early stage to suit their future function.[18,19]

The upper part of the bladder is derived from the yolk sac. The mucosa lining is derived from the endodermal lining of the vesicourethral canal; this epithelial layer (urothelium) is impermeable to water. The trigone and upper urethra are derived from the mesonephric ducts and are lined by cells of mesodermal origin; however, cells of endodermal origin later replace the trigonal surface.[9,10]

Connective tissue

The connective tissue of the bladder and urethra is derived from mesodermally derived mesenchyme.[12]

The connective tissue content of the bladder increases and matures with growth of the fetus;[20,21] this, in turn, increases the compliance of the fetal bladder, as has been demonstrated in the calf model (Fig. 9.7).[22,23] Compliance is maximal in the neonate and decreases with age.[23–26] It is the amount of type III collagen that correlates well with bladder elasticity, and it has been

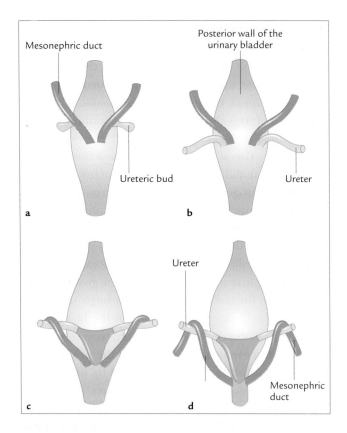

Figure 9.6. *Dorsal views of the developing bladder showing the relationship of the ureters and mesonephric ducts. Note the trigone formed by incorporation of the mesonephric ducts.*

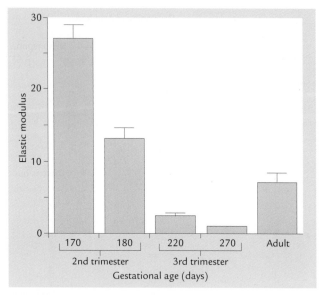

Figure 9.7. *Elastic (inverse of compliance) changes with gestational age in the fetal bovine bladder. Samples were taken across the range of gestations. A decrease in elastic modulus (an increase in compliance) coincides with the initial phase of urine production by the fetus.*

shown that the ratio of type III to type I collagen decreases with age (Fig. 9.8).[21,24,26] The proportion of collagen in the bladder decreases considerably during development: early fetuses have a 1:1 ratio of collagen to muscle, whereas at birth this ratio falls to 0.65 (Fig. 9.9).[24]

Elastin first appears in the bladder at around week 10.[27] Initially, the elastin fibres are fine and short but, with increasing gestation, the size, number and thickness increase. The total percentage of elastin in the bladder (throughout gestation) is of the order of 1–2%.[28]

Smooth muscle

Smooth muscle cells can be identified in the human bladder from as early as week 7.[29] The muscular development of the lower urinary tract has been described.[8,30–35] The smooth muscle of the bladder and urethra is formed from mesodermally derived mesenchyme;[12] although initially, it is undifferentiated and poorly organized, with time the organization increases in complexity.

The urothelium lining the bladder causes initiation and differentiation of the smooth muscle by way of cell-to-cell interactions between the bladder mesenchyme and the urothelium.[31] This process, which is similar to that of smooth muscle development in other parts of the body, is vital for the normal development of the bladder.[36]

Some authors suggest that the smooth muscle of the detrusor and urethra are of the same origin and form a continuous structure surrounding the bladder which can be thought of as a single tube.[8,33] However Dröes,[34] on examination of five male and six female fetuses, showed that the smooth muscle develops as three distinct structures – the detrusor, the trigonal system and the urethral smooth muscle.

In the fetus, the detrusor muscle surrounds the entire bladder and consists of three layers. It is fixed to surrounding structures by longitudinal bundles of fibres.

The trigonal muscle consists of an inner longitudinal layer and an outer circular layer and is continuous with the urethral musculature. Its fibres pass between bundles of the detrusor muscle; although they appear

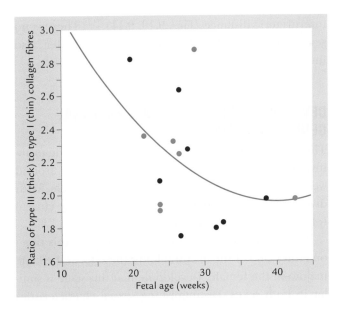

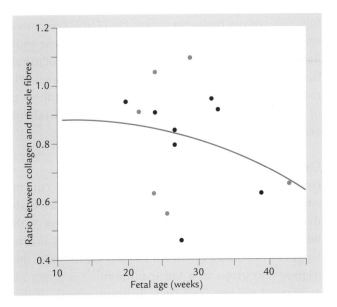

Figure 9.8. *Ratio of type III collagen (thick) to type I collagen (thin) as a function of age in the male (●) and female (●) human fetal bladder.*

Figure 9.9. *Ratio of collagen to muscle as a function of age in the male (●) and female (●) human fetal bladder.*

to intertwine, they are, in fact, distinct. The trigone musculature also completely encircles the proximal part of the urethra.

The third system is the smooth muscle of the urethra. It, too, consists of an outer circular and an inner longitudinal layer, completely surrounding the mid-part of the urethra in a circular fashion early in development; at term it surrounds the urethra in a horse shoe manner.

Striated muscle

The external urinary sphincter is composed of striated muscle. It is intrinsic to the urethral wall, acting like a sleeve closely applied to and surrounding the smooth muscle in the mid-portion of the urethra in the female (Fig. 9.4).[37] It is inserted into the trigonal region cranially (extending to the lower edge of the detrusor muscle) and into the lateral vaginal wall and perineal body caudally. The adult structures of the para-urethral and periurethral parts of the sphincter do not develop until the first or second year of life. The sphincter is horseshoe shaped, thickest anteriorly, surrounding the proximal part of the urethra and inserting into the trigonal region (Fig. 9.5). In the female, the striated muscle continues to develop, although the urethral smooth muscle largely disappears.

Bladder receptors

Little work has been done on the autonomic responses of the fetal bladder;[19,26,38] however, bladder receptors and the response of the bladder musculature to adrenergic and muscarinic stimulation have been studied in the animal model.[22,39–41] The response of the upper bladder segment to field stimulation initially is similar in manner to that of the lower segment; however, with increased length of gestation the upper segment response is greater.[22] Other data from animal models show that the lower segment exhibits an increasing degree of nitric oxide-induced relaxation than the upper segment;[22,42,43] this has been confirmed by studies in male fetuses.[44]

Receptors of the detrusor and urethral sphincter

A study[45] of autonomic receptors in human material has shown that cholinergic receptors are present in the detrusor and urethral sphincter as early as week 16. Although the density of receptors in the detrusor increases with gestation, the density in the urethral sphincter decreases. Alpha-adrenoceptors develop after 6 months, but only in the urethral sphincter; β-adrenoceptors are present only in the detrusor.

Bladder function

Urine formation starts at around week 10 of gestation.[46] Early in gestation, the bladder serves no storage function; with increasing gestation, the bladder increases its capacity and there is a decreasing pressure rise with increasing volume.[23] Indeed, the hourly amount of urine formed by the kidneys is approximately 5 ml at week 20, rising to 56 ml at term. The cycle of filling and emptying of the fetal bladder is maintained at a steady rate (about every 25 minutes) throughout gestation.[46]

Growth of the urinary tract

Growth of the lower urinary tract in the fetus occurs in a linear fashion.[30,47] The female urethra is shorter than that of the male, a difference that increases with increasing gestation. There are no differences in the length of the bladder between the sexes. Internally, the trigone also grows in a linear fashion;[30,47] it forms an equilateral triangle, and there is linear growth of the

interureteric distance (Figs. 9.10, 9.11).[30,47] There is no sex difference. The thickness of the bladder also increases in a linear manner until birth (Fig. 9.12).[20]

DEVELOPMENT OF THE FEMALE EXTERNAL GENITAL SYSTEM

The cloacal folds are derived from the cells of the primitive streak either side of the cloacal membrane around week 3,[16] and unite to form the genital tubercle. With division of the cloacal membrane at week 6, the cloacal folds divide into the urethral and anal folds.

The genital swellings become apparent at this time, on either side of the urethral folds; these form the labia majora in the female. Development at this stage is similar in both sexes. Distinguishing sexual characteristics

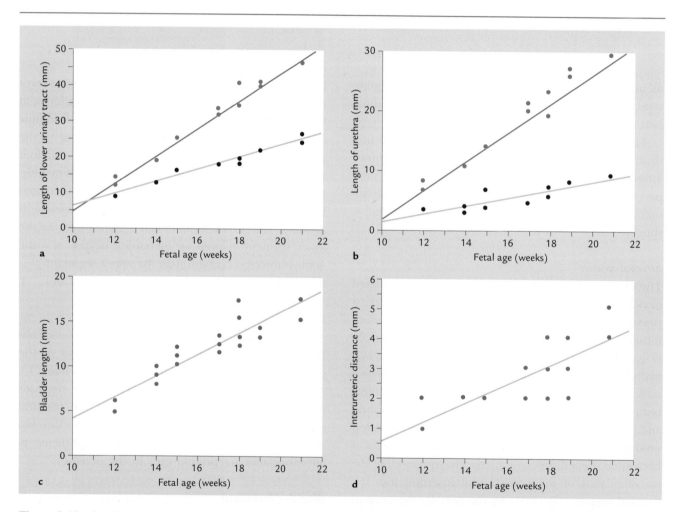

Figure 9.10. *Graphical representation of growth of the human male (•) and female (•) fetal lower urinary tract (a) lower urinary tract; (b) urethra; (c) bladder; (d) interureteric distance.*

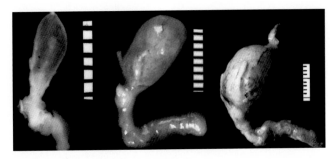

Figure 9.11. *Growth of the human fetal lower urinary tract: (a) 12-week male bladder; (b) 15-week male bladder; (c) 19-week male bladder. (Reprinted from ref. 47 by permission of Wiley-Liss Inc., a division of John Wiley & Sons, Inc.)*

begin to appear during week 9, and the external genitalia are fully differentiated by week 12.[10]

The genital tubercle elongates to form the clitoris, with the expanded glans at the distal end.[16] The urethral folds remain unfused in the female and form the labia minora.[10] The lower part of the urogenital sinus – the urogenital groove – forms the vestibule. It is thought that these developments are under the control of oestrogen. The genital tubercle in the female at this stage is larger than that in the male; however, its growth and development stop much earlier than in the male.

SUMMARY

The lower urinary tract is derived from several cell lines. The upper part of the bladder is derived from endoderm, whereas the trigone and upper urethra originate from the mesoderm of the mesonephric ducts. The bladder can be identified in the fetus from as early as week 6 of gestation, with urine production commencing at about week 10. Growth of the fetal lower urinary tract occurs in a linear manner. Although it is functional at birth, further differentiation and development continue until early adolescence.

REFERENCES

1. Moore KL, Persaud TVN. Beginning of human development. *The Developing Human. Clinically Orientated Embryology*, 5th edn. Philadelphia: Saunders, 1993; 14–39

2. Snell RS. Fertilization, cleavage, blastocyst formation, and implantation. *Clinical Embryology for Medical Students*, 3rd edn. Boston: Little, Brown and Co., 1983; 49–69

3. Moore KL, Persaud TVN. Formation of the bilaminar embryonic disc. *The Developing Human. Clinically Orientated Embryology*, 5th edn. Philadelphia: Saunders, 1993; 40–52

4. Moore KL, Persaud TVN. Formation of the embryo. *The Developing Human. Clinically Orientated Embryology*, 5th edn. Philadelphia: Saunders, 1993; 53–69

5. Sadler TW. Embryonic period. *Langham's Medical Embryology*, 7th edn. Philadelphia: Williams and Wilkins, 1995; 67–89

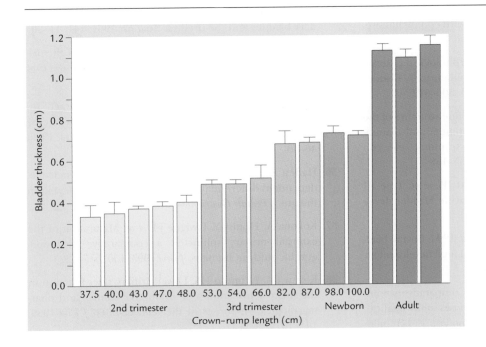

Figure 9.12. *Fetal and adult bovine bladder-wall thickness illustrating increase in bladder-wall size with increasing age.*

6. Moore KL, Persaud TVN. Development of tissues, organs and body form. *The Developing Human. Clinically Orientated Embryology*, 5th edn. Philadelphia: Saunders, 1993; 70–92

7. Snell RS. Urinary system. *Clinical Embryology for Medical Students*, 3rd edn. Boston: Little, Brown and Co., 1983; 197–214

8. Tanagho EA, Smith DR. Mechanism of urinary continence. 1. Embryological, anatomical and pathological considerations. *J Urol* 1968; 100: 640–646

9. Hamilton WJ, Mossman HW. The urogenital system. *Human Embryology*. Cambridge: Cambridge University Press, 1972; 377–437

10. Moore KL, Pesaud TVN. Urogenital system. *The Developing Human. Clinically Orientated Embryology*, 5th edn. Philadelphia: Saunders, 1993; 265–303

11. Sadler TW. Urogenital system. *Langham's Medical Embryology*, 7th edn. Philadelphia: Williams and Wilkins, 1995; 272–311

12. Vaughan ED, Middleton GW. Pertinent genitourinary embryology. *Urology* 1975; 6: 139–149

13. McLachlan J. The urinary system. *Medical Embryology*. Wokingham: Addison-Wesley, 1994; 323–338

14. Coplen DE. Prenatal intervention for hydronephrosis. *J Urol* 1997; 157: 2270–2277

15. Arant BS, Jr. Postnatal development of renal function during the first year of life. *Pediatr Nephrol* 1987; 1: 308–312

16. Mesrobian H-GJ, Sessions RP, Lloyd RA, Sulik KK. Cloacal and urogenital abnormalities induced by etretinate in mice. *J Urol* 1994; 152: 675–678

17. Moore KL. *Clinically Oriented Anatomy*, 3rd edn. Baltimore, Williams and Wilkins, 1992

18. Ayres PH, Shinohara Y, Frith CH. Morphological observations of the epithelium of the developing urinary bladder of the mouse and rat. *J Urol* 1985; 133: 506–512

19. Newman J, Antonakopoulos GN. The fine structure of the human fetal urinary bladder. Development and maturation: a light, transmission and scanning electron microscopy study. *J Anat* 1989; 166: 135–138

20. Baskin LS, Constantinescu S, Duckett JW *et al.* Type III collagen decreases in normal fetal bovine bladder development. *J Urol* 1994; 152: 688–691

21. Baskin L, Meaney D, Landsman A *et al.* 1994. Bovine bladder compliance increases with normal fetal development. *J Urol* 1994; 152: 692–695

22. Lee JG, Coplen D, Macarak E *et al.* Comparative studies on the ontogeny and autonomic responses of the fetal calf bladder at different stages of development: involvement

of nitric oxide on field stimulated relaxation. *J Urol* 1994; 151: 1096–1101

23. Coplen DE, Macarak EJ, Levin RM. Developmental changes in normal fetal bovine whole bladder physiology. *J Urol* 1994; 151: 1391–1395

24. Kim KM, Kogan BA, Massad CA, Huang YC. Collagen and elastin in the obstructed fetal bladder. *J Urol* 1991; 146: 528–531

25. Susset JG, Servot-Viguier D, Lamy F *et al.* Collagen in 155 human bladders. *Invest Urol* 1978; 53: 134–140

26. Kim KM, Kogan BA, Massad CA, Huang YC. Collagen and elastin in the normal fetal bladder. *J Urol* 1991; 146: 524–527

27. Escala JM, Keating MA, Boyd G *et al.* Development of elastin fibres in the upper urinary tract. *J Urol* 1989; 141: 969

28. Cortivo R, Pagano F, Passerini G *et al.* Elastin and collagen in the normal and obstructed urinary bladder. *Br J Urol* 1981; 53: 134–138

29. Matsuno T, Tokunaka S, Koyanagi T. Muscular development in the urinary tract. *J Urol* 1984; 132: 148–152

30. Wesson MB. Anatomical, embryological and physiological studies of the trigone and neck of bladder. *J Urol* 1920; 4: 279–315

31. Baskin LS, Hayward SW, Young P, Cunha GR. Role of mesenchymal–epithelial interactions in normal bladder development. *J Urol* 1996; 156: 1820–1827

32. Lapides J. Structure and function of the internal vesical sphincter. *J Urol* 1958; 80: 341–353

33. Woodbourne RT. The sphincter mechanism of the urinary bladder and the urethra. *Anat Rec* 1961; 141: 11–20

34. Dröes JTPM. Observations on the musculature of the urinary bladder and the urethra in the human fetus. *Br J Urol* 1974; 46: 179–185

35. Tanagho EA. Anatomy of the lower urinary tract. In: PC Walsh, RF Gittes, AD Perlmutter, TA Stamey (eds) *Campbell's Urology*, 5th edn. Philadelphia: Saunders, 1986; 46–60

36. Haffen K, Kedinger M, Simon-Assmann P. Mesenchyme-dependent differentiation of epithelial progenitor cells in the gut. *J Pediatr Gastroenterol Nutr* 1987; 6: 14–17

37. Kokoua A, Homsy Y, Lavigne J-F *et al.* Maturation of the external urinary sphincter: a comparative histotopographic study in humans. *J Urol* 1993; 150: 617–622

38. Kogan BA, Iwamoto HS. Lower urinary tract function in the sheep fetus: studies of autonomic control and pharmacological responses of the fetal bladder. *J Urol* 1989; 141: 1019–1024

39. Lee JG, Wein AJ, Levin RM. Distribution and function of the adrenergic and cholinergic receptors in the fetal calf bladder during mid-gestational age. *Neurourol Urodyn* 1993; 12: 599–602

40. Levin RM, Keating MA, Potter L, Wein AJ Ontogeny of purinergic function in the rabbit bladder. *Neurourol Urodyn* 1989; 8: 386–387

41. Saeki H, Okazaki T, Kadowaki H *et al.* The development of the autonomic innervation and contractile response of the rat urinary bladder. *Neurourol Urodyn* 1989; 8: 338–341

42. Persson K, Andersson KE. Nitric oxide and relaxation of the pig lower urinary tract. *Br J Pharmacol* 1992; 106: 416–418

43. Persson K, Igawa Y, Mattiasson A, Andersson KE. Effects of inhibition of the L-arginine/nitric oxide pathway in the rat lower urinary tract in vivo and in vitro. *Br J Pharmacol* 1992; 107: 178–181

44. Dixon JS, Jen PYP. Development of nerves containing nitric oxide synthase in the human male urogenital organs. *Br J Urol* 1995; 76: 719–725

45. Mitolo-Chieppa D, Schonauer S, Grasso G *et al.* Ontogenesis of autonomic receptors in detrusor muscle and bladder sphincter of human fetus. *Urolology* 1983; 21: 599–603

46. Rabinowitz R, Peters MT, Vyas S *et al.* Measurement of fetal urine production in normal pregnancy by real-time ultrasonography. *Am J Obstet Gynecol* 1989; 161: 1264

47. Cutner A, Moscoso G, Cardozo LD *et al.* Growth of the normal human lower urinary tract from 12 to 21 weeks gestation. *Anat Rec* 1992; 234: 568–574

10

Female urethral embryology with clinical applications

S. A. Zderic

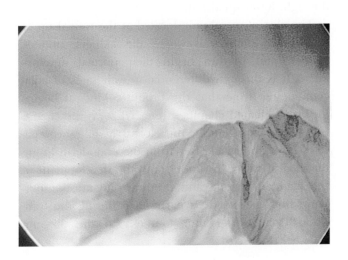

INTRODUCTION

The two major goals of this chapter are (1) to review the steps in the normal fetal development of the female urethra, and (2) to demonstrate several clinical applications of this material in the assessment of the incontinent female patient. This review might be more appropriately entitled 'The normal development of the female perineum', for to isolate normal female fetal urethral embryology from the genesis of the bladder, trigone, vagina and rectum would be impossible.

EARLY EMBRYOGENESIS

Following conception, the normal embryo undergoes a series of divisions leading to implantation of the zygote within the endometrial wall of the uterine cavity. With further growth, unknown molecular mechanisms dictate differentiation of these cells into the various germ layers, and by 22 days, the embryo is a disc-shaped structure containing ectoderm, and mesoderm with a large adjoining yolk sac (Fig. 10.1a). With normal embryogenesis at 28 days (3 mm crown–rump length), this disc is folded, and the entire intestinal tract formation begins with tubularization of the yolk sac (Fig. 10.1b).[1] Over the course of the ensuing 6 weeks, this tube differentiates into the stomach, small intestine and large intestine. The developing intestine is extruded into the umbilical cord for a while, and then returns to the intestinal cavity while undergoing a 245-degree anticlockwise rotation about the superior mesenteric artery. This process, which is complete by week 10 of embryonic development, explains why the caecum is located in the right lower quadrant.

The cloacal membrane located at the caudal tip of the human embryo is where the kidneys, ureters, bladder and urethra begin their normal development. It is through differential growth rates of adjacent mesenchyme that the primitive hindgut begins to form a dilated chamber, referred to as the cloaca. In early embryogenesis, the cloacal membrane separates the ectodermal layer from the endoderm lining the cloacal cavity. To understand the development of the bladder, trigone and urethra, one must understand how the cloaca is partitioned during the transition from the 4 mm (4-week) to the 36 mm (10-week) embryo.

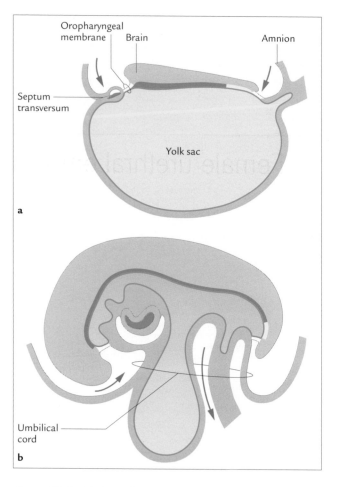

Figure 10.1. *(a) Sagittal section of the discoid 22-day-old embryo, showing the relationship of the yolk sac to the neural and mesenchymal layers prior to the folding. The arrows show the direction of the subsequent folding that takes place by day 28. The oropharyngeal membrane and cloacal membranes are already developing at the cranial and caudal ends of the neural tube. (b) Sagittal section of the embryo at day 28, showing the residual yolk sac contained within the developing umbilical cord. The second smaller extension of the yolk sac into the cord (which forms the basis of the allantois) can be seen. The cloacal membrane is just to the right of the umbilical cord.*

PARTITIONING OF THE CLOACA

At the 4 mm stage of development the dilated distal hindgut forms the internal cloaca, lined with endoderm derived from the yolk sac. It is separated from the external cloaca (which is composed of ectoderm) by the cloacal membrane.[2] During this stage of embryogenesis, one fold of yolk sac (the allantois) extends anteriorly from the cloaca towards the umbilicus (Fig. 10.2a), which forms the embryological basis of the urachus. This anterior extension of the internal cloaca (the allantois) will also contribute to parts of the future bladder and urethra. However, in order for these structures to form, the internal cloaca must be partitioned. The internal cloaca is partitioned by the caudal migration of the urorectal septum, which begins at the 4-week stage and is complete by the 6-week stage. The exact mechanism by which this takes place is debated: Torneaux claimed that the septum is a crescent-shaped body that descends caudally until it meets the cloacal membrane; in contrast, the opinion of Rathke was that the urorectal septum formed from

the medial migration of (and fusion in the midline of) two mesodermal folds. Irrespective of which mechanism predominates, embryologists agree that there is a progressive craniocaudal progression of the urorectal septum such that, by 6 weeks of development, the internal cloaca has been fully partitioned into an anterior urogenital sinus and a posterior rectum. Upon completion of this partitioning, the cloacal membrane ruptures, allowing communication between the internal and external cloaca (Fig. 10.2b).

By 6 weeks, the distal-most extension of the urorectal septum has met the cloacal membrane, which ruptures – thus completing the division of the internal cloaca. At this point, the external cloaca must undergo partitioning for the normal perineum to develop. The external cloaca is partitioned by the development of the uroanal septum, which has two components – deep and superficial. The deep component of the uroanal septum is a small distal extension of the urorectal septum. The superficial component is composed of inward migration of the genital folds which then fuse in the midline, ultimately to create the perineal body and raphe (Fig. 10.2c, d). It is at this point in embryogenesis that major differences begin to take place in external sexual differentiation – with males developing a longer perineal body, an anterior deflection of the proximal urethra, and fusion of the genital folds to form the scrotum. Internally, within the male fetus, the müllerian ducts involute under the influence of müllerian inhibitory substance and the wolffian ducts differentiate into the vasa deferentia under the influence of testosterone. This same time point in embryogenesis also marks the onset of müllerian differentiation in the female.

MÜLLERIAN DIFFERENTIATION

Differentiation of the müllerian duct system begins by week 6.[3] These ducts form the basis of the right and left fallopian tubes. Fusion of these two ducts in the midline produces the uterus, cervix and proximal two-thirds of the vagina. The müllerian ducts begin as solid cords which undergo canalization during their differentiation. Apoptosis is the probable molecular mechanism for the formation of these tubular structures. The distal-most müllerian ducts unite to form the proximal two-thirds of the vagina; these fuse with, and penetrate, the posterior aspect of the urethra at week 7 to form

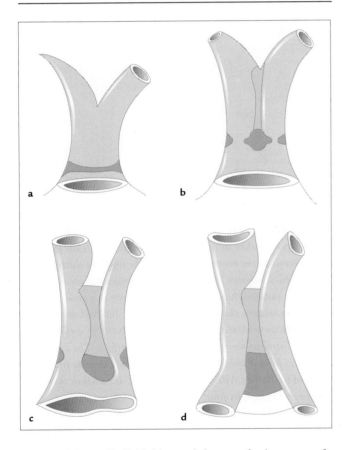

Figure 10.2. *(a) Undivided internal cloaca at the 4 mm stage of development. The developing urorectal septum separates the allantois from the hindgut. The allantoic extension to the left leads to the umbilical cord and the future navel; this extension forms the basis of the urachal remnant. (b) Division of the internal cloaca is completed in this sequence, and the cloacal membrane has now ruptured, allowing for communication between the internal and external cloacal chambers. (c) With further growth, the external cloaca is partitioned by an extension of the urorectal septum and an ingrowth of the genital folds. (d) Fusion of the genital folds in the midline completes the separation of the urethra anteriorly from the rectum posteriorly.*

the urogenital sinus (Fig. 10.3). The müllerian ducts are guided to the posterior urethra by the right and left wolffian ducts.

It is extremely important to appreciate the interaction between the müllerian and wolffian systems leading to formation of the urogenital sinus. The wolffian ducts serve to guide the proximal two-thirds of the vagina into the posterior urethra; the ducts are then carried towards the perineum in the lateral walls of the vagina where, in the course of normal differentiation, they undergo involution. In some instances, however, the wolffian ducts fail to involute completely, and remain as small cysts within the lateral vaginal wall. Occasionally, these remnants become larger and infected, and present clinically as Gartner's duct cysts. This embryology is also clinically relevant because the ureteral buds arise from the wolffian system; therefore, rare ectopic ureteral insertions into the lateral vaginal wall may be present in a woman with a long-standing history of urinary incontinence.

THE TRIGONE AND URETERS

Near week 4, the wolffian ducts penetrate the internal cloaca near the cloacal membrane; this point of convergence (also referred to as Müller's tubercle) is where the müllerian structures will enter the urethra to create the urogenital sinus. The trigone[4] begins to form when the wolffian ducts penetrate the internal cloaca. In week 5, the ureteral buds develop while the distal wolffian ducts are absorbed within the cloaca. With distal dilatation of the ureteral buds, the ureters are finally incorporated into their spots within the trigone. Buds arising from the correct portion of the mesonephros are incorporated into the right spot within the trigone. In contrast, ureteral buds that arise low along the mesonephric duct produce a ureter that is very lateral to the trigone and will reflux. Those ureteral buds that develop high along the mesonephros, ultimately are carried outside the bladder and into ectopic positions, usually within the urethra. These ureteric buds also penetrate the mesonephric blastema and the process of renal differentiation begins in full. By week 9, fetal urine production begins; the ability of the developing bladder to undergo mechanical distension is crucial for normal development. Clinically, the bladder may be imaged by ultrasonography at week 14 of gestation, and bladder cycling is observed even at this point. The

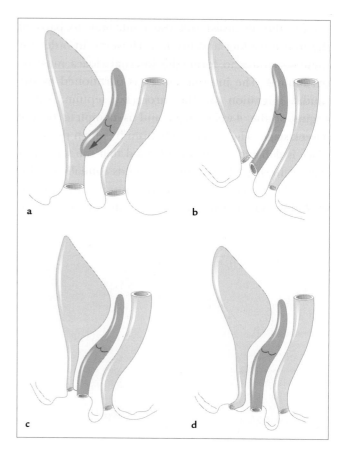

Figure 10.3. *(a) The müllerian ducts migrate to and penetrate the posterior urethra at week 7. The müllerian ducts are guided to this point in the posterior urethra by the wolffian ducts. (b) The ducts migrate caudally, and the urogenital sinus becomes a shallow channel. At this point there is a good separation between the urethra and vagina. (c) With continued growth the urogenital sinus disappears, as both the urethra and vaginal introitus are now at the perineal surface. The distal vagina is formed from sinus epithelium which streams into the vaginal vault. (d) With continued growth, the urethra turns anteriorly to reach its final location.*

importance of bladder cycling and fetal bladder distension is illustrated by the rare cases of bilateral ectopic ureters which arise only in female patients. These ectopic ureters often insert into the urethra, although vaginal and perineal insertions are also possible. This is clinically significant, because these women are incontinent of urine owing to the ureteric malpositioning distal to the striated external sphincter. In addition, their incontinence management is complicated by a malformed bladder neck and very tiny non-compliant bladders.

SMOOTH AND STRIATED MUSCLE DIFFERENTIATION

The developing urethra and bladder contain no muscle in the early stages of development. By week 7–8, muscle fibres begin to appear within the primitive mesenchyme that composes the bladder and urethra. What triggers this differentiation of mesenchyme into muscle in the bladder and urethra? Experimentally, Baskin has shown that urothelium is required if explants of primitive mesenchyme are to express smooth muscle-specific α-actin in nude mice.[5] Furthermore, this differentiation may be triggered by other epithelial surfaces (such as respiratory or intestinal epithelium, albeit not as efficiently), implying that these epithelial surfaces secrete a hormone or growth factor that is required for this transformation of mesenchyme into muscle. The sequence of events in the development of the female urethra has been outlined primarily in descriptive terms for this chapter; however, future treatises on this topic will draw on a growing body of sophisticated molecular studies. Future work in experimental models, 'knockout' or transgenic mice, and step sections of human embryos will allow the tools of molecular biology to be applied to (a) gain a better understanding of how the normal bladder and urethra develop and (b) understand how these molecular signals go awry, leading to congenital problems such as ectopic ureters or urogenital sinus anomalies.

The urethrovesical junction forms a sphincter that is under autonomic (involuntary) control; it is analogous to the shutter of a camera which is maintained in a closed position until the moment of exposure, when it must open for the proper amount of time.[6] By analogy, the smooth muscle of the bladder neck must remain in a closed position until such time as micturition is initiated, at which point it must open to allow for the expulsion of urine at low pressures. From the urethrovesical junction, smooth muscle fibres develop within the mesenchyme of the urethra in three layers – longitudinal (innermost), transverse (middle) and a second longitudinal layer (outermost).[7] These smooth muscular fibres have been reported to run the entire length of the urethra. Studies of human female fetuses at 20 and 23 weeks' gestation have also confirmed the presence of a striated 'external sphincter' that is located in the distal one-third of the urethra.[8] In contrast, the female fetus studied at 14 weeks had no identifiable striated external sphincter. Immunohistochemical studies in the female fetus have shown evidence of somatic innervation of the urethra by nerves carried in the anterior and lateral vaginal wall.[9]

CLINICAL EXAMPLES

Three examples serve to illustrate the clinical relevance of the preceding material in understanding the female patient with urinary incontinence.

Urogenital sinus

Patients with a urogenital sinus present with a normally functioning rectum that is often anteriorly displaced and with one common channel into which the urethra and vagina converge. Often, the site of this convergence is low and near the perineum; however, on occasion, the urogenital sinus may be long. In some cases, the voided urine may be trapped within the vagina, resulting in hydrocolpos. These infants present with a palpable pelvic mass, and decompression is required in the neonatal period. Today, most of these patients are diagnosed by prenatal sonography. These patients may rarely present as young children who develop infections within the pool of trapped urine, or with overflow incontinence. The embryological basis for this anomaly is apparent, bearing in mind how the müllerian systems fuse with the urethra and then migrate caudally during the course of normal perineal development. Failure of this distal migration means that the urethra and vagina will remain fused in a Y-type configuration, with only one channel emptying to the perineal surface. On physical examination the vaginal introitus is absent from these children (although the labia majora and minora will be normal in appearance) and a single opening in the urethral position. This diagnosis is confirmed radiographically by a retrograde injection of contrast into the urogenital sinogram (genitogram).[10] For low lesions, a perineal approach will allow for interposition of a perineal skin flap to complete a vaginoplasty, taking advantage of the dilated vaginal walls.[11] For high lesions, a combined abdominal–perineal approach may be required, although in recent years a posterior sagittal approach has been used more often.[12]

Ureterocele

In the female, extravesical ureteroceles will extend across the bladder neck and down into the urethra.

107

During the endoscopic approach to the bladder neck, an extravesical ureterocele will be apparent as a large cyst, usually at the 6 o'clock position. For many ureteroceles, the portion extending across the bladder neck and into the urethra is small; however, for some large extravesical ureteroceles, the large cystic cavity produces a great deal of distortion of the bladder neck and posterior urethra. This disruption of the bladder neck and urethra poses a challenge to paediatric urologists seeking to excise such large ureteroceles, because it requires a successful reconstruction of the urethra and bladder neck. The difficulties associated with this operation lead some urologists to suggest that the initial management of ureteroceles associated with duplex systems (and in some instances the only management) should consist of partial nephrectomy. This approach has been used with much success for well-selected patients, although in the long run 30–50% of these patients require reimplantation for residual reflux.[13]

Ewalt *et al.*[14] observed that, of patients treated by partial nephrectomy alone, 10% subsequently developed stress urinary incontinence, despite the absence of any bladder neck or urethral surgery.[14] This observation is of interest because it points out that large ureteroceles are capable of significantly distorting the developing bladder neck and urethra. Could it be that the developing 'hammock', as hypothesized by DeLancey,[15] is also distorted to a degree that makes normal urethral coaptation and function unlikely once this large tense cystic cavity is deflated? Normal urethral function might seem less likely in such a setting for two reasons: (1) a large ureterocele will distort the bladder neck, which will then not close properly at rest (the shutter mechanism will not close completely); (2) once the tense ureterocele is deflated, the urethra will not be suspended properly in relation to the pubis, further lowering intrinsic urethral resistance (an inadequate hammock).

Ectopic ureter

During the course of ureteral bud formation from the mesonephric duct, the potential exists for an ectopic orifice insertion. A ureteral bud that develops very low along the mesonephric duct is ultimately incorporated into the bladder wall far away from the trigone. This ureter has lateral ectopia, and often has significant vesicoureteral reflux associated with it. In contrast, a ureteral bud that develops very high along the mesonephric duct will miss being incorporated into the trigone and will usually insert within the urethra. These ectopic ureters may be obstructed because the ureter passes through the bladder neck; however, during micturition, the bladder neck relaxes and the hydronephrotic system drains. This forms the basis for the cyclic voiding cystourethrogram: 70–80% of ectopic ureters will reflux if the bladder is cycled sufficiently to empty the ectopic ureter; this will then lower the resistance and allow for retrograde flow of the contrast.

The major significance of ectopic ureters is that they may account for a lifelong history of urinary incontinence in women. This diagnosis must always be suspected in the female patient who has never been dry day or night; in younger patients, parents may recall that they never changed a dry nappy. The diagnosis may often be made in older women as well, and the presenting symptoms may relate more to infection than incontinence if the associated renal function is poor.[16] Today, most ectopic ureters are diagnosed by prenatal sonography, because most are associated with a significant degree of hydronephrosis, making such delayed presentations less likely. A far greater challenge faces the physician treating a female patient with bilateral ectopic ureters: these women have a hypoplastic bladder neck, total urinary incontinence and a small and non-compliant bladder. The data would suggest that these patients will require a bladder-neck reconstruction, bladder augmentation and appendicovesicostomy to achieve urinary continence.[17]

REFERENCES

1. Moore KL, Persaud TVN. *The Developing Human. Clinically Oriented Embryology*, 5th edn. Philadelphia: Saunders, 1993

2. Douglas Stephens F, Smith ED, Hutson JM. Normal embryology of the cloaca. *Congenital Anomalies of the Urinary and Genital Tracts.* Oxford: Isis Medical Media, 1996; 3–12

3. Douglas Stephens F, Smith ED, Hutson J.M. Müllerian and Wolffian anomalies. *Congenital Anomalies of the Urinary and Genital Tracts.* Oxford: Isis Medical Media, 1996; 50–55

4. Douglas Stephens F, Smith ED, Hutson JM. Morphology and embryology of the bladder. *Congenital Anomalies of the Urinary and Genital Tracts.* Oxford: Isis Medical Media, 1996; 141–144

5. Disandro MJ, Li Y, Baskin IS *et al.* Mesenchymal epithelial interactions in bladder smooth muscle differentiation: epithelial specificity. *J Urol* 1998; 160: 1040–1046

6. Zderic SA, Levin RM, Wein AJ. Voiding function: relevant anatomy, physiology, pharmacology, and molecular aspects. In: Gillenwater JY, Grayhack JT, Howards SS, Duckett JW (eds) *Adult and Pediatric Urology*, 3rd edn. Chicago: Mosby Year Book, 1996; 1159–1165

7. Colleselli K, Stenzl A, Eder R *et al.* The female urethral sphincter: a morphological and topographical study. *J Urol* 1998; 160: 49–54

8. Kokoua A, Homsy Y, Lavigne JF *et al.* Maturation of the external urinary sphincter: a comparative histotopographic study in humans. *J Urol* 1993; 150: 617–622

9. Borirakchanyavat S, Abouseif SR, Carroll PR *et al.* Continence mechanism of the isolated female urethra: an anatomical study of the intrapelvic somatic nerves. *J Urol* 1997; 158: 822–826

10. Jaramillo D, Lebowitz RL, Hendren WH. The cloacal malformation: radiologic findings and imaging recommendations. *Radiology* 1990; 177: 441–448

11. Rink RC, Pope JC, Kropp BP *et al.* Reconstruction of the high urogenital sinus: early perineal prone approach without division of the rectum. *J Urol* 1997; 158: 1293–1297

12. Domini R, Rossi F, Ceccarelli PL, DeCasto R. Anterior sagittal transanorectal approach to the urogenital sinus in adrenogenital syndrome: a preliminary report. *J Pediatr Surg* 1997; 32: 714–719

13. Caldamone AA, Snyder HM, Duckett JW. Ureteroceles in children: followup of management with the upper tract approach. *J Urol* 1984; 131: 1130–1133

14. Husmann DA, Ewalt DH, Glenski WJ, Bernier PA. Ureterocele associated with ureteral duplication and a nonfunctioning upper pole segment: management by partial nephrectomy alone. *J Urol* 1995; 154: 723–726

15. DeLancey JOL. Structural support of the urethra as it relates to stress urinary incontinence: the hammock hypothesis. *Am J Obstet Gynecol* 1994; 170: 1713–1723

16. Leonovicz PF, O'Connell BJ, Uehling DT. Vaginal ectopic ureter with Gartner's duct cyst. *J Urol* 1997; 158: 2235–2236

17. Jayanthi VR, Churchill BM, Khoury AE, McLorie GA. Bilateral single ectopic ureteral ectopia: difficulty attaining continence using standard bladder neck repair. *J Urol* 1997; 158: 1933–1936

11

Anatomy

J. O. L. DeLancey

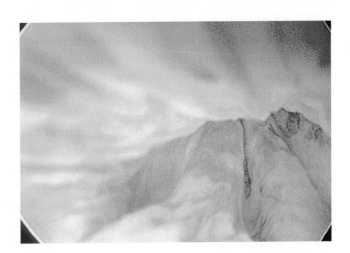

GENERAL EMBRYOLOGY

Development of the bladder and urethra

During early development, beginning about 15 days after fertilization, three layers (endoderm, mesoderm and ectoderm) form the embryo. A gap in this three-layered arrangement occurs in the caudal end of the embryo where the endoderm and ectoderm fuse without an intervening mesoderm. This region forms the cloacal membrane, which lies just caudal to the body stalk. A reservoir develops above the cloacal membrane formed by the junction of the hindgut and the allantois. The ventral allantois is a tubular endodermal outgrowth of the yolk sac, which starts to form 17–19 days after fertilization and which lies in the body stalk; at its caudal end it is fused with the hindgut.

The wedge of tissue that lies at the junction of the allantois and the hindgut is called the urorectal septum. It grows caudally between the allantois and hindgut until it reaches the cloacal membrane, thereby dividing the cloaca into an anterior urogenital sinus and posterior anorectum. This also divides the cloacal membrane into the urogenital membrane and anal membrane. The urorectal septum will become the perineal body in the adult.

At about this time, the mesodermal borders of the cloacal membrane thicken. Lateral to the cloaca these thickenings form the urethral folds and, at the cranial end of the membrane, the genital tubercle. Further growth of the urethral folds and genital tubercle leads to the formation of the penis and urethra in the male and of the labia and clitoris in the female.

As the cloaca is being partitioned, the mesonephric ducts enter into the ventral wall of the cloaca. This point of entry into the urogenital sinus is continuous with the allantois and is called the vesicourethral canal; it will form the urethra and bladder in the adult. The sinus below the mesonephric ducts is destined to become the vaginal vestibule.

As previously mentioned, the cloacal membrane lies adjacent to the body stalk. Ingrowth of tissue from the lateral aspects of the body wall separates these structures and is responsible for the lower portion of the abdominal wall. Failure of this ingrowth gives rise to bladder exstrophy.

Four embryological primordia within the urogenital sinus (those of the detrusor muscle, trigonal muscle,

urethral smooth muscle and urethral striated muscle) develop into the female urethra and bladder. Although the urethra and bladder form a single continuous mass on gross inspection, microscopically and functionally there are important differences in the musculature from one region to another, explicable in terms of their different embryological derivations. In both the male and female there is a fifth prostatic primordium; however, in the female this fails to provide any significant structure in the adult and is not discussed here.

FUNCTIONAL ANATOMY OF THE LOWER URINARY TRACT

The inseparable relationship between structure and function in living organisms is one of the common themes found in biology. The anatomy and clinical behaviour of the lower urinary tract exemplify this immutable link. The following descriptions are intended to offer a brief overview of some clinically relevant aspects of lower urinary tract structure that help us understand the normal and abnormal behaviour of this system. Because of the importance of the pelvic floor to lower urinary tract function, comments on the structure of the lower urinary tract organs are followed by a section describing the structure of the pelvic floor as it relates to micturition, continence and pelvic organ support.

The lower urinary tract can be divided into the bladder and urethra. At the junction of these two continuous, yet discrete, structures lies the vesical neck. This hybrid structure represents that part of the lower urinary tract where the urethral lumen traverses the bladder wall before becoming surrounded by the urethral wall. It contains portions of the bladder muscle, and also elements that continue into the urethra.

The vesical neck is considered separately because of its functional differentiation from the bladder and the urethra. The spatial relationships of this region are illustrated in Figure 11.1 and described in Table 11.1.

Bladder

The bladder consists of the detrusor muscle, covered by an adventitia and serosa over its dome, and lined by a submucosa and transitional cell epithelium. The muscular layers of the detrusor are not discrete; nevertheless, in general, the outer and inner layers of the

Table 11.1. *Topography of urethral and para-urethral structures**

Approximate location[†]	Region of the urethra	Para-urethral structures
0–20	Intramural urethra	Urethral lumen traverses the bladder wall
20–60	Midurethra	Sphincter urethrae muscle Pubovesical muscle Vaginolevator attachment
60–80	Perineal membrane	Compressor urethrae muscle Urethrovaginal sphincter muscle
80–100	Distal urethra	Bulbocavernosus muscle

* Smooth muscle of the urethra was not considered.
[†] Expressed as a percentage of total urethral length.
Reproduced from ref. 4 with permission.

detrusor musculature tend to be longitudinal, with an intervening circular–oblique layer.

Two prominent bands on the dorsal aspect of the bladder form one of the prominent landmarks of detrusor musculature.[1] They are derived from the outer longitudinal layer and pass beside the urethra to form a loop on its anterior aspect, called the detrusor loop. On the anterior aspect of this loop, some detrusor fibres leave the region of the vesical neck and attach to the pubic bones and pelvic walls; these are called the pubovesical muscles and are discussed below.

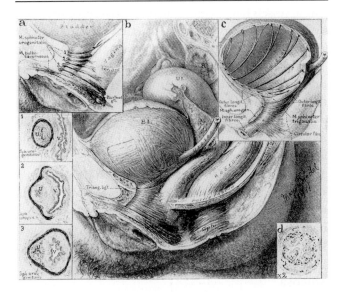

Figure 11.1. *The lower urinary tract, including the striated urogenital sphincter muscle.*

Trigone

Within the bladder there is a visible triangular area known as the vesical trigone. The two ureteral orifices and the internal urinary meatus form its apices. The base of the triangle, the interureteric ridge, forms a useful landmark in cystoscopic identification of the ureteric orifices. This triangular elevation is caused by the presence of a specialized group of smooth muscle fibres that lie within the detrusor, and arise from a separate embryological primordium. They are continuous above with the ureteral smooth muscle;[2] below, they continue down the urethra. In addition to their visible triangular elevation, these muscle fibres form a ring inside the detrusor loop at the level of the internal urinary meatus[3] (Fig. 11.2). Some fibres continue down the dorsal surface of the urethra and lie between the ends of the U-shaped striated sphincter muscles of the urethra. These smooth muscle fibres of the trigone are clearly separable from those of the detrusor by the smaller size of their fascicles and greater density of surrounding connective tissue. The mucosa over the trigone frequently undergoes squamous metaplasia and therefore differs from that in the rest of the bladder. The circumferential distribution of the trigonal ring fibres at the vesical neck might contribute to closure of the lumen of the vesical neck in this area, but its role has yet to be fully elucidated.

113

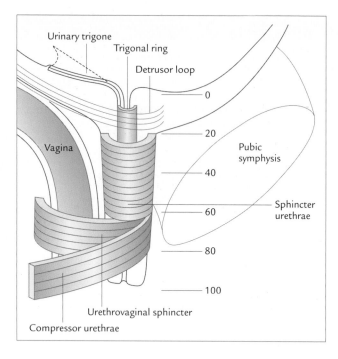

Figure 11.2. *Schematic diagram of the striated urogenital sphincter muscle and trigonal musculature within the bladder base and urethra (cut in sagittal section). The ruler indicates the locations of structures along the urethral length.*

Urethra

The urethra holds urine in the bladder and is therefore an important structure that helps determine urinary continence. It is a complex tubular viscus extending below the bladder. In its upper third it is clearly separable from the adjacent vagina, but its lower portion is fused with the wall of the latter structure. Embedded within its substance are a number of elements that are important to lower urinary tract function; their locations are summarized in Table 11.1.[4]

Striated urogenital sphincter

The outer layer of the urethra is formed by the muscle of the striated urogenital sphincter (Figs 11.3, 11.4) which is found from about 20% to 80% of the total urethral length (measured as a percentage of the distance from the internal meatus to the external meatus). In its upper two-thirds, the sphincter fibres lie in a primarily circular orientation; distally, they leave the confines of the urethra and either encircle the vaginal wall as the urethrovaginal sphincter or extend along the inferior pubic ramus above the perineal membrane (urogenital

diaphragm) as the compressor urethrae. This muscle is composed largely of slow-twitch muscle fibres,[5] which are well suited to maintaining the constant tone exhibited by this muscle. In addition, voluntary muscle activation increases urethral constriction during times when increased closure pressure is needed. In the distal urethra, this striated muscle compresses the urethra from above; proximally, it constricts the lumen. Studies of skeletal muscle blockade suggest that this muscle is responsible for approximately one-third of resting urethral closure pressure.[6]

Urethral smooth muscle

The smooth muscle of the urethra is contiguous with that of the trigone and detrusor, but can be separated from these other muscles on embryological, topographical and morphological grounds.[3,7] It has an inner longitudinal layer, and a thin outer circular layer, with the former being by far the more prominent of the two (Fig. 11.5). The layers lie inside the striated urogenital sphincter muscle, and are present throughout the upper four-fifths of the urethra. The configuration of the circular muscle suggests a role in constricting the lumen, and the longitudinal muscle may help to shorten and funnel the urethra during voiding.

Submucosal vasculature

Lying within the urethra is a surprisingly well-developed vascular plexus that is more prominent than one would expect for the ordinary demands of so small an organ.[8] These vessels have been studied in serial reconstruction by Huisman,[3] who has demonstrated the presence of several specialized types of arteriovenous anastomoses. They are formed in such a way that the flow of blood into large venules can be controlled to inflate or deflate them. This would assist in forming a watertight closure of the mucosal surfaces, and offer the possibility of rapid increases in their filling from the pressure on the abdominal vessels that supply them. Occlusion of the arterial inflow to these venous reservoirs has been shown to influence urethral closure pressure.[6] In addition, these appear to be hormone sensitive,[3] which may help to explain some individuals' response to oestrogen supplementation.

Mucosa

The mucosal lining of the urethra is continuous above with the transitional epithelium of the bladder and

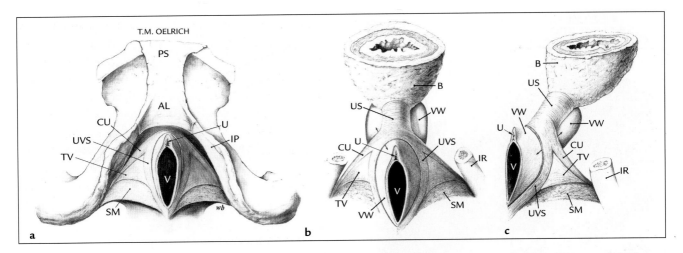

Figure 11.3. *Striated urogenital sphincter muscle seen from below after removal of the perineal membrane (a) and pubic bones (b, c). US, urethral sphincter; UVS, urethrovaginal sphincter; CU, compressor urethrae; B, bladder; IR, ischiopubic ramus; TV, transverse vaginal muscle; SM, smooth muscle; U, urethra ; V, vagina; VW, vaginal wall. (Reproduced from ref. 28 with permission.)*

below with the non-keratinizing squamous epithelium of the vestibule. This mucosa shares a common derivation from the urogenital sinus with the lower vagina and vestibule. Like these other areas, its mucosa is hormonally sensitive and undergoes significant change, depending on its state of stimulation.

Connective tissue

In addition to the contractile and vascular tissue of the urethra, there is a considerable quantity of connective tissue interspersed within the muscle and the submucosa. This tissue contains both collagenous and elastin fibres. Studies that have sought to abolish the active aspects of urethral closure have suggested that the non-contractile elements contribute to urethral closure.[3] However, it is difficult to study the function of these tissues because there is no specific way to block their action pharmacologically or surgically.

Glands

A series of glands are found in the submucosa, primarily along the dorsal (vaginal) surface of the urethra.[9] They are most concentrated in the lower and middle thirds, and vary in number. The location of urethral diverticula (which are derived from cystic dilatation of these glands) follows this distribution, being most common distally and usually originating along the dorsal surface of the urethra. In addition, their origin within the submucosa indicates that the fascia of the urethra

must be stretched and attenuated over their surface, and indicates the need for its approximation after diverticular excision.

Vesical neck

The term 'vesical neck' is both a regional and a functional one, as previously discussed. It does not refer to a single anatomical entity; it denotes that area, at the base of the bladder, where the urethral lumen passes through the thickened musculature of the bladder base. Therefore, it is sometimes considered as part of the bladder musculature, but it also contains the urethral lumen studied during urethral pressure profilometry. It is a region where the detrusor musculature, including the detrusor loop, surrounds the trigonal ring and the urethral meatus.

The vesical neck has come to be considered separately from the bladder and urethra because it has unique functional characteristics. Specifically, sympathetic denervation or damage of this area results in its remaining open at rest;[10] when this happens in association with stress incontinence, simple urethral suspension is often ineffective in curing this problem.[11]

Functional terms

A number of terms have been used to describe functional units within the vesicourethral unit, based upon

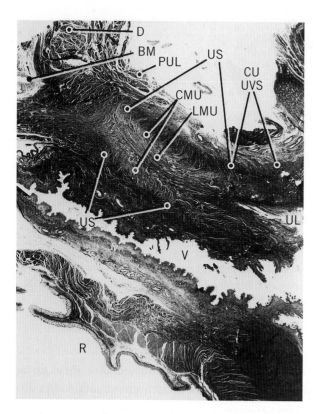

Figure 11.4. *Sagittal section from a 29-year-old cadaver, cut just lateral to the midline and not quite parallel to it. The section contains tissue nearer the midline in the distal urethra where the lumen can be seen than at the vesical neck. BM, bladder mucosa; CMU, circular smooth muscle of the urethra; CU, compressor urethrae; D, detrusor muscle; LMU, longitudinal smooth muscles of the urethra; PB, perineal body; PS, pubic symphysis; PUL, pubourethral ligament; PVM, pubovesical muscle; R, rectum; T, trigonal ring; UL, urethral lumen; US, urethral sphincter; UVS, urethrovaginal sphincter; V, vagina. (Reproduced from ref. 4 with permission.)*

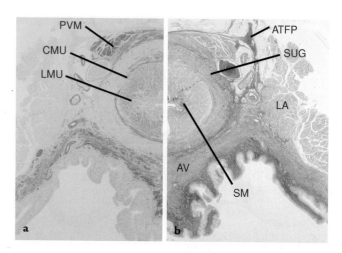

Figure 11.5. *Axial midurethral actin immunoperoxidase histological section for smooth muscle (a) and mirrored Mallory Trichrome histological section (b) from the same specimen. A few small blood clots are identified in the submucosa (SM). The longitudinal (LMU) and circular (CMU) smooth muscle of the urethra, the pubovesical muscle (PVM) and the smooth muscle layer of the anterior vaginal wall (AV) are easily identified on the actin-stained immunoperoxidase preparation whereas the striated urogenital sphincter muscle (SUG) does not stain with actin. ATFP, arcus tendineus fasciae pelvis; LA, levator ani muscles.*

radiographic observations of the activities of these viscera. The term 'extrinsic continence mechanism' or 'external sphincteric mechanism' usually refers to that group of structures that respond when an individual is instructed to stop the urine stream. The two phenomena observed during this effort are a constriction of the urethral lumen by the striated urogenital sphincter and an elevation of the vesical neck, caused by contraction of the levator ani muscles, as described below. The intrinsic continence mechanism then consists of the structures which lie within the vesical neck, and which are not specifically activated by contraction of the voluntary muscles. It is this system that fails in patients whose vesical neck can be seen to be open at rest.

PELVIC FLOOR

The position and mobility of the bladder and urethra are recognized as important to urinary continence.[12] Because these two organs are limp and formless when removed from the body, they must depend upon attachments to the pelvic floor for their shape and position. Fluoroscopic examination has shown that the upper portions of the urethra and vesical neck are normally mobile structures, whereas the distal urethra remains fixed in position.[13,14] The pelvic floor muscles and fasciae determine these aspects of support and fixation.

The pelvic floor consists of several components lying between the pelvic peritoneum and the vulvar skin. These are (from above downwards), the peritoneum, viscera and endopelvic fascia, levator ani muscles, perineal membrane and external genital muscles. The eventual support for all of these structures comes from their connection to the bony pelvis and its attached muscles. The viscera are often thought of as being supported by the pelvic floor; however, they are actually a part of it. Through such structures as the cardinal and uterosacral ligaments and the pubocervical fascia, the viscera have an important role in forming the pelvic floor.

Endopelvic fascia

The viscerofascial layer

The top layer of the pelvic floor is provided by the endopelvic fascia that attaches the pelvic organs to the pelvic walls, thereby suspending the pelvic organs.[15–17] Because this layer is a combination of the pelvic viscera and the endopelvic fascia, it is referred to here as the *viscerofascial* layer. It is common to speak of the fasciae and ligaments alone, separate from the pelvic organs as if they had a discrete identity; however, unless these fibrous structures have something to attach to (the pelvic organs), they can have no mechanical effect.

On each side of the pelvis the endopelvic fascia attaches the uterus and vagina to the pelvic wall (Figs 11.6–11.8). This fascia forms a continuous sheet-like mesentery, extending from the uterine artery at its cephalic margin to the point at which the vagina fuses with the levator ani muscles below. The part that attaches to the uterus is called the *parametrium* and that which attaches to the vagina, the *paracolpium*.

The parametria are made up of what are clinically referred to as the cardinal and uterosacral ligaments,[18,19] and which are two different parts of a single mass of tissue. The uterosacral ligaments are the visible and palpable medial margin of the cardinal–uterosacral ligament complex.

Although these tissues are termed 'ligaments' and 'fasciae', they are *not* the same type of tissue as that seen in the 'fascia' of the rectus abdominis muscle or in the ligaments of the knee, both of which are composed of dense, regular, connective tissue. These supportive tissues consist of blood vessels, nerves and fibrous connective tissue, and can be thought of as mesenteries that supply the genital tract bilaterally. Their composition

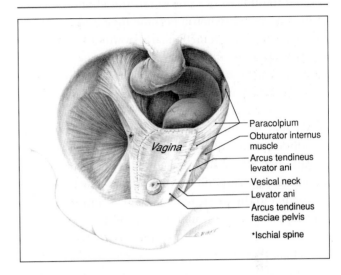

Figure 11.7. *Vagina and supportive structures drawn from dissection of a 56-year-old cadaver after hysterectomy. The paracolpium extends along the lateral wall of the vagina. (From ref. 17 with permission.)*

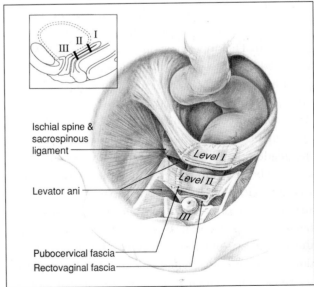

Figure 11.8. *Level I (suspension) and level II (attachment). In level I the paracolpium suspends the vagina from the lateral pelvic walls. Fibres of level I extend both vertically and also posteriorly towards the sacrum. In level II, the vagina is attached to the arcus tendineus fasciae pelvis and superior fascia of levator ani. (From ref. 17 with permission.)*

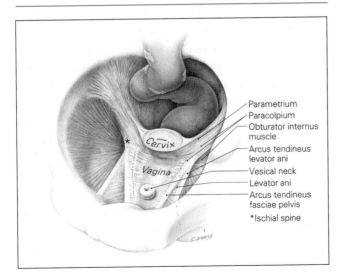

Figure 11.6. *Supportive tissues of the cervix and upper vagina. Bladder has been removed above the vesical neck (©1999, JOL DeLancey).*

reflects their combined function as neurovascular conduits as well as supportive structures.

The structural effect of this arrangement is most evident when the uterine cervix is pulled downwards with a tenaculum, as occurs during dilatation and curettage, or pushed downwards, as during laparotomy. After a certain amount of descent within the elastic range of the fascia, the parametria become tight and arrest the further cervical descent. Similarly, downward descent of the vaginal apex after hysterectomy is resisted by the paracolpia. The fact that these ligaments do not limit the downward movement of the uterus in normal healthy women is attested to by the observation that the cervix may be drawn down to the level of the hymen with little difficulty.[20]

Although it is traditional to focus attention on the ligaments that suspend the uterus, the attachments of the vagina to the pelvic walls are equally important and are responsible for normal support of the vagina, bladder and rectum, even after hysterectomy. The location of damage to these supports determines whether a woman has a cystocele, rectocele, or vaginal vault prolapse; understanding the different characteristics of this support helps understanding of the different types of prolapse that can occur.

After hysterectomy the upper two-thirds of the vagina is suspended and attached to the pelvic walls by the paracolpium.[17] This paracolpium has two portions (Fig. 11.8). The upper portion (level I) consists of a relatively long sheet of tissue that suspends the vagina by attaching it to the pelvic wall. In the mid-portion of the vagina, the paracolpium attaches the vagina laterally and more directly to the pelvic walls (level II). This attachment stretches the vagina transversely between the bladder and rectum and has functional significance. The structural layer that supports the bladder ('pubocervical fascia') is composed of the anterior vaginal wall and its attachment through the endopelvic fascia to the pelvic wall. It is not a layer separate from the vagina, as sometimes suggested, but is a combination of the anterior vaginal wall and its attachments to the pelvic wall. Similarly, the posterior vaginal wall and endopelvic fascia (rectovaginal fascia) form the restraining layer that prevents the rectum from protruding forwards, blocking formation of a rectocele. In the distal vagina (level III) the vaginal wall is directly attached to surrounding structures without any intervening paracolpium: anteriorly it fuses with the

urethra, posteriorly with the perineal body and laterally with the levator ani muscles.

Damage to the upper suspensory fibres of the paracolpium causes a type of prolapse that differs from damage to the mid-level supports of the vagina: defects in the support provided by the mid-level vaginal supports (pubocervical and rectovaginal fasciae) result in cystocele and rectocele, whereas loss of the upper suspensory fibres of the paracolpium and parametrium is responsible for development of vaginal and uterine prolapse. These defects occur in varying combinations and this variation is responsible for the diversity of clinical problems encountered within the overall spectrum of pelvic organ prolapse

Pelvic diaphragm

Subjecting it to constant force may stretch any connective tissue within the body. Skin expanders used in plastic surgery stretch the dense and resistant dermis to extraordinary degrees, and flexibility exercises practised by dancers and athletes elongate leg ligaments with as little as 10 minutes of stretching a day. Both of these observations underscore the malleable nature of connective tissue when subjected to force over time. If the ligaments and fasciae within the pelvis were subjected to the continuous stress imposed on the pelvic floor by the great weight of abdominal pressure, they would stretch; this stretching does not occur because the pelvic floor muscles close the pelvic floor and carry the weight of the abdominal and pelvic organs, preventing constant strain on the ligaments.

Below the viscerofascial layer is the levator ani group of muscles[21] (Fig. 11.9). They have a connective-tissue covering on both superior and inferior surfaces, known as the superior and inferior fasciae of the levator ani, respectively. When these muscles and their fasciae are considered together, the combined structure is termed the pelvic diaphragm.

The levator ani consists of two portions – the pubovisceral muscle and the iliococcygeus muscle.[22,23] The pubovisceral muscle is a thick U-shaped muscle, the ends of which arise from the pubic bones on either side of the midline and which passes behind the rectum, forming a sling-like arrangement. This portion includes both the pubococcygeus and puborectalis portions of the levator ani. Laterally, the iliococcygeus arises from a fibrous band on the pelvic wall (arcus tendineus levator

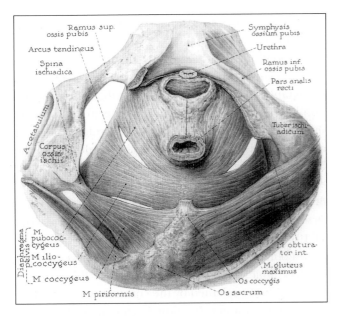

Figure 11.9. *Levator ani muscles seen from below. That portion of the pubococcygeus which inserts into the rectum and forms a 'U' behind it is termed the puborectalis. (Reproduced from Anson B.* Atlas of Human Anatomy, *Philadelphia: Saunders, 1950, with permission.)*

ani; ATLA) and forms a relatively horizontal sheet that spans the opening within the pelvis and provides a shelf on which the organs may rest.

The pubovisceral muscle has several components. The pubococcygeus muscle is the most cephalic portion of the levator; it passes from the pubic bones to insert on the inner surface of the coccyx. This comprises only a small portion of the overall levator complex. Clinicians have often referred to the entire pubovisceral muscle as the pubococcygeus. The pubococcygeus portion of the levator ani muscles actually connects two relatively immovable structures (pubis and coccyx) and, therefore, could not be expected to contribute substantially to supporting the pelvic organs. The pubovisceral muscle passes beside the vagina; the lateral vaginal walls are attached to it. The muscle then continues dorsally, where some fibres insert into the rectum between the internal and external sphincter while others pass behind the anorectal junction. The vagina attaches to the medial portion of the pubovisceral muscle and the fibres between the vagina and pubic bone are referred to as the pubovaginalis muscle. These muscle fibres are responsible for elevating the urethra during pelvic muscle contrac-

tion, but muscle fibres of the levator have no direct connection to the urethra itself.

The opening within the levator ani muscle through which the urethra and vagina pass (and through which prolapse occurs) is called the *urogenital hiatus* of the levator ani. The rectum also passes through this opening; however, because the levator ani muscles attach directly to the anus, it is not included in the name of the hiatus. The hiatus, therefore, is bounded ventrally (anteriorly) by the pubic bones, laterally by the levator ani muscles and dorsally (posteriorly) by the perineal body and external anal sphincter. The normal baseline activity of the levator ani muscle keeps the urogenital hiatus closed: it squeezes the vagina, urethra and rectum closed by compressing them against the pubic bone and it lifts the floor and organs in a cephalic direction.

The levator ani muscles have constant activity,[24] like that of other postural muscles. This continuous contraction is similar to the continuous activity of the external anal sphincter muscle and closes the lumen of the vagina in a way similar to that by which the anal sphincter closes the anus. This constant action eliminates any opening within the pelvic floor through which prolapse could occur and forms a relatively horizontal shelf on which the pelvic organs are supported.[25,26]

The interaction between the pelvic floor muscles and the supportive ligaments is critical to pelvic organ support. As long as the levator ani muscles function properly, the pelvic floor is closed and the ligaments and fascia are under no tension; the fasciae simply act to stabilize the organs in their position above the levator ani muscles. When the pelvic floor muscles relax or are damaged, the pelvic floor opens and the vagina lies between the high abdominal pressure and low atmospheric pressure; in this situation it must be held in place by the ligaments. Although the ligaments can sustain these loads for short periods of time, if the pelvic floor muscles do not close the pelvic floor then the connective tissue must carry this load for long periods and will eventually fail to hold the vagina in place.

This support of the uterus has been likened to a ship in its berth, floating on the water attached by ropes on either side to a dock.[27] The ship is analogous to the uterus, the ropes to the ligaments and the water to the supportive layer formed by the pelvic floor muscles. The ropes (ligaments) function to hold the ship (uterus) in the center of its berth as it rests on the water (pelvic floor muscles). If, however, the water level were to fall so far that the ropes would be required to hold the ship without the support of the water, the ropes would break. The analogous situation in the pelvic floor involves the pelvic floor muscles supporting the uterus and vagina that are stabilized in position by the ligaments and fasciae: once the pelvic floor musculature becomes damaged and no longer holds the organs in place, the connective tissue fails because of significant overload.

Perineal membrane and external genital muscles

In the anterior portion of the pelvis, below the pelvic diaphragm, is a dense triangular membrane containing a central opening called the perineal membrane (urogenital diaphragm). This lies at the level of the hymenal ring and attaches the urethra, vagina and perineal body to the ischiopubic rami. Just above the perineal membrane are the compressor urethrae and urethrovaginal sphincter muscles, previously discussed as part of the striated urogenital sphincter muscle.

The term 'perineal membrane' replaces the old term 'urogenital diaphragm', reflecting more accurate recent anatomical information.[28] Previous concepts of the urogenital diaphragm show two fascial layers, with a transversely orientated muscle between them (the deep transverse perineal muscle). Observations based on serial histology and gross dissection, however, reveal a single connective tissue membrane, with muscle lying immediately above. The correct anatomy explains the observation that pressures during a cough are greatest in the distal urethra,[29,30] where the compressor urethrae and urethrovaginal sphincter can squeeze the lumen in anticipation of a cough.[31]

Position and mobility of the urethra

When the importance of urethral position to determining urinary continence was recognized, anatomical observations revealed an attachment of the tissues around the urethra to the pubic bones. These connections were referred to as the pubourethral ligaments[32] and were found to be continuous with the connective tissue of the perineal membrane.[33] Further studies[31,34,35] have expanded these observations and revealed several separate structural elements contained within these tissues that have functional importance to urinary continence.

As mentioned earlier in this chapter, urethral support is dynamic rather than static. Fluoroscopic and topographic observations[13,14] suggest that urethral position is determined both by attachments to bone and by those to the levator ani muscles. The role of the connection between the ureteral supports and those to the levator ani is probably more important than previously thought, for the following reasons. The resting position of the proximal urethra is high within the pelvis, some 3 cm above the inferior aspect of the pubic bones[36] (Fig. 11.10) and above the insertion of the 'posterior pubourethral ligaments' which attach near the lower margin of the pubic bones.[32] Maintenance of this position would be best explained by the constant muscular activity of the levator ani. In addition, the upper two-thirds of the urethra is mobile[13,14,37] and under voluntary control. At the onset of micturition, relaxation of the levator ani muscles allows the urethra to descend and obliterates the posterior urethrovesical angle (Fig. 11.10). Resumption of the normal tonic contraction of the muscle at the end of micturition returns the vesical neck to its normal position.

The anterior vaginal wall and urethra arise from the urogenital sinus and are intimately connected. The support of the urethra does not depend on attachments of the urethra itself to adjacent structures, but on the con-

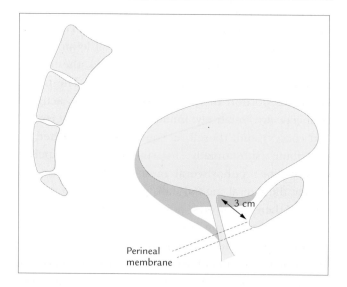

Figure 11.10. *Topography and mobility of the normal proximal urethra and vesical neck based upon resting ( ) and voiding (■) in nulliparae.*

nection of the vagina and periurethral tissues to the muscles and fasciae of the pelvic wall. Surgeons are most familiar with seeing this anatomy through the space of Retzius, and this view is also helpful in understanding urethral support (Fig. 11.11). On either side of the pelvis, the arcus tendineus fasciae pelvis (ATFP) is found as a band of connective tissue attached at one end to the lower one-sixth of the pubic bone, 1 cm from the midline, and at the other end to the ischial spine. The anterior portion of this band lies on the inner surface of the levator ani muscle that arises some 3 cm above the ATFP. Posteriorly, the levator ani arises from a second arcus, the ATLA, which fuses with the ATFP near the ischial spine.

The layer of tissue that provides urethral support has two lateral attachments – a fascial attachment and a muscular attachment (Fig. 11.12). The fascial attachments of the urethral supports connect the periurethral tissues and anterior vaginal wall to the ATFP and have been termed the paravaginal fascial attachments.[34] The muscular attachment connects these same periurethral tissues to the medial border of the levator ani muscle. These attachments allow the normal resting tone of the levator ani to maintain the position of the vesical neck, supported by the fascial attachments (Fig. 11.13). When the muscle relaxes at the onset of micturition, it allows the vesical neck to rotate downwards to the limit of the elasticity of the fascial attachments; at the end of micturition, contraction allows it to resume its normal position.

Also within this region are the pubovesical muscles, which are extensions of the detrusor muscle.[1,38,39] They lie within connective tissue; when both muscular and fibrous elements are considered together they are termed the pubovesical ligaments, in much the same way that the smooth muscle of the ligamentum teres is referred to as the round ligament (Figs 11.4, 11.5, 11.11, 11.12). Although the terms 'pubovesical ligament' and 'pubourethral ligament' have sometimes been considered to be synonymous, the pubovesical ligaments are different structures from the urethral supportive tissues. Fibres of the detrusor muscle are able to undergo great elongation and these weak tissues are, therefore, not suited to maintain urethral position under stress. In addition, they run in front of the vesical neck rather than underneath it, where one would expect supportive tissues to be found. It is not surprising, therefore, that these detrusor fibres do not differ,

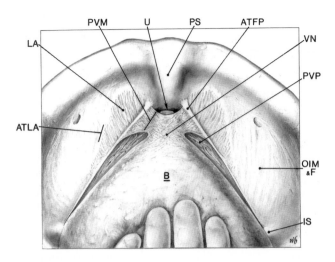

Figure 11.11. *Space of Retzius (drawn from cadaver dissection). Pubovesical muscle (PVM) can be seen going from vesical neck (VN) to arcus tendineus fasciae pelvis (ATFP) and running over the para-urethral vascular plexus (PVP). ATLA, arcus tendineus levator ani; B, bladder; IS, ischial spine; LA, levator ani muscles; OIM&F, obturator internus muscle and fascia; PS, pubic symphysis; U, urethra. (Reproduced from ref. 39 with permission.)*

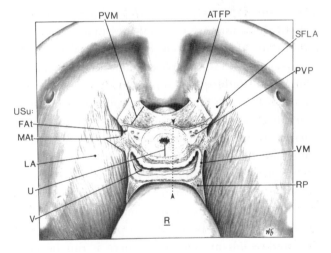

Figure 11.12. *Relationship of the supportive tissues of the urethra (USu) to the pubovesical muscles (PVM). Cross-section of the urethra (U), vagina (V), arcus tendineus fasciae pelvis (ATFP) and superior fascia of levator ani (SFLA) just below the vesical neck (drawn from cadaver dissection). The PVM lie anterior to the urethra, and anterior and superior to the para-urethral vascular plexus (PVP). The USu ('the pubourethral ligaments') attach the vagina and vaginal surface of the urethra to the levator ani (LA) muscles (MAt, muscular attachment) and to the superior fascia of the LA (FAt, fascial attachment). Additional abbreviations: R, rectum; RP, rectal pillar; VM, vaginal wall muscularis. (Reproduced from ref. 39 with permission.)*

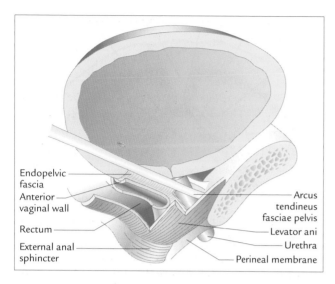

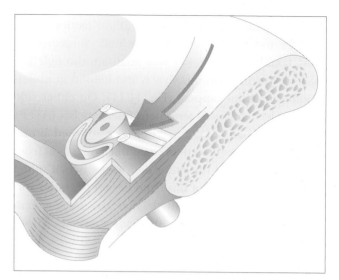

Figure 11.13. *Lateral view of the pelvic floor structures related to urethral support, seen from the side in the standing position cut just lateral to the midline. Note that windows have been cut in the levator ani muscles, vagina and endopelvic fascia, so that the urethra and anterior vaginal walls can be seen.*

Figure 11.14. *Lateral view of pelvic floor with the urethra, vagina and fascial tissues transected at the level of the vesical neck, drawn from three-dimensional reconstruction indicating compression of the urethra by downward force (arrow) against the supportive tissues indicating the influence of abdominal pressure on the urethra (arrow).*

in stress-incontinent patients, from those in patients without this condition.[40] The tissues that support the urethra are separated from the pubovesical ligaments by a prominent vascular plexus, and are easily parted from them. Rather than supporting the urethra, the pubovesical muscles may be responsible for assisting in vesical neck opening at the onset of micturition by contracting to pull the anterior vesical neck forwards, as some have suggested.[41]

This mechanism influences incontinence by determining not how high or how low the urethra is but how it is supported. In examining anatomical specimens, simulated increases in abdominal pressure reveal that the urethra lies in a position where it can be compressed against the supporting hammock by rises in abdominal pressure (Fig. 11.13). In this model, it is the stability of this supporting layer under the urethra rather than the height of the urethra that determines stress continence. In an individual with a firm supportive layer, the urethra would be compressed between abdominal pressure and pelvic fascia (Fig. 11.14) in much the same way that the flow of water through a garden hose can be stopped by stepping on and compressing it against underlying paving. If, however, the layer under the urethra becomes unstable and does not provide a firm backstop against which the urethra can be

compressed by abdominal pressure, the opposing force that causes closure is lost and the occlusive action is diminished. This latter situation is similar to an attempt to stop the flow of water through a garden hose by stepping on it while it lies on soft soil.

The structural and functional aspects of the body must always be in agreement. As new functional observations are made of the lower urinary tract, it will be necessary to re-examine our anatomical concepts; doubtless, some of the structural arrangements described in this chapter will be corrected, expanded upon and improved. This will continue to enhance our ability to understand the variety of patients with lower urinary tract dysfunction, and will improve our ability to restore normal urinary control.

REFERENCES

1. Gil Vernet S. *Morphology and Function of the Vesico-prostato-urethral Musculature*. Italy: Edizioni Canova Treviso, 1968

2. Woodburne RT. The ureter ureterovesical junction and vesical trigone. *Anat Rec* 1965; 151: 243–249

3. Huisman AB. Aspects on the anatomy of the female urethra with special relation to urinary continence. *Contrib Gynecol Obstet* 1983; 10: 1–31

4. DeLancey JOL. Correlative study of paraurethral anatomy. *Obstet Gynecol* 1986; 68: 91–97

5. Gosling JA, Dixon JS, Critchley HOD, Thompson SA. A comparative study of the human external sphincter and periurethral levator ani muscles. *Br J Urol* 1981; 53: 35–41

6. Rud T, Anderson KE, Asmussen M *et al.* Factors maintaining the intraurethral pressure in women. *Invest Urol* 1980; 17: 343–347

7. Dröes JTPM. Observations on the musculature of the urinary bladder and urethra in the human foetus. *Br J Urol* 1974; 46: 179–185

8. Berkow SG. The corpus spongiosum of the urethra: its possible role in urinary control and stress incontinence in women. *Am J Obstet Gynecol* 1953; 65: 346–351

9. Huffman J. Detailed anatomy of the paraurethral ducts in the adult human female. *Am J Obstet Gynecol* 1948; 55: 86–101

10. McGuire EJ. The innervation and function of the lower urinary tract. *J Neurosurg* 1986; 65: 278–285

11. McGuire EJ. Urodynamic findings in patients after failure of stress incontinence operations. *Prog Clin Biol Res* 1981; 78: 351–360

12. Hodgkinson CP. Relationships of the female urethra in urinary incontinence. *Am J Obstet Gynecol* 1953; 65: 560–573

13. Muellner SR. Physiology of micturition. *J Urol* 1951; 65: 805–810

14. Westby M, Asmussen M, Ulmsten U. Location of maximum intraurethral pressure related to urogenital diaphragm in the female subject as studied by simultaneous urethrocystometry and voiding urethrocystography. *Am J Obstet Gynecol* 1982; 144: 408–412

15. Ricci JV, Thom CH. The myth of a surgically useful fascia in vaginal plastic reconstructions. *Q Rev Surg Obstet Gynecol* 1954; 2: 261–263

16. Uhlenhuth E, Nolley GW. Vaginal fascia a myth? *Obstet Gynecol* 1957; 10: 349–358

17. DeLancey JOL. Anatomic aspects of vaginal eversion after hysterectomy. *Am J Obstet Gynecol* 1992; 166: 1717–1728

18. Range RL, Woodburne RT. The gross and microscopic anatomy of the transverse cervical ligaments. *Am J Obstet Gynecol* 1964; 90: 460–467

19. Campbell RM. The anatomy and histology of the sacrouterine ligaments. *Am J Obstet Gynecol* 1950; 59: 1–12

20. Bartscht KD, DeLancey JOL. A technique to study cervical descent. *Obstet Gynecol* 1988; 72: 940–943

21. Dickinson RL. Studies of the levator ani muscle. *Am J Dis Women* 1889; 22: 897–917

22. Lawson JON. Pelvic anatomy. I Pelvic floor muscles. *Ann R Coll Surg Engl* 1974; 54: 244–252

23. Lawson JON. Pelvic anatomy. II Anal canal and associated sphincters. *Ann R Coll Surg Engl* 1974; 54: 288–300

24. Parks AG, Porter NH, Melzak J. Experimental study of the reflex mechanism controlling muscles of the pelvic floor. *Dis Colon Rectum* 1962; 5: 407–414

25. Berglas B, Rubin IC. Study of the supportive structures of the uterus by levator myography. *Surg Gynecol Obstet* 1953; 97: 677–692

26. Nichols DH, Milley PS, Randall CL. Significance of restoration of normal vaginal depth and axis. *Obstet Gynecol* 1970; 36: 251–256

27. Paramore RH. The uterus as a floating organ. *The Statics of the Female Pelvic Viscera*. London: HK Lewis, 1918; 12–15

28. Oelrich TM. The striated urogenital sphincter muscle in the female. *Anat Rec* 1983; 205: 223–232

29. Hilton P, Stanton SL. Urethral pressure measurement by microtransducer: the results in symptom-free women and in those with genuine stress incontinence. *Br J Obstet Gynaecol* 1983; 90: 919–933

30. Constantinou CE. Resting and stress urethral pressures as a clinical guide to the mechanism of continence in the female patient. *Urol Clin North Am* 1985; 12: 247–258

31. DeLancey JOL. Structural aspects of the extrinsic continence mechanism *Obstet Gynecol* 1988; 72: 296–301

32. Zacharin RF. The anatomic supports of the female urethra. *Obstet Gynecol* 1968; 21: 754–759

33. Milley PS, Nichols DH. Relationship between the pubo-urethral ligaments and the urogenital diaphragm in the human female. *Anat Rec* 1971; 170: 81–83

34. Richardson AC, Edmonds PB, Williams NL. Treatment of stress urinary incontinence due to paravaginal fascial defect. *Obstet Gynecol* 1981; 57: 357–362

35. DeLancey JOL. Structural support of the urethra as it relates to stress urinary incontinence: the hammock hypothesis. *Am J Obstet Gynecol* 1994; 170: 1713–1720

36. Noll LE, Hutch JA. The SCIPP line – an aid in interpreting the voiding lateral cystourethrogram. *Obstet Gynecol* 1969; 33: 680–689

37. Jeffcoate TNA, Roberts H. Observations on stress incontinence of urine. *Am J Obstet Gynecol* 1952; 64: 721–738

38. Woodburne RT. Anatomy of the bladder and bladder outlet. *J Urol* 1968; 100: 474–487

39. DeLancey JOL. Pubovesical ligament: a separate structure from the urethral supports (pubo-urethral ligaments). *Neurourol Urodynam* 1989; 8: 53–62

40. Wilson PD, Dixon JS, Brown ADG, Gosling JA. Posterior pubo-urethral ligaments in normal and genuine stress incontinent women. *J Urol* 1983; 130: 802–805

41. Power RMH. An anatomical contribution to the problem of continence and incontinence in the female. *Am J Obstet Gynecol* 1954; 67: 302–314

12

Clinical physiology of micturition

J. L. Mostwin

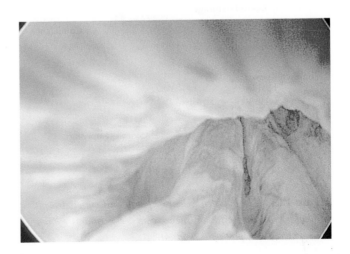

INTRODUCTION

Clinicians need a simple, practical concept of micturition to understand lower urinary tract symptoms, to plan and interpret objective studies in women with incontinence and voiding dysfunction, and to feel confident in their aproach to the patient. One such concept is that of the bladder cycle, incorporating all major elements of bladder function and continence into a continuous whole (Fig. 12.1).

The physiological basis of most components of the bladder cycle is understood. In the normal adult human, the bladder is constantly filled and periodically emptied. There is conscious awareness of filling and the eventual need to void, subliminal guarding against involuntary leakage by recruitment of external sphincter activity, and sustained bladder contraction and sphincteric relaxation coordinated by a set of spinally mediated reflexes.

Clinical urodynamic testing to evaluate bladder function begins at one part of this cycle, usually at the start of filling when the bladder is emptied naturally or by catheter, and progresses to the point where urine is discharged by normal or abnormal means (including clinical incontinence). An experienced urodynamic examiner can study only selected elements of the bladder cycle yet still emerge with a comprehensive understanding of the patient's function. In addition to a physiological approach, mastery of urodynamic practice also requires an understanding of lower urinary tract musculature and the major neuroanatomical pathways regulating it.

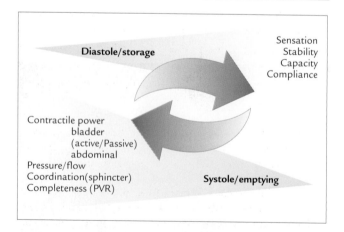

Figure 12.1. *The bladder cycle incorporates all major elements of bladder function and continence into a continuous conceptual whole. PVR, post-void residual.*

This chapter reviews the important experimental and clinical work that has given rise to modern concepts of bladder function. The selections have been chosen for their relevance to clinical work. Anatomical concepts relevant to understanding lower urinary tract function are also reviewed, and finally, essential clinical events of the bladder cycle are described. Many comprehensive reviews of bladder physiology may be found in major textbooks[1-3] and in the clinical and scientific literature. The recent report of the World Health Organization *1st International Consultation on Incontinence*[4] provides the most up-to-date summary of information in the field.

EARLY PHYSIOLOGICAL STUDIES: EXPERIMENTAL WORK

Early physiological studies focused on resting activity of the bladder, reflexes underlying voiding physiology produced by bladder filling or urethral manipulation, and the relative roles of the sympathetic and parasympathetic nervous systems in controlling these reflexes.

Sherrington's animal experiments at the end of the 19th century first showed that the bladder was spontaneously active, governed by rhythmic pacemaker activity which could be influenced by stimulation of spinal nerve roots. It was already known that the mammalian bladder had a parasympathetic motor innervation arising from anterior sacral roots 2, 3 and 4 carried in pelvic nerves, and a sympathetic motor innervation arising from the mid-lumbar roots carried in the hypogastric nerves. Both nerves merged presacrally to form a pelvic plexus from which postganglionic fibres were distributed to lower pelvic viscera. Sherrington[5] was the first to study the effect of nerve stimulation on the bladder by the volumetric methods developed previously by two clinicians, Mosso and Pellicani,[6] replacing the previous method of visual inspection by which activation of the bladder muscle upon nerve stimulation was determined. Sherrington knew that Mosso and Pellicani had previously recorded spontaneous fluctuations of intravesical pressures in conscious patients. He observed that stimulating either group of roots resulted in a distinctly unilateral contraction of the bladder, which varied in strength and character depending upon which roots were stimulated: sacral roots caused rapid, powerful contractions of brief duration; lumbar roots produced a weaker, longer-lasting contraction of longer latency. He noted that lumbar root stimulation produced a contraction difficult to distinguish from spontaneously occurring rhythmic contraction. He tried to abolish spontaneous activity by cutting the spinal cord, its roots and peripheral nerves in various combinations: spontaneous activity always persisted. Even after the bladder was removed from the animal and placed in a warm saline bath at an intravesical pressure of $2–4\,cmH_2O$, activity persisted. He was finally able to distinguish between lumbar and sacral efferent stimulation by eliminating spontaneous activity with large doses of morphine and chloralose. He concluded:

> It seems therefore justifiable to suppose that here . . . just as . . . in the middle third of the ureter . . . the rhythmic action of the monkey's bladder arises in its own muscular wall. Its 'beat', like that of the heart, is of intrinsic origin.

The recognition of spontaneous bladder activity has still not found a place in clinical neurourological practice, but continues to have a role in experimental work.

The first thorough description of reflex bladder activity was provided by Barrington.[7-9] He studied volumetric changes produced in the urethra and bladder of the cat in response to nerve stimulation, and described seven reflexes, as follows:

1. a hindbrain reflex evoked by distending the bladder, producing contraction of the bladder, having afferent and efferent paths in the pelvic nerves;
2. a hindbrain reflex evoked by running water through the urethra, producing bladder contraction, having afferent paths in pudendal and efferent paths in pelvic nerves;
3. a spinal reflex evoked by distending the proximal urethra, producing slight transient contraction, having afferent and efferent paths in hypogastric nerves;
4. a spinal reflex evoked by running water through the urethra, producing relaxation of the urethra, having afferent and efferent paths in the pudendal nerve;
5. a spinal reflex evoked by bladder distension, producing urethral relaxation, having afferents in pelvic and efferents in pudendal nerves;
6. a spinal reflex evoked by bladder distension, producing relaxation of the proximal urethra, having afferents and efferents in pelvic nerves;
7. a spinal reflex evoked by running water through the urethra, producing bladder contraction, having both paths in the pelvic nerves.

Barrington's reflexes form the core of most modern thinking about clinical neurourology, and are of particular interest to the clinician dealing with women's incontinence.

Langworthy *et al.*[10] experimentally localized the voiding centre to the brain stem. They created stereotactically controlled thermal lesions in the cat brain; recorded voiding behaviour, bladder and urethral function; and then performed post-mortem examinations to correlate physiological behaviour with locations of the brain lesions. Various areas of the cortex and cut brain stem were also stimulated. The most vigorous contraction of the bladder and the greatest associated intravesical pressure rise was produced by stimulating areas just lateral to the posterior commissure, and anterior and lateral to the aqueduct of Sylvius. They concluded:

> We have localized areas of the cerebral cortex of cats which on stimulation produced or stopped micturition. The bladder becomes hyperirritable to stretch stimuli after removal of the motor cortices. Reflex mechanisms in the midbrain appear to control tone in the vesical muscle.

It would take many years for Langworthy's observations to be accepted into general neurourological practice, replacing the widely held opinion that the voiding centre was located in the sacral cord.

Two additional important studies of bladder function were performed in conscious subjects prior to the Second World War. Denny-Brown and Robertson[11] studied the events of voiding and the volumetric changes of the bladder in relation to sphincter activity. They found spontaneous waves of pressure in the bladder during filling. As these increased in amplitude, subjective sensations of fullness or urinary urgency developed in the subjects. The subjects, when asked, could voluntarily suppress the summation of these pressure waves. Among their conclusions, those authors noted the following:

> Apart from a faint background of maintained tonic activity, spontaneous vesical activity takes the form of waves of contraction appearing in rhythmical progressions.

> Willed effort to micturate can evoke powerful contractions of the bladder with very brief latency of development. These contractions in their form and rhythm differ in no way from the spontaneous reaction of the viscus.

> Voluntary restraint of micturition has a direct effect on the contraction of the bladder, so that spontaneous nervous

discharges responsible for vesical contractions can be completely inhibited with ease.

Relaxation of the musculature of the perineum appears to be inseparably associated with the voluntary development of micturition.

The internal (involuntary) sphincter contracts and relaxes in reciprocal relationship with the detrusor muscle of the wall of the bladder.

The other study conducted before the Second World War was by Learmonth,[12] an Irish surgeon working at the Mayo Clinic. He observed the effects of direct hypogastric nerve stimulation and division on the urinary tract of conscious patients undergoing open pelvic operations. Unilateral stimulation resulted in contraction of the ipsilateral ureteral orifice; tightening of the trigone; contraction of the internal sphincter; and contraction of the musculature of the prostate, seminal vesicles and ejaculatory ducts. Sectioning the hypogastric nerve produced relaxation of the ureteral orifice, trigone and internal sphincter, with no appreciable effect on the dome or the lateral walls of the bladder. He cited two cases of low spinal cord injury in which the pelvic nerve supply to the bladder had been interrupted and voiding could not be accomplished until division of the hypogastrics had been performed. He concluded:

> ... the results of sympathetic neurectomy in the two cases cited in which inability to empty the bladder resulted from functional impairment of the parasympathetic system, the sympathetic system remaining intact, seems to me almost to force acceptance of the hypothesis that sympathetic influences act as a brake on contractions of the detrusor.

These historical studies treated the urinary bladder as an organ for the storage and expulsion of urine, much as a modern urodynamicist would, concentrating on hydrodynamics and integration by central and peripheral reflexes. Several conclusions emerged from these early studies, which remain valid today: (1) the bladder muscle is capable of rhythmic and spontaneous contraction *in* and *ex vivo*; (2) there is reciprocal innervation of the component parts of micturition mediated by sympathetic, parasympathetic and somatic pathways, and stimulation of each of the pathways produces effects specific for certain regions of the lower urinary tract; (3) the sensory events of micturition are represented at the cortical level and overall coordination and facilitation of voiding is regulated by the higher centres of the central nervous system.

More recent studies have reinforced and extended these early observations. Plum[13, 14] confirmed the persistence of autonomous bladder activity in animals and patients under general and spinal anaesthesia, even with pharmacological ganglionic blockade. El-Badawi and other anatomists have identified an extensive intramural network of ganglia in the various layers of the bladder,[15–18] and deGroat and co-workers have described local ganglionic responses to sensory stimulation of the bladder and identified several reflex pathways using electrophysiological techniques.[19, 20] Most interestingly, in view of Learmonth's observations on spinally injured patients, they have demonstrated that stimulation of bladder wall afferents results in reciprocal sympathetic inhibition of pelvic nerve efferent firing until a certain threshold of sensory stimulation is reached.

EARLY URODYNAMIC STUDIES: CLINICAL PHYSIOLOGY

The need to manage a large population of spinal cord injuries surviving the Second World War led to many detailed studies using water cystometry, radiography and clinical examination. Such studies led to the comprehensive classification of Bors and Comarr,[21] in which bladder dysfunction was classified by clinical signs and symptoms, correlated with whatever lesions were known to be present. Bors and Comarr borrowed the terms 'upper motor neuron' and 'lower motor neuron', used to describe skeletal muscle behaviour in high and low spinal injury, to describe two characteristic patterns of bladder activity that emerged after the period of spinal shock. The former, frequently associated with suprasacral injury, was characterized by a spastic bladder of small capacity, responding to filling with strong involuntary contractions, usually resulting in incontinence and often associated with simultaneous spastic, obstructing contractions of the external sphincter. The latter, frequently associated with sacral cord injury or pelvic crush injury, was associated with a larger flaccid bladder or a thickened, poorly compliant bladder incapable of generating contraction, and patulous internal and relaxed external sphincters, resulting in overflow incontinence. The 'spastic' and 'flaccid' nature of the two patterns of injury resulted in an appealing but incorrect analogy with skeletal muscle behaviour in similar conditions. It was generally assumed – and the idea was much popularized in urology[22] – that a sacral cord micturition centre was responsible for the voiding reflex, subject only to conscious inhibition by higher centres. Release of inhibition by suprasacral injury resulted in an 'uninhibited bladder', much as skeletal spasticity was due to damage to corticospinal tracts. Destruction of the sacral centre resulted in a flaccid bladder, much as lower cord or peripheral nerve injury resulted in flaccid skeletal muscle injury.

The terms 'upper and lower motor neuron' were misnomers: only pudendal nerves carry the axons of true motor neurons having cell bodies in the anterior horn, and which are involved in control of micturition. Pudendal nerves provide afferent and efferent pathways only to the external sphincter. (Poliomyelitis, in which anterior horn cells are damaged, is not generally associated with bladder dysfunction.) The motor supply to the bladder originates from neurons having their cell bodies in the intermediolateral cell column. None the less, the concept of a sacral micturition centre under the inhibition of higher centres was popular in urology from the 1950s to the mid-1970s.

The era of modern clinical urodynamics began with the work of Hinman and Miller in the 1950s.[23, 24] These authors investigated normal voiding, measured intravesical and intra-urethral pressure and urinary flow rate, and simultaneously observed cineradiographic changes in the bladder. They showed that a fall in urethral pressure and a radiographic sign of opening of the posterior urethra were the first events in normal voiding. In some women, they could see that a fall in urethral pressure alone was sufficient to achieve voiding; in men, higher intravesical pressures were required to overcome urethral resistance. These techniques were then successfully adopted at the Middlesex Hospital in London[25] to study patients with a large variety of voiding complaints.[26,27] Patterns of dysfunctional voiding, such as those with urinary outflow obstruction from benign prostatic hyperplasia or bladder-neck contracture, were identified in patients without overt neurological disease. Bladder overactivity found in patients without overt neurological disease was termed 'idiopathic detrusor instability'. The Middlesex group widely disseminated the urodynamic approach for the investigation and management of many patients with voiding complaints and was successful in focusing attention on the role of urinary tract function in everyday urology.

In the United States, urodynamic techniques were used by several groups to study adults[28,29] and children.[30] Of particular interest were studies of children with no neurological abnormalities but with functional incoordination of bladder and sphincters.[31] In children, non-neurological abnormalities such as posterior urethral valves led to prenatal and neonatal obstruction, and also resulted in eventual voiding abnormalities based on permanent bladder changes, even after surgical ablation of obstructing valves.[32] Studies such as these underscored the importance of obstruction alone as a cause of bladder overactivity and dysfunction. Voiding dysfunction in other congenital anomalies such as prune-belly syndrome[33] and bladder exstrophy[34] have also been studied. These investigations have resulted in a growing appreciation by clinicians of the integration of the various components of micturition and their clinical abnormalities.

CONTEMPORARY STUDIES

The most recent studies of bladder function have focused on the distribution and pharmacology of autonomic receptors in the urinary tract, their significance in the control of motility, the function of the smooth muscle of the bladder itself, the cellular and molecular control of voiding reflexes and the details of the function and integration of neuroanatomical pathways. Extensive work has shown that most mammalian bladder, urethral and prostate tissue is invested with homogeneously distributed muscarinic receptors, but that adrenergic receptors are unevenly distributed.[35,36] The bladder neck (internal sphincter) and urethra (especially in males) have a dense distribution of α-adrenoceptors, and the bladder dome contains β-adrenoceptors in a lesser density than α. There is now great interest in the plasticity of these receptor populations and reflexes because they are affected by obstruction, ageing and other sources of pathology. These findings have been utilized in several ways:

1. Krane and Olsson[37,38] first demonstrated that the bladder neck in spinal cord injury patients behaves autonomously; it is dependent on α-adrenergic stimulation; it is related to the syndrome of 'autonomic

dysreflexia', and it can be controlled by pharmacological α-adrenergic blockade.

2. Caine *et al.*[39] first studied the role of α-adrenoceptors in the prostate and bladder neck. This work has led to successful treatment of prostatic obstruction and acute urinary retention[40,41] and forms a cornerstone of modern management of prostatic obstruction.

3. Receptor populations may change after trauma or hormonal manipulation.[42] Increased α-adrenergic bladder innervation after spinal injury or obstruction may contribute to bladder instability.

4. Neural populations regulating reflex bladder function may undergo changes under the influence of urethral outflow obstruction or neural degeneration.[43] Hyperreflexia in patients with obstruction or lower urinary tract symptoms can be due in part to changes in these reflexes and may require pharmacological treatment specific for neurotransmission.[44]

5. Today, these developments have led to a widely utilized neurourological pharmacopoeia[44–47] to enhance or diminish contractility in the bladder or urethra.

These historical, urodynamic and pharmacological studies form the basis of our current concepts of urinary tract motility, as presented in the major urological textbooks and monographs dealing with this subject.[1–3,48–53] The degree of control theoretically predicted by urodynamic, physiological and pharmacological studies, however, remains disappointing.[46,54] Clinical studies tend to lag considerably behind the experimental ones on which most drug recommendations are based. Many clinicians consider the results of pharmacological treatment of voiding disorders disappointing. Attempts to denervate surgically or control pharmacologically, in particular, the uninhibited bladder have met with only partial success.[55] Among the reasons put forward are lack of understanding of normal physiological events associated with voiding and lack of understanding of basic pathophysiological changes in abnormal voiding, including the possible contributions of unknown non-adrenergic, non-cholinergic (NANC) neurotransmitters. Candidates for such a transmitter have included ATP, vasoactive intestinal polypeptide, prostaglandins and, most recently, nitric oxide.[56]

STRUCTURAL FEATURES RELEVANT TO FUNCTION

The bladder is mostly composed of interdigitating fibres of smooth muscle[57,58] which can stretch to almost four times resting length without increasing linear tension. This creates a hollow muscular viscus capable of storing increasing amounts of urine for prolonged periods of time at continuously low pressure until evacuation can be conveniently initiated. In contrast to intestinal smooth muscle, bladder smooth muscle is not organized into distinct inner longitudinal and outer circular layers except in the region of the urethra. These smooth muscle bundles act as interdigitating slings originating near the urethra, traversing the spherical dimensions of the bladder and coursing back to the urethra. The narrow portion of the internal urethral meatus, or bladder neck, provides sphincteric closure of the urethra by its very muscular arrangement. At the proximal urethra, which is the region of highest intraluminal pressure and, hence, of continence at rest, there is an inner longitudinal arrangement of muscular fibres, representing direct continuation of these muscle bundles, and a sleeve of outer circular muscle. In addition, a sleeve of circular striated muscle surrounds the urethra at this point, forming the external sphincter (rhabdosphincter).

The arrangement of smooth muscles at the internal urethral meatus, or proximal urethra, favours tonic closure at rest.[57,59,60] Although it is known that a fall in urethral pressure and radiographic signs of opening of the proximal urethra are the earliest signs of the initiation of normal micturition,[61] there is no general agreement on whether this takes place because the urethra is 'pulled open' (i.e. the longitudinal fibres extending into the urethra from the bladder shorten, pulling apart the circular fibres while the sphincter relaxes), or whether the urethral muscles themselves cease tonic activity. Various NANC transmitters have been proposed as mediators of the activity; the most recent of which is nitric oxide.[56]

Thickness and suppleness of muscle fibres and the collagen composition of the interstitium also affect storage compliance. Obstructive and neuropathic conditions such as myelodysplasia are associated with increased collagen deposition in the interstitium, probably secreted by the smooth muscle cells themselves in response to injury or obstruction.[62,63] The increasing presence of collagen may affect the distensibility of the bladder at higher filling volumes and may account for a loss of compliance and higher intravesical pressures during end-filling states. This can threaten an already compromised sphincter (as in myelodysplasia), produce vesicoureteral reflux and lead to increased urgency or trigger unstable contractions. Muscle thickness increases in lower cord myelodysplasia and hypertrophy following obstruction. Thicker muscle bundles are less distensible and less compliant and may lead to the same difficulties as stiffness due to collagen deposition.

THE BLADDER CYCLE

At birth, the bladder stores and discharges urine in a rhythmic manner independent of cortical control. This pattern gradually comes under voluntary control some time during the first 5 years of life. The development of voluntary control probably requires: development of sufficient strength and maturity of pelvic somatic musculature; cortical appreciation of proprioceptive signals regarding bladder fullness; cortical regulation of somatosensory pathways; and the ability to link the inhibition of voiding to voluntary contraction of the external urinary sphincter. When parental supervision is added to this 'toilet-training' period, the basic elements for early biofeedback training are in place. Similar methods are used in biofeedback and behavioural training programmes for incontinent adults to re-educate and restore these same reflexes. The technique of sacral stimulation of somatosensory pathways in the pudendal nerve for treatment of urge incontinence also relies on this form of reflex inhibition.

Bladder cycle I – diastole: the filling phase

The bladder cycle consists mostly of: time spent storing urine; accommodating to an increasing volume at low pressure; inhibiting contraction by giving rise to gradual awareness of filling; activating a reciprocal guarding reflex by rhabdosphincter contraction; and generating reciprocal inhibition of bladder parasympathetic stimulation. The important clinical elements of the filling phase, which can be measured during urodynamic testing, are sensation, stability, compliance, capacity and (although not usually considered to a great extent) recruitment of external sphincter activity. Each of these elements can vary independently and each may be studied by conventional clinical urodynamic techniques.

Sensation

Bladder sensation consists of several different sources of nervous information. *Proprioception,* the sensation of visceral distension, is transmitted by long-latency C-fibres in parasympathetic afferents travelling in the pelvic nerves to sacral segments 2, 3 and 4, and is then carried along the dorsal columns to the pons where it is integrated into processing centres that supply the cortex with a conscious sensation of bladder filling. *Nociception,* under normal conditions, transmits information about temperature and pain from the bladder mucosa. *Somatosensory perception* transmits information through sacral segments 2, 3 and 4 via the pudendal nerve about the state of the external sphincters and the distension or movement of fluid through the urethra. In the normal human, bladder sensation is never painful; it distinguishes warm from cold, and leads to increasing conscious awareness of filling. Conventional urodynamic testing distinguishes four distinct sensory phases during filling: (1) a first desire to void; (2) a sense of fullness; (3) a strong desire to void; (4) imminent voiding or urgency. Throughout this increasing awareness of voiding, the bladder should store urine at low pressures and there should be no leakage. Other than by evoked cortical potential studies, there is no objective way to evaluate sensation except by direct contact with the subject during a urodynamic test.

Bladder filling is not a purely passive phenomenon. Electromyographic recording (needle or surface) from the pelvic floor or the external sphincter show gradual recruitment of muscle activity, the so-called 'guarding reflex'. This indicates that cortical activity is taking place during filling, activating somatosensory pathways which increase sphincter contraction, increasing sphincteric resistance and also activating reciprocal inhibitory pathways which reduce bladder muscle contractility.

Sensation can be diminished selectively by disease such as diabetic or alcoholic neuropathy, tabes dorsalis or subacute combined deficiency (vitamin B12 and folate deficiency). Pain or dysaesthesia can be produced by inflammation, bladder stone, infection, radiation or interstitial cystitis. Abnormal sensation may be produced by altered spinal cord reflexes, learned behaviour or pelvic muscle spasm, none of which directly involves the bladder itself but all of which can lead to urgency, urge incontinence, pain or reduced storage capacity. This particular area of disordered sensation is an important area of contemporary research.

Cortical lesions affecting sensation (brain tumour, stroke, Alzheimer's disease) may reduce cortical awareness and thus inhibition, and may permit incontinence despite a normal lower urinary tract.

Stability

Absence of involuntary bladder contraction during filling is considered to be a hallmark of normal adult function. During filling, bladder capacity is normally reached with increasing awareness of fullness but without phasic increases in bladder pressure. Phasic increases in bladder pressure can occur with or without the individual's awareness that something is happening in the bladder. Involuntary contractions may occur with or without a sensation of urgency or impending urination, during the filling phase or only at capacity, and with or without associated changes in bladder compliance. The International Continence Society has arbitrarily decided that phasic contractions equivalent to a pressure of $15 \, cmH_2O$ or more may be defined as unstable bladder contraction. In clinical practice this value serves only as a guideline, and many problems related to stability remain unsolved.

Instability can be produced or elicited by rapid filling of the bladder (a rate exceeding $100 \, ml/min$) or the use of gas or cold water as a filling medium. More common causes are obstruction and neurological injury/illness. The greatest problem in clinical neuro-urology is relating the findings of stability during cystometry to the clinical presence of urgency and urge incontinence. Many patients with urge incontinence are presumed to have bladder overactivity and unstable contractions, even if testing conditions fail to demonstrate them.

However, there is a significant problem relating the sensory symptom of urgency and urge incontinence to the urodynamic finding of instability. Exactly how urgency and motor instability are related is not clear. If some historical background is considered, bladder instability was first characterized in patients with spinal injury; because these men often suffered from urgency and urge incontinence, it was assumed that instability and urgency were related. Then, the Middlesex group showed that prostatic obstruction was associated with urgency and urodynamic evidence of bladder instability, resolving in up to 75% of affected patients after prostatectomy.[64] These kinds of observations led to the hypothesis that urgency is a symptom of underlying

unstable contractions: as bladder pressure rises, the patient experiences an impending need to void, sometimes with expulsion of urine: *urge incontinence*. Animal experiments also supported this hypothesis: partial urethral obstruction, similar to prostatic obstruction, resulted in bladder muscle hypertrophy and unstable contractions during cystometry *in vivo*.[65] However, more recent animal work has shown that experimental urethral obstruction produces new neurological reflexes associated with increased frequency of voiding and evidence of unstable contractions on cystometry. In a rat model of partial urethral obstruction, the number of sensory nerve cell bodies in the dorsal ganglia increases, as do the neurological events associated with reflex voiding.[66] Nerve growth factor secreted by the smooth muscle cells of the bladder after obstruction may initiate the proliferation of sensory and sympathetic neurons and the development of these increased reflexes.[67] Thus, it has been suggested that the emergence of new spinal reflexes may lead to urgency and frequency in the absence of direct bladder abnormalities. It is, therefore, important for the clinician to keep separate the concepts of motor bladder instability as demonstrated on cystometry and the clinical symptoms of urgency, frequency and urge incontinence, which have recently been brought together under the acronym LUTS (lower urinary tract symptoms).[68]

In summary, there is experimental evidence that instability can be due to either sensory or motor changes in the bladder. During filling cystometry it is not possible to distinguish between the two; that is why it is essential to determine whether contractions are associated with abnormal sensation.

Compliance

Compliance is a measure of bladder elasticity or tone, mathematically described as change in volume with respect to pressure. During normal filling, bladder pressure remains low. A bladder demonstrating decreased compliance during filling is described as hypertonic. The compliance of a normal bladder is almost infinite until capacity is reached: graphic representation of pressure as a function of volume (the cystometrogram) is essentially flat. The flatness of this curve is due to (a) reciprocal inhibitory pathways, (b) anatomical arrangement and great stretching potential of smooth muscle of the bladder, and (c) absence of restriction by collagen. Disturbance of any of these three factors can significantly alter compliance, increasing pressure during filling. Increased pressure during filling at lower volumes is a clinical finding of extreme importance. At resting intravesical pressures greater than 40 cmH$_2$O, the ability of the ureters to propel urine from the renal pelvis is compromised, hydrostatic pressures are transmitted to the upper tracts and renal deterioration commences.[69] Increased intravesical pressures at lower volumes may also work against a sphincter which is compromised by intrinsic deficiency or poor support, increasing the chances of incontinence due to sphincteric opening at a volume lower than would be seen otherwise.

Causes of reduced compliance include bladder muscle hypertrophy, which results from bladder outlet obstruction, most typically seen in adult men with prostatic obstruction and boys with posterior urethral valves. In adult women it is most likely to be seen following iatrogenic obstruction following surgery for stress incontinence. Hypertrophied muscle is less elastic than normal detrusor smooth muscle and it has also synthesized increased amounts of collagen, further increasing stiffness. Decentralization of the bladder – as in myelodysplasia or spinal cord injury, or after such operations as cytolysis – may also lead to hypertrophic musculature and increased collagen deposition. Age alone may lead to a partial replacement of bladder smooth muscle by collagen.

Changes in compliance and stability may be found together in the presence of neurological injury or disease, physical damage to the bladder by radiation or fibrosis, or after prolonged catheter drainage leading to increased compliance. In this setting, the phasic changes of instability are superimposed upon the rising slope of tonicity. Thus a bladder may be both hypertonic and hyperactive.

Capacity

Capacity is the volume to which the bladder will fill until voiding commences voluntarily or involuntarily due to contraction, sphincteric relaxation, sphincteric incompetence or rising intravesical pressure which overcomes sphincteric resistance. Absolute capacity is limited at its maximum by the viscoelastic properties of the bladder, the physical limits of smooth muscle stretch and the resistance of the outflow. Relative functional capacity can be affected by sensation, stability or decreased compliance. Residual urine can alter functional capacity by functioning as storage 'dead space', which limits the amount of urine the bladder will store during the voiding interval. A large bladder, which may hold 1000 ml or more, may void only 200 ml at a time, so that the functional capacity is only 200 ml. Normal values for capacity in adults have not been determined; however, generally accepted values range between 280 and 600 ml.

Bladder cycle II – systole: the emptying phase

The important elements of the emptying phase are (a) sources of power for bladder emptying, (b) urethral opening and sphincteric coordination, and (c) urinary flow rate and pattern, voiding pressure and completeness of emptying.

Young and Wesson, after cystopic examination of men while voiding, suggested that the trigonal muscle contracted and appeared to flatten the elevated ridge of bladder neck muscle. They proposed this as a mechanism of urethral opening.[70]

Hutch studied anatomical dissections of trigone and proximal urethra and observed voiding using fluoroscopy. He proposed that voiding commenced when the trigone flattened and the urethra funnelled to permit passage of urine.[60] This observation was remarkably similar to that in women with stress incontinence, studied by Jeffcoate and Roberts,[71] who, on the basis of lateral cystourethrograms, concluded:

> the most characteristic anatomical change, present in four out of five cases of incontinence, is loss of the posterior vesico-urethral angle so that the urethra and the trigone tend to come into line.

Hinman and Miller, as described earlier, observed that opening of the urethra was the first event in normal bladder emptying. McGuire[61] has also reported opening of the bladder neck (proximal urethra) as the first videourodynamic sign of normal voiding or bladder contraction; it is usually associated with cessation of electrical activity of the sphincter. These findings are remarkably consistent with Barrington's observation, made more than 50 years ago.

Although it is generally agreed that the urethra opens during the first phase of normal micturition, there is no agreement about whether this is an active or passive phenomenon. Innervation and relaxation of the proximal urethra independent of bladder contraction was suggested by earlier studies of Tanagho, in which bladder neck and proximal urethra were surgically separated from the bladder body.[72] The presence and pharmacological response of α-adrenoceptors in the smooth muscle of the trigone and proximal urethra of both men and women would suggest a role for these receptors in the initiation of normal voiding; however, men who have undergone sympathectomy after retroperitoneal lymph node dissection for testis tumour and have lost seminal emission do not show voiding dysfunction. Recent evidence suggests that nitric oxide may mediate active relaxation of proximal urethral smooth muscle.[73,74] A purely mechanical explanation for urethral opening by bladder contraction is suggested by the anatomical arrangement of smooth muscle of the urethra. The interdigitating bundles of the bladder form more distinct longitudinal bundles continuous with the urethra. The proximal urethra and the bladder form one organ. The proximal urethral portion, surrounded by skeletal muscle fibres of the voluntary sphincter, is the very area that shows opening on videourodynamic studies. Relaxation of a contracted external sphincter associated with shortening of detrusor muscle might explain the sort of events that are seen during the initiation of voiding. The relative roles of this kind of passive opening of the urethra and a more active relaxation of the smooth muscle component remain to be determined.

The source of power for urinary evacuation is normally a sustained contraction of detrusor smooth muscle fibres. It has been suggested that, during contraction, there is a synchronization of spontaneous subclinical contractions leading to a sustained contraction of the whole organ with successful emptying. This may take place by coordinated release of acetylcholine released from parasympathetic postganglionic nerve terminals in the bladder. There is probably a depolarization of smooth muscle cells with an inward flow of calcium current. Isolated electrical events in bladder muscle may spread to surrounding cells, spreading the wave of contraction. As more cells are depolarized, calcium is released from intracellular stores in individual muscle cells and made available to the actin/myosin complex in the muscle. This leads to shortening, which continues until the calcium is returned to the intracellular stores. The cellular events are dependent on energy from ATP produced by the mitochondria. A bladder forced to contract against obstruction, or

thickened by prolonged obstruction, shows decreased biochemical energy production, limiting its ability to sustain contraction. Whether abnormalities of bioenergetics are found in ageing alone has not yet been determined, but the clinical findings of detrusor hyperactivity with impaired contractility in the elderly suggest that this is possibile.[75]

In some patients, gravity alone may lead to expulsion of urine when the sphincter is relaxed, as Hinman and Miller demonstrated. In others, voluntary straining (Valsalva) or manual pressure on the bladder (Credé) can be used to enhance or replace diminished intrinsic bladder contraction. Throughout emptying there is normally a sensation of urine passing through the urethra, as Barrington found. During urodynamic testing it is possible to determine the relative contribution of abdominal and intrinsic forces to the expulsion of urine, and the sensation that accompanies it.

Sphincteric coordination

Electromyographic activity recorded by simple external electrodes ceases during voiding and is usually associated with urethral relaxation as the first sign of normal voiding. This coordination undergoes changes in spinal cord disease/injury, most typically in quadriplegia or multiple sclerosis. Pathological contraction of the external sphincter during bladder contraction, termed detrusor sphincter dyssynergia (DSD), may be partial or total and, unless it represents a voluntary form of extreme attempts to prevent urination (such as in Hinman syndrome), is almost always associated with neurological disease. The effect of DSD on the bladder is similar to that of outlet obstruction.[29, 76]

Sphincteric relaxation and initiation of voiding is subject to powerful cortical influence, so clinical urodynamic testing can often be confounded by embarrassment or unpleasant or unfamiliar testing circumstances. This is an issue with which all urodynamicists must contend.

Flow rate and pattern

Urinary flow can be measured by recording the rate at which urinary volume accumulates in a receptacle, on a scale displaying the first derivative of volume with respect to time, dV/dt. Other flow meters use different techniques to produce a similar tracing. The maximum flow rate achieved during the expulsion of urine is generally considered the most important variable. The other important aspect of the flow rate is the pattern of the tracing. When normal, it appears as an abrupt rise in flow rate during the early phase of voiding, followed by a gradual return to zero. An abnormal pattern might show a slower rise to a lower maximum value followed by a long plateau phase, suggesting obstruction or weak contraction of the bladder. An intermittent or sawtooth pattern may suggest intermittent straining to overcome limited contractility or intermittent obstruction such as would occur with DSD. Most nomograms have been compiled to assist interpreting maximum urethral flow-rate values in men with infravesical obstruction.[77] The Liverpool nomograms have included women.[78]

Pressure–flow studies

Only simultaneous recording of intravesical and intra-abdominal pressure during voiding with flow rate and pattern can determine whether diminished flow is due to motor failure of the bladder or high-pressure voiding against an obstruction.[79] Nomograms relating intravesical pressure and flow rate have been established to aid in the clinical diagnosis of obstruction.[80] Much controversy regarding the correlation of predictions derived from these nomograms and clinical results from relief of obstruction still exists in urology.

COMPLETENESS OF EMPTYING

The presence of residual urine at the completion of voiding is considered abnormal. Functionally, it represents intravesical dead space, similar to an increased functional residual capacity in chronic obstructive pulmonary disease. It means that the bladder cycle is already partially through its filling phase before it has even begun.

Residual urine may be due to anatomical shunts such as diverticula, dilated refluxing ureters or cystoceles. A normal bladder contracting against high outlet resistance may fail to empty completely; however, in the absence of a shunt, a more likely cause is a partially decompensated bladder, which may fail to empty at all against an outlet obstruction or empty only partially after the obstruction has been relieved.

CONCLUSIONS

Further progress in neurourology will require an understanding of the basic mechanisms underlying contractility of the smooth muscle and the reflexes that coordinate and integrate the various components of the urinary tract and the central nervous system. The practitioner, however, can rely on the simple concept of the bladder cycle to incorporate all basic elements of bladder function and continence into a single whole, creating a useful framework for everyday work.

REFERENCES

1. Bradley WF. Physiology of the urinary bladder. In: Walsh PC, Gittes RE, Perlmutter AD, Stamey TA (eds) *Campbell's Urology*, 5th edn. Philadelphia: Saunders, 1986; 129–185

2. Steers WD. Physiology of the urinary bladder. In: Walsh PC, Retik AB, Stamey TA, Vaughn E Jr (eds) *Campbell's Urology*, 6th edn. Philadephia: Saunders, 1992; 142–176

3. Steers WD, Persson K. Neurophysiology of bladder and urethral function. In: Whitfield HN, Hendry WF, Kirby RS *et al.* (eds) *Textbook of Genitourinary Surgery*, 2nd edn. Oxford: Blackwell Science, 1998;

4. Abrams P, Khoury S, Wein A. *Incontinence (1st International Consultation on Incontinence of the World Health Organization).* Plymouth: Health Publications, 1999

5. Sherrington CS. Notes on the arrangment of some motor fibres in the lumbo-sacral plexus. *J Physiol (Lond)* 1892; 13: 621–772

6. Mosso A, Pellicani P. [Observations]. *Arch Biol (Paris)* 1882; 1: 97, 291

7. Barrington FJF. The nervous mechanism of micturition. *Q J Exp Physiol* 1915; 8: 33–71

8. Barrington FJF. The component reflexes of micturition in the cat. Parts I and II. *Brain* 1931; 54: 177–188

9. Barrington FJF. The component reflexes of micturition in the cat. Part III. *Brain* 1941; 64: 239–243

10. Langworthy OR, Kolb LC, Lewis LG. *Physiology of Micturition.* Baltimore: Williams and Wilkins; 1940

11. Denny-Brown D, Robertson EG. On the physiology of micturition. *Brain* 1933; 56: 149–190

12. Learmonth JR. A contribution to the neurophysiology of the urinary bladder in man. *Brain* 1931; 54: 147–176

13. Plum F. Autonomous urinary bladder activity in man. *Arch Neurol Psychiatry* 1960; 2: 497–503

14. Plum F, Cofelt RH. The genesis of vesical rhythmicity. *Arch Neurol Psychiatry* 1960; 2: 487–503

15. El-Badawi A, Schenk EA. Dual innervation of the mammalian urinary bladder. *Am J Anat* 1966; 119: 405–428

16. El-Badawi A, Schenk EA. A new theory of innervation of

bladder musculature. Part I: morphology of intrinsic vesical innervation apparatus. *J Urol* 1968; 99: 585–587

17. El-Badawi A, Schenk EA. A new theory of innervation of bladder musculature. Part 4: innervation of the vesicourethral junction and external sphincter. *J Urol* 1974; 111: 613–615

18. Dixon JS, Gilpin SA, Gilpin CJ *et al.* Intramural ganglia of the human urinary bladder. *Br J Urol* 1983; 55: 195–198

19. DeGroat WC, Saum WR. Synaptic transmission in parasympathetic ganglia in the urinary bladder of the cat. *J Physiol (Lond)* 1976; 256: 137–158

20. DeGroat WC. Mechanisms underlying recurrent inhibition in the sacral parasympathetic outflow to the urinary bladder. *J Physiol (Lond)* 1976; 257: 503–513

21. Bors E, Comarr AE. *Neurological Urology.* Baltimore: University Park Press, 1971

22. Lapides J, Diokno A. Urine transport, storage and micturition. In: Lapides J (ed) Philadelphia: Saunders, 1976; 190–241

23. Hinman F Jr, Miller GM, Nickel E *et al.* Vesical physiology demonstrated by cineradiography and serial roentgenography. *Radiology* 1954; 62: 713–719

24. Hinman F Jr, Miller GM, Nickel E *et al.* Normal micturition – certain details as shown by serial cystograms. *California Med* 1955; 82: 6–7

25. Abrams P, Blaivas JG, Stanton SL *et al.* The standardisation of terminology of lower urinary tract function. The International Continence Society Committee on Standardisation of Terminology. *Scand J Urol Nephrol Suppl* 1988; 5–19

26. Turner-Warwick RC, Whiteside CG. Clinical urodynamics. *Urol Clin North Am* 1979; 6: 1–293

27. Turner-Warwick RC, Whiteside CG. Urodynamic studies and their effect upon management. In: Chisholm G, Williams DI (eds) *Scientific Foundations of Urology.* London: William Heinemann, 1982; 442–257

28. Blaivas JG, Fisher DM. Combined radiographic and urodynamic monitoring: advances in techniques. *J Urol* 1981; 125: 693–694

29. Blaivas JG, Sinha HP, Zayed AAH *et al.* Detrusor external dyssynergia: a detailed electromyographic study. *J Urol* 1981; 125: 545–548

30. Cook WS, Firlit C, Stephens FD. Techniques and results of urodynamic evaluation in children. *J Urol* 1977; 117: 346–349

31. Allen TD. The non-neurogenic, neurogenic bladder. *J Urol* 1977; 117: 232–238

32. Bauer SB, Dieppa RA, Labib KK *et al.* The bladder in boys with posterior urethral valves: a urodynamic assessment. *J Urol* 1979; 121: 769–773

33. Cromie W, Duckett J. Urodynamics in childhood. *Urol Clin North Am* 1979; 6: 227–236

34. Toguri AG, Churchill BM, Schillinger JF *et al.* Continence in cases of bladder exstrophy. *J Urol* 1978; 119: 538–540

35. Edvardsen P, Setekleiv J. Distribution of adrenergic receptors in the urinary bladder of cats, rabbits and guinea pigs. *Acta Pharmacol Toxicol Scand* 1968; 26: 437–445

36. Awad SA, Bruce AW, Cano-Ciampi G *et al.* Distribution of alpha and beta adrenoceptors in the human urinary bladder. *Br J Pharmacol* 1974; 50: 525–529

37. Krane R, Olsson C. Phenoxybenzamine in neurogenic bladder dysfunction. I: A theory of micturition. *J Urol* 1973; 110: 650–652

38. Krane R, Olsson C. Phenoxybenzamine in neurogenic bladder dysfunction. II: Clinical considerations. *J Urol* 1973; 110: 653–656

39. Caine M, Raz S, Ziegler M. Adrenergic and cholinergic receptors in the human prostate, prostatic capsule and bladder neck. *Br J Urol* 1975; 47: 193–202

40. Caine M, Pfam S, Perlberg S. The use of alpha-adrenergic blockade in benign prostatic obstruction. *Br J Urol* 1976; 48: 252–255

41. Christmas TJ, Kirby RS. Alpha-adrenoceptor blockers in the treatment of benign prostatic hyperplasia. *World J Urol* 1991; 9: 36–40

42. Sundin T, Dahlstrom A. The sympathetic innervation of the bladder and urethra in the normal state and after parasympathetic denervation at the spinal root level. *Scand J Urol Nephrol* 1973; 7: 131–149

43. Steers WD, De Groat WC. Effect of bladder outlet obstruction on micturition reflex pathways in the rat. *J Urol* 1988; 140: 864–871

44. De Groat WC, Downie JW, Levin RM *et al.* Basic neurophysiology and neuropharmacology. In: Abrams P, Khoury S, Wein A (eds) *Incontinence (1st International Consultation on Incontinence of the World Health Organization).* Plymouth: Health Publications, 1999; 105–154

45. Wein AJ. Pharmacology of the bladder and urethra. In: Mundy AR, Stephenson T, Wein AJ (eds) *Urodynamics: Principles, Practice and Applications.* Edinburgh: Churchill Livingstone, 1983; 26–41

46. Milroy E. Pharmacologic management of common urodynamic problems. *Urol Clin North Am* 1979; 6: 265–272

47. Hald T, Andersen JT. Pharmacology of the lower urinary tract. In: Whitfield HN, Hendry WF, Kirby RS *et al.* (eds) *Textbook of Genitourinary Surgery*, 2nd edn. Oxford: Blackwell Science, 1998; 458–464

48. Bissada NK, Finkbeiner AE. *Lower Urinary Tract Function and Dysfunction: Diagnosis and Management*. New York: Appleton-Century-Crofts, 1978

49. Hald T, Bradley WF. *The Urinary Bladder: Neurology and Dynamics*. Baltimore: Williams and Wilkins, 1982

50. Yalla SV, McGuire EJ, Elbadawi A *et al. Neurourology and Urodynamics: Principles and Practice*. New York: Macmillan, 1988

51. McGuire EJ. *Clinical Evaluation and Treatment of Neurogenic Vesical Dysfunction*. Baltimore: Williams and Wilkins, 1984

52. Mundy AR. Clinical physiology of the bladder, urethra and pelvic floor. In: Mundy AR, Stephenson T, Wein AJ (eds) *Urodynamics: Principles, Practice and Applications*. Edinburgh: Churchill Livingstone, 1983

53. Smith JC. The function of the bladder. In: Blandy J (ed) *Urology*. Oxford: Blackwell, 1976

54. Benson T. Drug therapy for voiding disorders: why all the confusion? In: Barrett DM, Wein AJ (eds) *Controversies in Neuro-Urology*. Edinburgh: Churchill Livingstone, 1981; 253–259

55. Mundy AR. The surgical treatment of detrusor instability. *Neurourol Urodyn* 1986; 4: 357–365

56. Lee JG, Wein AJ, Levin RM. Comparative pharmacology of the male and female rabbit bladder neck and urethra: involvement of nitric oxide. *Pharmacology* 1994; 48: 250–259

57. Tanagho EA. Surgical anatomy of the genitourinary tract: anatomy of the lower urinary tract. In: Walsh PC, Retik AB, Stamey TA, Vaughn E Jr (eds) *Campbell's Urology*, 6th edn. Philadelphia: Saunders, 1992; 40–68

58. Gosling J, Alm P, Bartsch G *et al*. Gross anatomy of the lower urinary tract. In: Abrams P, Khoury S, Wein A (eds) *Incontinence (1st International Consultation on Incontinence of the World Health Organization)*. Plymouth: Health Publications, 1999; 21–56

59. Hutch JA, Amar AA. *Vesicoureteral Reflux and Pyelonephritis*. New York: Appleton-Century-Crofts, 1972

60. Hutch JA. *Anatomy and Physiology of the Bladder, Trigone and Urethra*. New York: Appleton-Century-Crofts, 1972

61. McGuire EJ. *Clinical Evaluation and Treatment of Neurogenic Vesical Dysfunction*. Baltimore: Williams and Wilkins, 1984

62. Murakumo M, Ushiki T, Koyanagi T *et al*. Scanning electron microscopic studies of smooth muscle cells and their collagen fibrillar sheaths in empty, distended and contracted urinary bladders of the guinea pig. *Arch Histol Cytol* 1993; 56: 441–449

63. Murakumo M, Ushiki T, Abe K *et al*. Three-dimensional arrangement of collagen and elastin fibres in the human urinary bladder: a scanning electron microscopic study. *J Urol* 1995; 154: 251–256

64. Turner-Warwick RT, Whiteside CG, Arnold EP. A urodynamic view of prostatic obstruction and the results of prostatectomy. *Br J Urol* 1973; 45: 631–645

65. Brading AF, Mostwin JL, Sibley GN *et al*. The role of smooth muscle and its possible involvement in diseases of the lower urinary tract. *Clin Sci* 1986; 70: 7s–13s

66. Steers WD, Ciambotti J, Etzel B *et al*. Alterations in afferent pathways from the urinary bladder of the rat in response to partial urethral obstruction. *J Comp Neurol* 1991; 310: 401–410

67. Steers WD, Kolbeck S, Creedon D *et al*. Nerve growth factor in the urinary bladder of the adult regulates neuronal form and function. *J Clin Invest* 1991; 88: 1709–1715

68. Jackson S, Donovan J, Brookes S *et al*. The Bristol Female Lower Urinary Tract questionnaire: development and psychometric testing. *Br J Urol* 1996; 77: 805–812

69. Wan J, McGuire EJ, Bloom DA *et al*. Stress leak point pressure: a diagnostic tool for incontinent children. *J Urol* 1993; 150: 700–702

70. Young HH, Wesson MB. The anatomy and surgery of the trigone. *Arch Surg* 1921; 3: 1–37

71. Jeffcoate TNA, Roberts H. Observations on stress incontinence of urine. *Am J Obstet Gynecol* 1952; 64: 721–738

72. Tanagho EA, Smith DR. Anatomy and function of the bladder neck. *Br J Urol* 1966; 38: 54

73. Bennett BC, Vizzard MA, Booth AM *et al*. Role of nitric oxide in reflex urethral sphincter relaxation during micturition. *Soc Neurosci Abstr* 1993; 19: 511

74. Thornbury KD, Hollywood MA, McHale NG. Mediation by nitric oxide of neurogenic relaxation of the urinary bladder neck muscle in sheep. *J Physiol (Lond)* 1992; 451: 133–144

75. Brading AF, Fry CH, Maggi CA *et al*. Cellular biology. In: Abrams P, Khoury S, Wein A (eds) Incontinence *(1st International Consultation on Incontinence of the World Health Organization)*. Plymouth: Health Publications, 1999; 57–104

76. Bushman W, Steers WD, Meythaler JM. Voiding dysfunction in patients with spastic paraplegia: urodynamic evaluation and response to continuous intrathecal baclofen. *Neurourol Urodyn* 1993; 12: 163–170

77. Siroky MB, Krane RJ, Olsson CA. The flow rate nomogram. I. Development. *J Urol* 1979; 122: 665–668

78. Haylen BT, Ashby D, Sutherst JR *et al*. Maximum and average urine flow rates in normal male and female

populations – the Liverpool nomograms. *Br J Urol* 1989; 64: 30–38

79. Chancellor MB, Balivas JG, Kaplan SA *et al.* Bladder outlet obstruction versus impaired detrusor contractility: the role of uroflow. *J Urol* 1991; 145: 810–812

80. Schafer W. Analysis of bladder-outlet function with the linearized passive urethral resistance relation, linPURR, and a disease-specific approach for grading obstruction: from complex to simple. *World J Urol* 1995; 13: 47–58

13

Pharmacology of the bladder

K.-E. Andersson, K. Waldeck

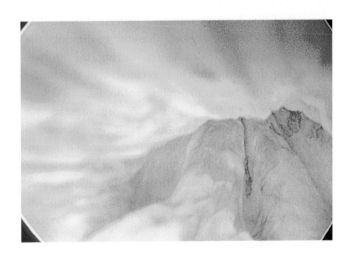

INTRODUCTION

Pharmacological treatment of urinary incontinence is a main option, and several drugs with different modes and sites of action have been tried with varying degrees of success.[1-4] However, to be able to optimize treatment, knowledge about the mechanisms of micturition and of the targets for treatment is necessary.

The lower urinary tract is controlled by a complex interplay between the central and peripheral nervous systems and local regulatory factors.[5,6] Malfunction at various levels may result in micturition disorders, which can be roughly classified as disturbances of storage or emptying. Failure to store urine can lead to various forms of incontinence (mainly urge and stress incontinence), and can theoretically be improved by agents that decrease detrusor activity and increase bladder capacity, and/or increase outlet resistance.

This chapter is a brief review of the normal nervous control of the lower urinary tract and of some targets for treatment of urinary incontinence.

NERVOUS MECHANISMS FOR BLADDER EMPTYING AND URINE STORAGE

The nervous mechanisms for bladder emptying and urine storage involve a complex pattern of efferent and afferent signalling in parasympathetic, sympathetic and somatic nerves (Fig. 13.1). These nerves constitute reflex pathways which either maintain the bladder in a relaxed state, enabling urine storage at low intravesical pressure, or which initiate micturition by relaxing the outflow region and contracting the bladder smooth muscle. Under normal conditions, there is a reciprocal relationship between the activity in the detrusor and the activity in the outlet region. During voiding, contraction of the detrusor muscle is preceded by a relaxation of the outlet region, thereby facilitating the bladder emptying.[7-9] Conversely, during the storage phase, the detrusor muscle is relaxed, and the outlet region is contracted to maintain continence.

Contraction of the detrusor smooth muscle and relaxation of the outflow region result from activation of *parasympathetic* neurons located in the sacral parasympathetic nucleus in the spinal cord at the level of S2–S4.[3,10] The axons pass through the pelvic nerve and synapse with postganglionic nerves in the pelvic plexus, in ganglia on the surface of the bladder (vesical ganglia), or within the walls of the bladder and urethra

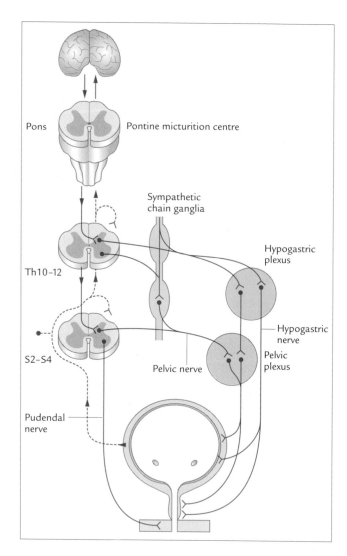

Figure 13.1. *Innervation of the lower urinary tract. The bladder and urethra receive parasympathetic (pelvic nerve), sympathetic (hypogastric nerve), as well as somatic (pudendal nerve) innervation. Sensory afferents can be found in the pelvic and hypogastric nerves as well as in the pudendal nerves.*

(intramural ganglia).[11] Preganglionic neurotransmission is mediated predominantly by acetylcholine acting on nicotinic receptors, although the transmission can be modulated by adrenergic, muscarinic, purinergic and peptidergic presynaptic receptors.[3] The postganglionic neurons in the pelvic nerve mediate the excitatory input to the human detrusor smooth muscle by releasing acetylcholine which acts on muscarinic receptors. However, an atropine-resistant component has been demonstrated in functionally and morphologically altered human bladder tissue.[5,12] It has been suggested that this atropine-resistant contraction is mediated by ATP.[13,14] In contrast, the bladder of several animal species has a notable non-adrenergic, non-cholinergic (NANC) contractile component.[15,16] It has been demonstrated that ATP is one important mediator of these contractions,[17] although the involvement of other transmitters cannot be ruled out.[5] The pelvic nerve also conveys parasympathetic fibres to the outflow region and the urethra. These fibres exert an inhibitory effect and thereby relax the outflow region. This is mediated partly by nitric oxide,[18] although other transmitters might be involved.[19–21]

Most of the *sympathetic* innervation of the bladder and urethra originates from the intermediolateral nuclei in the thoracolumbar region (T10–L2) of the spinal cord. The axons travel either through the inferior mesenteric ganglia (IMF) and the hypogastric nerve, or pass through the paravertebral chain and enter the pelvic nerve. Thus, sympathetic signals are conveyed in both the hypogastric nerve and the pelvic nerve.[11] Preganglionic sympathetic transmission, like the parasympathetic preganglionic transmission, is predominantly mediated by acetylcholine acting on nicotinic receptors. Some preganglionic terminals synapse with postganglionic cells in the paravertebral ganglia or in the IMF, while others synapse closer to the pelvic organs, and short postganglionic neurons innervate the target organs. Thus, the hypogastric and pelvic nerves contain both pre- and postganglionic fibres.[11] The predominant effects of the sympathetic innervation of the lower urinary tract in humans are inhibition of the parasympathetic pathways at spinal and ganglion levels, and mediation of contraction of the bladder base and the urethra. However, in several animals, adrenergic innervation of the detrusor is believed to inactivate the contractile mechanisms in the detrusor directly.[22] Noradrenaline is apparently released in response to electrical stimulation of detrusor tissues *in vitro*,[23] and the normal response of detrusor tissues to released noradrenaline is relaxation.[24,25]

Most of the *sensory* innervation of the bladder and urethra reaches the spinal cord via the pelvic nerve and dorsal root ganglia. In addition, some afferents travel in the hypogastric nerve. The sensory nerves of the striated muscle in the rhabdosphincter travel in the pudendal nerve to the sacral region of the spinal cord.[11] The most important afferents for the micturition process are myelinated Aδ-fibres and unmyelinated C-fibres

travelling in the pelvic nerve to the sacral spinal cord,[26] conveying information from receptors in the bladder wall to the spinal cord. The Aδ-fibres respond to passive distension and active contraction, thus conveying information about bladder filling.[27] The activation threshold for Aδ-fibres is 5–15 cmH$_2$O, which is the intravesical pressure at which humans report the first sensation of bladder filling.[3] C-fibres have a high mechanical threshold and respond primarily to chemical irritation of the bladder mucosa[28] and to cold.[29] Following chemical irritation, the C-fibre afferents exhibit spontaneous firing when the bladder is empty and increased firing during bladder distension.[28] These fibres are normally inactive and are therefore termed 'silent fibres'.

The storage phase

During the storage phase the bladder has to relax in order to maintain a low intravesical pressure. This relaxation is in part enabled by a spinal reflex pathway triggered by vesical afferent activity in the pelvic nerves, which initiates sympathetic firing from the lumbar region of the spinal cord. The sympathetic firing has an inhibitory effect on bladder ganglia, thereby decreasing excitatory parasympathetic inputs to the bladder.[3] In contrast to what has been found in several animal species, there is little evidence for a functionally important sympathetic innervation of the human detrusor. The sympathetic innervation of the human bladder is found mainly in the outlet region, where it mediates contraction during the storage phase. Hence, distension of the human bladder is enabled by the intrinsic properties of the bladder smooth muscle and the quiescence of the parasympathetic efferent pathways.[3,30] Thus, under normal conditions bladder distension during the filling phase activates Aδ-fibres which stimulate sympathetic efferents in the spinal cord. Thus, the Aδ-afferents and the sympathetic efferent fibres constitute a vesicospinovesical storage reflex which maintains the bladder in a relaxed mode while the proximal urethra and bladder neck are contracted.

The emptying phase

Vesicobulbovesical micturition reflex

Bladder filling leads to increased activation of tension receptors within the bladder wall and thus to increased afferent activity in Aδ-fibres. These fibres project onto spinal tract neurons mediating increased sympathetic firing to maintain continence as discussed above (storage reflex). In addition, the spinal tract neurons convey the afferent activity to more rostral areas of the spinal cord and the brain. One important receiver of the afferent information from the bladder is the pontine micturition centre (PMC) in the rostral brain stem. The PMC receives information both from afferent neurons in the bladder and from more rostral areas in the brain (i.e. the cerebral cortex and hypothalamus). This information is integrated in the PMC, which also controls the descending pathways in the micturition reflex. Thus, the PMC can be seen as a switch in the micturition reflex, inhibiting parasympathetic activity in the descending pathways when there is low activity in the afferent fibres, and activating the parasympathetic pathways when the afferent activity reaches a certain threshold.[3] The threshold is believed to be set by the inputs from more rostral regions in the brain. In cats, lesioning of regions above the inferior colliculus usually facilitates micturition by elimination of inhibitory inputs from the more rostral areas; on the other hand, transections at a lower level inhibit micturition. Thus, the PMC seems to be under tonic inhibitory control. Variation of the inhibitory input to the PMC results in variation of bladder capacity. Experiments in rats have shown that the micturition threshold is regulated by GABA-ergic inhibitory mechanisms in the PMC neurons[31] (see later).

Vesicospinovesical micturition reflex

Spinal lesions rostral to the lumbosacral level interrupt the vesicobulbovesical pathway and abolish the supraspinal and voluntary control of micturition. This results initially in an areflexic bladder accompanied by urinary retention.[3] An automatic vesicospinovesical micturition reflex develops slowly, although voiding is generally insufficient owing to bladder sphincter dyssynergia (i.e. simultaneous contraction of bladder and urethra). It has been demonstrated experimentally in cats with chronic spinal lesions that the afferent limb of this reflex is conveyed through unmyelinated C-fibres which usually do not respond to bladder distension,[28] suggesting changed properties of the afferent receptors in the bladder. Accordingly, the micturition reflex in cats with chronic spinal lesions is blocked by capsaicin, a neurotoxin which is believed to block part of the C-fibre-mediated neurotransmission (see Sensory nerves, page 145).[32,33]

TARGETS FOR PHARMACOLOGICAL INTERVENTION

CNS targets

Anatomically, several central nervous system (CNS) regions may be involved in micturition control: these include not only supraspinal structures – such as the cortex and diencephalon, midbrain and medulla – but also spinal structures.[3] Several transmitters are involved in the micturition reflex pathways described above and may be targets for drugs designed for control of micturition. However, few drugs with a CNS site of action have been developed.

GABA

GABA (γ-aminobutyric acid) is a major inhibitory neurotransmitter in the CNS and, at least in some species, the supraspinal micturition reflex pathway is under tonic GABA-ergic inhibitory control.[3,34] Both $GABA_A$ and $GABA_B$ receptor agonists can suppress spinal and supraspinal components of the micturition reflex. Baclofen, a $GABA_B$ agonist considered to depress monosynaptic and polysynaptic motor neurons and interneurons in the spinal cord, effectively inhibited the micturition reflex when administered intrathecally to rats.[35] The drug has been used in voiding disorders, including detrusor hyperreflexia secondary to lesions of the spinal cord.[4] Thus, intrathecal baclofen was shown to be useful in patients with spasticity and bladder dysfunction.[36,37] When administered orally, the drug was also effective in the treatment of idiopathic detrusor overactivity.[38] Enhancement of GABA-ergic transmission by, for example, inhibition of GABA reuptake or of GABA transaminase, which is the therapeutic target of some of the new antiepileptic drugs,[39] may also have therapeutic potential in the treatment of bladder overactivity.

Serotonin

The serotonergic control mechanism of the lower urinary tract is complex and may involve modulation of sympathetic, parasympathetic and somatic efferent pathways. Thus, the lumbosacral autonomic, as well as the sphincter motor nuclei, receive a dense serotonergic input from the raphe–spinal pathway.[6] Drugs interfering with serotonin or with serotonin receptors (for example the selective serotonin reuptake inhibitors) have not been systematically tested as a treatment of the overactive bladder in humans. Whether imipramine (which, among other effects, blocks the reuptake of serotonin) depresses bladder overactivity by this mechanism,[40] has not been established. Duloxetine, a combined noradrenaline and serotonin reuptake inhibitor, has been shown, in animal experiments, to increase the neural activity to the external urethral sphincter and to increase bladder capacity through effects on the CNS.[41] Promising clinical experiences with duloxetine in the treatment of stress incontinence have been reported.[42]

Noradrenaline

The role of noradrenergic CNS pathways for micturition control has not been established. Noradrenergic neurons in the brain stem project to the autonomic and somatic nuclei in the lumbosacral spinal cord. Bladder activation through these bulbospinal noradrenergic pathways may involve excitatory α_1-adrenoceptors.[34] In rats undergoing continuous cystometry, doxazosin given intrathecally, decreased micturition pressure, both in normal rats and in animals with postobstruction bladder hypertrophy.[43] The effect was much more pronounced in animals with hypertrophied/overactive bladders. Doxazosin given intrathecally, but not intraarterially, to spontaneously hypertensive rats exhibiting bladder hyperactivity normalized bladder activity.[44] It was suggested that doxazosin has a site of action at the level of the spinal cord and ganglia.

Dopamine

Patients with Parkinson's disease may have detrusor hyperreflexia, possibly as a consequence of nigrostriatal dopamine depletion and failure to activate inhibitory D1 receptors.[45] However, other dopaminergic systems may activate D2 receptors, facilitating the micturition reflex. Sillén *et al.*[46] showed that apomorphine, which activates both D1 and D2 receptors, induced bladder overactivity in anaesthetized rats via stimulation of central dopaminergic receptors. The effects were abolished by infracollicular transection of the brain, and by prior intraperitoneal administration of the centrally acting dopamine receptor blocker spiroperidol. Kontani *et al.*[47,48] suggested that the bladder overactivity induced by apomorphine in anaesthetized rats resulted from synchronous stimulation of the micturition centres in the brain stem and spinal cord, and that the response was elicited by stimulation of both dopamine D1 and

D2 receptors. Blockade of central dopamine receptors may be expected to influence voiding; however, the therapeutic potential of drugs with this action has not been established.

Peripheral targets

Possible peripheral targets for pharmacological intervention may be (a) the efferent neurotransmission, (b) the smooth muscle itself – including various receptors, ion channels and intracellular second-messenger systems – and (c) the afferent neurotransmission. Although many effective drugs are available for these target systems, most of them are not useful in the clinical situation, owing to the lack of selectivity for the lower urinary tract, which may result in intolerable side effects. Thus, a main task is to find systems or receptors, specific for the lower urinary tract, that can be manipulated without disturbing other systems in the body; an alternative is to design drugs in a way that results in higher tissue concentrations in the lower urinary tract than elsewhere in the body.

Muscarinic receptors

Both normal bladder contractions and contractions in hyperactive bladders are predominantly mediated by acetylcholine acting on muscarinic receptors.[5] A NANC component, responsible for part of the electrically induced contraction has been demonstrated in studies *in vitro* using tissue specimens from functionally disturbed bladders,[5,12] but its clinical significance is not known. Muscarinic receptor antagonists are currently the most important drugs for treatment of bladder hyperactivity. Five muscarinic receptor subtypes, M_1–M_5, have been cloned and pharmacologically defined.[49,50] The human bladder contains M_2 and M_3,[51–53] with a predominance of M_2 receptors. Both M_2 and M_3 receptors are G-protein coupled, but activate different second-messsenger systems: generally, activation of M_2 receptors leads to decreased cAMP levels and to the closing of potassium channels, whereas M_3 receptors are believed to activate the phosphoinositide system.[49] It has been demonstrated that the response of isolated human bladder smooth muscle to muscarinic agonists is increased phosphoinositide turnover.[54] In addition, experiments with cultured human bladder smooth muscle cells showed that increased phosphoinositide turnover is caused by stimulation of the M_3 receptor,[55] suggesting that the M_3 receptors are important media-tors of contraction in the human bladder. The role for M_2 receptors in the bladder is still unclear.[48,56] The fact that exogenous cAMP relaxes bladder smooth muscle *in vitro*, and the existence of β-adrenoceptors in the bladder, have led to speculation that activation of M_2 receptors could reverse a relaxant effect mediated by β-adrenoceptors, since M_2 receptors and β-adreno-ceptors have opposite effects on cAMP formation. This hypothesis is supported by results from experiments in rats in which stimulation of M_2 receptors was able to mediate bladder contractions both *in vitro* and *in vivo*, probably by reversing β-adrenoceptor-mediated relaxations.[56]

Muscarinic receptors are also located on nerve ter-minals, modulating transmitter release both in ganglia and at the neuromuscular junction. Studies on rat blad-ders have shown that M_2 receptors have an inhibitory effect on transmitter release, whereas stimulation of presynaptic M_1 receptors enhances acetylcholine release.[57,58] In these experiments, the effect of the inhibitory M_2 receptors dominated, but it has been argued that facilitatory M_1 receptors can be activated during the high-frequency parasympathetic nerve dis-charge that occurs during micturition.

β-Adrenoceptors

β-Adrenoceptor agonists, such as isoprenaline, have a potent relaxant effect on isolated human bladder.[5] It has been speculated that β-adrenoceptors might have a physiological role as mediators of bladder relaxation during the filling phase. If this is true, a disturbance in this system could contribute to bladder overactivity. The inhibitory effect of isoprenaline on electrically induced contractions was shown to be weaker in detrusor muscle strips from patients with bladder instability than in muscle strips from patients with a normal bladder. How-ever, agonist-induced contractions in both normal and hyperactive bladders were similarly relaxed by isopre-naline.[59] In addition, no difference in β-adrenoceptor density was seen in receptor-binding studies on normal and hyperactive bladders.[60]

It has been suggested that an atypical β-adrenocep-tor subtype might be present in the human bladder, since the non-selective β-adrenoceptor antagonist pro-pranolol inhibited agonist-induced effects, whereas antagonists with selectivity towards $β_1$- or $β_2$-adrenocep-tors were less effective.[61,62] However, other studies have demonstrated favourable effects on bladder hyperactiv-ity of selective $β_2$-adrenoceptor agonists such as terbu-taline and clenbuterol, although treatment with these agents has been limited by side effects.[1,4] Recently, Igawa *et al.*[63,64] demonstrated that mRNAs for $β_1$-, $β_2$- and $β_3$-adrenoceptors were present in both normal and neu-rogenic human bladders. A relaxant effect was mediated primarily by the $β_3$-adrenoceptor. Thus, CGP-12177A, a partial $β_3$-adrenoceptor agonist and $β_1$/$β_2$-adrenoceptor antagonist, had a pronounced relaxant effect.[63,64] Evi-dence for $β_3$-mediated detrusor relaxation has also been obtained from experiments on rat bladder. Oshita *et al.*[65] demonstrated that isolated rat-bladder strips were more sensitive to BRL 3744, a $β_3$ agonist, than to isoprenaline. Furthermore, experiments with propranolol and a selective $β_2$ antagonist (ICI 118551) indicated that more than one receptor subtype was involved. These results could not be confirmed in rabbit bladder, indicating a species variation in β-adrenoceptor subtypes.[65]

α-Adrenoceptors

The normal human detrusor responds to noradrenaline by relaxing,[24,25] probably because of effects on both α- and β-adrenoceptors. Stimulation of $α_2$-adrenoceptors on cholinergic neurons may lead to a decreased release of acetylcholine, and stimulation of postjunctional β-adrenoceptors to relaxation of the detrusor muscle.[5,66]

Drugs stimulating α-adrenoceptors have hardly any contractile effects in isolated, normal, human detrusor muscle. However, there is evidence that this may change in bladder hyperactivity associated with, for example, hypertrophic bladder and outflow obstruction[25] and in neurogenic bladders.[5] It seems well established that α-adrenoceptor antagonists can ameliorate lower urinary tract symptoms in men with benign prostatic hyperpla-sia, and in women,[67-69] and occasionally can abolish detrusor hyperactivity in these patients.[25,70,71]

Ion channels

Ion channels are important regulators of cell function. Located within the plasma membrane, they control the permeability to different ions. The two most thoroughly investigated classes of ion channels are calcium chan-nels and potassium channels.

Calcium channels

Calcium is a key component for function in many cells: in smooth muscle, an increased intracellular calcium concentration activates the contractile mechanisms; in nerve terminals, calcium influx in response to action potentials is an important mechanism for neurotransmitter release. Calcium channels can be divided into at least four different subtypes – L, N, P and Q. The calcium channels present in smooth muscle are L-type (dihydropyridine-sensitive) calcium channels and appear to be involved in contraction of the human bladder, irrespective of the mode of activation.[72] A decrease of the membrane potential (depolarization) increases the tendency for calcium channels to open, thereby increasing the calcium influx. Thus, the channel function is dependent on the membrane potential and the channels are termed voltage-operated calcium channels (VOCCs). Elevated intracellular calcium levels are also believed to initiate release of calcium from intracellular stores, a mechanism called calcium-induced calcium release.[73,74] Apparently, regulation of the intracellular calcium concentration in smooth muscle cells is one conceivable way to modulate bladder contraction. Dihydropyridines, such as nifedipine, have a potent inhibitory effect on isolated detrusor muscle.[5] Inhibitory effects have also been demonstrated on experimentally induced contractions under conditions *in vivo* in rats,[75] and clinically in patients with bladder hyperactivity.[1]

If bladder hyperactivity is caused by increased calcium permeability, changes in functional properties or in the number of calcium channels might be expected in bladders exhibiting this property. However, this could not be verified in a study bladder tissues from children with myelodysplasia, a condition frequently associated with detrusor hyperreflexia.[76]

Potassium channels
Potassium channels represent another mechanism to modulate the excitability of the smooth muscle cells. Under normal conditions, the resting membrane potential in smooth muscle cells is determined predominantly by the membrane conductivity to potassium ions. Increased potassium conductivity will lower the membrane potential by increasing the potassium efflux. As a consequence, this will increase the threshold for opening of VOCCs. There are several different types of potassium channels and at least two subtypes have been found in the human detrusor – ATP-sensitive potassium channels (K_{ATP}) and large conductance calcium-activated potassium channels

(BK_{Ca}). Studies on isolated human detrusor muscle and bladder tissue from several animal species have demonstrated that potassium-channel openers reduce spontaneous contractions as well as contractions induced by carbachol and electrical stimulation.[5] However, the lack of selectivity of currently available potassium-channel openers for the bladder versus the vasculature has thus far limited the use of these drugs. The first generation of K_{ATP}-channel openers, such as cromakalim and pinacidil, were found to be 8–200 times more potent as inhibitors of vascular preparations than of detrusor muscle.[77,78] No effects of cromakalim or pinacidil on the bladder were found in studies in patients with spinal cord lesions or detrusor instability secondary to outflow obstruction.[79,80] However, new K_{ATP}-channel openers have been developed, claimed to have selectivity towards the bladder.[81,82] One of these, ZD6169, which activates K_{ATP}-channels in human bladder cells, has been shown to reduce micturition frequency in rats at doses that produced no cardiovascular effects.[81,83] The mechanism for this selectivity is unclear, as no selectivity was observed *in vitro*.[77] It has been suggested that one mechanism of action might be suppression of capsaicin-sensitive afferents in the bladder.[84]

Sensory nerves
As mentioned above, appropriate bladder function is dependent on intact afferent signalling from the bladder to the CNS. This signalling conveys information about bladder filling and the status of the tissue, such as the presence of infectious agents. The afferent nerves consist of small, slowly conducting, myelinated Aδ-fibres and slowly conducting, unmyelinated C-fibres. The former are excited by mechanoreceptors and convey information about bladder filling, while C-fibres mediate painful sensations recognized by chemoreceptors. Capsaicin is a neurotoxin obtained from the red pepper (*Capsicum*) and is a useful tool to distinguish pharmacologically different subsets of afferent nerves. Capsaicin is believed to interact with vanilloid receptors[85,86] and thereby to mediate an initial excitation and release of neuropeptides followed by desensitization of the nerve endings. Nerves responding to capsaicin treatment are termed capsaicin sensitive and correspond generally to C-fibres. Capsaicin has been used to demonstrate that C-fibres may modulate the afferent signalling in the

micturition reflex. Maggi *et al.*[87] instilled capsaicin intravesically ($0.1–10\,\mu mol/l$) in patients with hypersensitivity disorders: it was found that capsaicin treatment resulted in a concentration-dependent decrease of the volume required to elicit the first desire to void, decreased bladder capacity and decreased pressure threshold for micturition. All patients reported disappearance or marked attenuation of their symptoms a few days after administration of capsaicin. Intravesical capsaicin, at considerably higher concentrations ($1–2\,mmol/l$), has since been used with success in patients with bladder overactivity due to neurological disorders, such as multiple sclerosis or traumatic chronic spinal lesions; the effect of treatment may last for 2–7 months.[88–90] Under normal conditions, C-fibres do not seem to be involved in the micturition reflex; however, spinal cord injury might change this pattern, as demonstrated in animal experiments in which the voiding reflex was mediated by unmyelinated C-fibres and could be blocked by capsaicin.[91]

It has been suggested that capsaicin-sensitive nerves, in addition to conveying sensory information, may also have a local effect on the smooth muscle by local release of peptides from the sensory nerve terminals.[92,93] Immunohistochemical experiments have demonstrated several peptides in sensory bladder nerves, such as substance P, neurokinin (NK) A and calcitonin gene-related peptide. Local release of these peptides has been shown to produce diverse biological effects – such as smooth muscle contraction, facilitation of neurotransmitter release from nerves, vasodilatation and increased plasma permeability[94] – effects that may initiate bladder overactivity. If this is the case, blockade of NK receptors would be an interesting therapeutic principle.

Prostanoids

Prostanoids are synthesized from the common precursor, arachidonic acid, a process catalysed by the enzyme cyclooxygenase (COX). This process occurs locally in both bladder muscle and mucosa,[95–97] and is initiated by various physiological stimuli such as stretching of the detrusor muscle, but also by injuries of the vesical mucosa, nerve stimulation, and by agents such as ATP and mediators of inflammation.[98] There appear to be species variation in the spectrum of prostanoids and the relative amounts synthesized and released by the urinary bladder. Biopsy specimens from the human

bladder were shown to release prostanoids in the following quantitative order: prostaglandin (PG)I_2 > PGE$_2$ > PGF$_{2\alpha}$ > thromboxane A$_2$.[97] PGF$_{2\alpha}$, PGE$_1$ and PGE$_2$ contract isolated detrusor muscle, whereas PGE$_1$ and PGF$_{2\alpha}$ relax (or have no effect on) urethral smooth muscle.[5] Even if prostaglandins have contractile effects on the human bladder, it is still unclear whether they contribute to the pathogenesis of unstable detrusor contractions. Prostanoids may affect the excitation–contraction coupling in the bladder smooth muscle in two ways – directly by effects on the smooth muscle and/or indirectly by effects on neurotransmission.[98] Probably, prostanoids act not as true effector messengers along the efferent arm of the micturition reflex but rather as neuromodulators of efferent and afferent neurotransmission.[98,99] An important physiological role might be sensitization of sensory nerves. A possible mechanism for prostanoid-induced sensitization of nociceptive afferents has been presented by Gold *et al.*[100] who demonstrated an increase in tetrodotoxin-resistant sodium currents in response to PGE$_2$ application to cells from rat dorsal ganglia. Evidence for a sensitizing effect of PGE$_2$ has also been demonstrated *in vivo*. It was shown in the rat urinary bladder that intravesical instillation of PGE$_2$ lowered the threshold for reflex micturition, an effect that was blocked by systemic capsaicin desensitization. Indomethacin pretreatment and systemic capsaicin increased the micturition threshold without affecting the amplitude of the micturition contraction.[98] As intravesical PGE$_2$ did not reduce the residual volume in capsaicin-pretreated animals, it was suggested that endogenous prostanoids enhance the voiding efficiency through an effect, direct or indirect, on sensory nerves.

Prostanoids may also be involved in the pathophysiology of different bladder disorders. As pointed out by Maggi,[98] in cystitis there may be an exaggerated prostanoid production leading to intense activation of sensory nerves, increasing the afferent input.

COX is the pivotal enzyme in prostaglandin synthesis. It has recently been established that this enzyme exists in two isoforms, one constitutive (COX-1) and one inducible (COX-2).[101] The constitutive form is responsible for normal physiological biosynthesis, whereas the inducible COX-2 is activated during inflammation.[102,103] It has recently been demonstrated that the expression of COX-2 is increased during bladder obstruction.[104] If prostaglandins generated by COX-2 contribute to bladder overactivity, selective inhibitors of COX-2 would, theoretically, be one possible target for pharmacological therapy. Whether available selective COX-2 inhibitors would be useful as treatment for bladder overactivity remains to be established.

CONCLUSIONS

To control bladder activity effectively and to treat urinary incontinence caused by bladder overactivity, identification of suitable targets for pharmacological intervention is necessary. Such targets may be found in the CNS or peripherally. Drugs specifically directed at control of bladder activity are in development and will, it is hoped, lead to improved treatment of urinary incontinence.

ACKNOWLEDGEMENT

The authors acknowledge the support of the Swedish Medical Research Council (grant no. 6837).

REFERENCES

1. Andersson KE. Current concepts in the treatment of disorders of micturition. *Drugs* 1988; 35: 477–494

2. Nasr SZ, Ouslander JG. Urinary incontinence in the elderly. *Drugs Aging* 1998; 12: 349–360

3. Owens RG, Karram MM. Comparative tolerability of drug therapies used to treat incontinence and enuresis. *Drug Safety* 1998; 19: 123–139

4. Wein AJ. Pharmacology of incontinence. *Urol Clin North Am* 1995; 22: 557–577

5. Andersson K-E. Pharmacology of lower urinary tract smooth muscles and penile erectile tissues. *Pharmacol Rev* 1993; 45: 253–308

6. De Groat WC, Booth AM, Yoshimura N. Neurophysiology of micturition and its modification in animal models of human disease. In: Maggi CA (ed) *Nervous Control of the Urogenital System.* London: Harwood Academic, 1993; 227–290

7. Asmussen M, Ulmsten U. Simultaneous urethrocystometry with a new technique. *Scand J Urol Nephrol* 1976; 10: 7–11

8. Low JA. Urethral behaviour during the involuntary detrusor contraction. *Am J Obstet Gynecol* 1977; 128: 32–42

9. Tanagho EA, Miller ER. Initiation of voiding. *Br J Urol* 1970; 42: 175–183

10. Fletcher TF, Bradley WE. Neuroanatomy of the bladder–urethra. *J Urol* 1978; 119: 153–160

11. Lincoln J, Burnstock G. Autonomic innervation of the urinary bladder and urethra. In: Maggi CA (ed) *Nervous Control of the Urogenital System.* London: Harwood Academic, 1993; 33–68

12. Sjögren C, Andersson KE, Husted S *et al.* Atropine resistance of transmurally stimulated isolated human bladder muscle. *J Urol* 1982; 128: 1368–1371

13. Hoyle CH, Chapple C, Burnstock G. Isolated human bladder: evidence for an adenine dinucleotide acting on P2X-purinoceptors and for purinergic transmission. *Eur J Pharmacol* 1989; 174: 115–118

14. Ruggieri MR, Whitmore KE, Levin RM. Bladder purinergic receptors. *J Urol* 1990; 144: 176–181

15. Ambache H, Zar MA. Non-cholinergic transmission by postganglionic motor neurons in the mammalian bladder. *J Physiol (Lond)* 1970; 210: 761–783

16. Burnstock G, Dumsday B, Smythe A. Atropine resistant excitation of the urinary bladder: the possibility of transmission via nerves releasing a purine nucleotide. *Br J Pharmacol* 1972; 44: 451–461

17. Burnstock G, Cocks T, Kasakov L, Wong HK. Direct evidence for ATP release from non-adrenergic, non-cholinergic ('purinergic') nerves in the guinea-pig taenia coli and bladder. *Eur J Pharmacol* 1978; 49: 145–149

18. Andersson KE, Persson K. The L-arginine/nitric oxide pathway and non-adrenergic, non-cholinergic relaxation of the lower urinary tract. *Gen Pharmacol* 1993; 24: 833–839

19. Bridgewater M, Brading AF. Evidence for a non-nitrergic inhibitory innervation in the pig urethra. *Neurourol Urodyn* 1993; 12: 357–358

20. Hashimoto S, Kigoshi S, Muramatsu I. Nitric oxide-dependent and -independent neurogenic relaxation of isolated dog urethra. *Eur J Pharmacol* 1993; 231: 209–214

21. Werkstrom V, Persson K, Ny L *et al.* Factors involved in the relaxation of female pig urethra evoked by electrical field stimulation. *Br J Pharmacol* 1995; 116: 1599–1604

22. Van Arsdalen K, Wein A. Physiology of micturition and continence. In: Krane RJ, Siroky M (eds) *Clinical Neurourology.* New York: Little Brown, 1998; 25–82

23. Mattiasson A, Andersson KE, Elbadawi A *et al.* Interaction between adrenergic and cholinergic nerve terminals in the urinary bladder of rabbit, cat and man. *J Urol* 1987; 137: 1017–1019

24. Åmark P, Nergardh A, Kinn AC. The effect of noradrenaline on the contractile response of the urinary bladder. An in vitro study in man and cat. *Scand J Urol Nephrol* 1986; 20: 203–207

25. Perlberg S, Caine M. Adrenergic response of bladder muscle in prostatic obstruction. Its relation to detrusor instability. *Urology* 1982; 20: 524–527

26. Kuru M. Nervous control of micturition. *Physiol Rev* 1965; 45: 425–494

27. Janig W, Morrison JF. Functional properties of spinal visceral afferents supplying abdominal and pelvic organs, with special emphasis on visceral nociception. *Prog Brain Res* 1986; 67: 87–114

28. Habler HJ, Janig W, Koltzenburg M. Activation of unmyelinated afferent fibres by mechanical stimuli and inflammation of the urinary bladder in the cat. *J Physiol* 1990; 425: 545–562

29. Fall M, Lindstrom S, Mazieres L. A bladder-to-bladder cooling reflex in the cat. *J Physiol* 1990; 427: 281–300

30. Andersson K-E. Pathways for relaxation of detrusor smooth muscle. In: Baskin L, Hayward SW (eds) *Advances in Bladder Research*. New York: Kluwer Academic/Plenum, 1999; 241–252

31. Mallory BS, Roppolo JR, de Groat WC. Pharmacological modulation of the pontine micturition center. *Brain Res* 1991; 546: 310–320

32. de Groat WC, Nadelhaft I, Milne RJ et al. Organization of the sacral parasympathetic reflex pathways to the urinary bladder and large intestine. *J Auton Nerv Syst* 1981; 3: 135–160

33. Maggi CA. The dual sensory and 'efferent' function of the capsaicin-sensitive primary sensory neurons in the urinary bladder and urethra. In: Maggi CA (ed) *Nervous Control of the Urogenital System*. London: Harwood Academic, 1993; 383–422

34. de Groat WC, Vizzard MA, Araki I, Roppolo J. Spinal interneurons and preganglionic neurons in sacral autonomic reflex pathways. *Prog Brain Res* 1996; 107: 97–111

35. Igawa Y, Mattiasson A, Andersson K-E. Effects of GABA-receptor stimulation and blockade on micturition in normal rats and rats with bladder outflow obstruction. *J Urol* 1993; 150: 537–542

36. Bushman W, Steers WD, Meythaler JM. Voiding dysfunction in patients with spastic paraplegia: urodynamic evaluation and response to continuous intrathecal baclofen. *Neurourol Urodyn* 1993; 12: 163–170

37. Steers WD, Meythaler JM, Haworth C et al. Effects of acute bolus and chronic continuous intrathecal baclofen on genitourinary dysfunction due to spinal cord pathology. *J Urol* 1992; 148: 1849–1855

38. Taylor MC, Bates CP. A double-blind crossover trial of baclofen – a new treatment for the unstable bladder syndrome. *Br J Urol* 1979; 51: 504–505

39. Perucca E. The new generation of antiepileptic drugs: advantages and disadvantages. *Br J Clin Pharmacol* 1996; 42: 531–543

40. Maggi CA, Borsini F, Lecci A et al. Effect of acute or chronic administration of imipramine on spinal and supraspinal micturition reflexes in rats. *J Pharmacol Exp Ther* 1989; 248: 278–285

41. Thor KB, Katofiasc MA. Effects of duloxetine, a combined serotonin and norepinephrine reuptake inhibitor, on central neural control of lower urinary tract function in the chloralose-anesthetized female cat. *J Pharmacol Exp Ther* 1995; 274: 1014–1024

42. Zinner N, Sarshik S, Yalcin I et al. Efficacy and safety of duloxetine in stress urinary incontinent patients: double-blind, placebo-controlled multiple dose study. (Abstr. 225.) Proceedings, ICS 28th Annual Meeting, Jerusalem, Israel, September 14–17, 1998; 173–174

43. Ishizuka O, Persson K, Mattiasson A et al. Micturition in conscious rats with and without bladder outlet obstruction – role of spinal alpha(1)-adrenoceptors. *Br J Pharmacol* 1996; 117: 962–966

44. Persson K, Pandita RK, Spitsbergen JM et al. Spinal and peripheral mechanisms contributing to hyperactive voiding in spontaneously hypertensive rats. *Am J Physiol* 1998; 275: R1366–1373

45. Yoshimura N, Mizuta E, Kuno S et al. The dopamine D1 receptor agonist SKF 38393 suppresses detrusor hyperreflexia in the monkey with parkinsonism induced by 1-methyl-4-phenyl-1,2,3,6-tetrahydropyridine (MPTP). *Neuropharmacology* 1993; 32: 315–321

46. Sillén U, Rubenson A, Hjalmas K. On the localization and mediation of the centrally induced hyperactive urinary bladder response to L-dopa in the rat. *Acta Physiol Scand* 1981; 112: 137–140

47. Kontani H, Inoue T, Sakai T. Dopamine receptor subtypes that induce hyperactive urinary bladder response in anesthetized rats. *Jpn J Pharmacol* 1990; 54: 482–486

48. Kontani H, Inoue T, Sakai T. Effects of apomorphine on urinary bladder motility in anesthetized rats. *Jpn J Pharmacol* 1990; 52: 59–67

49. Eglen RM, Hegde SS, Watson N. Muscarinic receptor subtypes and smooth muscle function. *Pharmacol Rev* 1996; 48: 531–565

50. Caulfield MP, Birdsall NJM. International Union of Pharmacology: XVII. Classification of muscarinic acetylcholine receptors. *Pharmacol Rev* 1998; 50: 279–290

51. Yamaguchi O, Shishido K, Tamura K et al. Evaluation of mRNA encoding muscarinic receptor subtypes in human detrusor muscle. *Neurourol Urodyn* 1994; 13: 464–465

52. Yamaguchi O, Shishido K, Tamura K *et al.* Evaluation of mRNAs encoding muscarinic receptor subtypes in human detrusor muscle. *J Urol* 1996; 156: 1208–1213

53. Wang P, Luthin GR, Ruggieri MR. Muscarinic acetylcholine receptor subtypes mediating urinary bladder contractility and coupling to GTP binding proteins. *J Pharmacol Exp Ther* 1995; 273: 959–966

54. Andersson KE, Holmquist F, Fovaeus M *et al.* Muscarinic receptor stimulation of phosphoinositide hydrolysis in the human isolated urinary bladder. *J Urol* 1991; 146: 1156–1159

55. Harriss DR, Marsh KA, Birmingham AT, Hill SJ. Expression of muscarinic M3-receptors coupled to inositol phospholipid hydrolysis in human detrusor cultured smooth muscle cells. *J Urol* 1995; 154, 1241–1245

56. Hegde SS, Choppin A, Bonhaus D *et al.* Functional role of M-2 and M-3 muscarinic receptors in the urinary bladder of rats in vitro and in vivo. *Br J Pharmacol* 1997; 120: 1409–1418

57. Somogyi GT, de Groat WC. Evidence for inhibitory nicotinic and facilitatory muscarinic receptors in cholinergic nerve terminals of the rat urinary bladder. *J Auton Nerv Syst* 1992; 37: 89–98

58. Somogyi GT, Tanowitz M, de Groat WC. M1 muscarinic receptor-mediated facilitation of acetylcholine release in the rat urinary bladder. *J Physiol (Lond)* 1994; 480: 81–89

59. Eaton AC, Bates CP. An in vitro physiological study of normal and unstable human detrusor muscle. *Br J Urol* 1982; 54: 653–657

60. Restorick JM, Mundy AR. The density of cholinergic and alpha and beta adrenergic receptors in the normal and hyper-reflexic human detrusor. *Br J Urol* 1989; 63: 32–35

61. Larsen JJ. Alpha- and beta-adrenoceptors in the detrusor muscle and bladder base of the pig and beta-adrenoceptors in the detrusor muscle of man. *Br J Pharmacol* 1979; 65: 215–222

62. Nergardh A, Boreus LO, Naglo AS. Characterization of the adrenergic beta-receptor in the urinary bladder of man and cat. *Acta Pharmacol Toxicol* 1977; 40: 14–21

63. Igawa Y, Nishizawa O, Yamazaki Y *et al.* Functional and molecular biological evidence of β3-adrenoceptors in the human detrusor. *J Urol* 1997; 157: 175

64. Igawa Y, Yamazaki Y, Takeda H *et al.* Functional and molecular biological evidence for a possible β3-adrenoceptor in the human detrusor muscle. *Br J Pharmacol* 1999; 126: 819–825

65. Oshita M, Hiraoka Y, Watanabe Y. Characterization of beta-adrenoceptors in urinary bladder – comparison between rat and rabbit. *Br J Pharmacol* 1997; 122: 1720–1724

66. Andersson K-E. The overactive bladder: pharmacological basis of drug treatments. *Urology* 1997; 50 (Suppl 6A): 74–84

67. Andersson KE, Lepor H, Wyllie MG. Prostatic alpha-1 adrenoceptors and uroselectivity. *Prostate* 1997; 30: 202–215

68. Jollys JV, Jollys JC, Wilson J *et al.* Does sexual equality extend to urinary symptoms? *Neurourol Urodyn* 1993; 12: 391–392

69. Lepor H, Machi G. Comparison of the AUA symptom index in unselected males and females between 55 and 79 years of age. *Urology* 1993; 42: 36–40

70. Caine M. The present role of alpha-adrenergic blockers in the treatment of benign prostatic hyperplasia. *J Urol* 1986; 136: 1–4

71. Eri LM, Tveter KJ. α-Blockade in the treatment of symptomatic benign prostatic hyperplasia. *J Urol* 1995; 154: 923–934

72. Forman A, Andersson KE, Henriksson L *et al.* Effects of nifedipine on the smooth muscle of the human urinary tract in vitro and in vivo. *Acta Pharmacol Toxicol* 1978; 43: 111–118

73. Ganitkevich VY, Isenberg G. Contribution of Ca(2+)-induced Ca2+ release to the [Ca2+]i transients in myocytes from guinea-pig urinary bladder. *J Physiol (Lond)* 1992; 458: 119–137

74. Isenberg G, Wendt-Gallitelli MF, Ganitkevich V. Contribution of Ca(2+)-induced Ca2+ release to depolarization-induced Ca2+ transients of myocytes from guinea-pig urinary bladder myocytes. *Jpn J Pharmacol* 1992; 58: 81P–86P

75. Diederichs W, Sroka J, Graff J. Comparison of Bay K 8644, nitrendipine and atropine on spontaneous and pelvic-nerve-induced bladder contractions on rat bladder in vivo. *Urol Res* 1992; 20: 49–53

76. Shapiro E, Tang R, Rosenthal E, Lepor H. The binding and functional properties of voltage dependent calcium channel receptors in pediatric normal and myelodysplastic bladders. *J Urol* 1991; 146: 520–523

77. Barras M, Van der Graf PH, Christophe P, Itzchak A. Relaxant efficacy of potassium channel openers in rabbit isolated bladder and mesenteric artery. *Eur Urol* 1996; 30: 240

78. Edwards G, Henshaw M, Miller M, Weston AH. Comparison of the effects of several potassium-channel openers on rat bladder and rat portal vein in vitro. *Br J Pharmacol* 1991; 102: 679–680

79. Hedlund H, Mattiasson A, Andersson KE. Effects of pinacidil on detrusor instability in men with bladder outlet obstruction. *J Urol* 1991; 146: 1345–1347

80. Komersova K, Rogerson JW, Conway EL *et al.* The effect of

levcromakalim (BRL 38227) on bladder function in patients with high spinal cord lesions. *Br J Clin Pharmacol* 1995; 39: 207–209

81. Howe BB, Halterman TJ, Yochim CL *et al.* Zeneca ZD6169: a novel KATP channel opener with in vivo selectivity for urinary bladder. *J Pharmacol Exp Ther* 1995; 274: 884–890

82. Masuda N, Uchida W, Shirai Y *et al.* Effect of the potassium channel opener YM934 on the contractile response to electrical field stimulation in pig detrusor smooth muscle. *J Urol* 1995; 154: 1914–1920

83. Pandita RK, Persson K, Andersson K-E. Effects of the K+ channel opener, ZD6169, on volume and PGE2-stimulated bladder activity in conscious rats. *J Urol* 1998; 158: 2300–2304

84. Yu YB, Fraser MO, de Groat WC. Effect of intravesical administration of ZD6169 on the micturition reflex and on C-fos expression in the spinal cord induced by noxious bladder stimulation in the rat. *Soc Neurosci* 1996; 22: 93

85. Szallasi A. The vanilloid (capsaicin) receptor: receptor types and species differences. *Gen Pharmacol* 1994; 25: 223–243

86. Szallasi A, Conte B, Goso C *et al.* Vanilloid receptors in the urinary bladder: regional distribution, localization on sensory nerves, and species-related differences. *Naunyn Schmiedebergs Arch Pharmacol* 1994; 347: 624–629

87. Maggi CA, Barbanti G, Santicioli P *et al.* Cystometric evidence that capsaicin-sensitive nerves modulate the afferent branch of micturition reflex in humans. *J Urol* 1989; 142, 150–154

88. Chandiramani VA, Peterson T, Duthie GS, Fowler CJ. Urodynamic changes during therapeutic intravesical instillations of capsaicin. *Br J Urol* 1996; 77: 792–797

89. Fowler CJ, Beck RO, Gerrard S *et al.* Intravesical capsaicin for treatment of detrusor hyperreflexia. *J Neurol Neurosurg Psychiatry* 1994; 57: 169–173

90. Geirsson G, Fall M, Sullivan L. Clinical and urodynamic effects of intravesical capsaicin treatment in patients with chronic traumatic spinal detrusor hyperreflexia. *J Urol* 1995; 154: 1825–1829

91. de Groat WC, Kawatani M, Hisamitsu T *et al.* Mechanisms underlying the recovery of urinary bladder function following spinal cord injury. *J Auton Nerv Syst* 1990; 30: S71–77

92. Maggi CA. The role of peptides in the regulation of the micturition reflex: an update. *Gen Pharmacol* 1991; 22: 1–24

93. Maggi CA, Meli A. The role of neuropeptides in the regulation of the micturition reflex. *J Auton Pharmacol* 1986; 6: 133–162

94. Maggi CA. Tachykinins and calcitonin gene-related peptide (CGRP) as co-transmitters released from peripheral endings of sensory nerves. *Prog Neurobiol* 1995; 45: 1–98

95. Brown WW, Zenser TV, Davis BB. Prostaglandin E2 production by rabbit urinary bladder. *Am J Physiol* 1980; 239: F452–8

96. Downie JW, Karmazyn M. Mechanical trauma to bladder epithelium liberates prostanoids which modulate neurotransmission in rabbit detrusor muscle. *J Pharmacol Exp Ther* 1984; 230: 445–449

97. Jeremy JY, Tsang V, Mikhailidis DP *et al.* Eicosanoid synthesis by human urinary bladder mucosa: pathological implications. *Br J Urol* 1987; 59: 36–39

98. Maggi CA. Prostanoids as local modulators of reflex micturition. *Pharmacol Res* 1992; 25: 13–20

99. Andersson K-E, Sjögren C. Aspects on the physiology and pharmacology of the bladder and urethra. *Prog Neurobiol* 1982; 19: 71–81

100. Gold MS, Reichling DB, Shuster MJ, Levine JD. Hyperalgesic agents increase a tetrodotoxin-resistant Na+ current in nociceptors. *Proc Natl Acad Sci USA* 1996; 93: 1108–1012

101. Feng L, Sun W, Xia Y *et al.* Cloning two isoforms of rat cyclooxygenase: differential regulation of their expression. *Arch Biochem Biophys* 1993; 307: 361–368

102. Pairet M, Engelhardt G. Distinct isoforms (COX-1 and COX-2) of cyclooxygenase: possible physiological and therapeutic implications. *Fundam Clin Pharmacol* 1996; 10: 1–17

103. Vane JR, Botting RM. Mechanism of action of anti-inflammatory drugs. *Scand J Rheumatol Suppl* 1996; 102: 9–21

104. Park JM, Yang T, Arend LJ *et al.* Cyclooxygenase-2 is expressed in bladder during fetal development and stimulated by outlet obstruction. *Am J Physiol* 1997; 273: F538–F544

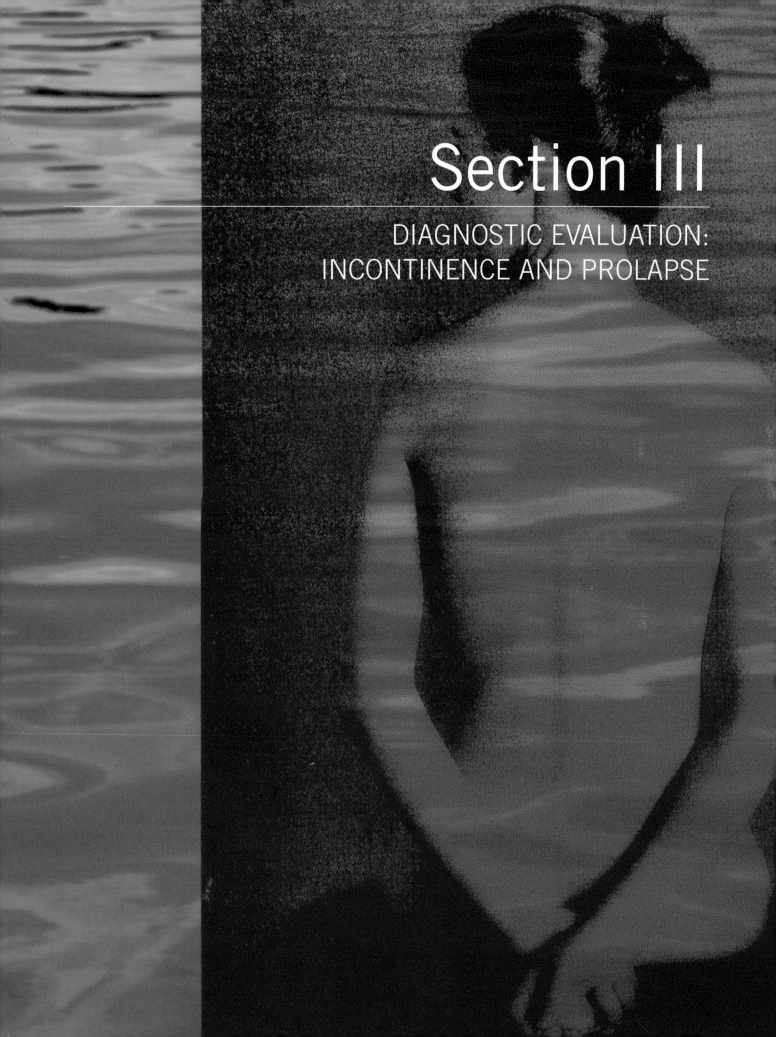

Section III

DIAGNOSTIC EVALUATION:
INCONTINENCE AND PROLAPSE

14

History and examination

V. Khullar, L. Cardozo

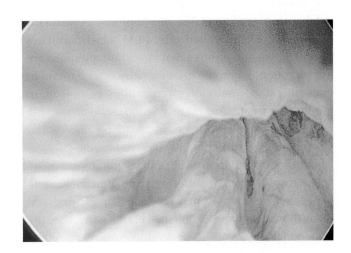

INTRODUCTION

Listening to any patient is important and a history should be obtained in a methodical manner. Urinary symptoms in a woman are the product of lower urinary tract dysfunction and a woman's adaptation to her environment to ameliorate her symptoms.

Alterations in lifestyle can lead to a reduction in quality of life. A woman who is suffering from urinary frequency may not perceive this as a problem if she is always near a toilet; however, once she no longer has easy access to a toilet the urinary symptoms may become very troublesome. The impact of urinary symptoms may be reduced by using protective pads or frequent visits to the toilet to keep the bladder empty.

There are a number of ways by which a woman can alter her urinary symptoms through behaviour: for example, she can drink less.[1] By restricting the fluid intake to less than 500 ml fluid in 24 hours, urinary frequency may not appear to be severe; however, if she subsequently drinks a litre of fluid a day, she may develop very severe frequency, nocturia and urge incontinence.

The volume of urine voided depends not only on fluid intake but also on whether the urinary fluid output is controlled. Thus, if there is an abnormality of the excretion of antidiuretic hormone, this can lead to an increase in urine output which the woman then has to match by an increased fluid intake. Antidiuretic hormone has been found to have a reversed circadian rhythm in some women complaining of nocturia[2] and in children with nocturia or nocturnal enuresis.[3]

History

The history enables the woman's own words to be translated into a graduated list of symptoms. A standard questionnaire can be used (Fig. 14.1), which facilitates history taking and ensures that important questions are not forgotten. Later, the questionnaire can be useful in evaluating the results of investigations as well as in monitoring treatment. History is not useful as the sole method of diagnosis; diagnosis based on history and examination is correct in only 65% of women.[4]

Urinary symptoms are valuable in guiding the management of a woman suffering from urinary incontinence, as investigations may produce a diagnosis that is inconsistent with the problems complained of by the woman. History may also be used to evaluate the effect

URINARY SYMPTOMS – DIRECT QUESTIONING

to be completed with the doctor

Daytime frequency ☐   Night-time ☐
Volume range

INCONTINENCE SYMPTOMS

stress incontinence ☐	urgency ☐
urge incontinence ☐	wet at rest ☐
wet on standing ☐	wet at night ☐
unaware of wetness ☐	pads/pants ☐

VOIDING CHARACTERISTICS

poor stream ☐	unable to interrupt flow ☐
post-micturition dribble ☐	strain to void ☐
incomplete emptying ☐	☐

OTHER SYMPTOMS

cough ☐	constipation ☐
leg weakness ☐	rectal soiling ☐
perineal discomfort ☐	enuresis after school age ☐
pain on micturition ☐	pain on intercourse ☐
	leakage on intercourse ☐

0 = no problem, 1 = occasionally, 2 = frequently
Pain on micturition 0 = nil, 1 = urethral, 2 = perineal,
3 = suprapubic, 4 = loin
Pain on intercourse 0 = no pain, 1 = superficial, 2 = deep

Figure 14.1. *Standard questionnaire for urinary symptoms.*

of treatment and guide the investigator about the urodynamic tests to be performed and the degree of provocation to be used.

The woman's urinary problems should be described in her own words. Thus, stress incontinence, although used to describe the urinary leakage associated with increase in intra-abdominal pressure, does not indicate the severity of the leakage or impact on the woman's quality of life. The length of time that the woman has had the problem will discriminate between the transient and established symptoms and this also allows the deterioration in quality of life to be assessed over time. A questionnaire is useful in eliciting urinary symptoms,

Table 14.1. *Classification of urinary symptoms into groups*
Abnormal storage
Incontinence urge, stress
Frequency/nocturia
Nocturnal enuresis
Abnormal voiding
Straining to void
Hesitancy
Incomplete emptying
Poor stream
Post-micturition dribble
Abnormal sensation
Urgency
Dysuria
Absent sensation
Painful bladder

especially where the woman is too embarrassed to describe them herself. The questions can be grouped into three main areas: the first group comprises disorders of abnormal storage, the second group includes symptoms associated with the abnormal voiding, and those in the final group are associated with abnormal sensation (Table 14.1). The woman should be questioned about each symptom, as she may not be able to describe (or may be too embarrassed to mention) them.[5] It is particularly important to recognize that urinary symptoms are a taboo subject and that only 10% of spouses know of their partner's incontinence.[6]

It should be recognized that different conditions can cause the same urinary symptoms: for example, overflow incontinence and detrusor instability (DI) can both produce urinary frequency and leakage. The former condition induces urinary frequency secondary to a reduced functional bladder capacity as the bladder never completely empties; DI causes urinary frequency due to a reduced bladder capacity because of an overactive detrusor; thus, the same symptom can be produced by two different mechanisms. Symptoms of mixed incontinence are found in a large proportion of women in all diagnostic categories: 55% of women with urethral sphincter incompetence and 35% of women with DI will have these symptoms.[7] Multiple symptoms have been amalgamated in an attempt to improve the accuracy of diagnosis. Even when complex scoring systems (such as those of the American Urological Association or visual analogue scores) are used, none of these methods suffi-ciently discriminates between genuine stress incontinence (GSI) and DI to be of diagnostic value.[8]

URINARY SYMPTOMS

Frequency

Frequency is the number of times a woman voids during her waking hours. The normal daytime frequency is between four and seven voids per day. The range of daytime urinary frequency in a symptomatic population is much greater (Fig. 14.2). Frequency is not diagnostic for GSI[9] or for DI,[10] even though women with DI void more frequently. Multiple voids occurring at a particular time of day may suggest a cause such as congestive cardiac failure or the ingestion of large volumes of fluid or of diuretics. Abnormal urinary frequency may occur for many reasons, as listed in Table 14.2. Women who void infrequently can be at risk of developing voiding difficulties.[11]

Daytime urinary frequency does not increase with age, as can be seen from data collected from our symptomatic population (Table 14.3).

Nocturia

Nocturia is defined as rising from sleep to void more than once a night. This symptom should be

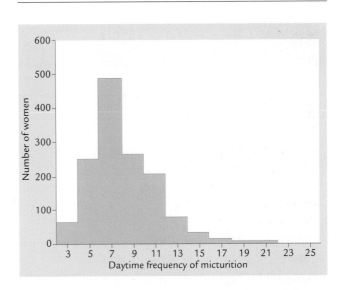

Figure 14.2. *Daytime frequency of micturition in a symptomatic population.*

Table 14.2. *Causes of abnormal urinary frequency*

Increased fluid intake and urine output; normal bladder capacity

- Osmotic diuresis, e.g. diabetes mellitus
- Abnormal antidiuretic hormone production, e.g. diabetes insipidus
- Polydipsia; often the woman enjoys drinking a favourite beverage and only rarely is the behaviour psychotic

Reduced functional bladder capacity

- Inflamed bladder increasing bladder sensation, e.g. acute bacterial cystitis, interstitial cystitis
- Detrusor instability
- Habit or fear of urinary incontinence
- Urinary residual secondary to detrusor hypotonia or outlet obstruction (rare)
- Increased bladder sensation in normal bladder, e.g. anxiety

Reduced structural bladder capacity

- Fibrosis after infection, e.g. tuberculosis
- Non-infective cystitis, e.g. interstitial cystitis, carcinoma
- Irradiation fibrosis, e.g. for bladder or cervical carcinoma
- Post surgery, e.g. partial cystectomy
- Detrusor hypertrophy

Decreased urinary frequency

- Detrusor hypotonia
- Impaired bladder sensation, e.g. diabetic neuropathy
- Reduced fluid intake

Table 14.3. *Effect of age on daytime urinary frequency in a symptomatic population*

| Age (years) | n | Urinary frequency | |
		Mean	Interquartile range
< 20	23	4.9	2–8
20–29	93	5.1	2–7
30–39	250	6.5	4–9
40–49	445	5.9	1–8
50–59	393	5.7	1–8
60–69	266	5.4	1–8
70–79	177	5.5	2–8
80–89	62	5.0	2–7
Over 90	5	4.8	2–8

Table 14.4 *Effect of age on night-time frequency in a symptomatic population*

| Age (years) | n | Urinary frequency | |
		Mean	Interquartile range
< 20	23	1.3	0–2
20–29	93	1.7	0–3
30–39	250	1.9	1–3
40–49	445	1.8	1–3
50–59	393	2.0	1–3
60–69	266	2.2	1–3
70–79	177	2.6	1–4
80–89	62	3.2	0–4
Over 90	5	4.1	2–5

differentiated from increased voiding by a woman because she is already awake. Up to the age of 70 years more than a single void at night is considered abnormal. After this age every extra decade increases the normal upper limit of nocturnal voids by one: thus, a normal 85-year-old woman may void three times at night. This change is probably related to an increased incidence of subclinical cardiac failure, where the extracellular fluid returns to the vascular compartment at night and is excreted by the kidneys.[2] This increase in nocturia can be seen in the symptomatic population we investigated (Table 14.4); the percentage of women referred with nocturia also increases with age. Reduction of fluid intake in the evening does not appear to alter nocturia.[12]

URINARY INCONTINENCE

Questions about urinary incontinence should help to determine not only the situation in which it occurs but also the amount and sensations felt during the loss, as this helps to determine the cause of the urinary leakage. Urinary incontinence is defined as the involuntary loss of urine that is a social or hygienic problem and is objectively demonstrable. Urine loss can either be extra-urethral incontinence (i.e. not through the urethra)[13] or urethral. It is important to recognize that the type of urinary incontinence is not a diagnosis but is a symptom or a sign. Severe urinary incontinence pro-

Table 14.5. *Causes of urinary incontinence*

Urethral sphincter incompetence

- Sphincter dysfunction
- Abnormal bladder-neck support

Detrusor overactivity

- Idiopathic detrusor instability
- Detrusor hyperreflexia, e.g. multiple sclerosis, spinal trauma

Mixed incontinence

Urethral diverticula

Congenital abnormalities, e.g. epispadias, ectopic ureter, bladder extrophy, spina bifida occulta

Transient incontinence

- Urinary tract infection
- Restricted mobility
- Constipation
- Excessive urine production
  - diuretic therapy
  - diabetes mellitus
  - diabetes insipidus
  - cardiac failure
  - hypercalcaemia
- Confusion, e.g. dementia, acute illness
- Atrophic urethritis and vaginitis

Pharmacological causes, e.g. diuretics, tranquillizers, cholinergic agents, prazosin

Fistulae, e.g. urethral, vesical, ureteral

Overflow incontinence

- Hypotonic detrusor
- Rarely urethral obstruction

Urethral instability

Functional

duces many symptoms common to different diagnostic categories. Although there are many causes of urinary incontinence they can grouped into 11 categories (Table 14.5).

The pattern of urine loss should be determined; it may be continuous or intermittent. Continuous urine loss is rare, occurring particularly at night, and is associated with fistulae or, occasionally, ectopic ureters. Fistulae are mainly a result of pelvic surgery, malignant disease or radiotherapy. Obstetric fistulae are seen in

women in developing countries. Women who complain that they are never dry tend to suffer from severe intermittent urinary incontinence rather than a continuous loss of urine. This may be seen after failed continence operations resulting in a fixed fibrosed 'drain pipe' (type 3) urethra.[14] A woman who complains of urine loss 'all the time' may have severe DI.

The pattern of urinary incontinence should be linked to any associated activity, such as laughing, physical exercise, sexual intercourse or putting the key in the front door. The severity of the urinary incontinence can be quantified not only by the volume and frequency of episodes but also by the numbers of pads or changes of underwear required in a 24-hour period and the magnitude of the provoking stimulus. There is often little relationship between the findings of urodynamic tests and the symptoms described by the woman in her daily activities. This reflects the modification in behaviour and lifestyle that she has made to ameliorate the effect of urinary incontinence on her life. This does not, however, reduce the importance of symptoms, as they may still be impairing her quality of life.

Often, women will not admit to incontinence but state that they 'leak'. This should be borne in mind when taking the history.

Stress incontinence

Stress incontinence is the involuntary loss of urine with an increase in intra-abdominal pressure such as coughing, sneezing, running and lifting. There is no associated urgency. The urine is often lost in small, discrete amounts.[15,16] This must be differentiated from urge incontinence. Only 39% of women complaining of stress incontinence actually have GSI.[17]

Urge incontinence

Urge incontinence occurs with the symptom of urgency (a strong, sudden desire to void). Often, women will describe an inability to get to the toilet in time. The quantity of urine lost can be a few drops prior to voiding or the entire contents of the bladder, and the woman may describe at least one occasion where the urine has poured down her legs uncontrollably. There may be many triggers for urge incontinence, such as changes in temperature, opening the front door, hearing running water and, occasionally, during sexual intercourse at orgasm. As the main coping strategy for this symptom is increasing voiding frequency, pad usage or incontinent episodes are not very useful in assessing the severity of the condition. The symptom of urge incontinence has a limiting sensitivity of 78% and a specificity of 39% in the diagnosis of DI.[4] This contrasts with the findings of Farrar *et al.*[18] where women with urge incontinence were found to have DI in 80% of cases.

Mixed incontinence

Mixed urinary incontinence, where the woman often has symptoms of stress and urge incontinence, is very common. It is important to determine the balance between the two symptoms and which troubles her the most. The length of time the two symptoms of stress and urge incontinence have existed has prognostic value in determining the success of continence surgery: Scotti[19] found that women with stress incontinence preceding urgency had a cure rate of 78.6% (22/28) for urge incontinence compared with 22.2% (4/18) of women with antecedent urge incontinence.

Coital incontinence

Urinary incontinence can occur during sexual intercourse either on penetration or during orgasm. Urinary leakage on penetration is more likely to occur in women with urethral sphincter incompetence and an anterior vaginal wall prolapse.[20] The urinary incontinence is not associated with urgency. Urinary incontinence can also occur with orgasm. The leakage is associated with urgency and is thought to be related to DI.[21,22]

Giggle incontinence

Giggle incontinence, where the bladder empties when the subject laughs, is found in young women. It has a clear history and is difficult to reproduce while under investigation. The problem usually resolves as the woman matures.

Nocturnal enuresis

Nocturnal enuresis is urinary loss during sleep; this must be differentiated from waking with urgency and then leaking before arriving at the toilet, which is urge incontinence. Nocturnal enuresis can be primary or secondary; primary nocturnal enuresis starts in childhood and can persist into adulthood, the woman never having been consistently dry at night;[23] secondary nocturnal enuresis is when the incontinence restarts in adulthood following a period of night-time continence, even if it resolved as a child. The causes for this can be abnormal circadian secretion of antidiuretic hormone, DI, abnormal control of the micturition reflex or abnormal sleep pattern. A family history should be sought and the presence of diurnal symptoms noted.

Urgency

Urgency is a strong and sudden desire to void that is inappropriate and which, if not relieved, can result in urge incontinence. If this symptom is recorded more often than once a week it may be considered abnormal.

VOIDING DIFFICULTIES

Voiding difficulties may present with a variety of symptoms.

Hesitancy

Occasional hesitancy is common in women but only 7% of women complaining of persistent hesitancy are found to be obstructed.[17] Hesitancy is a delay in the starting of the urinary stream when the woman wishes to void. The symptom of hesitancy with a full bladder can indicate that there is an obstruction when voiding, either because the urethral sphincter is not relaxing when the detrusor contracts (detrusor sphincter dyssnergia), or due to a stricture of the urethra. This symptom may also occur as a result of an acontractile detrusor muscle or psychological inhibition of the voiding reflex. Hesitancy does not discriminate between these problems. Women with DI may complain of hesitancy and poor stream and this is related to the small volumes of urine passed frequently in response to urgency.

Straining to void

The intra-abdominal pressure is increased by a Valsalva manoeuvre, which also increases the intravesical pressure, and this can improve bladder emptying. If the urinary stream is impaired and is intermittent, each transient increase in flow is associated with an increase in intra-abdominal pressure. This pattern of voiding preoperatively is associated with urinary retention after incontinence surgery, especially with sling procedures.

Incomplete emptying

The sensation that urine is left in the bladder after micturition can be due to fluid remaining in the bladder, or secondary to an abnormality of bladder sensation, or due to after-contractions of the bladder; these women do not always have increased post-micturition urinary residual volumes. The sensation of incomplete emptying is also associated with an open bladder neck at rest, as seen on videocystourethrography.

Women with prolapse can develop functional obstruction and may retain residual urine. A cystocele can also act as a sump and a rectocele can press anteriorly on the urethra in women who void by straining, preventing complete emptying of the bladder.

Post-micturition dribble

After voiding is completed, a woman may complain of intermittent urinary loss; this symptom may be related to a urethral diverticulum, a cystourethrocele or DI, the dribble being associated with fluid left in the bladder after voiding or a separate fluid collection. Where detrusor contractions occur after the completion of voiding, urgency will often accompany the urinary leakage. Post-micturition dribble should be distinguished from terminal dribble, which is continuous with the main flow of urine.

Poor stream

Decreased urinary stream may be described as 'decreased force'. The urine flow rate is dependent on the volume of urine passed, the pressure generated to empty the bladder and a low urethral resistance. To assess this symptom adequately, the volumes of urine voided should be recorded and then assessed and compared with a frequency/volume chart. A reduced urine flow can be due to a reduced voided volume, bladder outflow obstruction (rare in women) or decreased bladder contractility; the latter can be neuropathic (lower motor neuron lesions) or myopathic.

Bladder/urethral pain

Dysuria

Dysuria (pain on passing urine, experienced in the urethra) is often described as 'burning on passing urine' and can be aggravated by sexual intercourse. As an isolated symptom it is associated with urinary tract infections or urethritis.

Endometriosis on the bladder may cause dysuria that is present at certain times in the menstrual cycle. Pelvic inflammatory disease may cause dysuria, usually with coexistent symptoms of vaginal discharge and pyrexia.

Bladder pain

Suprapubic pain is associated with inflammation of the bladder, bladder stones or tumour. The pain more commonly occurs after micturition as the bladder mucosa closes down. Some women complain of pain after voiding and have DI; the pain has been found to coincide with contractions. The presence of bladder pain is an indication for cystoscopy and bladder biopsy. Suprapubic pain can be associated with pathology outside the bladder but within the pelvis.

Loin pain

Loin pain originates in the flank and radiates to the ipsilateral groin. The pain is referred from the sensory nerves innervating the kidney and urethra. There are many causes of such pain: for example, acute or chronic obstruction of the urinary tract can cause pain that becomes more acute as the pressure generated within the urinary tract increases; women with DI may complain of loin pain associated with urgency, and this can be due to vesicoureteric reflux.

Haematuria

Blood in the urine should always be investigated and should never be ignored. In women it is often due to urinary tract infections.

NEUROLOGICAL HISTORY

Women should be questioned about any alteration in sensation and motor power in the legs or perineum. The latter may be described as altered sensation during sexual intercourse or an inability to feel the urinary stream during micturition. Faecal incontinence is described as diarrhoea which causes staining of underwear or urgency to defecate. Increasing back pain with urinary and neurological symptoms must be treated rapidly and seriously as these may indicate a worsening central intervertebral disc prolapse. Neurological symptoms can also be a result of peripheral neuropathy associated with diabetes mellitus, cerebrovascular accidents, Parkinson's disease or multiple sclerosis.

GYNAECOLOGICAL SYMPTOMS

The lower urinary tract has receptors to oestrogen;[24] it is therefore important to enquire about changes in urinary symptoms during the menstrual cycle and to note the presence of the menopause. The majority of women complaining of urological symptoms have coexisting gynaecological pathology.[25] As vaginal prolapse alters the range of treatments for urinary incontinence, enquiries about symptoms of vaginal prolapse and prolapse affecting micturition and defecation should be made. Over 40% of women with urethral sphincter incompetence will also have significant cystoceles,[7] making this an important symptom affecting management of female urinary incontinence. A vaginal prolapse can mask urethral sphincter incompetence;[26] it is, therefore, important to identify any prolapse before a urodynamic test, so that a vaginal ring can be inserted during the provocative phase of such a test to expose any underlying urethral sphincter incompetence. Previous continence operations have an important influence on the future success of continence surgery, as the urethral sphincter may be altered by scarring and damage to sphincter innervation by previous vaginal surgery, as well as by distortion and narrowing of the bladder neck. Operations on the uterus may interfere with the innervation of the bladder, particularly after radical hysterectomy for carcinoma. Pelvic radiotherapy has profound effects, such as fibrosis, on the bladder; this can produce the symptoms of urgency and frequency.

PAST MEDICAL HISTORY

It is important to record all previous major abdominal and pelvic surgery, and urinary complications as a result of the surgery should be noted. The postoperative course can often be revealing, particularly when women have been unable to void spontaneously and have required catheterization; this could indicate prolonged overdistension, which can lead to voiding difficulties due to detrusor hypotonia.[27] Surgery to the spine and neurological impairment after this must be recorded, particularly in relation to any possible nerve damage. Operations on the large bowel, particularly those involving dissection at the side wall of the pelvis, such as abdominoperineal resection of the rectum, may result in denervation. Conditions increasing abdominal pressure, such as chronic cough or constipation, can produce the symptom of stress incontinence and make a minor problem more severe; such conditions are also implicated in the development of vaginal prolapse.[28] Cardiac and renal failure can produce frequency and nocturia through polyuria. Endocrine disorders such as diabetes mellitus or diabetes insipidus may lead to polyuria and polydipsia. Chronic diabetes mellitus can produce frequency as a result of overflow incontinence secondary to a hypotonic detrusor and impaired bladder sensation.

There appears to be an association between schizophrenia and DI.[29] Additionally, women suffering from dementia may not empty their bladders frequently and may not be aware of the need to void.

The number of proven urinary tract infections during the past 2 years should be recorded. Childhood enuresis is particularly important, as often these patients have DI.

The obstetric history should include parity, length of labour, mode of delivery and weight of the largest infant, although such information has not been shown to be very useful as the details of labour are not recalled accurately. Caesarean section or epidural block during labour and the retention of urine *post partum* are possible precursors of voiding difficulties.[30,31]

DRUG HISTORY

Many drugs affect the lower urinary tract. Diuretics can produce urgency, frequency and urge incontinence.[32] Benzodiazepines sedate and may cause confusion and secondary incontinence, particularly in elderly patients. Alcohol impairs mobility, produces diuresis and can alter the perception of bladder filling. Anticholinergic drugs impair detrusor contractility and may cause urinary retention with secondary overflow incontinence: such drugs include antipsychotics, anti-

Table 14.6. *Drugs that improve bladder storage*

Musculotrophic drugs

- Oxybutynin chloride
- Flavoxate hydrochloride
- Dicyclomine chloride
- Tolterodine
- Propiverine

Anticholinergic drugs

- Emepronium bromide/carrageenate
- Propantheline bromide
- Trospium chloride

Calcium antagonists

- Nifedipine
- Flunarizine

Tricyclic antidepressants

- Imipramine
- Doxepin

β-Adrenoceptor agonists

- Terbutaline
- Salbutamol

Prostaglandin synthetase inhibitors

- Flurbiprofen
- Indomethacin

Neurotoxins

- Capsaicin

Drugs reducing urine production

- Desmopressin

Drugs increasing urethral resistance

- α-Adrenergic agonists
  - Phenylpropanolamine hydrochloride
  - Midodrine
  - NS-49
- β-Adrenergic antagonist
  Propranolol

Oestrogens

Table 14.7. *Drugs that improve bladder emptying*

Increased detrusor contractility

- Cholinergic drugs
  - Bethanecol
  - Carbachol
- Anticholinesterase
- Prostaglandins
  - E_2
  - $F_{2\alpha}$

Decreased outlet resistance

- α-Adrenoceptor antagonists
  - Phenoxybenzamine
  - Phentolamine
  - Prazosin
- Striated muscle relaxants
  - Baclofen
  - Dantrolene
  - Diazepam

depressants, opiates, antispasmodics and antiparkinsonian drugs.

Drugs improving bladder storage are shown in Table 14.6. Sympathomimetic drugs, which are often found in cold remedies, can increase the urethral sphincter resistance and produce voiding difficulty. Drugs improving bladder emptying are shown in Table 14.7. Prazosin, a postsynaptic α-adrenergic blocker used to treat hypertension, has been found to cause urethral relaxation and urinary incontinence.[33] Caffeine, found in coffee and tea, is a diuretic; the combination of caffeine and the fluid can lead to frequency, urgency and urge incontinence. However, caffeine as a tablet without fluid does not appear to affect the bladder.[34]

EXAMINATION

Before examining the woman it is important to reassure her about the possibility of urinary leakage and explain that she should not be embarrassed as a result of it. The woman's mobility and mental state affect her ability to react to her incontinence problem and may influence management. An abridged test of her mental state (Mini Mental Status Exam) can be conducted, as well as an assessment of her motivation and manual dexterity, as these may influence her compliance with treatment and follow-up.

It is important to perform a screening neurological examination testing the tone, strength and movement of the lower limbs. It is particularly useful to test the abduction and spreading of toes, as the innervation for the lateral abductors comes from S3. Anal tone should be assessed and gentle tapping of the clitoris will produce a reflex contraction of the anal sphincter (bulbo-cavernosus reflex). Additionally, a voluntary cough should cause a reflex contraction of the anal sphincter. An intact sacral reflex can be tested by stroking the skin lateral to the anus, which should elicit a contraction of the external anal sphincter.

GYNAECOLOGICAL EXAMINATION

The condition of the vulval skin is important as there may be signs of excoriation, oedema or erythema due to exposure of the skin to urine on the vulva for prolonged periods of time, and to concomitant candidiasis. Vaginal atrophy, particularly in women more than 10 years after the menopause, may be noted.

Any cystocele, rectocele, or uterine or vault descent should be assessed as this can alter the patient's urinary symptoms.[26] Genital prolapse can be best assessed in the Sims' (left lateral) position on coughing and straining, using a Sims' speculum. Digital examination of vaginal prolapse is best assessed with the woman standing, legs abducted and performing a Valsalva manoeuvre. Baden and Walker described a vaginal prolapse grading system where the prolapse was classified according to points halfway down the vagina and at the hymenal ring;[35] this method of classifying genital prolapse has been superseded by the International Continence Society (ICS) method.[36] All measurements use a ruler and are relative to the hymenal ring. The measurements along the anterior, posterior and superior parts of the vagina are recorded during a maximum Valsalva manoeuvre. Additional measurements of the vaginal introitus and perineal body are recorded and the figures are written in a grid to help note keeping (Fig. 14.3). The ICS pelvic organ prolapse quantification score (POP-Q) has good inter- and intra-observer reliability,[37] and the level of agreement was found to be higher between two observers using kappa statistics than using the traditional genital prolapse grading system.[38]

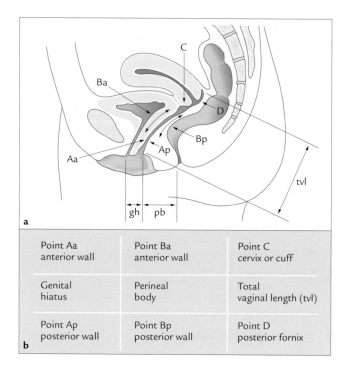

Point Aa anterior wall	Point Ba anterior wall	Point C cervix or cuff
Genital hiatus	Perineal body	Total vaginal length (tvl)
Point Ap posterior wall	Point Bp posterior wall	Point D posterior fornix

Figure 14.3. *International Continency Society assessment of prolapse: (a) points of measurement (gh, genital hiatus; pb, perineal body; tvl, total vaginal length) and (b) method of notation of the measrements.*

To demonstrate stress incontinence, the woman should have a full bladder;[39] often, she will have emptied her bladder prior to gynaecological examination, thus making it impossible to demonstrate stress incontinence.

Bonney[40] described a test of bladder-neck elevation which, he claimed, indicated the likelihood of curing stress incontinence with a vaginal repair. The procedure is as follows:

The patient, whose bladder should not recently have been emptied, is told to cough violently and the escape of urine is noted. The index and middle finger of the examiner's hand should be inserted into the vagina and the anterior vaginal wall pressed against the sub-public angle but without pressing on the urethra. The patient is now told to cough again. If the pressure of the fingers prevents the leak, the operation of anterior colporrhaphy, if properly carried out, will cure her.

However, this test produces occlusion of the urethra, which is not reproduced surgically; thus, Bonney's test is positive, irrespective of the urodynamic diagnosis and cause of the urinary leakage, and is of no practical use.[41,42]

If the woman is likely to need incontinence surgery, vaginal mobility and scarring should be assessed. The urethra should be examined for any discharge, inflammation or fixation. If the patient is complaining of a discharge, or has had a recent onset of symptoms of urgency and frequency, it may be useful to obtain swabs to culture for chlamydia and gonococcus.

The anterior vaginal wall should be examined for any mass that may be a urethral diverticulum or a urethral or vaginal cyst, and a bimanual examination should be performed to exclude abnormal pelvic organs, masses, uterine impaction or a large postmicturition urinary residual.[43] Pelvic masses such as ovarian cysts, and uterine enlargement greater than 12-weeks size, can cause pressure symptoms resulting in frequency; often, the symptoms resolve once the mass has been removed.

Finally, rectal examination is not routinely performed but is particularly important in the elderly to exclude faecal impaction, which can aggravate urinary incontinence or impair voiding.

Q-tip test

The mobility of the urethra and bladder neck can be evaluated by inserting a sterile, lubricated, 'Q-tip' cotton bud into the urethra to the level of the bladder neck. The patient is then asked to strain. The rotational movement of the bladder neck around the symphysis pubis causes the Q-tip to move, cranially. The angle of the Q-tip is measured relative to the horizontal, using an orthopaedic goniometer. The resting and straining angles are measured and the difference between the two angles is calculated; a change of more than 30 degrees is thought to represent a hypermobile urethra. Although this test does not establish the diagnosis of stress incontinence[44] and does not add any extra information to history and examination,[45-47] it is thought by some clinicians to indicate the most appropriate continence procedure when GSI has been diagnosed, and may predict failure of incontinence surgery.[48]

CONCLUSIONS

History and examination alone cannot diagnose female urinary disorders but can guide future investigation and management. In some cases a very obvious cause can be found and dealt with, avoiding the need for further investigations that may be embarrassing, expensive and invasive.

REFERENCES

1. Griffiths DJ, McCracken PN, Harrison GM, Gormley EA. Relationship of fluid intake to voluntary micturition and urinary incontinence in geriatric patients. *Neurourol Urodyn* 1993; 12: 1–7

2. Carter PG, McConnell AA, Abrams P. The significance of atrial natriuretic peptide in nocturnal urinary symptoms in the elderly. *Neurourol Urodyn* 1992; 11: 420–421

3. Norgaard JP. Pathophysiology of nocturnal enuresis. *Scand J Urol Nephrol* 1991; Suppl 140: 7–31

4. Sand PK, Ostergard DR. Incontinence history as a predictor of detrusor stability. *Obstet Gynecol* 1988; 71: 257–259

5. Khullar V, Damiano R, Toozs-Hobson P, Cardozo LD. Prevalence of faecal incontinence among women with urinary incontinence. *Br J Obstet Gynaecol* 1998; 105: 1211–1213

6. Brocklehurst JC. Urinary incontinence in the community – analysis of a MORI poll. *Br Med J* 1993; 306: 832–834

7. Cardozo LD, Stanton SL. Genuine stress incontinence and detrusor instability – a review of 200 patients. *Br J Obstet Gynaecol* 1980; 87: 184–188

8. Wise BG, Cutner A, Cardozo LD *et al.* Do detailed symptom questionnaires negate the need for urodynamic investigation? *Neurourol Urodyn* 1992; 11: 353–355

9. Larsson G, Victor A. The frequency/volume chart in genuine stress incontinent women. *Neurourol Urodyn* 1992; 11: 23–31

10. Larsson G, Abrams P, Victor A. The frequency/volume chart in detrusor instability. *Neurourol Urodyn* 1991; 10: 533–543

11. Swinn MJ, Lowe E, Fowler CJ. The clinical features of non-psychogenic urinary retention. *Neurourol Urodyn* 1998; 17: 383–384

12. Hill S, Cardozo LD, Khullar V. Does evening fluid restriction improve nocturia? *Int Urogynecol J* 1995; 6: 242

13. Bates P, Bradley WE, Glen E *et al.* First report on the standardisation of terminology of lower urinary tract function.

Urinary incontinence. Procedures related to the evaluation of urine storage – cystometry, urethral closure pressure profile, units of measurement. *Br J Urol* 1976; 48: 39–42

14. Blaivas JG, Appell RA, Fantl JA *et al.* Definition and classification of urinary incontinence: recommendations of the Urodynamic Society. *Neurourol Urodyn* 1997; 16: 149–151

15. James ED, Flack FC, Caldwell KPS, Martin MR. Continuous measurement of urine loss and frequency in incontinent patients. *Br J Urol* 1971; 43: 233–237

16. James ED. The behaviour of the bladder during physical activity. *Br J Urol* 1978; 50: 387–394

17. Abrams P. The clinical contribution of urodynamics. In: Abrams P, Feneley R, Torrens M (eds) *Urodynamics.* Berlin: Springer-Verlag, 1983; 118–174

18. Farrar DJ, Whiteside CG, Osborne JL, Turner-Warwick RT. A urodynamic analysis of micturition symptoms in the female. *Surg Gynecol Obstet* 1975; 141: 875–881

19. Scotti RJ, Angell G, Flora R, Greston WM. Antecedent history as a predictor of surgical cure of urgency symptoms in mixed incontinence. *Obstet Gynecol* 1998; 91: 51–54

20. Kelleher CJ, Cardozo LD, Wise BG, Cutner A. The impact of urinary incontinence on sexual function. *Neurourol Urodyn* 1992; 11: 359–360

21. Field SM, Hilton P. The prevalence of sexual problems in women attending for urodynamic investigation. *Int Urogynecol J* 1993; 4: 212–215

22. Sutherst JR. Sexual dysfunction and urinary incontinence. *Br J Obstet Gynaecol* 1979; 86: 387–388

23. Foldspang A, Mommsen S. Adult female urinary incontinence and childhood bedwetting. *J Urol* 1994; 152: 85–88

24. Iosif CS, Batra S, Ek A *et al.* Estrogen receptors in the human female lower urinary tract. *Am J Obstet Gynecol* 1981; 141: 817–820

25. Benson JT. Gynecologic and urodynamic evaluation of women with urinary incontinence. *Obstet Gynecol* 1985; 66: 691–694

26. Rosenzweig BA, Pushkin S, Blumenfeld D, Bhatia NN. Prevalence of abnormal urodynamic test results in continent women with severe genitourinary prolapse. *Obstet Gynecol* 1992; 79: 539–542

27. Hinman F. Postoperative overdistension of the bladder. *Surg Gynecol Obstet* 1976; 142: 901–902

28. Spence-Jones C, Kamm MA, Henry MM, Hudson CN. Bowel dysfunction: a pathogenic factor in uterovaginal prolapse and urinary stress incontinence. *Br J Obstet Gynaecol* 1994; 101: 147–152

29. Bonney W, Gupta S, Arndt S *et al.* Neurobiological correlates of bladder dysfunction in schizophrenia. *Neurourol Urodyn* 1993; 12: 347–349

30. Kerr-Wilson RHJ, Thompson SW, Orr JW *et al.* Effect of labor on the postpartum bladder. *Obstet Gynecol* 1984; 64: 115–118

31. Kerr-Wilson RHJ, McNally S. Bladder drainage for Caesarean section under epidural analgesia. *Br J Obstet Gynaecol* 1986; 93: 28–30

32. Fantl JA, Wyman JF, Wilson M *et al.* Diuretics and urinary incontinence in community-dwelling women. *Neurourol Urodyn* 1990; 9: 25–34

33. Hoffman BB, Lefkowitz RJ. Adrenergic receptor antagonists. In: Gilman AG, Rall TW, Nies AS, Taylor P (eds) *Goodman and Gilman's The Pharmacological Basis of Therapeutics*, 8th edn. New York: Pergamon Press, 1990; 221–243

34. Creighton SM, Stanton SL. Caffeine: does it affect your bladder? *Br J Urol* 1990; 66: 613–614

35. Baden WF, Walker TA. Physical diagnosis in the evaluation of vaginal relaxation. *Clin Obstet Gynecol* 1972; 15: 1055–1059

36. Bump RC, Mattiasson A, Bø K *et al.* The standardization of terminology of female pelvic organ prolapse and pelvic floor dysfunction. *Am J Obstet Gynecol* 1996; 175: 10–17

37. Hall AF, Theofrastous JP, Cundiff GW *et al.* Interobserver and intraobserver reliability of the proposed International Continence Society, Society of Gynecologic Surgeons, and American Urogynecologic Society pelvic organ prolapse classification system. *Am J Obstet Gynecol* 1996; 175: 1467–1470

38. Athanasiou S, Hill S, Gleason C *et al.* Validation of the ICS proposed pelvic organ prolapse descriptive system [Abstr]. *Neurourol Urodyn* 1995; 14: 414–415

39. Robinson H, Stanton SL. Detection of urinary incontinence. *Br J Obstet Gynaecol* 1981; 88: 59–61

40. Berkeley C, Bonney V. *A Textbook of Gynaecological Surgery.* 3rd edn. London: Cassell, 1935

41. Migliorini GD, Glenning PP. Bonney's test – fact or fiction? *Br J Obstet Gynaecol* 1987; 94: 157–159

42. Bhatia NN, Bergman A. Urodynamic appraisal of the Bonney test in women with stress urinary incontinence. *Obstet Gynecol* 1983; 62: 696–699

43. Norton PA, Peattie AB, Stanton SL. Estimation of residual urine by palpation. *Neurourol Urodyn* 1989; 8: 330–331

44. Bergman A, McCarthy TA, Ballard CA, Yanai J. Role of the Q-tip test in evaluating stress urinary incontinence. *J Reprod Med* 1987; 32: 273–275

45. Fantl JA, Hurt WG, Bump RC *et al.* Urethral axis and sphincteric function. *Am J Obstet Gynecol* 1986; 155: 554–558

46. Walters MD, Diaz K. Q-tip test: a study of continent and incontinent women. *Obstet Gynecol* 1987; 70: 208–211

47. Walters MD, Shields LE. The diagnostic value of history, physical examination and the Q-tip cotton swab test in women with urinary incontinence. *Am J Obstet Gynecol* 1988; 159: 145–149

48. Bergman A, Koonings PP, Ballard CA. Negative Q-tip test as a risk factor for failed incontinence surgery in women. *J Reprod Med* 1993; 34: 193–197

15

Voiding diary

M.-A. Harvey, E. Versi, J. P. Weiss

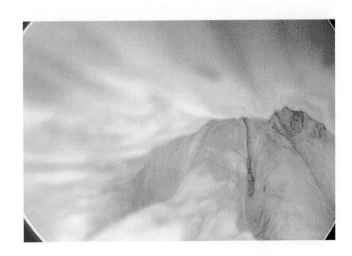

WRITTEN VOIDING DIARY

History (including a report from recollection of the frequency, nocturia and incontinence episode) and physical examination to visualize urine loss and to document the presence of prolapse are paramount in the evaluation of urinary incontinence, and have been covered in the preceding chapter. The voiding diary (also referred to as frequency/volume chart, urinary or incontinence diary, bladder or voiding record) is an important adjunct in the assessment of the incontinent patient, as it allows the following:

1. quantification of total fluid (liquid and food) intake (as judged by the total output);
2. semi-objective evaluation of severity of voluntary diurnal frequency and nocturia;
3. global estimation of severity of the condition (number of incontinence episodes and the size of the leak);
4. association of an event (incontinence, urgency) to a specific provocation (cough, running water, etc.);
5. bladder retraining as therapeutic intervention for detrusor instability (DI)/sensory urgency.

Voiding diaries are widely used in clinical as well as research settings to assess evolution of subjective symptoms before and after therapy. As a technique of confirming a patient's complaints, this is a prospective method that is unbiased by patient's recall. However, it may increase awareness of bladder behaviour, which may in itself influence the data collected – the so-called 'Heisenberg uncertainty' principle.

Although the concept of the diary has inspired a substantial amount of writing, the characteristics of diary collection have not been standardized in terms of duration or types of event noted (timing, type and quantity of fluid intake; circumstances associated with the incontinence and/or void such as urgency, dysuria or activities leading to increased intra-abdominal pressure such as coughing).

Obviously, it is important to establish normal diary patterns before using this instrument to evaluate abnormal patterns in patients. Larsson and Victor[1] and, more recently, Kassis and Schick[2] have used a voiding diary in normal women in an attempt to develop norms. Table 15.1 summarizes their findings: the average diurnal frequency was less than six times, but the upper limits of the range were 10.03[1] and 9.41.[2] Usually, seven times daily is regarded as the upper limit of normal; in these studies this was true for 80%[1] and 86%[2] of the normal subjects. With regard to the frequency for 97.7% (mean + 2 SD) of the population studied, the diurnal frequency was 8.62[1] and 8.15.[2]

Elements of a voiding diary

The basic frequency/volume chart, as the name implies, consists of a record of the time that a void took place and the volume voided. However, the information gathered from a voiding diary varies widely from one author to another, and may include the following:

- number of incontinence episodes;
- magnitude of incontinence episodes;
- associated events (type of incontinence, urgency);
- activity;

Table 15.1. *Findings on the frequency/volume chart in normal females**

Variable	Kassis and Schick (ref. 2) n = 33		Larsson and Victor (ref. 1) n = 151 24 h
	(Daytime)	(Night-time)	
Mean voided volume (ml)	237 (67)	379 (132)	250 (79)[†]
Frequency	5.63 (1.26)	0.08 (0.16)	5.8 (1.41)
Total voided volume (ml)	1005 (497)	409 (130)	
Output/24 h (ml)	1473 (386)		1430 (487)

* Values are means with standard deviations (SD) in parentheses.
Adapted from refs. 1 and 2.
† Night-time: 370 ml.

- provocative manoeuvre (sneeze, running tap);
- time and quantity of fluid intake;
- number of pads used per day.

Bailey *et al.*[3] compared five different charts and reported a good patient acceptability in recording associated events and provocative manoeuvres. Figure 15.1 illustrates an example of a voiding diary such as that used in our unit. The value of recording the quantity of fluid imbibed is limited, as much of the water intake is in the form of food. When constructing a diary, it must be appreciated that there is a trade-off between the quantity of the information collected and its quality, as patients often experience 'diary fatigue', with consequent corruption of the data collected.

Duration of the diary

The duration of a voiding diary has not been standardized. Abrams and Klevmark[4] support the use of a 7-day diary, as it includes a variety of activities and covers work and leisure time, and both weekdays and weekend days, thus providing a global 'snapshot' of a patient's problem. Wyman *et al.*[5] performed a test–retest variability analysis and found that a 1-week diary was as reliable as a 2-week diary. Others have suggested optimal periods of 48 hours[1,2] and 3 days.[6] Larsson and Victor[1] found a significant correlation from day 1 to day 2 when tested consecutively in a 48-hour diary and concluded that for 'scientific value, the observation time may be prolonged to strengthen the reliability of the recordings'. Similarly, when the patient repeated a 48-hour diary at a later date, a significant correlation with the week-long diary was maintained, implying that a 48-hour record could suffice, thus limiting the demand on the patient. Barnick[7] reported a significant correlation for all values recorded on a 5-day diary when compared with a 1-day diary (the first day of the 5-day diary). However, the 1-day diary tended to overestimate consistently the maximum voided volume, indicating a bias.

In the light of these arguments, it seems reasonable to have patients keep diaries for a period longer than 24 hours, but it should be appreciated that the compliance with the diary decreases with longer duration.[8]

Validity

Validity expresses the relation between observed measurements and the true state of the entity being studied.[9] To be valid, a test (voiding diary) has to be reproducible and must agree with the true state of the entity being measured (e.g. diurnal frequency, nocturia, functional capacity).[9] As it is difficult to assess with certainty the true state of a patient's symptomatology (as it would require an independent observer following the patient all the time for 2, 5 or 7 days), the best approximation is the reported symptoms from history (for frequency and nocturia) or from objective measurement from cystometry or cystoscopy (for maximal capacity).

Several studies[5,10,11] have examined the agreement between voiding diary and symptoms but no consensus is forthcoming. In a study involving history, a 2-week diary and urodynamic studies, Wyman *et al.*[5] found a significant correlation between the history-based diurnal and nocturnal frequencies and the diary ($r = 0.57$ and 0.63, respectively; $p < 0.001$). Similarly, there was a concurrence of 71% for the number of incontinent episodes on history data. In a more recent comparative study,[10] the same group also showed a significant correlation between the two methods for the number of incontinent episodes and use of absorptive pads when comparing history recall and diary data. In this study, Elser *et al.*[10] did not report on frequency or nocturia. Finally, McCormack *et al.*[11] found very similar diurnal and nocturnal frequencies between two methods of data gathering – questionnaire and cystoscopy versus diary evaluation. They also found that patients tended to report a greater frequency in questionnaires than in the diary. The latter has been corroborated by Abrams and Klevmark,[4] and it is thought that self-reported frequency may be influenced by the patient's emotional subjectivity.

The maximum voided volume is regarded as the functional capacity. The validity of the diary in assessing the functional capacity has been established by comparing diary-recorded volumes and cystometric capacity[12] or cystoscopic capacity.[11] The mean largest volume voided (483 ml) correlated with the mean cystometric capacity (377 ml) ($r = 0.493$; $p < 0.01$) but not with cystoscopic maximum capacity. Endoscopic determination of mean maximal capacity was 382.38 ± 149.10 ml when the frequency/volume chart reported

Brigham & Women's Hospital
Division of Urogynecology   MR# _____

24 Hours Voiding Diary

Name: _____ Date: ____ / ____ / ____ Tel # H: _____ W: _____

Directions:

1) Enter the time (including nighttime) in Column 1
2) On the same line as the time, write
   (a) The amount you urinate (ounces or cc's) in the toilet in Column 2
   OR
   (b) If you have a strong urge to urinate, put a ✔ in Column 3
   OR
   (c) If you accidentally leak, put a ✔ in Column 4 (S = small amount—drops, M = medium amount—wet pad or underwear, L = large—soaking)
   (d) Comment on what you were doing when you leaked urine in Column 6
   OR
   (e) The amount of liquid you drink in Column 7

2) Put a star * next to the time you go to bed and the time you get up.

1	2	3	4	5	6	7
Time	Amount in toilet	Urge to urinate (✔ if present)	Leak (✔ if present)	Amount of urine leakage (S, M or L)	Comments	Amount of fluid drunk

Figure 15.1. *Voiding diary used at the Continence Center for Women, Brigham & Women's Hospital, Boston, MA, USA.*

a mean diurnal and nocturnal capacity of 175.56 ± 64.29 and 232.5 ± 129.64 ml, respectively. The maximal functional bladder capacities, as calculated from the diary, were 374.22 ml for the diurnal and 633.09 ml for the nocturnal capacity. Consequently, the cystometric maximal capacity seems to underestimate the functional maximal bladder capacity. The obvious problem is the choice of variable chosen from the voiding diary: the average voided volume does not correspond to the maximum voided volume, as most people might void at or shortly after the 'first sensation' and rarely wait to be at their maximum tolerable limit. Furthermore, the presence of a foreign body (cystoscope) in the urethra, the use of analgesia/anaesthesia, the rate of filling and the temperature of the filling medium may also alter the results found at time of cystoscopy and/or cystometry.

The statistical technique used in most studies, using the correlation coefficient, is questionable. The latter, *r,* measures the strength of the relationship between two variables, not the agreement between them. It is highly possible that two tests disagree, despite a high degree of correlation.[13] The correlation coefficient does not provide reliable information with regard to reproducibility or the true variation of the test.

In summary, notwithstanding the above caveats, the voiding diary can be considered as reasonably valid in determining the diurnal and nocturnal frequencies and the functional capacity.

Reliability

Reliability reflects the capacity of a test to differentiate among the individuals studied, in particular, diseased individuals from normal ones.[9] Larsson *et al.*[1,14,15] reported on the reliability of the voiding diary in differentiating patients with DI[14] or genuine stress incontinence (GSI)[15] from normal subjects (Table 15.2). He concluded that the overlap between normal patients and patients with DI was great for all parameters, and he reached the same conclusion regarding patients with GSI. Accordingly, the diary is not a reliable test for diagnostic discrimination between either condition and normal bladder function.

Instructions to patients on chart completion

It has been shown[8] that providing a patient with a diary, together with minimal written instructions (similar to that depicted in Figure 15.1) gave similar results to a diary obtained following intense verbal instruction, provided that a certain minimum level of comprehension on the part of the patient (Mini Mental Status Exam ≥ 24) was guaranteed. Consequently, it is reasonable to expect a patient to fill out a diary prior to the initial consultation visit, and this is expected to increase the efficiency of patient evaluation.

In one study examining patient compliance,[16] patients who failed to complete a voiding diary mailed

Table 15.2. *Differences in variables from voiding diaries in normal subjects and in patients with detrusor instability (DI) or genuine stress incontinence (GSI)*			
Variable	Normal[†] (n = 151)	DI[†] (n = 62)	GSI[†] (n = 81)
Total voided volume (ml/24 h)	1430 (630, 2580)	1490 (630, 2390)	1550 (750, 2800)*
Frequency/24 h	5.8 (3.5, 9.0)	9.5 (5.5, 14.0)[§]	6.5 (4.0, 10.5)**
Mean voided volume	250 (120, 430)	170 (70, 210)[§]	220 (110, 430)
Largest single voided volume (ml)	460 (200, 1000)	330 (150, 700)[§]	500 (200, 850)*

[†] Values are means, with 2.5 and 97.5 percentiles in parentheses.
p values refer to comparisons with normal subjects: *$p < 0.05$; **$p < 0.01$; [§]$p < 0.001$
Adapted from refs. 1, 14 and 15.

prior to the visit were more likely to be non-Caucasian and complaining of pelvic organ prolapse, not of urinary symptoms. The authors also noted that non-completion of a diary before the visit was not a good predictor for the absence of urinary symptoms or a normal urodynamic study.[16]

COMPUTERIZED VOIDING DIARY

Computerized diaries have been developed to overcome the lack of compliance that is occasionally seen, and to increase motivation.[17] Matched asymptomatic and incontinent women were asked to fill out a written diary for 7 days followed by a week using a computerized diary; the patients' impressions of the use of the two systems were recorded. Preliminary results suggest that patients felt that their symptoms were more accurately reflected by the computerized version (92.6 vs 14.8%); they were more motivated to provide data (92.6 vs 14.8%) and the computerized version was easier to remember (100 vs 12.2%). In a subsequent study, the same group documented an increased volume of data and greater patient compliance in reporting bladder symptoms and events with the computerized diary.[18] However, the two methods were not comparable, as the computerized diary prompted more data entry (urgency, urgency with leak, intake) than the written diary, where patients were only asked to mark the time of a normal void and intake, with no space for any other information. It is interesting to note that, despite the skeletal nature of the conventional diary, patients still found it easier to comply with the computerized diary.

SUMMARY

Although limited by its poor reliability in differentiating normal from abnormal voiding patterns, the diary remains valid for the determination of frequency and functional capacity, as well as in demonstrating frequency and severity of urinary incontinence. It is easy to complete and this can be done by the patient prior to the consultation; the diary can thus be used to assess the extent of the symptomatology presented at the initial visit. It can also be used to triage care to determine the urgency and complexity of the consultation. A computerized form of the diary shows promise but corroboration and a greater volume of data are needed to assess its validity.

REFERENCES

1. Larsson G, Victor A. Micturition patterns in a healthy female population, studied with a frequency/volume chart. *Scand J Urol Nephrol Suppl* 1988; 114: 53–57

2. Kassis A, Schick E. Frequency–volume chart pattern in a healthy female population. *Br J Urol* 1993; 72: 708–710

3. Bailey R, Shepherd A, Tribe B. How much information can be obtained from frequency/volume charts? *Neurourol Urodyn* 1990; 9: 382–383

4. Abrams P, Klevmark B. Frequency volume charts: an indispensable part of lower urinary tract assessment. *Scand J Urol Nephrol Suppl* 1996; 179: 47–53

5. Wyman JF, Choi SC, Harkins SW *et al.* The urinary diary in evaluation of incontinent women: a test–retest analysis. *Obstet Gynecol* 1988; 71: 812–817

6. Sommer P, Bauer T, Nielsen KK *et al.* Voiding patterns and prevalence of incontinence in women: a questionnaire survey. *Br J Urol* 1990; 66: 12–15

7. Barnick C. Frequency/volume charts. In: Cardozo L (ed) *Urogynecology: the King's Approach.* New York: Churchill Livingstone, 1997: 104

8. Robinson D, McClish DK, Wyman JF *et al.* Comparison between urinary diaries completed with and without intensive patient instructions. *Neurourol Urodyn* 1996; 15: 143–148

9. Kahn KS, Chien PFW, Honest MR, Norman GR. Evaluation measurement variability in clinical investigations: the case of ultrasonic estimation of urinary bladder volume. *Br J Obstet Gynaecol* 1997; 104: 1036–1042

10. Elser DM, Fantl JA, McClish DK *et al.* Comparison of 'subjective' and 'objective' measures of severity of urinary incontinence in women. *Neurourol Urodyn* 1995; 14: 311–316

11. McCormack M, Infante-Rivard C, Schick E. Agreement between clinical methods of measurement of urinary frequency and functional bladder capacity. *Br J Urol* 1992; 69: 17–21

12. Diokno AC, Wells TJ, Brink CA. Comparison of self-reported voided volume with cystometric bladder capacity. *J Urol* 1987; 137: 698–700

13. Bland JM, Altman DG. Statistical methods for assessing agreement between two methods of clinical measurement. *Lancet* 1986; i: 307–310

14. Larsson G, Abrams P, Victor A. The frequency/volume chart in detrusor instability. *Neurourol Urodyn* 1991; 10: 533–543

15. Larsson G, Victor A. The frequency/volume chart in genuine stress incontinent women. *Neurourol Urodyn* 1992; 11: 23–31

16. Heit M, Brubaker L. Clinical correlates in patients not completing a voiding diary. *Int Urogynecol J Pelvic Floor Dysfunct* 1996; 7: 256–259

17. Rabin JM, McNett J, Badlani GH. Computerized voiding diary. *Neurourol Urodyn* 1993; 12: 541–554

18. Rabin JM, McNett J, Badlani GH. A computerized voiding diary. *J Reprod Med* 1996; 41: 801–806

16

Pad tests

M.-A. Harvey, E. Versi

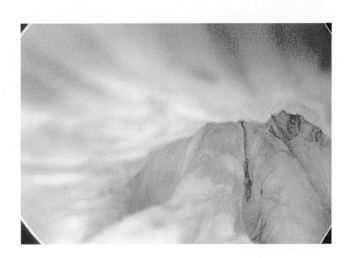

INTRODUCTION

The objective demonstration of urinary incontinence is of paramount importance in its definition and diagnosis.[1] However, the patient's perception of neither incontinence[2] nor its severity[3] are well correlated with urodynamic measures; a quantification method was therefore required. Over the past 25 years, several methods have been proposed to reach this goal. The work was pioneered by James *et al.*[4] with the use of the Urilos nappy (diaper) test. It was followed by the use of perineal pads, first referred to by Caldwell in 1974;[5] this technique is now the most widely used and studied. Other innovative methods were developed, going from the urethral electrical conductance test[6–8] to temperature-sensitive devices,[9] and included simpler methods such as the quantitative paper towel test[10] and the pyridium test.[11]

These techniques have been developed for, and used in, different settings. First, they have been used to quantify urine loss, thus allowing objective evaluation of severity of the condition and effect of treatment in a non-invasive way. Secondly, specially designed pads have allowed detection of urine leakage during ambulatory cystometry, where it is not possible (as during office cystometry) to visualize directly urine loss from the external urethral meatus.

URILOS

James *et al.*[4] first described a 'nappy' (diaper) consisting of an interleaved pair of electrodes embedded in an absorbent cloth, having the capacity to monitor and quantify urine loss as a function of time. A low-voltage (50 mV) alternating current was used to detect the variation in electrical conductivity resulting from the contact of urine with the electrodes.

Initially, the Urilos (N.H. Eastwood & Son, Ltd, London, UK) was said to be able to detect volumes from less than 1 ml to approximately 100 ml, with a variation of up to 20% when repeated. Subsequent studies[2,12] have attempted to assess the reliability of the Urilos system. The difference in volume recorded between different nappies varied between 13[2] and 25%;[12] when nappies from different boxes were compared, the variation between them was as much as 68%.[12] Because of its lack of precision, the Urilos test never gained widespread popularity.

PERINEAL PADS

Although referred to by Caldwell in 1974,[5] the method of perineal pad weight testing in the ambulatory patient was not described until 1981.[13] The following decade produced most of the literature on the subject. Several protocols were studied and can, in the main, be divided into short-term or long-term pad tests. Short-term protocols include the 1-hour and 2-hour pad tests: the 1-hour pad test was standardized by the International Continence Society (ICS) in 1983[14] (Table 16.1) and includes staging of the severity of incontinence (Table 16.2). Long-term protocols consist of home pad tests of 12, 24 and 48 hours and have not, as yet, been subject to standardization.

Table 16.1. *Standardized 1-hour pad test*

Time (minutes)	Procedure/activities	
	Tester	Patient
0	Apply pre-weighed pad	Drink 500 ml sodium-free liquid Sit and rest
30		Walking, stair-climbing
45		Sit/stand × 10 Cough × 10 Run on the spot × 1 minute Pick up objects from floor Wash hands under running water × 1 minute
60	Collect and weigh pad	Patient voids (volume measured by tester)

Adapted from ref. 14.

Table 16.2. *Categorization of urinary incontinence according to weight gain in the 1-hour pad test**

Category	Weight gain (g)
Dry	< 2
Slight to moderate	2–10
Severe	10–50
Very severe	> 50

* According to International Continence Society classification (ref. 1).

Short-term pad test

Reliability

Reliability reflects the capacity of a test to differentiate among the individuals studied, in particular, diseased individuals from normal ones.[15]

The first report of a normal threshold in a 1-hour pad test in continent women was by Sutherst *et al.*[13] When results from 50 women with urinary control were compared with those from 100 women referred for incontinence, a maximum weight change of the pad of 1 g was measured in all the continent patients vs a mean of 12.2 g in incontinent women. Versi and Cardozo[16] compared the 1-hour pad test with videourodynamic studies in continent and incontinent (genuine stress incontinence, GSI) patients: in 90 patients without incontinence and with normal videourodynamic studies, the mean pad weight gain was 0.39 g, with a 99% upper confidence limit of 1.4 g. The ICS fixed the threshold at 2 g.

Validity

Validity expresses the relation between observed measurements and the true state of the entity being studied.[15]

Validity of the pad test can be reflected by the accuracy of the measured volume lost and its sensitivity in detecting such a loss. If the sensitivity is poor, the test will not detect the true state of the entity, namely the presence of incontinence. However, as there is currently no means of detecting the true amount of urine leak with each incontinence episode, the validity of the pad test will be reflected in its ability to demonstrate incontinence in a patient who complains of urinary incontinence.

Overall, the sensitivity of the pad test in screening for GSI is poor. Versi *et al.*[17] assessed the value of the pad test as a screening tool in 311 patients, for which the diagnosis was subsequently made by multichannel videourodynamics. These authors found a 68% sensitivity, and a false-negative rate of 32%. Similar false-negative rates, 14–35%,[18,19] were found in other studies, which contrasts with the absence of false negatives reported by Hahn and Fall.[20] If the pad test was used as an adjunctive test to uroflowmetry and cystometry, the sensitivity for diagnosis of GSI increased to 81%, but the false-negative rate remained high at 19%.[17] When a more provocative test protocol was used, the sensitivity was increased to 94%.[19]

Reproducibility

Reproducibility represents the capacity of a test to demonstrate similar results on the same patient when performed either at a different point in time (intraobserver) or by different investigators (interobserver). Several studies have investigated this aspect with variable results when the bladder volume is fixed[20–24] and when it is not.[19,25–28]

Studies evaluating the reproducibility of the 1-hour pad test without controlling for bladder volume reported an overall acceptable, though variable, correlation. Correlation coefficients (r) were calculated to be between 0.68 and 0.77 when tests were performed in the same department.[19,25] Notable exceptions to this were one study[25] reporting a correlation coefficient of only 0.1 (when comparing the test performed in different departments on the same patient) and another[28] on only 16 patients, which showed a very high correlation of 0.91. In a further two studies, a clinically significant intra-individual variation of 50–150% was found.[26,27] Given these results, assessment of the severity of a patient's condition based on ICS criteria (Table 16.2) would be rather variable. Indeed, analysis of the data shows a change in the severity stage status in up to 30%[26] or 44%,[27] depending on the dataset.

The 1-hour pad test as described by the ICS is reasonably reproducible; however, its validity in differentiating between different severity stages is poor.[26,27]

With controlled bladder volume, test–retest correlation depends on the volume infused. With the subjects' bladders filled to capacity (as measured on the cystometrogram), two studies have shown good correlation coefficients in patients with GSI (Table 16.3). In women with detrusor instability (DI), the correlation was slightly less at 0.84.[23] If the bladder volume at which the test is performed decreases, the correlation remains reasonable

Table 16.3. *Reproducibility of pad tests in women with GSI, when their bladders are filled to capacity*		
	Ref. 20 (n = 50)	Ref. 23 (n = 67)
Mean volume (ml) at capacity (± SD or range)	273 (150–400)	356 (± 92.8)
Test–retest correlation (Pearson's correlation, *r*)	0.94	0.97

Table 16.4. *Regimen of more provocative exercises*
Stair-climbing equivalent to 100 steps up and down
Coughing strongly 10 times
Running on the spot for 1 minute
Washing the hands under running water for 1 minute
Jumping on the spot for 30 seconds with feet together
Jumping on the spot for 30 seconds with feet alternately apart and together (star jumps)

Adapted from ref. 20.

($r = 0.74$ at 75% of capacity;[24] $r = 0.97$ at 50% of bladder capacity[22]), although variable between studies. Jakobsen et al.[21] compared pad testing at 50% v 75% of maximum capacity in 70 randomized patients: test–retest analysis showed no difference when performed at 50% of bladder capacity; however, when the test was conducted at 75%, the pad weight gain was significantly greater during the second test. Furthermore, more patients in the 50% group found that the test was representative of their daily experience.

On the basis of the available data, it is not possible to make assumptions about the best technique for performing the 1-hour pad test. Furthermore, the statistical technique used in most studies – the correlation coefficient – is questionable: as previously stated, *r* measures the strength of the relationship between two variables, not the agreement between them; it is highly possible that two tests may disagree, despite a high correlation.[29] The correlation coefficient does not provide reliable information with regard to reproducibility or the true variation of the test. Bland and Altman[29] have illustrated this concept, using test–retest data with high correlation (Pearson's). A plot of the difference between the two methods on the *y*-axis, against the mean of the two methods on the *x*-axis for each patient, may display considerable lack of agreement. Good agreement is demonstrated when the mean of the methods is within two standard deviations (2 SD) of the average difference between the tests.

To conclude, the 1-hour pad test is poor as a screening test as it has a high false-negative rate. None the less, it remains useful as an adjunct to urodynamic testing. Its reproducibility is reasonable and appears to be improved by a standardized bladder volume and a more provocative exercise regimen, such as that shown in Table 16.4.

Home pad test

In view of the high false-negative rate found in the 1-hour pad test, a home pad test, with increased test duration, was advocated. The 1-hour pad test was criticized because of its artificial setting and short duration. The first preliminary report of such a home test was presented by Sutherst's group at the ICS annual meeting in 1983,[30] in which a 12-hour home pad test was compared with a 1-hour test in 20 patients. The authors demonstrated a good correlation between the 1-hour test and any 1 hour of the home test. Since then, other reports have been published.[18,31–33]

Versi et al.[33] performed a 48-hour home test on 24 continent patients and determined the normal threshold as a weight gain of less than 15 g/48 h (8 g/24 h). Validity was also evaluated by comparing the home pad test with videourodynamic studies on 156 patients. The sensitivity of the pad test was 92% with false-negative and false-positive rates of 8 and 28%, respectively, for the diagnosis of GSI. It is of interest to note that eight of 12 patients with a false-positive pad test (i.e. normal urodynamic study) were subsequently found to have DI on repeat urodynamic studies. The authors proposed that such a test could be an adjunct to conventional cystometry for detecting occult DI.

Reproducibility of the 48-hour home pad test has been reported as very good. Versi et al.[33] found a correlation coefficient of 0.94 between two 48-hour pad tests on 112 patients and, on the basis of the analysis proposed by Bland and Altman,[29] a difference between the mean of the two tests of 1.6%. Victor et al.[31] noted a similar result, with a correlation coefficient of 0.90 between two 48-hour tests.

In order to decrease the length of the test and ease its execution, a 24-hour home test has been evaluated. The normal range in 23 continent patients tested twice was determined to be below $8\,g/24\,h$;[18] Versi *et al.*[33] found similar results in normal subjects during the 48-hour test. The 24-hour pad test was consistently found to be reproducible ($r = 0.82$;[18] $r = 0.90$;[33] $r = 0.92$[34]). When compared with the 48-hour test, it showed no statistical difference in terms of reproducibility.[33,34] Consequently, a 24-hour home pad test seems to be adequate clinically for detecting and quantifying urinary incontinence, and possibly for detecting occult DI.

One-hour pad test versus home pad test

Only a few studies compared the home test with the 1-hour pad test, but they consistently showed poor correlation between the two tests.[18,31,34] The home pad test was positive in more patients complaining of incontinence than was the 1-hour pad test. The largest reported series included 31 women with incontinence:[18] 23 patients had GSI and eight had mixed incontinence. Each patient performed a 1-hour pad test at a fixed bladder volume (filled at time of cystometry) followed by a 24-hour home pad test. According to the 1-hour pad test, 18 patients were incontinent ($\geq 2\,g$) versus 28 patients on the 24-hour home pad test ($\geq 8\,g$), giving a false-negative rate of 39% when compared with the 24-hour home pad test. No correlation was found between the two tests ($r = 0.22$; $p > 0.05$). Similarly, Victor *et al.*[31] found a poor correlation between the results of the 48-hour or the 1-hour pad tests ($r = 0.10$; $p > 0.05$) when studied in 17 patients with urinary incontinence (the type was not specified in the report). Finally, Thind *et al.*[34] obtained comparable results on 25 women (14 with symptoms of stress, five with urge and six with mixed incontinence), with a rate of false negatives of 36% with the 1-hour pad test and a low correlation ($r = 0.35$; $p < 0.1$).

In a series of 48 patients with varied causes of incontinence, comparing 1-hour and 48-hour pad tests (unpublished data), we obtained a false-positive rate of 17%, with eight patients being wrongly identified as incontinent with the 1-hour pad test, and a false-negative rate of 16%. In the subgroup of 22 patients with symptoms of stress incontinence only, the 1-hour pad test had a false-positive rate of 23% and a false-negative rate of 9%.

These studies suggest that the home pad test is more sensitive than the 1-hour pad test, at no cost to reproducibility, especially in detecting urge and mixed incontinence.

PAPER TOWEL TEST

Most of the methods objectively quantifying urine loss preclude detection of small volumes, as these may overlap with perspiration and vaginal secretions. A simple non-invasive test was developed to detect such losses associated with stress incontinence.[10] While a tri-fold brown paper towel is held under the perineum, the patient is asked to cough three times. The surface of the wetted area is calculated using the ellipse formula (πxy, x and y being the orthogonal axes of the area), and this is then converted to the volume of urine lost (using a standard curve). The relationship between the measured area and a known fluid volume was found to have a very strong correlation ($r = 0.998$). In a test–retest evaluation within the same visit and between visits, the authors also noted a high correlation coefficient and concluded that the quantitative paper towel test was accurate and reliable in detecting small losses of urine due to stress incontinence. However, this test has not been validated against a 'gold-standard' diagnostic method such as multichannel videourodynamics; consequently, the sensitivity and specificity of this diagnostic method is currently unknown.

PYRIDIUM TEST

Phenazopyridine hydrochloride (Pyridium) ingestion results in the dye being excreted by the kidney with consequent colouring (orange) of the urine, and this has been used by clinicians to detect incontinence. Wall *et al.*[11] reported the sensitivity and specificity of Pyridium as a qualitative test in incontinent patients. In a study comparing this method with a standardized 1-hour pad test in asymptomatic women and those with GSI (diagnosed by subtracted cystometry), the sensitivity and specificity of the Pyridium pad test were 100% and 48%, respectively. The poor specificity was due to a high false-positive rate in asymptomatic patients. This may be explained by staining of the perineum at the time of a previous void, resulting in tinting of a subsequent pad on vulvar contact or by a minimal, clinically insignificant, loss of urine in normal women. These results were subsequently confirmed in a study testing continent (self-reported) women, during exercise,[35] in which Nygaard and Zmolek reported nearly 100% pyridium staining after physical activity, with a mean pad weight of 4.59 ± 3.55 g (outdoor exercise) or 1.33 ± 0.97 g (indoor exercise). Pyridium staining was minimal, with a mean stained area of 2.66 mm (range 0–11 mm). No cut-off limit in the pad weight has been previously established to define a normal pad test during exercise, given that there would be a greater weight gain due to perspiration alone.

In the light of these reports, the use of Pyridium in detecting transurethral incontinence can be perceived as unreliable and non-specific. None the less, it remains useful in the diagnosis of extra-urethral urine loss (e.g. fistulae).

URETHRAL ELECTRICAL CONDUCTANCE

The urethral electric conductance test was developed by Plevnik *et al.*[36] It is based on the knowledge that impedance of the urothelium is greater than that of urine. Mounted on a 7F catheter, two 1 mm electrodes, placed 1 mm apart, carry a low non-stimulatory voltage (20 mV).[37] The electrical conductance between the electrodes increases as the milieu increases in ionic content. Thus, when urine enters the urethra, the ionic content of the milieu is changed, resulting in a decrease in electrical impedance. This is measurable by a change in electrical current (in mA) between the two plates.

This technique, known as the distal urethral electric conductance (DUEC) test, was adapted to assess sphincter incompetence by detecting the presence of urine 1.5 cm proximal to the external urethral meatus. In a preliminary report presented at the ICS in 1985,[38] the test was positive (i.e. increase in electrical current $\geq 2.5\,\mu$A) in 27 of 36 symptomatic women and was more sensitive than physical examination in detecting stress incontinence. However, it has not been compared in sufficient numbers with the standardized 1-hour pad test and the sensitivity and specificity of this diagnostic method are unknown. In addition, this method does not quantify urine loss. None the less, it is a promising technique that merits further study

TEMPERATURE-SENSITIVE DEVICES

Temperature-sensitive devices can be employed to detect urine loss during ambulatory urodynamic studies. The technique relies on detection of a difference in urinary and perineal temperature by diode temperature sensors.[9] When such a device was studied in continent and incontinent women and compared with pad weight results, the sensitivity and specificity were found to be 95.2% and 90.6%, respectively. However, it was not possible with this technique to quantify urine loss; consequently, it cannot be used to assess severity of incontinence and response to treatment.

SUMMARY

To date, the perineal pad test is still the most useful objective urine loss test in clinical practice. A short version has been standardized to a certain degree by the ICS, rendering its use more uniform for collection of research data. However, the bladder volume at the beginning of the 1-hour test remains to be standardized. The short-term pad test has been found to be reliable in differentiating normal from abnormal continence mechanisms; however, its validity is somewhat limited as it has a significant false-negative rate. The 1-hour pad test has been found to have good reproducibility, which apparently is improved by a standardized bladder volume and a more provocative exercise regimen. Finally, the short-term pad test (≤ 1 hour) has been found to be a poor method by which to categorize severity of incontinence.

The long-term pad test (≥ 24 hours), on the other hand, has been found to be a valid method of detecting incontinence, with excellent sensitivity and a low false-negative rate. The reproducibility was similarly noted to be good for both a 48-hour and a 24-hours test period. Hence, a 48-hour home pad test is a good tool for detection of incontinence, particularly for the detection of occult DI missed on urodynamic studies, which is an advantage over the 1-hour pad test.

More data are required to determine the sensitivity and validity of the paper towel test, the DUEC test and the temperature-sensitive devices; however, these methods remain interesting for objective determination of incontinence. Urilos is of historical interest and the Pyridium test has a false-positive rate that is too high to make it useful for routine clinical practice.

REFERENCES

1. Abrams P, Blaivas JG, Stanton SL *et al.* The standardization of terminology of lower urinary tract function. *Scand J Urol Nephrol Suppl* 1988; 114: 5–19

2. Stanton SL, Ritchie D. Urilos: the practical detection of urine loss. *Am J Obstet Gynecol* 1977; 128: 461–463

3. Frazer MI, Haylen BT, Sutherst JR. The severity of urinary incontinence in women: comparison of subjective and objective data. *Br J Urol* 1989; 63: 14–15

4. James ED, Flack FC, Caldwell KPS, Martin MR. Continuous measurement of urine loss and frequency in incontinent patients. *Br J Urol* 1971; 43: 233–237

5. Caldwell KPS. Clinical use of the recording nappy. *Urol Int* 1974; 29: 172–173

6. Plevnik S, Vrtacnik P, Janez J. Detection of fluid entry into the urethra by electric impedance measurement: electric fluid bridge test. *Clin Phys Physiol Meas* 1983; 3: 309–313

7. Peattie AB, Plevnik S, Stanton SL. The use of bladder neck electric conductance (BNEC) in the investigation and management of sensory urge incontinence in the female. *J R Soc Med* 1988; 81: 442–444

8. Plevnik S, Brown M, Sutherst JR, Vrtacnik P. Tracking of fluid in urethra by simultaneous electric impedance measurement at three sites. *Urol Int* 1983; 38: 29–32

9. Eckford SD, Finney R, Jackson SR, Abrams P. Detection of urinary incontinence during ambulatory monitoring of bladder function by a temperature-sensitive device. *Br J Urol* 1996; 77: 194–197.

10. Miller JM, Ashton-Miller JA, DeLancey JOL. The quantitative paper towel test for measuring stress-related urine loss. *Proc Am Urogynecologic Soc, 18th annual meeting.* Chicago: American Urogynecologic Society, 1997; 44

11. Wall LL, Wang K, Robson I, Stanton SL. The pyridium pad test for diagnosing urinary incontinence. *J Reprod Med* 1990; 35: 682–684

12. Wilson PD, Al Samarrai MT, Brown DG. Quantifying female incontinence with particular reference to the Urilos System. *Urol Int* 1980; 35: 298–302

13. Sutherst J, Brown M, Shawer M. Assessing the severity or urinary incontinence in women by weighing perineal pads. *Lancet* 1981; i: 1128–1130

14. Bates P, Bradley W, Glen E *et al. Fifth Report on the Standardization of Terminology of Lower Urinary Tract Function.* Bristol: International Continence Society Committee on Standardization of Terminology, 1983

15. Khan KS, Chien PFW, Honest MR, Norman GR. Evaluating measurement variability in clinical investigations: the case of ultrasonic estimation of urinary bladder volume. *Br J Obstet Gynaecol* 1997; 104: 1036–1042

16. Versi E, Cardozo L. Perineal pad weighing versus videographic analysis in genuine stress incontinence. *Br J Obstet Gynaecol* 1986; 93: 364–366

17. Versi E, Cardozo L, Anand D. The use of pad tests in the investigation of female urinary incontinence. *J Obstet Gynecol* 1988; 8: 270–273

18. Lose G, Jørgensen L, Thunedborg P. 24-Hour home pad weighing test versus 1-hour ward test in the assessment of mild stress incontinence. *Acta Obstet Gynecol Scand* 1989; 68: 211–215

19. Jørgensen L, Lose G, Andersen JT. One-hour pad-weighing test for objective assessment of female urinary incontinence. *Obstet Gynecol* 1987; 69: 39–42

20. Hahn I, Fall M. Objective quantification of stress urinary incontinence: a short, reproducible, provocative pad test. *Neurourol Urodyn* 1991; 10: 475–481.

21. Jakobsen H, Kromann-Andersen B, Nielsen KK, Maegaard E. Pad weighing tests with 50% or 75% bladder filling: does it matter? *Acta Obstet Gynecol Scand* 1993; 72: 377–381

22. Lose G, Rosenkilde P. Gammelgaard J, Schroeder T. Pad-weighing test performed with standardized bladder volume. *Urology* 1988; 32: 78–80

23. Fantl JA, Harkins SW, Wyman JF *et al.* Fluid loss quantitation test in women with urinary incontinence: a test–retest analysis. *Obstet Gynecol* 1987; 70: 739–743

24. Kinn AC, Larsson B. Pad test with fixed bladder volume in urinary stress incontinence. *Acta Obstet Gynecol Scand* 1987; 66: 369–371

25. Christensen SJ, Colstrup H, Hertz JB *et al.* Inter- and intra-departmental variations of the perineal pad weighing test. *Neurourol Urodyn* 1986; 5: 23–28.

26. Mundt-Pettersen B, Mattiasson A, Sundin T. Reproducibility of the 1 hour incontinence test proposed by the ICS standardization committee. *Proc. International Continence Society, 14th annual meeting.* Innsbruck: International Continence Society, 1984; 90–91

27. Lose G, Gammelgaard J, Jørgensen TJ. The one-hour pad-weighing test: reproducibility and the correlation between the test result, the start volume in the bladder, and the diuresis. *Neurourol Urodyn* 1986; 5: 17–21

28. Klarskov P, Hald T. Reproducubility and reliability of urinary incontinence assessment with a 60 min test. *Scand J Urol Nephrol* 1984; 18: 293–298

29. Bland JM, Altman DG. Statistical methods for assessing agreement between two methods of clinical measurement. *Lancet* 1986; i: 307–310

30. Ali K, Murray A, Sutherst J, Brown M. Perineal pad weighing test: comparison of one hour ward pad test with twelve hours home pad test. *Proc. International Continence Society, 13th Annual Meeting.* Aachen: International Continence Society, 1983: 380–382

31. Victor A, Larsson G, Åsbrink AS. A simple patient-administered test for objective quantitation of the symptom of urinary incontinence. *Scand J Urol Nephrol* 1987; 21: 277–279.

32. Rasmussen A, Mouritsen L, Dalgaard A, Frimodt-Møller C. Twenty-four hour pad weighing test: reproducibility and dependency of activity level and fluid intake. *Neurourol Urodyn* 1994; 13: 261–265

33. Versi E, Orrego G, Hardy E *et al*. Evaluation of the home pad test in the investigation of female urinary incontinence. *Br J Obstet Gynaecol* 1996; 103: 162–167

34. Thind P, Gerstenberg TC. One-hour ward test vs. 24-hour home pad weighing test in the diagnosis of urinary incontinence. *Neurourol Urodyn* 1991; 10: 241–245

35. Nygaard I, Zmolek G. Exercise pad testing in continent exercisers: reproducibility and correlation with voided volume, pyridium staining and type of exercise. *Neurourol Urodyn* 1995; 14: 125–129

36. Plevnik S, Brown M, Sutherst JR, Vrtacnik P. Tracking of fluid in urethra by simultaneous electric impedance measurement at three sites. *Urol Int* 1983; 38: 29–32

37. Plevnik S, Holmes DM, Janez J *et al*. Urethral electric conductance (UEC) – a new parameter for evaluation of urethral and bladder function: methodology of the assessmant of its clinical potential. *Proceeedings of the 15th Annual Meeting of the International Continence Society*, London 1985; 90–91

38. Holmes DM, Plevnik S, Stanton SL. Distal urethral electric conductance (DUEC) test for the detection of urinary leakage. *Proc. International Continence Society 15th Annual Meeting*. London: International Continence Society, 1985; 94–95

17

Uroflowmetry

B. Haylen

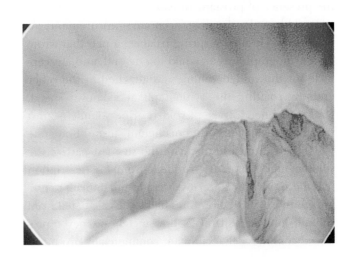

INTRODUCTION

One of the core aims of urodynamic testing is to screen for the presence of voiding difficulty, i.e. abnormally slow and/or incomplete micturition. Uroflowmetry, or the measure of urine flow over time, allows the simple and non-invasive analysis of the normality or otherwise of urine flow, while the complementary measurement of residual urine volume will indicate the completeness or otherwise of micturition.

Abnormal urine flow rates or patterns in women will generally require the further investigation of voiding cystometry in order to determine the cause. Pressure–flow analysis will allow discrimination between the presence of one of the two main causes of abnormally slow urine flow – bladder outflow obstruction and a hypotonic or atonic bladder

It is important clinically to diagnose or eliminate the diagnosis of voiding difficulty in women presenting for assessment of symptoms of lower urinary tract dysfunction. Surgical treatment of genuine stress incontinence (GSI) and drug treatment of detrusor instability (DI) both have the potential to cause voiding difficulty. Pre-existing voiding difficulty will prejudice these treatments, leading to the possibility of acute or chronic retention.

HISTORY OF UROFLOWMETRY

The first attempt to obtain an objective measurement of the urine flow rate was made in 1897 by Rehfisch (Ryall and Marshall)[1] using a poorly detailed method employing an air-displacement principle. In the opinion of Ballenger *et al.*,[2] the cast distance of urinary stream (voiding distance) might be a useful clinical guide to the presence of prostatic disease.

Drake[3] made the first accurate measurements of urine flow. He used a spring balance; a pen that wrote on a kymograph was attached to one end, and a receptacle for the voided volume was attached to the other end. By rotating the kymograph at a known speed, Drake obtained a trace of voided urine volume against time. He calculated the maximum urine flow rate (MUFR) by a measurement of the steepest part of the volume–time curve. It is evident from his description that the apparatus was relatively crude and difficult to use. Furthermore, urine flow rates had to be calculated from volume–time data. Drake's flow meter was never produced commercially. Kaufman[4] commercially produced

a modification of Drake's flow meter that was more refined but, similarly, made no direct recording of urine flow rate.

The advent of electronics in medical instrumentation allowed the mass production of accurate and reliable recording devices. Von Garrelts[5] designed the first of the electronic urine flow meters, which consisted of a tall urine-collecting cylinder with a pressure transducer in the base. The pressure transducer measured the pressure exerted by an increasing column of urine as the patient voided. Since a direct relationship existed between the volume voided and the pressure recorded, von Garrelts was able to produce a direct recording of urine flow rate by electronic differentiation with time.

DEFINITION OF URINE FLOW RATE MEASUREMENTS

In any field of scientific measurement, it is important that all workers use standardized terminology. Urine flow rates are measured in millilitres per second. Figure 17.1 denotes the definitions for urine flow rate measurements as suggested by the Standardization Committee of the International Continence Society (ICS), as follows:

- Flow rate is the volume of fluid expelled via the urethra per second.
- Voided volume is the total volume expelled via the urethra.

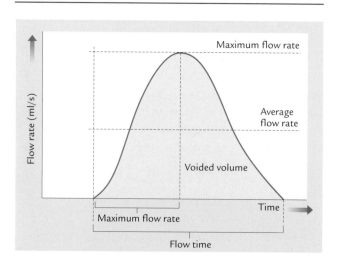

Figure 17.1. *Urine flow rates (International Continence Society definitions).*

- Maximum flow rate is the maximum measured value of the flow rate.
- Flow time is the time over which measurable flow occurs. Flow time is easily measured if flow is continuous, unless there is lengthy terminal dribble that may be noted but not included in the flow time. If urine flow is intermittent, the time intervals between flow episodes are not included.
- Average flow rate is the volume voided divided by the flow time. The voided volume may be calculated from the area beneath the flow–time curve.

METHODS OF URINE FLOW RATE MEASUREMENT

Numerous physical principles have been employed over the years in an attempt to develop what Backman and von Garrelts[7] and von Garrelts and Strandell[8] would see as an ideal uroflowmeter:

- High level of accuracy at different voided volumes and urine flow rates;
- Easy-to-read and rapidly available permanent tracings;
- Unobtrusive and not distracting to the patient by appearance or sound;
- Easy to clean.

Many methods have been used for urine flow measurement, from measuring the time to void a given volume through audiometric and radioisotope methods to include even high-speed cinematography. Figures 17.2a–d take a light-hearted look at these methods, none of which is currently popular. The most common method has been that of Drake[3] modified by von Garrelts and Strandell[8] – the measurement of urine weight.

In addition, flow meters have been produced that use the principles of air displacement, differential resistance to gas flow, electromagnetism, photoelectricity, electrical capacitance and a rotating disc.

Flow meters employing the principles of weight transduction, a rotating disc and a capacitance transducer are the best known and the most completely tested and validated of the flow meters available.

The weight transducer type of flow meter (Fig. 17.3a) weighs the voided urine and, by differentiation with time, produces an 'on-line' recording of urine flow rate (FR):

$$FR = dV/dT$$

where dV is the change in volume of urine over change in time, dt.

The rotating-disc flow meter (Fig. 17.3b) depends on a servometer maintaining the rotation of the disc at a constant speed. Urine hits the disc, and the extra power required to maintain the speed is electronically converted into a measurement of flow rate.

The capacitance flow meter is the simplest of the three flow meters, and consists of a funnel leading urine into a collecting vessel. The transducer is in the form of a dipstick made of plastic and coated with metal, which dips into the vessel containing the voided urine (Fig. 17.3c).

All three types of flow meter perform accurately and efficiently. For clinical purposes, the measured and indicated flow rate should be accurate to within $\pm 5\%$ of the clinically significant flow rate range.[9] The capacitance (dipstick) flow meter is the least expensive to buy and has the advantage of no moving parts, which means that mechanical breakdowns are eliminated. Rotating-disc flow meters have the advantage of not requiring priming with fluid. Automatic start and stop facilities in some modern flow meters assist by minimizing patient and staff involvement during the uroflowmetry.

CLINICAL MEASUREMENT OF URINE FLOW RATES

The environment for patient flow-rate recording is of considerable importance. Female patients usually void in circumstances of almost complete privacy. It is essential in the clinical situation that every effort is made to make the patient feel comfortable and relaxed. If these requirements are ignored, psychological factors are introduced and a proportion of patients will fail to void in a representative way. Ideally, all free uroflowmetry studies should be performed in a completely private uroflowmetry room/toilet, lockable from the inside, and out of hearing range of other staff and patients. As crouching over a toilet seat causes a 21% reduction in the average urine flow rate,[10] patients should be encouraged to sit to void. When video studies are combined with pressure–flow recordings in a radiology department, up to 30% of women may fail to void.

A patient should be encouraged to attend for uroflowmetry with her bladder comfortably full. It is

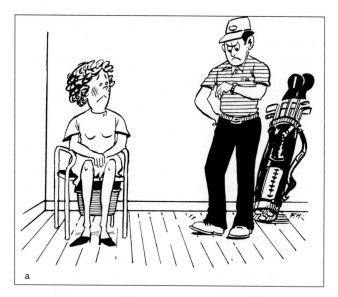

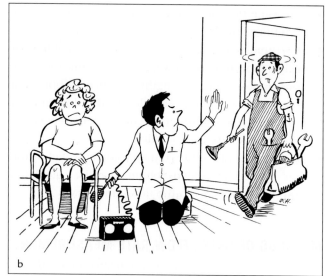

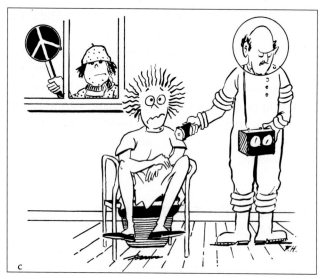

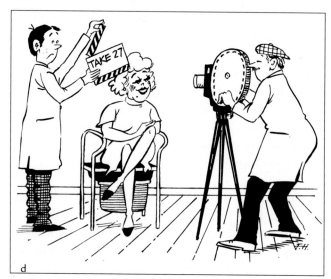

Figure 17.2. *(a) Time to void a given volume; (b) audiometric uroflowmetry; (c) radioisotope uroflowmetry; (d) high-speed cinematography. (Courtesy of Mr Frank Harris, Cartoonist, Liverpool Echo.)*

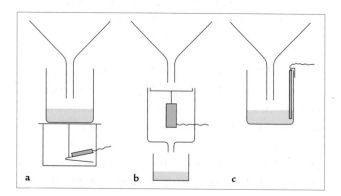

Figure 17.3. *Urine flow meters. (a) weight transducer; (b) rotating disc; (c) capacitance (dipstick).*

desirable that the measured urine flow rates should be for a voided volume within the patient's normal range. This range can be determined if, in the week before the flow study, the patient completes a frequency–volume chart (urinary diary). On this chart, the patient enters the volumes of fluid consumed and the volumes of urine voided. Recent nomograms, however, provide normal reference ranges for urinary flow rates over a wide range of voided volumes. There is generally no need for multiple uroflowmetry in most women. Abnormal or unusual flow curves and urinary flow rates, however, merit repetition of the study.

URINE FLOW RATES IN NORMAL (ASYMPTOMATIC) WOMEN

The MUFR and average urinary flow rate (AUFR) are the two most important uroflowmetry parameters. They are both numerical representations of the urine flow curve. The clinical usefulness of urine flow rates had been attenuated by the lack of absolute values defining normal limits.[11] As urine flow rates are known to have a strong dependence on voided volume,[3,12] these normal limits need to be over a wide range of voided volumes, ideally in the form of nomograms.

Studies on normal values for urine flow rates in women include those of Peter and Drake,[13] Scott and McIhlaney,[14] Backman,[15] Susset *et al.*,[16] Walter *et al.*,[17] Drach *et al.*,[12] Bottacini and Gleason,[18] Fantl *et al.*[19] and Rollema *et al.*[20] Data and/or statistical analyses in these studies have not allowed construction of effective nomograms. Difficulties have included small patient numbers,[16–20] the use of outmoded or less-well-evaluated equipment[12,13] and the incompleteness of data at lower voided volumes,[12,15] due in part to the inaccuracy of some equipment at lower voided volumes.[12]

The MUFR has been studied most. Recommended lower limits of normality range between 12 and 20 ml/s. Most commonly, a minimum rate of 15 ml/s is quoted for the same parameter if at least 150 ml (or sometimes 200 ml) has been voided. The practice of artificially imposing minimum limits for the voided volume is difficult to justify,[21] and very often is impractical. Women with certain states of lower urinary tract dysfunction – those in whom the flow rate might be most important – may not be able to hold 200 ml. Because of the strong dependency of urine flow rate on voided volume, a normal urine flow rate at 200 ml might not also be normal at 400 ml.

In a study in 1989, Haylen *et al.*[22] studied 249 female volunteers (aged 16–63 years), all of whom were deemed normal by denying specific urinary symptomatology, and who underwent uroflowmetry studies. Each women voided once in a completely private environment over a calibrated rotating disc-type uroflowmeter; 46 voided on a second occasion. The MUFR and AUFR of the first voids were compared with the respective voided volumes. By using statistical transformations of both voided volumes and urine flow rates, relationships between the two variables were obtained. This allowed the construction of nomo-

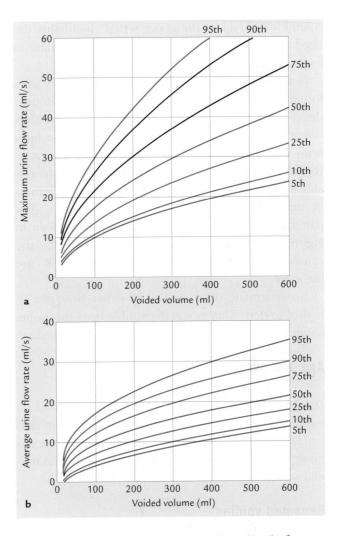

Figure 17.4. *Liverpool maximum (a) and average (b) flow-rate nomogram for women. Curves are centiles.*

grams, which, for ease of interpretation, have been displayed in centile form. Figures 17.4a and b show the 'Liverpool' nomograms for the maximum and average flow rates, respectively, in women.

CLINICAL FACTORS INFLUENCING URINE FLOW RATES IN NORMAL (ASYMPTOMATIC) WOMEN

Voided volume

The use of nomograms overcomes the dangers of referencing flow rates to any one voided volume. A maximum flow rate of 15 ml/s might fall just within the 5th centile curve at 200 ml voided volume, although well below the same curve at 400 ml. The median voided volume of 171 ml in the above series[22] highlights the need for normal reference ranges to include data at lower voided volumes.

Both the MUFR and AUFR in the above study were found to have a strong and essentially equal dependence on voided volume. The clinical use of either flow rate is equally valid. However, the centile lines onto which the MUFR and AUFR fall for the same voided volume (centile rankings) are not interchangeable in an individual instance, owing to wide variations in urine flow patterns. The closer the urine flow pattern comes to the 'ideal' flow–time curve seen in Figure 17.1 the more chance there will be that the centile rankings for the MUFR and AUFR are the same.

No systematic deterioration of either flow rate at higher voided volumes was discernible from this population study. The same may not be true for an individual.

Age and parity

Drach *et al.*,[12] Fantl *et al.*[19] and Haylen *et al.*[22] found no significant age dependence of urine flow rates in normal women. The same studies also found that there was no significant effect of parity on urine flow rates in normal women.

Repeated voiding

There was a remarkable consistency in the centile rankings of the paired first and second voids in the study of Haylen *et al.*[22] This consistency is further witnessed in the multiple voids from a single 25-year-old normal female volunteer (Fig. 17.5). Fantl *et al.*[19] found no significant difference between the first and up to the sixth void in the 60 women that they tested.

Clinically, in the majority of normal women, the centile rankings of successive voids will not differ widely. It is uncertain, at present, whether this is also true for women with lower urinary tract dysfunction. As suggested previously, abnormal or unusual urine flow rates or curves merit repetition of the study.

Presence of a catheter

The nomograms described above refer to free flowmetry voids; they are not applicable where pressure from another catheter is present in the urethra. All urethral

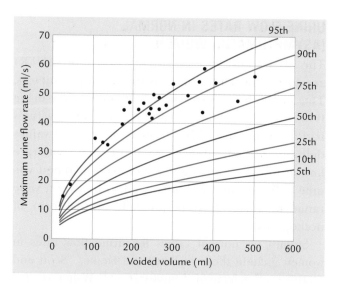

Figure 17.5. *Maximum flow rates from a large number of voids by a 25-year-old female volunteer superimposed on the relevant Liverpool nomogram.*

catheters can be expected to have the effect of decreasing urine flow rates for the equivalent voided volume. Part of this reduction may be physical obstruction, with pressure catheters varying from 6FG (microtransducer) to 10FG (water-filled). By necessity, potentially unfavourable environmental and psychological factors are introduced when catheterization uroflowmetry is performed. Ryall and Marshall[23] suggested that the reduction in MUFR caused by the fine (diameter = 2 mm) urethral catheter used in their study of 147 symptomatic men was of the order of several ml/s. Although small, this reduction was enough to change the diagnostic categorization of one-third of their subjects.

Normal male vs normal female urine flow rates

Urine flow rates in women are higher than those in men.[7,12,22] Women's MUFR values are on average 0.19 times greater than those of young men and 0.39 times greater than those of older men.[22] Urethral length (4 vs 20 cm) should account for all the intersex difference.[7,22]

URINE FLOW RATES IN WOMEN WITH SYMPTOMS OF LOWER URINARY TRACT DYSFUNCTION

Between 1958 and 1990, there were four studies on urine flow rates in symptomatic women (those with symptoms of lower urinary tract dysfunction), three of which were small.[12,13,18] The other study[24] was limited to the effect of final urodynamic diagnosis on urine flow rates. Three studies[13,18,24] indicated that symptomatic women had slower urine flow rates than normal women, with one study[12] showing no difference.

In 1995, Haylen *et al.*[25] completed a further study of 250 women who were consecutive referrals for urogynaecological assessment including urodynamics because of symptoms of lower urinary tract dysfunction. The flow data for these women were converted to centiles from the Liverpool nomograms for the following analyses of their median values.

Comparison of the urine flow rates of symptomatic and asymptomatic women

Table 17.1 shows that the median centiles of the MUFR and AUFR of the urogynaecology (symptomatic) patients were significantly reduced compared with those of the asymptomatic population. There was close agreement between the 1990 and 1995 studies of Haylen *et al.*,[24,25] performed in different countries.

Table 17.1. *Urine flow rates of symptomatic and asymptomatic women*

Flow rate	Population*	
	Symptomatic	Asymptomatic
Median centile maximum urine flow rate	32 (31)	50
Median centile average urine flow rate	26 (26)	50

*Data from ref. 24 in parentheses.

Effect of the presence of genital prolapse on urine flow rates in symptomatic women

As seen in Table 17.2, there is a generally progressive decline in the MUFR and AUFR (median centiles) of symptomatic women with increasing grades of genital prolapse. The most significant decline occurs in the presence of uterine prolapse, closely followed by cystocele and enterocele. There is a smaller effect in the presence of a rectocele.

Effect of hysterectomy on urine flow rates in symptomatic women

A significant decline has been found in the urine flow rates of symptomatic women (median centiles) who have had a hysterectomy (Table 17.3), the effect being the same for both vaginal and abdominal hysterectomy. The urine flow rates for those symptomatic women without hysterectomy were found to be the same as those for the asymptomatic female population.

Further analysis suggests that, in women who have had a hysterectomy and have intercurrent genital prolapse, there is a cumulative decline in urine flow.

Effect of age and parity on urine flow rates in symptomatic women

In symptomatic women, unlike asymptomatic women, there is a significant effect of age on the MUFR and AUFR, as shown in Table 17.4.

Figure 17.6 depicts the decline in urine flow rates with age in patients with no previous hysterectomy or intercurrent genital prolapse (top line); the presence of either (centre line) or both (bottom line) of these

Table 17.2. *Effect of genital prolapse on urine flow rates* in symptomatic women*

Genital prolapse grade	Cystocele		Uterine		Rectocele		Enterocele	
	MUFR	AUFR	MUFR	AUFR	MUFR	AUFR	MUFR	AUFR
0	42	30	49	37	43	32	35	20
1	35	32	32	32	24	16	11	10
2/3	20	11	17	11	32	27	17	12
p	0.0010	0.0049	0.0001	0.001	0.0030	0.0831	0.0012	0.0054

*AUFR, average urine flow rate; MUFR, maximum urine flow rate.

Table 17.3. *Effect of hysterectomy on urine flow rates* in symptomatic women*

History	Number of women	MUFR	AUFR
No hysterectomy	124	50	31
Abdominal hysterectomy	71	23	18
Vaginal hysterectomy	25	23	20
p		0.014	0.0357

*Abbreviations as in Table 17.2.

Table 17.4. *Effect of age on urine flow rates* in symptomatic women*

Age (years)	Number of women	MUFR	AUFR
< 49	71	48	34
49–62	82	38	24
> 62	67	20	11
p		0.0001	0.0004

*Abbreviations as in Table 17.2.

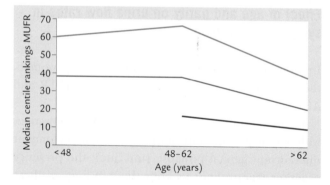

Figure 17.6. *Urine flow rate centiles declining with age in patients who have or have not had a previous hysterectomy or intercurrent genital prolapse: (—) neither; (—) either; (—) both; MUFR, maximum urine flow rate.*

factors is seen to contribute to increasing deterioration of urine flow rates with age.

There is a decline in the urine flow rates of symptomatic women with increasing parity, although this effect is not statistically significant.

Table 17.5. *Effect of final urodynamic diagnosis* on the maximum and average urine flow rates (MUFR and AUFR) of symptomatic women*

Diagnosis	Number of women	MUFR	AUFR
GSI	107	48	40
DI	14	38	32
VD	7	1	6
GSI plus DI	39	34	32
GSI plus VD	22	3	2
DI plus VD	14	3	2
GSI plus VD plus DI	10	4	7
Normal	7	70	52

*GSI, genuine stress incontinence; DI, detrusor instability; VD, voiding difficulties.

Effect of final urodynamic diagnosis on the urine flow rates of symptomatic women

Median urine flow rate centiles of the urogynaecology patients categorized according to the final urodynamic diagnosis are given in Table 17.5. All categories of diagnoses have median centiles below those for the normal female population (50 by definition). Voiding difficulty appears to be the diagnosis for which urine flow rates might have the best discriminatory ability. Further analysis shows that the 10th centile of the Liverpool nomogram[22] for the MUFR has the best discriminatory ability (sensitivity 81%, specificity 92%) with respect to diagnosing the presence or absence of the final diagnosis of voiding difficulty, either as a solitary or a mixed diagnosis.

OTHER FACTORS INFLUENCING URINE FLOW RATES

Urine flow depends on the relationship between the bladder and urethra during voiding. The situation during voiding is the antithesis of the situation required for continence: continence depends on intra-urethral pressure being higher than intravesical pressure; for voiding to occur, intravesical pressure must exceed intra-urethral pressure.

Enhorning,[26] and, later, Asmussen and Ulmsten,[27] showed clearly that, before any rise in intravesical pressure, a fall in intra-urethral pressure occurred. This suggests that the urethra actively relaxes during voiding rather than being passively 'blown open' by the detrusor contraction. Soon after the urethra has relaxed and pelvic floor descent has occurred, the detrusor contracts. The detrusor normally contrives to contract until the bladder is empty, producing a continuous flow curve. Many women void by urethral relaxation alone, with minimal or no detrusor involvement. This method of voiding is common in women with GSI.

Changes in intra-abdominal pressure also influence urine flow. Some women appear to void entirely by increasing intra-abdominal pressure (that is, by contraction of the diaphragm and anterior abdominal wall muscles).

It follows from this discussion that the urine flow may differ from normal as a result of abnormalities of the urethra or the detrusor.

Urethral factors

Anatomical factors
The urethra may be abnormally narrow, or the urethra may not be straight. The narrowest part of the urethra, as shown by video studies of voiding, is usually the middle zone. However, the urethra may become narrowed and the most common site is at the external meatus, associated with oestrogen deficiency in postmenopausal women. Bladder-neck obstruction in the female is extremely rare.[28] The female urethra is usually straight, and deviation from this state is most common in anterior vaginal wall prolapse and higher degrees of uterine and vaginal vault prolapse. The data in Table 17.2 confirm the adverse effect of such prolapse on urine flow rates. Vaginal repair of the prolapse has been thought not to produce a significant alteration in postoperative flow rates, irrespective of whether stress incontinence was present preoperatively.[29] However, correction of anterior vaginal wall prolapse by a colposuspension does lead to deterioration in urine flow rates.[30]

Pathological factors
Unusual congenital conditions, such as urethral duplication, urethral diverticula or urethral cysts, may obstruct voiding. Infective lesions, as in urethritis or infected para-urethral cysts, may lead to voiding difficulty. Post-traumatic strictures and urethral neoplasms will have a similar effect. Intravaginal abnormalities, such as prolapse or foreign bodies, may also obstruct micturition.

Functional factors
Abnormal urethral behaviour during voiding may lead to alteration in the urine flow rate recording. Urethral closure may be due to contraction of the intra-urethral striated muscle or to contraction of the pelvic floor. In the neurologically abnormal patient, contraction of the intra-urethral striated muscle with or without the pelvic floor is known as detrusor sphincter dyssynergia. In the nervous and anxious but neurologically normal patient, the urethra may be closed by pelvic floor contraction, and this may be termed detrusor pelvic floor dyssynergia.

Detrusor factors

Contractility
It is well known that, when neurological disease occurs, bladder behaviour may be altered. However, in patients with no neurological disease, poor detrusor contractility may be responsible for a slow flow rate. Such patients may have urinary tract infections or urinary retention. These patients have normal urethral function, as judged by pressure profilometry or radiology; their reduced flow rates are secondary to a weak and poorly sustained detrusor contraction. A proportion of this clinical group goes on to demonstrate classical neurological disease such as multiple sclerosis.

Innervation
Normal detrusor behaviour depends on normal innervation. Bladder contractions are preserved if the sacral reflex arc is intact even when the upper motor neurons are damaged; however, if the sacral reflex arc is damaged, bladder contractions are generally absent. The only form of contractile activity possible when the lower motor neuron is damaged is locally mediated – the 'autonomous' bladder. The urine flow rates produced by the abnormally innervated bladder are usually reduced and interrupted.

Pathological factors
Although little specific literature on the subject exists, it is evident that gross disease of the detrusor will result in abnormal urine flow rates. The fibrosis resulting from

irradiation, tuberculosis, cystitis or interstitial cystitis is likely to impair detrusor contractility.

URINARY FLOW PATTERNS

Urine flow curves are complementary to flow rates in the assessment of voiding. Because flow curves cannot be represented numerically (except by urine flow rates), they are less useful for clinical comparisons than flow rates. Several patterns of flow curves can, however, be recognized.

Normal

The normal flow trace (Fig. 17.7a, b) shows a symmetrical peak with MUFR generally achieved within

5 seconds of the beginning of voiding. The MUFR is generally 1.5–2 times the AUFR.

A low normal (suboptimal) flow trace (Fig. 17.8a) shows no symmetrical peak. MUFR, somewhere between the 5th and 25th centile, occurs early, then the flow

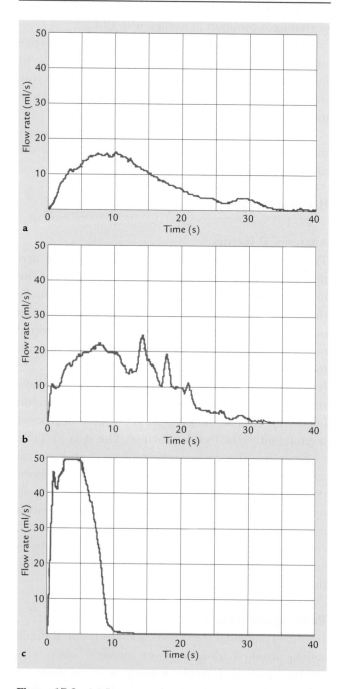

Figure 17.8. *(a) Low normal (suboptimal) urine flow pattern (voided volume 261 ml; MUFR 17.0 ml/s); (b) abdominal strain pattern (voided volume 353 ml; MUFR 25.7 ml/s); (c) high take-off urine flow pattern (voided volume 336 ml; MUFR 53.8 ml/s).*

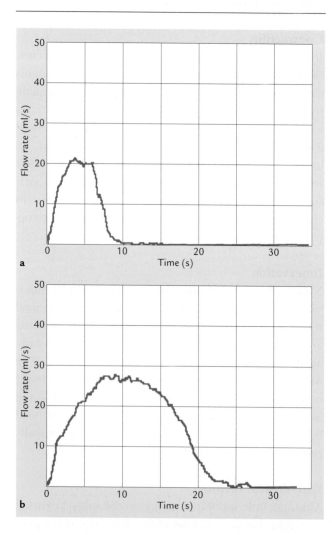

Figure 17.7. *Normal flow curves for voided volume of (a) 121 ml (MUFR 21.2 ml/s) and (b) 345 ml (MUFR 24.7 ml/s).*

trails off. An abdominal strain pattern (Fig. 17.8b) shows the influence of generally intermittent abdominal strain during the void: this manifests itself as irregular, moderately rapid accelerations in MUFR. A high take-off pattern (Fig. 17.8c) shows a very rapid acceleration to a high MUFR. A higher incidence of such traces has been noted in both men and women with DI.

Abnormal: continuous flow

Urine flow curves reflected in flow rates below the 5th centile may generally be regarded as abnormal; abnormality can be suspected in those curves with flow rates between the 5th and 10th centile.

A reduced urine flow rate may be due either to urethral obstruction or to poor detrusor contraction

(Fig. 17.9a, b). It is necessary to perform full pressure–flow studies to demonstrate the cause of a reduced urine flow rate.

Abnormal: interrupted flow

An abdominal pressure voiding pattern (Fig. 17.10a) is where abdominal straining provides the pressure behind the voiding: little detrusor activity is present and the result is irregular interrupted peaks of flow. The MUFR is more than twice the AUFR.

A voluntary sphincter contraction urine flow pattern (Fig. 17.10b) occurs as the anxious, nervous patient closes her distal urethral sphincter mechanism. The flow rate may decrease or stop. Characteristically, the rate of change of flow rate is rapid, indicating sphincter

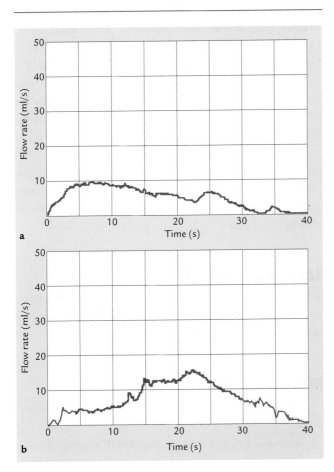

Figure 17.9. *(a) Reduced urine flow pattern caused by bladder outflow obstruction (maximum detrusor voiding pressure 54 cmH$_2$0; voided volume 210 ml; MUFR 10.5 ml/s); (b) reduced urine flow pattern caused by detrusor underactivity (maximum detrusor voiding pressure 15 cmH$_2$0; voided volume 245 ml; MUFR 15.0 ml/s).*

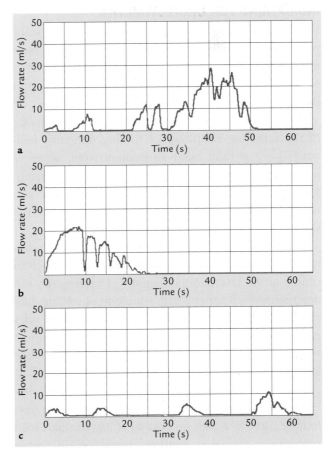

Figure 17.10. *(a) Abdominal pressure voiding pattern (voided volume 357 ml; MUFR 28.8 ml/s); (b) voluntary sphincter contraction urine flow pattern (voided volume 272 ml; MUFR 23.2 ml/s); (c) detrusor sphincter dyssynergia flow pattern (voided volume 161 ml; average flow rate 2.9 ml/s; MUFR 10.6 ml/s).*

closure. The fluctuations due to detrusor underactivity would be much slower than those seen here.

Detrusor sphincter dyssynergia is an involuntary phenomenon in which the expected coordination of the detrusor contraction and urethral relaxation is lost. Despite an effective detrusor contraction, the urethral mechanism remains closed for longer periods of time (up to several minutes). Detrusor sphincter dyssynergia may result in a large volume of residual urine, together with upper tract dilatation and renal failure and is often associated with repeated infection. Detrusor sphincter dyssynergia occurs only in neurologically abnormal patients, most classically in high spinal cord trauma. The flow rate produced by detrusor sphincter dyssynergia (Fig. 17.10c) is usually reduced and always interrupted.

INDICATIONS FOR UROFLOWMETRY

Uroflowmetry should be regarded as a screening test for voiding difficulties in all women with symptoms of lower urinary tract dysfunction. In this role, uroflowmetry is complementary to symptoms of voiding difficulty and the measurement of the residual urine volume. Of apparently normal women, 30% will describe at least one of the following symptoms of voiding difficulty: hesitancy; poor stream; need to strain to void; sense of incomplete emptying, or the need to revoid immediately. This compares with 70% and 53% of urodynamic patients who will admit to at least one or at least two of the same symptoms, respectively.[31]

Up to 26% of women referred for urodynamic studies will have an abnormally slow MUFR (under the 10th centile of the Liverpool nomogram). Uroflowmetry will determine which patients with symptoms of voiding difficulty require further investigation. If urine flow rates prove to be normal in this group, further investigation of voiding function is unnecessary. However, if flow rates are low, pressure–flow studies are indicated.

Abnormal results from urine flow studies are less common in female than in male patients. This is because, in male patients, a high proportion of lower urinary tract problems is related to outflow obstruction; in female patients, the incidence of outflow obstruction is low, whereas the incidence of incontinence and associated abnormalities of bladder behaviour is high.

Flow studies are preliminary to cystometry, which is necessary to define the urodynamic abnormality responsible for the symptom complex of frequency,

nocturia, urgency and urge incontinence. Anticholinergic medication will exacerbate any tendency towards urinary retention in patients with the combined diagnoses of DI and voiding difficulty.

Flow studies are an important preoperative investigation in women awaiting surgery for GSI. Assuming that GSI has been urodynamically confirmed, a normal flow rate reassures the surgeon that long-term voiding difficulty is much less likely to follow the operation to cure the stress incontinence. As effective surgery usually results in an increase in urethral resistance, in women with poor preoperative flow rates, incomplete emptying or even persistent failure to void may follow surgery;[32] therefore, urine flow studies, with or without pressure–flow studies, are to be recommended before surgery.

Voiding problems in patients with neuropathic lower urinary tract dysfunction consist of three main types: (1) patients may experience incontinence as a result of bladder instability; (2) the main problem may be the failure to empty the bladder because of a poorly sustained detrusor contraction; (3) detrusor sphincter dyssynergia may prevent an effective detrusor contraction from emptying the bladder, with the consequent possible complications of recurrent infections or renal failure. Urine flow studies may suggest the origin of the problems experienced by this group of patients, although video pressure–flow studies are desirable in almost every case.

ACKNOWLEDGEMENTS

The contribution of Professor Paul Abrams to earlier chapters co-authored with the current author on the same subject is acknowledged.

REFERENCES

1. Ryall RL, Marshall VR. Measurement of urinary flow rate. *Urology* 1983; 22: 556–564

2. Ballenger EG, Elder OF, McDonald HP. Voiding distance decrease as important early symptom of prostatic obstruction. *South Med J* 1932; 25: 863

3. Drake WM. The uroflowmeter: an aid to the study of the lower urinary tract. *J Urol* 1948; 59: 650–658

4. Kaufman J. A new recording uroflowmeter: a simple automatic device for measuring voiding velocity. *J Urol* 1957; 78: 97–102

5. Von Garrelts B. Analysis of micturition: a new method of recording the voiding of the bladder. *Acta Chir Scand* 1956; 112: 326

6. International Continence Society. Second report on the standardisation of terminology of lower urinary tract function. *Br J Urol* 1977; 49: 207–210

7. Backman K-A, Von Garrelts B. Apparatus for recording micturition. *Acta Chir Scand* 1963; 126: 167–171

8. Von Garrelts B, Strandell P. Continuous recording of urinary flow rate. *Scand J Urol Nephrol* 1972; 6: 224–227

9. Rowan D, James ED, Kramer AEJL *et al.* Urodynamic equipment: technical aspects. International Continence Society Working Party on Urodynamic equipment. *J Med Eng Technol* 1987; 11: 57–64

10. Moore KH, Richmond DH, Sutherst JR *et al.* Crouching over the toilet seat: prevalence among British gynaecological outpatients and its effect upon micturition. *Br J Obstet Gynaecol* 1991; 98: 569–572

11. Marshall VR, Ryall RI, Austin ML, Sinclair GR. The use of urinary flow rates obtained from voided volumes less than 150 ml in the assessment of voiding ability. *Br J Urol* 1983; 55: 28–33

12. Drach GW, Ignatoff J, Layton T. Peak urine flow rate: observations in female subjects and comparison to male subjects. *J Urol* 1979; 122: 215–219

13. Peter WP, Drake WM Jr. Uroflowmetric observations in gynecologic patients. *J Am Med Assoc* 1958; 166: 721–724

14. Scott R, McIhlaney JG. Voiding rate in normal adults. *J Urol* 1961; 128: 429–432

15. Backman K-A. Urinary flow during micturition in normal women. *J Urol* 1965; 137: 497–499

16. Susset JG, Picker P, Kretz M, Jorest R. Clinical evaluation of uroflowmeters and analysis of normal curves. *J Urol* 1973; 109: 874–878

17. Walter S, Olesen KP, Nordberg J, Hald T. Bladder function in urologically normal middle aged females. *Scand J Urol Nephrol* 1979; 13: 249–258

18. Bottacini MR, Gleason DJ. Urodynamic norms in women: normals versus stress incontinents. *J Urol* 1980; 124: 659–661

19. Fantl JA, Smith PJ, Schneider V *et al.* Fluid weight uroflowmetry in women. *Am J Obstet Gynecol* 1982; 145: 1017–1024

20. Rollema HJ, Griffiths DJ, Jones U. Computer-aided uroflowmetry. Normal values in healthy women and applications in gynaecological patients. *Proceedings of the International Continence Society, London*, 1985; P210–211

21. Ryall RL, Marshall VR. Normal peak urinary flow rate obtained from small voided volumes can provide a reliable assessment of bladder function. *J Urol* 1982; 127: 484–487

22. Haylen BT, Ashby D, Sutherst JR *et al.* Maximum and average urine flow rates in normal male and female populations – the Liverpool nomograms. *Br J Urol* 1989; 64: 30–38

23. Ryall RL, Marshall VR. The effect of a urethral catheter on the measurement of maximum urinary flow rate. *J Urol* 1982; 128: 429–432

24. Haylen BT, Parys BT, Anyaegbunam WI *et al.* Urine flow rates in male and female urodynamic patients compared with the Liverpool nomograms. *Br J Urol* 1990; 65: 483–487

25. Haylen BT, Law MG, Frazer MI, Schulz S. Urine flow rates and residual urine volumes in urogynecology patients. *Int Urogynecol J* 1999; 6: 378–383

26. Enhorning G. Simultaneous recording of intravesical and intraurethral pressure. *Acta Chir Scand (Suppl)* 1961; 276: 1–68

27. Asmussen M, Ulmsten U. Simultaneous urethrocystometry with a new technique. *Scand J Urol Nephrol* 1976; 10: 7–11

28. Turner Warwick R, Whiteside CG, Worth PH *et al.* A urodynamic view of the clinical problems associated with bladder neck dysfunction and its treatment by endoscopic incision and trans-trigonal posterior prostatectomy. *Br J Urol* 1973; 45: 44–59

29. Stanton SL, Hilton P, Norton C, Cardozo L. Clinical and urodynamic effects of anterior colporrhaphy and vaginal hysterectomy for prolapse, with and without incontinence. *Br J Obstet Gynaecol* 1982; 89: 459-463

30. Stanton SL, Cardozo L Williams JE *et al.* Clinical and urodynamic features of failed incontinence surgery in the female. *Obstet Gynaecol* 1978; 51: 515–520

31. Haylen BT. *Screening for Voiding Difficulties in Women*. MD Thesis, University of Liverpool, 1988; 105

32. Stanton SL, Cardozo L, Chaudhury N. Spontaneous voiding after surgery for urinary incontinence. *Br J Obstet Gynaecol* 1978; 83: 149–152

18

Cystometry

P. N. Hughes, P. Abrams

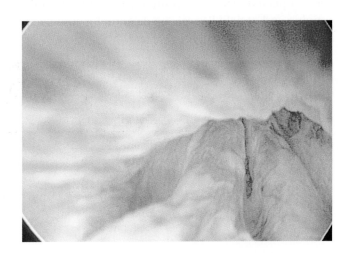

DEFINITION

Cystometry is the method by which the pressure–volume relationship of the bladder is measured. The measurements are taken during the filling and voiding phases of micturition.

AIMS

Cystometry is performed clinically as part of urodynamic investigations to help make a diagnosis and hence to plan suitable treatment or further appropriate investigations. Cystometry aims to evaluate detrusor and urethral function during the storing (or filling) and voiding cycles of micturition. It is essential that diagnoses made at the time of cystometry are related to the patient's symptoms and physical findings at the time of examination. The aim is to reproduce the patient's symptoms and provide a pathophysiological explanation of the patient's problems. Cystometry can also be used for research purposes or to provide objective measurements following particular treatments.

INDICATIONS

Ideally, all patients with lower urinary tract symptoms suggesting a bladder or urethral disorder should undergo urodynamic studies. The bladder is known as the 'unreliable witness': urinary symptoms alone do not always allow the correct diagnosis to be made and inappropriate treatment may be given.[1–5] However, with limited resources and access to such a service, patients with 'clear-cut' symptoms can initially be managed empirically, for example with pelvic floor exercises for suspected stress incontinence, and bladder training and anticholinergic medication for suspected detrusor instability (DI). Urodynamic tests should be conducted in patients:

- with mixed symptomatology (e.g. urgency, frequency and stress incontinence);
- with a suspected voiding disorder;
- being considered for bladder-neck surgery;
- with previous unsuccessful incontinence surgery;
- with neuropathic bladder disorders;
- in whom conservative measures have failed (e.g. physiotherapy for symptoms of stress incontinence, and anticholinergic drug treatment and bladder training for symptoms of urgency).

PREPARING FOR CYSTOMETRY

Quality control during cystometry

Quality control is vital to allow accurate, reproducible and interpretable pressure readings and to allow identification of artefacts. The International Continence Society (ICS) has defined these steps in a technical report:

- Setting zero at atmospheric pressure: this must be done prior to inserting the catheters; before zero is set, the manometer tubing connecting the transducers must be flushed;
- Calibrating the transducers: they should be calibrated at $0–100\,cmH_2O$; the bladder p_{ves} (intravesical pressure) and rectal p_{abd} (intra-abdominal pressure) lines should be in the positive range $+5$ to $+50$ cmH_2O; the p_{det} (detrusor pressure) should be slightly above zero, range -5 to $+15\,cmH_2O$;

Table 18.1. *Lower urinary tract function according to urethral and detrusor action during the filling and voiding cycles of micturition, and the possible diagnoses*

Cycle	Detrusor	Urethra	Diagnosis
Filling	Relaxed Normal Overactive	Contracted Incompetent Incompetent	Normal Stress incontinence Detrusor instability
Voiding	Contracted Underactive High pressure	Relaxed Normal Normal	Normal ?Idiopathic Obstructive cause

• Establishing a reference level for pressure: the superior border of the symphysis pubis is the fixed reference level for external and fluid-filled catheter systems; the transducers should be levelled to this horizontal plane.

During the investigation, quality control is ensured by asking the patient to cough at regular (1 minute) intervals (see Fig.18.5.) Before recording is started, the patient is asked to cough and the p_{ves} and p_{abd} traces are observed. An equal rise in the two pressure lines must be observed and a complete subtraction of these two pressures should result in no change of the p_{det} line. (Sometimes a small artefactual biphasic blip is seen, but this also indicates acceptable subtraction.) The patient should cough before and after voiding to ensure quality control again and that no displacement of catheters has occurred. During filling, the p_{ves} and p_{abd} lines should not decline.

Patient position

For convenience, the catheters are put in position with the patient supine (see Fig.18.1.) Cystometry should then be done in the upright position, because this is the physiological position and the majority of women complain of symptoms when upright and active. It is convenient to ask the patient to sit on a commode with a flow meter situated below to measure any leakage of urine during the test. Some women complain of leakage when changing position (e.g. on bending over or getting up from the sitting position); these changes in posture can be mimicked during the test to try to reflect everyday stresses on the bladder and to provoke leakage. Whenever the patient's position is altered, the position of the transducer must be readjusted to the pressure reference level of the upper border of the symphysis pubis.

With the catheters in position, the filling catheter is connected to a suitable filling medium. The rest of the equipment should be close to the patient for convenience and, if a computer screen is available, then this should be in a position viewable by the patient so that explanations can be given during the test.

If there is severe DI that prevents proper filling even at a reduced rate (10–20 ml/s), then filling in the supine position may be required in order for any useful information to be gathered from cystometry.

Reduced mobility or severe disablement of patients by neurological disease, may necessitate cystometry in the supine position.

Filling medium

Water or 0.9% (normal) saline are the fluids most frequently used as they are cheap and convenient, and mimic urine in consistency. The fluid is commonly used at room temperature (22°C); however, body temperature (37°C) may be more physiological. Cystometry has been performed with the filling medium warmed to body temperature and no difference in results was noticed;[6] however, this has not yet been scientifically investigated and standardization is required. It is known that ice-cold infusion fluid can stimulate bladder contractility at low bladder volumes[7] and therefore should not be used in routine cystometry.

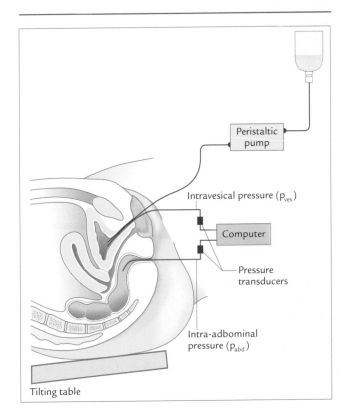

Peristaltic pump

Intravesical pressure (p_{ves})

Computer

Pressure transducers

Intra-adbominal pressure (p_{abd})

Tilting table

Figure 18.1. *Schematic diagram of catheter position.*

In the past, carbon dioxide has been used in gas cystometry[8] but it is not now recommended as it is not a physiological medium for the bladder, it dissolves in urine to form irritant carbonic acid and it can cause pain in hypersensitive bladders; furthermore, capacity measurement is inaccurate as the gas is both compressible and soluble in urine.[9] In addition, after gas cystometry it is not possible to obtain a pressure–flow analysis of the voiding phase of micturition.

Filling rates

Three filling rates are defined by the ICS:[10]

1. Slow-fill cystometry up to 10 ml/min;
2. Medium-fill cystometry between 10 and 100 ml/min;
3. Fast-fill cystometry when the rate is greater than 100 ml/min.

We recommend a filling rate of 50 ml/min, which, although convenient in the setting of a busy urodynamic unit, is not so fast as to be grossly unphysiological; it also allows time to discuss symptoms with the patient and to assess whether those symptoms have been successfully reproduced. The rate can be reduced to 30 ml/min in a patient with a very hypersensitive or overactive bladder.

Slow-fill cystometry is indicated in patients with neuropathic bladders. Rapid filling is rarely used but can be a further provocative test for DI.

Equipment

Multichannel cystometry requires a urine flow meter, two transducers, an electronic subtraction unit to derive p_{det} ($p_{ves} - p_{abd}$), a recorder with a printout, and an amplifying unit (see Fig. 18.2.) All measurements are made in centimetres of water (cmH$_2$O).

The bladder pressure is measured using either:

- a fluid-filled line (a 1 mm diameter fluid-filled catheter, such as an epidural catheter, is inserted into the bladder and connected to an external pressure transducer; see Fig. 18.3), or
- a solid micro-tip pressure transducer (a transducer is mounted on the tip of this solid 7F catheter and hence is an internal pressure transducer system; see Fig. 18.4). This catheter-mounted transducer

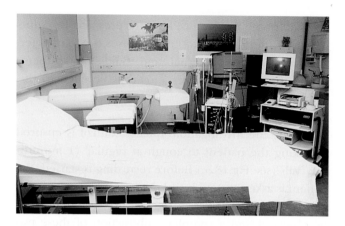

Figure 18.2. *Equipment: couch/cystometry unit/patient unit and flow meter.*

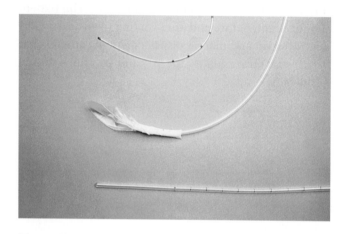

Figure 18.3. *From top to bottom: epidural catheter, rectal line, filling catheter.*

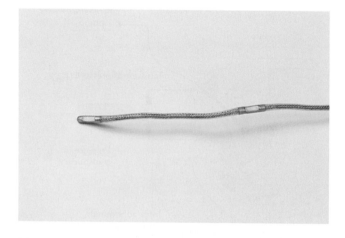

Figure 18.4. *Solid catheter-tip transducer (Gaeltec).*

eliminates artefacts arising from the fluid-filled system which needs to be connected to an external transducer.

Abdominal pressure is measured with a rectal (or occasionally vaginal)[11] catheter (a 2 mm diameter catheter covered with a finger stall to prevent blockage by faeces) which is inserted into the rectum to a distance approximately 10–15 cm above the anal margin. This line is taped to the patient's buttock close to the anal verge to prevent any slippage during the test. The tubing must be flushed from the transducer end before recording is commenced.

The zero reference for all measurements is taken as being approximately level with the upper edge of the pubic symphysis

A filling catheter (8F) is inserted into the bladder via the urethra (or, occasionally, by the suprapubic route).

The catheters are fixed in place by tape close to the external urethral meatus or anal verge on the medial aspect of the thigh or buttock.

MEASUREMENTS

The following measurements are made (Fig.18.5):

1. p_{ves} is measured with the bladder transducer via a urethral or suprapubic catheter;
2. p_{abd} is taken as the pressure around the bladder and measured with the rectal (or occasionally a vaginal) line;
3. p_{det} is obtained by subtracting the abdominal from the intravesical pressure ($p_{det} = p_{abd} - p_{ves}$) and represents the pressure generated by the bladder wall, usually as detrusor contractions;
4. The volume infused into the bladder is recorded;
5. The urine flow rate as leakage during filling and flow during voiding is recorded.

Measuring bladder and intra-abdominal pressure simultaneously ensures that any pressure changes observed can be interpreted correctly. A rise in the bladder pressure line could be due to detrusor activity or due to abdominal straining being transmitted to the bladder. The electronic subtraction allows detrusor pressure to be measured and any change in pressure seen on the traces to be attributed appropriately.

Detrusor function is assessed directly from observation of the pressure changes. Urethral function must be inferred from the pressure changes within the bladder

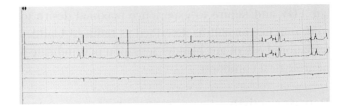

Figure 18.5. *Normal cystometrogram with coughs showing equal rises on intravesical pressure (p_{ves}) and intra-abdominal pressure (p_{abd}) (p_{det}, detrusor pressure).*

and by measuring any leakage during filling, and urine flow during voiding.

METHOD

The test should be fully explained to the patient; in particular, the importance of her expressing her sensations during the test, as they happen, should be emphasized. The symptoms can then be used to annotate the cystometry trace and help with interpretation. Before cystometry is performed, the patient undergoes flowmetry. Any residual urine on subsequent catheterization is then measured.

Filling cystometry

Bladder sensation, detrusor activity, bladder compliance, bladder capacity and urethral function can all be assessed during this procedure.

Bladder sensation

During the filling phase the patient is asked to indicate:

- her first desire to void (FDV) – this sensation may not be truly representative, owing to the interfering presence of the catheter;
- the strong desire to void (SDV);
- any urgency (an urgent desire to void with fear of leakage or fear of pain).

These volumes are noted. The above terminology has been defined by the ICS.[10]

Bladder sensation may be normal, absent, decreased or increased. Bladder hypersensitivity (increased bladder sensation) is a condition where there is an early FDV at less than 100 ml and this persists and worsens, limiting the bladder capacity to 250 ml. Conversely, a late FDV and failure to experience maximal desire to void, urgency or pain is described as reduced bladder sensation. Lack of any bladder sensation may indicate a neurological condition.

Detrusor activity

Detrusor activity is described as normal/'stable' or abnormal/'unstable'/'overactive'. The presence of involuntary phasic detrusor contractions is diagnosed by detecting a rise in the detrusor pressure line; the patient should be asked whether there is associated urgency. Precipitating factors such as coughing or running water, used to provoke symptoms, may also induce detrusor activity and are noted. Any rise in detrusor pressure during filling and on standing is recorded.

The detrusor that is shown by cystometry to contract spontaneously or with provocation while the patient is trying to inhibit voiding is known as the unstable detrusor (overactive bladder). Some women will not experience any symptoms at the time of these contractions, in which case the significance of bladder overactivity is unknown.

When there is a known neurological condition (e.g. multiple sclerosis), overactivity of the detrusor may be seen and is termed detrusor hyperreflexia.

DI has been defined[10] as phasic contractions in which the pressure rises and then falls (see Fig.18.6.) The ICS does not quantify the pressure changes that might be involved; however, in practice, pressure changes of less than 5 cmH$_2$O are ignored.

Bladder compliance

The term bladder compliance describes the relationship between pressure and volume in the bladder and is measured in ml/cmH$_2$O. As a normal bladder fills there is very little or no change in the pressure (i.e. the bladder is a low-compliance system). Filling rates can alter bladder compliance; hence, the filling rate of the cystometry must always be documented. In neurologically normal women, reduced compliance is usually artefactual owing to the bladder being filled excessively fast. Fast filling may mask bladder overactivity, producing apparent low compliance in its place.

Urethral function

During the filling phase in a normal women, the urethral closure pressure remains positive (i.e. it is greater than the intravesical pressure), even at times of increased intra-abdominal pressure; hence, continence is maintained. To allow voiding, closure pressure falls as the urethra relaxes. If involuntary loss of urine is seen without detrusor activity, then the urethral closure mechanism is said to be incompetent. A diagnosis of genuine stress incontinence can be made if this leakage is associated with an increase in intra-abdominal pressure that causes the intravesical pressure to exceed the intra-urethral pressure and the absence of a detrusor contraction (see Fig. 18.7.)

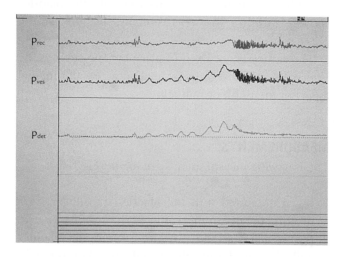

Figure 18.6. *Cystometrogram showing detrusor instability and urge incontinence: p_{rec}, rectal (intra-abdominal) pressure; p_{ves}, intravesical pressure; p_{det}, detrusor pressure.*

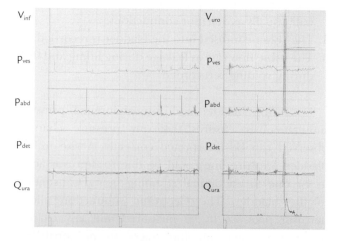

Figure 18.7. *Cystometrogram showing stress incontinence with coughing: Q_{ura}, flow rate (ml/s); p_{det}, detrusor pressure; p_{abd}, intra-abdominal pressure; p_{ves}, intravesicular pressure; V_{inf}, infusion volume; V_{uro}, volume voided (ml).*

Voiding cystometry

At the end of filling, the bladder-filling catheter is removed to avoid any artefacts during voiding due to urethral obstruction. If leakage has not been noted during the filling phase the patient is asked to cough a few times. If leakage is still not noted at this time, then the patient is asked to stand and given provocative instructions (stand with legs apart and cough, star jumps, squatting, hand washing) to try to induce leakage.

The patient, now back on the commode with the intravesical and rectal pressure catheters still *in situ*, is instructed to void and the detrusor pressure and urine flow rate are recorded simultaneously. Voiding pressure at maximum flow ($p_{det}Q_{max}$) and flow rate are recorded.

Voluntary initiation of a detrusor contraction is required for normal micturition and this is sustained until the bladder is empty. The pressure rise is dependent on the outlet resistance and on the contraction of the detrusor itself: if the detrusor pressure is low with low flow rates, the detrusor is defined as underactive; if the pressure is high with low or normal flow rates, this may be indicative of an obstructive problem. If the detrusor muscle is functioning normally then abdominal straining should not be required.

A further rise in detrusor pressure after the completion of voiding or an 'after contraction' is sometimes seen at the end of a completed void; however, the significance of this finding is unknown.

PITFALLS OF CYSTOMETRY

To ensure accurate measurements, the bladder line, rectal line and all tubing should be flushed to ensure that all bubbles have been removed before recording begins. In addition, all connections should be tight, as any leak will cause errors in the pressure measurements recorded. Pressure values will tend to be lower if there are bubbles or leaks in the pressure system.

Rectal contractions can sometimes be seen on the recording trace and these artefacts may be misinterpreted; it is, therefore, important to be aware of rectal activity. If possible the patient should have an empty rectum. If the rectal line slips slowly during the recording, the p_{abd} line will be seen to drift downwards, which could be incorrectly interpreted as a rise in the detrusor pressure and reduced compliance. Careful examination of the intravesical line shows the bladder pressure to be constant and should allow this false reading to be noticed.

Quality control at the start of each cystometry is vital, and should be repeated intermittently during the test and again at the end of the test to ensure that good pressure transmission is continuing. This is done by asking the patient to cough and seeing an equal rise in the abdominal and vesical line and no rise (or a small biphasic deflection in a fluid-filled system) on the detrusor line.

The transducers must be zeroed at atmospheric pressure to ensure reliable detrusor pressure readings. It is important that, after any movement or change of the patient's position, this is checked and readjusted accordingly. The reference point for fluid-filled systems is taken as the level of the superior edge of the symphysis pubis.

NORMAL CYSTOMETRY

Cystometry of a normal bladder shows the following:

1. Residual urine of less than 50 ml;
2. FDV between 150 and 200 ml;
3. Capacity (taken as SDV) of greater than 400 ml;
4. Little or no detrusor pressure rise on filling (see Fig. 18.8);
5. Absence of detrusor contractions during the filling phase;
6. No leakage on coughing;

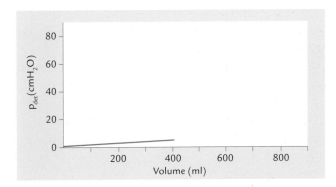

Figure 18.8 *Normal filling cystometrogram showing minimal increase in detrusor pressure (p_{det}) The filling speed is 50 ml/min, the patient is seated, the bladder capacity is 403 ml and the first desire to void is at 135 ml.*

7. No detrusor contraction provoked by coughing or running water (precipitating factors);

8. A maximum voiding detrusor pressure of less than 50 cmH$_2$O, with a maximum flow rate greater than 15 ml/s for a volume greater than 150 ml.

CONCLUSIONS

Cystometry is a component of urodynamic studies to investigate lower urinary tract dysfunction. It is vital that women are assessed with a proper history and examination and the findings of the cystometric findings evaluated in the light of the symptomatology. The majority of women will have their symptoms explained, and/or further management decisions can be made from conventional cystometry. Further cystometry can be performed using ambulatory monitoring over a longer period of time and, in more natural circumstances, together with videocystourethrography for simultaneous assessment of the anatomy (see chapters 24 and 25).

REFERENCES

1. Cardozo LD, Stanton SL. Genuine stress incontinence and detrusor instability – a review of 200 patients. *Br J Obstet Gynaecol* 1970; 42: 714–723

2. Shepherd AM, Powell PH, Ball AJ. The place of urodynamic studies in the investigation and treatment of female urinary tract symptoms. *J Obstet Gynecol* 1982; 3: 123–125

3. Largo-Janssen FM, Debruyne FMJ, Van Weel C. Value of the patient's case history in diagnosing urinary incontinence in general practice. *Br J Urol* 1991; 67: 569–572

4. Jarvis GJ, Hall S, Stamp S *et al.* An assessment of urodynamic examination in incontinent women. *Br J Obstet Gynaecol* 1980; 87: 893–896

5. Byrne DJ, Hamilton Stewart PA, Gray BK. The role of urodynamics in female urinary stress incontinence. *Br J Urol* 1987; 59: 228–229

6. Abrams P. Urodynamic techniques – cystometry. *Urodynamics*, 2nd edn. London: Springer Verlag, 1997; 17–117

7. Aslund K, Rentzhogh L, Sandstromb G. Effects of ice cold saline and acid solution in urodynamics. Proc. 18th Annual Meeting of the International Continence Society, Oslo, Norway. Oslo: ICS, 1988; 1–2

8. Torrens MJ. A comparative evaluation of carbon dioxide and water cystometry and sphincterometry. *Proc Int Cont Soc Portoroz* 1977; 7: 103–104

9. Wein AJ, Hanno PM, Dixon DO *et al.* The reproducibility and interpretation of carbon dioxide cystometry. *J Urol* 1978; 120: 205–206

10. Abrams P, Blaivas JG, Stanton SL *et al.* The International Continence Society Committee on Standardisation of Terminology; the standardisation of terminology of lower urinary tract function. *Scand J Urol Nephrol Suppl* 1988; 114: 5–19

11. James ED. The vagina as an alternative to the rectum in measuring abdominal pressure during urodynamic investigations. *Br J Urol* 1987; 60: 212–216

19

The pressure–flow plot in the evaluation of female incontinence

A. Wagg, J. Malone-Lee

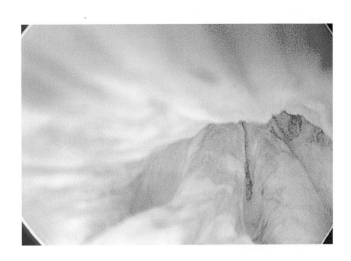

THE PRESSURE–FLOW PLOT

The physiology of the pressure–flow plot

The voiding pressure–flow plot is a record of the voiding phase of the filling and voiding cystometrogram. These graphs plot the detrusor pressure during voiding and the associated flow rate over time, typically delayed chronologically to allow synchrony between pressure and flow (see later). The plot is commonly used to assess the presence or absence of significant bladder outlet obstruction in men, with a view to surgical intervention. It is also of value in the assessment of disordered detrusor contractile function. A schematic pressure–flow tracing, presented stage by stage, is shown in Figure 19.1. The pressure–flow plot illustrates the relationship between the contracting detrusor, the driving force to empty the bladder, and the modulation of that force by the outflow tract. Analysis of the pressure–flow plot requires an understanding of the muscle mechanics involved in bladder emptying and knowledge of the properties of the urethra during voiding.

The bladder

The mechanical properties of smooth muscles, such as the detrusor, have not been explored as thoroughly as those of striated muscle but the general principles as applied to striated muscle appear to be a valid approximation.

Muscle contraction is dependent upon the tension within it and upon the speed at which the muscle can shorten. The amount of force that smooth muscle can generate is dependent upon the magnitude of stretch of the muscle above its resting length (Fig.19.2). However, the maximum isometric force (when there is no shortening allowed) is dependent only upon the velocity of shortening of the muscle in a similar manner to that described by Hill[1] for striated muscle (Fig.19.3).

The equation that describes this relationship, is:

$$(F/F_{iso} + a/F_{iso})(u + b) = (1 + a/F_{iso})\,b$$

where b and a/F_{iso} are constants, which are independent of the degree of extension, F_{iso} is the isometric force of the bladder, F/F_{iso} is the ratio of observed force of contraction to isometric force and u is the speed of shortening.

For the bladder, the Hill equation has been evolved into the bladder output relation (BOR) by Griffiths[2]

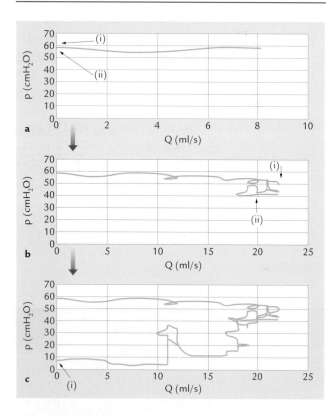

Figure 19.1. *The evolution of the pressure (p)–flow (Q) plot. (a) Start of micturition: (i) detrusor pressure rises; (ii) sphincter opens and flow starts (p_{det,open}). (b) Maximum flow (Q_{max}): (i) pressure and flow are synchronous; the urethral sphincter is maximally dilated; (ii) the 'passive' phase of micturition begins. (c) End of micturition: (i) micturition ceases at the lowest detrusor pressure that allows flow (p_{det,clos}).*

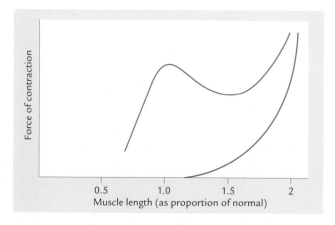

Figure 19.2. *The length–tension relationship for smooth muscle: — maximum tension; — resting tension.*

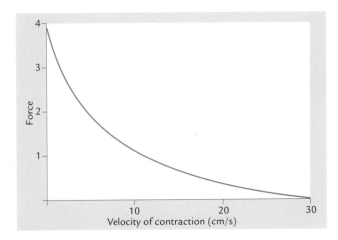

Figure 19.3. *The Hill plot for striated muscle: muscle length 8 cm.*

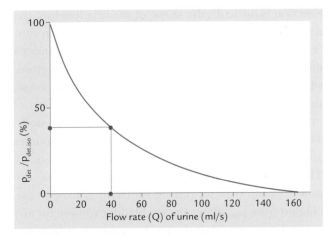

Figure 19.4. *The bladder output relation (BOR): p_{det}, detrusor pressure; $p_{det,iso}$ isovolumetric detrussor pressure; Q, flow rate from bladder; Q* (volume-dependent measure of the speed of shortening of the bladder muscle) = 40 ml/s; intercept (4Q*) = 160 ml/s.*

(Fig.19.4), relating detrusor pressure to urinary flow. This is achieved by mathematically relating the changes in a single strip of bladder to the changes occurring in the complete bladder.

If the bladder is treated as a simple sphere of radius R, then the detrusor pressure, p_{det}, is given by

$$p_{det} = T/\pi R^2$$

where T is the total tension across the bladder circumference and R is the radius of the sphere. This relates detrusor pressure, measured clinically, to the tension measured in muscle strips in laboratory experiments.[3]

Likewise, a relationship between linear speed of shortening of a bladder strip and flow rate from the bladder may be derived:

$$(p_{det}/p_{det,iso} + a/F_{iso})(Q + Q^*) = (1 + a/F_{iso})\,Q^*$$

where Q is the flow rate from the bladder and Q* is a volume-dependent measure of the speed of shortening of the bladder muscle.[4]

The detrusor pressure is dependent upon both the volume of urine within the bladder and the urinary flow rate. This dependence on the flow rate is described by the bladder output relation: the higher the rate of flow, the lower the bladder pressure. During any single void, the plot of pressure versus flow moves sequentially through points on curves described by the BOR, depending upon the volume of urine remaining within the bladder (Fig.19.5). The isovolumetric detrusor pressure is largely volume independent and may be used to assess the contractile function

of the bladder. The stop test – voluntary cessation of voiding – may be performed to determine a value for isovolumetric pressure ($p_{det.iso}$). Using the values on the pressure–flow plot just before and just after the stop test, a straight line may be plotted to give an approximate value for Q*, which is reasonably accurate provided that the detrusor pressure during flow is more than half of the $p_{det.iso}$. Because of the volume dependence of Q*, the bladder volume should be above 200 ml. In practice, assessment of detrusor contractile

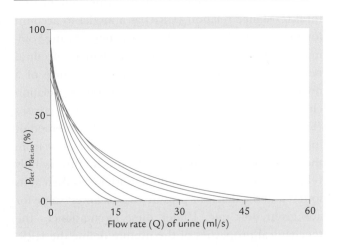

Figure 19.5. *The voiding pattern follows the BOR in a volume-dependent manner: bladder volumes for the curves depicted (from right to left) are 500, 400, 300, 200, 100, 50 and 25 ml. Abbreviations as in Figure 19.4.*

function is difficult: the shape of the relationship, the dependence upon bladder volume and variation during voiding all complicate the process. Schäfer's method divides the pressure–flow plot into regions, which describe the contraction as very weak, weak, normal or strong. The region into which the point of maximum flow falls indicates contraction strength. These regions may be incorporated into urodynamics analysis software for easy graphical interpretation.[5] The variable 'Watts factor', which represents the power of the bladder during shortening, may be calculated from p_{det}, flow rate and bladder volume for any point during a void. It does not require any additional manoeuvres to be performed by the patient to obtain additional variables, but is quite difficult to calculate.[6]

The urethra

The properties of the urethra interact with the contracting detrusor throughout micturition. Thus, the urethral outlet resistance modulates the performance of the bladder and influences what may be measured clinically. Flow through the urethra has been modelled mathematically, treating the urethra as an elastic, distensible tube, the properties of which alter throughout the time course of voiding. Despite the changes in appearance of the urethra, which are observable on fluoroscopy, it has become apparent that the flow-controlling zone of the urethra remains and continues to govern urethral resistance. Griffiths formulated the urethral resistance relation (URR) as a model to account for the known changes in hydrodynamics during voiding.[3] Given no significant functional changes, urethral resistance remains fixed during the time course of a normal micturition while the bladder output relation changes as the volume within the bladder decreases (Fig.19.6). Abdominal straining, or another method of increasing urinary flow, causes a deviation away from the URR during voiding. Ideally, the urethra is fully relaxed during voiding; urethral resistance is then at its lowest and the detrusor pressure has its lowest value for any given flow rate. Under these circumstances the mechanical properties of the urethra define the URR. This relationship is called the passive URR (PURR).

Urethral activity can only increase the detrusor pressure above the value defined by the PURR. Any deviation of the pressure–flow plot from the PURR

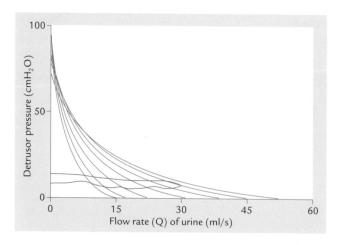

Figure 19.6. *The urethral resistance relation (—) during voiding: the red lines show the bladder output relation for various bladder volumes, as depicted in Figure 19.5.*

towards higher pressures is considered to be a result of activity of the urethral or periurethral musculature. Because the data provided by any single void are a resolution of both the BOR and the URR, the URR is difficult to interpret clinically. This has led to the development of other, simpler methods to quantify bladder outlet resistance in a quantitative fashion.[7–13]

Generating the data

The need to manipulate the data to allow for the delay in the recording of flow rate can be illustrated by the marked alteration in the form of the pressure–flow plot when subjected to increasing delay (Fig.19.7). Interpretation of the pressure–flow plot might then be significantly different, especially at the start and end of voiding, if this delay is not allowed for. In the clinical situation, asking the patient to stop voiding, and then timing the delay between this and the cessation of recorded flow may make an estimation of this interval. If this time interval is accurately pre-set on the urodynamics software, then, as the flow rate falls, a marked rise in detrusor pressure should occur at the same time. During voiding, the detrusor pressure and corresponding flow are probably only in synchrony towards the maximal flow rate from the bladder. In the female subject with a relatively short urethra, the true delay has been estimated as 0.4 seconds in the sitting position, but as much as 1.1 seconds when standing during videourodynamic studies.[14] In the clinical situation, the

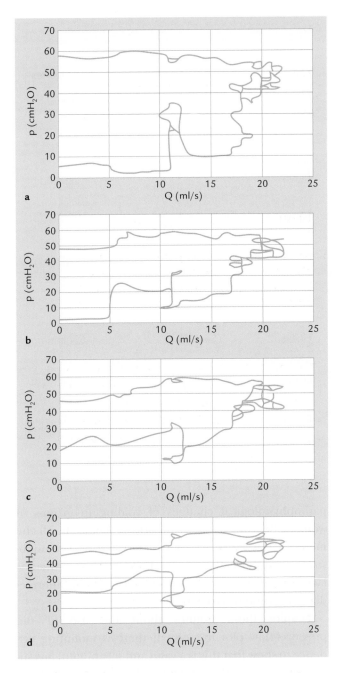

Figure 19.7. *Effect of varying delays in the recording of flow rate on pressure (p) and flow (Q) data: (a) no delay; (b) 1 s; (c) 1.5 s; (d) 2 s.*

pressure–flow plot produces extremely complex shapes, often depending upon functional, pathological and psychological factors. The technique produces reproducible results, test–retest variability being in the region of 2 cmH$_2$O detrusor pressure in 87% of men and similarly consistent in women.[15,16]

As the use of an intra-urethral pressure catheter could itself alter the dynamics of voiding, the smallest diameter catheter should be used to record intravesical pressure. One study, however, reports an 8F catheter as having no effect upon the resulting pressure–flow plot variables when compared with an epidural catheter (external diameter 1.1 mm).[17] Our practice is to use an epidural catheter alone, the urethral filling catheter being removed prior to voiding. The International Continence Society standardization committee has produced guidelines for data acquisition, use of terminology and data analysis for pressure–flow studies.[18]

ANALYSIS OF THE PRESSURE–FLOW PLOT

The simplest shapes of pressure–flow plot are produced when the urethral resistance does not change throughout voiding. Because the time course of each void cannot be derived from the plot, it is necessary to use the raw curves of pressure and flow data to identify the start of voiding. In addition, reference to the source data is required to eliminate artefacts, for instance those caused by abdominal straining or abnormal respiration, prior to further analysis. The need to classify the severity of bladder outlet obstruction in males has led to the development of a number of nomograms, which use a variety of variables based upon the pressure–flow plot to achieve this (see Table 19.1).[7–13] There is much debate about the use of these methods to classify true obstruction, and no clear agreement about the physiological validity of any of them, although each has its ardent exponents. Each classification has been produced from clinical observations of voiding in men; none has used female data. Despite this, some workers have applied standard nomograms to female data, although the validity of doing so is questionable. The incidence of significant bladder outlet obstruction from such studies appears to be low – around 4%.[19] True (anatomical) obstruction in women is often iatrogenic, following surgery for stress incontinence. There are, however, data from studies of women and men with neurogenic bladder dysfunction which have reported the incidence of high-pressure, low-flow voiding patterns, which may mimic an obstructed void.[20]

Each method differs in the variables used to classify the plot and how and whether they are combined. Some methods grade urethral resistance on a continuous scale; others grade it in a small number of classes

Table 19.1. *Classification of the pressure–flow plot*

Method	Aim	No. of data points	Shape of urethral resistance relation	No. of variables	Categories
Abrams / Griffiths nomogram	Diagnosis of obstruction	1	–	–	3
Spangberg nomogram	Diagnosis of obstruction	1	–	–	3
URA	Quantification of resistance	1	Curve	1	Continuum
linPURR	Quantification of resistance	1	Linear	1	7
Schäfer PURR	Quantification of resistance	Multiple	Curve	2	Continuum
CHESS	Quantification of resistance	Multiple	Curve	2	16
OBI	Quantification of resistance	Multiple	Linear	1	Continuum
DAMPF	Quantification of resistance	2	Linear	1	Continuum
Abrams/ Griffiths number	Quantification of resistance	1	Linear	1	Continuum

From refs. 7–13.

(Table 19.1). If there are few classes, small changes in resistance may not be detected; however, in a continuous scheme, small changes may be detected that have no clinical relevance. Some methods of analysis result in a single measure of obstruction; others result in two or more. A single variable enables easy comparison with other measurements but represents an unacceptable simplification of data and sacrifices accuracy and validity. A larger number of variables makes comparison more difficult but potentially gives higher accuracy and validity. Too many variables makes comparison between tests difficult and suffers from the inherent problems of reproducibility of the technique.

Some of the methods are intended primarily to quantify urethral resistance. These may have more potential for use in women, although none has been used as such. These methods may avoid the semantics that have been associated with the use of other measures, which are intended only for the diagnosis of obstruction. Methods that quantify urethral resistance on a scale may be useful for describing pathophysiological changes of voiding in groups of women. Because of their underlying similarity, all the methods classify clearly obstructed and clearly unobstructed pressure–flow studies consistently, but there is lack of agreement in a minority of cases with 'intermediate' urethral resistance.

Despite these doubts about the use of the pressure–flow plot in women, there is mounting evidence to show that this is a valid and meaningful investigation.[21,22] The pathophysiological information that may be derived from the plot may aid diagnosis and management of women with lower urinary tract symptoms. For example, using variables derived from the pressure–flow plot, urethral function can be seen to decline in association with greater age (Fig.19.8).[23] This is in line with the findings based upon urethral pressure profile measurements.[24]

The detrusor pressure at the start of voiding ($p_{det.open}$) has been found to be significantly higher in women with detrusor instability (DI) and hyperreflexia, regardless of age. Those women with detrusor

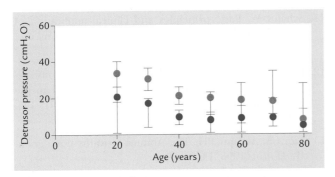

Figure 19.8. *Change in detrusor pressure at urethral opening (● $p_{det.open}$) and urethral closure (● $p_{det.clos}$) in association with greater age in women with stable bladders; horizontal bars show medians and 95% confidence intervals. For $p_{det.open}$, p = 0.045; for $p_{det.clos}$, p = 0.22*

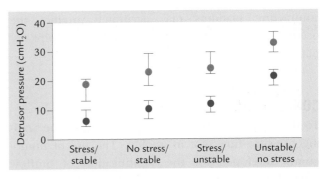

Figure 19.9. *Variation in detrusor pressure at urethral opening (●, $p_{det.open}$) and (●, $p_{det.clos}$) in women with lower urinary tract symptoms, according to urodynamic diagnosis; horizontal bars show medians and 95% confidence intervals.*

hyperreflexia have significantly higher values of $p_{det.open}$ than those with idiopathic DI. Similarly, this variable is significantly lower in women with stress incontinence than in women with none (Fig.19.9).[23] This finding has been replicated, although using a different approach to the calculation of urethral resistance.[25] In the absence of objective spontaneous detrusor activity during the filling phase of the cystometrogram, therefore, finding a high $p_{det.open}$ provides corroborative evidence for the existence of DI. However, this measure has yet to be validated through a clinical intervention study.

The gradient or slope of the pressure–flow plot can give useful information about the viscoelastic properties of the urethra during voiding. If urethral resistance does not change throughout micturition, then the gradient of the low-pressure flank of the plot follows the URR. In general, the higher the pressure for a given flow rate, and/or the steeper or more sharply curved upward the low-pressure flank of the plot, the higher the urethral resistance. A slope that is near horizontal, as occurs in the majority of women, indicates an elastic urethra. The more positive the gradient (dp/dQ), the 'stiffer' the urethra, large changes in detrusor pressure making very little difference to the observed flow rate. Urethral stiffness measured in this fashion increases in association with greater age.[23] This is in accordance with other methodology and with histological analysis of cadaveric urethras.[26,27] The application of the PURR developed by Schäfer is one method by which a measure of these urethral properties may be made.[5] This involves fitting a curve to the

low-pressure flank of the pressure–flow plot with its intercept at the lowest value of detrusor pressure that allows urinary flow. Once again, there are assumptions made for the derivation of this analysis that may not be valid in real life. This is particularly the case when the cross-sectional area of the urethra changes widely during voiding or when there is urethral activity. As previously stated, urethral activity can only increase the detrusor pressure above the value defined by the PURR; therefore, as with the URR, any deviation of the pressure–flow plot from the PURR towards higher pressures is considered to be a result of activity of the urethral or periurethral muscles. The linPURR, a further development of this technique, utilizes a straight-line fit to quantify urethral resistance.[28]

The detrusor pressure at the cessation of flow ($p_{det.clos}$) has also been found to be useful diagnostically in women. This pressure is equivalent to the minimal pressure required to allow urinary flow in the urethra when completely relaxed. This variable is smaller in association with greater age in women with lower urinary tract symptoms. $p_{det.clos}$ is higher in women with either idiopathic DI or detrusor hyperreflexia.[23] A study into the use of pressure–flow plot variables in voiding efficiency in women revealed that Q*, detrusor shortening velocity, detrusor pressure at urethral closure and the pressure–flow plot gradient were able to discriminate between effective and ineffective voiding. In addition, these variables were found to vary independently of one another.[20]

There are also data that suggest that Q*, which is able to discriminate between 'fast' and 'slow' contracting bladders may accurately predict the occurrence of voiding difficulty following colposuspension for stress incontinence.[29]

CONCLUSIONS

To date there has been little application of the voiding pressure–flow plot in women. The use of nomograms developed for the identification of outflow tract obstruction in men may not be valid in women. However, data are accumulating that suggest that the pressure–flow plot can give useful information about physiological changes in urinary tract function and the variation of urethral resistance with disease, and clinically useful data relating to detrusor contractile function.

REFERENCES

1. Hill AV. The heat of shortening and the dynamic constants of muscle. *Proc R Soc Lond [Biol]* 1938; 126: 136–195

2. Griffiths DJ. *Urodynamics: The Mechanics and Hydrodynamics of the Lower Urinary Tract.* Medical Physics Handbooks 4. Bristol: Adam Hilger, 1980

3. Griffiths DJ. Urethral resistance to flow: the urethral resistance relation. *Urol Int* 1975; 30: 28–32

4. Van Mastrigt R, Griffiths DJ. Clinical comparison of bladder contractility parameters calculated from isometric contractions and pressure–flow studies. *Urology* 1987; 29: 102–106

5. Griffiths DJ. Assessment of detrusor contraction strength or contractility. *Neurourol Urodyn* 1991; 10: 1–18

6. Schäfer W. The contribution of the bladder outlet to the relation between pressure and flow rate during micturition. In: Hinman F Jr (ed) *Benign Prostatic Hypertrophy.* New York: Springer-Verlag, 1983; 470–496

7. Griffiths DJ. Constantinou CE, van Mastrigt R. Urinary bladder function and its control in healthy females. *Am J Physiol* 1986; 251: R225

8. Abrams PH, Griffiths DJ. The assessment of prostatic obstruction from urodynamic measurements and from residual urine. *Br J Urol* 1979; 51: 129–134

9. Spangberg A. Estimation of urethral resistance by curve fitting in the pressure–flow plot. *World J Urol* 1995; 13: 65–69

10. Höfner K, Kramer AEJL, Tan HK *et al.* Chess classification of urethral obstruction based upon pressure–flow analysis. *Neurourol Urodyn* 1993; 12: 414–415

11. Schäfer W. Basic principles and clinical application of advanced analysis of bladder voiding function. *Urol Clin North Am* 1990; 17: 553–566

12. Kranse M, Van Mastrigt R. The derivation of an obstruction index from a three-parameter model fitted to the lowest part of the pressure–flow plot. *J Urol* 1991; 145: 261A

13. Lim CS, Abrams PH. The Abrams–Griffiths nomogram. *World J Urol* 1995; 13: 34–39

14. Kranse R, van Mastrigt R, Bosch R. Estimation of the lag time between detrusor pressure and flow rate signals. *Neurourol Urodyn* 1995; 14: 217–229

15. Rosier PFWM, de la Rosette JJMCH, Koldewijn EL *et al.* Variability of pressure–flow analysis parameters in repeated cystometry in patients with benign prostatic hyperplasia. *J Urol* 1995; 150: 1520–1525

16. Sorenson S, Knudsen U, Kirkeby H, Djurhuus J. Urodynamic investigations in healthy fertile females during the menstrual cycle. *Scand J Urol Nephrol Suppl* 1988; 114: 28–34

17. Reynard JM, Lim C, Swami S, Abrams P. The obstructive effect of a urethral catheter. *J Urol* 1996; 155: 901–903

18. Abrams P, Blaivas JG, Stanton SL, Andersen JT. The standardisation of terminology of lower urinary tract function. The International Continence Society Committee on Standardisation of Terminology. *Scand J Urol Nephrol Suppl* 1988; 114: 5–19

19. Massey JA, Abrams PH. Obstructed voiding in the female. *Br J Urol* 1988; 61: 36–39

20. Sakakibara R, Hussein IF, Swinn MJ *et al.* Flow–pressure study in patients with neurological diseases – a preliminary report. *Neurourol Urodyn* 1998; 17: 304–305

21. Wagg AS, Malone-Lee JG. Pressure–flow plot analysis and voiding inefficiency in women with lower urinary tract symptoms. *Neurourol Urodyn* 1997; 16: 435–437

22. Wagg AS, Gray R, Malone-Lee JG. Pressure–flow plot analysis in women with detrusor instability and genuine stress incontinence. *Neurourol Urodyn* 1995; 14: 439–440

23. Wagg AS, Lieu PK, Ding YY, Malone-Lee JG. A urodynamic analysis of age-associated changes in urethral function in women with lower urinary tract symptoms. *J Urol* 1996; 156: 1984–1988

24. Rud T. Urethral pressure profile in continent women from childhood to old age. *Acta Obstet Gynecol Scand* 1980; 59: 331–335

25. Bosch R, Groen J. Urethral resistance is related to type of incontinence: changing etiologic concepts in female incontinence. *Neurourol Urodyn* 1998; 17: 386–387

26. Brocklehurst JC. Aging of the human bladder. *Geriatrics* 1972; 27: 154

27. Peruchchini D, DeLancey JOL, Ashton-Miller JA. Regional striated muscle loss in the female urethra: where is the striated muscle vulnerable? *Neurourol Urodyn* 1997; 16: 407–408

28. Schäfer W. Analysis of bladder outlet function with the linearized passive urethral resistance equation, linPURR, and a disease-specific approach for grading obstruction: from complex to simple. *World J Urol* 1995; 13: 47–58

29. Boos K, Cardozo L, Anders K, Malone-Lee JG. The calculation of detrusor muscle velocity to explain voiding difficulties after Burch colposuspension. *Proceedings of the International Continence Society Annual Meeting* 1996; abstr 281. Athens: International Continence Society

20

Urethral pressure measurements

G. Lose

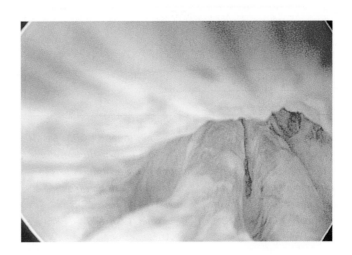

INTRODUCTION

Urethral pressure measurements have been used for more than 75 years to assess urethral closure function.[1]

The urethral pressure and the urethral closure pressure are idealized concepts which aim to represent the ability of the urethra to prevent leakage. As long as the intra-urethral pressure exceeds the proximal fluid pressure, urine cannot leak and so the subject should be continent.

CIRCUMSTANCES AND TYPES OF MEASUREMENTS

Intraluminal urethral pressure may be measured (a) with the subject at rest, with the bladder at any given volume, (b) during coughing or straining, and (c) during the process of voiding.[2]

Measurements can be made at one point in the urethra over a period of time (continuous urethral pressure recording) (Fig. 20.1) or as a urethral pressure profile (UPP) (Fig. 20.2).

Urethral pressure profilometry is the measurement of intraluminal pressure along the length of the urethra. A mechanical retracting puller (Fig. 20.3) that is synchronized with the chart or digital recorder allows measurement of anatomical distances in the profile.

Two types of UPP may be measured:

1. Resting UPP (Fig. 20.2), with the bladder and subject at rest;
2. Stress UPP (Fig. 20.2), with a defined applied stress (e.g. cough, strain or Valsalva manoeuvre).

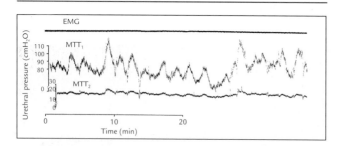

Figure 20.1. *Pressure variations recorded from a healthy female volunteer. The registration was done with a micro-tip transducer catheter (MTT) (5F). The orientation of the transducer was in an anterior position. MTT$_1$ is the pressure variation recorded at maximum urethral closure pressure, MTT$_2$ 1 cm distally. (Reproduced from ref. 25 with permission. Copyright ©1986 John Wiley & Sons).*

The simultaneous recording of both intra-urethral (p_{ura}) and intravesical (p_{ves}) pressure enables calculation of urethral closure pressure i.e. $p_{ura} - p_{ves}$ (Fig. 20.2).

TECHNIQUES

The three main methods for UPP measurement are (1) perfused catheters with side holes (Fig. 20.4a), (2) catheter-tip transducer catheters (Fig. 20.4b) and (3) balloon catheters (Fig. 20.4c).

Perfused catheters with side holes

The technique is mainly based on the description by Brown and Wickham.[3] The system measures the pressure needed to force water or gas slowly through one or more side or end holes in a round catheter. The perfusion rate should be at least 2 ml/min,[4] in order to avoid blockage of the catheter apertures by the urethral mucosa. The technique is relatively simple. It has been documented that water-filled perfusion catheters fulfil the demands for recording cough-produced variations.[5] The catheters are relatively cheap and are disposable.

Catheter-tip transducer catheters

This technique was popularized by Asmussen and Ulmsten.[6] In fact, the transducer measures not the hydrostatic pressure but the normal stress component on its surface. Because of the rapid-frequency response of around 2000 Hz, the technique is suitable for recording very rapid changes in intra-urethral pressure, such as those occurring during coughing. The technique is also ideal for long-term measurements. The stiffness of the catheters may lead to an interaction between the transducer and the urethral wall, resulting in a directional artefact.[7–9] This means that conventional UPP parameters at rest and during coughing provide different results, depending on the orientation of the transducer.[7–9] The results obtained with the transducer in the lateral orientation (9 or 3 o'clock) compared with the anterior position seem to be most in accordance with the clinical situation in women with stress incontinence.[7]

The surface area of a pressure transducer is very small (approximately 1 mm). Obviously, the 'pressure'

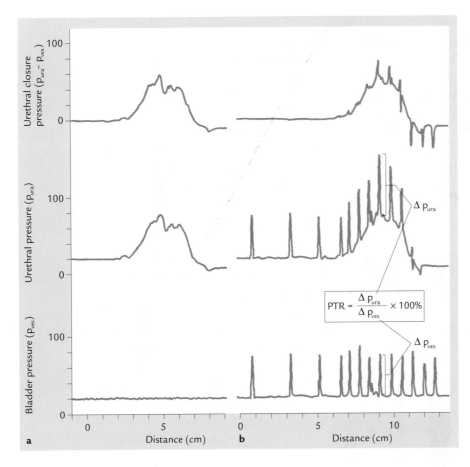

Figure 20.2. *Urethral pressure profiles at rest (a) and during coughs (b) in a continent woman: 7F dual sensor tip transducer catheter, supine position, 200 ml bladder volume. PTR, pressure transmission ratio (= [$\Delta p_{ura}/\Delta p_{ves}$] × 100%).*

$$PTR = \frac{\Delta p_{ura}}{\Delta p_{ves}} \times 100\%$$

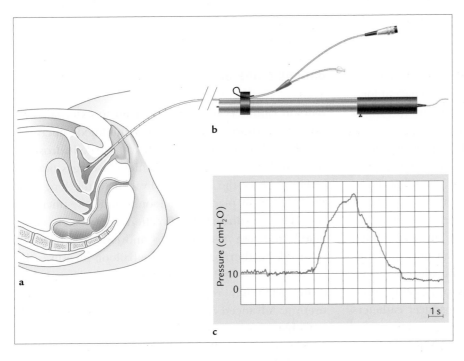

Figure 20.3. *Urethral pressure profilometry (a) technique for urethral pressure measurement; (b) puller device for retraction of catheter during profilometry (Medtronic, Dantec, Urology); (c) urethral pressure profile trace at rest.*

217

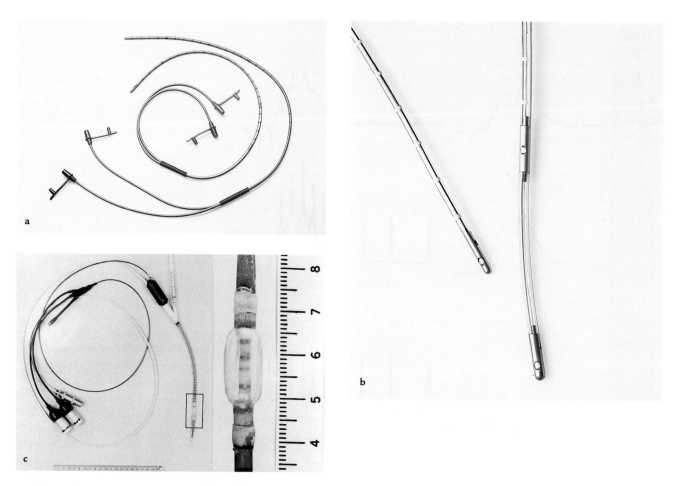

Figure 20.4. *(a) Two-lumen catheters (10F) for urethral pressure profilometry (Medtronic, Dantec, Urology). (b) A single (6F) and a dual (8F) sensor tip transducer catheter (Medtronic, Dantec, Urology). (c) Balloon catheter, mounted on a double micro-tip transducer catheter. The proximal pressure sensor is placed inside the balloon.*

measured in a small area in a given direction may not always be indicative of the pressure in an adjacent location and hence may not be representative of the state of the entire urethra.

In combined bladder and urethral pressure measurements, micro-tip transducers may record pressures that differ from those of liquid-perfused catheters because of the difference in the height of the bladder, and urethral transducers are not cancelled out by the siphon effect in saline-filled catheters with external pressure transducers. Thus, the vertical distance between two transducers during measurement should be taken into account when data are analysed. The micro-tip transducer catheters are relatively costly.

Balloon catheters

Balloon catheters may be connected to external pressure transducers[10] or may be modified micro-tip transducer catheters[11, 12] (Fig. 20.4c). A true hydrostatic pressure is measured. The technique averages out the variations over the length equivalent to the length of the balloon. By placing a balloon around the micro-tip pressure transducer, the directional artefact is eliminated and the sensitivity to movement artefact is reduced. Furthermore, since the balloon measures the pressure over 1 or 1.5 cm length of the urethra, it may more accurately represent the state of the entire urethra. Advanced catheters[12] are not yet commercially available.

RELIABLILITY OF MEASUREMENTS

Reliability of measurements depends on accuracy (validity) and reproducibility (precision) of the test results. The available information shows that UPP parameters are subject to a certain amount of inter- and intra-individual variation.[4,13–16] This variation is due to methodological and biological factors.

The variation because of pure intrinsic instrumental factors is generally low, of the order of a few per cent.[4,14,17] Measurements *in vivo*, however, are subject to significant variation because of methodological differences in terms of size, type of catheter (perfusion, micro-tip, balloon or optic), rate of perfusion, retraction, posture of the patient and content of the bladder.

Furthermore, the urethral pressure at a given point in the urethra is not constant: it is subject to significant normal physiological fluctuations of the order of 40 cmH$_2$0 (Fig. 20.1) due to changes in the activity of smooth muscle[18] and/or striated muscle.[19] In this context it is important to be aware that the patient often is unable to relax her pelvic floor during urethral pressure measurement, especially during the first profile.

The reliability of measurements also depends on the quality of the urodynamic practice, routine and expertise.

Finally, all techniques imply the introduction of a probe and hence opening of the urethral lumen, which introduces a systematic artefact for all measurements.

Consequently, the accuracy (validity) of urethral pressure data is difficult to establish since the true urethral pressure is unknown. The test–retest variation is significant (i.e. low reproducibility) because of the influence of so many different factors. At the moment there is no consensus on how to standardize the technique of urethral profilometry. It is recommended that authors specify their technique according to the International Continence Society (ICS)[2] and provide reproducibility data (or indicate their absence).

CLINICAL MEASUREMENTS AND PARAMETERS

The Standardization Committee of the ICS has defined the parameters in common use (Fig. 20.5). Recordings of profile parameters must be repeated several times to verify reproducibility.

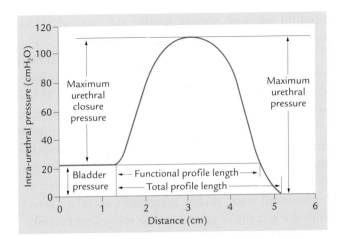

Figure 20.5. *Definition of terms in urethral pressure profilometry.*

Static measurements in the resting urethra

The static parameters relate to the permanently acting closure forces along the urethra.[20]

Since the results of urethral pressure measurements are so highly dependent on the technique used and the circumstances of measurement, it is recommended that each laboratory should draw up its own frame of reference. The magnitude of some reference values reported[10,16,18,21–24] is shown in Table 20.1.

In long-duration measurements, the urethral pressure shows considerable variation in patients and healthy women.[19] Sørensen *et al.*[25] found urethral pressure variations from 3 to 66 cmH$_2$O during 1-hour's continuous recording in healthy women. These pressure variations seem to be genuine;[26] however, during ambulatory urodynamic monitoring the urethral pressure may decrease to zero without leakage, because of artefacts and methodological problems attendant on the use of micro-tip transducer catheters.[27] Consequently, it has been recommended that ambulatory monitoring of

Table 20.1. *Magnitude of reference values of conventional static urethral presure parameters reported in the literature*

Parameter	Value
Maximum urethral pressure	50–80 cmH$_2$O
Maximum closure pressure	40–70 cmH$_2$O
Functional length	3 cm

urethral pressure should involve the use of a leak detector.[27]

Maximum urethral pressure (MUP), like maximum urethral closure pressure (MUCP), declines as a function of age,[10,22,28] and both MUP and MUCP are reduced in stress-incontinent women.[10,18,21,23] However, since the overlap between the values from continent and incontinent women is so great, it has been impossible to define a cut-off level that allows differentiation between women with and without stress incontinence.

Standard static profile parameters correlate poorly with the severity of genuine stress incontinence (GSI).[29] Successful surgical treatment of stress incontinence is not associated with significant changes in the resting parameters.[30,31]

Conventional urethral pressure measurement yields a single pressure at a given site in the urethra. This pressure depends on the cross-sectional area (CA) of the probe used.[20] If the CA of the urethra is changed consecutively, a pressure–CA relationship is outlined (Fig. 20.6). This relationship, given by the equation $p_{ura} = E \times CA + p_0$, characterizes the urethral sphincter function, since p_0 describes the pressure at which the urethra opens and elastance ($E = d_{pura}/dCA$) is the

Table 20.2. Magnitude of special static midurethral parameters reported in the literature	
Parameter	Value
p_0	55–60 cmH$_2$O
Elastance	1.10–1.25 cmH$_2$O/mm^2

resistance against dilatation. The maintenance of continence depends on the ability of the closure mechanism to produce a p_0 that is higher than p_{ves} and/or a high elastance in order to prevent opening and subsequent dilatation of the urethra, both at rest and during stress episodes. Reference values have been reported by several authors[20,32,33] (Table 20.2). Elastance and p_0 can be estimated by conventional techniques if measurements are performed with different size catheters.[34] The usability of these parameters remains to be documented.

An MUCP value less than 20 cmH$_2$O ('low-pressure urethra') has been considered predictive of poor outcome of conventional bladder-neck suspension operations,[35] and has been the most popular single predictor of intrinsic sphincter deficiency (ISD). It can be seen from Figure 20.7 that urethral pressure depends on the CA of the measuring probe, and, for instance, if a probe with a CA of 11 mm^2 (=12F) is used, the same pressure will be obtained in the patient with hyperlaxity and the

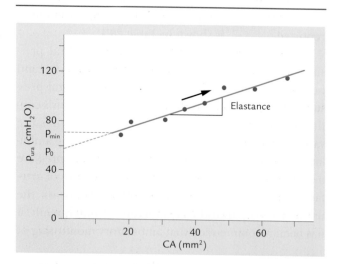

Figure 20.6. *Related values of urethral pressure (p_{ura}) and cross-sectional area (CA) in a healthy volunteer. Measurement is performed 0.75 cm from the bladder neck with the subject in the supine position with an empty bladder. The solid line is the regression line ($p_{ura} = dp_{ura}/dCA$) CA + p_0, where p_0 is the theoretical uninstrumented urethral pressure. The slope of the curve dp_{ura}/dCA is the elastance, where elastance is the reciprocal of compliance (a measure of the increase in [e.g. airway] pressure for a given increase in volume of [e.g.] gas or air).*

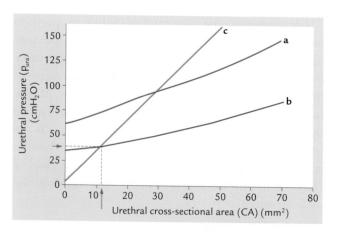

Figure 20.7. *The p_{ura}–CA relationship in (a) a normal woman, (b) a stress-incontinent woman with urethral hyperlaxity and (c) a stress-incontinent woman with intrinsic sphincter deficiency. The figure shows that the pressure measured with a probe with CA of 11 mm^2 (~12F) (indicated by arrows) would yield the same pressure in patients b and c.*

patient with ISD. Measurement of MUCP does not allow for the differentiation between a rigid malfunctioning urethra and hyperlaxity. This can be done by estimation of elastance and p_0.[20]

Dynamic measurements in the resting urethra

Conventional methods measure the urethral pressure at a fixed CA given by the dimensions of the probe. Urinary stress incontinence however, is a dynamic event with forced opening of the urethra. The dynamic urethral pressure response to a simulated urine ingression has been studied by several authors (Fig. 20.8a).[32,33,36–38] The pressure response represents an integrated stress response from the surrounding tissues, which may reflect the viscoelastic properties of the involved structures (Fig. 20.8b). Bagi *et al.*[37] have found that striated muscle fibres are of dominating significance for the pressure response. Pudendal nerve blockade affects urethral stress relaxation significantly by a reduction in the fast time constant, $\tau\beta$.[39] Data show that the stress relaxation response is significantly changed at the bladder neck and midurethrally in patients with stress incontinence (Fig. 20.8b), indicating that the resistance against dilatation of the urethra by ingression of urine is decreased.[20,32,36,40]

Thind[38] has estimated that urethral viscoelasticity may account for 25% of the urethral resistance to dilatation.

Measurements during coughing and voluntary contraction of the pelvic floor

Stress incontinence normally occurs in relation to an increase in abdominal pressure such as during coughing. Consequently, it seems relevant to test the urethral closure function during coughing. Furthermore, it has been shown that changes in static pressure-profile parameters measured in the resting urethra do not necessarily reflect changes in cough-produced profile data.[41] Therefore, it seems relevant to supplement resting profile results with measurements during stress episodes to assess urethral competence.

The parameters commonly in use are the cough profile, pressure transmisson ratio (PTR), leak-point pressure, and time separation during coughing.

Cough profile

If every cough along the urethral closure pressure profile generates a negative spike that reaches the zero zone (i.e. pressure equalization), the test is considered 'positive' and hence suggests the diagnosis of GSI (Fig. 20.1). Thus, the concept is defined as an 'all-or-nothing' phenomenon. However, the test may be 'negative' in patients with GSI and 'positive' in situations where urine loss does not occur.[7,27,42] The test result may vary within the individual woman, according to the size of the cough.[43] Cough profile parameters correlate poorly with the severity of GSI.[29] Reproducibility of the test has not been established. Richardson[42] has reported the predictive value of a positive test to be 82–86% and the predictive value of a normal test to be 57–58% in the diagnosis of GSI in

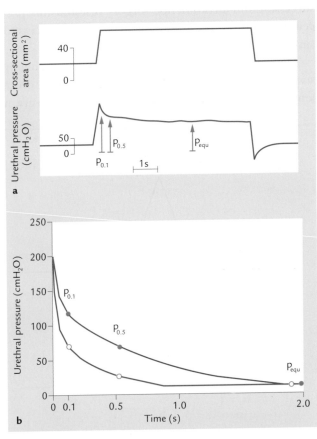

Figure 20.8. *(a) Simultaneous measurement of urethral pressure and cross-sectional area during forced dilatation; measurement at the bladder neck in a healthy 28-year-old female volunteer. The pressures 0.1 s and 0.5 s after dilatation and at equilibrium were used for calculation. (b) Schematic illustration of urethral stress relaxation with pressure decay following forced dilation in a continent* —•— *and a stress incontinent* —•— *woman.*

women with lower urinary tract symptoms. The reliabilty (and hence the usefulness) of cough profilometry using conventional micro-tip transducer catheters is dubious.

Pressure transmission ratio (PTR)

The concept of the PTR, defined as the increment in urethral pressure during coughing as a percentage of the simultaneously recorded increment in bladder pressure, has received considerable attention. However, it remains unclear what is really recorded. It has been suggested that the urethral pressure spike represents the sum of passively and actively generated closure forces, which may explain why the PTR can exceed 100%. Data indicate that differences in PTR between continent and stress-incontinent women are due to differences in the actively created forces.[44]

Pressure studies have shown that the pressure created inside the urethal lumen is higher than the pressure outside the urethra during coughing.[43,45] Thus, the the term 'pressure transmission' is misleading, as there appears to be a pressure gradient from inside to outside the urethra.

Clinically, Bump *et al.*[46] found that a PTR value of less than 90% in the proximal urethra had a positive predictive value of 53% and a negative predictive value of 97%.

As previously stated, test results may vary within the individual woman, according to the intensity of the cough.[47] Studies have shown that PTR measurement is subject to marked variation and that the overlap between normal and stress-incontinent values is so great that PTR is of limited value in predicting whether the urethral mechanism is competent or incompetent.[23,48-50]

Leak-point pressure

Valsalva or cough leak-point pressure has been introduced as a quantifiable measure of urethral sphincter function.[51] According to some authors, the test is remarkably reproducible;[52] however, others have found significant test–retest variation.[53] The cough leak-point pressure has been found to show a moderate degree of inverse correlation with pad-test data.[54,55] At the moment the test is not standardized. The test result depends on the size of the catheter and vesical volumes.[56] Although leak-point pressure measurement may be useful in quantifying urethral sphincter competence, the test cannot disclose the underlying

pathophysiology, and thus cannot differentiate between stress incontinence due to hypermobility and that due to ISD.

Dynamic urethral pressure parameters are generally affected by surgery.[30,57] However, the association between the result and the change in the parameter used is not straigthtforward.[57]

Time separation during coughing

Several authors have studied the time separation between changes in bladder and urethral pressure during coughing.[11,58,59] In continent women, urethral pressure has been found to rise approximately 200 ms before pressure in the bladder begins to rise during coughing (Fig. 20.9), whereas this preceding increase in urethral pressure is lacking in stress-incontinent women.[11,59] A recent study found that successful anti-incontinence surgery restored this preceding urethral pressure rise, whereas unsuccessful surgery did not.[60]

The cough urethral pressure profile is highly suspectible to artefacts and pitfalls. The main problem is that micro-tip transducer catheters measure a

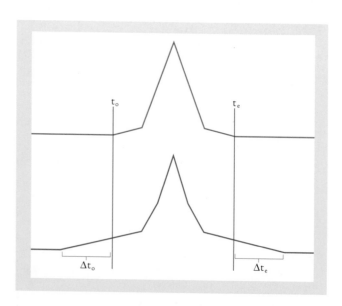

Figure 20.9. *Schematic drawing of normal pressure variations in bladder (top line) and urethra (bottom line) during a stress episode: t_o, time of onset of pressure increase in the bladder; t_e, time at the end of pressure increase in the bladder; Δt_o, time difference between the onset of pressure increase in the urethra and that in the bladder; Δt_e, time difference between the end of pressure increase in the urethra and that in the bladder.*

unidirectional force instead of a true pressure. Artefacts occur because of catheter stiffness, weight and movement.[8,9,61]

Contraction of the pelvic floor

Urethral pressure measurement has been used to assess the effect of pelvic floor contraction.[10,16,32,62] Significant differences have been found between stress-incontinent and healthy women.[10,62,63] Advanced techniques enable measurement of the effect of the urethral closure function in terms of power generation during coughing and voluntary contraction of the pelvic floor.[62] In women with GSI, the mean power generation during such contraction is reduced by approximately 50% all along the urethra, while the mean power generation during coughing is reduced by 25% midurethrally.[63]

Urethral pressure measurement during contraction may have potential in the investigation of pelvic floor function and in the assessment of the effect of intervention.

Detrusor and urethral instability

Urethral pressure measurement may have a role in the identification of the chronological sequence of bladder and urethral pressure changes in order to differentiate between different pathophysiological entities. Incontinence may occur because of a urethral pressure decrease without a detrusor contraction;[27] this appears to be a rare entity, which has been termed unstable urethra. The simultaneous measurement of urethral and bladder pressures in patients with detrusor instability reveals two different patterns: one type is characterized by an uninhibited bladder contraction followed by urethral relaxation; the other comprises a detrusor contraction preceded by urethral relaxation.[64] This differentiation may have therapeutic relevance.

Local pathology in the urethra

Urethral pressure measurements may be useful to disclose local pathology in the urethra, such as diverticula and strictures.[65-67] New techniques can localize the exact site of an obstructive area in the urethra.[20]

Impaired bladder emptying

Impaired bladder emptying may be suspected in women with low flow rate or significant post-micturition residual urine. A pressure–flow study can differentiate between infravesical obstruction and detrusor hypoactivity. In obstructed and equivocal cases, urethral investigation may add important diagnostic information. Conventional urethral pressure profilometry during rest may reveal a stricture. More advanced techniques, such as urethral pressure profilometry during urination,[68] or measurement of related values of pressure and cross-sectional area along the urethra,[20,69,70] may be useful to assess the mechanical properties of the urethra and detect local areas of obstruction. Thus, urethral investigation may be helpful in planning the correct treatment in women with impaired bladder emptying, and may prevent inappropriate urethrotomy in cases of poor detrusor function, which potentially may damage the closure apparatus and lead to stress incontinence.

Research tool

Although all parameters show a certain degree of interindividual variability, they may still be useful when large series of women are studied for the understanding of normal physiological and pathophysiological mechanisms. In the individual subject some parameters are fairly reproducible, which implies that they may be especially useful in sequential measurements (e.g. before and after intervention in the individual patient).

There is no doubt that the 'urethral pressure' is of significant importance for the continence mechanism. However, urethral pressure is a complex measure.[71] It is important to improve the quality of our techniques of measurement and our concepts of interpretation instead of merely increasing the quantities of data based on standard questionable urodynamic measurements.

CONCLUSIONS

- Urethral pressure measurement with conventional techniques is of limited value in assessment of urethral sphincter function. The 'standard' parameters do not (a) discriminate between stress incontinence and other disorders, (b) provide a precise measure of the severity of the condition, or (c) return to normal after successful incontinence surgery.

- Urethral pressure measurements may be useful in disclosing local pathology such as strictures or diverticula and in targeting the intervention of specific conditions (e.g. 'low-pressure urethra').
- Urethral pressure measurements may be useful as a research tool to study normal physiological and pathophysiological mechanisms and changes after intervention (e.g. pharmacological treatment) in the individual patient.

Urethral pressure measurements should not be perfomed automatically with the current equipment but should be based on good urodynamic practice in terms of (a) careful indication and selection of test parameters and procedures, (b) precise measurement with data quality control and complete documentation and (c) accurate analysis and critical reporting of results.

REFERENCES

1. Bonney V. On diurnal incontinence of urine in women. *J Obstet Gynaecol Br Emp* 1923; 30: 358–365

2. Abrams P, Blaivas JG, Stanton SL, Andersen JT. The standardization of terminology of the lower urinary tract. *Scand J Urol Nephrol Suppl* 1988; 114: 5–19

3. Brown M, Wickham JEA. The urethral pressure profile. *Br J Urol* 1969; 41: 211–217

4. Abrams PH, Martin S, Griffiths DJ. The measurement and interpretation of urethral pressure obtained by the method of Brown and Wickham. *Br J Urol* 1978; 50: 30–38

5. Thind P, Bagi P, Lose G, Mortensen S. Characterization of pressure changes in the lower urinary tract during coughing with special reference to the demands of the pressure recording equipment. *Neurourol Urodyn* 1994; 13: 219–225

6. Asmussen M, Ulmsten U. Simultaneous urethrocystometry and urethral pressure profile measurement with a new technique. *Acta Obstet Gynecol Scand* 1975; 54: 385–386

7. Anderson RS, Shepherd AM, Feneley RCL. Microtransducer urethral profile methodology in variations caused by transducer orientation. *J Urol* 1983; 130: 727–728

8. Plevnik S, Janez J, Vratcnik P, Brown M. Directional differences in urethral pressure recording: contributions from the stiffness and weight of recording catheter. *Neurourol Urodyn* 1985; 4: 117–128

9. Schäfer W. Regarding 'directional differences in urethral pressure recording: contributions from the stiffness and weight of recording catheter'. *Neurourol Urodyn* 1986; 5: 119–120

10. Enhörning G. Simultaneous recording of intravesical and intra-urethral pressure: a study of urethral closure in normal and stress incontinent women. *Acta Chir Scand Suppl* 1961; 276: 1–68

11. Van der Kooi JB, Van Wanroy PJA, De Jonge MC, Kornelis JA. Time separation between cough pulses in bladder, rectum and urethra in women. *J Urol* 1984; 132: 1275–1278

12. Lose G, Colstrup H, Saksager K, Kristensen JK. New probe for measurement of related values of cross-sectional area and pressure in a biological tube. *Med Biol Eng Comput* 1986; 24: 488–492

13. Hilton P. The urethral pressure profile at rest: an analysis of variance. *Neurourol Urodyn* 1982; 1: 303–311

14. Lose G, Schroeder T. Pressure/cross-sectional area probe in the assessment of urethral closure function. *Urol Res* 1990; 18: 143–147

15. Meyhoff HH, Nordling J, Walter S. Short and long term reproducibility of urethral closure pressure profile parameters. *Urol Res* 1979; 7: 269–271

16. Plante P, Susset J. Studies of female urethral pressure profile. Part I. The normal urethral pressure profile. *J Urol* 1980; 123: 64–69

17. Ghoneim MA, Rottenbourg JL, Fretin J, Susset JG. Urethral pressure profile. *Urology* 1975; 5: 632–637

18. Sørensen S. Urethral pressure variations in healthy and incontinent women. *Neurourol Urodyn* 1992; 11: 549–591

19. Kulseng-Hanssen S. Urethral pressure variation. *Int Urogynecol J* 1993; 4: 366–372

20. Lose G. Simultaneous recording of pressure and cross-sectional area in the female urethra: a study of urethral closure function in healthy and stress incontinent women. *Neurourol Urodyn* 1992; 11: 55–89

21. Hilton, P, Stanton SL. Urethral pressure measurement by microtransducer: the results in symptom free women and in those with genuine stress incontinence. *Br J Obstet Gynaecol* 1983; 90: 919–933

22. Rud T. Urethral pressure profile in continent women from childhood to old age. *Acta Obstet Gynecol Scand* 1980; 59: 331–335

23. Versi E, Cardozo L, Studd J, Cooper D. Evaluation of urethral pressure profilometry for the diagnosis of genuine stress incontinence. *World J Urol* 1986; 4: 6–9

24. Lose G. Mechanical properties of the urethra in healthy female volunteers. Static measurements in the resting urethra. *Neurourol Urodyn* 1989; 8: 451–459

25. Sørensen S, Kirkeby HJ, Stødkilde–Jørgensen H, Djurhuus JC. Continuous recording of urethral activity in healthy female volunteers. *Neurourol Urodyn* 1986; 5: 5–16

26. Colstrup H, Lose G, Jørgensen L. Pressure variation in the female urethra measured by the infusion technique: is it an artefact? *Neurourol Urodyn* 1988; 7: 457–460

27. Kulseng-Hanssen S. Ambulatory urodynamic monitoring of women. *Scand J Urol Nephrol Suppl* 1996; 30: 27–37

28. Diokno AC, Normolle DP, Brown MB, Herzog AR. Urodynamic tests for female geriatric urinary incontinence. *Urology* 1990; 36: 431–439

29. Meyer S, De Grandi P, Schmidt N *et al.* Urodynamic parameters in patients with slight and severe genuine stress incontinence: is the stress profile useful? *Neurourol Urodyn* 1994; 13: 21–28

30. Henriksson L, Ulmsten U. A urodynamic evaluation of the effect of abdominal urethrocystopexy and vaginal sling urethroplasty in women with stress incontinence. *Am J Obstet Gynecol* 1987; 131: 77–82

31. Bergman A, McCarthy TA. Urodynamic changes after successful operation for stress urinary incontinence. *Am J Obstet Gynecol* 1983; 147: 325–327

32. Colstrup H. Closure mechanism of the female urethra. *Neurourol Urodyn* 1987; 6: 271–298

33. Thind P. The significance of smooth and striated muscles in the sphincter function of the urethra in healthy women. *Neurourol Urodyn* 1995; 14: 585–618

34. Thind P, Lose G, Colstrup H. How to measure urethral elastance in a simple way. Elastance: definition, determination and complications. *Urol Res* 1991; 19: 241–244

35. Sand PK, Bowen LW, Panganiban R, Ostergard DR. The low pressure urethra as a factor in failed retropubic urethropexy. *Obstet Gynecol* 1987; 68: 399–402

36. Lose G, Colstrup H. Mechanical properties of the urethra in healthy and stress incontinent females: dynamic measurements in the resting urethra. *J Urol* 1990; 144: 1258–1262

37. Bagi P, Thind P, Norsten M. Passive urethral resistance to dilatation in healthy women: an experimental simulation of urine ingression in the resting urethra. *Neurourol Urodyn* 1995; 14: 115–123

38. Thind P. An analysis of urethral viscoelasticity with particular reference to the sphincter function in healthy women. *Int Urogynecol J* 1995; 6: 209–228

39. Thind P, Bagi P, Mieszczak C, Lose G. Influence of pudendal nerve blockade on stress relaxation in the female urethra. *Neurourol Urodyn* 1996; 15: 31–36

40. Thind P, Lose G. Urethral stress relaxation phenomenon in healthy and stress incontinent women. *Br J Urol* 1992; 69: 75–78

41. Thind P, Lose G, Colstrup H, Andersson K-E. The effect of pharmacological stimulation and blockade of autonomic receptors on the urethral pressure and power generation during coughing and squeezing of the pelvic floor in healthy females. *Scand J Urol Nephrol* 1993; 27: 519–525

42. Richardson DA. Value of the cough pressure profile in the evaluation of patients with stress incontinence. *Am J Obstet Gynecol* 1986; 155: 808–811

43. Bunne G, Öbrink A. Urethral closure pressure with stress. A comparison between stress incontinent and continent women. *Urol Res* 1978; 6: 127–134

44. Lose G. Urethral pressure and power generation during coughing and voluntary contraction of the pelvic floor in females with genuine stress incontinence. *Br J Urol* 1991; 67: 580–585.

45. Papa Petros PE, Ulmsten U. Urethral pressure increase on effort originates from within the urethra and continence from musculovaginal closure. *Neurourol Urodyn* 1995; 14: 337–350

46. Bump RD, Copeland WE, Hurt WG, Fantl JA. Dynamic urethral pressure/profilometry pressure transmission ratio determinations in stress-incontinent and stress-continent subjects. *Am J Obstet Gynecol* 1988; 159: 749–755

47. Swift SE, Rust PF, Ostergard DR. Intrasubject variability of pressure-transmission ratio in patients with genuine stress incontinence. *Int Urogynecol J* 1996; 7: 312–316

48. Richardson DA, Ramahi A. Reproducibility of pressure transmission ratios in stress incontinent women. *Neurourol Urodyn* 1993; 12: 123–130

49. Lose G, Thind P, Colstrup H. The value of pressure transmission ratio in the diagnosis of stress incontinence. *Neurourol Urodyn* 1990; 9: 323–324

50. Rosenzweig BA, Bhatia NN, Nelson AL. Dynamic urethral pressure profilometry pressure transmission ratio: what do the numbers really mean? *Obstet Gynecol* 1991; 777: 586–590

51. McGuire ES, Fitzpatrick CC, Wan J *et al.* Clinical assessment of urethral sphincter function. *J Urol* 1993; 150: 1452–1454

52. Bump RC, Elser DM, McClish DK. Valsalva leak point pressures in adult women with genuine stress incontinence: reproducibility effect of catheter caliber and correlations with passive urethral pressure profilometry. *Neurourol Urodyn* 1993; 12: 307–308

53. Siltberg H, Larsson G. Victor A. The reproducibility of a new method to measure leak point pressure in patients with GSI. *Neurourol Urodyn* 1994; 13: 456–458

54. Theofrastous JP, Bump RC, Elser DM *et al.* Correlation of urodynamic measures of urethral resistance with clinical measures of incontinence severity in women with pure genuine stress incontinence. The Continence Program for Women Research Group. *Am J Obstet Gynecol* 1995; 173: 407–412

55. Siltberg H, Larsson G, Victor A. Reproducibility of a new method to determine cough-induced leak-point pressure in women with stress urinary incontinence. *Int Urogynecol J* 1996; 7: 13–19

56. Bump RC, Elser DM, Theofrastous JP, McClish DK. Valsalva leak point pressures in women with genuine stress incontinence: reproducibility, effect of catheter caliber and correlations with other measures of urethral resistance. *Am J Obstet Gynecol* 1995; 173: 551–557

57. Sayer TR, Hosker GL, Warrell DW. Does successful bladder neck surgery alter urethral closure? *Neurourol Urodyn* 1991; 10: 448–449

58. Faysal MH, Constantinou CE, Rother LF, Govan DA. The impact of bladder neck suspension on the resting and stress urethral pressure profile: a prospective study comparing controls with incontinent patients preoperatively and postoperatively. *J Urol* 1981; 125: 55–60

59. Thind P, Lose G, Jørgensen L, Colstrup H. Urethral pressure increment preceding and following bladder pressure elevation during stress episode in healthy and stress incontinent women. *Neurourol Urodyn* 1991; 10: 177–183

60. Pieber D, Zivkovic F, Tamussino K. Timing of urethral pressure pulses before and after continence surgery. *Neurourol Urodyn* 1998; 17: 19–23

61. Richardson DA. Reduction of urethral pressure response to stress: relationship to urethral mobility. *Am J Obstet Gynecol* 1986; 155: 20–25

62. Lose G, Golstrup H. Urethral pressure and power generation during coughing and voluntary contraction of the pelvic floor in healthy females. *Br J Urol* 1991; 67: 573–579

63. Susset J, Plante P. Studies of female urethral pressure profile. Part II: Urethral pressure profile in female incontinence. *J Urol* 1980: 123: 70–74

64. Elia G, Bergman A. Urethral pressure changes in women with detrusor instability. *Int Urogynecol J* 1994; 5: 98–101

65. Højsgaard A. The urethral pressure profile in female patients with meatal stenosis. *Scand J Urol Nephrol* 1976; 10: 97–99

66. Summitt RH, Stovall TG. Urethral diverticula: evaluation by urethral pressure profilometry, cystourethroscopy and voiding cystourethrogram. *Obstet Gynecol* 1992; 80: 695–699

67. Bhatia NN, McCarthy TA, Ostergard DR. Urethral pressure profiles in women with diverticula. *Obstet Gynecol* 1981; 58: 375–378

68. Sullivan MP, Yalla SV. Micturition profilometry. In: Raz S (ed) *Female Urology*. Philadelphia: Saunders, 1996; 132–142

69. Regnier CH. Direct static measurement of obstruction. *Neurourol Urodyn* 1986; 5: 251–257

70. Susset IG, Ghoniem GM, Regnier CH. Abnormal urethral compliance in females: diagnosis, results and treatment. *J Urol* 1983; 129: 1063–1065

71. Golstrup H, Lose G, Thind P. Urethral pressure – which one? *Urol Res* 1992; 20: 169–172

21

Leak-point pressures

E. J. McGuire, W. W. Leng

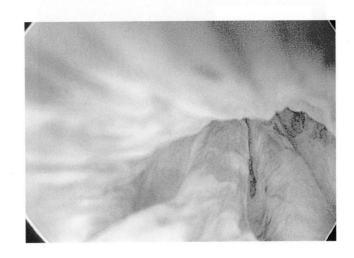

DETRUSOR PRESSURE AS AN EXPULSIVE FORCE

Historical note

Detrusor pressures required to drive urine across the urethra in neurogenic conditions are very closely related to outcome with respect to the upper urinary tract.[1,2] This relationship was first described in myelodysplastic children at two centres – Yale and the University of New Mexico. In those studies, a group of children with myelodysplasia were followed with routine videourodynamic evaluation and periodic upper tract surveillance (Fig. 21.1). When these data were analysed it became clear that detrusor pressures at the instant of leakage of $40\,cmH_2O$ or more were associated with a 100% risk of upper tract injury if untreated[2] (Fig. 21.2). Most of these children had an areflexic bladder and relatively fixed urethral resistance at the level of the external sphincter. The internal sphincter is completely non-functional and the bladder outlet always open in such cases[3,4] (Fig. 21.3). Resistance to detrusor pressure (p_{det}) as an expulsive force by the 'external sphincter' is fixed since the sphincter does not have the requisite neural mechanism to adjust to changes in bladder activity or volume. Urethral closing pressure profiles (UPPs) then measure urethral pressure in a relatively static environment and the p_{det} measured at the time of leakage is equal to the maximum urethral closing pressure.

As Schäfer, Griffiths and many others have shown, p_{det} during voiding (or leakage where p_{det} is the expulsive force) reflects the outlet resistance and not the quality or strength of the detrusor musculature.[5,6] In

normal voiding, or neurogenic conditions associated with reflex detrusor contractility, profound changes in urethral resistance and pressures occur throughout the voiding cycle. UPP values measured prior to detrusor

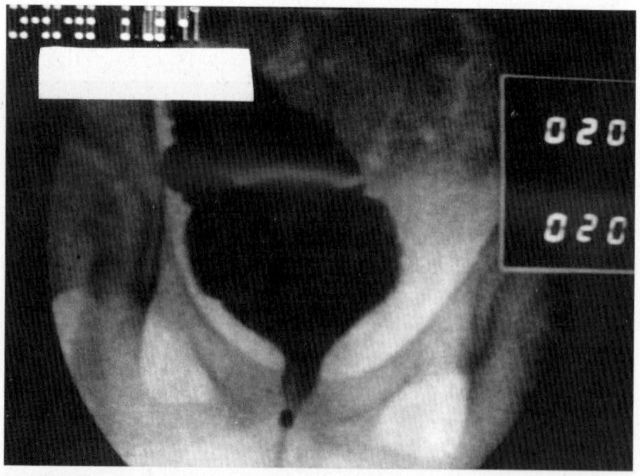

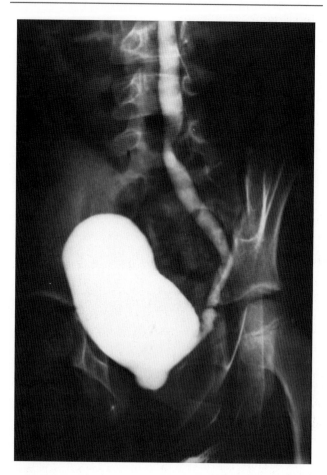

Figure 21.2. *Upper urinary tract deterioration resulting from long-standing increased detrusor storage pressures.*

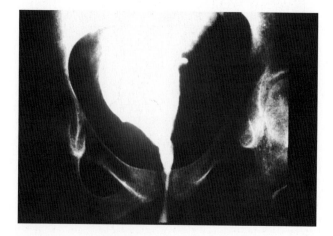

Figure 21.1. *Myelodysplastic bladder demonstrating open bladder neck at rest.*

Figure 21.3. *Myelodysplastic bladder with open bladder neck and fixed external sphincter.*

reflex contractility are then not related to outlet resistance at the time of urinary flow. Because, during flow, urethral resistance is difficult to measure directly, it has been calculated from p_{det} and flow data (Fig. 21.4).[7]

Neurogenic conditions

Detrusor leak-point pressures have been measured in myelodysplastic patient populations and in patients with spinal cord injury. A predictable series of changes occurs in circumstances where abnormal outlet resistance is maintained in the face of detrusor expulsive efforts. First, there is an elevated detrusor pressure at the time of voiding or leakage; secondly, there is gradual deterioration of detrusor compliance.[8,9] If this condition is untreated, compliance continues to deteriorate and ambient bladder storage pressures gradually rise. If storage pressures approach 40 cmH$_2$O for any significant period of time, or continuously,

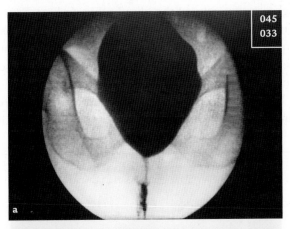

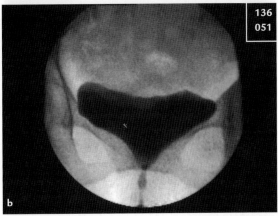

Figure 21.4 (a, b). *Two different urodynamic studies showing that maximal urethral pressure does not correlate with outlet resistance at the onset of urinary flow.*

upper tract dilatation and vesicoureteral reflux and transmission of p_{det} to the renal papillae occur.[2]

Identical findings have been reported by various workers in cases of obstructive uropathy related to non-neurogenic conditions, such as benign prostatic hypertrophy. Thus, renal damage and ureteral damage have been associated with high-pressure chronic retention in patients with obstructive prostatism.[10] Abnormal compliance is a sign of advanced obstruction or tissue injury (Fig. 21.5); this finding makes treatment mandatory.[11] In situations where obstructive uropathy is a possibility (such as prostatism or neurogenic conditions) abnormal compliance is a derivative finding of considerable significance. In the first place, abnormal compliance is induced by elevated or abnormal outlet resistance; secondly, abnormal compliance is intrinsically dangerous. Currently, we do not know precisely how abnormal outlet resistance initiates the cascade of events that leads to altered compliance and the morphological changes which accompany it; however, we know that several growth factors are certainly involved.[12–14]

Treatment

Treatment can be directed at the outlet, for example, by prostatectomy, sphincterotomy or sphincter dilatation.[15,16] The beneficial effect of lowered outlet resistance on compliance and altered morphology has been demonstrated.[16] This type of effect may not always be achievable and it seems likely that, at some point, irre-

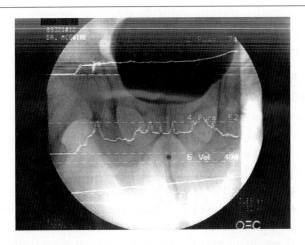

Figure 21.5. *Obstructive uropathy due to benign prostatic hypertrophy. This urodynamic study provides evidence of very poor compliance and no urinary flow despite a fully relaxed sphincter and contracting bladder. p$_{ves}$, 74; p$_{ura}$, 52; EMG off.*

versible damage occurs to the detrusor as a result of obstructive processes – neurogenic or structural. As an example, not all bladders recover reasonable storage and expulsive function after posterior urethral valve ablation or prostatectomy.

Treatment can also be directed at the bladder; indeed, intermittent catheterization with or without anticholinergic agents, if implemented early in an obstructive process, seems to prevent the development of altered compliance.[8,9,17,18] Alternatively, the bladder can be surgically enlarged and emptied periodically by intermittent catheterization. In females, compliance abnormalities are more commonly encountered as a result of direct tissue injury (for example, from radiation therapy or chemotherapy) than from obstructive conditions; however, occasionally, radical hysterectomy and/or abdominal perineal resection may result in decentralization of the bladder with fixed sphincteric resistance and development of altered compliance.[17]

Patients who have conditions that could be associated with altered compliance should be studied to determine whether that condition exists, before any urethral treatment for stress incontinence is contemplated; this is because altered compliance introduces a detrusor expulsive component that will complicate therapy of incontinence directed at urethral sphincteric deficiency.

Summary

In situations where the expulsive force is the detrusor, the outlet directly controls detrusor pressure and there is a proportional linear relationship between these two.

ABDOMINAL PRESSURE AS AN EXPULSIVE FORCE

In certain situations, abdominal pressure (p_{abd}) is also an expulsive force. Normally, leakage does not result from abdominal pressure excursions and, if leakage is produced by abdominal pressure, some problem with urethral function generally exists. Although the measurement of intraluminal pressures within the urethra has some bearing on the detrusor pressure to cause leakage, that kind of relationship does not exist when abdominal pressure is the expulsive force.[19] Consider for example, a 'neourethra' constructed from the appendix or a short segment of tubularized ileum. This

neourethra is anastomosed to the bladder end-to-side with no effort to tunnel or construct a valvular mechanism, and the distal end is simply sutured to the skin of the lower abdomen.[20] These neourethra units work very well and leakage occurs only when detrusor pressure rises and forces urine into the appendix. Incontinence associated with abdominal pressure excursions does not occur (Fig. 21.6).

This neourethra has no neural mechanism to protect it, and it has no 'external sphincter' to contract to prevent leakage with activity (for example, coughing, straining or lifting). Indeed, intraluminal pressures at rest within the neourethra are very low, only slightly higher than those measured simultaneously in the urinary reservoir. These findings have considerable significance with respect to our concept of urethral sphincter function *vis-à-vis* abdominal pressure as an expulsive force.

Urine is normally held securely at the bladder neck during stressful manoeuvres and does not enter the proximal urethra, bearing down (as it were) on the high-pressure zone of the 'distal sphincter' mechanism (Fig. 21.7).[21] These findings suggest that urethral resistance to abdominal pressure is largely passive and mechanical and occurs in the proximal urethral segment, resulting in incontinence at the bladder neck.

When urethral leakage is driven by abdominal pressure, some problem with urethral function must exist,

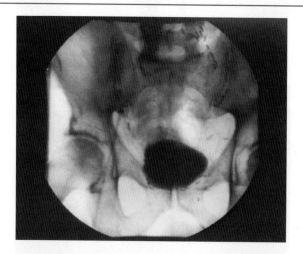

Figure 21.6. *An example of an unmodified appendix used as a neourethra or appendicovesicostomy. Note the urodynamic catheter exiting from the right lower quadrant abdominal stoma. At a moderate volume (200 ml) there is no leakage with straining or effort; leakage occurs only when detrusor pressure rises with a detrusor contraction.*

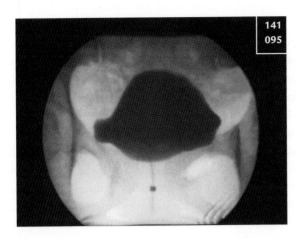

Figure 21.7. *Cystogram showing a normally closed bladder neck at the time of Valsava straining.*

teric deficiency (ISD).[22–24] In the original descriptions, open non-functional internal sphincter mechanisms were noted, often in the presence of demonstrable reflex and volitional 'external sphincter' contractility. Absence of, or weakness of, internal sphincter coaptation leads to leakage driven by relatively low abdominal pressures. In other words, a urethra open at rest in the face of normal detrusor pressure is a 'bad' urethra that will leak easily at modest abdominal pressures and with modest effort or exercise (Fig. 21.9). This occurs in patients incontinent after prostatectomy, in myelodysplastic patients, as a result of certain kinds of spinal cord injury or spinal cord infarction, and in women with type III stress incontinence.[18,25,26]

provided that detrusor pressure is 'normal'. A bladder that exhibits poor compliance will, at certain volumes, force urine into the proximal urethra; at that point, detrusor pressure and proximal urethra pressures become isobaric. When that situation occurs, very small changes in abdominal pressure are associated with considerable urethral leakage. The expulsive force here is, however, not abdominal pressure but primarily detrusor pressure (Fig. 21.8).

Historical findings

Videourodynamic studies led to the description of type III stress urinary incontinence (SUI) or intrinsic sphinc-

URETHRAL PRESSURE PROFILES AND URETHRAL FUNCTION

Some closing pressure is required for normal urethral resistance to abdominal pressure. Using fluoroscopy and recorded urethral pressures with precise localization of the pressure-sensing aperture, it is possible to infer poor urethral function from certain findings. Obviously, if there is no pressure at all the urethra will not function as an organ of continence. If urethral closing pressure in the proximal 1.5 cm of the female urethra is zero, type III SUI (ISD) is present and leakage can be expected to occur at low abdominal pressures (Fig. 21.10).[27] However a 'normal' high-pressure zone pressure is not indicative of a competent

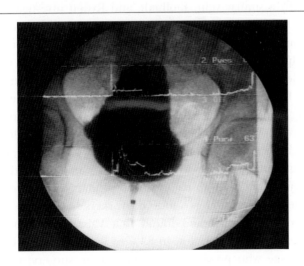

Figure 21.8. *Rising detrusor pressure in a poorly compliant bladder forces the bladder neck open and fills the proximal urethra. p_{ura}, 63; EMG off.*

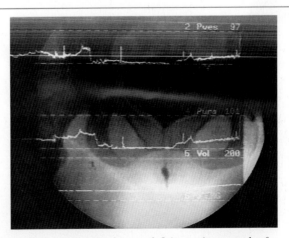

Figure 21.9. *Intrinsic sphincter deficiency. An example of a fixed open sphincter mechanism in a 68-year-old woman who had undergone anterior colporraphy with retropubic suspension. She leaked in any position with minimal effort. p_{ves}, 97; p_{ura}, 101; EMG off.*

sphincter, nor is a low-pressure urethra necessarily associated with incontinence.

Maximum urethral closing pressure (MUCP) values decline with age and may be statistically lower in subjects with stress incontinence than in those without; however, a single UPP value, high or low, has no particular significance for an individual patient. For example, Salinas and co-workers conducted a videourodynamic study of 50 females undergoing urethropexy for SUI:[28] they found that urethral pressures did not correlate with the clinical findings or the urodynamic demonstration of urinary incontinence after urethropexy. Similarly, Swift and Ostergard attempted to determine the sensitivity and specificity of urodynamic testing methods in the diagnosis of genuine stress incontinence (GSI) in 108 patients:[29] of this group, 60% were found to have GSI by one measure or another. Those authors concluded that observation of urine loss with cough during multichannel urodynam-

ics was the best examination for diagnosing stress incontinence. They found pressure transmission ratios and pressure equalization ratios to be relatively insensitive, but stress leak-point pressure was specific and relatively sensitive.

In another study, Khullar and co-workers treated 34 elderly women with collagen injections and found 77% at 2 years to be symptomatically cured.[30] Despite this, the UPP values were unchanged in these patients when compared with the preoperative studies in the same patients. A similar study was conducted by Bennett and co-workers in Atlanta, on 12 patients with ISD caused by spinal cord injury or myelodysplasia.[31] They found that the injection of glutaraldehyde cross-linked collagen raised the abdominal leak-point pressure, on average, by 57 cmH$_2$O and improved continence function. Thus, failure to demonstrate a change in UPP values despite subjective and objective cure, and the coincident finding of an elevated abdominal leak-point pressure, suggests that measurement of intra-urethral closing pressures is not synonymous with definition of urethral resistance to abdominal pressure as an expulsive force. These findings were discussed by Lose in a paper in 1997: he found that urethral pressure measurement and UPP parameters were of limited value in the assessment of urethral sphincter function, as the parameters 'do not discriminate stress incontinence from other disorders,' nor provide a measure of severity of the condition, nor do they return to normal after successful incontinence surgery.[32]

In a similar vein, Kjolhede and Ryden investigated in 1994 the clinical and urodynamic characteristics of women with recurrent incontinence after a Burch colposuspension.[33] This group (which is known on videourodynamic study to have a very high incidence of ISD) was investigated by such methods as pad testing, cough stress testing, cystometry and urethral pressure profilometry. They were found to have a very low incidence of a 'low-pressure urethra' by UPP testing; in fact, a low-pressure urethra was less common in this group than it was in patients with primary stress incontinence. Cummings and co-workers[34] studied 57 women with SUI and found that Valsalva leak-point pressures were very low in 83% of women with severe leakage who previously had undergone surgery; they concluded that women with very severe leakage and previous bladder-neck surgery are very likely to have urethral dysfunction as demonstrated by Valsalva leak-

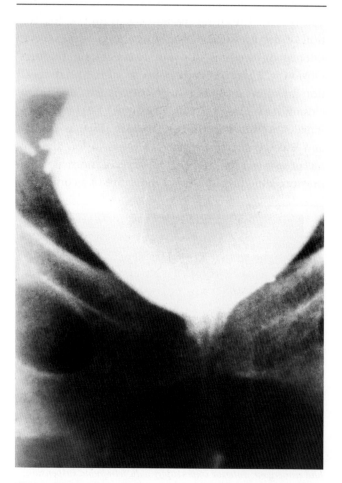

Figure 21.10. *Cystourethrogram showing the open bladder neck at rest.*

point pressure testing.[33] These data are in keeping with results of earlier videourodynamic studies.[34] In a similar study, Swift and Ostergard compared stress leak-point pressures and MUCP in 59 patients with GSI.[35] They found a poor clinical relationship between stress leak-point pressure and MUCP. Although the authors accepted the fact that a low urethral closing pressure was diagnostic of ISD, their findings actually support the conclusion that one cannot make that diagnosis with UPP values alone.[29]

Leak-point pressures

Within certain well-defined limits, measurement of the abdominal pressure required to cause leakage provides qualitative and quantitative information on the relative strength or weakness of the urethral sphincter mechanism during the storage mode of bladder activity. Such measurements must be taken in the upright position and in adults at volumes between 200 and 300 ml. Detrusor compliance must be normal. Genital prolapse of any kind renders leak-point pressure testing somewhat inaccurate; this is proportional to the degree of prolapse (Fig. 21.11). Many persons with genital prolapse do not have the symptom 'stress incontinence', but they do have videourodynamic evidence of that condition, such evidence including urethral mobility and/or actual leakage when the prolapse is reduced. In these instances, symptomatic stress incontinence is masked by the condition of prolapse, but may be unmasked when the prolapse is repaired.[36–38]

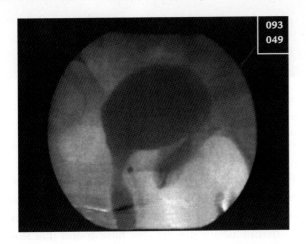

Figure 21.11. *Oblique view of a cystogram showing severe cystocele prolapse.*

Leak-point pressures are not, in themselves, very useful without considerable ancillary information, which includes measurement of bladder compliance and assessment (in the upright position) of the presence or absence of urethral mobility and/or prolapse of any genital structure – vaginal vault, enterocele, cystocele, rectocele or uterus. For a number of technical reasons, and because of the quality of information, testing an upright subject, with the bladder filled with contrast under fluoroscopy, is the most exacting and useful method of evaluation of women with 'stress incontinence symptoms'.[25,39,40]

'A normal urethra'

The finding of a normal urethra is valuable; by contrast, urodynamic assessment of altered detrusor control mechanisms leading to motor urge incontinence is much less accurate. Although urodynamic studies are advocated to rule out detrusor instability (DI), they cannot actually do that. If in the upright position at a bladder volume of 250 ml with good-to-excellent effort generating an abdominal pressure of 150 cmH$_2$O or more, no leakage occurs; presumptive evidence of 'no stress incontinence or normal urethral function' exists (Fig. 21.7). The finding of a 'normal urethra' means that the cause of leakage is elsewhere and usually this means the detrusor, or its control mechanism. The converse, a 'normal' cystometrogram (CMG), does not provide any evidence that the aetiology of the incontinence is urethral.

In males, after radical prostatectomy, a 10F catheter may occlude a rigid but open small-bore urethral anastomosis and lead to inadequate assessment of urethral function. That is, the catheter may obstruct the urethra, and leak-point pressure testing may not demonstrate incontinence when, in fact, that condition does exist. If the findings do not 'fit' the clinical situation the catheter can be removed and the study repeated. Under video observation, patients strain repetitively to the same abdominal pressure.

Types of stress incontinence by leak-point pressure testing

Urethral dysfunction suitable for injectable agents
Urinary leakage that occurs with very little effort at low abdominal pressures when there is little or no urethral

mobility will often respond to collagen injection.[41,42] Stress incontinence in elderly women that occurs in association with slight motion at higher pressures, 80–110 cmH$_2$O, is also suitable for collagen treatment (Fig. 21.7).

Urethral leakage associated with mobility

Urethral leakage associated with urethral mobility is potentially correctable by procedures that stabilize the urethra: these include retropubic suspensions, needle-type suspensions, and slings (Fig. 21.12). Slings may be more robust over time than the other procedures, but the outcome data are not derived from randomized double-blind studies and, generally, the precise condition treated in each patient reported is not clearly defined. Conclusions drawn from long-term outcome data segregated by operative procedure are suspect.[43,44]

A high failure rate over time has been reported for various non-sling operations. This information is not actually very useful unless it is known precisely (a) what condition was treated in an individual patient and (b) with what condition failure was noted; in most such reports, that is not the case. Videourodynamic data conclusively demonstrate that stress incontinence is not one condition and only complete pre- and postoperative information will enable treatment to be modified to improve outcome. It is clear that leakage occurring with little or no effort at very low abdominal pressures is not reliably repaired by suspension procedures other than slings. Five-year outcomes for slings in these patients are better than those for standard procedures in patients with primary stress incontinence.[43,44]

Prolapse and the videourodynamic assessment of urethral function

Major genital prolapse – a grade III–IV cystocele, for instance – has a protective effect on the urethra. As has been noted by many workers, repair of genital prolapse may be followed by unmasking of severe stress incontinence if the urethra is not suspended or treated with a sling or some other form of repair at the time of the surgery for the prolapse.[36,37]

Preoperatively, urethral mobility associated with or without stress incontinence symptoms on a video study in subjects with significant prolapse is presumptive

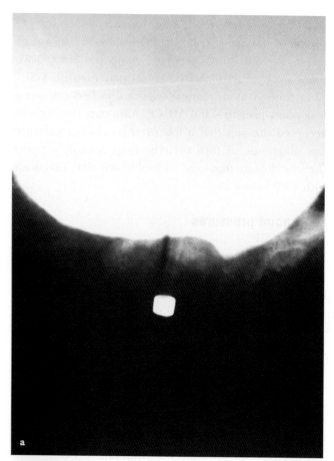

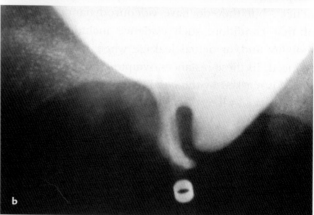

Figure 21.12. *(a) 'Rest' and (b) 'strain' sequence showing hypermobile urethra characteristic of type II stress urinary incontinence.*

evidence of the stress incontinence condition even if there are no symptoms.[19] Ability to demonstrate urethral leakage despite prolapse indicates that severe urethral dysfunction is present. We have found that slings stabilize the anterior vaginal wall securely in cases of prolapse and provide superior long-term results when compared with other suspension procedures (e.g. needle suspensions), with respect to both stress incontinence and recurrent prolapse or enterocele development. Leak-point pressure testing in this circumstance provides some information but is not useful in selecting a type of operation, as the values do not reflect the relative strength of the urethra.

Validation of leak-point pressure testing

McGuire and co-workers in 1993 studied 125 women with stress incontinence using videourodynamics and compared MUCP with leak-point pressures.[19] Patients with type III ISD on video evaluation had low Valsalva leak-point pressures but such patients were not reliably identified by UPP testing. Wan and co-workers in 1993 studied myelodysplastic children and demonstrated that detrusor leak-point pressures and abdominal leak-point pressures were different, despite the fixed nature of the urethra in such individuals.[45] Bump and co-workers, in a study of 159 women with pure GSI, found that a Valsalva leak-point pressure of 52 cmH$_2$O or less, and certain urethral axis abnormalities, were associated with ISD.[46] They also found that low MUCP was related to ISD. Haab and co-workers evaluated 50 patients with stress incontinence with leak-point pressure testing and they noted that bladder volume had a significant effect on leak-point pressures:[47] with increasing volume, a diminution of leak-point pressure values was noted. They concluded that a vesical leak-point pressure measured at 200 ml constituted a reference value in view of its sensitivity and specificity. Carr and co-workers used low leak-point pressure values to select elderly patients for sling surgery: they found slings to be effective in these patients.[48] This method of identification of patients for sling surgery has been reported by several groups.[49–51] In addition, Gormley and co-workers[52] evaluated patients with leak-point pressure testing before and after pubovaginal sling procedures. Slings raised the abdominal pressure to induce leakage to infinity, but did not change the detrusor leak-point pressure.

LEAK-POINT PRESSURES AND OTHER URODYNAMIC TESTS

Leak-point pressures are useful as part of a total evaluation of patients with incontinence. As noted above, lack of leakage at 'high' abdominal pressures in the absence of prolapse suggests that the urethra is not the problem. If leakage does occur during an excursion of abdominal pressure, the pressure at which that takes place has some bearing on the degree of urethral dysfunction and how that problem might be corrected medically or surgically.

The traditional evaluation of women with SUI is by two-channel subtraction cystometry.[53] That method is based on the assumption that a lack of unstable detrusor activity suggests the diagnosis of GSI or leakage driven by abdominal pressure without a detrusor component. For a number of technical reasons the two-channel subtraction CMG will not actually do what it is intended to do: these reasons include poor sensitivity and specificity of the test (CMG) for the condition DI.[54–56] In addition, there are now clear data to indicate that DI in many patients with overt SUI is actually caused by the latter condition; thus, an attempt to rule out bladder instability is not likely to be very helpful in such patients.[57] In addition, although all workers agree that persistent bladder instability after surgery for SUI is a clinical problem of considerable significance, it is not clear that preoperative urodynamic testing helps to avoid or prevent this problem postoperatively: for instance, lack of overt bladder instability does not mean freedom from urge incontinence or bladder instability postoperatively; nor does a positive CMG in the preoperative setting indicate that failure will occur as a result of persistent DI. Stanton, in a review of outcome 10–20 years after retropubic suspension,[58] for instance, found that preoperative bladder instability was not a prognostic factor with respect to failure. Although most publications relating to sling procedures note a 7–15% incidence of persistent bladder instability or symptomatic urge incontinence in the immediate postoperative period, the occurrence of that problem is not predicted by preoperative cystometry.[38,57]

It seems reasonable, then, to establish in each patient that stress incontinence is present, not present, or potentially present in women with prolapse; this can be achieved by upright leak-point pressure testing supplemented, if necessary, by video observation. This kind of testing is best done after a careful pelvic examination and will provide prospective data, from which better treatment plans can be formulated, in the awareness of the outcome of a specific surgical procedure with reference to the condition actually treated.

REFERENCES

1. McGuire EJ, Woodside JR, Borden TA *et al.* Prognostic value of urodynamic testing in myelodysplastic patients. *J Urol* 1981; 126: 205

2. McGuire EJ, Woodside JR, Borden TA *et al.* Upper tract deterioration in patients with myelodysplasia and detrusor hypertonia: a follow-up study. *J Urol* 1983; 129: 823

3. McGuire EJ, Wang SC, Usitalo A *et al.* Modified pubovaginal sling in girls with myelodysplasia. *J Urol* 1986; 135: 94

4. McGuire EJ. Myelodysplasia: pathophysiology, neuroanatomy, and correlations with urologic manifestations. *J Pediatr Neurosci* 1985; 1: 4

5. Griffiths DJ. Urodynamic assessment of bladder function. *Br J Urol* 1977; 49: 29

6. Schäfer W. Eine Physiologische Methode zur Beschreiburg der Druk-Flow-Beziehung Wahrend der Miktion. *Biomed Tech* (*Berlin*) 1971; 21: 11

7. Schäfer W. Urethral resistance? Urodynamic concepts of physiological and pathological bladder outlet function during voiding. *Neurourol Urodyn* 1986; 4: 161

8. Wang SC, McGuire EJ, Bloom DA. A bladder pressure management system for myelodysplasia: clinical outcome. *J Urol* 1989; 142: 1504

9. Ghoniem GM, Roach MD, Lewis VH *et al.* The value of leak-point pressure and bladder compliance in the urodynamic evaluation of meningomyelocele patients. *J Urol* 1990; 144: 1440

10. O'Reilly PH, Brooman PJC, Farah NB *et al.* High pressure chronic retention: incidence, aetiology, and sinister implications. *Br J Urol* 1986; 58: 644

11. McGuire EJ. Interaction of bladder filling behavior and ureteral function. *World J Urol* 1990; 8: 194

12. Steers WD. Neuroplasticity secondary to infravesical obstruction. *Neurourol Urodyn* 1990; 9: 559

13. Steers WD, Tuttle J, Creedon D. Hyperplastic and activity-related changes in nerve growth factor in the urinary bladder. *J Urol* 1990; 143: 367A

14. Uvelius B, Arner A, Malmgren A. Contractile and cytoskeleton proteins in detrusor muscle from obstructed rat and human bladder. *Neurourol Urodyn* 1989; 8: 396

15. Chancellor M, Rivas DA. Current management of detrusor-sphincter dyssynergia. *Urology* 1995; 8: 291

16. Bloom DA, Knechtel JM, McGuire EJ. Urethral dilation improves bladder compliance in children with meningomyelocele and high leak-point pressures. *J Urol* 1990; 144: 430

17. Chamberlain DH, Hopkins MP, Roberts JA *et al.* Effects of early removal of indwelling urinary catheter after radical hysterectomy. *Gynecol Oncol* 1991; 43: 98

18. McGuire EJ, Noll F, Maynard FA. Pressure management system for the neurogenic bladder after spinal cord injury. *Neurourol Urodyn* 1991; 10: 223

19. McGuire EJ, Fitzpatrick CC, Wan J *et al.* Clinical assessment of urethral sphincter function. *J Urol* 1993; 150: 1452

20. English SF, Pisters LL, McGuire EJ. Use of appendix as a continent catheterizable stoma. *J Urol* 1998; 159: 747

21. McGuire EJ. Urethral sphincter mechanisms: another evaluation of incontinence. In: Pollack HM, McClennan BL (eds) *Clinical Urography*. Philadelphia: Saunders, 1998

22. McGuire EJ. Combined radiographic and manometric assessment of urethral sphincter function. *J Urol* 1977; 118: 632

23. McGuire EJ, Woodside JR. Diagnostic advantages of fluoroscopic monitoring during urodynamic evaluation. *J Urol* 1981; 125: 830

24. Blaivas JG. A modest proposal for the diagnosis and treatment of urinary incontinence in women. *J Urol* 1987; 138: 597

25. Gudziak MR, McGuire EJ, Gormley EA. Urodynamic assessment of urethral sphincter function in postprostatectomy incontinence. *J Urol* 1996; 156: 1131

26. McGuire EJ. Urodynamic evaluation of stress incontinence. *Urol Clin North Am* 1995; 22: 657

27. McGuire EJ. Urodynamic findings after failure of stress incontinence operations. In: Zinner N, Sterling A (eds) *Female Incontinence*. New York: A.R. Liss, 1981; 385–390

28. Salinas CJ, Virseda CM, Hermeda GI, Esteban F *et al.* The need for an adequate urodynamic study in the assessment of stress incontinence following urethropexy. *Arch Esp Urol* 1990; 49: 970

29. Swift SE, Ostergard DR. Evaluation of current urodynamic testing methods in the diagnosis of genuine stress incontinence. *Obstet Gynecol* 1995; 86: 85

30. Khullar V, Cardozo CD, Abbott D. GAX collagen in the treatment of urinary incontinence in elderly women. *Br J Obstet Gynaecol* 1997; 104: 96

31. Bennett JK, Green BG, Foote JE *et al.* Collagen injections for intrinsic sphincter deficiency in the neuropathic urethra. *Paraplegia* 1995; 33: 697

32. Lose C. Urethral pressure measurement. *Acta Obstet Gynecol Scand Suppl* 1997; 166: 39

33. Kjolhede P, Ryden G. Prognostic factors and long term results of the Burch operation: a retrospective study. *Acta Obstet Gynecol Scand* 1994; 73: 642

34. Cummings M, Boullier JA, Parra RO *et al*. Leak-point pressures in women with urinary stress incontinence: correlations with patient history. *J Urol* 1997; 157: 818

35. Swift SE, Ostergard DR. A comparison of stress leak-point pressure and maximal urethral closure pressure in patients with genuine stress incontinence. *Obstet Gynecol* 1995; 85: 704

36. McGuire EJ, Gardy M, Elkins T *et al*. The treatment of incontinence with pelvic prolapse. *Urol Clin North Am* 1991; 18: 349

37. Gardy M, Kozminski M, DeLancey JOL *et al*. Stress incontinence and cystoceles. *J Urol* 1991; 145: 1211

38. Cross CA, Cespedes RD, McGuire EJ. Treatment results using pubovaginal slings in patients with large cystoceles and stress incontinence. *J Urol* 1997; 158: 431

39. Song JT, Rozanski T, Belville W. Stress leak-point pressure: a simple and reproducible method utilizing a fiberoptic microtransducer. *Urology* 1995; 46: 81

40. Nitti VW, Coombs AJ. Correlation of Valsalva leak-point pressure with subjective degree of stress incontinence. *J Urol* 1996; 155: 281

41. Homma Y, Kawabe K, Kageyama S *et al*. Injection of glutaraldehyde cross-linked collagen for urinary incontinence: 2-year efficacy by self-assessment. *Int J Urol* 1996; 3: 124

42. Faerber GM. Endoscopic collagen injection therapy in elderly women with type I stress incontinence. *J Urol* 1996; 155: 512

43. Blaivas JG, Jacobs BZ. Pubovaginal sling in the treatment of complicated stress incontinence. *J Urol* 1991; 145: 1214

44. Haab F, Zimmern PE, Leach GE. Female stress urinary incontinence due to intrinsic sphincter deficiency: recognition and management. *J Urol* 1996; 156: 3

45. Wan J, McGuire EJ, Bloom DA, *et al*. Stress leak-point pressure: a diagnostic tool for incontinent children. *J Urol* 1993; 150: 1452

46. Theofractous JP, Cundiff GW, Harris RL *et al*. The effect of vesical volume on Valsalva leak-point pressure in women with genuine stress incontinence. *Obstet Gynaecol* 1996; 87: 711

47. Haab F, Dmochowski R, Zimmern P. The Valsalva leak-point pressure as a function of volume. *Prog Urol* 1997; 7: 422

48. Carr LK, Walsh PJ, Abraham VE *et al*. Favorable outcome of pubovaginal slings for geriatric women with stress incontinence. *J Urol* 1997; 157: 125

49. Curtis MR, Gormley EA, Latini JM *et al*. Prospective development of a cost-effective program for the pubovaginal sling. *Urology* 1997; 49: 41

50. Govier FB, Gibbons RD, Correa RJ *et al*. Pubovaginal slings using fascia lata for the treatment of intrinsic sphincter deficiency. *J Urol* 1997; 157: 117

51. Mason RC, Roach M. Modified pubovaginal sling for treatment of intrinsic sphincter deficiency. *J Urol* 1996; 156: 1620

52. Gormley EA, Bloom DA, McGuire EJ *et al*. Pubovaginal slings for the management of urinary incontinence in female adolescents. *J Urol* 1994; 152: 822

53. Peatie AB, Stanton SL. The Stamey operation in the older woman. *Br J Obstet Gynaecol* 1989; 96: 983

54. Van Waalwijk Van Doorn ES, Remmus A, Janknegt RA. Extramural ambulatory urodynamic monitoring during natural filling and normal daily activities: evaluation of 100 patients. *J Urol* 1991; 146: 124

55. Porru D, Usai E. Standard and extramural ambulatory urodynamic investigation for the diagnosis of detrusor instability-correlated incontinence and micturition disorders. *Neurourol Urodyn* 1994; 13: 237

56. Bhatia NN, Bradley WE, Haldeman S. Urodynamics continuous monitoring. *J Urol* 1982; 128: 963

57. Langer R, Ron-El R, Bukovsky I *et al*. Colposuspension in patients with stress urinary incontinence and detrusor instability. *Eur Urol* 1988; 14: 437

58. Alcalay M, Monga AK, Stanton SL. Burch colposuspension: a ten to twenty year follow up. *Br J Obstet Gynaecol* 1995; 102: 740–746

22

Electromyography

D. B. Vodušek, C. J. Fowler

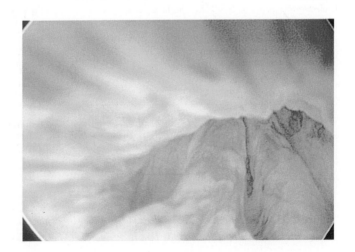

INTRODUCTION

Modern electromyography (EMG) began in 1929 with the introduction of the concentric needle electrode (CNE),[1] the design of which has remained largely unchanged (Fig. 22.1). Few clinical EMG studies of the pelvic floor were conducted until the 1970s,[3,4] when several important papers were published.[5–8] Subsequently, EMG has been used increasingly in urogynaecology, neurourology and proctology research and often forms part of a routine diagnostic investigation.

EMG may be performed for two quite distinct although complementary purposes: (1) the 'behaviour' patterns of activity of a particular muscle can be identified; (2) EMG can also be used to demonstrate whether a muscle is normal, myopathic or denervated/reinnervated. The former is called 'kinesiological EMG' and the latter 'motor unit' EMG, but more usually both types of examination are referred to simply as EMG.

THE MOTOR UNIT

The bioelectrical activity generated by muscle fibres is recorded extracellularly in EMG. Action potentials are generated by depolarization of single muscle fibres, but the innervation of muscle is such that a single muscle fibre does not contract on its own but, rather, in concert with other muscle fibres that are part of the same motor unit (i.e. innervated by the same motor neuron).

Motor neurons innervating striated muscle lie in the anterior horn of the spinal cord. To allow rapid conduction of impulses they have relatively large cell bodies with large-diameter axonal processes, which are myelinated. The neurons that innervate the sphincters, however, are relatively smaller than those innervating skeletal limb and trunk muscles. The motor axon tapers within the muscle and then branches to innervate muscle fibres scattered throughout the muscle (Fig. 22.2). It is unlikely that fibres that are part of the same motor unit will be adjacent to one another. This dispersion of muscle fibres is said to be non-random, although the stage of development at which it occurs and the factors determining the arrangement are not known.

The number of muscle fibres innervated by an axon is known as the 'innervation ratio'. This parameter cannot be easily estimated, nor can the number of motor units per muscle. The muscle fibres making up a motor unit determine the contraction properties of the unit. Muscle fibres can be classified according to their twitch tension, speed of contraction and histochemical staining properties. The majority of muscle fibres in the pelvic floor and sphincters are type 1, although regional variation can occur.[9,10] Motor units that fire for prolonged periods of time at lower firing frequencies (i.e. 'tonically'; see below), are made up of fatigue-resistant type 1 fibres. Type 2 fibres make up motor units that fire briefly and in rapid bursts (i.e. 'phasically'). No clinical electrophysiological method is available, unfortunately, to estimate the proportion of motor units of different muscle fibre types.

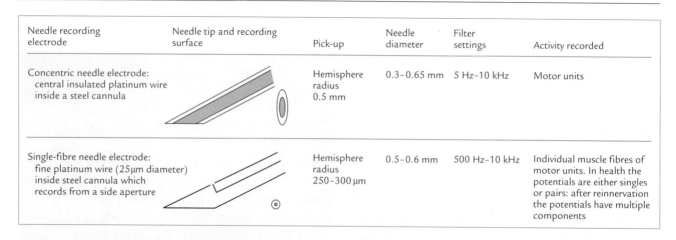

Needle recording electrode	Needle tip and recording surface	Pick-up	Needle diameter	Filter settings	Activity recorded
Concentric needle electrode: central insulated platinum wire inside a steel cannula		Hemisphere radius 0.5 mm	0.3–0.65 mm	5 Hz–10 kHz	Motor units
Single-fibre needle electrode: fine platinum wire (25 μm diameter) inside steel cannula which records from a side aperture		Hemisphere radius 250–300 μm	0.5–0.6 mm	500 Hz–10 kHz	Individual muscle fibres of motor units. In health the potentials are either singles or pairs: after reinnervation the potentials have multiple components

Figure 22.1. *The concentric needle electrode and the single-fibre needle electrode, their physical characteristics, the filter settings required for use and the nature of the activity that each records. (Modified from ref. 2.)*

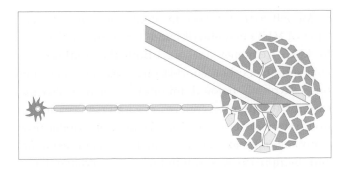

Figure 22.2. *Schematic diagram of a motor unit, showing the motor neuron which is located in the anterior horn of the spinal cord (Onuf's nucleus in the case of the sphincters) and the motor axon, which travels in the peripheral nerve to the muscle. Here it divides, innervating a number of muscle fibres, most of which are not adjacent.*

KINESIOLOGICAL EMG

Method

The qualitative and quantitative description of a muscle's activity over time can be obtained through prolonged recording of its bioelectrical activity. Such techniques have an application in rehabilitation and sports medicine to study movement. Meaningful kinesiological EMG requires an innervated muscle. If the lower motor neuron integrity of a particular muscle is questioned, 'motor unit' EMG analysis (see page 243) has to be performed first.

The aims of the investigation will determine the choice of muscle for EMG examination. Routine EMG as part of urodynamic studies usually employs a single channel for recording from the urethral or anal sphincter muscle. It is assumed that, as the sphincters are small circular muscles, the two sides react in a similar fashion, although this may not always be the case, as was shown for the levator ani.[11]

If the pattern of activity of an individual muscle is required, the technique should ideally provide a selective recording, uncontaminated by neighbouring muscles, but recording activity within the muscle under study. Unfortunately, both objectives are difficult to achieve simultaneously and the purpose of the investigation will suggest an acceptable compromise. Overall detection from the bulk of a muscle can be achieved only with non-selective electrodes; selective recordings

from small muscles can be made only with intramuscular electrodes with small detection surfaces. Contamination is possible with non-selective recordings, while selective recordings may fail to detect activity in all parts of the source muscle. Meaningful recordings from deep muscles can be accomplished only by invasive techniques.

Truly selective recording from sphincter muscles can probably be obtained only by intramuscular electrodes, usually the CNE. This electrode is widely available, sturdy, easy to introduce and adjustable in position, and has a standardized active surface. However, pain on movement of the source muscle can occur and the electrode can easily be dislodged. Instead, two thin isolated/bare-tip wires (with a hook at the end) can be introduced into the muscle with a cannula; the latter is then withdrawn, and the wires stay in place. The advantages of this type of recording are good positional stability and painlessness once the wires are inserted, although their position cannot be adjusted to any great extent.

To reduce the invasiveness of EMG recording, various surface-type electrodes have been devised. Small skin-surface electrodes can be applied to the perineal skin; for intravaginal placement a disposable electrode set on a vinyl foam pad is available;[12] other special intravaginal recording devices have been described.[13] Anal plugs can be used for recording from the anal sphincter, and catheter-mounted ring electrodes to record from the urethral sphincter.[14] Surface electrodes are apt to produce recordings with more artefacts and these may be less easily identified. Critical on-line assessment of the 'quality' of the EMG signal is mandatory in kinesiological EMG, and this requires either auditory or oscilloscope monitoring of the raw signal. Integration of high-quality EMG signals may help in quantification of results, as can automatic analysis of the interference pattern.[15]

Findings in normal and abnormal conditions

At rest, the normal kinesiological sphincter EMG shows some continuous activity (this may be increased voluntarily or reflexly) (Fig. 22.3). This activity can be recorded for up to 2 hours[7] and even after a subject has fallen asleep during the examination.[6,16] Such physiological spontaneous activity may be called 'tonic' and consists of prolonged firing of tonic motor units,

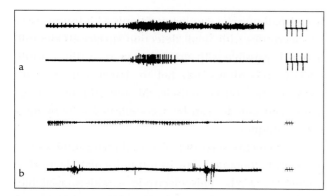

Figure 22.3. *Kinesiological EMG recordings from the pubococcygeal muscles (recording with intramuscular wires: right, upper traces; left, lower traces). (a) Recordings from a 33-year-old nulliparous woman (50 μV/division). Continuous firing of motor unit potentials is seen on the right with a gradual recruitment on voluntary contraction. On the left, no ongoing activity is present. Symmetrical recruitment on voluntary contraction is present. (b) Recordings from a 52-year-old woman with stress urinary incontinence (20 μV/division). Some ongoing muscle activity can be seen in both pubococcygeal muscles. On voluntary contraction, recruitment can be seen only on the left. On the right, there is actually a decrease in firing of motor units on voluntary contraction.*

not rapidly interchanging activation and inactivation of different motor units.[16]

The uptake area of the electrode will determine the quantity of activity recorded (Fig. 22.1). Using a CNE, activity from one to five motor units is usually recorded per detection site at rest. 'Tonic' activity is encountered in a large number of detection sites of the levator ani muscle;[17] it typically consists of low-amplitude motor unit potentials (MUPs), which fire rather regularly at low frequencies. A study of 39 such motor units from the anal sphincter in 17 subjects (inclusion criterion was rhythmic spontaneous firing for 2 minutes before onset of measurement) showed that the range of discharge rates was 2.5–9.4 Hz (mean ± SD 5.3 ± 1.8 Hz).[18] Any reflex or voluntary activation procedure is mirrored first by an increase in the firing frequency of the motor units; then, with any stronger activation or increase in abdominal pressure, new, so-called 'phasic' motor units are recruited (Fig. 22.3). These are usually of higher amplitude and their discharge rates are higher and irregular. Also encountered are a small percentage of motor units with an 'intermediate' activation pattern.[18]

As well as differences in amplitude, the different types of MUPs may also differ in duration, as evidenced by EMG frequency analysis.[19] Both the urethral and anal sphincters show short-lasting voluntary activation times (typically below 1 minute),[20] which is also the case for the pubococcygeus.[17] All EMG activity in the urethral sphincter ceases on voiding prior to a detrusor contraction. Lesions between the lower sacral segments and the upper pons result in loss of coordinated detrusor sphincter activity; detrusor contractions are then accompanied by an increase in sphincter EMG activity.[21] This pattern of activity is termed detrusor sphincter dyssynergia. On the basis of the temporal relationship between urethral sphincter and detrusor contractions, three types of dyssynergia have been described.[22] Differentiation is needed between this neurogenic uncoordinated sphincter behaviour and 'voluntary' contractions, which may occur in the so-called 'non-neuropathic voiding disorders'. The latter may be a learned abnormality of behaviour,[23] and may be encountered in women with dysfunctional voiding.[24]

Urethral sphincter contraction (or, at least, failure of relaxation) during involuntary detrusor contractions has also been reported in patients with Parkinson's disease.[25] The normal physiological behaviour of the striated anal sphincter is characterized by its relaxation on defecation,[26] and a paradoxical sphincter activation during defecation has been described in Parkinson's disease, so-called 'anismus'.[27]

The pubococcygeus in the healthy female reveals similar patterns of activity to those found in the urethral and anal sphincters at most detection sites (i.e. continuous activity at rest, some increase in activity during bladder filling and a reflex increase in activity during any activation manoeuvre such as talking, deep breathing or coughing). Relaxation occurs during voiding and, in health, the muscles on both sides act in concert.[17] In women with stress incontinence, the physiological patterns of activation as well as the coordination between the two sides may be lost[11] (Fig. 22.3).

Little is known about the normal activity patterns of different pelvic floor muscles (i.e. urethral sphincter, urethrovaginal sphincter, anal sphincter muscle, different parts of the levator ani), but it is generally assumed that they act in a coordinated fashion as one, although differences have been demonstrated even between the intra-urethral and periurethral sphincter in normal females.[28] Disease states often result in loss of the coordinated behaviour – as has been shown, for instance, for the levator ani and the urethral and anal sphincters.[5,29] Using the kinesiological EMG recording as a biofeedback signal has allowed modification of disturbances in pelvic floor muscle activity.[30]

Diagnostic usefulness of kinesiological EMG

Indirect proof of the integrity of respective neural pathways is given by demonstration of voluntary and reflex activation of pelvic floor muscles. Kinesiological EMG recordings of sphincter muscles, either urethral or anal, can be obtained to determine sphincter behaviour during bladder filling and voiding. Generally, simultaneous studies of detrusor and sphincter activity are obtained only in patients with suspected detrusor sphincter dyssynergia. External anal sphincter EMG can be used in the assessment of anorectal dysfunction.[26] The diagnostic contribution of kinesiological EMG is not yet established other than in the polygraphic urodynamic recordings to diagnose detrusor sphincter dyssynergia.

EMG METHODS TO DIFFERENTIATE NORMAL FROM PATHOLOGICAL MUSCLE

Needle EMG may help to differentiate between normal, denervated and reinnervated and possibly myopathic muscle; this type of EMG has also been termed 'motor unit' EMG. The needle electrode must be appropriately placed in the target muscle. The levator ani muscle is reached transcutaneously after location by transrectal or transvaginal palpation. The urethral sphincter is anatomically separate from the pelvic floor musculature[31] and can be approached either perineally with a needle insertion 0.5 cm laterally to the urethral orifice, or it can be reached transvaginally using a Simms' speculum to retract the posterior vaginal wall. The latter approach is less uncomfortable.[32] The position of the needle should be adjusted in a systematic way in order to avoid repeated analysis of the same motor unit.

Normal fiFndings using a concentric needle EMG electrode

The CNE is most commonly used in EMG and consists of a central insulated platinum wire encased within a steel cannula. The tip is ground to give an elliptical area of 580 × 150 mm (Fig. 22.1). This type of electrode has

the recording characteristics necessary to record spike activity from about 20 muscle fibres. The number of motor units recorded therefore depends upon both the local arrangement of muscle fibres within the motor unit and the level of contraction of the muscle.

The following information can be provided using CNE EMG:[4,33] insertion activity, abnormal spontaneous activity, MUPs and interference pattern. Initial placement of the needle in healthy skeletal muscle elicits a short burst of 'insertion activity', which is due to mechanical stimulation of excitable membranes. Insertion activity is recorded at a sensitivity setting of 50 μV per division, which is also the gain used to record spontaneous activity. At rest, tonic MUPs are the only normal activity recorded, but phasic MUPs can be activated reflexly or voluntarily. MUPs should be analysed at a sensitivity setting that allows their full display. The commonly used time scale is 5 or 10 ms per division, with an amplitude gain of 50–500 μV per division (Fig. 22.4). The commonly used amplifier filter settings for

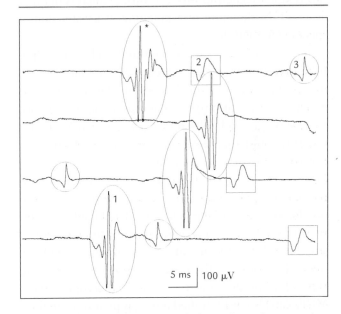

Figure 22.4. *Concentric needle EMG recording of motor unit potentials (MUPs) from the urethral sphincter of a 35-year-old stress-incontinent female, several years after second vaginal delivery. At this detection site three MUPs are continuously firing and can be analysed. It can be seen that the MUP with the asterisk differs from the others of similar overall shape. Further analysis of such a signal is needed to ascertain whether it is a superimposition of two individual MUPs or an instability within a complex of MUPs. The use of trigger and delay facility is advantageous to solve such questions (see Fig. 22.5).*

concentric needle EMG (CN EMG) are 5–10,000 Hz. The activity of those muscle fibres closest to the recording electrode largely determine the amplitude of an MUP. Other fibres within 0.5 mm radius of the recording electrode contribute little to the amplitude, but in a normal motor unit there are unlikely to be more than two or three fibres belonging to the same motor unit.[2] Amplitude is highly sensitive to needle position and very minor adjustments of the electrode will result in major changes: e.g. a change in position by 0.5 mm alters the amplitude 10–100-fold.

The duration of an MUP is the time between the first deflection and return to baseline of the waveform. The number of muscle fibres within the motor unit controls this time, which is little affected by the proximity of the recording electrode to the nearest fibre. Defining the exact point of return to the baseline is difficult in this measurement. The phases of an MUP are defined by the number of times the potential crosses the baseline; a unit that has four phases or more is said to be polyphasic. Related to this is a 'turn', which is defined as a shift in direction of a potential of greater than a specified amplitude.

Individual MUPs can be captured and their amplitude and duration measured using the standard recording facilities available on all modern EMG machines. It is necessary to capture the same potential repeatedly, using a trigger and delay line, to ensure that MUPs are identified and that the late components of complex potentials are not due to superimposition of several MUPs (Fig. 22.5). When an incoming signal achieves a particular pre-set value, the trigger device starts the oscilloscope sweep. The delay line has the effect of displaying the triggering signal, not from the moment of triggering but after an interval of some 1–5 milliseconds; this results in the triggering potential appearing repeatedly in the centre of the oscilloscope screen. MUPs can also be identified if they appear repeatedly in a prolonged recording of EMG activity. Both of these approaches favour identification of relatively large MUPs and become less reliable on stronger activation of muscle; these failings are absent from certain computer averaging programs for MUPs. Instead of MUP analysis, an automatic quantitative analysis of the interference pattern using the turns/amplitude plot has been suggested,[15] but it has yet to be demonstrated to be of greater value in assessment of reinnervation than individual motor unit analysis.

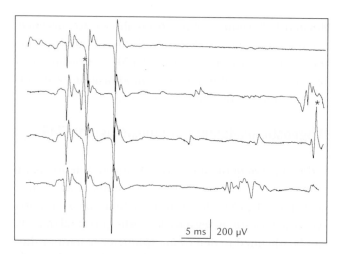

Figure 22.5. *A concentric needle EMG recording from the urethral sphincter of an 18-year-old nulliparous female 4 years after a partial cauda equina injury. A trigger and delay facility is used. A complex motor unit potential (MUP) with prolonged duration is shown. Superimposition of another individual MUP (asterisk) may be falsely interpreted as instability of the potential.*

In general, MUPs are below 1 mV and, in the case of the normal urethral and anal sphincter, below 2 mV. The majority are less than 7 milliseconds in duration and less than 15% are above 10 milliseconds; most are bi- and triphasic, but up to 15% (possibly up to 33%) may be polyphasic. The shape of normal MUPs is stable on repetitive recording.[20,28,34–38]

In addition to 'tonic' firing motor units of the sphincters, new MUPs are recruited voluntarily and reflexly. The numbers of recruited motor units are estimated by such manoeuvres. Normally, MUPs should intermingle to produce a 'full interference' pattern on the oscilloscope (i.e. loss of the baseline when the muscle is contracted powerfully or during a strong cough).

Single-fibre EMG: method and normal findings

The external proportions of the single-fibre EMG (SFEMG) electrode are similar to those of a CNE, being made of a steel cannula 0.5–0.6 mm in diameter with a bevelled tip. However, instead of the recording surface being at the end, the SFEMG has a fine insulated platinum or silver wire embedded in epoxy resin, which is exposed through an aperture on the side, 1–5 mm behind the tip (Fig. 22.1). The diameter of the platinum wire is 25 mm and will pick up activity from within a hemispherical volume 300 mm in diameter. This is much smaller than the uptake area of the CNE, which is 1 mm diameter. Because of the arrangement of muscle fibres in a normal motor unit, an SFEMG needle will record only one to three single muscle fibres from the same motor unit. In addition, the amplifier filters are set in such a way that low-frequency activity is eliminated (500 Hz to 10 kHz). Thus, the contribution of each muscle fibre appears as a biphasic positive–negative action potential.

The SFEMG parameter that reflects motor unit morphology is termed 'fibre density' (FD), and is the mean number of muscle fibres belonging to an individual motor unit per detection site. Recordings from 20 different detection sites are necessary to measure FD (Fig. 22.6), the number of component potentials to each motor unit being recorded and averaged. The normal FD for the anal sphincter is below 2.0.[39–41] Small changes with age have been reported; the FD in women is significantly greater than that in men (1.52 ± 0.5 vs 1.43 ± 0.14).[41]

Instability of MUPs – the 'jitter' – can also be measured using the SFEMG electrode.[2,42]

The SFEMG electrode is able to record even small changes occurring in motor units due to reinnervation, but is less suitable to detect changes due to denervation itself, such as abnormal insertion and spontaneous activity.

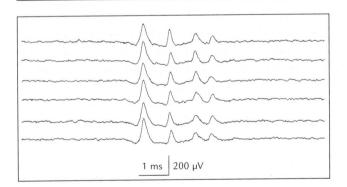

Figure 22.6. *Single-fibre EMG recording from the anal sphincter of a 51-year-old nulliparous female with an extrapyramidal syndrome and recent development of poor bladder emptying accompanied by stress incontinence. The fibre density in the anal sphincter was found to be 3.7 and a diagnosis of multiple system atrophy was suggested. Further development of the clinical picture supported the diagnosis.*

EMG findings due to denervation and reinnervation

All motor unit activity ceases after complete denervation and there may be electrical silence for several days. 'Insertion activity' becomes more prolonged at 10–20 days following a denervating injury, and abnormal spontaneous activity in the form of short biphasic spikes ('fibrillation potentials') and biphasic potentials with prominent positive deflections ('positive sharp waves') appears. MUPs appear again after axonal reinnervation; the first are short bi- and triphasic; these soon become polyphasic, serrated and of prolonged duration.[43]

Complete denervation can be observed in perineal muscles after traumatic lesions to the lumbosacral spine and damage to the cauda equina. Most lesions will, however, cause only partial denervation. In partially denervated muscle, some MUPs remain and mingle, eventually giving rise to abnormal spontaneous activity. As the MUPs in sphincter muscles are also short and mostly bi- or triphasic, it requires considerable experience with EMG to recognize abnormal spontaneous activity in the presence of a few surviving motor units. Abnormal spontaneous activity has been described as the most specific marker for degeneration of Onuf's nucleus occurring in patients with multiple system atrophy (MSA).[44]

A peculiar type of abnormal insertion activity occurs in long-standing partially denervated muscle – the so-called 'repetitive discharges'. These are made up of repetitively firing groups of potentials with so little jitter between the potentials that it is thought that the activity must be due to ephaptic or direct transmission of impulses between muscle fibres.[45,46] However, the striated muscle of the urethral sphincter without any other evidence of neuromuscular disease may show this activity; it has been suggested that such activity causes impaired relaxation of the muscle when spontaneous and profuse.[47]

There is, by definition, a loss of the number of motor units in partially denervated muscle. The amount is difficult to estimate, however, as the amount of motor unit activity recorded depends on needle position and voluntary activation.[48] In partially denervated muscle, collateral reinnervation takes place and, provided that there are still some intact motor units within the muscle, surviving motor nerves will sprout and grow out to reinnervate those muscle fibres that have lost their nerve supply, resulting in a change in the arrangement of muscle fibres within the unit. Unlike healthy muscle (where it is unusual for two adjacent muscle fibres to be part of the same motor unit), following reinnervation, several muscle fibres all belonging to the same motor unit come to be adjacent to one another. During the early stages of reinnervation the newly outgrown motor sprouts are thin and therefore conduct slowly. This is reflected by prolongation of the waveform of the muscle action potential which may have small, late components (Fig. 22.5). Neuromuscular transmission in these newly grown sprouts may also be insecure, so that the motor unit may show instability. With time, and provided there is no further deterioration in innervation, in skeletal muscle the reinnervating axonal sprouts increase in diameter and thus increase their conduction velocity so that activation of all parts of the reinnervated motor unit becomes more synchronous; this has the effect of increasing the amplitude and reducing towards normal the duration of the MUPs measured with a CNE. This phenomenon may differ in the sphincter muscles, where long-duration MUPs appear to remain a prominent feature of reinnervated motor units.[49]

Several conditions exist in which gross changes of reinnervation may be detected in motor units of the pelvic floor. Following a cauda equina lesion, the MUPs are likely to be prolonged and polyphasic;[36] similar marked changes are seen in patients with lumbosacral myelomeningoceles.

Neuropathic changes can be recorded in sphincter muscles of patients with MSA.[49] This condition is a progressive neurodegenerative disease which, particularly in its early stages, is often mistaken for Parkinson's disease, but is poorly responsive to anti-parkinsonian treatment. Autonomic failure, causing postural hypotension, and unsteadiness and clumsiness due to cerebellar ataxia, may be additional features. Urinary incontinence occurs early in this condition in both men and women, often some years before the onset of obvious neurological features.[50] As part of the neurodegenerative process, loss of motor units occurs in Onuf's nucleus, so that partial but progressive denervation of the sphincter results and recorded motor units show changes of reinnervation, becoming markedly prolonged. Sphincter EMG is of value in distinguishing between idiopathic Parkinson's disease and MSA,[49,51] but may not be obvious in the early stages of the disease.[52] Similar changes of chronic reinnervation may be found in other parkinsonian syndromes such as progressive supranuclear palsy.[53] These changes can also be demonstrated as an increase in fibre density on SFEMG.[38]

EMG changes in genuine stress incontinence

Denervation is thought to be involved in the genesis of genuine stress incontinence (GSI); consequently, EMG techniques have been used to look at the extent of nerve damage following childbirth and in the assessment of women with GSI.[54] An increase in FD in the external anal sphincter has been demonstrated using SFEMG in women with urinary stress incontinence.[55] One study looked at the relationship between stress incontinence, genitourinary prolapse and partial denervation of the pelvic floor.[56] Results showed that women with normal urinary control who were parous had an increase in FD in the pubococcygeus with age that was slightly higher than that of age-matched nulliparous women. Women with stress incontinence without prolapse had much higher FDs than did comparable age-matched control subjects. Similar FDs were noted in women with stress incontinence with prolapse and in those with prolapse alone; FDs were significantly higher than those in asymptomatic women. It was concluded that the pubococcygeus is partially denervated and then reinnervated in women with stress incontinence, genital prolapse or both. Using a CNE to examine the pubococcygeus following childbirth, the same group found a significant increase in duration of individual motor units following labour and vaginal delivery.[57] The changes were most marked in women who had urinary incontinence 8 weeks after delivery and who had had a prolonged second stage and had given birth to heavier babies.

The CNE EMG changes found in these studies were more subtle than those following a cauda equina lesion or in MSA. The control group in any study of GSI that uses an EMG technique should be carefully defined and an adequate sample of relevant EMG parameters obtained from each subject.

EMG changes in women with urinary retention and obstructed voiding

It had been assumed that isolated urinary retention in young women was either due to psychogenic factors or the first symptom of onset of multiple sclerosis.[58] CNE EMG in this group, however, has demonstrated that a number of these patients have profuse complex repetitive discharges (CRDs) and decelerating burst (DB) activity in the urethral sphincter muscle.[59] It was proposed that this pathological spontaneous activity leads to sphincter contraction, which endures during micturition and causes obstruction flow. Recent proof of this has been demonstrated by combined CNE EMG and kinesiological EMG analysis of a group of female subjects with dysfunctional voiding.[24] CRDs have a very characteristic sound quality over the loudspeaker on the EMG machine, like a helicopter or motorcycle engine. It is the DBs that produce a myotonic-like sound, which has been likened to underwater recordings of whales. CRDs may be difficult to distinguish from chronically reinnervated motor units except that the jitter of the potentials is very much less.[47] Why this activity occurs is not known, but the syndrome has been associated with polycystic ovaries.[59] It is probable that an as yet unidentified hormonal abnormality to which the striated muscle is peculiarly sensitive is involved. Loss of stability of membranes within the striated muscle allows ephaptic transmission to manifest as the CRDs. Typically, patients with this syndrome are pre-menopausal, and the condition has its maximum incidence in women under the age of 30. The clinical presentation of what is primarily a disorder of sphincter relaxation depends on the secondary effect it has on the detrusor: instability or failure of contractility can occur.

Detrusor instability with this disorder of sphincter relaxation presents as urgency and frequency and possibly incomplete emptying. Detrusor failure is associated with urinary retention with a bladder capacity in excess of 1 litre without previous urgency having occurred. This implies that the condition has been partial, but asymptomatic, for some time and that chronic retention has damaged the afferent innervation of the bladder, causing loss of the sensation of urgency. Fluctuations in the condition may occur and, although it may have a spontaneous onset in some, it can also follow an event such as administration of general anaesthesia. It is hypothesized that the precipitating event may have an adverse effect on a precariously compromised detrusor muscle and, by tipping the balance, may cause retention. Preliminary results of the response to treatment by neuromodulation of urinary retention due to the sphincter abnormality appear promising.

It has been argued that CNE EMG is mandatory in women with urinary retention because it can detect both changes of denervation and reinnervation that occur with a cauda equina lesion, as well as abnormal spontaneous activity.[60] It should certainly be carried out before a woman is stigmatized as having 'psychogenic urinary retention'.

EMG changes in primary muscle disease

EMG changes reflect pathological changes in the structure of the motor unit. More subtle are changes in EMG due to disease of the muscle fibres. Although in skeletal muscle the 'typical' features of myopathy are said to be showers of small, low-amplitude polyphasic units recruited at mild effort, such changes in the pelvic floor have not been reported, even in patients known to have generalized myopathy.[61] Pelvic floor muscle involvement in limb-girdle muscular dystrophy in a nulliparous female has been reported, but CNE, EMG of her urethral sphincter was reported as normal.[62]

Scant information is available on the effects on EMG recording from muscle which has been subject to a severe stretch injury such as occurs during childbirth. There may well be changes reflecting rupture of individual muscle fibres and injury to small intramuscular nerves.

Diagnostic usefulness of EMG methods

CNE EMG and SFEMG have both been employed in neurourological, urogynaecological and proctological research. SFEMG determination of FD provides a quantifiable parameter to measure the reinnervation changes in sphincter muscle, but little else of clinical relevance can be learnt. The use of CNE EMG, however, allows rapid confirmation of the normality or abnormality of the muscle examined simply by 'observing' the motor unit activity on the oscilloscope screen. This may be one reason why quantified determination of MUP parameters by CNE EMG is not as widely used as it might be expected, although quantified CNE EMG does provide the same information on reinnervation changes in muscle as the SFEMG parameter of FD.[16,38] In the authors' experience the CNE is preferable for routine diagnostics in uroneurology as the whole spectrum of changes in the course of denervation/reinnervation and spontaneous activity can be observed. The electrophysiological method of choice in routine examination of skeletal muscle is CNE EMG. It should be logical to extend an EMG examination from, for example, the lumbar and upper sacral myotomes to the lower sacral myotomes in a child with myelomeningocele or in an adult after a cauda equina lesion. Furthermore, the CNE can be employed at the same diagnostic session for recording motor evoked responses, and/or reflex responses.[18]

One caveat is that it is a common misconception that EMG can accurately measure the amount of partial denervation that has occurred. As explained in the preceding sections, denervation causes fibrillation activity and a reduction in the total number of motor units; however, fibrillations in the pelvic floor are difficult to identify with certainty. Unfortunately, a good method does not currently exist for estimating the number of lost or remaining motor units. By analysing MUPs, however, changes due to reinnervation may be identified.

CONCLUSIONS

Our understanding of pelvic floor, lower urinary tract and bowel function in health and disease has been greatly assisted through kinesiological and 'motor unit' EMG, but there is still much research to be done. Better-defined age-stratified control values are needed for wider application of diagnostic EMG in patients with suspected neurogenic dysfunction.

REFERENCES

1. Adrian ED, Bronck DW. The discharge of impulses in motor nerve fibres. Part II. The frequency of discharge in reflex and voluntary contractions. *J Physiol (Lond)* 1929; 67: 119–151

2. Fowler CJ. Electromyography: normal and pathological findings. In: Osselton JW, Binnie CD, Cooper R, Fowler CJ, Mauguière F, Prior PF (eds) *Clinical Neurophysiology. EMG, Nerve Conduction and Evoked Potentials*. Oxford: Butterworth–Heinemann, 1995; 76–102

3. Franksson C, Petersén I. Electromyographic investigation of disturbances in striated muscle of urethral sphincter. *Br J Urol* 1955; 27: 154–161

4. Chantraine A. Electromyographie des sphincters striés urétal et anal humains. Etude descriptive et analytique. *Rev Neurol (Paris)* 1966; 115: 396–403

5. Vereecken RL, Verduyn H. The electrical activity of the paraurethral and perineal muscles in normal and pathological conditions. *Br J Urol* 1970; 42: 457–463

6. Jesel M, Isch-Treussard C, Isch F. Electromyography of striated muscle of anal urethral sphincters. In: Desmedt JE (ed) *New Developments in Electromyography and Clinical Neurophysiology*, Volume 2. Basel: Karger, 1973; 406–420

7. Chantraine A, Leval J, Onkelinx A. Motor conduction velocity in the internal pudendal nerves. In: Desmedt JE (ed) *New Developments in Electromyography and Clinical Neurophysiology*, Volume 2. Basel: Karger, 1973; 433–438

8. Blaivas JG, Labib KB, Bauer SB, Retik B. A new approach to electromyography of the external urethral sphincter. *J Urol* 1977; 117: 773–777

9. Gilpin S, Gosling J, Smith A, Warrell D. The pathogenesis of genitourinary prolapse and stress incontinence of urine. A histological and histochemical study. *Br J Obstet Gynaecol* 1989; 96: 15–23

10. Heit M, Benson T, Russell B, Brubaker L. Levator ani muscle in women with genitourinary prolapse. *Neurourol Urodyn* 1996; 15: 17–29

11. Deindl F, Vodušek DB, Hesse U, Schüssler B. Pelvic floor activity patterns: comparison of nulliparous continent and parous urinary stress incontinent women. A kinesiological EMG study. *Br J Urol* 1994; 73: 413–417

12. Lose G, Tanko A, Colstrup H, Andersen JT. Urethral sphincter electromyography with vaginal surface electrodes: a comparison with sphincter electromyography recorded via periurethral coaxial, anal sphincter needle and perianal surface electrodes. *J Urol* 1985; 133: 815–818

13. Smith A, Hosker G, Warrell D. The role of pudendal nerve damage in the aetiology of genuine stress incontinence in women. *Br J Obstet Gynaecol* 1989; 96: 29–32

14. Nordling J, Meyhoff H, Walter S, Andersen J. Urethral electromyography using a new ring electrode. *J Urol* 1978; 120: 571–573

15. Aanestad Ø, Flink R, Stålberg E. Interference pattern in perineal muscles: I. A quantitative electromyographic study in normal subjects. *Neurourol Urodyn* 1989; 8: 1–9

16. Vodušek DB. A neurophysiological study of human sacral reflexes. MSc Thesis. Ljubljana: University E. Kardelj, 1982; 1–55 (in Slovene)

17. Deindl FM, Vodušek DB, Hesse U, Schüssler B. Activity patterns of pubococcygeal muscles in nulliparous continent women. *Br J Urol* 1993; 72: 46–51

18. Vodušek DB. Electrophysiology. In: Schüßler B, Laycock J, Norton P, Stanton S (eds) *Pelvic Floor Re-education, Principles and Practice*. London: Springer-Verlag, 1994; 83–97

19. Vereecken RL, Ketelaer P, Joossens J, Leruitte A. Frequency analysis of the electromyographic activity in striated pelvic floor muscles. *Eur Neurol* 1977; 3: 333–336

20. Vereecken RL, Derluyn J, Verduyn H. Electromyography of the perineal striated muscles during cystometry. *Urol Int* 1975; 30: 92–98

21. Blaivas JG, Sinha HP, Zayed AAH, Labib KB. Detrusor–external sphincter dyssynergia. *J Urol* 1981; 125: 542–544

22. Chancellor MB, Kaplan SA, Blaivas JG. Detrusor–external sphincter dyssynergia. In: Bock G, Whelan J (eds) *Neurobiology of Incontinence.* (Ciba Foundation Symposium 151). Chichester: John Wiley, 1990; 195–206

23. Rudy DC, Woodside JR. Non-neurogenic neurogenic bladder: the relationship between intravesical pressure and the external sphincter electromyogram. *Neurourol Urodyn* 1991; 10: 169–176

24. Deindl FM, Vodušek DB, Bischof C, Hartung R. Zwei verschiedene Formen von Miktionsstörungen bei jungen Frauen: Dyssynerges Verhalten im Beckenboden oder Pseudomyotonie im externen urethralen Sphinkter? *Aktuel Urol* 1997; 28: 88–94

25. Pavlakis AJ, Siroky MB, Goldstein I, Krane RJ. Neurourologic findings in Parkinson's disease. *J Urol* 1983; 129: 80–83

26. Read NW. Functional assessment of the anorectum in faecal incontinence. In: Bock G, Whelan J (eds) *Neurobiology of Incontinence.* (Ciba Foundation Symposium 151). Chichester: John Wiley, 1990; 119–138

27. Mathers SE, Kempster PA, Law PJ *et al.* Anal sphincter dysfunction in Parkinson's disease. *Arch Neurol* 1989; 46(10): 1061–1064

28. Chantraine A, De Leval J, Depireux P. Adult female intra- and peri-urethral sphincter-electromyographic study. *Neurourol Urodyn* 1990; 9: 139–144

29. Nordling J, Meyhoff HH. Dissociation of urethral and anal sphincter activity in neurogenic bladder dysfunction. *J Urol* 1979; 122: 352–356

30. O'Donnell PD, Doyle R. Biofeedback therapy technique for treatment of urinary incontinence. *Urology* 1991; 37: 432–436

31. Gosling JA. Anatomy. In: Stanton SL (ed) *Clinical Gynecologic Urology.* St Louis: Mosby, 1984; 3–12

32. Lowe EM, Fowler CJ, Osborne JL, DeLancey JOL. Improved method for needle electromyography of the urethral sphincter in women. *Neurourol Urodyn* 1994; 13: 29–33

33. Petersén I, Franksson C, Danielson CO. Electromyographic study of the muscles of the pelvic floor and urethra in normal females. *Acta Obstet Gynaecol Scand* 1955; 34: 273–285

34. Bartolo DCC, Jarratt JA, Read NW. The cutaneo-anal reflex: a useful index of neuropathy? *Br J Surg* 1983; 70: 660–663

35. Vodušek DB, Light JK. The motor nerve supply of the external urethral sphincter muscles. *Neurourol Urodyn* 1983; 2: 193–200

36. Fowler CJ, Kirby RS, Harrison MJG *et al.* Individual motor unit analysis in the diagnosis of disorders of urethral sphincter innervation. *J Neurol Neurosurg Psychiatry* 1984; 47: 637–641

37. Varma JS, Smith AN, McInnes A. Electrophysiological observations on the human pudendo-anal reflex. *J Neurol Neurosurg Psychiatry* 1986; 49: 1411–1416

38. Rodi Z, Vodušek DB, Denislic M. Clinical uro-neurophysiological investigation in multiple sclerosis. *Eur J Neurol* 1996; 3: 574–580

39. Neill ME, Swash M. Increased motor unit fibre density in the external anal sphincter muscle in ano-rectal incontinence: a single fibre EMG study. *J Neurol Neurosurg Psychiatry* 1980; 43: 343–347

40. Vodušek DB, Janko M. SFEMG in striated sphincter muscles (abstr). *Muscle Nerve* 1981; 4(3): 252

41. Jameson JS, Chia YW, Kamm MA *et al.* Effect of age, sex and parity on anorectal function. *Br J Surg* 1994; 81: 1689–1692

42. Stålberg E, Trontelj JV. *Single Fiber Electromyography: Studies in Healthy and Diseased Muscle,* 2nd edn. New York: Raven Press, 1994

43. Brown FW. *The Physiological and Technical Basis of Electromyography.* London: Butterworth, 1984

44. Schwarz J, Kornhuber M, Bischoff C, Straube A. Electromyography of the external anal sphincter in patients with Parkinson's disease and multiple system atrophy: frequency of abnormal spontaneous activity and polyphasic motor unit potentials. *Muscle Nerve* 1997; 20: 1167–1172

45. Trontelj J, Stålberg E. Bizarre repetitive discharges recorded with single fibre EMG. *J Neurol Neurosurg Psychiatry* 1983; 46: 310–316

46. Fowler CJ. Pelvic floor neurophysiology. In: Osselton JW, Binnie CD, Cooper R, Fowler CJ, Mauguière F, Prior PF (eds) *Clinical Neurophysiology. EMG, Nerve Conduction and Evoked Potentials.* Oxford: Butterworth–Heinemann, 1995; 233–252

47. Fowler CJ, Kirby RS, Harrison MJG. Decelerating bursts and complex repetitive discharges in the striated muscle of the urethral sphincter associated with urinary retention in women. *J Neurol Neurosurg Psychiatry* 1985; 48: 1004–1009

48. Siroky MB. Electromyography of the perineal floor. In: Boone TB (ed) *Urodynamics I. The Urologic Clinics of North America,* Volume 23. Philadelphia: Saunders, 1996; 299–307

49. Palace J, Chandiramani VA, Fowler CJ. Value of sphincter EMG in the diagnosis of multiple system atrophy. *Muscle Nerve* 1997; 20: 1396–1403

50. Beck RO, Betts CD, Fowler CJ. Genitourinary dysfunction in multiple system atrophy: clinical features and treatment in 62 cases. *J Urol* 1994; 151: 1336–1341

51. Eardley I, Quinn NP, Fowler CJ *et al.* The value of urethral sphincter electromyography in the differential diagnosis of parkinsonism. *Br J Urol* 1989; 64: 360–362

52. Stocchi F, Carbone A, Inghilleri M *et al.* Urodynamic and neurophysiological evaluation in Parkinson's disease and multiple system atrophy. *J Neurol Neurosurg Psychiatry* 1997; 62: 507–511

53. Vallderiola F, Valls-Solè J, Tolosa ES, Marti MJ. Striated anal sphincter denervation in patients with progressive supranuclear palsy. *Mov Disord* 1995; 9: 117–121

54. Snooks SJ, Badenoch DF, Tiptaft RC, Swash M. Perineal nerve damage in genuine stress incontinence. *Br J Urol* 1985; 57: 422–426

55. Anderson R. A neurogenic element to urinary genuine stress incontinence. *Br J Urol* 1984; 91: 41–45

56. Smith ARB, Hosker GL, Warrell DW. The role of partial denervation of the pelvic floor in aetiology of genitourinary prolapse and stress incontinence of urine. A neurophysiological study. *Br J Obstet Gynaecol* 1989; 96: 24–28

57. Allen R, Hosker G, Smith A, Warrell D. Pelvic floor damage and childbirth: a neurophysiological study. *Br J Obstet Gynaecol* 1990; 97: 770–779

58. Siroky M, Krane R. Functional voiding disorders in women. In: Krane R, Siroky M (eds) *Clinical Neuro-Urology.* Boston: Little Brown, 1991; 445–457

59. Fowler CJ, Christmas TJ, Chapple CR *et al.* Abnormal electromyographic activity of the urethral sphincter, voiding dysfunction, and polycystic ovaries: a new syndrome? *Br J Med* 1988; 297: 1436–1438

60. Fowler CJ, Kirby RS. Electromyography of the urethral sphincter in women with urinary retention. *Lancet* 1986; i: 1455–1456

61. Caress J, Kothari M, Bauer S, Shefner J. Urinary dysfunction in Duchenne muscular dystrophy. *Muscle Nerve* 1996; 19: 819–822

62. Dixon PJ, Christmas TJ, Chapple CR. Stress incontinence due to pelvic floor muscle involvement in limb-girdle muscular dystrophy. *Br J Urol* 1990; 65: 653–660

23

Nerve conduction studies

C. J. Fowler, D. B. Vodušek

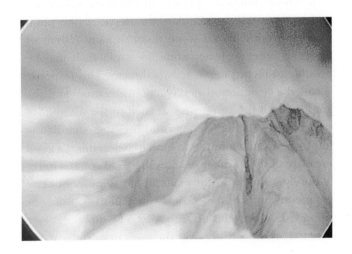

INTRODUCTION

Clinical neurophysiological tests consist of electrical recordings from muscles (i.e. electromyography [EMG]; see chapter 22) and nerve conduction studies. The latter examine the capacity of a nerve to transmit a test electrical stimulus along its length. If motor function is present in the nerve being tested, responsiveness can be measured by stimulating at a proximal point and recording an elicited muscle response (Fig. 23.1). The time taken for the muscle to contract can be measured, in addition to the amplitude of the muscle response (known as the compound muscle action potential or 'M' response).[1] The amplitude depends on the number of intact individual motor fibres, unlike measures of latency (i.e. time to onset of response) and conduction velocity, which reflect the conduction speed of the single fastest motor fibre. Because of this, measures of latency are a poor indicator of integrity or level of innervation. The amplitude of the evoked muscle response is a better guide; however, because this measurement depends so heavily on the configuration of the electrodes employed, amplitude is not as valuable as theoretically expected. Under ideal circumstances, to measure the potential amplitude of a compound muscle action the active recording reference should be placed over the motor end-plate (i.e. the point of entry of nerve into muscle) and the reference electrode over an insertion tendon. In the case of a strap-shaped muscle, the former can be identified as midway along its anatomical length; in more anatomically complex muscles, such as exist in the pelvis, the motor end-plate region is virtually impossible to identify and it is difficult to record well-formed compound muscle action potentials.

If sensory fibres are present in the nerve under test and it is possible to stimulate the nerve at one point with electrodes placed some distance away (10 cm or more, in order to lessen stimulus artefact), it may be possible to record nerve activity directly. This response is called a 'compound nerve action potential' and the amplitude of the response is related to the number of nerve fibres being depolarized by the stimulating impulse. When measured in limb muscles, this is a good measure of the number of active nerve fibres. If a nerve is purely sensory, as, for example, in some peripheral cutaneous branches, electrical stimulation (possibly by using ring electrodes around a finger) stimulates sensory nerves. Recording over the median or ulnar nerve

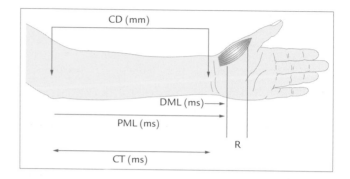

Figure 23.1. *Measurements to be made in calculating motor conduction velocity (CV): CD, conduction distance; CT, conduction time; PML, proximal motor latency; DML, distal motor latency; R, recording electrodes. CV = CD/CT.*

at the wrist and using the technique of 'averaging', will result in a discernible response known as a sensory action potential. Unfortunately, with the possible exception of recording from the dorsal nerve of the penis, for anatomical reasons, recording of sensory action potentials is not possible in the pelvis.

Thus, many of the nerve conduction studies carried out in the sacral region have developed on the basis of principles that are suited to the stimulating and recording conditions of the limbs but which adapt less well to the neuroanatomical arrangements of the pelvis.

NEUROPHYSIOLOGY OF THE SACRAL MOTOR SYSTEM

To evaluate limb motor nerves, motor conduction velocity is routinely measured. However, access to stimulation of the nerve at two separate points is required, with measurement of the distance between them (Fig. 23.1); this is not possible in the pelvis. Measurement of the terminal motor latency of a muscle response requires a shorter length of motor nerve to be accessible.[1] Terminal motor latency of the pudendal nerve can be measured by recording with a concentric needle electrode from the bulbocavernosus, anal or urethral sphincter muscles in response to bipolar stimulation of the perianal or perineal surface. The latencies of muscle evoked potentials (MEPs) from the perineal muscles obtained in this way are between 4.7 and 5.1 ms.[2] Similar latencies have been obtained recording from the anal sphincter and using the same method of stimulation.[3,4]

The pudendal terminal motor latency is more often measured using stimulation with a special 'surface electrode assembly' attached to a gloved index finger. This method, developed at the St Mark's Hospital, London,[5] is often referred to as the 'St Mark's stimulator'. A bipolar stimulating electrode is fixed to the tip of the gloved finger and a recording electrode pair placed 3 cm proximally on the base of the finger (Fig. 23.2a). The finger is inserted into the subject's rectum and stimulation is performed close to the ischial spine. The terminal motor latency for the anal sphincter 'M wave' is typically around 2 ms with this form of stimulator (Fig. 23.2b). Responses from the urethral sphincter can also be obtained if a catheter-mounted electrode is used. Unfortunately, amplitudes of the 'M wave' response have not proved contributory. No explanation is forthcoming for the difference in latencies obtained by the 'perineal' and 'transrectal' methods.

Cadaveric studies have shown that the levator ani or pubococcygeus muscle receives innervation direct from sacral nerve roots S2–4 before the formation of the pudendal nerve trunk.[6] In theory, therefore, these should not contract with stimulation of the pudendal nerve at the level of the ischial spine. However, Smith et al.[7] and subsequently Allen et al.[8] were both able to record the latency of pelvic floor responses by stimulating at this point. Certain studies have shown that the pudendal terminal motor latency increases with age,[9,10] but others contradict this.[11] The St Mark's group initially showed that perineal latency was abnormally prolonged in patients with urinary stress incontinence,[12] a finding which was confirmed by the Manchester group.[7] Working on the hypothesis that the pudendal nerve was

stretched and injured during childbirth, several studies examined the pudendal or perineal latency immediately *post partum*. Using a concentric needle electrode, Allen et al.[8] demonstrated that damage had occurred to the innervation of the pubococcygeus in some women *post partum*; however, no prolongation of the latency to stimulation of that muscle was noted when women were examined 2 months *post partum*. Snooks et al.[13] observed a significant increase in the mean pudendal nerve terminal motor latency at 48–72 hours after vaginal delivery, but this returned to normal in 60% of women after 2 months. A 5-year follow-up of 14 multiparous women from this group found that the mean pudendal motor latency was prolonged on both sides; fibre density of the anal sphincter was increased, and anal manometry showed a reduction in anal canal pressure during maximal squeeze contraction.[14] On this basis, it was concluded that occult damage to the pudendal innervation of the external anal sphincter had persisted and worsened over the 5-year period and possibly had been exacerbated by abnormal straining patterns of defecation.

Although Sultan et al.[15] demonstrated a small (0.1 ms) but statistically significant increase in pudendal nerve latency following vaginal delivery, using anal endosonography they demonstrated a defect of either the internal or external anal sphincter or both in 35% of women after vaginal delivery. There was also a strong association between these defects and the development of bowel symptoms. It was suggested that, rather than a causal relationship between the two, this reflected a traumatic cause common to both. No correlation of

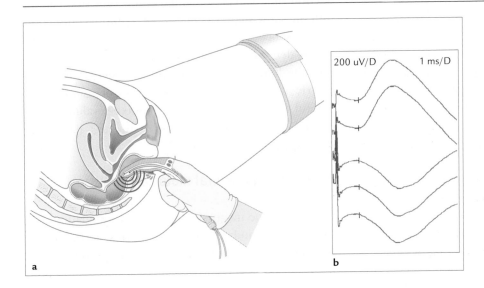

a   b

200 uV/D   1 ms/D

Figure 23.2. *The St Mark's stimulator. (a) Use of the stimulator in the rectum. The ischial spine is palpated and pudendal nerve stimulated. (b) Typical responses recorded using the stimulator. The upper two traces are recorded from the left side and the lower three from the right. The latencies are within normal limits (1.9–2.2 ms)*

pudendal nerve terminal latency to parity was found in another study.[9] Measurement of the pudendal terminal latency has demonstrated a prolongation in primiparae and multiparae after delivery (Fig. 23.3), and an association with an occurrence of pelvic instability and the use of vacuum extraction.[16] Significantly increased pudendal terminal latency was observed in women with urinary incontinence;[16] this has also been found in women with pelvic floor prolapse;[17,18] with a further lengthening of the latency following vaginal dissection for repair or suspension procedures.[18]

The term 'pudendal neuropathy' is an established term, which is particularly used by coloproctologists. It should be noted that pudendal motor latency is not a measure of denervation of the muscles innervated by the pudendal nerve, because prolongation of latency is a poor measure of denervation. It is unlikely that a pathological process affecting a nerve so that it causes a increase in latency of less than 1.0 ms over a 5 cm distance could possibly interfere significantly with the timing of reflex responses, such as those involved with the recruitment of motor units on coughing or sneezing (i.e. manoeuvres that cause stress incontinence).

It is true that an abnormality of this latency must indicate some sort of pathology of the pudendal nerve, but the full significance of these findings remains to be explained. It may be that, unlike the situation in the carpal tunnel syndrome (where conduction slowing is in the main trunk), in patients with neurogenic lesions affecting the innervation of the pelvic floor, damage to the nerve occurs distally at sites where the motor nerve is branching within the muscle.[8]

Anterior sacral root (cauda equina) stimulation

Development of special electrical[19] and magnetic[20] stimulators has allowed transcutaneous stimulation of deeply situated nervous tissue. Stimulation of mainly the roots at the exit from the vertebral canal occurs when these stimulators are applied over the spine.[21] Various reports have been published of these techniques applied to the sacral roots.[22,23] It remains controversial as to whether parasympathetic efferents can be stimulated magnetically. It has been claimed that MEPs from detrusor can be produced by magnetic stimulation of the cauda equina;[24] however, others have demonstrated inhibition of detrusor hyperreflexia following sacral root stimulation.[25] Needle EMG rather than non-selective surface electrodes should be used to record MEPs to electrical or magnetic stimulation because both depolarize underlying neural structures in a non-selective fashion and there may be activation of several muscles innervated by lumbosacral segments. Responses from gluteal muscles have been shown to contaminate attempts to record from the sphincters, resulting in inaccuracies.[26] Recording of MEPs with magnetic stimulation has been less successful than with electrical stimulation, and there is often a large stimulus artefact.[27,28] This can be decreased by positioning the ground electrode between the recording electrodes and the stimulating coil[29] (Fig. 23.4). A peripheral conduction time can be obtained using root stimulation, with the subsequent calculation of a central conduction time (see below).[27]

The demonstration of a perineal MEP on stimulation over the lumbosacral spine and recorded with a concentric needle EMG electrode may occasionally be helpful, but an absent response has to be evaluated with caution and the clinical value of the test has yet to be established.

Assessment of central motor pathways

Using the same magnetic or electrical stimulation, it is possible to stimulate the motor cortex and record a response from the pelvic floor. Magnetic stimulation is less unpleasant, and cortical electrical stimulation is no

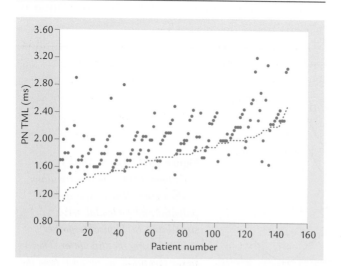

Figure 23.3. *Pudendal nerve terminal motor latency (PNTML) measured in 146 women during pregnancy (●) and 3 months after delivery (●).*

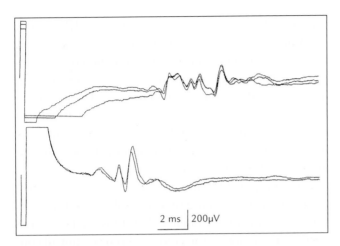

Figure 23.4. *Concentric needle EMG recording from the anal sphincter, showing responses on 'strong' electrical stimulation with surface electrodes over the back (upper trace at level L1; lower trace at level S3). Digitimer stimulator; stimulus duration 0.50s, stimulus amplitude 50%). Three and two consecutive responses are superimposed, respectively.*

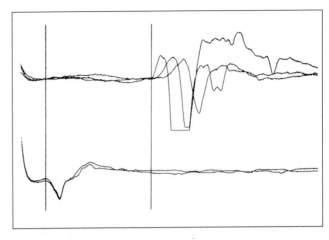

Figure 23.5. *Recording from the urethral sphincter with a concentric needle electrode in response to magnetic stimulation over the lower lumbar spine (lower trace; latency 6.5 ms) and the motor cortex (upper trace; latency 25.4 ms). The effect of 'facilitation' (i.e. a slight voluntary contraction) on shortening the latency of the response following cortical stimulation is evident.*

longer used in awake subjects. MEPs in anal[26] and urethral[30] sphincters and in the bulbocavernosus[26] muscles were reported using electrical stimulation over the motor cortex of healthy subjects. If no 'facilitatory manoeuvre' was used, mean latencies were between 30 and 35 ms; if, however, stimulation was performed during a period of slight voluntary contraction of the muscle, the latencies of MEPs shortened significantly (for up to 8 ms) (Fig. 23.5).

By applying stimulation to both the scalp and the back (at level L1), and subtracting the latency of the respective MEPs, a 'central conduction time' can be obtained. Central conduction times of approximately 22 ms without, and about 15 ms with, the facilitation (i.e. slight voluntary contraction), have been reported.[27]

It has been observed that patients with multiple sclerosis and spinal cord lesions have substantially longer central conduction times than do healthy controls;[31] however, as these patients all had clinically recognizable cord disease, the diagnostic contribution of the method remains doubtful.

Because of the significant influence of voluntary contraction, the variability of both total and central conduction times makes the method somewhat clinically unreliable. A well-formed sphincter MEP with a normal latency in a patient with a functional disorder, or in a medicolegal case, may on occasion be helpful, but there is no established clinical use for this type of test.

NEUROPHYSIOLOGY OF THE SACRAL SENSORY SYSTEM

Cerebral somatosensory evoked potentials (SEPs)

The pudendal response following electrical stimulation of the clitoral nerve is easily recorded.[27,32–36] This SEP is highly reproducible and of highest amplitudes at the central recording site ([Cz−2 cm: Fz] of the International 10–20 EEG System; i.e. 2cm behind the central point [Cz], which is derived by measuring a subject's skull and dividing it into tenths [the International 10–20 EEG system]; Fz is the central front of the electrode).[37] Amplitudes of the P40 measure between 0.5 and 12 μV.[33] The first positive peak at 41 ± 2.3 ms[33] (termed P1 or P40) is usually clearly defined in healthy subjects, using a stimulus two to four times the sensory threshold current strength[33,36] (Fig. 23.6). Subsequent negative (at around 55 ms) and then further positive waves are interindividually quite variable in expression and amplitude and, in addition, have little known clinical relevance.

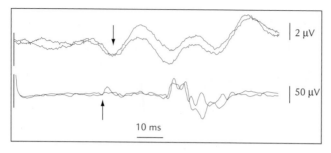

Figure 23.6. *Cerebral somatosensory evoked potential (SEPs) (above) and bulbocavernosus reflex (below) on dorsal penile nerve stimulation (rectangular electric pulses, 0.2 ms long, at 1 Hz) in a 37-year-old woman with a compressive fracture of L1, difficulties in starting voiding but no neurological deficit. SEP is recorded with surface electrodes (Cz− 2 cm: Fz); the bulbocavernosus reflex is recorded from the anal sphincter with surface electrodes. Two consecutive averages of 128 responses are superimposed. The P40 of the SEP and the first component of the bulbocavernosus reflex are indicated. The first reflex component is spurious at the applied stimulation strength, which was two-times sensory threshold; the second (late) reflex component is obvious.*

Pudendal SEP recordings have been widely employed in patients with neurogenic bladder dysfunction due to multiple sclerosis,[31] but more recent findings show that the tibial cerebral SEPs are more often abnormal than the pudendal SEP.[38] Only in exceptional cases is the pudendal SEP abnormal but the tibials normal, pointing to an isolated conus involvement.[38] Cerebral SEPs on clitoral stimulation were reported as a potentially valuable intra-operative monitoring method in patients with cauda equina or conus at risk of a surgical procedure.[39,40]

One study found that pudendal evoked potentials in investigations of urogenital symptoms due to neurological disease were of less value than a clinical examination looking for signs of spinal cord disease in the lower limbs (i.e. lower limb hyperreflexia and extensor plantar responses).[41] Circumstances may exist, such as loss of bladder or vaginal sensation in a patient, when it is reassuring to be able to record a normal pudendal evoked response.

Electrical stimulation of urethra, bladder and anal canal

Cerebral SEPs can also be obtained on stimulation of bladder mucosa.[42] It is essential to use bipolar stimulation in the bladder or proximal urethra when making such measurements, otherwise somatic afferents will be depolarized.[30,43,44] A maximum amplitude over the midline (Cz− 2 cm: Fz) has been demonstrated with such

cerebral efferents;[44] however, the potential is of low amplitude (1 μV or less) and variable configuration, and may be difficult to identify in some control subjects.[44,45] The typical latency of the most prominent negative potential (N 1) is about 100 ms.[44,45] The responses are of more relevance to neurogenic bladder dysfunction than the pudendal SEP, as the Aδ sensory afferents from the bladder and proximal urethra accompany the autonomic fibres in the pelvic nerves.[44]

Another possible stimulation site in the perineal region is the anal canal. This can result in cerebral SEPs with a slightly longer latency than those obtained following stimulation of the clitoris;[28] however, not all control subjects demonstrate this response. The rectum and sigmoid colon have also been stimulated, with two types of cerebral SEPs being recorded: one was similar in shape and latency to the pudendal SEP, and the other to the SEP recorded on stimulation of the bladder/ posterior urethra.[46]

SACRAL REFLEXES

Physiological background, methods and terminology

Electrophysiologically recordable responses of the perineal/pelvic floor muscles to (electrical) stimulation in the urogenitoanal region are referred to as 'sacral reflexes'. The two reflexes commonly elicited in the lower sacral segments are the anal and the bulbocavernosus reflexes. Both of these have the afferent and efferent limb of their reflex arc in the pudendal nerve, and are centrally integrated at the S2–S4 cord levels (Fig. 23.6). Electrophysiological correlates of these reflexes have been described. It is possible to use electrical,[2,47–50] mechanical[51] or magnetic[28] stimulation. Whereas the latter two modalities have been applied only to the clitoris, electrical stimulation can be applied at various sites, such as the dorsal clitoral nerve,[2,36,52,53] perianally,[39,54] or bladder neck/proximal urethra, using a catheter-mounted ring electrode.[43,55] Bradley, one of the pioneers of uroneurophysiology, termed this 'electromyelography',[55] but (fortunately) this term did not persist. Depending on which muscle the reflex response is recorded from, the terms 'vesicourethral' and 'vesicoanal' are applied to these reflexes.[56] Needle electrodes applied transperineally[54] or the 'St Mark's electrode',[55] may be used to stimulate the pudendal nerve itself; and the term 'deep pudendal reflex' has been suggested.[54]

Consistent mean latencies of between 31 and 38.5 ms have been reported for sacral reflexes obtained following electrical stimulation of the clitoral nerve.[2,36,47–50,52,53,58] Sacral reflex responses obtained on perianal or bladder neck/proximal urethra stimulation have latencies between 50 and 65 ms.[2,53,57] This more prolonged response is thought to be due to the afferent limb of the reflex being conveyed by thinner myelinated nerves with slower conduction velocities than the thicker myelinated pudendal afferents. The contraction of the anal sphincter on stimulation of the perianal region – the 'anal reflex' – also has a longer latency possibly due to thinner myelinated fibres in its afferent limb as it is produced by a noxious stimulus. On stimulation perianally, a short-latency potential can also be recorded as a result of depolarization of motor branches to the anal sphincter.[2,3] This 'M wave' has been mistaken for a reflex response.

Sacral reflex on electrical stimulation of clitoris

The 'bulbocavernosus reflex', which is the sacral reflex evoked on dorsal penile or clitoral nerve stimulation, is a complex response, often formed by two components.[2,50,59] The first component (with typical latency of about 33 ms) is that most often termed the 'bulbocavernosus' reflex. It is thought to be an oligosynaptic reflex response, as the variability of single motor neuron discharges within this reflex is similar to that of the first component of the blink reflex.[59] The second component has a similar latency to the sacral reflexes evoked by stimulation perianally or from the proximal urethra. Single motor neuron reflex responses within this component have much greater variability, as is typical for a polysynaptic reflex,[59] and discrete responses are not always demonstrable.[51] Different properties of the two components of the reflex may be noted in control subjects and patients: whereas, in normal subjects, the first component usually has a lower threshold, in patients with partially denervated pelvic floor muscles the first reflex component cannot be obtained with single stimuli, but on strong stimulation the later reflex component does occur.[50] Confusion can result and greatly 'delayed' reflex responses may be recorded in patients, as a result of overlooking the possibility that it is not a delayed first component but an isolated second component of the reflex that has been recorded. Double stimuli can help to clarify the situation by revealing more clearly the first component, which was not obvious on stimulation with single stimuli.[51,60]

Separate analyses of sacral reflex responses recorded with needle or wire electrodes are possible for each side of the anal sphincter;[50] this is important because unilateral or asymmetrical lesions are common. Unilateral stimulation of the clitoris is not possible, however. Sacral reflex responses on stimulation of the clitoral nerve have been proposed to be useful in patients with cauda equina and lower motor neuron lesions,[48] although a reflex with a normal latency does not exclude the possibility of an axonal lesion in its reflex arc. Most reports deal with abnormally prolonged sacral reflex latencies; however, the possibility of a tethered cord has been suggested from a very short reflex latency,[61] the shorter latency being attributed particularly to the low location of the conus. Shorter latencies of sacral reflexes in patients with suprasacral cord lesions have also been reported.[53] Continuous intraoperative recording of sacral reflex responses on clitoral stimulation is feasible if double pulses[62,63] or a train of stimuli are used.

Sacral reflex testing should be a part of the 'diagnostic battery' of which central needle EMG exploration of the pelvic floor muscles is the most important part. Measurement of sacral reflexes is established universally and, apart from EMG, is the most time-honoured uroneurophysiological diagnostic procedure. Nevertheless, it is unrealistic to expect that, with measurement of sacral reflexes, a single, easily learned test could distinguish between neurogenic and non-neurogenic sacral dysfunction. Although testing reflex responses is a valid and useful method to assess integrity of reflex arcs, and electrophysiological assessment of sacral reflexes is a more quantitative, sensitive and reproducible way of assessing the S2–S4 reflex arcs than any of the clinical methods, uncritical interpretation of such results should be discouraged.

Sacral reflex on mechanical stimulation

Although, in both men and women, mechanical stimulation has been used to elicit the bulbocavernous reflex;[64] experience in female patients is, as yet, limited. Either a standard commercially available reflex hammer or a customized electromechanical hammer can be used.[65] Such stimulation is painless and can be used in children, or in patients with pacemakers in whom electrical stimulation is contraindicated.

AUTONOMIC NERVOUS SYSTEM

The uroneurophysiological methods discussed so far assess only the thicker myelinated fibres, whereas it is the autonomic nervous system – the parasympathetic component in particular – that is most relevant to sacral organ function. It has been argued that local involvement of the sacral nervous system (such as in trauma or compression) will usually involve somatic and autonomic fibres simultaneously. However, certain local pathological conditions (for example, mesorectal excision of carcinoma or radical hysterectomy) can result in purely isolated lesions and require a method by which the parasympathetic and sympathetic nervous systems innervating the pelvic viscera can be assessed directly. Although cystometry can provide some information on parasympathetic bladder innervation, from a clinical neurophysiological point of view direct electrophysiological testing would be preferable. In cases when a general involvement of thin fibres is expected, assessment of the function of thin sensory fibres is an indirect way to examine autonomic fibres. As unmyelinated afferent fibres transmit temperature sensation and pain, unmyelinated fibre neuropathy can be identified by testing thermal sensitivity. Thin (visceral sensory) fibres are tested by stimulating the proximal urethra or bladder, and recording sacral reflex responses or cerebral SEPs.

Sympathetic skin response

Sweat gland activity in the skin is mediated by the sympathetic nervous system. Changes in sweat gland activity lead to changes in skin resistance – a sympathetic skin response (SSR). 'Stressful stimulation' results in a shift in potential, which can be recorded with surface electrodes from the skin of palms and soles; this is thought to be useful in assessment of neuropathy involving unmyelinated nerve fibres.[66] The SSR can also be recorded from perineal skin.[67,68] The SSR is a reflex arc consisting of myelinated sensory fibres, a complex central integrative mechanism and a sympathetic efferent limb (with postganglionic non-myelinated C-fibres).

The stimulus used in clinical practice is usually an electric pulse delivered to the upper or lower limb (to mixed nerves), but the genital organs can also be stimulated.[67] Latencies of 1.5–2.3 s of SSR on the penis following stimulation of a median nerve at the wrist have been reported;[67,68] these could be obtained in all normal subjects with a large variability (Fig. 23.7). No control data exist in women as yet. The responses are easily habituated and depend on a number of endogenous and exogenous factors, including skin temperature, which should be at least 28°C. Only an absent SSR can be taken as abnormal.

CONCLUSIONS

Neurophysiology has proved valuable in supporting the hypothesis that the nervous system is involved in a proportion of patients with sacral dysfunction, as for instance patients with stress urinary and idiopathic faecal incontinence.[5,13] Tests have helped to establish the function of the sacral nervous system in patients with suprasacral spinal cord injury,[69] to reveal the consequences of particular types of surgical intervention[70] and to elucidate the innervation of pelvic floor muscles.[71,72] A recent introduction is the technique of intraoperative monitoring, where studies of evoked

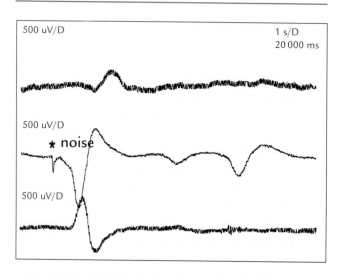

Figure 23.7. *Sympathetic skin responses recorded from the foot at 2.3 s (upper trace), from the penis at 1.52 s (middle trace) and from the hand (lower trace) with silver–silver chloride surface electrodes in response to a sudden noise. The possible value of the equivalent potentials recorded in women has not yet been examined.*

potentials have helped to prevent lesions of the neural structures at risk from the surgical procedure.[39,62,73] Further research applications of uroneurophysiological methods are expected, as elucidation of many of the neurological aspects of urological, gynaecological and proctological problems is still necessary.

REFERENCES

1. Fowler CJ. Electromyography: normal and pathological findings. In: Osselton JW, Binnie CD, Cooper R, Fowler CJ, Mauguière F, Prior PF (eds). *Clinical Neurophysiology. EMG, Nerve Conduction and Evoked Potentials.* Oxford: Butterworth–Heinemann, 1995; 76–102

2. Vodušek DB, Janko M, Lokar J. Direct and reflex responses in perineal muscles on electrical stimulation. *J Neurol Neurosurg Psychiatry* 1983; 46: 67–71

3. Bartolo DCC, Jarratt JA, Read NW. The cutaneo-anal reflex: a useful index of neuropathy? *Br J Surg* 1983; 70: 660–663

4. Pedersen E, Klemar B, Schroder HD *et al.* Anal sphincter responses after perianal electrical stimulation. *J Neurol Neurosurg Psychiatry* 1982; 45: 770–773

5. Kiff ES, Swash M. Normal proximal and delayed distal conduction in the pudendal nerves of patients with idiopathic (neurogenic) faecal incontinence. *J Neurol Neurosurg Psychiatry* 1984; 47: 820–823

6. Junemann K-P, Lue T, Schmidt R, Tanagho E. Clinical significance of sacral and pudendal nerve anatomy. *J Urol* 1988; 139: 74–80

7. Smith A, Hosker G, Warrell D. The role of pudendal nerve damage in the aetiology of genuine stress incontinence in women. *Br J Obstetr Gynaecol* 1989; 96: 29–32

8. Allen R, Hosker G, Smith A, Warrell D. Pelvic floor damage and childbirth: a neurophysiological study. *Br J Obstet Gynaecol* 1990; 97: 770–779

9. Jameson JS, Chia Y W, Kamm MA *et al.* Effect of age, sex and parity on anorectal function. *Br J Surg* 1994; 81: 1689–1692

10. Laurberg S, Swash M. Effects of aging on the anorectal sphincters and their innervation. *Dis Colon Rectum* 1989; 32: 737–742

11. Barret JA, Brocklehurst JC, Kiff ES *et al.* Anal function in geriatric patients with faecal incontinence. *Gut* 1989; 30: 1244–1251

12. Snooks SJ, Badenoch DF, Tiptaft RC, Swash M. Perineal nerve damage in genuine stress incontinence. *Br J Urol* 1985; 57: 422–426

13. Snooks SJ, Swash M, Setchell M, Henry MM. Injury to the pelvic floor sphincter musculature in childbirth. *Lancet* 1984; ii: 546–555

14. Snooks SJ, Swash M, Mathers SE, Henry MM. Effect of vaginal delivery in the pelvic floor: a 5-year follow-up. *Br J Surg* 1990; 77: 1358–1360

15. Sultan A, Kamm M, Hudson C *et al.* Anal-sphincter disruption during vaginal delivery. *N Engl J Med* 1993; 329: 1905–1911

16. Tetzschner T, Soerensen M, Joensson L *et al.* Delivery and pudendal nerve function. *Acta Obstet Gynaecol Scand* 1997; 76: 294–299

17. Smith ARB, Hosker GL, Warrell DW. The role of partial denervation of the pelvic floor in aetiology of genitourinary prolapse and stress incontinence of urine. A neurophysiological study. *Br J Obstet Gynaecol* 1989; 96: 24–28

18. Benson T, McClellan E. The effect of vaginal dissection on the pudendal nerve. *Obstet Gynaecol* 1993; 82: 387–389

19. Merton PA, Morton HB. Stimulation of the cerebral cortex in the intact human subject. *Nature* 1980; 285: 227

20. Barker AT, Jalinous R, Freeston IL. Non-invasive magnetic stimulation of the human motor cortex. *Lancet* 1985; i: 1106–1107

21. Mills KR, Murray NMF. Electrical stimulation over the human vertebral column: which neural elements are excited? *Electroencephalogr Clin Neurophysiol* 1986; 63: 582–589

22. Swash M, Snooks SJ. Slowed motor conduction in lumbosacral nerve roots in cauda equina lesions: a new diagnostic technique. *J Neurol Neurosurg Psychiatry* 1986; 49: 809–816

23. Vodušek DB. Electrophysiology. In: Schuessler B, Laycock J, Norton P, Stanton S (eds) *Pelvic Floor Re-education, Principles and Practice.* London: Springer-Verlag, 1994; 83–97

24. Bemelmans BLH, Van Kerrebroeck PEV, Debruyne FMJ. Motor bladder responses after magnetic stimulation of the cauda equina. *Neurourol Urodyn* 1991; 10(4): 380–381

25. Sheriff MKM, Shah PJR, Fowler CJ *et al.* Neuromodulation of detrusor hyper-reflexia by functional magnetic stimulation of the sacral roots. *Br J Urol* 1996; 78: 39–46

26. Vodušek DB, Zidar J. Perineal motor evoked responses. (Proceedings of the 18th Annual Meeting of the International Continence Society, Oslo.) *Neurourol Urodyn* 1988; 7: 236–237

27. Opsomer RJ, Caramia MD, Zarola F *et al.* Neurophysiological evaluation of central, peripheral sensory and motor pudendal fibres. *Electroencephalogr Clin Neurophysiol* 1989; 74: 260–270

28. Loening-Baucke V, Read NW, Yamada T, Barker AT. Evaluation of the motor and sensory components of the pudendal nerve. *Electroencephalogr Clin Neurophysiol* 1994; 93: 35–65

29. Jost WH, Schimrigk K. A new method to determine pudendal nerve motor latency and central motor conduction time to the external anal sphincter. *Electroencephalogr Clin Neurophysiol* 1994; 93: 237–239

30. Thiry AJ, Deltenre PF. Neurophysiological assessment of the central motor pathway to the external urethral sphincter in man. *Br J Urol* 1989; 63: 515–519

31. Eardley I, Nagendran K, Lecky B *et al.* The neurophysiology of the striated urethral sphincter in multiple sclerosis. *Br J Urol* 1991; 67: 81–88

32. Haldeman S, Bradley WE, Bhatia N. Evoked responses from the pudendal nerve. *J Urol* 1982; 128: 974–980

33. Vodušek DB. Pudendal somatosensory evoked potential and bulbocavernosus reflex in women. *Electroencephalogr Clin Neurophysiol* 1990; 77: 134–136

34. Haldeman S, Bradley WE, Bhatia N, Johnson BK. Cortical evoked potentials on stimulation of pudendal nerve in women. *Urology* 1983; 6: 590–593

35. Tackmann W, Vogel P, Porst H. Somatosensory evoked potentials after stimulation of the dorsal penile nerve: normative data and results from 145 patients with erectile dysfunction. *Eur Neurol* 1987; 27: 245–250

36. Vodušek DB. Pudendal somatosensory evoked potentials. *Neurologija* 1990; 39(Suppl 1): 149–155

37. Guerit JM, Opsomer RJ. Bit-mapped imaging of somatosensory evoked potentials after stimulation of the posterior tibial nerves and dorsal nerve of the penis/clitoris. *Electroencephalogr Clin Neurophysiol* 1991; 80: 228–237

38. Rodi Z, Vodušek DB, Denislic M. Clinical uro-neurophysiological investigation in multiple sclerosis. *Eur J Neurol* 1996; 3: 574–580

39. Vodušek DB, Deletis V, Abbott R, Turndorf H. Prevention of iatrogenic micturition disorders through intraoperative monitoring. (Proceedings of the ICS 20th Annual Meeting, Aarhus, Denmark,12–15 September 1990.) *Neurourol Urodyn* 1990; 9(4): 444–445

40. Cohen BA, Major MR, Huizenga BA. Pudendal nerve evoked potential monitoring in procedures involving low sacral fixation. *Spine* 1991; 16(Suppl 8): 375–378

41. Delodovici ML, Fowler CJ. Clinical value of the pudendal somatosensory evoked potential. *Electroencephalogr Clin Neurophysiol* 1995; 96: 509–515

42. Badr GG, Carlsson CA, Fall M *et al.* Cortical evoked potentials following the stimulation of the urinary bladder in man. *Electroencephalogr Clin Neurophysiol* 1982; 54: 494–498

43. Sarica Y, Karacan I. Bulbocavernosus reflex to somatic and visceral nerve stimulation in normal subjects and in diabetics with erectile impotence. *J Urol* 1986; 138: 55–58

44. Hansen MV, Ertekin C, Larsson LE. Cerebral evoked potentials after stimulation of the posterior urethra in man. *Electroencephalogr Clin Neurophysiol* 1990; 77: 52–58

45. Gänzer H, Madersbacher H, Rumpl E. Cortical evoked potentials by stimulation of the vesicourethral junction: clinical value and neurophysiological considerations. *J Urol* 1991; 146: 118–123

46. Loening-Baucke V, Read NW, Yamada T. Further evaluation of the afferent nervous pathways from the rectum. *Am J Physiol* 1992; 25: G927–G933

47. Rushworth G. Diagnostic value of the electromyographic study of reflex activity in man. *Electroencephalogr Clin Neurophysiol* 1967; (Suppl 25): 65–73

48. Ertekin C, Reel F. Bulbocavernosus reflex in normal men and patients with neurogenic bladder and/or impotence. *J Neurol Sci* 1976; 28: 1–15

49. Vacek J, Lachman M. The bulbocavernosus reflex in diabetics with erectile dysfunction: a clinical and EMG study. *Cas Lek Cesk* 1977; 33: 1014–1017 (in Czech)

50. Krane RJ, Siroky MB. Studies on sacral evoked potentials. *J Urol* 1980; 124: 872–876

51. Vodušek DB. Neurophysiological Study of Bulbocavernosus Reflex in Man. DSc Thesis, University of Ljubljana,1988; 1–129 (in Slovene)

52. Varma JS, Smith AN, McInnes A. Electrophysiological observations on the human pudendo-anal reflex. *J Neurol Neurosurg Psychiatry* 1986; 49: 1411–1416

53. Bilkey WJ, Awad EA, Smith AD. Clinical application of sacral reflex latency. *J Urol* 1983; 129: 1187–1189

54. Contreras Ortiz O, Bertotti AC, Rodriguez Nuñez JD. Pudendal reflexes in women with pelvic floor disorders. *Zentralbl Gynäkol* 1994; 116: 561–565

55. Bradley WE. Urethral electromyelography. *J Urol* 1972; 108: 563–564

56. Fowler CJ, Betts CD. Clinical value of electrophysiological investigations of patients with urinary symptoms. In: Mundy AR, Stephenson TP, Wein AJ (eds) *Urodynamics: Principles, Practice and Application*, 2nd edn. Edinburgh: Churchill Livingstone, 1994; 165–181

57. Pedersen E, Harving H, Klemar B *et al.* Human anal reflexes. *J Neurol Neurosurg Psychiatry* 1978; 41: 813–818

58. Vereecken RI, De Meirsman J, Puers B *et al.* Electrophysiological exploration of the sacral conus. *J Neurol* 1982; 227: 135–144

59. Vodušek DB, Janko M. The bulbocavernosus reflex. A single motor neuron study. *Brain* 1990; 113: 813–820

60. Rodi Z, Vodušek DB. The sacral reflex studies: single versus double pulse stimulation. (Proceedings of the 25th Annual Meeting of the International Continence Society, Sydney, Australia,17–20 October 1995.) *Neurourol Urodyn* 1995; 14: 496–497

61. Hanson P, Rigaux P, Gilliard C, Bisset E. Sacral reflex latencies in tethered cord syndrome. *Am J Phys Med Rehabil* 1993; 72: 39–43

62. Vodušek DB, Deletis V, Abbott R *et al.* Intraoperative monitoring of pudendal nerve function. In: Rother M, Zwiener U (eds). *Quantitative EEG Analysis – Clinical Utility and New Methods.* Jena: Universitatsverlag Jena, 1993; 309–312

63. Deletis V, Vodušek DB. Intraoperative recording of the bulbocavernosus reflex. *Neurosurgery* 1997; 40(1): 88–92

64. Dystra D, Sidi A, Cameron J *et al.* The use of mechanical stimulation to obtain the sacral reflex latency: a new technique. *J Urol* 1987; 137: 77–79

65. Podnar S, Vodušek DB, Trsinar B, Rodi Z. A method of uroneurophysiological investigation in children. *Electroencephalogr Clin Neurophysiol* 1997; 104: 389–392

66. Shahani BT, Halperin JJ, Boulu P, Cohen J. Sympathetic skin response – a method of assessing unmyelinated axon dysfunction in peripheral neuropathies. *J Neurol Neurosurg Psychiatry* 1984; 47: 536–542

67. Opsomer RJ, Pesce Fr, Abi Aad A *et al.* Electrophysiologic testing of motor sympathetic pathways: normative data and clinical contribution in neurourological disorders. (Proceedings of the 23rd Annual Meeting of the International Continence Society, Rome.) *Neurourol Urodyn* 1993; 12: 336–338

68. Daffertshofer M, Linden D, Syren M *et al.* Assessment of local sympathetic function in patients with erectile dysfunction. *Int J Impot Res* 1994; 6: 213–225

69. Koldewijn EL, van Kerrebroeck PEV, Bemelmans BLH *et al.* Use of sacral reflex latency measurements in the evaluation of neural function of spinal cord injury patients: a comparison of neuro-urophysiological testing and urodynamic investigations. *J Urol* 1994; 152: 463–467

70. Liu S, Christmas TJ, Nagendran K *et al.* Sphincter electromyography in patients after radical prostatectomy and cystoprostatectomy. *Br J Urol* 1992; 69: 397

71. Vodušek DB, Light JK. The motor nerve supply of the external urethral sphincter muscles. *Neurourol Urodyn* 1983; 2: 193–200

72. Percy JP, Neill ME, Swash M *et al.* Electrophysiological study of motor nerve supply of pelvic floor. *Lancet* 1980; i:16–17

73. Gearhart JP, Burnett A, Owen JH. Measurement of pudendal evoked potentials during feminizing genitoplasty: technique and applications. *J Urol* 1995; 153: 486

24

Videourodynamics

S. Herschorn

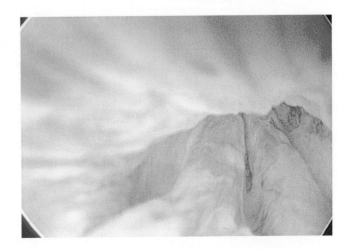

INTRODUCTION

Urodynamics were first synchronized with cineradiography in the early 1950s through the pioneering efforts of E. R. Miller.[1,2] The initial goal was to minimize the radiation exposure to the patient during cystourethrography. Originally, the patient exposure was high when 'movies' were taken; however, with the advent of image intensifiers, video transduction and, later, videotape recording of the images, patient exposure was reduced. This permitted bursts of continuous activity to be recorded during critical phases of lower urinary tract activity without overexposing the patient. Today most studies can be accomplished with less than 1 minute of fluoroscopy time.[3] These developments have contributed a wealth of information to our knowledge about lower urinary tract function and dysfunction. Modern videourodynamic techniques incorporate fluoroscopy with the evolution of the urodynamic machine from a strip chart recorder to a microcomputer.

Videourodynamic studies are not necessary in every patient and simpler studies frequently provide enough information to delineate and treat the dysfunction adequately. Videourodynamic studies are beneficial when simultaneous evaluation of physiology and anatomy is needed to provide detailed information about the whole or parts of the storage and emptying phases. Complex incontinence where the history does not fit with the findings on preliminary investigations, incontinence for which there has been previous surgical intervention, and incontinence in the face of a neurological abnormality, are well suited for videourodynamic evaluation.

The cost involved in the technique, as a result of the time and effort of the personnel and the expense of the machinery, can be justified by its utility in solving complicated problems. The cost also restricts the technique to larger centres where a sufficiently large patient base justifies the expense. In this chapter the procedures are outlined, examples of the applications are provided and the limitations are discussed.

COMPONENTS OF VIDEOURODYNAMICS

A typical arrangement for videourodynamic studies is shown in Figure 24.1. The fluoroscopic table is used in both the supine and upright positions. A video recorder may be used to record the studies for future review.

TESTS PERFORMED

Uroflow

Although the urodynamic catheters have less effect on voiding patterns in females than males, it is still useful to obtain a urine flow (uroflow) reading on arrival of the patient, which may be compared with the flow data generated during the urodynamic study. After the

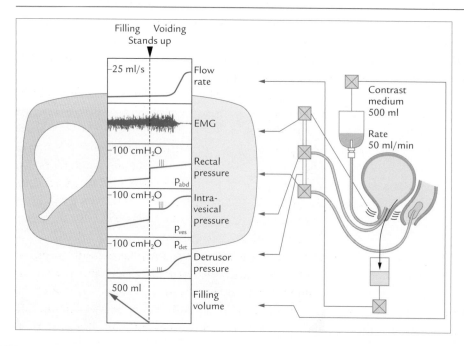

Figure 24.1. *Schematic diagram of videourodynamic set-up.*

uroflow reading has been obtained, the patient's post-void residual can be determined on introduction of the urodynamic catheters.[4]

Cystometry

The first part of the study is cystometry, the method by which the pressure–volume relationship of the bladder is measured.[5] It is used to assess detrusor activity, sensation, capacity and compliance. The detrusor pressure (p_{det}) is calculated by subtraction of the abdominal pressure (p_{abd}), as measured by a rectal balloon, from the total intravesical pressure (p_{ves}). The subtracted detrusor pressure reflects the activity and pressures generated by the detrusor muscle alone. However, artefacts in the p_{det} may be produced by intrinsic rectal contractions.[5]

Overactive detrusor function is characterized by spontaneous or provoked involuntary contractions which the patient cannot completely suppress.[5] Any such contraction seen while the patient is attempting to inhibit micturition is termed *detrusor instability*. Although originally defined as a minimum pressure rise of 15 cmH$_2$O[6] the same diagnosis can be made if the patient's symptoms are reproduced by lesser rises of pressure.[7,8] *Motor urgency* is caused by overactive detrusor function and *sensory urgency* by a hypersensitive bladder;[5] however, it is possible that these are both conditions in the same spectrum and that patients with sensory urgency are able to inhibit the unstable contractions during cystometry but not during activities of normal living.[9] The term *detrusor hyperreflexia* is used to describe the uninhibited contractions when there is objective evidence of an associated neurological disorder.[5]

Another type of overactive bladder dysfunction is reduced compliance. *Bladder compliance* is defined as the change in pressure for a given change in volume.[3] It is calculated by dividing the volume change by the change in detrusor pressure during that change in bladder volume, and is expressed in ml/cmH$_2$O.[5] Normal bladder compliance is high and, in the laboratory, the normal pressure rise is less than 6–10 cmH$_2$O.[3] Low bladder compliance implies a poorly distensible bladder. The actual numerical values to indicate normal, high or low compliance are not yet defined.[5]

The finding of bladder overactivity on cystometry is important if it relates to the clinical condition of the patient. Bladder instability has been reported in 30–35% of patients with stress incontinence undergoing surgery. It resolves in the majority following repairs and does not have a significant impact on outcomes.[10,11] On the other hand, if the patient's symptoms are primarily from bladder overactivity, or if other factors predisposing to abnormal bladder behaviour are present, the cystometric findings will influence treatment. These factors include a history of radiation, chronic bladder inflammation, indwelling catheter, chronic infection, chemotherapy, voiding dysfunction following pelvic surgery and other neurological conditions.

Leak-point pressures

The Valsalva or abdominal leak-point pressure (VLPP) tests the strength of the urethra and is the total abdominal pressure (p_{ves} or p_{abd}) at which leakage occurs during a progressive Valsalva manoeuvre or cough in the absence of a bladder contraction.[12] The study is performed with the subject sitting or standing with approximately 150–200 ml of fluid in the bladder. A VLPP of less than 60 cmH$_2$O is evidence of significant intrinsic sphincter deficiency (ISD) and correlates well with severe leakage; a VLPP of between 60 and 90 cmH$_2$O suggests a component of ISD, and a VLPP of more than 90 cmH$_2$O suggests minimal ISD, with leakage mainly due to hypermobility.[3] A cystocele may produce inferior pressure on an incompetent urethra which will prevent incontinence and falsely elevate the VLPP. When a cystocele is present, the VLPP should be repeated with the prolapse reduced by insertion of a vaginal pack. The VLPP has been shown to be reproducible[13] but has not yet been standardized.

The detrusor or bladder leak-point pressure (LPP) is the detrusor pressure at which urethral leakage occurs during bladder filling on cystometry. This parameter is used to investigate and follow-up patients with neurogenic and low-compliance bladders. In general, patients with a detrusor LPP of more than 25–30 cmH$_2$O are at risk for upper tract deterioration from reflux or obstruction;[8,14] in these patients it is necessary to assess compliance as well. A high detrusor LPP indicates poor compliance with urethral obstruction whereas a low detrusor LPP is seen in patients with incompetent urethras. In order to demonstrate poor compliance in these patients, filling may be done with a Foley catheter to obstruct the outlet.[15] If both the compliance and the detrusor LPP are low, treatment has to be directed to the bladder as well as the outlet.

Electromyography

Sphincter electromyography (EMG) during videourodynamics is used to examine striated sphincter activity during filling and voiding. These are termed kinesiological studies and can be performed with surface electrodes, vaginal or anal probes, and needles. Normal sphincter EMG activity has a characteristic audio quality which may be monitored simultaneously. Its most important role is the identification of abnormal sphincter activity in patients with neurogenic bladder dysfunction and in those with voiding dysfunction of behavioural origin.[16] EMG recordings are not necessary in routine videourodynamics for incontinence in females who have no neurological abnormalities.

Pressure–flow studies

Pressure–flow studies are designed to provide dynamic information on the emptying phase of lower urinary tract function. Obstruction is not common in females,[17] but may be found after surgical correction of stress

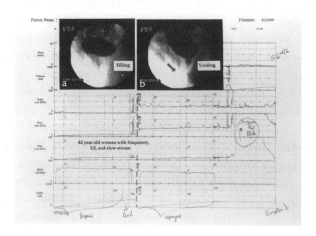

Figure 24.2. *Videourodynamic study of a 62-year-old woman with lower urinary tract irritative symptoms following multiple urethral dilatations. The study shows a stable bladder on filling. Her voiding pressure exceeds 170 cmH₂O and her flow rate is low. There is a urethral stricture visible (arrow in b) with proximal dilatation. p_{abd}, abdominal pressure; p_{ves}, intravesical pressure; p_{det}, detrusor pressure; I_{H_2O}, infusion rate of water; V_{H_2O}, volume of water.*

urinary incontinence and less commonly with detrusor sphincter dyssynergia, with pseudodyssynergia[18] and, rarely, with stricture disease. Interference with voiding may also be associated with pelvic organ prolapse. Although there are no established nomograms to depict pressure/flow in women as there are in men, a pattern of high detrusor pressure and low urinary flow indicates obstruction (Fig. 24.2). Simultaneous cystography can demonstrate the level.

Detrusor pressure during voiding is characteristically low in females. A preoperative study which demonstrates a low detrusor pressure with a low flow rate, if the free flow rate is low as well, may aid in counselling the patient about postoperative urinary retention after stress incontinence surgery.

URODYNAMIC EQUIPMENT REQUIRED

Uroflowmeters

Flow meters are commonly of one of three types: weight, electronic dipstick, or rotating disc.[7] The first measures the weight of the collected urine; the second measures the changes in electrical capacitance of a dipstick mounted in the collecting chamber; the third measures the power required to keep a rotating disc rotating at a constant speed while the urine, which tends to slow it down, is directed towards it. All three can provide high sensitivity and reproducibility of data.

Multichannel recorder

As the procedure involves measuring simultaneous pressures during both phases of lower urinary tract function and flow during the voiding phase, a multichannel recorder is necessary. Many systems are available,[19] most of which have dispensed with a strip-chart output in favour of a television monitor display of the procedure.

The actual choice of components of the study is up to the individual clinician. Figure 24.1 illustrates the possible inclusions. The channels demonstrating volume of fluid instilled and volume voided are helpful but not essential, as these can be measured manually. The EMG channel is not necessary for routine clinical practice but can be helpful if many patients with neurological disease are seen; its inclusion introduces another level of complexity and sophistication. Furthermore, the fluoroscopy component will demonstrate detrusor external sphincter dyssynergia in patients with suprasacral lesions and will show urethral obstruction in patients with dysfunctional voiding.

Controversy exists regarding the use of subtracted detrusor pressure versus intravesical pressure. Bladder pressure can be recorded only via the pressure line in the bladder. This pressure is affected by intra-abdominal pressure, which can be measured separately by a rectal catheter. Increases in intra-abdominal pressure can result from straining, the upright position, and other provocative activities such as coughing, jumping and heel jouncing. In order to get an accurate recording of bladder pressure and to eliminate the effect of intra-abdominal pressure, Bates *et al.*[20] emphasized the value of electronically subtracting the intra-abdominal pressure from the intravesical pressure. However, even with the patient quiescent and totally cooperative, artefacts may be produced by intrinsic rectal contractions,[5] since the bladder pressure is derived from the electronic subtraction. On the other hand, McGuire *et al.*[21] do not measure rectal or abdominal pressure with a separate catheter, but monitor urethral pressure together with bladder pressure through two lumens of the same catheter. They state that urethral pressure reflects rectal or abdominal pressure, allowing them to differentiate bladder contractions from abdominal straining. In our unit, we use the technique of subtracted detrusor pressure.

Fluoroscopy

Any good-quality fluoroscopy unit with a high-resolution image intensifier and a table that can function in both supine and erect positions is satisfactory. Fluoroscopic images are obtained selectively during the filling and voiding study and are either superimposed on the pressure–flow tracing or displayed on a separate screen. The fluoroscopic images can be stored and reproduced individually or as continuous clips during key parts of the study. A recording of the procedure can be made for subsequent review.

Since the contrast medium instilled into the bladder is unlikely to be absorbed, we generally use the less-expensive high-osmolality contrast media. A dilute solution of one litre of Hypaque is prepared by the pharmacy and supplied in sterile bags for intravenous use.

VIDEOURODYNAMIC TECHNIQUE

The patient reports for the examination with a full bladder, and a flow rate is obtained. The patient is then catheterized with the urodynamics catheters and may be fitted with the EMG recording devices, if this procedure is to be performed. The equipment is then zeroed. Two 8F (38 cm) infant-feeding tubes – one for filling, which is removed prior to the voiding study, and one for pressure measurements – are inserted into the bladder. Residual urine is measured. The rectal catheter is a 14F (42 cm) with a balloon over the tip.

A supine or semi-oblique filling study is carried out and various measurements are taken during the study and responses to actions such as Credé or Valsalva manoeuvres, or coughing, are recorded. The filling is usually at a medium rate of 50–75 ml/min.[5] The bladder is filled, emptied and then refilled in the patient's usual voiding position (lying, sitting or standing). Two bladder fillings are usually done since decreased compliance may be a result of the medium filling rate[22] and a second test verifies it. The upright position of the second filling is also a provocative test for instability.[5] Additional responses to Credé, and Valsalva manoeuvres and cough are again recorded.

During the study, recordings are made of bladder images in the filling phase in the supine and/or in the upright positions. Anteroposterior (AP) and oblique views are obtained. The AP position permits documentation of reflux and its extent; in the oblique position, the course of the urethra can be seen separate from a cystocele. Note is made of the bladder outline and its position relative to the symphysis and appearance of the bladder neck at rest and with straining and coughing. Leakage of urine with instability, or decreased compliance, or with various stress manoeuvres is recorded. In the upright position, the presence of a cystocele and its relationship to the urethra are also noted. The voiding phase (or parts of it) are recorded if the patient can void in front of the camera, when the pressures and flow are recorded together with the fluoroscopic image. If the patient cannot void with the catheters in place they are removed and the uroflow may be measured; the voided volume is also measured. Total fluoroscopy time is usually less than a minute.

The recorded study provides an opportunity for the case to be reviewed and discussed. All of the events of the study are recorded and displayed on the monitor during the study. The urodynamic machine is usually equipped with the capability of compressing the study so that it can be viewed on an ordinary letter-size sheet of paper.

INDICATIONS AND EXAMPLES

Urinary incontinence

The main advantage of fluoroscopic imaging during the urodynamic study is to obtain an anatomical view of the function or dysfunction. The technique is ideally suited to the evaluation of incontinence. A useful anatomical/radiological classification of female incontinence is given in Table 24.1.[23] We use this classification to describe the radiological abnormality and add to it the information from the VLPP and the position of the urethra in relation to the cystocele to describe the functional problem. Each of the urodynamic tracings in the figures is shown in full with annotations made during the study. The video recordings depicting crucial parts of the studies were obtained from an image printer connected to the fluoroscope.

Type I abnormalities are illustrated in Figures 24.3 and 24.4. The patient in Figure 24.3 leaks with a VLPP of 62 cmH$_2$O, indicating a probable component of ISD in her incontinence. The patient in Figure 24.4 also has a high VLPP of more than 120 cmH$_2$O on straining during upright filling. At the end of filling, a cough causes a large leak without much hypermobility and appears to be accompanied by a small bladder contraction; this indicates that she has stress incontinence as well as cough-induced instability.

Figures 24.5–24.8 demonstrate type IIa abnormalities. The patient in Figure 24.5 has a high VLPP indicating primarily a hypermobile urethra without any appreciable cystocele. In Figure 24.6, the patient has an unstable contraction with incontinence in the upright position; she also has a high VLPP. The patient shown in Figure 24.7 has a grade II cystocele that appears with straining; she probably has mainly a lateral defect.[24]

The patient in Figure 24.8 complained primarily of urgency incontinence. Although she has a type IIa defect, no leakage was demonstrated (type 0). She has small contractions at the end of the upright filling, showing bladder instability.

Type IIb abnormalities are shown in Figures 24.9–24.11. The bladder neck in Figure 24.9 is seen well below the lower margin of the symphysis and is associated with a grade 2 cystocele. Since the bladder neck is

---

Table 24.1 *Radiological types of stress incontinence (Blaivas classification)*

Type	Features
0	Vesical neck and proximal urethra closed at rest and situated at or above the lower end of the symphysis pubis. They descend during stress but incontinence is not seen.
I	Vesical neck closed at rest and is well above the inferior margin of the symphysis. During stress the vesical neck and proximal urethra open and descend less than 2 cm. Incontinence is seen.
IIa	Vesical neck closed at rest and is above the inferior margin of the symphysis. During stress the vesical neck and proximal urethra open and descend more than 2 cm. Incontinence is seen.
IIb	Vesical neck closed at rest and is at or below the inferior margin of the symphysis. During stress there may or may not be further descent but the proximal urethra opens and incontinence is seen.
III	Vesical neck and proximal urethra are open at rest. The proximal urethra no longer functions as a sphincter. There is obvious urinal leakage with minimal increases in intravesical pressure.

From ref. 23.

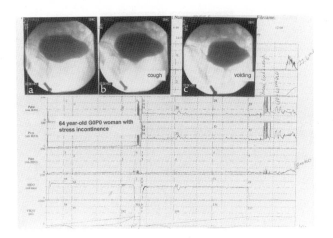

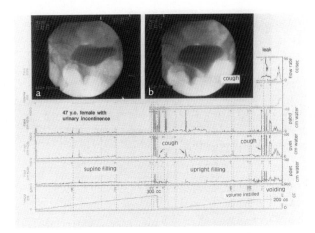

Figure 24.3. *Videourodynamic study of a 64-year-old G4P4 woman with type I stress incontinence. She has a normal bladder capacity. The bladder neck is slightly open at rest (a). With coughing (b) there is a small amount of descent and her Valsalva leak-point pressure is 62 cmH₂O. She has no apparent cystocele and her voiding phase (c) is normal. Abbreviations as in Figure 24.2.*

Figure 24.5. *Videourodynamic study of a 47-year-old G1P1 woman with type IIa stress incontinence. Her bladder neck is open at rest (a). Leakage and hypermobility are seen with coughing (b). Abbreviations as in Figure 24.2.*

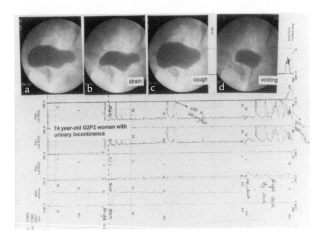

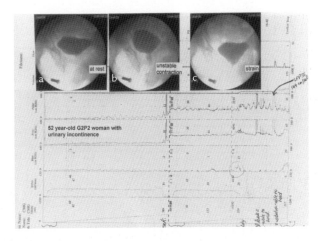

Figure 24.4. *Videourodynamic study of a 74-year-old G2P2 woman with type I stress incontinence. Her bladder neck is slightly open at rest (a). In the upright position (b) she leaks with straining and a Valsalva leak-point pressure of 122 cmH₂O. She also leaks with coughing (c) that is followed by a detrusor contraction (arrow). Her voiding is normal (d). Abbreviations as in Figure 24.2.*

Figure 24.6. *Videourodynamic study of a 52-year-old G2P2 woman with a type IIa abnormality who complains of both stress and urgency incontinence. The bladder neck is slightly open at rest (a). She has an unstable contraction (arrow) on upright filling that results in incontinence (b). With straining she leaks with a Valsalva leak-point pressure of more than 140 cmH₂O (c). Abbreviations as in Figure 24.2.*

above the base of the cystocele, the patient probably has a combined central and lateral defect. In Figure 24.10 the grade 2–3 cystocele is not associated with demonstrable stress incontinence, despite coughing and straining pressures of more than 100 cmH₂O; it appears to be primarily a central defect. Clinical examination must include reducing the cystocele and checking for stress incontinence. The patient in Figure 24.11 has a

combined central and lateral defect. She has marked bladder instability with urgency incontinence but stress incontinence is not demonstrated because of the compressive effect of the cystocele.

Type III incontinence or pure ISD is demonstrated by the patient in Figure 24.12. Her bladder neck is open at rest, no appreciable descensus is seen with coughing or straining, and her VLPP is low at 59 cmH₂O.

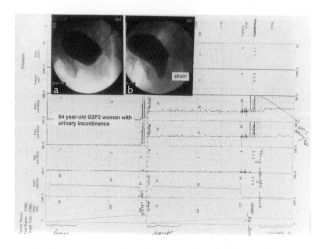

Figure 24.7. *Videourodynamic study of a 64-year-old G2P2 woman with type IIa stress incontinence. Her bladder neck is well supported on upright filling (a) and with straining (b) she leaks with a Valsalva leak-point pressure of 144 cmH2O and a cystocele is demonstrated It is probable that she has mainly a lateral defect. Abbreviations as in Figure 24.2.*

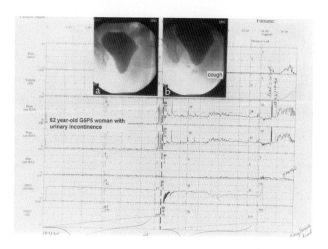

Figure 24.9. *Videourodynamic study of a 62-year-old G5P5 woman with type IIb stress incontinence. Her bladder neck (arrow) on filling (a) is below the symphyseal margin and a cystocele is seen. It is most likely that she has a combined central and lateral defect. She has leakage with coughing (b) and a Valsalva leak-point pressure of 62 cmH2O on straining. Abbreviations as in Figure 24.2.*

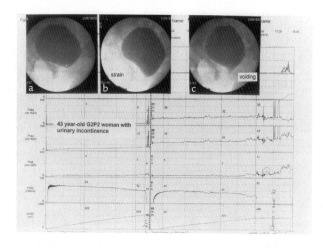

Figure 24.8. *Videourodynamic study of a 43-year-old G2P2 woman complaining of urge incontinence. Filling is normal and the bladder neck is well supported (a). On straining (b), she has type IIa descent but no incontinence is seen (type 0). She has unstable contractions at the end of upright filling (arrows). Her voiding is normal (c). Abbreviations as in Figure 24.2.*

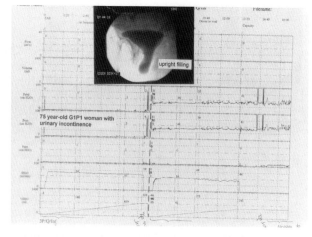

Figure 24.10. *Videourodynamic study of a 75-year-old G1P1 woman with a grade 2–3 cystocele (upright filling). Although she complains of stress incontinence it is not visible on this study. Her bladder neck (arrow) is at the lower margin of the symphysis. The cystocele appears primarily to be a central defect. Clinical evaluation must include reducing the cystocele and testing for stress incontinence. She may need a suspension in addition to the cystocele repair if surgery is opted for. Abbreviations as in Figure 24.2.*

Neurogenic bladder dysfunction

Videourodynamics can be helpful in assessing patients with neurogenic bladders. Since incontinence and upper tract dilatation can be prevented and treated by achieving a low-pressure storage and emptying system,[14,25] the study provides a framework for treatment. Anatomical abnormalities can be correlated with pressure changes.

Examples of neurogenic problems are shown in Figures 24.13–24.15. As the flow rate is not measured in

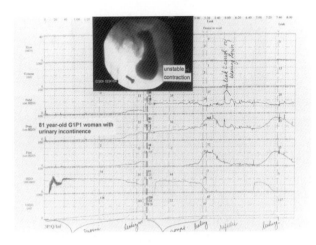

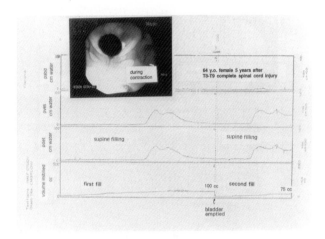

Figure 24.11. *Videourodynamic study of an 81-year-old G1P1 woman with a central and lateral defect. The bladder neck is below the symphysis (arrow). She has marked instability on supine and upright filling (open arrows). Although she complains of stress, in addition to urge incontinence, it is not demonstrated on this study. Abbreviations as in Figure 24.2.*

Figure 24.13. *Videourodynamic study of a 64-year-old woman 5 years after a T8–9 spinal cord injury following a motor vehicle accident. She has left vesicoureteral reflux (open arrow) seen during hyperreflexic contractions (arrows). Abbreviations as in Figure 24.2.*

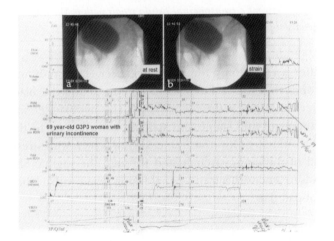

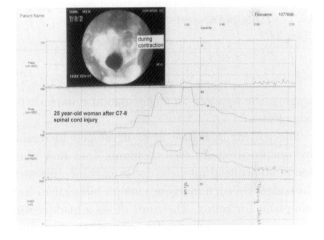

Figure 24.12. *Videourodynamic study of a 69-year-old G3P3 woman with type III abnormality. Her bladder neck is open at rest (arrow in a). On straining (b) there is no hypermobility and her Valsalva leak-point pressure is 59 cmH₂O. She has had two previous stress incontinence repairs. Abbreviations as in Figure 24.2.*

Figure 24.14. *Videourodynamic study of a 25-year-old woman with a C7–8 lesion 16 months after spinal cord injury following a motor vehicle accident. She needed an indwelling catheter for repeated attacks of autonomic dysreflexia and her upper tracts showed marked bilateral hydronephrosis. Her bladder is markedly trabeculated and during a contraction her external sphincter remains tight, consistent with detrusor sphincter dyssynergia. She was subsequently treated with an ileal augmentation cystoplasty and a continent abdominal stoma. Abbreviations as in Figure 24.2.*

Figures 24.13 and 24.14, fewer channels are used during the study.

The patient in Figure 24.13 has a small-capacity hyperreflexic but compliant bladder with grade 1 left vesicoureteral reflux. Her main problem was incontinence between catheterizations and treatment is with anticholinergics and monitoring of her upper tracts. The patient in Figure 24.14 has a markedly trabeculated hyperreflexic bladder with filling pressures of more than 100 cmH₂O. The study demonstrates detrusor external sphincter dyssynergia with an open bladder neck and tight sphincter. She also had bilateral hydronephrosis, as shown on upper tract

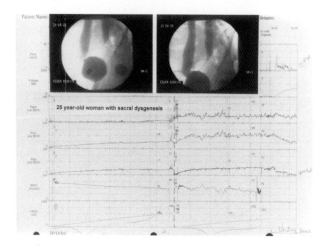

Figure 24.15. *Videourodynamic study of a 25-year-old woman with sacral dysgenesis. She had an artificial sphincter inserted for urinary incontinence at age 14 years and then developed bilateral vesicoureteral reflux unresponsive to multiple ureteral reimplantations. The study shows decreased bladder compliance on filling (arrows). She has gross bilateral reflux and a small-capacity bladder. She subsequently underwent augmentation ileal cystoplasty and bilateral reimplants. Abbreviations as in Figure 24.2.*

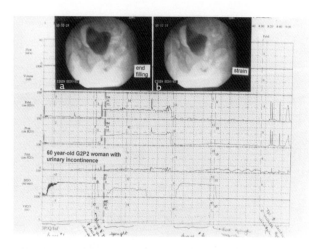

Figure 24.16. *Videourodynamic study of a 60-year-old G2P2 woman who underwent an ileal neobladder to urethra after cystectomy for muscle-invasive carcinoma of the bladder. The study was conducted with a Foley catheter blocking the urethra to test compliance (a), which is normal. All of the leakage was demonstrated to exit the fistula at the anastomosis (arrow in b). She underwent a transvaginal fistula repair with a Martius labial fat-pad flap. Abbreviations as in Figure 24.2.*

imaging; she required an augmentation cystoplasty for management.

The patient in Figure 24.15 developed increasing hydronephrosis and raised creatinine level after insertion of an artificial sphincter for urinary incontinence. She had previously undergone multiple bilateral ureteral reimplants for reflux. The study shows a bladder with poor compliance and gross bilateral reflux. The refluxing ureters probably dampen the bladder pressure, thus improving the appearance of the compliance curve. She was also treated with an augmentation cystoplasty.

Other urodynamic problems

Obstruction

Although outflow obstruction is uncommon in female patients,[17] it is occasionally seen. The patient in Figure 24.2 had an iatrogenic and functionally significant urethral stricture that was treated by visual internal urethrotomy.

Complex problems

The patient in Figure 24.16 had a fistula at the anastomosis between an ileal neobladder and the urethra

after a cystectomy for bladder cancer. The study was conducted with a Foley catheter obstructing the bladder neck to test the compliance. The neobladder was compliant and stable and was not contributing to the incontinence. No urethral leakage was seen with stress; all of the contrast emanated through the vagina. She was treated with a transvaginal fistula repair with a labial fat-pad flap.

PITFALLS OF VIDEOURODYNAMICS

In order that a meaningful and relevant study can be conducted, the patient has to be relaxed and compliant. Occasionally, apprehensive patients will faint when the table is moved from the supine to the upright position and the study cannot be completed. Furthermore, with an apprehensive patient, stress incontinence may not be demonstrated. Of 1103 studies that we have reviewed in our laboratory for neurologically normal women whose chief complaint was stress incontinence, we were unable to demonstrate stress incontinence on fluoroscopy in 239 (21.7%). It is also difficult for many patients to void in front of the camera, with catheters in the bladder and rectum and observers watching them. In our series, only 585 patients (53%) were able to void, and some of these did so with abdominal straining; the others were unable to void during the procedure and the voiding data were obtained from the uroflow study.

The position of the patient has to be correct to optimize visibility of the lower urinary tract on fluoroscopy. Visibility may be poor or absent with very obese patients. The clinician also has to maintain a dialogue with the patient to image crucial events, as the patient must relay changes in sensation during filling and may be the first to sense incontinence.

The radiation equipment must be well maintained and undergo regular maintenance and safety inspections. Since fluoroscopy time is short, radiation exposure to the patient should not be a problem; however, the clinician should use recommended radiation protection such as aprons and thyroid shields.

The other pitfalls relate to the urodynamic aspects and are similar to those previously outlined by O'Donnell.[26] Standardized terminology to communicate results and concepts should always be used. The testing procedures and equipment should be compatible with commonly accepted methodologies. The value and limitations of each measurement must be realized: for example, the VLPP may not be useful in the presence of a grade 3 cystocele. To confirm reliability within a particular laboratory it is necessary to have a high test–retest correlation of studies. The validity of a test refers to its ability to measure what it is supposed to measure. The clinician must always be aware of how the test compares with a 'gold-standard' test, which, in urodynamics, may be difficult to establish. The urodynamic studies should correlate with other clinical data: the voiding history, the physical examination, the endoscopic examination, the urodynamic evaluation and, in this case, the radiological studies, should serve to validate one another and strengthen the clinical assessment. Finally, any failure to maintain equipment may lead to inaccurate results.

CONCLUSIONS

Videourodynamic techniques have evolved over the years, with improvements in technology and refinements in the concepts of lower urinary tract structure, function and treatment. There are exciting developments in other newer imaging technogies. Ultrasonography can be used during urodynamic studies but the vaginal probe alters the position of the bladder neck,

and perineal probes are undergoing investigation.[27] Magnetic resonance imaging has provided significant advances in knowledge about the pelvic floor,[28] but it is carried out in the supine position and interventional magnetic resonance has not been adapted to the technique. The tests, therefore, are as relevant today, for the appropriate indications, as when they were first conceptualized almost 50 years ago.

REFERENCES

1. Miller E. The beginnings. *Urol Clin North Am* 1979; 6: 7–9

2. Enhörning G, Miller ER, Hinman F Jr. Urethral closure studied by cine-roentgenography and simultaneous bladder–urethra pressure recording. *Surg Gynecol Obstet* 1964; 118: 507–516

3. Webster GD, Kreder KJ. The neurourologic evaluation. In: Walsh PC, Retik AB, Vaughan ED Jr Wein AJ (eds) *Campbell's Urology*, 7th edn. Philadelphia: Saunders, 1998; 927–952

4. Abrams P, Torrens M. Urine flow studies. *Urol Clin North Am* 1979; 6: 71–79

5. Abrams P, Blaivas JG, Stanton SL, Andersen JT. Standardisation of terminology of lower urinary tract function. *Neurourol Urodyn* 1988; 7: 403–427

6. Bates P, Bradley WE, Glen E *et al.* First report on the standardization of terminology of lower urinary tract function. *Br J Urol* 1976; 48: 39–42

7. Massey A, Abrams P. Urodynamics of the female lower urinary tract. *Urol Clin North Am* 1985; 12: 231–246

8. Blaivas JG. Cystometry. In: Blaivas JG (ed) *Atlas of Urodynamics.* Baltimore: Williams and Wilkins, 1996; 31–47

9. Creighton SM, Pearce JM, Robson I *et al.* Sensory urgency: how full is your bladder? *Br J Obstet Gynaecol* 1991; 98: 1287–1289

10. Awad SA, Flood HD, Acker KL. The significance of prior anti-incontinence surgery in women who present with urinary incontinence. *J Urol* 1988; 140: 514–517

11. McGuire EJ. Bladder instability in stress incontinence. *Neurourol Urodyn* 1988; 7: 563

12. McGuire EJ, Fitzpatrick CC, Wan J *et al.* Clinical assessment of urethral sphincter function. *J Urol* 1993; 150: 1452–1454

13. Heritz DM, Blaivas JG. Reliability and specificity of the leak point pressure. *J Urol* 1995; 153: 492A

14. McGuire EJ, Woodside JR, Borden TA, Weiss RM. Prognostic value of urodynamic studies in myelodysplastic children. *J Urol* 1981; 126: 205–209

15. Woodside JR, McGuire EJ. Technique for detection of detrusor hypertonia in the presence of urethral sphincteric incompetence. *J Urol* 1982; 127: 740-743

16. Fowler C. Electromyography. In: Blaivas JG (ed) *Atlas of Urodynamics*. Baltimore: Williams and Wilkins, 1996; 60–76

17. Farrar D, Turner-Warwick R. Outflow obstruction in the female. *Urol Clin North Am* 1979; 6: 217–225

18. Wein, AJ, Barrett, DM. Other voiding dysfunctions and related topics. In: Wein AJ, Barrett DM (eds) *Voiding Function and Dysfunction*. Chicago: Medical Year Book, 1988; 274–301

19. Blaivas JG. Deciding on the right urodynamic equipment. In: Blaivas JG (ed) *Atlas of Urodynamics*. Baltimore: Williams and Wilkins, 1996; 19–28

20. Bates CP, Whiteside G, Turner-Warwick R. Synchronous cine/pressure/flow cysto-urethrography with special reference to stress and urge incontinence. *Br J Urol* 1970; 42: 714–723

21. McGuire EJ, Cespedes RD, Cross CA, O'Connell HE. Videourodynamic studies. *Urol Clin North Am* 1996; 23: 309–321

22. Webb RJ, Styles RA, Griffiths CJ *et al.* Ambulatory monitoring of patients with low compliance as a result of neurogenic bladder dysfunction. *Br J Urol* 1989; 64: 150–154

23. Blaivas JG, Olsson CA. Stress incontinence: classification and surgical approach. *J Urol* 1988; 139: 727–731

24. Raz S, Stothers L, Chopra A. Vaginal reconstructive surgery for incontinence and prolapse. In: Walsh PC, Retik AB, Vaughan ED Jr, Wein AJ (eds) *Campbell's Urology*, 7th edn. Philadelphia: Saunders, 1998; 1059–1094

25. Barkin M, Dolfin D, Herschorn S. The urologic care of the spinal cord injured patient. *J Urol* 1983; 129: 335–339

26. O'Donnell PD. Pitfalls of urodynamic testing. *Urol Clin North Am* 1991; 18: 257–268

27. Virtanen HS, Kiilhoma PJA. Ultrasound urodynamics. In: Blaivas JG (ed) *Atlas of Urodynamics*. Baltimore: Williams and Wilkins, 1996; 117–125

28. Yang A, Mostwin JL, Rosenshein N, Zerhouni EA. Pelvic floor descent in women: dynamic evaluation with fast MR imaging and cinematic display. *Radiology* 1991; 179: 25–33

25

Ambulatory urodynamics

S. Salvatore, V. Khullar, L. Cardozo

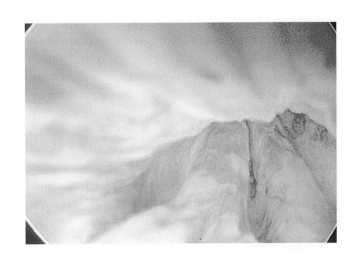

INTRODUCTION

Laboratory urodynamics is currently the 'gold standard' in the objective assessment of urinary symptoms. However, it is necessarily unphysiological because it measures pressures during retrograde bladder filling using a fast filling rate and during voiding.

In the past, attempts have been made to monitor lower urinary tract function on a long-term basis and in an ambulant patient. The aim was to overcome some of the problems encountered in standard urodynamics.

The first problem is physiological: when monitoring detrusor function using standard urodynamics, fast retrograde bladder filling is employed, which is necessarily provocative. The second is environmental: incontinence is a benign condition, and reliance is placed on the person's symptoms as evidence of disease; many of these symptoms are related to acts of everyday life, all of which are removed in a laboratory atmosphere. Thirdly, throughout the period of time during which the standard urodynamic tests are being conducted, the individual is the focus of attention and is asked to respond to certain commands; this may lead to cortical suppression of detrusor activity.

The first description of a bladder-pressure measurement in an ambulant patient was reported by Mackay[1] using radiotelemetry, followed by many other methods. To allow an individual to be mobile, the system must employ telemetry, long cables or portable recording units. In the first systems, telemetry was used.[2–5] A pressure-sensitive radio pill was inserted into the bladder, allowing intravesical pressure to be monitored without the presence of a foreign body in the urethra. However, the cost, limited range of transmission and occasional difficulty in retrieval prevented its widespread use.

In standard urodynamics the lines used are fluid filled. A study of natural filling in spinal injury patients[6] demonstrated increased phasic activity. However, in general, fluid-filled lines are not recommended as they are prone to movement artefact and the pressures measured are dependent on the relative position of the pressure transducer to the tip of the fluid-filled line; thus, the baseline measurement alters as the woman changes position. Air is not subject to the same movement artefact, and air-filled tubes have been used in ambulatory urodynamics.[2] In this system, one end of the tube is filled by a meniscus of urine and the other is covered by a compliant balloon to prevent fluid travelling down the tube and thus producing artefact. In this set-up, the position of the catheter relative to the transducer is unimportant; unfortunately, however, changes in the temperature can alter pressure measurement.

As time has progressed, tape-recording systems have been used. Initially, these systems had a limited capacity which enabled pressures to be recorded only above a certain pre-set threshold.[7] If the patient became symptomatic during the test, but the threshold had not been met, then the pressure was unrecorded and therefore no substantive diagnosis was provided. Subsequently, Griffiths[8] has developed an ambulatory system using micro-tip pressure transducers and a digital solid-state recorder. In this system the information is recorded digitally, transferred and then reviewed at the end of the test. The trace can then be compressed or expanded without loss of information.

EQUIPMENT

There are three main components to an ambulatory system (Figs 25.1–25.3): these are (1) the transducers; (2) the recording unit, and (3) the analysing system.

The transducers are solid state and are mounted on a 7F bladder and rectal catheter, to measure the pressure impinging on it. Most transducers have the pressure-sensitive membrane a few millimetres beyond the tip of the catheter and therefore pressure changes are recorded when the tip touches the side of the bladder. This can be overcome by inserting two

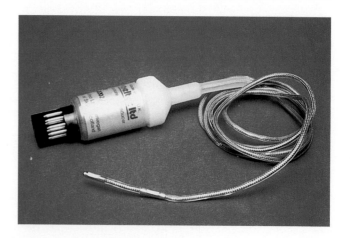

Figure 25.1. *Bladder pressure catheter.*

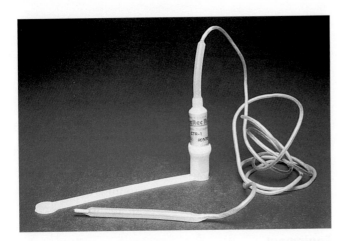

Figure 25.2. *Rectal pressure catheter.*

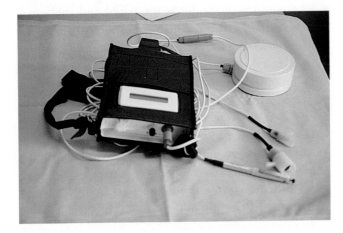

Figure 25.3. *Ambulatory urodynamic equipment.*

catheters, and the intravesical pressure change is deemed significant only if it is recorded on both transducers. The rectal catheter is covered with silicone in order to protect it from deformation.[9] There can be problems with drift of the transducer, but this is usually less than $3\,cmH_2O$ within the 4-hour test.[8]

The recording system must be portable and, ideally, battery powered to allow freedom of movement. Sampling of the pressures should be at 4 Hz and the memory should be digital, allowing the trace to be compressed and expanded. A trace should not be interpreted in isolation: a recording unit should have some means of marking events during the test – the simpler the better, as patients often find multiple buttons confusing and pressing the wrong button can confuse the interpretation. As well as marking the event, it is helpful if there is some mechanism of timing, either by having an in-built timer in the unit or by asking the

patient to record the time. The recorder should have an option to be connected to an electronic 'nappy' (diaper), allowing accurate information about urine loss. In addition there should be a connector to a gravimetric flow meter that will calculate pressure–flow curves and check when detrusor instability has occurred.

The pressure traces are downloaded onto a computer, which can then analyse detrusor and urethral function. There are a variety of different formats. The software available today enables the trace to be expanded or compressed, the scales to be changed, a pressure–flow study to be analysed and a computerized archive of the tests performed to be maintained. It is important to choose the appropriate scale for the pressure and time measurements; the patient's diary and trace should be reviewed with the patient. This allows further information to be gleaned, which a simple system of pushing buttons might have missed.

The urine loss itself needs to be evaluated. Using a weighed perineal pad for the length of the test gives some idea of the severity of the incontinence, but gives little information about when the loss occurred. If the timing of the loss can be calculated, then the manometric changes leading to incontinence can be interpreted and may be helpful in determining the cause of urinary leakage. There are three ways of achieving this. The first is the Urilos (Exeter) (Fig. 25.4) electronic nappy, which has already been alluded to. It has elongated, interleaved electrodes embedded in absorbent material. A 50 mV (low-voltage) alternating current is passed between the two

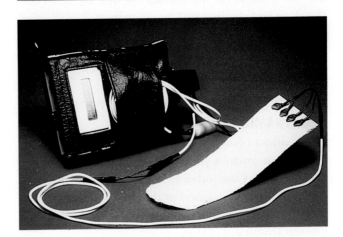

Figure 25.4. *'Urilos' pad connected to the recording unit.*

electrodes; as the urine loss increases, so does this current. Obviously, this depends on the electrodes being within the urine, which is definitely not guaranteed, and so the pad has to be preloaded with a known volume of electrolyte solution. This method is suitable only for volumes between 1 and 100 ml and is reproducible within 20%.

The second method is to measure perineal temperature, which is usually 30–40°C. Urine has a higher temperature than that of the body, 37°C. When there is leakage of urine there is a transient rise in temperature which then falls rapidly, allowing effective detection of distinct episodes of urine loss. The rate of the temperature increase may correlate well with the quantity of leaked urine. A single temperature detector is ineffective, as the position of the detector in relation to the leaked urine changes; hence, a parallel array of diodes has been used with a separate reference diode. Problems of interpretation can occur if the patient has her legs together when seated, as the perineal temperature may then rise.

The third method relies on a catheter placed within the urethra. Two electrodes are mounted on the catheter and an electrical current is passed between them. If urine is passed, either voluntarily or involuntarily, there is increased conduction and a larger current passes across the electrodes. It is vital that the electrodes are placed correctly: for instance, with the electrode in the proximal urethra, a change in the electrical current would indicate the presence of urine; however, this may not have originated from urinary leakage, as this can occur with urethral instability. Conversely, if the electrodes are not in the urethra, then no leakage would be detected. Distal urethral electrical conductance is not used clinically in ambulatory urodynamics, but is mainly a research tool.

METHOD OF CONDUCTING AN AMBULATORY URODYNAMIC STUDY

The conduct of ambulatory urodynamic studies differs in different units. A specific International Continence Society (ICS) Committee is now working on the standardization of the method of this dianostic test.

The following protocol is that employed at the King's College Hospital, London.

Preparation

- All patients should be informed that the procedure will take at least 4 hours.
- They should be asked to wear loose comfortable separate clothing (e.g. track suit).
- If the patient wishes to empty her bowels, it is better to do so before the test.
- Patients are asked to drink 180 ml of fluid (equivalent to a cupful) every hour. This amount is estimated on the basis of a daily fluid intake of about 2 litres.

Equipment

- The equipment should be prepared and calibrated in accordance with the manufacturer's instructions.
- The catheters should be zeroed to air prior to insertion. Failure to do this often leads to the recording going out of range.
- Transducers are stored in a moist environment until required, then sterilized in Cidex and rinsed in sterile water before insertion.
- All transducers and equipment are used with an aseptic technique.
- A Urilos quantitative urine leakage detector is worn by the patient. The size of the Urilos can be comparable to a commercially available sanitary towel[9] and can be fixed to the patient's underpants by adhesive wings.

Set-up

- The reasons for the test and all the procedures should be explained in full; patient compliance is essential.
- Urinary tract infection should be excluded before the test.
- Catheters are inserted using an aseptic technique. Both bladder transducers are placed in the bladder in order to exclude artefacts during analysis (Figs 25.5–25.7). The rectal catheter is inserted into the rectum inside a non-lubricated condom, to prevent contamination of the silicone coating.
- Once inserted, the catheters are taped to the inner thigh close to the labia, (as close to the urethra as possible) using several pieces of 5 cm micropore tape. The lines are then brought forward, over the abdomen, and arranged to be accessible through the clothing.

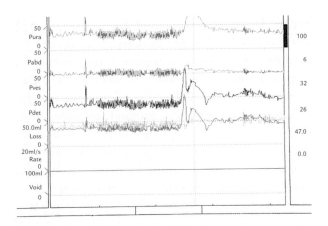

Figure 25.5. *Ambulatory urodynamic trace showing abnormal detrusor activity with pressure rise on the detrusor line and on both the 'intravesical' transducers in the presence of leakage.*

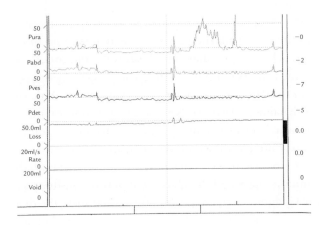

Figure 25.6. *Ambulatory urodynamic trace showing an artefact on the urethral line.*

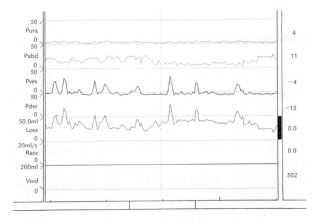

Figure 25.7. *Ambulatory urodynamic trace showing an artefact on the bladder line.*

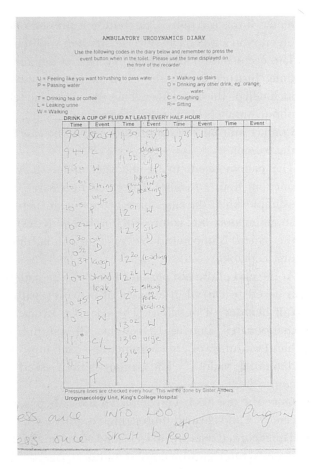

Figure 25.8. *Ambulatory urodynamic diary filled in by a woman.*

- The previously calibrated ambulatory box is then connected to the catheters and arranged for maximum patient comfort.

Procedure

- Once the set-up is completed the read-out can be checked on the real-time trace. If the trace is satisfactory the test may proceed.
- The patient is instructed in the use of the diary (Fig. 25.8). This will provide information of activity during the test. It is essential that the woman understands the diary as this is very important in the analysis. The diary should be checked frequently to ensure compliance.
- The patient should not use her own watch but the timer on the ambulatory box.
- She is instructed on how to use the flow-rate machine and the event button, if unable to return to the flow

meter. If this is required, the button is pressed once on entry to a toilet, and once again when void starts. The event button should not be used at any other time. Instructions for the event button should be included on the diary sheet, as are the names and telephone numbers of the test coordinators.

- Contact with the test coordinator should be easy for the patient.
- The patient needs to be checked on-line at least once an hour (or more if deemed necessary), for example when the lines have come out, if there is an ambulatory box failure (such as low batteries), if the patient is uncomfortable, or if the test becomes unacceptable.
- At the end of the test period (4 hours), the patient is asked to carry out a series of activities, with a full bladder (if possible). The use of provocative manoeuvres such as 10 coughs, 10 star jumps, hand-washing or heel-bouncing, can improve diagnostic yield.[10,11] The patient is then asked to void.
- Once the test has been completed the catheters are removed and cleaned thoroughly.
- The recorded data are down loaded according to the manufacturer's instructions (4 minutes/page).
- The traces are then reviewed by the test coordinator, interpreting the diary with the patient present. If possible, another observer should also be present.
- After the test the patient is warned that she may have a stinging sensation in her urethra and bladder for up to 12 hours. For this reason, fluid intake should be maintained and, if symptoms of cystitis are present or the urine becomes offensive, she should seek advice from her doctor.
- Women who are known to have residuals, reflux, recurrent urinary tract infection or diabetes should be given antibiotic cover.

Comments

As previously mentioned, although the above protocol is that currently used at the King's College Hospital, London, in other units the procedure of ambulatory urodynamics may differ: for example, the bladder catheter can be inserted with a single transducer intravesically and the other in the midurethra, at the point of maximal urethral closure pressure. This would allow recording of both the bladder and the urethral

function. However, this method has two major drawbacks: (a) it is not possible to detect artefacts that are due to the contact of the intravesical transducer membrane with the bladder wall; (b) because of patient movements, the urethral transducer can move and give unreliable information on urethral pressure. Some units have tried to overcome the last problem by stitching the catheter to the labia minora, but this may be too uncomfortable and offputting to many women. Furthermore, the most important current clinical application for ambulatory urodynamics is the exclusion of abnormal detrusor contractions, the study of urethral function being of secondary importance.

The bladder catheter can also be inserted suprapubically. Although this could be acceptable for some men, we do not believe there is any advantage of doing this in women.

In our opinion, it is mandatory to interpret the trace and the diary with the patient present at the end of the study. The use of a diary emphasizes the importance of linking urinary symptoms with the investigation; this is as valid for laboratory urodynamics as it is for ambulatory urodynamics. Urinary symptoms are important, as abnormal detrusor activity cannot be diagnosed unless it is associated with symptoms such as urgency or urge incontinence. In a recent study,[12] we found that both the symptom diary and the placement of two transducers in the bladder can decrease, by almost two-thirds, the diagnosis of pathological detrusor activity on ambulatory urodynamics, by minimizing possible artefacts.

CLINICAL STUDIES

Asymptomatic volunteers

The clinical use of ambulatory urodynamics is limited by the high prevalence (38–69%) of abnormal detrusor contractions detected with this method in asymptomatic volunteers.[5,13–15] These results call ambulatory urodynamics and its validity into question, suggesting that it is oversensitive in the diagnosis of detrusor instability. Van Waalwijik van Doorn[14] proposed an equation, the detrusor activity index, to distinguish 'abnormal' from 'physiological' detrusor contractions. The mean detrusor activity index is calculated as the sum of the number of uninhibited contractions per hour multiplied by 10, the mean amplitude and the mean duration of these contractions. In a prospective study[16] of 26 asymptomatic women we showed that the diagnosis of 'detrusor instability' is highly dependent on trace interpretation and the technique used to conduct the test. In our population of asymptomatic volunteers, the prevalence of abnormal detrusor contractions varied from 76.9 to 11.5%, according to the definition used of an abnormal event, the use of the diary with the woman present during interpretation and the placement of two transducers in the bladder. We defined abnormal detrusor contraction as when a simultaneous detrusor pressure rise on both bladder lines occurred, but only if associated with symptoms (urgency or leakage), in line with the ICS definition of detrusor instability. According to our definition of abnormal detrusor contraction, ambulatory urodynamic findings are normal in almost 90% of asymptomatic women, which is similar to the rate of normal findings in laboratory urodynamic studies. This definition is also applied during our laboratory urodynamic tests, indicating that ambulatory urodynamics does not need new diagnostic standards or methods. Laboratory urodynamics involves the careful observation of urinary symptoms correlated with the cystometric trace. Ambulatory urodynamics does not differ in this respect, and the process becomes even more important in the correct diagnosis of abnormal detrusor contraction.

Variables recorded on ambulatory urodynamics

Voided volume

Many authors have reported that the volume voided during ambulatory urodynamic studies is less than during laboratory urodynamics.[13,17–19] There may be various reasons for this:

- The irritation of the catheter in an ambulant patient may exacerbate the desire to void.
- During conventional urodynamics we usually try to reach the maximum functional bladder capacity; presumably, this does not happen in ambulatory urodynamics, with the patient voiding at a comfortable bladder fullness.

Detrusor pressure

It is not possible to detect low bladder compliance using ambulatory urodynamics.[20] Both abnormal detrusor contractions and the maximum detrusor pressure

during the voiding phase are greater in ambulatory urodynamic than in conventional urodynamic studies.

Flow rate

The flow rate is higher in ambulatory urodynamic than in laboratory urodynamic studies.[21]

CLINICAL APPLICATIONS

Inconclusive urodynamics

A proportion of women complaining of urinary symptoms can have an inconclusive laboratory urodynamic evaluation. In our unit, 10.9% of 5000 symptomatic women did not have any urodynamic abnormality on provocative videocystourethrography. Similarly, Vereecken and Van Nuland[19] showed abnormalities on ambulatory urodynamics in 20 of 28 subjects with urinary symptoms but with an inconclusive laboratory urodynamics result.

Poor correlation between symptoms and conventional urodynamics

One hundred patients[22] complaining of urinary symptoms underwent ambulatory urodynamics after having a laboratory urodynamic result that did not correlate with their symptoms or after unsuccessful incontinence surgery. The ambulatory urodynamic studies diagnosed detrusor instability twice as often as laboratory urodynamics. The test was described as normal in 32 patients undergoing laboratory urodynamics, but in only five undergoing ambulatory urodynamics. The latter test diagnosed only eight patients as having urethral sphincter incompetence, compared with 13 on laboratory urodynamics.

In another study,[10] 52 patients underwent a laboratory urodynamic study, with poor symptom correlation. All of them also underwent ambulatory urodynamics, which showed detrusor instability in 31 patients with a conventional urodynamic diagnosis of a stable bladder. Of these 31 patients, 11 had detrusor instability only after provocative manoeuvres, emphasizing the need to carry out this part of the test. This study also showed that incontinence was detected more frequently on ambulatory urodynamics using a Urilos nappy.

Anders *et al.*[23] compared the diagnosis obtained by ambulatory urodynamics with that obtained by conventional urodynamics in 475 symptomatic women. Ambulatory urodynamics proved to be more sensitive than laboratory urodynamics in the diagnosis of detrusor instability, but less sensitive to genuine stress incontinence.

Low compliance

Low bladder compliance is defined as a steep detrusor pressure rise during the filling phase on laboratory urodynamics, giving a detrusor pressure rise greater than $10 \, cmH_2O$ to $300 \, ml$ or greater than $15 \, cmH_2O$ to $500 \, ml$ bladder volume. The significance of this is debated: some feel that this is a passive phenomenon related to the reduced elasticity of the bladder wall, others that the increase in pressure is associated with a tonic detrusor contraction. In the former, the pressure rise should not decrease at the end of filling; in the latter, the detrusor pressure should decay exponentially as the contracting detrusor relaxes. In a series of patients with neuropathic bladders,[20] who developed an increase in detrusor pressure of more than $25 \, cmH_2O$ at a filling rate of $100 \, ml/min$, during ambulatory urodynamics there was a much smaller increase in detrusor pressure on orthograde filling than when these patients underwent cystometry using faster filling rates; however, the frequency of phasic detrusor instability correlated well with the magnitude of the pressure increase during conventional cystometry. It was also found that the greater number of phasic detrusor contractions during ambulatory monitoring correlated well with the presence of a dilated upper renal tract. However, the diagnosis of low compliance on filling during laboratory urodynamics did not correlate with upper tract dilatation.

Preoperative evaluation

Incontinence surgery is indicated in cases of genuine stress incontinence. Detrusor instability should be excluded prior to surgery, as it is an important cause of operative failure. However, detrusor instability can appear after an incontinence operation (such as Burch colposuspension) and is referred to as *de novo*. It is still debated whether this could be due to an excessive dissection during the operation, or that detrusor instability was not diagnosed prior to surgery. Ambulatory

urodynamics has been used to predict the appearance of *de-novo* detrusor instability after incontinence surgery in two studies.[24,25] It appears that preoperative ambulatory urodynamics did, indeed, predict those women who would develop postoperative detrusor instability.

Pressure–flow study

Ambulatory urodynamics can be useful to assess the voiding phase in patients who are unable to void during conventional urodynamic studies because of embarrassment, or in those who experience suprapubic pain after voiding. The latter can be associated with a post-void uninhibited detrusor contraction, which should be treated as detrusor instability; however, these patients also require cystoscopy and bladder biopsy.

Sensory urgency

A conventional urodynamic diagnosis of sensory urgency requires cystoscopy and biopsies. Where histology is inconclusive it may be appropriate to perform ambulatory urodynamics.

CONCLUSIONS

Ambulatory urodynamics is a relatively new diagnostic tool in the evaluation of lower urinary tract dysfunction. However, its place in daily clinical practice is still to be defined, in part because there is no standard terminology and technique for this diagnostic test. Various studies have confirmed the greater sensitivity of ambulatory urodynamics than that of laboratory tests in detecting detrusor overactivity. Now that progress is being made towards understanding the presence of abnormal detrusor contractions in asymptomatic volunteers, and 'normal parameters' are about to be defined, ambulatory urodynamics promises to become an important diagnostic tool in the assessment of the overactive bladder.

AMBULATORY SYSTEMS

Dantec

Dantec Tempo can record up to six channels. The system will record for up to 24 hours and can be connected to a flow meter, allowing pressure–flow studies. The recorder unit has two event marker buttons and downloads to a personal computer.

Gaeltec

The Gaeltec MPR2 can record seven channels for over 24 hours. The box has a built-in clock display. It is possible to connect the system to a gravimetric flow meter and Urilos pad for detecting urinary leakage. A single-event marker is available. Data are downloaded onto a personal computer which needs at least 2 MB of random access memory. Analysis software is provided in the package.

MMS

The UPS-2020 is a multipurpose ambulatory system; it can record for up to 24 hours, and five event markers are available. The system can also record leakage detection and electromyography. Data are downloaded onto a personal computer which requires at least 2 MB of random access memory. Zoom facility and colour graphics are part of the software.

Synetics

This ambulatory system can record up to six channels for over 24 hours. The system has a memory capacity of 4 MB and data are downloaded to a standard personal computer.

Weist

Camsys 6300 can record three pressure channels and one electromyographic channel for over 24 hours. Three event-marker buttons are available. The data are downloaded onto a personal computer. This system can be used with a Windows operating system.

REFERENCES

1. Mackay RS. Radiotelemetering from within the human body. *Institute of Radio Engineers Transactions on Medical Electronics* (ME6) 1959; 11: 100–105

2. Warrell DW, Watson BW, Shelley T. Intravesical pressure measurements in women during movement using a radio-pill and an air-probe. *J Obstet Gynaecol Br Commonw* 1963; 70: 959–967

3. Miyagawa I, Nakamura I, Ueda M *et al.* Telemetric cystometry. *Urol Int* 1993; 41: 263–265

4. Vereecken RL, Puers B, Das J. Continuous telemetric monitoring of bladder function. *Urol Res* 1983; 11: 15–18

5. Thuroff JW, Jonas V, Frohneberg D *et al.* Telemetric urodynamic investigation in normal males. *Urol Int* 1980; 35: 427–434

6. Tsuji I, Kuroda K, Nakajima F. Excretory cystometry in paraplegic patients. *J Urol* 1960; 83: 839–844

7. Bhatia NN, Bradley WE, Haldeman S, Johnson BK. Continuous monitoring of bladder and urethral pressure: new technique. *Urology* 1981; 18: 207–210

8. Griffiths CJ, Assi MS, Styles RA *et al.* Ambulatory monitoring of bladder and detrusor pressure during natural filling. *J Urol* 1989; 142: 780–784

9. German K, MacLachlan D, Johnson S *et al.* Improvements in the design of equipment used for ambulatory urodynamics. *Br J Urol* 1994; 74: 377–378

10. Webb RJ, Ramsden PD, Neal DE. Ambulatory monitoring and electronic measurement of urinary leakage in the diagnosis of detrusor instability and incontinence. *Br J Urol* 1991, 68: 148–152

11. Athanasiou S, Anders K, Salvatore S *et al.* Short-term provocative ambulatory urodynamics. *Neurourol Urodyn* 1996; 4: 276–278

12. Salvatore S, Khullar V, Anders K, Cardozo LD. Reducing artefacts in ambulatory urodynamics. *Br J Urol* 1998; 81: 211–214

13. Robertson AS, Griffiths CJ, Ramsden PD, Neal DE. Bladder function in healthy volunteers: ambulatory monitoring and conventional urodynamic studies. *Br J Urol* 1994; 73: 242–249

14. Van Waalwijk Van Doorn ESC, Remmers A, Janknegt RA. Conventional and extramural ambulatory urodynamic testing of the lower urinary tract in female volunteers. *J Urol* 1992; 47: 1319–1326

15. Heslington K, Hilton P. Ambulatory monitoring and conventional cystometry in asymptomatic female volunteers. *Br J Obstet Gynaecol* 1996; 103: 434–441

16. Salvatore S, Khullar V, Cardozo L *et al.* Ambulatory urodynamics: what's normal? *Neurourol Urodyn* 1997; 5: 512–513

17. Styles RA, Neal DE, Ramsden PD. Comparison of long-term monitoring and standard cystometry in chronic retention of urine. *Br J Urol* 1986; 58: 652–656

18. Yeung CK, Godley ML, Duffy PG, Ransley PG. Natural filling cystometry in infants and children. *Br J Urol* 1995; 75: 531–537

19. Vereecken RL, Van Nuland T. Detrusor pressure in ambulatory versus standard urodynamics. *Neurourol Urodyn* 1998; 17: 129–133

20. Webb RJ, Styles RA, Griffiths CJ *et al.* Ambulatory monitoring of bladder pressures in patients with low compliance as a result of neurogenic bladder dysfunction. *Br J Urol* 1989; 64: 150–154

21. Webb RG, Griffiths CJ, Zacharin KK, Neal DE. Filling and voiding pressures measured by ambulatory monitoring and conventional studies during natural and artificial bladder filling. *J Urol* 1991; 91: 815–818

22. Van Waalwijk Van Doorn ESC, Remmers A, Janknegt RA. Extramural ambulatory urodynamic monitoring during natural filling and normal daily activities: evaluation of 100 patients. *J Urol* 1992; 146: 124–131

23. Anders K, Khullar K, Cardozo L *et al.* Ambulatory urodynamic monitoring in clinical urogynaecological practice. *Neurourol Urodyn* 1997; 5: 510–512

24. Khullar V, Salvatore S, Cardozo LD *et al.* Ambulatory urodynamics: a predictor of de-novo detrusor instability after colposuspension. *Neurourol Urodyn* 1994; 13: 443–444

25. Heslington K, Hilton P. The incidence of detrusor instability by ambulatory monitoring and conventional cystometry pre and post colposuspension. *Neurourol Urodyn* 1995; 14: 416–417

26

Radiology and urogynaecology

D. Rickards, A. Rockall

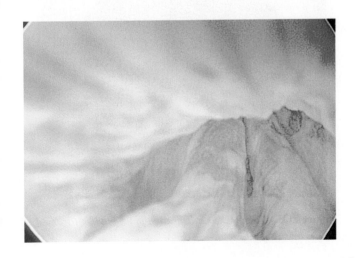

INTRODUCTION

In radiological urogynaecology, plain films, excretory urography (EU) and contrast studies are the diagnostic procedures available. Interventional techniques are directed predominantly towards ureteric obstruction and injury.

PLAIN FILM STUDIES

Bladder calcification

Bladder wall calcification is rare. Tuberculosis, radiation cystitis, amyloidosis and most commonly throughout the world, schistosomiasis[1] (Fig. 26.1) are common causes. Bladder adenocarcinomas and, rarely, treated transitional cell malignancy can calcify.

Emphysematous cystitis

Emphysematous cystitis occurs mostly in diabetic patients.[2] Gas is seen within the bladder wall, within the bladder lumen and occasionally within the pelvicalyceal system.

Dermoid tumours and other pelvic lesions

Dermoid tumours are characteristic mass lesions, often containing teeth (Fig. 26.2), and surrounded by a lucency which is due to fat within the lesion. Such tumours account for 20% of ovarian neoplasms. Uterine fibroids commonly calcify, are often multiple and

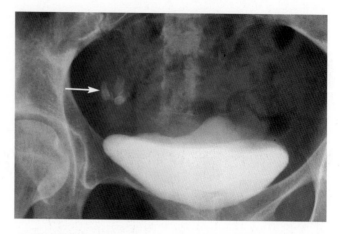

Figure 26.2 *Coned view of the pelvis during excretory urography. Note the teeth in the right hemipelvis (arrow). This appearance is characteristic of a dermoid.*

have a characteristic appearance. Bony lesions secondary to pelvic malignancy should be sought; they are usually lytic and destructive and become sclerotic following radiotherapy.

Spinal anomalies

Many spinal abnormalities are associated with lower urinary tract dysfunction, specifically spina bifida and sacral agenesis (Fig. 26.3).

Foreign bodies

Foreign bodies are commonly seen, even in the best-regulated circles (Fig. 26.4)!

EXCRETORY UROGRAPHY

EU demonstrates the anatomy of the urinary tract non-invasively and rapidly. Its role in the investigation of disorders of the lower urinary tract includes the demonstration of congenital anomalies, the relationship of the ureters and bladder to pelvic masses, abnormalities caused by trauma and the demonstration of filling defects and fistulae.

Technique

Following a plain radiograph of the abdomen and pelvis, an iodinated contrast medium is injected intravenously as a rapid bolus. Low-osmolality, non-ionic

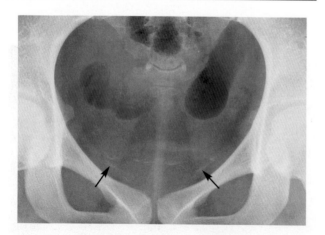

Figure 26.1. *Thin-walled calcification of the bladder (arrowed) characteristic of schistosomiasis.*

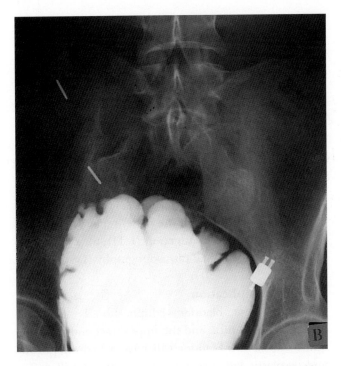

Figure 26.3. *Cystogram showing a neuropathic type of bladder. Note the sacral agenesis.*

contrast media are generally well tolerated by patients and have virtually no side effects. Once obstruction has been ruled out on the 5-minute renal area film, ureteric compression can be applied, at the level of the pelvic brim, for a further 5 minutes; this ensures retention of contrast in the pelvicalyceal systems. A full-length film is then taken immediately following release of compression, to demonstrate the ureters and the bladder. Oblique positioning may be used to demonstrate a specific abnormality, such as the ectopic insertion of a ureter. Fluoroscopy with spot films may also be useful. A film taken following micturition may be used to demonstrate residual urine and constant filling defects in distal ureters and bladder, as well as certain urethral abnormalities. The addition of uroflowmetry allows for physiological information.

Congenital anomalies

Duplex ureters

The most common ureteric anomaly is ureteric duplication, occurring in 0.8% of the population. Unilateral duplication is six times more frequent than bilateral.[3,4] EU demonstrates the insertion of the distal ureters, which will be ectopic. The upper moiety ureter usually

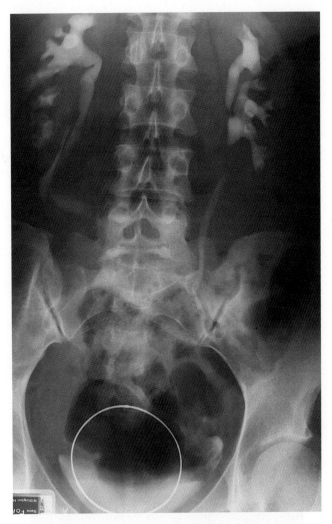

Figure 26.4. *Film from an excretory urography series demonstrating bilateral duplex kidneys. The circular metallic structure is a bracelet within the vagina.*

inserts medial and distal to the lower pole moiety. Vesicoureteric reflux occurs in the lower pole moiety, whereas the upper pole moiety is more commonly obstructed because of its longer vesical submucosal course.[5] Reflux may occur into the upper moiety if its insertion is into the bladder neck or urethra. The more distal the insertion, the more likely that the patient may present with continuous dribbling incontinence from birth.

About one-third of ectopic ureters insert at the bladder neck or at the level of the distal sphincter; one third insert into the vaginal vestibule. More rarely, an ectopic ureter may insert at the level of the cervix or uterus. Difficulties may arise in demonstrating the position of an

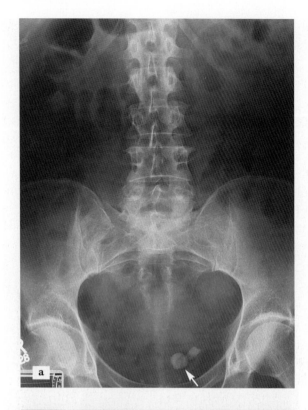

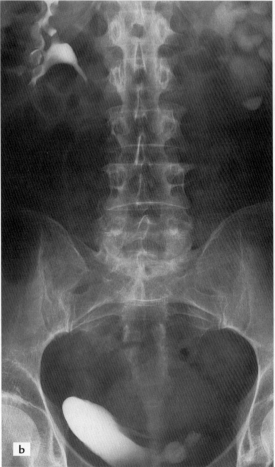

ectopic ureter, particularly if there is a poorly functioning upper moiety.

Ureterocele

A ureterocele, a cystic dilatation of the intravesical ureter, is more common in females and is usually associated with the insertion of the upper pole moiety of a complete ureteric duplication. The characteristic EU appearance is a 'cobra head' filling defect in the bladder, often associated with a calculus (Fig. 26.5), or at another ectopic site of insertion such as the bladder base or urethra. Although the patient may present with recurrent urinary tract infection (UTI), the diagnosis is often made on prenatal ultrasonography (US).

Bladder reduplication

When complete, bladder reduplication is associated with a single urethra, and the upper tract ending in the blind side of the bladder will have a hydronephrotic and dysplastic kidney. Cystography and US will define the anatomy.

Urethral diverticula

Urethral diverticula may be demonstrated on the postmicturition film of an EU, although this is not the investigation of choice.

Acquired bladder lesions

Pelvic masses

Displacement of the ureters and bladder by pelvic masses may be clearly demonstrated on EU. The level of associated ureteric obstruction will also be defined, but rarely will the cause be evident. It is useful to know, before surgical intervention, the position of the ureters in relation to a mass. Causes include a large fibroid uterus, ovarian masses (Fig. 26.6) or haematoma following surgery or trauma.

Figure 26.5. *On the plain film (a) there is a calculus in the left inferior hemipelvis (arrowed). On the 40 min full-length film (b) there is dilatation of the left upper tract. The stone is within a simple ureterocele, one that is not associated with a duplex ureter.*

following pelvic surgery is seen as a loss of contiguity of the distal ureter with the bladder, and leak of contrast into the retroperitoneum or peritoneal cavity. Trauma to the bladder may follow blunt or penetrating injuries or may be secondary to iatrogenic interventions such as surgery (open or endoscopic) or cystography. Although gross bladder rupture will be demonstrated on EU, small tears may not be seen and EU alone cannot be relied upon to rule out bladder rupture. Bladder rupture is most commonly extraperitoneal (Fig. 26.7). Contrast is characteristically seen anteriorly and laterally with flame-shaped strands restricted to the perivesical tissues. Intraperitoneal rupture will result in contrast

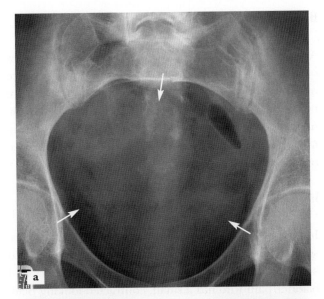

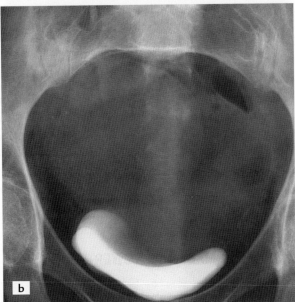

Figure 26.6. *Plain film of an excretory urogram showing (a) a well-defined pelvic mass (arrows) which is compressing the superior aspect of the bladder; however, (b) the ureters are normal. The well-defined nature of the lesion suggests an ovarian cyst, but ultrasonography would be needed to confirm this.*

Trauma

EU examination following surgical or non-surgical trauma defines the integrity of the ureters and bladder, assuming adequate renal function, and is the first step in the diagnostic pathway. Transection of a distal ureter

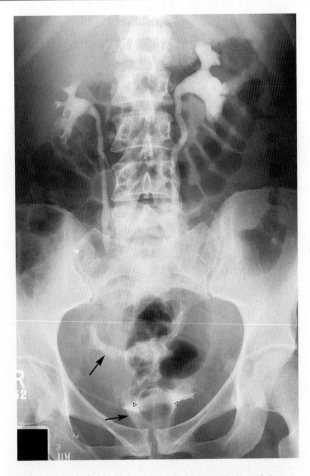

Figure 26.7. *Excretory urography following blunt pelvic trauma. There is a Foley's catheter in the bladder (arrowheads). There is slight dilatation of both ureters and extraperitoneal bladder rupture (upper arrow). This study strongly suggests that the ureters are involved, a suspicion that would be confirmed only on retrograde or antegrade pyelography. Contrast is demonstrated in the vagina, confirming a vesicovaginal fistula (lower arrow).*

spilling freely between loops of bowel. Combined extraperitoneal and intraperitoneal rupture is seen in 10% of cases. Pelvic trauma may cause a massive pelvic haematoma which will compress the bladder, elongating it and elevating or displacing the bladder base (Fig. 26.8).

Filling defects

The wide differential of filling defects demonstrated in the distal ureters or bladder on EU does depend on the clinical presentation. EU provides preliminary information concerning position and size of a filling defect but, if tumour is suspected, then direct visualization at cystoscopy and ureteroscopy is indicated. Ureteroceles, stones and haematoma can often be further assessed with US to confirm the diagnosis.

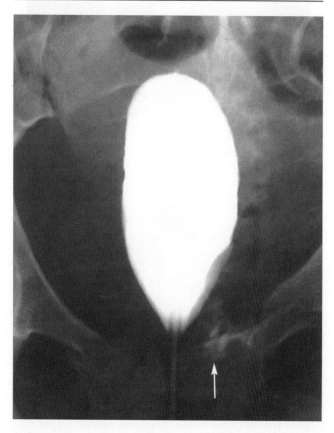

Figure 26.8. *Following pelvic trauma (note fractures of the pubic rami bilaterally), the bladder on the cystogram is compressed owing to pelvic haematoma. There is extraperitoneal extravasation of contrast (arrow).*

Bladder diverticula

Acquired diverticula are usually associated with outflow obstruction, whether associated with urethral stricture or detrusor sphincter dyssynergia. Diverticula are numerous, usually small (unlike congenital diverticula), are covered by urothelium on the outside and contain no smooth muscle. They often fail to empty, as seen on the post-micturition film.

Interstitial cystitis

Interstitial cystitis is more common in women with non-specific radiographic findings, but the diagnosis should be considered in any patient with gross frequency and bladder pain who has a small, contracted-looking bladder on EU.[6] Differential diagnosis would be with radiation cystitis.

Fistula

EU may non-invasively demonstrate vesicovaginal and ureterovaginal fistulae. Urethrovaginal fistulae may rarely be demonstrated on the post-micturition film; however, a false-positive result may arise owing to urethrovaginal reflux during micturition. EU is less likely to demonstrate fistulae to the bowel, owing to higher pressures.

DIAGNOSTIC IMAGING OF LOWER TRACT: FISTULAE

Urine leaking into the vagina or perineum, or onto the skin surface, or the presence of pneumaturia, all indicate a fistula from the lower urinary tract. There are a number of iatrogenic, neoplastic and inflammatory causes. The immediate diagnostic problem is locating the anatomical site of the fistula. This is normally done using a combination of EU, cystography, micturating cystourethography, barium or water-soluble contrast enemas, computed tomography (CT), magnetic resonance (MR) and sinography. Antegrade pyelography will definitively identify the level and cause of ureteric lesions. Which study method is used, and in which order, depends upon close clinical cooperation between clinician and radiologist, the suspected site of the fistula and the availability of imaging modalities.

Vesicovaginal fistulae

Vesicovaginal and uterovesical fistulae are the result of instrumentation, malignancy or radiotherapy (particularly that for cervical carcinoma). A combination of EU and cystography demonstrates most vesicovaginal fistulae (Fig. 26.9), although it is unusual to define the exact site and extent of the connection. Lateral projections are crucial, as contrast within the vagina or uterus can be masked by the contrast-distended bladder. Small fistulae may be missed even with adequately distended bladders and good radiography. When clinical suspicion remains high despite negative imaging, a variation is to insert a tampon into the vagina before EU and, when all films have been exposed, to remove the tampon and examine it radiographically to see if it has absorbed any contrast. False-positive results will be seen on post-micturition films when there is urethrovaginal reflux.

Ureterovaginal fistulae

Ureterovaginal fistulae arise as a complication of pelvic surgery, following necrosis of the ureter secondary to radiotherapy and after ureteroscopy. Although a ureterovaginal fistula may not be demonstrated on EU, it cannot be excluded: if the EU is normal and subsequent cystography is found to be normal, then either retrograde or antegrade pyelography is necessary.

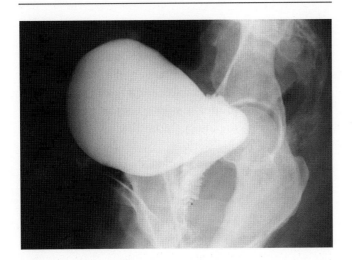

Figure 26.9. *Cystogram showing a vesicovaginal fistula.*

Urethrovaginal fistulae

Urethrovaginal fistulae are usually due to ischaemic necrosis of the vaginal and urethral walls following anterior colporrhaphy or infection after excision of urethral diverticula. They are often very difficult to diagnose and differentiate from urethrovaginal reflux. Good voiding urethrography offers the best hope and depends upon the patient being able to void at good flow rates under fluoroscopic control (Fig. 26.10). Positive-pressure urethrography is contraindicated where urethral trauma is suspected.

Colovesical, colovaginal or colouterovaginal fistulae

Patients with colovesical, colovaginal or colouterovaginal fistulae present with pneumaturia and UTI. Contrast enemas or cystography afford the best chance of demonstrating a fistula using barium, Gastrografin or ionic contrast (Fig. 26.11). Fistulous connection is seen in less than 70% of patients studied by barium enema; air is visible in the bladder in about 30%. Contrast studies do confirm the presence of underlying colonic disease, such as diverticular disease (the most common cause; Fig. 26.12) and excludes other potential causes such as Crohn's disease or colon carcinoma.

Urethrocutaneous fistulae

Most urethrocutaneous fistulae are urethral duplications, but these are very rare in females. Sinography is usually the imaging modality of choice.

INTERVENTIONAL RADIOLOGY AND LOWER TRACT FISTULA

Ureteric injuries

Ureteric injuries, whether partial or complete, inevitably result in urinary extravasation or urinoma formation, assuming continuing renal function. Once the level has been identified (Fig. 26.13), surgical correction or diversion is needed. Percutaneous nephrostomy (PCN) will divert most of the urine, but not all. Various techniques to ensure complete diversion have

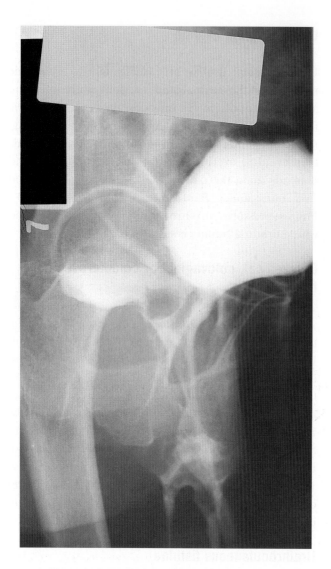
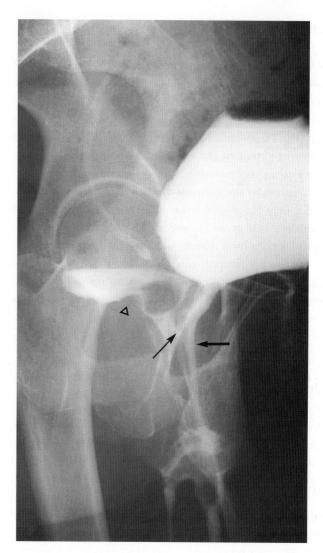

Figure 26.10. *Combined excretory urogram and cystogram demonstrating a urethrovaginal fistula (thin arrow). The ureter (thick arrow) is intact and contrast is pooling in the vagina (arrowhead).*

been tried, from balloons obstructing the ureter proximal to the injury to embolization of the ureteric lumen with coils. Catheters are manufactured that drain the pelvicalyceal system and attempt to occlude the proximal ureter with an intrinsic tail that sits within the ureteric lumen. PCN is always very difficult in these cases because the collecting system is decompressed and abdominal surgery renders it difficult for the patient to be prone or prone–oblique upon the fluoroscopy table. Nevertheless, PCN offers the best hope of urinary diversion in the short term.

Manipulation of the ureteric injury is possible whereby a double-J stent can be passed across the lesion (Fig. 26.14). If this can be achieved without further injuring the ureter, corrective surgery can be avoided, but it is wise to drain the upper tract as well to divert urine away from the injury, permitting ureteric recovery around the double-J stent.

Where urinoma have formed, drainage under US or CT control is valuable, especially where the urinoma has become infected, more likely where there is associated bowel trauma.

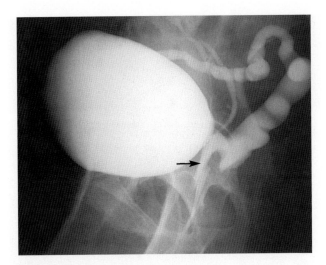

Figure 26.11. *Gastrografin enema demonstrating a colovaginovesical fistula. The vagina (arrow) is seen between the rectum and bladder.*

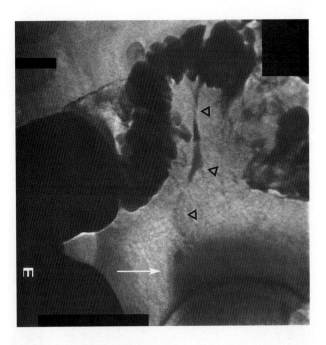

Figure 26.12. *Barium enema showing diverticular disease and a fistulous tract (arrowheads) communicating with the bladder (arrow).*

DIAGNOSTIC RADIOLOGY AND INTERVENTIONAL TECHNIQUES IN URINARY DIVERSION AND BLADDER AUGMENTATION

Urinary diversion

Irrespective of the type of diversion, and whatever underlying pathology has culminated in surgery, imaging aims to assess the integrity of the diversion, its relationship to the upper tracts and complications of either. Some complications can be relieved using interventional radiological techniques. The general principles involved are common to most types of diversion. Only some types are discussed here.

Ileal loop diversion

Loopography is a simple retrograde procedure. A 10–14F Foley catheter is inserted into the loop and inflated with 5–10 cm^3 of air to ensure that infused contrast does not reflux out of the loop. Under fluoroscopic control, contrast is injected by hand to distend the loop adequately and achieve reflux up the ureters, which occurs in 95% of patients. Under normal circumstances, the loop will be of normal calibre and probably will show peristalsis; reflux will occur up both ureters, which may be slightly dilated. Abnormal findings are as follows:

- No reflux up one or both ureters. This implies obstruction at the ureteroenteric anastomosis;
- Where reflux occurs, ureteric strictures with proximal dilatation suggest significant obstruction;
- Filling defects in the upper tracts which can be due to tumour, stone, blood clot or mucus;
- A rigid, non-peristaltic loop of poor calibre suggests loop ischaemia;
- Focal narrowing of the loop with proximal dilatation suggests a significant loop stenosis;
- Extravasation from the loop in the immediate postoperative stage is an indication of acute loop ischaemia, stitch dehiscence or poor surgical technique (Fig. 26.15);
- Dilatation of the loop and upper tracts suggests a stomal stricture;
- Filling defects within the loop due to stone etc.

Where doubt exists as to whether a ureteric stricture, usually at the anastomosis of the ureter with the loop, is significant is not determined by the degree of proximal dilatation, because dilatation does not equate to obstruction nor does a normal system exclude obstruction. If the clinical suspicion is one of obstruction (decreasing urine output, decreasing renal function), a

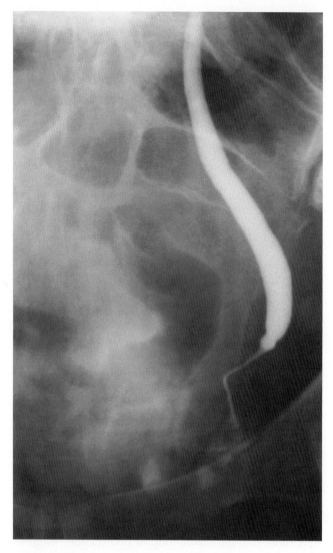

Figure 26.13. *At surgery, the ureter has been transected, with flow of contrast into the pelvis. The upper tract was drained percutaneously to divert urine away from the injury.*

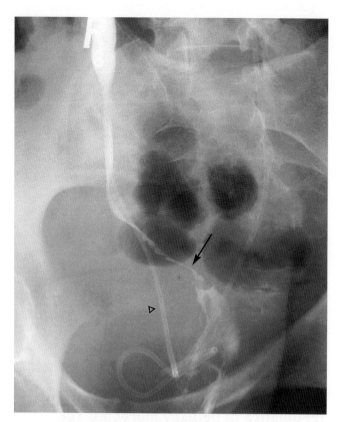

Figure 26.14. *The ureter was damaged at surgery and extravasation can be seen on an antegrade study (arrow). The true lumen of the ureter was manipulated and a double-J stent inserted across the defect (arrowhead).*

Whitaker test should be performed. This test demands the insertion of a catheter percutaneously into the pelvicalyceal system which is capable of both perfusion and pressure monitoring. While perfusing the upper tracts with dilute contrast medium at 10 ml/min and continuously recording the pelvicalyceal pressure, a pressure rise of more than $22 \, cmH_2O$ is diagnostic of obstruction and a pressure rise of less than $15 \, cmH_2O$ excludes obstruction. Between 15 and $22 \, cmH_2O$ is a grey area and it is appropriate to monitor the patient's clinical status.

Where obstruction in the ureter has been proved and the level and probable cause identified, balloon dilatation to 8 mm combined with antegrade double-J

stenting using 22 cm 8F stents has a good chance of curing the stricture, especially when the cause is one of ischaemia.[7] The stricture can also be held open with self-expanding metal stents which become incorporated into the urothelium, but they are complicated by interstitial hyperplasia. Such techniques are attractive because they are minimally invasive and surgery is difficult in the postoperative abdomen. Long-term success rates are disappointing.

A novel approach to these strictures is to use a special cautery catheter which cuts through the stricture; when this is followed by temporary stenting it can achieve a long-term resolution of the stricture in 70% of cases at 4 years.

Loop stenoses can also be treated by balloon dilatation via the stoma.

Colonic loop

If small bowel cannot be used, large bowel is employed and all imaging techniques for ileal loop imaging apply.

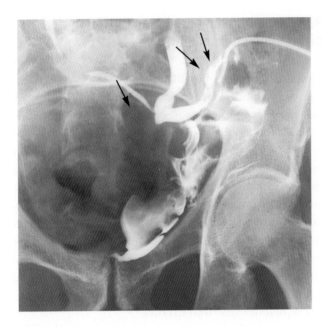

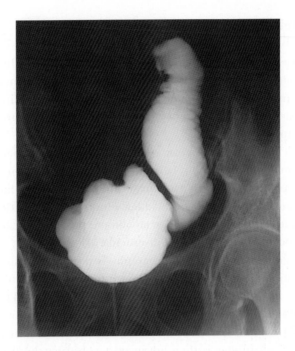

Figure 26.15. *Loopogram of an ileal loop diversion (arrowed) showing gross extravasation from the loop, but the loop in continuity with the ureters, in which reflux of contrast is seen.*

Figure 26.16. *Cystogram showing a caecocystoplasty without any complications.*

Ureterosigmoidostomy

Although ureterosigmoidostomy avoids the use of a stomal bag, it is complicated by the reflux of bowel contents into the upper tracts and an increased incidence of colon cancer.[8] Retrograde imaging by barium or Gastrografin enema and antegrade stenting are contraindicated. Ureterosigmoidostomy is a technique no longer used, but a population of patients who underwent the procedure in the past still occasionally present for imaging. EU is the only radiographic procedure of use.

Continent pouches

Access to the surgically formed urinary reservoir is by way of a stoma, a Mitrofanoff procedure or the patient's own urethra. Catheterization and contrast studies as for an ileal loop are appropriate. Pouch calculi are a common problem, forming on exposed surgical clips; triple-phosphate stones are common.[9]

Bladder augmentation

Enterocystoplasty

Enterocystoplasty increases bladder capacity.[10–13] Assessment of the bladder is by cystography (Fig. 26.16) and the diagnosis and treatment of complications is the same as for an ileal loop. Urodynamic studies are of great importance in assessing the function of the augmented bladder. Enterocystoplasty includes caecocystoplasty, ileocystoplasty, ileocaecocystoplasty, sigmoidocystoplasty, gastrocystoplasty and enterourethroplasty.

DIAGNOSTIC RADIOLOGY AND THE URETHRA

Indications for imaging are (1) urethral trauma, (2) urethral diverticula, (3) bladder-neck position and (4) distal sphincter competence.

Urethral injuries

Urethral injuries occur in 4% of pelvic fracture injuries.[14] Diagnosis is difficult radiologically as instrumentation of the urethra should be avoided. If a suprapubic catheter is in place, voided cystourethrography can be performed, but is often inconclusive.[15] The diagnosis is usually made clinically or by cystourethroscopy. Missed trauma can lead to sepsis, incontinence or stricture. Strictures usually involve the distal sphincter region and the diagnosis can be made by descending urethrography via a suprapubic catheter.

Urethral diverticula

Diverticula are reported to occur in 6% of adult women.[16] Diagnosis can be made by US (performed transrectally immediately after voiding), MR, voiding cystourethrography or positive-pressure urethrography.[17]

The success of voiding cystourethrography is dependent upon the patient being able to void under fluoroscopic control once an adequate amount of contrast has been instilled into the bladder. Fluoroscopy with the patient erect and in the semi-oblique position can be expected to show 60% of diverticula[18] (Fig. 26.17).

Positive-pressure urethrography is performed using a double-balloon catheter. The catheter is passed into the bladder and the distal balloon inflated. The catheter is gently pulled back so that the distal balloon obstructs the bladder neck. A second balloon mounted on the catheter is then advanced to obstruct the urethral meatus. Through a port between the two obstructing balloons, contrast is gently injected under fluoroscopic control and relevant films exposed. Using a positive pressure, up to 95% of diverticula will be diagnosed, but the technique is painful and double-balloon catheters are not readily available.[19]

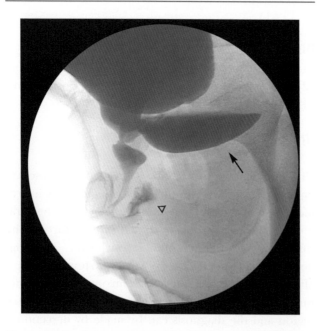

Figure 26.17. *Micturating cystogram showing huge urethral diverticulum (arrow). Note incidental urethrovaginal reflux during micturition (arrowhead).*

Bladder neck competence and position and distal sphincter competence

At cystography, an open bladder neck appears as a conical contrast-filled structure continuous with the bladder base. This can occur normally in nulliparous young females and as an indication of urinary continence is of limited value. On straining or coughing, the bladder base should not move inferiorly. A permanent record of this study can be achieved either by videotaping the study or by taking a rapid sequence of films using digital fluoroscopic equipment exposing films at two or four per second during straining or coughing. However, such images are of limited value to gynaecological surgeons but, where stress incontinence is seen and recorded, are of value in documenting the exact status of the bladder base and urethra.

REFERENCES

1. Pollack HM, Banner MP, Martinez LO. Diagnostic considerations in bladder wall calcifications. *Am J Roentgenol* 1981; 136: 791–797

2. Quint HJ, Drach GW, Rappaport WD, Hoffman CJ. Emphysematous cystitis: a review of the spectrum of disease. *J Urol* 1992; 147: 134–137

3. Campbell MF. Anomalies of the ureter. In: Campbell MF, Harrison JH (eds) *Urology*, 3rd edn. Philadelphia: Saunders, 1970: 1487–1542

4. Nation EF. Duplication of the kidney and ureter: a statistical study of 230 new cases. *J Urol* 1944; 51: 456–465

5. Frank JD, Snyder H McC. Congenital abnormalities of the ureter. In: Whitfield HN, Hendry WF, Kirby RS , Duckett JW (eds) *Textbook of Genitourinary Surgery*, 2nd edn. Oxford: Blackwell Science, 1998; 178–204

6. Holm-Bentzen M, Lose G. Pathology and pathogenesis of interstitial cystitis. *Urology* 1987; 29(Suppl 4): 8–13

7. Shapiro MJ, Banner MP, Amendola MA. Balloon dilatation of ureteroenteric strictures. *Radiology* 1988; 168: 385–387

8. Sakhuja V, Das T, Malik N, Chugh KS. A 55 year follow-up of a patient with bilateral ureterosigmoidostomy. *J Urol* 1992; 147: 1104–1106

9. Dangman BC, Lebowitz RL. Urinary tract calculi that form on surgical staples: a characteristic radiological appearance. *Am J Roentgenol* 1991; 157: 115–117

10. Kenny PH, Hamrick KM, Samuels LJ. Radiological evaluation of continent urinary resevoirs. *Radiographics* 1990; 10: 455–466

11. Ralls PW, Barakos JA, Skinner DG. Imaging of the Koch continent urinary reservoir. *Radiology* 1986; 161: 477–483

12. Ghoneim MA, Shaaban AA, Mahran MR, Koch NG. Further experience with the ureteral Koch pouch. *J Urol* 1992; 147: 361–365

13. Pagani JJ, Barbaric ZL, Cochran ST. Augmentation enterocystoplasty. *Radiology* 1979; 131: 321–326

14. Perry MO, Husmann DA. Urethral injuries in female subjects following pelvic fractures. *J Urol* 1992; 147: 139–143

15. Sandler CM, Corriere JN. Urethrography in the diagnosis of acute urethral injury. *Urol Clin North Am* 1989; 16: 283–289

16. Fortunato P, Schettini M, Galluci M. Diverticula of the female urethra. *Br J Urol* 1997; 80: 626–632

17. Coddington CC, Knab DR. Urethral diverticulum – a review. *Obstet Gynaecol Surv* 1983; 38: 357–363

18. Lang EK, Davis HJ. Positive pressure urethrography: a roentgenographic diagnostic method for urethral diverticula in the female. *Radiology* 1959; 72: 401–405

19. Greenberg M, Stone D, Cochran ST, Bruskewitz R. Female urethral diverticula: double balloon catheter study. *Am J Roentgenol* 1981; 136: 124–128

27

Ultrasonography

V. Khullar

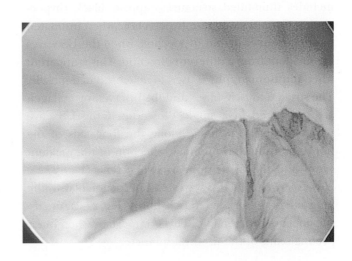

INTRODUCTION

Ultrasound (US) can be used to visualize fluid-filled structures without the use of a contrast medium. Urethral catheterization is not required to estimate post-micturition bladder volumes and this eliminates the risk of urinary tract infection (UTI). Ultrasonography allows soft tissues such as the kidney, urethra, urethral sphincter and bladder wall to be visualized and measured. The main advantage of US is that no ionizing radiation is used in imaging; thus, there is no risk to the woman or ultrasonographer from such radiation. The examinations can be repeated as frequently as required and there is no need for modifications to the rooms in which ultrasonography is performed. The installation and operating costs of US are significantly less than those of similar radiological equipment.

The main disadvantage of US is that the waves do not penetrate air and thus the probe always requires a coupling medium and direct contact in order to image structures. The US probe has a limited field of view, so that only certain parts of the urinary tract can be visualized at one time and, until recently, this was possible in only one plane. The advent of three-dimensional ultrasonography has made it possible to image a volume of tissue and review the image even when the woman is not present.[1–5] Many orientations that are not usually possible, and varying magnifications, can be reproduced. The disadvantage of this method of imaging is that it takes 4–5 seconds to scan the area of interest; thus, for dynamic images a clear picture may not be obtained.

The US image itself depends on the echogenicity of the tissues rather than on density; thus, tissues that have a high echogenicity (hyperechoic) appear white on the US image and those with a low echogenicity (and this includes fluid-filled structures) appear black (hypoechoic). Certain tissues are hyperechoic when insonated in one orientation and hypoechoic when the US waves are incident from a different direction. This is apparent when ultrasonography is used to image striated muscle. The striated muscle fibres and the intervening collagen are orientated in a single direction. If the US wave passes through the tissue along the long axis of the fibres, then there is minimal reflection of the incident waves and the tissue appears hypoechoic (Fig. 27.1). However, when the US waves pass perpendicular to the long axis of the striated muscle fibres (Fig. 27.2), the tissue appears hyperechoic. This is important when interpreting scans of the urethral sphincter.

The bony enclosure of the pelvis bone limits US imaging to the transabdominal, transvaginal, transrectal and transperineal approaches. The images rendered do require experience to interpret and each approach has limitations and advantages. The type of probe and frequency of the US wave (1–10 MHz) emitted determines what tissues are seen and the quality of the image obtained: the higher the US frequency, the better the resolution of the image; unfortunately, an increased frequency has a reduced depth of penetration due to

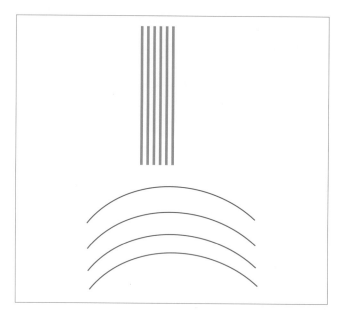

Figure 27.1. *Ultrasound waves passing through a structure with fibres running perpendicular to the ultrasound waves. This will appear hypoechoic (black).*

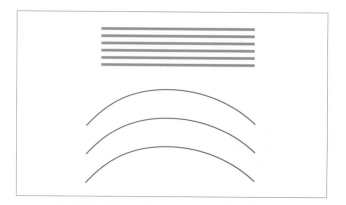

Figure 27.2. *The tissue orientation is such that ultrasound waves pass through the tissue parallel to the fibres. There are maximal reflective echoes and the structure appears hyperechoic (white).*

attenuation, so that 7.5 MHz is the highest frequency that can be used to image pelvic organs.

KIDNEYS

Kidneys are imaged with the woman lying supine. The right kidney is visualized using the liver as an acoustic window and the left kidney can be visualized using the spleen, particularly if there is splenomegaly. The left posterior lateral approach, with the woman rotated to 45 degrees, can be used to visualize the left kidney. Measurements can be made of the longest length by rotating the probe; the accuracy is within 1 cm,[6] and this is important for accurate measurement of the kidney as it is an ellipsoid.[7] Assessment of the entire kidney is performed by scanning the kidney in the transverse plane. The probe is moved from side to side to visualize the kidney adequately. The renal capsule is a well-defined hypoechoic structure. The inner edge of the renal parenchyma is not as well defined because there are multiple echoes from the pelvicalyceal fat.[8] The renal parenchyma is relatively hypoechoic and the medullary pyramids can be seen as hypoechoic oval areas adjacent to the pelvicalyceal system.[9] The parenchymal thickness should be measured, as a reduction may indicate scarring secondary to childhood pyelonephritis, reflux or infarcts. Sometimes the appearance of scarring may be imitated by fetal lobes which can persist into adulthood. This is easily differentiated, as the indentations between the fetal lobes are between the renal medullary pyramids.[10] The cortical thickness can be measured but the distance recorded is dependent on the approach and angulation of the probe as well as the size and age of the woman. Cortical thickness is measured from the capsule to the outer edge of the medullary pyramids. The parenchymal thickness is the measurement from the capsule to the outer edge of the pelvicalyceal fat echoes; this is reproducible and correlates well with measurements from intravenous urography.[6] The renal pelvis is usually filled with hyperechoic fat tissue; however, if there is dilatation of the collecting system, dark areas of fluid appear within the pelvis. Care must be taken in diagnosing dilatation as this may be seen if the bladder is full or if the patient is undergoing diuresis.[11] To exclude obstruction, a renal scan should be repeated after the patient has voided or when the patient is not having a significant diuresis. Ultrasonography is sensitive at detecting dilatation but it cannot determine the degree of obstruction, as severe obstruction can lead to only mild pelvicalyceal dilatation.

Dilatation of the pelvicalyceal system should be diagnosed only when an enlarged rounded renal pelvis obviously communicates with all the calyces. The dilatation may be reported as being mild, moderate or severe, but this can only be a qualitative description.[12,13] If there is marked long-standing obstructive dilatation, the renal parenchyma may be thinned.[14,15]

During pregnancy the collecting system is often dilated and this can be seen as early as 12 weeks' gestation.[12] With increasing gestation an increasing percentage of women have dilated collecting systems: by 36 weeks, over 60% of women have dilated pelvicalyceal systems. There is more dilatation of the right kidney than the left; within two days of delivery these changes can disappear. Possible reasons for the dilatation may be pressure of the enlarged uterus on the ureters, and the increased blood levels of progesterone causing smooth muscle relaxation and increased blood flow.[16]

Ultrasonography is also useful for detecting abnormalities of the upper urinary tract such as duplex, ectopic or horseshoe kidneys.

URETHRA AND SURROUNDING STRUCTURES

The normal anatomy of the proximal urethra has been imaged transabdominally using small mechanical sector scanners. The urethra has been described as having an anteroposterior (AP) diameter just inferior to the bladder of 1–1.5 cm and a transverse diameter[17] slightly larger than this; however, the quality of the image produced was reported to be poor, as the scans were performed with 3.5 MHz probes[17,18] and necessitated catheterization.[18] Catheters alter the position and mobility of the bladder neck and distort the urethral anatomy.[19] When the urethra is imaged abdominally in the transverse plane, the urethral sphincter has been described as an ovoid 'bull's eye'. The urethral sphincter has been imaged using the transabdominal approach and a 3.5 MHz transducer in volunteers who have been referred because of pelvic masses.[20] Unfortunately, neither urinary symptoms nor objective measures were recorded, but bladder filling and age did not affect the measurements. Transabdominal linear-array transducers are too large to allow good positioning or to obtain images of the bladder base and urethra posterior to the symphysis pubis in the sagittal plane; however, transrectal linear-array US scanners have been reported to achieve good images of the urethra and bladder neck.[21–26] The transrectal approach has been used to enable accurate placement of concentric needles into the striated muscle[27,28] and has also been used to measure the urethral sphincter in women with abnormal myotonic-like electromyographic activity. Ultrasonography is very sensitive in detecting urethral diverticula but differentiation from para-urethral cysts may be difficult if a connection cannot be visualized.[29,30]

Measurement of bladder volume

Ultrasonography allows the estimation of post-micturition residual urine volumes without the need for urethral catheterization and the concomitant risk of infection. It is particularly useful in the assessment and monitoring of patients with voiding difficulties. The transabdominal approach is the traditional method by which the pelvic organs are visualized. The full bladder allows all the pelvic organs to be visualized, and this is the ideal method of measuring bladder volume.[31–40] Many methods of calculating bladder volume have been proposed, most of which involve measuring bladder volume by imaging the maximal cross-sectional area in sagittal and transverse planes of the fluid within the bladder. The maximal AP, transverse and caudal–cranial diameters are measured. All of these calculations approximate the bladder to the volume of a sphere; thus, correction factors must be applied. The accuracy of bladder volume measurements is ±20%. At low volumes the bladder approximates to an ovoid structure with the major axis in the transverse plane; at larger volumes the bladder is more spherical in shape as the dome of the bladder distends, the trigone remaining fixed and unchanged. Below a volume of 50 ml, transvaginal scanning has been proposed as a more accurate method of measurement;[41–44] however, at larger volumes it is certainly as inaccurate as transabdominal scanning.[45]

Intravenous urography, used to investigate recurrent UTI in premenopausal women, has a low diagnostic yield and alters management in less than 2% of cases.[46,47] Transabdominal ultrasonography has been found to be more informative by demonstrating uterine and ovarian pathology, as well as post-micturition residuals where urography has been unhelpful.[48]

Bladder diverticula can be detected easily with transabdominal ultrasonography of a full bladder. Increased detrusor pressures can be due to detrusor instability (DI) or increased outflow resistance and can result in diverticula. Dynamic assessment of diverticula is important, as expansion of the pocket may occur during bladder filling and this distension may worsen during micturition. The efficiency of bladder emptying is then reduced, resulting in a post-micturition urinary residual. Calculi due to urinary stasis and transitional cell carcinoma within bladder diverticula occur in 5% of cases.[49] These diverticular contents can be detected or checked using ultrasonography, which may not be technically possible during cystourethroscopy. Calculi can be differentiated from carcinomas as they produce an acoustic shadow and move if the patient alters posture.

The majority of bladder cancers are exophytic and papillary in shape. This enables easy visualization on transabdominal ultrasonography with a filled bladder.[49] The major role of transabdominal ultrasonography is in the surveillance of selected patients with resected bladder tumours;[50] it has been shown to be successful over long periods of time. Transabdominal and transrectal ultrasonography have been used to replace flexible cystoscopy in the detection of recurrent bladder tumours. Although the majority of tumours can be identified by both techniques, in view of the invasive nature and morbidity associated with flexible cystoscopy,[51] ultrasonography may have a useful role in the follow-up of recurrent bladder tumours; it was preferred by the majority of patients.[50] Ultrasonography has been found to be the method of choice for imaging tumours of the trigone in women.[52]

TRANSVAGINAL ULTRASONOGRAPHY

The transvaginal approach allows the bladder, urethra and surrounding structures to be imaged clearly.[53] Higher frequencies (5 MHz and above) can be used to obtain high-resolution images. The abdominal approach, in contrast, does not allow the bladder neck to be visualized clearly or reproducibly,[17,54] and Q-tips, Foley catheters or paediatric feeding tubes have been used as markers. The urethra is seen as a hyperechoic line and urine entering the proximal urethra is seen as a dark area. The urethral sphincter can be seen as an ovoid structure around the urethra. The rhabdosphincter appears hypoechoic lateral to the urethra. During dynamic tests such as coughing, the vaginal probe can compress and easily distort the urethrovesical anatomy, preventing bladder-neck movement;[55] thus, results using this technique must be interpreted with care. Unfortunately, observation of urinary leakage and its timing in relation to a cough cannot be used to diagnose the cause of urinary incontinence, as DI cannot be diagnosed reliably. As the detrusor pressure is not measured during these provocative manoeuvres, and involuntary opening of the bladder neck can occur with DI, this test is unreliable.

The resting position of the bladder neck has been noted to be more caudal in women with stress incontinence than in continent women and during a Valsalva manoeuvre the bladder-neck has been noted to descend more in stress-incontinent than in healthy women.[56-58] However, women with uterovaginal prolapse have greater bladder-neck mobility than women who are incontinent.[54,59] Where anterior vaginal wall mobility has been assessed with the International Continence Society prolapse score,[60] this correlates well with bladder-neck movement.[61] This suggests that bladder-neck hypermobility is associated with vaginal prolapse. Increased antenatal bladder-neck mobility appears to be predictive of the development of postnatal stress incontinence if the bladder neck moves more than 10 degrees during a Valsalva manoeuvre.[62] Transvaginal ultrasonography has been used to assess incontinence procedures for genuine stress incontinence (GSI) postoperatively. The Burch colposuspension has been shown to increase the approximation of the bladder neck to the symphysis pubis and arrests the descent of the bladder neck during a Valsalva manoeuvre.[56,63] These features are not found in recurrent GSI. The Gittes and Stamey suspension procedures were also successful in arresting the descent of the bladder neck on Valsalva manoeuvre, but approximation of the bladder neck with the symphysis pubis did not occur.[56] Failure of the suspension procedure after initial success was associated with a return of mobility of the bladder neck observed on ultrasonography.

TRANSLABIAL ULTRASONOGRAPHY

An abdominal probe is used for the translabial approach. A US probe is covered with a disposable glove and gel is used to allow good contact between the surfaces. The probe is placed between the labia and the pelvis is imaged sagittally. A clear view of the bladder neck, urethra and vagina can be obtained but the symphysis pubis casts an acoustic shadow over the dome of a full bladder. The urethra appears as a hypoechoic tube and the rhabdosphincter is an ovoid hyperechoic structure around the urethra. Assuming that the urethral sphincter is an ellipsoid structure, the volume of the urethral sphincter can be calculated. Symptomatic women with urethral sphincter incompetence have smaller sphincters than asymptomatic women and these women in turn have smaller sphincters than women with DI.[64] This measurement may be a useful method of evaluating the urethral sphincter and may potentially predict the outcome of surgery.

Vaginal prolapse can be assessed using this method but only preliminary reports have been published.[65] This method of sonography does not impede movement of the bladder neck[59,66] or vaginal prolapse during a Valsalva manoeuvre or pelvic floor contraction. However, if uterovaginal prolapse is beyond the hymenal ring, then this technique impedes further descent of the prolapse. It has been suggested as a replacement for radiological screening[67] and a chair has been designed for scanning during voiding. The probe is fixed in a steerable mount controlled at a distance.[68] The position of the bladder neck before and after Burch colposuspension has been found to change when visualized with translabial ultrasonography.[69] Unfortunately, the postoperative position of the bladder neck does not predict cure after surgery.[69]

TRANSRECTAL ULTRASONOGRAPHY

Transrectal ultrasonography requires the patient to be in the left lateral or supine position. Urodynamic chairs have been developed so that the subject may sit and void while the bladder neck is being scanned. Acoustic coupling gel is put inside a condom which is used to protect the subject and the probe. The outside of the condom is also lubricated with gel prior to insertion. With the patient in this position, a sagittal view of the bladder neck is obtained anteriorly. The bladder, bladder base, bladder neck, urethra and symphysis pubis are visualized clearly. As the US waves are passing perpendicular to the urethra it appears hyperechoic; the surrounding rhabdosphincter appears hypoechoic laterally and hyperechoic anterior and posterior to the urethra. Occasionally, a good image is not obtained if the rectum is full of flatus or faeces. The probe can be used to measure post-void residuals and to visualize movement of the bladder neck.[23] Transrectal ultrasonography has been suggested as an alternative method of imaging during urodynamic studies and this has been compared with radiology.[22,26] The position of the probe in the rectum does not appear to alter the pressures measured during urodynamics;[21] however, the woman may be deterred from voiding because of sensation due to the probe.[21] A significant degree of rectal prolapse can cause the probe to move and the rectal probe can distort the bladder-neck movement, especially if the vagina is narrow and atrophic. Significant cystoceles or rectoceles can obscure the view of the urethra and bladder base.

This method of imaging is useful in urological patients who lack sensation in the anus and rectum. However, even with complete spinal cord transection the sacral cord reflexes may still be intact and the insertion of a probe into the anus may alter these reflexes. The bladder neck and proximal urethra have been visualized with transrectal ultrasonography during voiding and this has been found to aid diagnosis. The images are similar to those obtained during videocystourethrography[23,25] and have been used to diagnose catheter-induced hyperreflexia, posterior ledge at the bladder neck during voiding and false passages in the proximal urethra.[70-73] Occasionally, dilated ureters may be visualized and, although the ureteric urine jets can be visualized entering the bladder,[74] vesicoureteric reflux cannot be diagnosed.

INTRA-URETHRAL ULTRASONOGRAPHY

Images can be obtained from high-frequency US probes inserted into the urethra. The probe is shaped like a catheter and a 360-degree section perpendicular to the main axis of the intra-urethral probe is imaged. An oblique image through the urethra is obtained using intra-urethral ultrasonography; although this has been correlated with histology,[75] unfortunately this technique does not allow clear visualization of the outer border of the rhabdosphincter and thus the outer limits of the rhabdosphincter were not defined. The maximum cross-sectional area of the striated urethral sphincter has been found to be significantly smaller in women with urinary incontinence than in continent controls;[76] however, the high US frequencies used by the intra-urethral probe allow clear visualization of all the periurethral structures in only 60% of women studied. Artefacts associated with measurement can also occur if the urethra is not straight. The axis of the probe changes as the probe is drawn along the urethra and thus the plane imaged through the urethra is not constant. This limits the usefulness of this approach in viewing the periurethral structures.[76,77]

The function of the pelvic floor muscles has been indirectly assessed using ultrasonography by visualization of bladder-neck movement during pelvic floor contraction.[59,78-80] Transperineal imaging of the levator ani muscle is difficult, as only sections of the muscle are visualized when using two-dimensional ultrasonography.[79] Using a 5 MHz probe applied lateral to the posterior fourchette, the levator ani muscle has been described;[81,82] unfortunately, the structure imaged was less than 2 cm from the skin, suggesting that this was the deep transverse pernei muscles rather than the pelvic floor muscle, which is 3–4 cm from the skin.

THREE-DIMENSIONAL ULTRASONOGRAPHY

Three-dimensional ultrasonography allows images to be obtained in unlimited numbers through a selected volume and also at any angle to the US beam. The ability to image structures from any angle is particularly important when access is limited owing to the bony pelvis. Additionally, three-dimensional ultrasonography allows accurate volume measurements of the urethral sphincter, which is an irregular structure.

Imaging the urethra

The image of the urethra varies according to the approach. If US waves pass along the urethral axis, the longitudinal smooth muscle fibres and their surrounding collagen will appear hypoechoic and black, whereas the circular muscles will appear hyperechoic because the incident US waves are reflected as they travel perpendicular to the direction of the collagen fibres between the muscle fibres (Fig. 27.3). If, however, a transrectal/transvaginal approach is used, then the US waves pass perpendicular to the urethral axis, highlighting the longitudinal muscle fibres as hyperechoic and making the lateral parts of the rhabdosphincter hypoechoic (Fig. 27.4). Thus, the approach used depends upon which part of the urethral sphincter needs to be imaged.

Three-dimensional ultrasonography shows that the rhabdosphincter is thicker ventrally, thinning symmetrically at its lateral aspects and is thinnest on the dorsal surface. The transperineal approach visualizes the rhabdosphincter as a hyperechoic cylindrical structure around the urethra, with the hypoechoic core consisting of the longitudinal smooth muscle, urethral lumen and epithelium, and submucosal plexus; this has been confirmed by imaging cadaveric tissue, then comparing the histological measurements.[83] These ultrasonographic findings have also been validated using electromyography (EMG) of the urethral sphincter. The electrical activity of striated muscle was identified in the hypoechoic cylinder around the urethra.[27] This contrasts with the transvaginal approach, where the US waves pass perpendicular to the axis of the urethra, the

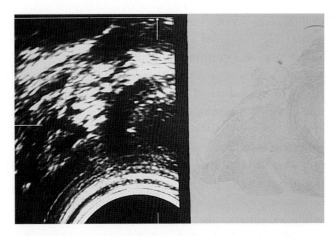

Figure 27.4. *Transvaginal approach to imaging the urethra. Note that the core of the urethra appears hyperechoic and the lateral fibres appear hypoechoic as they run perpendicular to the incident ultrasound waves.*

rhabdosphincter is hypoechoic around the urethra and the central core of the urethra is hyperechoic.

The urethra and urethral sphincter can be assessed at different levels. At the level of the bladder neck, the hyperechoic urothelium surrounded by the detrusor muscle fibres is seen, when the transvaginal approach is used. At the midurethral point, the rhabdosphincter can be clearly demonstrated surrounding the longitudinal smooth muscle. More distally, the urethral sphincter cross-sectional surface area decreases. This is mainly due to a reduction in the smooth muscle component rather than thinning of the striated muscle; thus, it is the smooth muscle that mainly contributes to the overall shape of the urethra.

In women with GSI there appears to be a thickening of the rhabdosphincter distally compared with that in women with DI. This correlates well with evidence of rhabdosphincter loss around the bladder neck with age.[84] To assess the volume of the urethral sphincter, a number of serial cross-sectional areas are measured along the urethral axis. To calculate the volume of the rhabdosphincter, the central 'core' volume is subtracted from the total urethral sphincter volume. The volume of the urethral sphincter has good inter- and intra-observer reproducibility and sections should be taken through the urethral sphincter at intervals no greater than 2 mm. In a study of 70 women with urinary symptoms, who had undergone urodynamic investigation, those with urethral sphincter incompetence had significantly smaller urethral sphincters than did

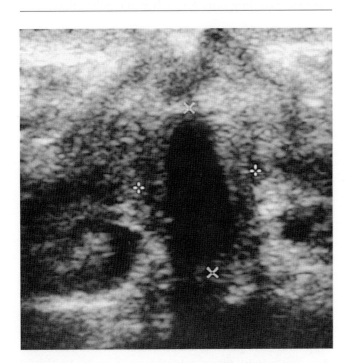

Figure 27.3. *Transperineal ultrasonography image of the urethra. The ultrasound waves pass along the long axis of the urethra. Longitudinal fibres do not produce any echo and appear hypoechoic (black).*

women with competent urethral sphincter mechanisms.[1] Their urethral sphincters were shorter and had a small maximal urethral sphincter cross-sectional area.

Childbirth is associated with the development of GSI. It has been postulated that damage to the pudendal nerve, which innervates the rhabdosphincter, leads to atrophy of the rhabdosphincter and reduction in sphincter volume.[85–87] Recently, evidence of reinnervation 6 months after vaginal delivery has indicated that this denervation process is temporary and another mechanism may be involved.[88] There is a reduction in sphincter volume after vaginal delivery,[89] which indicates that the bulk of the rhabdosphincter may be reduced during vaginal delivery; this may be a primary and most important cause of GSI.

The function of the urethral sphincter can be assessed with urethral pressure profilometry.[90–92] The urethral pressures are measured at rest and also during stress. It is thought that the resting urethral pressure profile (UPP) reflects the tone of the striated urethral sphincter. The volume of the urethral sphincter has been measured using three-dimensional ultrasonography and compared with the pressure measurements obtained during urethral pressure profilometry.[93] The length of the rhabdosphincter on ultrasonography was significantly correlated with the functional urethral length. Additionally, the distance from the proximal part of the sphincter to the plane of the maximal cross-sectional area, and the distance from the start of the UPP to the maximal urethral closure pressure (MUCP), were also significantly correlated. The area under the UPP curve was found to correlate well with the volume of the rhabdosphincter in most women except those who had undergone previous vaginal prolapse surgery, who were found to have higher MUCP values than would be suggested by the rhabdosphincter volume. This discrepancy is probably a result of scar tissue after vaginal surgery compressing the urethra, rather than any abnormality of the rhabdosphincter.

Although urethral pressure profilometry cannot be used to make the diagnosis of GSI, some authors have suggested that it may be used to plan the type of continence surgery and to predict the outcome. An MUCP of less than 20 cmH$_2$O has been shown to predict a poor outcome for incontinence surgery,[94,95] and it has been suggested that these women would benefit from a sling or perhaps even an artificial urinary sphincter.[94,96,97] However, one-third of all the patients whose surgical procedures have failed have a satisfactory preoperative MUCP. As suggested above, these women may have an elevated urethral closure pressure due to scar tissue rather than a damaged rhabdosphincter; thus, three-dimensional ultrasonography may, in the future, predict with greater accuracy successful continence surgery by measuring rhabdosphincter volumes.

EMG of the rhabdosphincter using a concentric needle is a difficult procedure that is uncomfortable for the patient, but it is useful in the investigation of patients with neurological disorders associated with lower urinary tract dysfunction.[98] As the technique is performed blind and the target site is a small volume of muscle tissue, it is not uncommon for it to take time to place the needle in the correct position – or even to fail to obtain a signal. Three-dimensional ultrasonography can be used to visualize the urethral sphincter to validate the correct position of the concentric needle EMG electrode.[27] The electrical activity is detected not only within the rhabdosphincter but also when the tip of the EMG needle has been clearly visualized outside the urethral sphincter; thus, it may be important in future to use three-dimensional ultrasonography to ensure that signals are recorded from the rhabdosphincter rather than surrounding muscles such as the pelvic floor.

The levator ani muscle

The pelvic floor is composed of a group of muscles termed the levator ani. This consists of two parts: the first makes up the diaphragm (ileococcygeus) and the second is a U-shaped band of muscle pulling the rectum anteriorly (pubococcygeus).[99] The pubococcygeus muscle arises from the inferior border of the pubic bone, extends dorsally and laterally, lateral to the vagina and then directs itself medially to interdigitate with its other half behind the anorectal junction. The medial edge of the pubococcygeus muscle leaves an opening through which the urethra, vagina and rectum can pass; this is termed the levator or urogenital hiatus.

The pubococcygeus is composed mainly of slow-twitch fibres which maintain constant tone and provide support for the pelvic and abdominal viscera. There are also fast-twitch fibres which are recruited during increases in intra-abdominal pressure such as coughing or sneezing.[100,101] Contraction of the pubococcygeus muscle compresses the rectum and vagina against the pubic bone, reducing the size of the levator ani hiatus and preventing possible prolapse of the pelvic organs.

There are two techniques for scanning the pelvic floor. The transperineal technique can scan the entire pelvic floor and, using three-dimensional ultrasonography, an image can be reconstructed perpendicular to the passage of the US waves through the tissues in the plane of the pelvic floor. This approach has the benefit of making the entire pubococcygeus muscle hyperechoic and the fibres can easily be seen passing dorsally around the anorectal junction (Fig. 27.5). Vaginal prolapse makes the transperineal approach difficult, as air trapped in the vagina impairs the image obtained.

If a 7.5 MHz transrectal probe is used, a transverse section of the pelvic floor can be obtained by inserting the probe vaginally. To image the levator hiatus correctly, the insertion of the levator ani muscle into the pubic bone should be identified. The insertion is 5 mm in width in the axial plane and can be used as a fixed point on both sides of the pubic bone. The posterior landmark is the anorectal angle, which can be identified in the transverse plane by determining where the rectum is most anterior. The medial margin of the pubococcygeus sling is demarcated clearly and the surface area and width of the levator ani hiatus can be measured. The widths of the levator hiatus are measured through the urethra, the midpoint of the vagina and

anterior to the rectum. If the US probe is moved more cranially, then the obturator internus can be seen and the attachment of the ileococcygeus muscle to the obturator fascia can also be demonstrated. Defects laterally in the vaginal walls can also be visualized using this technique. The area of the levator hiatus has been found to be larger in women with, than in those without, vaginal prolapse;[2] however, women who have GSI and prolapse appear to have the same-sized levator ani hiatus as women with prolapse alone. Conversely, women who do not have prolapse but have GSI do not have an enlarged levator ani hiatus. Thus, it appears that an enlarged levator ani hiatus is associated with the development of urogenital prolapse.

Additionally in this study,[2] the urethral sphincter volume was shown to be smaller in those women who had GSI and did not show any correlation in those women who had vaginal prolapse without GSI. It has also been noted, when imaging the urethral sphincter and the pelvic floor in women before and after delivery, that the levator ani surface area was increased in those women who had a vaginal delivery. However, there were no changes (in those women who were continent) in their maximal urethral sphincter volume and urethral sphincter length.

BLADDER WALL THICKNESS

The bladder wall can be measured in a reproducible manner using the transvaginal approach (Fig. 27.6). The bladder wall thins in response to bladder filling, but only once the intravesical volume has exceeded 50 ml.[102] Bladder wall thickness is best measured after the woman has voided and the intravesical volume has been measured as less than 50 ml. The bladder wall thickness is measured in the parasagittal plane, as the urethra sometimes obscures the dome of the bladder. Measurements are made at maximum magnification, perpendicular to the inner surface of the bladder at the dome, anterior wall and trigone. The mean of the three measurements is used as a test for detrusor overactivity. A pilot study comparing women with DI and GSI showed that those women diagnosed as having DI all had a mean bladder wall thickness greater than 5 mm. In an unselected group of 184 symptomatic women, 108 were found to have DI of whom 102 (94%) women had DI on videocystourethrography or ambulatory urodynamics; of 17 women with a bladder wall thickness of less than 3.5 mm, three were found to have DI.[102] Bladder wall thickness

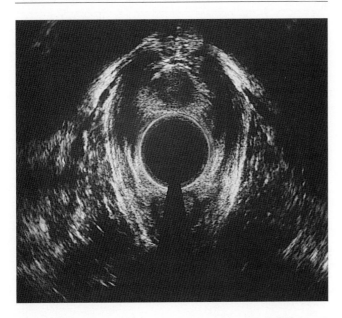

Figure 27.5. *Transvaginal ultrasonography scan of the levator ani hiatus, which is the inner margin of the levator ani muscle.*

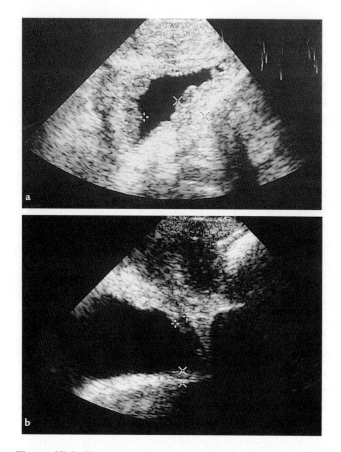

Figure 27.6. *Transvaginal ultrasonography of the post-micturition bladder. The bladder wall thickness is being measured (a) in a woman with detrusor instability and (b) in a woman with genuine stress incontinence.*

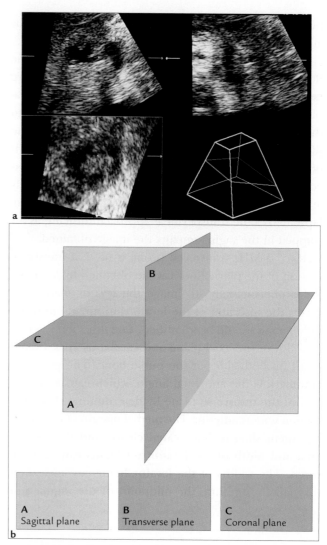

Figure 27.7. *(a) Three-dimensional ultrasound scan of the urethra and a urethral diverticulum using the transperineal approach. (b) Orientation of the three images to each other.*

has also been used in predicting the development of *de-novo* DI after Burch colposuspension. A mean bladder wall thickness preoperatively greater than 8 mm in women with GSI was associated with symptomatic urgency and urge incontinence postoperatively.

URETHRAL DIVERTICULA

Urethral diverticula are occasionally congenital but are usually acquired. They may occur as a result of childbirth, infection or instrumentation of the urethra. Their development is due to infection and obstruction of the periurethral glands, causing the formation of cystic structures that are mainly in the posterior wall of the distal urethra. The urethra can be imaged using X-rays with contrast. Because it is important to develop a positive pressure within the urethra, a positive-pressure double-balloon urethral (Trattner) catheter is used.

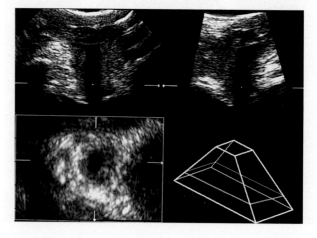

Figure 27.8. *The urethra after the suburethral diverticulum shown in Figure 27.7a had been removed.*

Diverticula can also be visualized using vaginal ultrasonography. The problem with using radiological techniques is that the soft tissue cannot be seen and the position of the ostium in relation to the urethral sphincter cannot be identified. This is important in counselling a patient and deciding which surgical approach should be used. With three-dimensional ultrasonography the urethral sphincter can be seen clearly and the ostium leading to the diverticulum can also be determined. The additional benefit of ultrasonography is that contents of the urethral diverticulum can be identified – for example, calculi or a soft tissue growth. The image of a urethral diverticulum is shown in Figure 27.7; the urethra after the diverticulum has been removed by subtotal diverticulectomy is depicted in Figure 27.8.

CONCLUSIONS

Ultrasonography offers a useful method by which the bladder, urethra and surrounding tissues may be studied and measured. At present, only measurements of urinary bladder volumes are of proven clinical value.

REFERENCES

1. Khullar V, Salvatore S, Cardozo LD *et al.* Three dimensional ultrasound of the urethra and urethral sphincter – a new diagnostic technique. *Neurourol Urodyn* 1994; 13: 352–354

2. Athanasiou S, Hill S, Cardozo LD *et al.* Three dimensional ultrasound of the urethra, periurethral tissues and pelvic floor (abstract). *Int Urogynecol J* 1995; 6: 239

3. Riccabona M, Nelson TR, Pretorius DH. Three-dimensional ultrasound: accuracy of distance and volume measurements. *Ultrasound Obstet Gynecol* 1996; 7: 429–434

4. Hamper UM, Trapanotto V, Sheth S *et al.* Three-dimensional US: preliminary clinical experience. *Radiology* 1994; 191: 397–401

5. Ng KJ, Gardener JE, Rickards D *et al.* Three-dimensional imaging of the prostatic urethra – an exciting new tool. *Br J Urol* 1994; 74: 604–608

6. Hederstrom E, Forsberg L. Accuracy of repeated kidney size estimation by ultrasonography and urography in children. *Acta Radiol Diagn* 1985; 26: 603–607

7. Hricak H, Lieto RP. Sonographic determination of renal volume. *Radiology* 1983; 148: 311–312

8. Rosenfield AT, Siegel NJ. Renal parenchymal disease. Histopathological-sonographic correlation. *Am J Roentgenol* 1981; 137: 793–798

9. Rosenfield AT, Taylor KJW, Grade M, DeGraaf CS. Anatomy and pathology of the kidney by grey-scale ultrasound. *Radiology* 1978; 128: 737–744

10. Marchal G, Verbeken E, Ogen R *et al.* Ultrasound of the normal kidney: a sonographic, anatomic and histologic correlation. *Ultrasound Med Biol* 1986; 12: 999–1009

11. Morin ME, Baker DA. The influence of hydration and bladder distension on the sonographic diagnosis of hydronephrosis. *J Clin Ultrasound* 1979; 7: 192–194

12. Malave SR, Neiman HL, Spies SM *et al.* Diagnosis of hydronephrosis: comparison of radionuclide scanning and sonography. *Am J Roentgenol* 1980; 135: 1179–1185

13. Dalla-Palma L, Bazzochi M, Pozzi-Mucelli RS *et al.* Ultrasonography in the diagnosis of hydronephrosis in patients with normal renal function. *Urol Radiol* 1983; 5: 221–226

14. Sanders RC, Bearman S. B-Scan ultrasound in the diagnosis of hydronephrosis. *Radiology* 1973; 108: 375–382

15. Ellenbogen PH, Scheible FW, Talner LB, Leopold GR. Sensitivity of grey scale ultrasound in detecting urinary tract obstruction. *Am J Roentgenol* 1978; 130: 731–733

16. Peake SC, Roxburgh HB, Langlois SleP. Ultrasonic assessment of the hydronephrosis of pregnancy. *Radiology* 1983; 146: 167–170

17. White RD, McQuown D, McCarthy TA, Ostergard DR. Real-time ultrasonography in the evaluation of urinary stress incontinence. *Am J Obstet Gynecol* 1980; 138: 235–237

18. Wexler JD, McGovern TP. Ultrasonography of female urethral diverticula. *Am J Roentgenol* 1980; 134: 737–740

19. Mouritsen L, Bach P. Ultrasonic evaluation of bladder neck position and mobility: the influence of urethral catheter, bladder volume and body position. *Neurourol Urodyn* 1994; 13: 637–646

20. De Gonzalez EL, Cosgrove DO, Joseph AE *et al.* The appearances on ultrasound of the female urethral sphincter. *Br J Radiol* 1988; 61: 687–690

21. Richmond DH, Sutherst J. Transrectal ultrasound scanning in urinary incontinence: the effect of the probe on urodynamic parameters. *Br J Urol* 1989; 64: 582–585

22. Brown MC, Sutherst JR, Murray A, Richmond DH. Potential use of ultrasound in place of X-ray fluoroscopy in urodynamics. *Br J Urol* 1985; 57: 88–90

23. Richmond DH, Sutherst JR, Brown MC. Screening of the bladder base and urethra using linear array transrectal ultrasound scanning. *J Clin Ultrasound* 1986; 14: 647–651

24. Shabsigh R, Fishman IJ, Krebs M. The use of transrectal longitudinal real-time ultrasonography in urodynamics. *J Urol* 1987; 138: 1416–1419

25. Shabsigh R, Fishman IJ, Krebs M. Combined transrectal ultrasonography and urodynamics in the evaluation of detrusor-sphincter dyssynergia. *Br J Urol* 1988; 62: 326–330

26. Bergman A, McKenzie CJ, Richmond J *et al.* Transrectal ultrasound versus cystography in the evaluation of anatomical stress urinary incontinence. *Br J Urol* 1988; 62: 228–234

27. Hill S, Khullar V, Cardozo LD *et al.* Ultrasound electromyography – a new technique (abstract). *Int Urogynecol J* 1995; 6: 243

28. Hasan ST, Hamdy FC, Schofield IS, Neal DE. Transrectal ultrasound guided needle electromyography of the urethral sphincter in males. *Neurourol Urodyn* 1995; 14: 359–364

29. Keefe B, Warshauer DM, Tucker MS, Mittelstaedt CA. Diverticula of the female urethra: diagnosis by endovaginal and transperineal sonography. *Am J Roentgenol* 1991; 156: 1195–1197

30. Abet L, Natho W, Schulze B *et al.* [Urethrography versus vaginal ultrasonography in urethral diverticula.] (In German.) *Gynakol Rundsch* 1990; 30 (Suppl 1): 238–241

31. Roehrborn CG, Peters PC. Can transabdominal ultrasound estimation of postvoiding residual (PVR) replace catheterisation? *Urology* 1988; 31: 445–449

32. Poston J, Joseph AEA, Riddle PR. The accuracy of ultrasound in the measurement of changes in bladder volume. *Br J Urol* 1983; 55: 361–363

33. Pedersen JF, Bartrum RJ, Grytter C. Residual urine determination by ultrasonic scanning. *Am J Roentgenol* 1975; 125: 474–478

34. McLean GK, Edell SL. Determination of bladder volumes by gray scale ultrasonography. *Radiology* 1978; 128: 181–182

35. Griffiths CJ, Murray A, Ramsden PD. Accuracy of and repeatability of bladder volume by means of ultrasonic B-mode scanning. *J Urol* 1986; 136: 808–812

36. Hartnell CG, Kiely EA, Williams G, Gibson RN. Real-time ultrasound measurement of bladder volume: a comparative study of three methods. *Br J Radiol* 1987; 60: 1063–1065

37. Beacock CJ, Roberts EE, Rees RWM, Buck AC. Ultrasound assessment of residual urine. A quantitative method. *Br J Urol* 1985; 57: 410–413

38. Rageth JC, Langer K. Ultrasonic assessment of residual urine volume. *Urol Res* 1982; 10: 57–60

39. Hakenberg OW, Ryall RL, Langlois SL, Marshal VR. The estimation of bladder volume by sonocystography. *J Urol* 1983; 130: 249–251

40. Roehrborn CG, Chinn HK, Fulgham PF *et al.* The role of transabdominal ultrasound in the preoperative evaluation of patients with benign prostatic hypertrophy. *J Urol* 1986; 135: 1190–1193

41. Haylen BT, Frazer MI, Sutherst JR, West CR. Transvaginal ultrasound in the measurement of bladder volumes in women. *Br J Urol* 1989; 63: 149–151

42. Haylen BT. Residual urine volumes in a normal female population: application of transvaginal ultrasound. *Br J Urol* 1989; 64: 347–349

43. Haylen BT. Verification of the accuracy and range of transvaginal ultrasound in measuring bladder volumes in women. *Br J Urol* 1989; 64: 350–352

44. Haylen BT, Frazer MI, MacDonald JH. Assessing the effectiveness of different urinary catheters in emptying the bladder: an application of transvaginal ultrasound. *Br J Urol* 1989; 64: 353–356

45. Baker KR, Drutz HP, Lemieux M-C. Limited accuracy of vaginal probe ultrasound in measuring residual urine volumes. *Int Urogynecol J* 1993; 4: 138–140

46. Fowler JE, Pulaski ET. Excretory urography cystography and cystoscopy in the evaluation of women with urinary tract infection. *N Engl J Med* 1981; 304: 462–465

47. Spencer J, Lindsell D, Mastorakou I. Ultrasonography compared with intravenous urography in the investigation of adults with haematuria. *Br Med J* 1990; 301: 1074–1076

48. McNicholas MMJ, Grifin JF, Cantwell DF. Ultrasound of the pelvis and renal tract combined with a plain film of the abdomen in young women with urinary tract infections: can it replace intravenous urography? *Br J Radiol* 1991; 64: 221–224

49. Fox M, Power RF, Bruce AW. Diverticulum of the bladder – presentation and evaluation in 115 cases. *Br J Urol* 1962; 34: 286–289

50. Davies AH, Mastorakou I, Dickinson AJ *et al.* Flexible cystoscopy compared with ultrasound in the detection of recurrent bladder tumours. *Br J Urol* 1991; 67: 491–492

51. Flannigan GM, Gelister JSK, Noble JG *et al.* Rigid versus flexible cystoscopy. A controlled trial of patient tolerance. *Br J Urol* 1988; 62: 537–540

52. Fernandez Fernandez A, Mayayo Dehesa T. Leiomyoma of the urinary bladder floor: diagnosis by transvaginal ultrasound. *Urol Int* 1992; 48: 99–101

53. Quinn MJ, Beynon J, Mortensen NJ, Smith PJB. Transvaginal endosonography: a new method to study the anatomy of the lower urinary tract in urinary stress incontinence. *Br J Urol* 1988; 62: 414–418

54. Bhatia NN, Ostergard DR, McQuown D. Ultrasonography in urinary incontinence. *Urology* 1987; 29: 90-4

55. Wise BG, Burton G, Cutner A, Cardozo LD. Effect of vaginal ultrasound probe on lower urinary tract function. *Br J Urol* 1992; 70: 12–16

56. Kil PJM, Hoekstra JW, van der Meijden APM *et al.* Transvaginal ultrasonography and urodynamic evaluation after suspension operations: comparison among the Gittes, Stamey and Burch suspensions. *J Urol* 1991; 146: 132–136

57. Weil EHJ, van Waalwijk van Doorn ESC, Heesakkers JPFA *et al.* Transvaginal ultrasonography: a study with healthy volunteers and women with genuine stress incontinence. *Eur Urol* 1993; 24: 226–230

58. Quinn MJ. Vaginal ultrasound and urinary stress incontinence. *Contemp Rev Obstet Gynaecol* 1990; 2: 104–110

59. Wise BG, Khullar V, Cardozo LD. Bladder neck movement during pelvic floor contraction and intravaginal electrical stimulation in women with and without genuine stress incontinence. *Neurourol Urodyn* 1992; 11: 309–311

60. Bump RC, Mattiasson A, Bø K *et al.* The standardization of terminology of female pelvic organ prolapse and pelvic floor adjustment. *J Am Obstet Gynecol* 1996; 175: 10–17

61. Boos K, Athanasiou S, Toozs-Hobson P *et al.* The dynamics of pelvic floor extrinsic continence mechanism before and after Burch colposuspension. *Neurourol Neurodyn* 1997 16: 411–412

62. King JK, Freeman RM. Is antenatal bladder neck mobility, a risk factor for postpartum stress incontinence? *Br J Obstet Gynaecol* 1998; 105: 1300–1307

63. Quinn MJ, Beynon J, Mortensen NN, Smith PJB. Vaginal endosonography in the post-operative assessment of colposuspension. *Br J Urol* 1989; 63: 295–300

64. Khullar V, Athanasiou S, Cardozo L *et al.* Urinary sphincter volume and urodynamic diagnosis. *Neurourol Urodyn* 1996; 15: 334–336

65. Creighton SM, Pearce JM, Stanton SL. Perineal video-ultrasonography in the assessment of vaginal prolapse: early observations. *Br J Obstet Gynaecol* 1992; 99: 310–313

66. Clark A, Creighton SM, Pearce M, Stanton SL. Localisation of the bladder neck by perineal ultrasound: methodology and applications. *Neurourol Urodyn* 1990; 9: 394–395

67. Koelbl H, Bernaschek G. A new method for sonographic urethrocystography and simultaneous pressure-flow measurements. *Obstet Gynecol* 1989; 74: 417–422

68. Schaer GN, Siegwart R, Perucchini D, DeLancey JO. Examination of voiding in seated women using a remote-controlled ultrasound probe. *Obstet Gynecol* 1998; 91: 297–301

69. Creighton SM, Clark A, Pearce JM, Stanton SL. Perineal bladder neck ultrasound: appearances before and after continence surgery. *Ultrasound Obstet Gynecol* 1994; 4: 428–433

70. Shapeero LG, Friedland GW, Perkash I. Transrectal sonographic voiding cystourethrography: studies in neuromuscular bladder dysfunction. *Am J Roentgenol* 1983; 141: 83–90

71. Perkash I, Friedland GW. Catheter-induced hyper-reflexia in spinal cord injury patients: diagnosis by sonographic voiding cystourethrography. *Radiology* 1986; 159: 453–455

72. Perkash I, Friedland GW. Posterior ledge at the bladder neck: crucial diagnostic role of ultrasonography. *Urol Radiol* 1986; 8: 175–183

73. Perkash I, Friedland GW. Ultrasonic detection of false passages arising from posterior urethra in spinal cord injury patients. *J Urol* 1987; 137: 701–702

74. Timor Tritsch IE, Haratz Rubinstein N, Monteagudo A *et al.* Transvaginal color Doppler sonography of the ureteral jets: a method to detect ureteral patency. *Obstet Gynecol* 1997; 89: 113–117

75. Schaer GN, Schmid T, Peschers U, DeLancey JO. Intraurethral ultrasound correlated with urethral histology. *Obstet Gynecol* 1998; 91: 60–64

76. Kirschner-Hermanns R, Klein H-M, Muller U *et al.* Intraurethral ultrasound in women with stress incontinence. *Br J Urol* 1994; 74: 315–318

77. Klein H-M, Kirschner-Hermanns R, Lagunilla J *et al.* Assessment of incontinence with intraurethral ultrasound: preliminary results (abstract). *Radiology* 1993; 187: 141–143

78. Schaer GN, Koechli OR, Schuessler B, Haller U. Perineal ultrasound for evaluating the bladder neck in urinary stress incontinence. *Obstet Gynecol* 1995; 85: 220–224

79. Peschers U, Schaer G, Anthuber C *et al.* Changes in vesical neck mobility following vaginal delivery. *Obstet Gynecol* 1996; 88: 1001–1006

80. Peschers UM, Schaer GN, DeLancey JO, Schuessler B. Levator ani function before and after childbirth. *Br J Obstet Gynaecol* 1997; 104: 1004–1008

81. Bernstein I, Juul N, Gronvall S *et al.* Pelvic floor muscle thickness measured by perineal ultrasonography. *Scand J Urol Nephrol* 1991; 137S: 131–133

82. Bernstein IT. The pelvic floor muscles: muscle thickness in healthy and urinary-incontinent women measured by perineal ultrasonography with reference to the effect of pelvic floor training. Estrogen receptor studies. *Neurourol Urodyn* 1997; 16: 237–275

83. Khullar V, Athanasiou S, Cardozo LD *et al.* Histological correlates of the urethral sphincter and surrounding

structures with ultrasound findings. *Int Urogynaecol J* 1996; 7: 16

84. Perucchini D, DeLancey JOL, Ashton-Miller JA. Regional striated muscle loss in the female urethra: where is the striated muscle vulnerable? *Neurourol Urodyn* 1997; 16: 407–408

85. Snooks SJ, Swash M, Henry MM, Setchell M. Risk factors in childbirth causing damage to the pelvic floor innervation. *Int J Colorectal Dis* 1986; 1: 20–24

86. Swash M, Snooks SJ, Henry MM. Unifying concept of pelvic floor disorders and incontinence. *J R Soc Med* 1985; 78: 906–911

87. Snooks SJ, Badenoch DF, Tiptaft RC, Swash M. Perineal nerve damage in genuine stress urinary incontinence. An electrophysiological study. *Br J Urol* 1985; 57: 422–426

88. Smith AR, Hosker GL, Warrell DW. The role of pudendal nerve damage in the aetiology of genuine stress incontinence in women. *Br J Obstet Gynaecol* 1989; 96: 29–32

89. Toozs-Hobson P, Athanasiou S, Khullar V *et al.* Why do women develop incontinence after childbirth? *Neurourol Urodyn* 1997; 16: 384–385

90. Versi E, Cardozo LD, Studd J. Distal urethral compensatory mechanisms in women with an incompetent bladder neck who remain continent, and the effect of the menopause. *Neurourol Urodyn* 1990; 9: 579–590

91. Hilton P, Stanton SL. Urethral pressure measurement by microtransducer: the results in symptom-free women and in those with genuine stress incontinence. *Br J Obstet Gynaecol* 1983; 90: 919–933

92. Tapp A, Cardozo L, Versi E *et al.* The effect of vaginal delivery on the urethral sphincter. *Br J Obstet Gynaecol* 1988; 95: 142–146

93. Khullar V, Salvatore S, Cardozo LD *et al.* Three dimensional ultrasound of the urethra and urethral pressure profiles (abstract.) *Int Urogynecol J* 1994; 5: 319

94. Sand PK, Bowen LW, Panganiban R, Ostergard DR. The low pressure urethra as a factor in failed retropubic urethropexy. *Obstet Gynecol* 1987; 69: 399–402

95. Bowen LW, Sand PK, Ostergard DR, Franti CE. Unsuccessful Burch retropubic urethropexy: a case-controlled urodynamic study. *Am J Obstet Gynecol* 1989; 160: 452–458

96. Koonings PP, Bergman A, Ballard CA. Low urethral pressure and stress urinary incontinence in women: risk factor for failed retropubic surgical procedure. *Urology* 1990; 36: 245–248

97. Blaivas JG, Olsson CA. Stress incontinence: classification and surgical approach. *J Urol* 1988; 139: 727–731

98. Fowler CJ, Kirby RS. Electromyography of urethral sphincter in women with urinary retention. *Lancet* 1986; 1: 1455–1457

99. Lawson JO. Pelvic anatomy. I. Pelvic floor muscles. *Ann R Coll Surg Engl* 1974; 54: 244–252

100. Gosling JA, Dixon JS, Humpherson JR. *Functional Anatomy of the Urinary Tract – An Integrated Text and Colour Atlas*. London: Gower, 1983

101. Gosling JA, Dixon JS, Critchley HOD, Thompson SA. A comparative study of the human external sphincter and periurethral levator ani muscles. *Br J Urol* 1981; 53: 35–41

102. Khullar V, Cardozo L, Salvatore S, Hill S. Ultrasound: a noninvasive screening test for detrusor instability. *Br J Obstet Gynaecol* 1996; 103: 904–908

28

Endoscopy

G. W. Cundiff

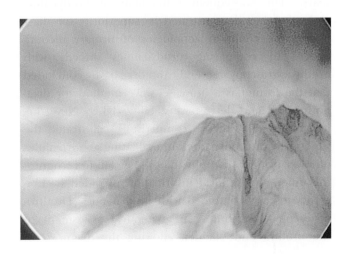

EVALUATION OF URINARY INCONTINENCE

Urinary incontinence is a non-specific symptom resulting from a variety of different conditions; the differential diagnosis of urinary incontinence in women is therefore broad and includes genuine stress incontinence (GSI), overactive bladder disorders, overflow incontinence, urinary tract fistulae and urethral diverticula. Distinguishing these different aetiologies is imperative, as each condition warrants a different therapeutic approach.

Prior to the advent of sophisticated diagnostic modalities, most physicians depended on historical information related to inciting events and associated symptoms combined with physical findings to determine the aetiology of incontinence. There is now a substantial body of literature addressing the inaccuracy of historical and physical findings.[1–3] Although physiological subtypes of urinary incontinence demonstrate significant population differences in the distribution of symptoms, the considerable overlap in symptoms limits predictive value in the individual patient. Attempts to improve this sensitivity by using pure symptoms or symptom complexes have proved to be equally inaccurate.[4] Consequently, although historical and physical examination findings are valuable to correlate findings with patient complaints, they are no more than a guide to the diagnosis of lower urinary tract disorders.

Recognition of the inaccuracy of symptomatology as the sole basis for diagnosing urinary incontinence fostered the development of new diagnostic modalities for better evaluation of the condition. Dynamic urethroscopy was initially proposed as a complete method for evaluating lower urinary tract dysfunction, and has been used in this capacity for more than 30 years.[5] The subsequent refinement of urodynamic evaluation has demonstrated its superiority for diagnosing the common aetiologies of urinary incontinence. In comparing urodynamics directly with urethrocystoscopy, several authors have concluded that the former is a more sensitive method for diagnosing GSI and detrusor instability (DI).[6,7] Nevertheless, although these comparisons illustrate the superiority of urodynamics in evaluating abnormalities of lower urinary tract physiology, they fail to recognize the unique anatomical information provided by urethrocystoscopy combined with urodynamics. Urethrocystoscopy contributes an anatomical assessment of the urethra and bladder, allowing the diagnosis of benign and malignant mucosal lesions that would remain undiagnosed by urodynamics alone.

Cundiff and Bent illustrated the value of urethrocystoscopy as an adjunct to urodynamics in a study of women undergoing combined urodynamics and urethrocystoscopy.[8] Urethrocystoscopy was considered important to 19% of the final diagnoses. Specifically, it provided new information in patients with anatomical abnormalities including intravesical lesions, intravesical foreign bodies, and urethral diverticula. Although not present in this series, urogenital fistula should be included in this category of anatomical lesions amenable to diagnosis by endoscopy.

INDICATIONS

The modern era of cost containment in medicine challenges physicians to determine a cost-effective approach to diagnosis that does not compromise the accuracy of the evaluation. In this context, it is important to define those women presenting with urinary incontinence who need the anatomical assessment provided by cystourethroscopy. There are several clear indications, which are addressed individually in the following sections.

Suspected anatomical lesions

Anatomical abnormalities, such as urogenital fistulae and urethral diverticula, might be suspected on the basis of history or urodynamics but require an anatomical assessment for confirmation. For example, a diverticulum can be suspected on the basis of a history of recurrent urinary tract infections, post-void dribbling, or pelvic pain. In such a patient a biphasic urethral pressure profile is virtually diagnostic of a urethral diverticulum; however, Leach and Bavendam found that only 72% of patients with a urethral diverticulum demonstrated a biphasic pattern.[9] This contrasts with the reported diagnostic accuracy for urethrocystoscopy of 84–90%.[10,11] Beyond diagnosis, urethrocystoscopy also provides important information about the size and location of the ostia, as well as the presence of multiple diverticula. The ability of cystourethroscopy to define the location, size and surrounding anatomical relationships pertains for urinogenital fistulae as well, and both Massee *et al.*[12] and Symmonds[13] consider it to be the simplest method for evaluating urinary tract fistulae.

Recurrent incontinence

Women with recurrent urinary incontinence following a therapeutic intervention comprise a complex group of patients that may suffer from preoperative misdiagnosis, failed intervention or a complication of the intervention. The fallibility of symptoms in determining the aetiology of incontinence is even greater in this group of patients, and they all deserve a thorough evaluation, including multichannel urodynamics as well as the anatomical assessment provided by cystourethroscopy.

When recurrent incontinence is associated with a urodynamic diagnosis of DI, the differential diagnosis includes new-onset DI, persistent but previously undiagnosed DI, obstruction-related DI, and mucosal irritation leading to DI. Mucosal irritation may be due to foreign bodies, such as a calculus, or an intravesical suture, which are easily diagnosed at cystourethroscopy. Outflow obstruction due to overzealous elevation of the urethrovesical junction (UVJ) at the time of retropubic urethropexy has also been shown to be a cause of DI in recurrent incontinence.[14] Cystourethroscopy is useful in these patients to achieve a visual evaluation of UVJ elevation and to eliminate other possible aetiologies in the differential diagnosis.

Recurrent GSI after continence surgery may result from persistent urethral hypermobility, or poor coaptation. Persistent urethral hypermobility occurs either from inadequate elevation of the UVJ or failed UVJ stabilization secondary to suture failure, poor tissue quality or excessive stress on the repair.[15] Poor coaptation, whether it is due to a damaged sphincter muscle, poor compressibility due to urethral fibrosis, or a lack of compressibility by surrounding organs, results in intrinsic sphincteric deficiency (ISD). These are women that clearly need an anatomical assessment such as that provided by cystourethroscopy.

INTRINSIC SPHINCTERIC DEFICIENCY

The Agency for Health Care Policy and Research defined ISD as a condition in which 'the urethral sphincter is unable to coapt and generate enough resistance to retain urine in the bladder.'[16] ISD is generally contrasted with the more common form of GSI, caused by bladder-neck hypermobility that results in a pressure transmission discrepancy between the bladder and urethra. Unfortunately, clinical criteria for ISD have not been standardized. Recent efforts to generate functional criteria for ISD have focused on leak-point pressures (LPPs) and maximum urethral closure pressures (MUCPs). Conventional surgical therapy for GSI due to hypermobility has been shown to have a high failure rate in patients with MUCP values of $20\ cmH_2O$ or less.[17,18] Outcome measures for LPP values are not currently available, yet discrepancies in the accuracy of both low MUCP and LPP have been demonstrated.[19,20] A substantial lack of concordance between low MUCP and low LPP has also been demonstrated. Moreover, low MUCP and LPP values are commonly associated with urethral hypermobility.[20]

In the absence of validated standard criteria for diagnosing ISD, an approach that combines historical risk factors with measures of incontinence severity, urodynamic evidence of poor urethral resistance and an anatomical evaluation of urethral coaptation seems to be warranted. Cystourethroscopy is perhaps the simplest approach to the anatomical evaluation of the UVJ. In comparing low MUCP with composite diagnostic criteria based on history, urodynamics and endoscopic appearance of the UVJ, Cundiff and Bent reported that low MUCP alone had a sensitivity of 20% and a positive predictive value of 40% for diagnosing ISD. They advocated a composite diagnosis that included the use of cystourethroscopy.[8]

The anatomical evaluation provided by cystourethroscopy can also be achieved using radiological techniques (see chapter 26). Transrectal and perineal ultrasonography (see chapter 27) have been used to evaluate women with urinary incontinence. Although most investigators have utilized ultrasonography to assess UVJ mobility,[21–23] others have advocated it as a means of differentiating between GSI and ISD.[24] This might be an alternative to urethroscopy for evaluating the UVJ but does not provide the mucosal evaluation of the lower urinary tract achieved with urethrocystoscopy. The same is true of fluoroscopy, although some authors feel that it is superior to cystourethroscopy for diagnosing ISD. Moreover, although videourodynamics can provide an equivalent anatomical evaluation of the UVJ, the cost of providing such a service is considerably higher than the cost of basic urethrocystoscopy.

Universal evaluation

There is general agreement that cystoscopy is indicated for patients complaining of irritative symptoms, persistent incontinence or voiding dysfunction following incontinence surgery. There is less agreement about the role of cystoscopy in the baseline evaluation of all women with urinary incontinence, and there are relatively few analyses to define its role in this capacity. However, one series suggests that, at the time of cystourethroscopy, up to 5% of patients presenting with urinary incontinence may have unsuspected neoplastic lesions, including bladder malignancies and potentially premalignant lesions such as cystitis glandularis.[8] Ideally, historical factors or urodynamic parameters could be used to distinguish those patients that merit urethrocystoscopy on the basis of risks for neoplastic lesions; nevertheless (in this relatively limited population), age over 60 years, symptoms of urgency, and a urodynamic diagnosis of DI were not predictive of these mucosal lesions. Moreover, common symptoms associated with mucosal lesions, such as pain and haematuria, were not present in these patients.

The annual age-adjusted incidence per 100 000 population for bladder cancer in women is reported as 6.2. It rises with increasing age, approaching 20 for age 55 years, and there are also regional variations.[25,26] Whether women presenting with urinary incontinence have a higher incidence of bladder cancer has not been determined. The benefits of combining cystourethroscopy with urodynamic evaluation for women presenting with urinary incontinence must, therefore, must be determined by individual clinicians.

INSTRUMENTATION

Rigid cystoscopy

There are three components to the rigid cystoscope – the telescope, the sheath and the bridge (Fig. 28.1) Each component serves a different function and is available with various options to facilitate its role under different circumstances.

Telescopes

The telescope transmits light to the bladder cavity as well as an image to the viewer. Today, virtually all rigid telescopes use a rod lens system. Telescopes designed for cystoscopy are available with several viewing angles including 0 degrees (straight), 30 degrees

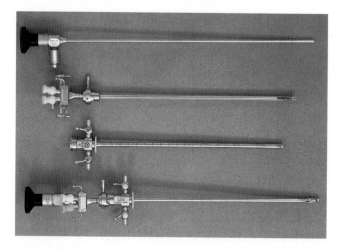

Figure 28.1. *Components of a rigid cystoscope: (from top to bottom) telescope, diagnostic (17F) sheath, bridge and assembled cystoscope.*

(forward–oblique), 70 degrees (lateral) and 120 degrees (retroview). The angled telescopes have a field marker that helps maintain orientation; it is visible as a blackened notch at the outside of the visual field and opposite the angle of deflection.

The different angles facilitate the inspection of the entire bladder wall. Although the 0-degree lens is essential to adequate urethroscopy, it is insufficient for cystoscopy. The 30-degree lens provides the best view of the bladder base and posterior wall, whereas the 70-degree lens permits inspection of the anterolateral walls. The retroview of the 120-degree lens is not usually necessary for cystoscopy of the female bladder but can be useful for evaluating the urethral opening into the bladder. For many applications, a single telescope is preferable. In diagnostic cystoscopy, the 30-degree telescope is usually sufficient, although a 70-degree telescope may be required in the presence of fixation of the UVJ. For operative cystoscopy, the 70-degree telescope is preferable.

Sheaths

The cystoscope sheath provides a vehicle for introducing the telescope and distending media into the vesical cavity. Sheaths are available in various calibres, ranging from 17 to 28F. When placed within the sheath, the telescope, which is 15F, only partially fills the lumen, leaving an irrigation–working channel. The smallest-diameter sheath is useful for diagnostic procedures; those of larger calibre provide space for the placement of instruments into the irrigation–working channel. The proximal end of the sheath has two irrigating ports, one for introduction of the distending media and another for its exit. The distal end of the cystoscope sheath is fenestrated to permit use of instrumentation in the angled field of view. It is also bevelled, opposite the fenestration, to increase the comfort of introduction of the cystoscope into the urethra. Bevels increase with the diameter of the cystoscope and larger-diameter sheaths may require an obturator for placement.

Bridges

The bridge serves as a connector between the telescope and sheath, and forms a water-tight seal with both. It may also have one or two ports for introduction of instruments into the irrigation–working channel. The Albarran bridge is a variation of the bridge that has a deflector mechanism at the end of an inner sheath. When placed within the cystoscope sheath, the deflector mechanism is located at the distal end of the inner sheath within the fenestra of the outer sheath. In this location, elevation of the deflector mechanism assists the manipulation of instruments within the field of view.

Urethroscopes vs cystoscopes

The architectural differences between the urethra and bladder place unique demands on the endoscopes used to evaluate these two structures. The narrow-calibre, straight lumen of the urethra is not adequately assessed by the angled cystoscope. The rigid urethroscope is a modification of the cystoscope, designed exclusively for evaluation of the urethra (Fig. 28.2). The urethroscope uses a telescope that is shorter and has a 0-degree viewing angle that provides a circumferential view of the urethral lumen as the mucosa in front of the urethroscope is distended by the distention media. The 0-degree lens is essential to adequate urethroscopy.

The urethroscope sheath is designed to maximize distension of the urethral lumen. The proximal end of the sheath, has a single irrigating port and the telescope only partially fills the sheath, leaving space for the irrigant to flow around it. Sheaths are available in 15 and 24F calibres. The larger-diameter sheath is useful, if tolerated, as it provides the best view of the urethral lumen by providing a more rapid fluid flow for maximal distension.

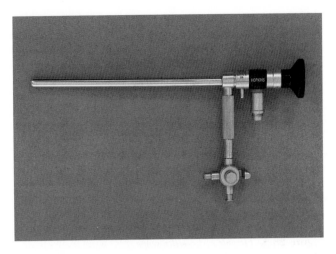

Figure 28.2. *Urethroscope.*

As the rigid urethroscope is primarily a diagnostic instrument, it does not have a bridge. Just as the cystoscope is inadequate for evaluation of the urethra, the urethroscope is inadequate for a complete assessment of the bladder. Alternatively, the urethrotomy scope utilized by urologists for the incision of uretral structures combines a 0-degree lens with a sheath which does not have a beaked end.

Flexible endoscopes

Unlike the rigid cystoscope, the flexible cystoscope combines the optical systems and irrigation–working channel in a single unit. The optical system consists of a single image-bearing fibre-optic bundle and two light-bearing fibre-optic bundles. The fibres of these bundles are coated, parallel, coherent optical fibres that transmit light even when bent. This permits incorporation of a distal tip-deflecting mechanism that will deflect the tip 290 degrees in a single plane. The deflection is controlled by a lever at the eyepiece. The optical fibres are fitted to a lens system that magnifies and focuses the image. A focusing knob is located just distal to the eyepiece. The irrigation–working port enters the instrument at the eyepiece opposite the deflecting mechanism. The coated tip is 15–18F in diameter and 6–7 cm in length, with the working unit comprising half the length (Fig. 28.3).

Because of the individual coating of the fibres, there is a small space between each fibre in the image guide. Consequently, the image appears somewhat granular. The delicate 5–10 μm diameter of the fibres makes them susceptible to damage that will further compromise the image or light transmission. Gentle handling

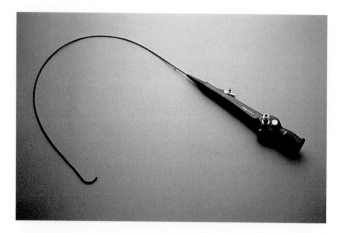

Figure 28.3. *Flexible cystourethroscope.*

is therefore essential to good visualization, not to mention the longevity of the instrument. The flow rate of the irrigation–working channel is approximately one-quarter that of a similar-size rigid cystoscope and is further curtailed by passage of instruments down this channel. Some tip deflection is also lost with use of the instrument channel.

In spite of these restrictions, several studies have compared rigid with flexible cystoscopy and found no compromise of diagnostic capabilities.[27,28] Many urologists prefer the flexible cystoscope because of improved patient comfort, but the improvement in patient comfort primarily applies to male patients, who often require general anaesthesia for diagnostic cystoscopy with a rigid instrument. The absence of a prostate gland and the short length of the female urethra make rigid cystoscopy well tolerated by women. This may offset any perceived advantage of flexible cystoscopy in female patients. Conversely, the ability to visualize the entire bladder and urethra without changing lenses increases the efficency of the flexible system.

ENDOSCOPIC TECHNIQUES

Because a complete endoscopic evaluation for urinary incontinence demands evaluation of both the bladder and urethra, diagnostic urethroscopy and cystoscopy are usually combined. Diagnostic cystourethroscopy in women is well tolerated as an office procedure without anaesthesia. Urethroscopy usually precedes the cystoscopic examination to prevent sheath-associated trauma from compromising the urethroscopic evaluation. Both rigid and flexible endoscopes will provide

adequate visualization of the lower urinary tract, but only rigid endoscopy is described here. The approach using a flexible cystoscope is similar to the technique described for rigid cystoscopy.

Dynamic urethroscopy

Sterile water or saline at room temperature are the most commonly used distending media. Instillation is by gravity through a standard intravenous infusion set with the bag at a height of 100 cm above the patient's pubic symphysis. The urethroscope has a 0-degree viewing angle (straight), ideal for viewing the urethral lumen directly in front of the urethroscope. The urethral meatus is cleansed with a disinfectant and, with the distension medium flowing, the urethroscope is introduced into the urethral meatus. The centre of the urethral lumen is maintained in the centre of the operator's visual field and the urethral lumen, distended by the infusing medium, is followed to the UVJ. The urethral mucosa is examined for redness, pallor, exudate and polyps as the urethroscope is advanced.

Dynamic urethroscopy, as originally described by Robertson,[29] provides a subjective evaluation of urethral function. With a bladder volume of at least 300 ml, the urethroscope is withdrawn until the UVJ closes one-third of the way, and the response of the UVJ to 'hold your urine' and 'squeeze your rectum' commands, as well as Valsalva manoeuvre and cough, are observed. The UVJ should close at all of these commands. The urethroscope is next withdrawn while a finger in the vagina obstructs the urethral lumen proximal to the urethroscope. This maximizes distension of the urethral lumen, providing the best possible view of the urethral mucosa. Gentle massage of the urethra against the scope 'milks' exudate from glands and diverticular openings, which helps to localize the ostia.

Diagnostic cystoscopy

Cystoscopy is performed using a 30-degree or 70-degree angled telescope in a 17F sheath. Topical anaesthetics should be avoided during urethroscopy, as they can affect the colour of the urethral mucosa; following urethroscopy, however, 1% lignocaine gel may be used as a lubricant and topical anaesthetic. The cystoscope is placed into the urethral meatus, with the blunt beak of the sheath directed posteriorly, and advanced to the bladder under direct visualization. An obturator is not usually necessary since downward pressure on the posterior urethral lumen with the blunt bleak of a 17F sheath fully opens the urethral lumen and is well tolerated by the majority of patients. The infusion of water is maintained at a slow rate until a volume of 300–400 ml is reached, or until the patient reports fullness. At this volume the flow may be stopped, unless it is required to improve the endoscopic view, in which case a small volume can be removed for patient comfort. Orientation is easily established by identifying an air bubble at the anterior dome of the bladder. This serves as a landmark during the remainder of the examination of the bladder mucosa. Beginning at the superior dome to the UVJ, the survey progresses in 12 sweeps, mimicking the points of a clock. Orientation is maintained by placing the field marker directly opposite that portion of the bladder to be inspected. Visualization of the bladder base can be difficult in patients with a large cystocele, although reduction of the prolapse with a finger in the vagina easily circumvents this problem. The mucosa is examined for colour, vascularity, trabeculation and abnormal lesions such as plaques or masses.

'Flat tyre' test

Endoscopic evaluation for urinary vaginal fistulae requires several modifications from the usual diagnostic technique. The 'flat tyre' technique permits differentiation of vesicovaginal and ureterovaginal fistulae, while also identifying the vaginal fistula opening. Prior to

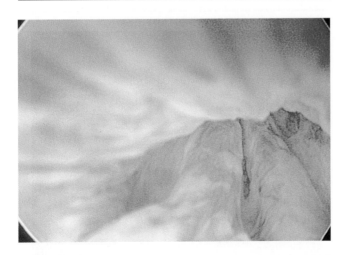

Figure 28.4. *Urethral lumen showing urethral crest and normal coaptation.*

cystoscopy, the vaginal vault is filled with 10% dextrose solution, and CO_2 gas is used in place of sterile water as a distending media through the cystoscope. The CO_2 distends the bladder and, if a vesicovaginal fistula is present, CO_2 bubbles into the water-filled vaginal vault, identifying the diverticular opening. Simultaneous administration of intravenous indigo carmine will identify a ureterovaginal fistula, as the dye seeps into the hypertonic fluid in the vagina. Vesicovaginal fistulae following hysterectomy are most commonly identified in the supratrigonal area of the bladder.

ENDOSCOPIC FINDINGS

Normal endoscopic findings

Normally, the urethral mucosa is pink and smooth with a posterior longitudinal ridge, known as the urethral crest (Fig. 28.4). The UVJ is typically round or an inverted horseshoe shape, and is completely coapted until the lumen is opened by the irrigant. The UVJ normally closes briskly and has minimal mobility on Valsalva manoeuvre.

In its normal state, the bladder mucosa has a smooth surface with a pale pink to glistening white hue. The translucent mucosa affords easy visualization of the branched submucosal vasculature. As the mucosa of the dome gives way to the trigone, it thickens and develops a granular texture. The reddened granular surface of the trigone is often covered by a white thickened membrane with a villous contour. Histological evaluation of the layer reveals squamous metaplasia, but it is usually referred to simply as metaplasia. The trigone is triangular, with the inferior apex directed toward the UVJ and the ureteral orifices forming the superior apices. As the cystoscope is advanced past the UVJ, the trigone is apparent at the bottom of the field. The interureteric ridge is a visible elevation that forms the superior boundary of the trigone, running between the ureteral orifices. The intramural portion of the ureters can often be seen as they course from the lateral aspect of the bladder towards the trigone and ureteral orifices. Although there is marked variation in the ureteral orifices, they are generally circular or slit-like openings at the apex of a small mound (Fig. 28.5). With efflux of urine, the slit opens and the mound retracts in the direction of the intramural ureter.

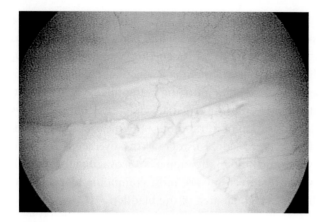

Figure 28.5. *Left ureteral orifice with squamous metaplasia overlying trigone. The interureteric ridge is also visible.*

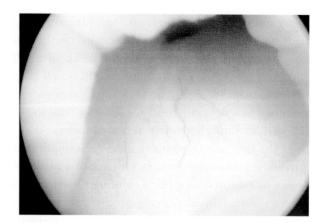

Figure 28.6. *Intrinsic sphincteric deficiency.*

When distended, the bladder is roughly spherical, but numerous folds of mucosa are evident in the empty or partially filled bladder. The uterus and cervix can usually be seen indenting the posterior wall of the bladder, which creates posterolateral pouches where the bladder drapes over the uterus into the paravaginal spaces. At times, visualization of the anterior portion of the bladder dome requires manual pressure on the lower abdomen.

Urethral hypermobility

During dynamic urethroscopy, the urethroscope visualizes the UVJ during straining, cough and pubococcygeal contraction. The urethral hypermobility typical of GSI causes the UVJ to open and descend in response to cough and a Valsalva manoeuvre, and the patient often will not be able to close the UVJ at the 'hold' and 'squeeze' commands.

Intrinsic sphincteric deficiency

Urethroscopic findings typical of the patient with ISD include a rigid, immobile urethra with poor coaptation (Fig. 28.6). In severe cases, the UVJ is unresponsive to commands and the lumen is visualized in its entirety from meatus to UVJ. DI should be suspected if there is uncontrollable urethral opening during filling.

Diverticula

Urethral diverticula occur in 1–3% of women, and are located along the posterolateral wall of the urethra as single or multiple outpouchings. Over one-half of the diverticular openings are at the midurethra, with a number more proximal and some more distal (Fig. 28.7). The urethroscopic diagnosis is most accurate when the bladder is filled, and the bladder neck or proximal urethra is occluded by a finger in the vagina. A steady flow of fluid is maintained into the urethra as the scope is withdrawn and urethra massaged by the finger pressing upward from below. This is one instance when CO_2 gas infusion is preferable to water or saline for urethroscopy.

Fistulae

Diagnosis is made in three steps after a fistula is suspected. Step one is to confirm that watery drainage is urine – phenazopyridine hydrochloride may be used for this purpose. The next step is to exclude urinary

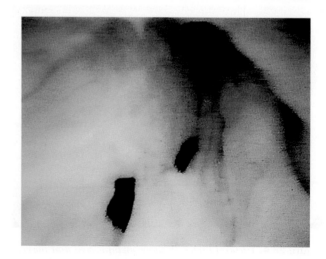

Figure 28.7. *Urethral diverticula.*

incontinence occurring from the urethra by filling the bladder and observing any loss from the urethra or vagina. Finally, the source of the fistula must be determined. This commences with a thorough speculum inspection, which may reveal a fistula site to the vagina. The double-contrast test is also useful, although cystoscopy and the 'flat tyre' test are the best way to visualize a fistula site in the bladder. A post-hysterectomy vesicovaginal fistula on the bladder side appears above the trigone medial to the ureters (Fig. 28.8); at vaginoscopy it is at the vaginal vault. Cystoscopy may show oedema and congestion, or even mucosal papillomatous hyperplasia in enterovesical fistulae. Sometimes, a ureteral catheter can be passed into a visible fistula opening to outline its path.

Foreign bodies

Intravesical foreign bodies may present with haematuria or as urge incontinence due to mucosal irritation. Bladder calculi may result from urinary stasis or the presence of a foreign body, or an inflammatory exudate may coalesce and serve as a nidus for stone formation (Fig. 28.9). Stones are of extremely variable cystoscopic appearance in terms of colour, size and shape, but generally have an irregular surface. Foreign bodies and stones are usually accompanied by varying degrees of general or localized inflammation. Cystourethroscopy can provide valuable information in making these diagnoses.

CONCLUSIONS

Endoscopy of the lower urinary tract is an invaluable tool to the physician treating women for urinary incontinence. Although it is not the best method for diagnosing GSI and DI, it does provide unique anatomical information with a simple, minimally invasive approach. Endoscopy is a useful adjunct to multichannel urodynamics in women with possible ISD, urethral diverticula, urogenital fistulae, foreign bodies or urothelial lesions.

REFERENCES

1. Largo-Janssen ALM, Debruyne FMJ, Van Weel C. Value of the patient's case history in diagnosing urinary incontinence in general practice. *Br J Urol* 1991; 67: 569–572

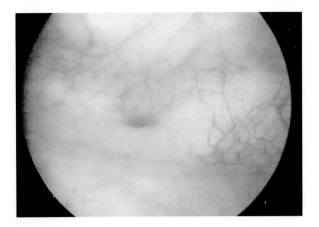

Figure 28.8. *Supratrigonal fistula.*

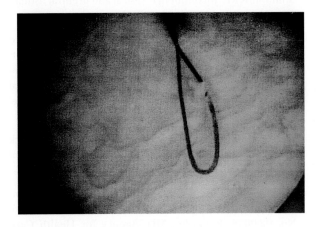

Figure 28.9. *Intravesical suture.*

2. Sand PK, Hill RC, Ostergard DR. Incontinence history as a predictor of detrusor stability. *Obstet Gynecol* 1988; 71: 257–259

3. Korda A, Krieger M, Hunter P, Parkin G. The value of clinical symptoms in the diagnosis of urinary incontinence in the female. *Aust N Z J Obstet Gynaecol* 1987; 27: 149–151

4. Cundiff GW, Harris RL, Coates KW, Bump RC. Clinical predictors of urinary incontinence in women. *Am J Obstet Gynecol* 1997; 177: 262–267

5. Robertson JR. Air cystoscopy. *Obstet Gynecol* 1968; 32: 328–330

6. Sand PK, Hill RC, Ostergard DR. Supine urethroscopic and standing cystometry as screening methods for detection of detrusor instability. *Obstet Gynecol* 1987; 70: 57–60

7. Scotti RJ, Ostergard DR, Guillaume AA, Kohatsu KE. Predictive value of urethroscopy as compared to urodynamics in the diagnosis of genuine stress incontinence. *J Reprod Med* 1990; 35: 772–776

8. Cundiff GW, Bent AE. The contribution of urethrocystoscopy to a combined urodynamic and urethrocysto-

scopic evaluation of urinary incontinence in women. *Int Urogynecol J* 1996; 7: 307–311

9. Leach GE, Bavendam TG. Female urethral diverticula. *Urology* 1987; 30: 407–415

10. Robertson JR. Urethral diverticula. In: Ostergard DR, Bent AE (eds) *Urogynecology and Urodynamics: Theory and Practice*, 3rd edn. Baltimore: Williams and Wilkins, 1991: 283–291

11. Drutz HP. Urethral diverticula. *Obstet Gynecol Clin North Am* 1989; 16: 923–929

12. Massee JS, Welch JS, Pratt JH, Symmonds RE. Management of urinary-vaginal fistula. *J Am Med Assoc* 1964; 190: 124–128

13. Symmonds RE. Incontinence: vesical and urethral fistulas. *Clin Obstet Gynecol* 1984; 27: 499–514

14. Bump RC, Hurt WG, Theofrastous JP *et al.* Randomized prospective comparison of needle colposuspension versus endopelvic fascia plication for potential stress incontinence prophylaxis in women undergoing vaginal reconstruction for stage II or IV pelvic organ prolapse. *Am J Obstet Gynecol* 1996; 175: 326–335

15. Bruskewitz R, Nielsen K, Graversen P *et al.* Bladder neck suspension material investigation in a rabbit model. *J Urol* 1989; 142: 1361

16. Urinary Incontinence Guideline Panel. *Urinary Incontinence in Adults: Clinical Practical Guidelines.* AHCPR Pub. No. 92-0038. Rockville, MD: Agency for Health Care Policy and Research, Public Health Service, U.S. Department of Health and Human Services, March 1992

17. Bergman A, Koonings PP, Ballard CA. Proposed management of low urethral pressure type of genuine stress urinary incontinence. *Gynecol Obstet Invest* 1989; 27: 155–159

18. Sand PK, Bowen LW, Panganiban R, Ostergard DR. The low pressure urethra as a factor in failed retropubic urethropexy. *Obstet Gynecol* 1987; 69: 399–402

19. Decter RM, Harpster L. Pitfalls in determination of leak point pressure. *J Urol* 1992; 148: 588–591

20. Bump RC, Coates KW, Cundiff GW *et al.* Diagnosing intrinsic sphincteric deficiency: comparing urethral closure pressure, urethral axis, and valsalva leak point pressures. *Am J Obstet Gynecol* 1997; 177: 303–310

21. Bergman A, McKenzie CJ, Richmond J *et al.* Transrectal ultrasound versus cystography in the evaluation of anatomical stress urinary incontinence. *Br J Urol* 1988; 62: 228–234

22. Chang HC, Chang SC, Kuo HC, Tsai TC. Transrectal sonographic cystourethrography: studies in stress urinary incontinence. *Urology* 1990; 36: 488–492

23. Gordon D, Pearce M, Norton P, Stanton S. Comparison of ultrasound and lateral chain urethrocystography in the determination of bladder neck descent. *Am J Obstet Gynecol* 1989; 160: 182–185

24. Weil EHK, van Waalwijk van Doorn ESC, Heesakkers JPFA *et al.* Transvaginal ultrasonography: a study with healthy volunteers and women with genuine stress incontinence. *Eur Urol* 1993; 24: 226–230

25. Young JL Jr, Percy CL, Asire AJ (eds) Surveillance, epidemiology, end results: incidence and mortality data, 1973–77. *Natl Cancer Inst Monogr* 1981; 57: 1–1082

26. Anton-Culver H, Lee-Feldstein A, Taylor TH. Occupation and bladder cancer risk. *Am J Epidemiol* 1992; 136: 89–94

27. Figueroa TE, Thomas R, Moon TD. A comparison of rigid with flexible instruments. *J La St State Med Soc*, 1987; 139: 26

28. Clayman RV, Reddy P, Lange PH. Flexible fiberoptic and rigid-rod lens endoscopy of the lower urinary tract: a prospective controlled comparison. *J Urol* 1984; 131: 715–716

29. Robertson JR. Endoscopic examination of the urethra and bladder. *Clin Obstet Gynecol* 1983; 26: 347–358

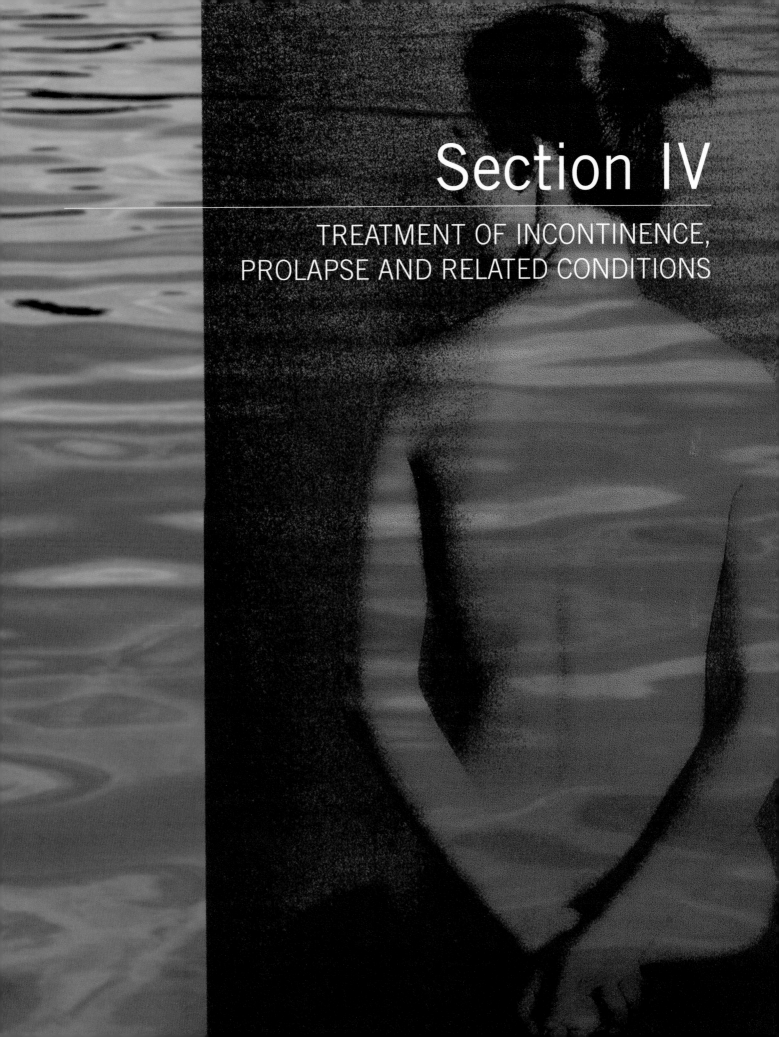

Section IV

TREATMENT OF INCONTINENCE,
PROLAPSE AND RELATED CONDITIONS

Outcomes of conservative treatment

D. Wilson, J. Hay-Smith, K. Bø

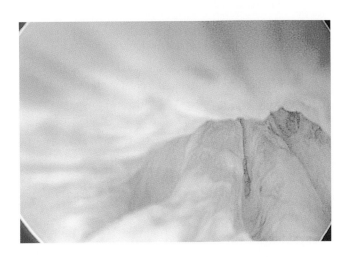

INTRODUCTION

This chapter reviews the outcomes of research investigating the principal types of conservative treatment of incontinence (lifestyle interventions, physical therapies, bladder retraining and anti-incontinence devices) and makes recommendations based on their efficacy to assist with the counselling of incontinent women regarding these treatment options. The recommendations are based on the best level of evidence currently available. At present this is provided by randomized controlled trials (RCTs) and, in particular, a meta-analysis (quantitative synthesis) of all available RCTs identified after a systematic review of the literature.[1] Where this is not available, then lesser levels of evidence are considered[2] (Table 29.1).

LIFESTYLE INTERVENTIONS

Lifestyle factors may play a role in either the pathogenesis or, later, the resolution of incontinence. Although published literature about lifestyle factors and incontinence is sparse, alterations in lifestyle are frequently recommended by healthcare professionals and lay people alike. To date, no RCT investigating the effect of lifestyle intervention(s) has been published. Most studies report associations only and do not assess the actual effect of applying or deleting the behaviour in question on incontinence.

Principal forms of lifestyle intervention include weight loss, reduction of physical forces (exercise, work), cessation of smoking, caffeine reduction and fluid management, relief of constipation and postural changes.

Weight loss

Obesity has been shown to be a risk factor for incontinence, with several studies reporting an association between increased weight and urinary incontinence.[3–9] Brown,[9] in her large multivariate analysis involving almost 8000 people, reported that the prevalence of daily incontinence increased by an odds ratio of 1.6 per 5 body mass index. However, only two published intervention studies have investigated incontinence after weight loss and these showed a reduction in incontinence after massive weight loss (mean 44 kg) in morbidly obese women.[10,11] Therefore, although weight loss would appear to be an appropriate treatment option for morbidly obese women, currently there is no information on the effect of weight loss in moderately obese women; one such trial is now ongoing.[12] Maintaining normal weight through adulthood may be an important factor in the prevention of incontinence; however, published data to substantiate this hypothesis are lacking. Given the high prevalence of both incontinence and obesity in women, the dual issues of weight loss and prevention of weight gain and their effect on incontinence should receive high research priority.

Physical forces (exercise, work)

Minimal stress incontinence is common in young exercising women,[13–15] and it is believed that strenuous exercise is likely to unmask the symptom of stress incontinence in otherwise asymptomatic women. There is little available information on whether strenuous exercise or activity causes the condition of incontinence in later life. In a study of former female Olympians, competitors in gymnastics or track and field were no more likely to report daily or weekly incontinence than were competitive swimmers.[16] Traumatic exercise may cause incontinence: a recent report described nine nulliparous infantry trainees who developed stress incontinence and pelvic floor defects for the first time during airborne training, which included parachute jumping.[17]

Table 29.1. Basis of recommendations for conservative treatment of incontinence

Level	Type of evidence
Ia	Evidence obtained from meta-analysis of randomized controlled trials.
Ib	Evidence obtained from at least one randomized controlled trial.
IIa	Evidence obtained from at least one well-designed controlled study without randomization.
IIb	Evidence obtained from at least one other type of well-designed quasi-experimental study.
III	Evidence obtained from well-designed non-experimental descriptive studies, such as comparative studies, correlation studies and case–control studies.
IV	Evidence obtained from expert committee reports or opinions and/or clinical experiences of respective authorities.

Adapted from ref. 2.

Surprisingly little information is available on workplace stressors. Danish nursing assistants, who were exposed to frequent heavy lifting, were 1.6 times more likely to undergo surgery for genital prolapse and/or incontinence than were women in the general population; however, the study did not control for parity.[18] Healthcare professionals commonly advise restricting exercise and heavy lifting following incontinence or prolapse surgery; however, there is no published evidence that this improves surgical outcome.

Given the large proportion of women employed in occupations that require heavy lifting and the paucity of scientific data about the association between exertion and incontinence, this should be investigated further. Specifically, research must establish whether heavy exertion is an aetiological factor in the pathogenesis of incontinence, and whether changing exertions can alleviate established incontinence or influence outcome of surgery for either incontinence or prolapse.

Smoking

There is no clear evidence to associate smoking with incontinence. The prevalence of incontinence was similar among smokers and non-smokers in one large study of 7949 women;[9] however, in a smaller study of 160 women,[19] smokers were more likely to report incontinence than were non-smokers. These trials had different study populations. Incontinent smokers were found to have stronger urethral sphincters and lower overall risk profiles than incontinent non-smokers;[20] therefore, it was proposed that more violent (and presumably more frequent) coughing promotes anatomical defects that allow incontinence. In addition, nicotine produces phasic contraction of isolated bladder muscle probes *in vitro*.[21,22]

No data have been reported regarding the effect of smoking cessation on the onset or resolution of incontinence.

Caffeine reduction and fluid management

No RCTs have assessed the efficacy of caffeine restriction, fluid management or dietary changes in the treatment of incontinence. On the basis of Brown's large multivariate analysis of almost 8000 women,[9] which showed no association between caffeine or alcohol drinking and daily incontinence,[9] caffeine is thought to

have a minor (if any) role in the pathogenesis of incontinence.[23] However, Creighton and Stanton[24] found that, following caffeine intake, women with detrusor instability (DI) had increased detrusor pressure on bladder filling whereas continent women had no such abnormality. Despite the fact that healthcare professionals commonly include limiting caffeine as part of the treatment plan, there is no published evidence that this intervention decreases incontinence. Caffeine consumption is pervasive in many societies and therefore RCTs to assess the effect of caffeine and other dietary factors are feasible and important.

A strong relationship between evening fluid intake, nocturia and nocturnal voided volume has been demonstrated in a geriatric population; this relationship was weaker for diurnal intake and voiding.[25] In incontinent women over 55 years of age, there was a modest positive relationship between fluid intake and severity of incontinence in women with stress incontinence; fluid intake accounted for 14% of the explained variability in the number of incontinent episodes.[26] No such correlation was found in women with DI.

However, as restriction of fluid intake may lead to urinary tract infections, constipation or dehydration, this intervention should be reserved for patients with abnormally high fluid intake and should be considered in the elderly with nocturia who have a high evening fluid intake.

Relief of constipation

There are data to suggest that chronic straining may be a risk factor for the development of incontinence. This is based on studies which found a positive association of straining at stool as a young adult,[27] and constipation,[28] with subsequent incontinence[27,28] and uterovaginal prolapse.[27] There also appears to be an association between straining and pudendal nerve function: the mean pudendal nerve terminal motor latency increased after straining, correlated with the amount of descent, and returned to resting by 4 minutes after a strain.[29] However, evidence of pudendal neuropathy was found in only 25% of women with abnormal perineal descent; in this large group of patients with defecation dysfunction, no relationship was seen between neuropathy and pelvic descent, leading to the conclusion that pelvic descent and neuropathy may be two independent findings.[30]

No intervention trials have addressed the effect of regulating bowel function on incontinence, and research is needed to determine whether eliminating straining by treating constipation improves incontinence. Further research is also needed to delineate the role of straining in the pathogenesis of incontinence. If this association holds, public education – particularly of parents and paediatricians – is needed to make an impact on the common problem of straining in children.

Postural changes and other lifestyle interventions

Urine loss during provocation can be significantly decreased by crossing the legs while coughing or by crossing the legs and bending forward.[31] However, no study has evaluated whether postural changes are a satisfactory form of treatment outside the laboratory setting, and they will be of limited value for women who are incontinent during exercise.

Many other lifestyle interventions for the treatment of urinary incontinence have been suggested by either healthcare professionals or the lay press but have not been evaluated in the non-geriatric population. Such interventions include reducing emotional stress, wearing non-restrictive clothing, utilizing a bedside commode, decreasing lower-extremity oedema, treating allergies and coughs, wearing cotton underwear and increasing sexual activity. Evidence concerning these interventions remains anecdotal and studies evaluating their effects are warranted. Although some lifestyle changes may prove beneficial for individuals, it is unlikely that manipulating these factors will have a major effect on the overall incontinence problem.

Conclusions

Most lifestyle intervention studies to date have reported associations only and have not assessed the actual effect of applying or removing the behaviour in question. Obesity seems to be an independent risk factor for the development of urinary incontinence and weight loss may be an appropriate treatment option for morbidly obese women. Chronic straining may also be a risk factor for the development of urinary incontinence; however, no intervention trials have examined the effect on incontinence of resolving constipation. Further research is needed to evaluate the effect of heavy exertion/exercise, smoking, caffeine and fluid intake on incontinence and whether their cessation can alleviate or prevent this condition.

PHYSICAL THERAPIES

Physical therapies include pelvic floor muscle (PFM) training (PFMT), biofeedback (BF), intravaginal resistance devices (IVRDs), vaginal cones (VCs) and electrical stimulation (ES), used singly or in combination. As three systematic reviews (with qualitative synthesis) of physical therapies for women with urinary incontinence are available,[23,32,33] the recommendations in this section are based solely on evidence from full published reports of RCTs.

Pelvic floor muscle training

PFMT programmes

In the trials reviewed there was a lack of consistency in PFMT programmes that implies an underlying lack of understanding of the physiological principles of rehabilitating PFM dysfunction, or differences in muscle-training philosophies. In general, many PFMT programmes were poorly reported, and other advice/education given concurrently was rarely detailed.

Success of PFMT will depend partly on ability to perform a correct voluntary PFM contraction (VPFMC) initially. Bump *et al.*[34] reported that 50% of women were unable to perform a correct VPFMC following brief verbal instruction, and as many as one-quarter were mistakenly performing a Valsalva manoeuvre. Therefore, it seems appropriate that all women should be examined and taught how to perform a correct VPFMC by a person with specialist training in this area before PFMT is undertaken.

Effective strength training relies on specificity (i.e. training reflects the functional activity of the muscle) and overload (i.e. increasing resistance to, frequency or duration of, muscle contraction). Effective overload strategies are likely to include maximal VPFMC, increased length of contraction, increased number of contractions and reduced rest periods. Strength training theory suggests that near-maximal contractions are the most significant factor in increasing strength[35] and that, ideally, contractions need to be sustained for

6–8 seconds in order to recruit an increasing number of motor units and fast-twitch fibres.[36] Extrapolation from strength training programmes for other skeletal muscles indicates that strength training of the PFM should include three sets of 8–12 slow maximal contractions, three to four times a week,[37] and that training should be continued for a minimum of 15–20 weeks.[35] However, indiscriminate use of this protocol may have adverse effects due to muscle fatigue, unless women are individually assessed to determine the strength/weakness of their PFM. Depending on assessment findings of fatiguability, a modified programme may be needed initially, progressing to meet the above recommendation.

Anecdotally, some clinicians report that compliance with PFMT programmes is poor. Three studies have used diaries to assess compliance with PFMT;[38–40] one study asked women to rate their compliance,[41] and another monitored class attendance.[42] The rates of compliance recorded were generally high, although they decreased over time.[39–41]

Two studies have investigated the effect of audiotapes on compliance.[43,44] Both studies investigated PFMT with and without supplementary audiotapes. Nygaard *et al.*[43] reported no differences between the groups with regard to compliance, whereas Gallo and Staskin[44] found that the tape increased levels of compliance.

PFMT vs no treatment

Four RCTs have reported significant improvements in PFMT groups when compared with controls.[38,41,42,45] Henalla *et al.*[45] studied a group of women with genuine stress incontinence (GSI); the other three trials included women with stress, mixed and urge incontinence.[38,41,42] There is level 1B evidence to suggest that, in groups of women with a range of urinary incontinence symptoms (stress, mixed, urge), PFMT is better than no treatment.

Reported cure/improvement rates at 3 months were remarkably consistent despite differences in the measures used. O'Brien *et al.*[42] and Lagro-Janssen *et al.*[41] stated that 68 and 74% of women, respectively, subjectively reported cure/improvement vs 5% and 3% of controls. Burns *et al.*[38] reported 68% (vs 18% of controls) cured/improved, measured by reduction in number of urine losses. Henalla *et al.*[45] used a pad test score and found that 65% of the PFMT group (vs no controls) were cured/improved. O'Brien and Long[46] reported findings from long-term follow-up (i.e. more

than 2 years): at 4 years, 68% of study participants had maintained their cure/improvement or improved further.

One abstract reported a trial of PFMT vs placebo PFMT:[47] no differences were found between the two groups. However, the placebo programme incorporated hip muscle activity, and hip muscles are known to co-contract with pelvic floor musculature.

Comparisons of PFMT programmes

A single trial investigating the effect of a home programme of PFMT vs a home programme with weekly PFMT group exercise class was found:[41] both groups showed significant improvements, with the exercise class group demonstrating significantly greater improvement on some measures (e.g. pad test). At 6 months, 60% of the exercise class group were judged to be continent or almost continent, compared with 17.3% of the home exercise only group. Long-term follow-up of the 'intensive' exercise group at 5 years[48] found that, although there had been a significant increase in urine loss over this period, 14 of the 20 women were satisfied with treatment and did not want further treatment.

In an abstract, Wilson *et al.*[49] reported a trial comparing 'standard' postnatal exercises (including VPFMC) with a specific home programme of PFMT and bladder retraining, in a sample of 734 postnatal women with urinary and/or faecal incontinence. At 12 months, 58% of the PFMT group and 68% of the 'standard' exercise group were still incontinent – a significant difference in improvement.

A single trial compared inpatient and outpatient conservative management of urinary incontinence in women.[50] Management included PFMT, bladder retraining and advice, and the researchers found that symptoms of both groups improved significantly, with no clear benefit of inpatient over outpatient treatment. Ramsay *et al.*[50] concluded that outpatient management was the more cost-effective option.

PFMT vs electrical stimulation

Five trials[45,51–54] have investigated the effect of ES in (genuine) stress incontinence. However, the trials were of poor-to-moderate methodological quality, had small sample sizes and used varied ES protocols.

Reported cure/improvement rates were variable and were measured by patient self-assessment at 6 weeks[51,52] or 6 months,[54] by pad test at 3 months,[45] or by a combined score at 4 months.[53] Hahn *et al.*,[54] Henalla *et al.*[45] and Hofbauer *et al.*[51] reported higher cure/improvement rates in the PFMT groups (100, 65, 63.6%, respectively) than in the ES groups (80, 32, 27.3%). Laycock and Jerwood[52] and Smith[53] found the reverse, with cure/improvement rates in the ES groups of 82.4 and 66%, respectively, versus 41.2 and 44% in the PFMT groups. Two of the trials reported findings from long-term follow-up:[55,52] less than one-half of the participants in the study by Laycock and Jerwood[52] responded, but Hahn *et al.*[55] followed-up 19 of the original 20 participants in their study and found that about one-half were further improved or their symptoms had not changed since completion of treatment.

Three abstracts of trials investigating PFMT vs ES were found:[56–58] Laycock[56] and Laycock *et al.*[58] suggested that there were no significant differences between treatment groups, whereas Wise *et al.*[57] reported significant improvement in both groups, with PFMT being significantly better than ES.

Owing to the lack of consistency in the trials, evidence for PFMT vs ES is unclear; however, to date, three of the five full published reports indicate that PFMT is of greater benefit.

PFMT vs medication, surgery and VCs

The effectiveness of PFMT vs medication, surgery or VCs is unclear. Only single RCTs have been found comparing PFMT and oestrogens,[45] PFMT and α–agonists,[40] PFMT and surgery,[59] and no full published reports of PFMT vs VCs were found.

PFMT vs medication

Two RCTs have investigated the effect of PFMT vs medication for stress incontinence: Henalla *et al.*[45] suggested that PFMT was superior to medication (vaginal oestrogen cream) in a group of women with GSI, reporting cure/improvement at 3 months in 65% of the PFMT group vs 12% of the medication group. Wells *et al.*[40] showed no differences between the medication (phenylpropanolamine hydrochloride) and PFMT groups in women with stress/mixed incontinence, with 84% cure/improvement after 4 weeks of medication and 77% after 6 months of PFMT.

PFMT vs surgery

One published RCT[59] compared PFMT with surgery for women with GSI, with significantly greater reduction in symptoms in the surgery group. One abstract of an RCT was found comparing 3 months of PFMT with Burch colposuspension for women with GSI:[60] the authors reported that two of 21 women from the PFMT group were objectively cured on urodynamic testing at 6 months, compared with 18 of 24 women following colposuspension.

PFMT vs vaginal cones

Although there have been no full published reports of RCTs comparing PFMT with VCs, three abstracts[57,61,62] have shown significant improvements in both treatment groups, with no significant differences between the groups.

PFMT in combination with other physical therapy adjuncts vs PFMT alone

PFMT is commonly used in combination with other adjuncts such as BF, IVRDs, ES and VCs.

PFMT with BF vs PFMT alone

Four RCTs compared PFMT with BF vs PFMT alone. All four trials[38,63–65] reported significant improvement in both treatment groups; however, only Glavind *et al.*[65] reported PFMT with BF to be superior to PFMT alone. There is level 1B evidence to suggest that PFMT with BF is no more effective than PFMT alone in women with (genuine) stress incontinence. It is important to stress, however, that this evidence should be used with caution in view of the small group sizes and the chance of type II error. There was also some variation in the types of BF used–all the studies used vaginal probes, with three studies using electromyographic (EMG) BF[38,64,65] and the other using pressure BF.[63]

Anecdotal evidence suggests that BF is used to particular effect in some subgroups (e.g. those women unable to perform a VPFMC on initial assessment). However, the role of BF in any subgroup is unclear, owing to a lack of published evidence to date. Clinicians may find occasions when BF would be a useful adjunct to treatment for the purposes of teaching, motivation and compliance.

PFMT with IVRD vs PFMT alone

To date, two RCTs[66,67] have found significant improvement in both groups but with no differences between the groups. Thus, the same conclusions regarding BF apply also to the use of IVRD with PFMT.

PFMT with ES or VCs vs PFMT alone

The effectiveness of PFMT in combination with ES[57] or VCs[68] compared with PFMT alone is as yet unclear, as only single RCTs with small sample sizes have been carried out to date. Both trials showed similar cure/improvement rates in the PFMT-only groups compared with the combination therapy groups.

Electrical stimulation

ES protocols

There was a wide variation in ES protocols used, with no consistent pattern emerging. Women with urinary incontinence have received a range of types of stimulation including faradism (low-frequency current with pulse duration of 1 ms or less), interferential therapy (two interfering medium-frequency currents) and specifically programmed neuromuscular electrical stimulation. In the trials included there was a lack of consistency in ES types and parameters that implies a lack of understanding of the physiological principles of rehabilitating PFM through ES, and this inconsistency makes direct comparison between studies inadvisable. In addition, the small group sizes mean that results may be affected by type II error.

ES vs no treatment or sham ES for (genuine) stress incontinence

With only a single RCT[45] with small sample size comparing ES with no treatment, there is insufficient evidence to determine whether ES is more effective than no treatment in women with (genuine) stress incontinence.

Six RCTs[51,52,69–72] have compared ES with sham ES in women with GSI, with four trials[51,52,69,70] finding significant improvement in the active-ES group only and the remaining two[71,72] finding no significant differences between the ES and sham-ES groups. The findings of the two highest-quality and most comparable studies[69,79] that investigated ES vs sham ES in women with GSI reported contradictory results – one study a positive outcome[69] and the other no effect.[72] Unfortunately, none of the ES studies included reported findings from medium- or long-term follow-up.

Anecdotal evidence suggests that ES is used with particular effect in some subgroups (e.g. those women unable to perform a VPFMC on initial assessment). However, the role of ES in any subgroup is not known, owing to a lack of published evidence. Some clinicians also differentiate between passive ES and active ES (where the patient tries to contract the PFM during ES), but the effect of these two approaches is also unknown.

ES vs no treatment or sham ES for urge incontinence

No trials comparing ES with no treatment for urge incontinence were found. A single trial indicated benefit of ES versus sham ES for women with DI: Brubaker *et al.*[71] compared ES with sham ES in women with urodynamically proven DI and found a significant reduction in detrusor overactivity in the active-ES group only. However, Abel *et al.*,[73] in an abstract of a RCT, compared ES with sham ES in women with urge incontinence and found subjective improvement in the active treatment group but no other differences between the two groups.

Further research is needed to investigate the effect of all aspects of the use of ES in the treatment of urinary incontinence.

Factors affecting outcomes of physical therapy interventions

Many of the factors traditionally supposed to affect outcomes of physical therapy interventions (e.g. age, severity of incontinence, previous pelvic surgery, prolapse and parity) may be less crucial than previously thought.[38,45,51,72] The single factor that appears to be most associated with positive outcome is greater motivation and/or compliance with physical therapy interventions.[39–42,55,65] It should be noted, however, that the association between compliance with physical therapy interventions and improvement may be due not to the effect of the intervention alone but to some other unknown factor. For example, trial participants who were compliant with active or placebo drug did better than those who were not compliant with either active or placebo medication.[74] Further investigation of all the above factors is required in high-quality RCTs before any real conclusions may be drawn.

DeLancey[64] makes a compelling argument for intervention for stress urinary incontinence to be based on accurate diagnosis of the underlying pathology, whether it be neurological, ligamentous/fascial or muscular. For example, he suggests that PFMT may be inappropriate where innervation of the muscles is not intact or where the muscles have been detached from their fascial connections. These hypotheses remain to be tested, and will rely in part on improving diagnostic accuracy. An abstract of an RCT[75] investigating the use of urodynamics prior to conservative treatment found that this did not improve outcome compared with treatment based on symptom-reporting only.

Conclusions

PFMT remains the mainstay of physical therapy treatment. There is level 1B evidence to suggest that, for women with a range of urinary incontinence symptoms (stress, mixed, urge), PFMT is better than no treatment. Specific PFMT targeted at women with GSI may optimize effectiveness and, for those women with mixed and urge incontinence, it may be appropriate to offer PFMT in combination with bladder retraining.

There is a marked lack of consistency in PFMT programmes. On the basis of extrapolation from the exercise science literature, PFM strength protocols should include three sets of 8–12 slow-velocity maximal contractions sustained for 6–8 seconds each, performed three or four times a week, and continued for at least 15–20 weeks. Prior to PFMT, women should be assessed by a person with specialist training to ensure that a correct VPFMC is being performed and to determine what protocol alterations, if any, are required to prevent muscle fatigue with over-vigorous exercise.

Expected rates of cure/improvement with PFMT in the short term may be in the range of 65–75%. However, in view of the failure of most studies to report cure and improvement rates separately, it is not possible to make a more specific estimate of effect, although it seems that improvement in the symptoms is a more common outcome than cure.

On the basis of the limited evidence currently available, there is no apparent difference in the effectiveness of PFMT with or without BF, or IVRD, although clinicians may find occasions when these would be useful adjuncts to treatment for the purposes of teaching, motivation and compliance.

Further research is needed, looking at all aspects of ES for urinary incontinence, as, to date, there is insufficient evidence to determine whether ES is better than no treatment for women with stress, mixed or urge incontinence. Similarly, the results of ES vs sham-ES for (genuine) stress incontinence are contradictory and further research is needed to evaluate the effect of ES on DI. Owing to the lack of consistency in the trials, evidence of effectiveness of PFMT vs ES for (genuine) stress incontinence is not clear, although three of the five trials show greater benefit of PFMT.

BLADDER RETRAINING

Bladder retraining (also referred to as bladder discipline, bladder drill, bladder training and bladder re-education) is a term used to describe the educational and behavioural process used to re-establish the control of urinary incontinence in adults. The recommendations in this section are based largely on one systematic review with qualitative synthesis of the available RCTs.[23]

Bladder retraining programmes typically involve several key elements: these are patient education on the mechanisms underlying continence and incontinence; a scheduled voiding regimen with gradually progressive voiding intervals; urgency control strategies using distraction and relaxation techniques; self-monitoring of voiding behaviour; and positive reinforcement provided by a clinician.[76] Bladder retraining requires a cognitively intact and motivated patient who is capable of independent toileting and can adhere to the scheduled voiding regimen.

This section focuses on the outcomes of bladder retraining in non-institutionalized women as either a sole therapy or concomitant with PFMT or drug therapy.

Bladder retraining programmes

At present, there are several variations related to the implementation of bladder retraining programmes. On the basis of extrapolation from the bladder-retraining literature,[23] an outpatient-retraining protocol should include an initial voiding interval typically beginning at 1 hour during waking hours only, which is increased by 15–30 minutes/week, depending upon tolerance of the schedule (i.e. fewer incontinent episodes than the previous week, minimal interruptions to the schedule, and the woman's feeling of control over urgency), until a 2–3-hour voiding interval is achieved. A shorter initial voiding interval (i.e. 30 minutes or less) may be necessary for women whose baseline voiding diaries reveal an average voiding interval of less than an hour. Education should be provided about normal bladder control and methods to control urgency, such as distraction and relaxation techniques and VPFMC. Self-monitoring of voiding behaviour using a voiding diary or treatment log should be included in order to determine adherence to the schedule, evaluate progress and determine whether the voiding interval should be changed. Clinicians should monitor progress, determine adjustments to the voiding interval and provide positive reinforcement to women undergoing bladder retraining at least weekly during the training period. If there is no reduction in incontinent episodes after 3 weeks of bladder retraining, the patient should be re-evaluated and other treatment options considered. Inpatient bladder retraining programmes may follow a more rigid scheduling regimen with progression of the voiding interval on a daily basis.

Bladder retraining vs no treatment

Bladder retraining as the sole therapy has been used in the treatment of DI, GSI, mixed incontinence and urge incontinence with a stable bladder.

Two RCTs reported significant improvements in the bladder retraining group compared with an untreated control group:[77,78] Jarvis and Millar[77] investigated the effect of bladder retraining in women with a diagnosis of DI, whereas, Fantl et al.[78] included women with GSI, DI and mixed incontinence. Reported cure/improvement rates varied between the two trials, which may have reflected the different follow-up periods, the type of outcome measures used or the bladder retraining protocol. Jarvis and Millar[77] reported that 90% of the treatment group were continent and 83.3% were symptom free at 6 months, whereas in the control group, 23.3% were continent and symptom free. The measurement of continence status (e.g. self-report, voiding diary etc.) was not specified. All women who were symptom free after treatment reverted to a normal cystometrogram. Fantl et al.[78] reported that 12% of the treatment group were continent and 76% had reduced their incontinent episodes by at least 50% or more at 6 weeks, as measured by a 7-day voiding diary; these results were maintained at 6 months. They also reported a 55% improvement in quality of life measured by a standardized questionnaire at 6 weeks, which was maintained over a 6-month period.[79] Significant reductions were also observed with diurnal and nocturnal frequency and volume of fluid lost on a pad test. Although some women did revert back to normal bladder function following training, no relationship was found between changes in urodynamic variables and the number of incontinent episodes.[80]

Seven clinical series[81–86] reported that bladder retraining effectively reduced incontinent episodes. In studies using a voiding diary to measure outcome, cure rates ranged from 50 to 86.6%, with improvement rates reported from 75 to 87.3% .

Bladder retraining vs PFMT

In a multicentre RCT, Wyman et al.[87] compared bladder retraining with PFMT augmented with BF and found that both interventions were equally effective in reducing incontinent episodes and improving quality of life in women with GSI, DI or both diagnoses. Cure rates determined by a 7-day voiding diary were 18 and 16% in the bladder retraining group at 3 and 6 months post-randomization, respectively, vs 13 and 20% in the PFMT group. Improvement rates (i.e. the percentage of patients achieving greater than 50% reduction of incontinent episodes) in the bladder training group were 52 and 46% at 3 and 6 months, respectively, vs 57 and 56% in the PFMT group.

Bladder retraining vs medication

Two RCTs[88,89] concluded that bladder retraining was superior to anticholinergic drug therapy in women with DI. Jarvis[88] found that inpatient bladder retraining was superior to an outpatient programme of combined drug therapy of flavoxate hydrochloride and imipramine. Cure/improvement rates in the bladder retraining group were 84% subjectively continent and 76% symptom free vs 56% continent and 48% symptom free in the drug therapy group. Patients who were symptom free at 4 weeks were able to maintain the effects at 12 weeks. Cystometric changes in both groups were related to the clinical changes. Columbo and associates[89] reported that a 6-week course of oxybutynin had a clinical cure rate similar to that of bladder retraining (74 vs 73%, respectively); a higher cure rate was noted in women with DI alone (74 vs 42%). However, the relapse rate at 6 months was higher for the oxybutynin group, those in the bladder-retraining group maintaining their results better. Changes in bladder stability corresponded to symptom improvement in both groups.

Bladder retraining in combination with other adjuncts

Bladder retraining with PFMT vs bladder retraining or PFMT alone

In a multicentre RCT, Wyman *et al.*[90] compared the combination therapy of bladder retraining and PFMT augmented with BF instruction in women with each treatment alone. The results suggest that bladder retraining is as effective as a combination intervention programme in reducing incontinence and improving quality of life when evaluation occurs 6 months from the initiation of treatment. Combination therapy was superior to bladder retraining alone at resolving incontinence episodes at 3 months (31 vs 18% cure rate). Subjects in the combination therapy group also had a superior improvement rate as determined by the percentage of subjects who achieved a 50% or greater reduction in incontinent episodes (70 vs 56% of subjects). However, by 6 months post-randomization, there were no significant differences between the three groups in either reduction of incontinent episodes or improvement of quality of life. Both cure and improvement rates in combination therapy had dropped (27 and 59%, respectively), whereas cure and improvement rates were better maintained in the bladder retraining group (16 and 41%, respectively). Women with GSI or DI with and without stress incontinence had similar reductions in incontinent episodes at the 3- and 6-month evaluations.

In another RCT, bladder retraining with PFMT was compared with brief psychotherapy or drug therapy (propantheline) in women with DI and sensory–urgency syndrome.[91] Incontinence episodes, as measured by a 7-day voiding diary, were significantly reduced in the psychotherapy group but not in the bladder retraining/PFMT or drug therapy groups at 12 weeks after the start of treatment. Improvements in the bladder retraining/PFMT group were associated with cystometric improvements in detrusor pressure.

An RCT that compared an inpatient with an outpatient programme of bladder retraining and PFMT reported that the outpatient programme was as effective as the impatient programme and could be conducted at less cost:[50] subjective cure/improvement rates were 63% in both groups; dry pad testing had similar rates in inpatients (70%) and outpatients (77%), and cure rates at 3 months (defined as no incontinent episodes on a voiding diary) were similar in inpatients (63%) and outpatients (53%).

Bladder retraining with drug therapy vs bladder retraining alone

Several studies have examined the efficacy of bladder retraining with the use of anticholinergic and/or sedative drug therapy in women with DI, urge incontinence with stable bladder, and sensory–urgency syndrome.[77,91–96] Of these, three are RCTs[88,91,96] and three are retrospective clinical series.[93–95] The results are inconsistent between studies, reflecting differences in the type of drug therapy, the drug dosage and the treatment outcomes evaluated. The majority of studies reported excellent short-term cure or improvement rates with bladder retraining added to the drug regimen (72–83.7%). One study reported a 50% cure rate at 3 years.[95]

Two studies comparing drug therapy plus bladder retraining, with bladder retraining plus placebo, did not find an additive benefit when bladder retraining was used in the protocol in the treatment of DI.[96,97] Szonyi *et al.*,[96] using a double-blind placebo-controlled parallel-group design, found no difference between the placebo group (bladder retraining and placebo) vs the drug group (oxybutynin with bladder retraining) in reducing incontinent episodes or nocturia.[96] However, the investigators concluded that the drug group was superior to the placebo (bladder retraining) group because it had greater subjective benefit (86 vs 55%). Wiseman *et al.*,[97] using a similar research design, reported no difference between the placebo and drug therapy (terodiline) groups[95] in reducing episodes of incontinence.

In contrast, Klarskov and co-workers found that drug therapy with bladder retraining was superior to bladder retraining and placebo.[98] Using a non-randomized double-blind placebo-controlled design, they found that terodiline with bladder training was superior to placebo and bladder training on both objective and subjective measures.

In a retrospective, two-group cohort design, Fantl et al.[94] found that 78.6% of patients receiving bladder retraining alone were subjectively cured (i.e. no further reports of incontinence and reported voidings occurring at 3–5-hour intervals without associated symptoms) and 21.5% were not cured, compared with 83.3% and 16.7%, respectively, in a group receiving combined bladder retraining and drug therapy.

Two retrospective studies reported an excellent initial response to an inpatient bladder retraining programme that included combination drug therapy (emepronium and fluphenazine/nortriptyline)[93,99] or oxybutynin.[95] Subjective cure/improvement rates were 85–88%. However, Ferrie and co-workers[99] found that the improvement rate dropped from 88% at the conclusion of treatment to 38% 6 months after hospital discharge. In a similar trial, subjective cure/improvement rates were not related to cystometric evidence of a stable bladder.[93]

In conclusion, bladder retraining appears to date to have benefits similar to those of drug therapy, and may have greater long-term benefit. Any additional benefit of combining bladder retraining with drug therapy was not consistently noted.

Factors affecting outcomes of bladder retraining

There is conflicting evidence on whether symptomatology, urodynamic diagnosis or urodynamic parameters affect treatment outcome. O'Brien et al.,[42] using a combination therapy approach, found that patients with mixed symptomatology did less well. Two RCTs found that urodynamic diagnosis (GSI, DI or both) had no effect on treatment outcome.[78,90] In contrast, Pengelly and Booth,[84] in a prospective clinical trial with historical controls, found that a poor result was associated with a strong ($>100 \, cmH_2O$ pressure) isometric contraction during voluntary interruption of micturition. Poor results were also noted with a history of nocturnal enuresis after 10 years of age and failure to show improvement after 2 weeks of treatment. Three retrospective clinical series reported that patients who were symptomatic but had stable bladders were more likely to respond better than those who had unstable bladder.[82,95,99] In a trial of bladder retraining with imipramine therapy, Castleden et al.[100] reported that decreased mental ability, decreased mobility and high detrusor pressure were associated with poorer outcomes. Another study reported that, although patients with reduced bladder compliance and idiopathic instability may initially do well, 40% of them will relapse.[95]

Compliance as a factor influencing outcome was mentioned in only one study.[90]

Conclusions

There appears to be level 1B evidence to suggest that, for women with urge, stress and mixed urinary incontinence, bladder retraining is more effective than no treatment. Evidence is inconsistent about expected cure rates, which may be dependent on when and how the outcome was measured or reflect differences in the bladder retraining protocol. Findings on objective (cystometric) changes do not always correspond to successful subjective change.

One RCT has indicated that bladder retraining and PFMT have similar efficacy, and this requires further investigation. Bladder retraining appears to have benefits similar to those of drug therapy to date, and may have greater long-term benefit. Similarly, the effectiveness of bladder retraining in combination with PFMT in comparison to either bladder retraining or PFMT alone is as yet unclear and further investigation is warranted. The one RCT available suggests that the long-term benefit of bladder retraining alone may be similar to that of bladder retraining combined with PFMT. Any additional benefit of combining bladder retraining with drug therapy was not noted consistently. Further RCTs are needed to compare bladder retraining alone and in combination with drugs and physical therapies.

ANTI-INCONTINENCE DEVICES

Urinary loss in the female patient may be the result of overactivity or underactivity of the detrusor or outlet, alone or in combination. Devices may act to correct, compensate for, or circumvent the pathophysiology of the detrusor or outlet in order to improve urinary storage and emptying. Varying levels of manual dexterity are required, depending on the device.

To date, few objective comparative clinical trials have involved devices for incontinence. This section examines the evidence for the management of urinary incontinence using devices.

Devices that treat incontinence secondary to failure to empty (detrusor underactivity/outlet overactivity) in non-neurogenic women

Nativ[101] published a descriptive report on a sphincter prosthesis composed of a self-retaining silicone catheter with a self-contained urinary pump (flow 10–12 ml/s), activated by a small hand-held control device. The study was descriptive and uncontrolled, and involved a small number (15) of patients, who utilized the device for varying periods (2 weeks to 16 months). Continence and bladder emptying were reported as good, with minimal morbidity. There were no specific comments on the effect of the device on urethral integrity.

On the basis of the data obtained from neurogenic patients, it seems that clean intermittent catheterization is superior to an indwelling catheter for long-term management in the ambulatory population. Technological developments utilizing indwelling mechanical urethal valves and pumps may provide an alternative. This should be identified as an important area for further research.

Devices that treat failure to store (outlet underactivity) in non-neurogenic ambulatory women

Failure to store secondary to decreased outlet activity may be manifested in the symptoms and signs of GSI. Treatment of this condition with devices involves (a) external urinary collection, (b) intravaginal support of the bladder neck, or (c) blockage of urinary leakage by occluding egress (i) at the external meatus or (ii) with an intra-urethral device.

External collection devices

Female external collecting devices are placed over the urethral meatus or within the introital area; they are secured by straps, adhesive or suction, and empty into a drainage bag. These devices have been developed and tested, and a few reports on their use have been published, but they have not been widely distributed or sold. Many of the published studies of devices are small descriptive studies performed on patients in a rehabilitation centre or nursing home rather than in the ambulatory population, and are not referenced.

No devices for the collection of urine have been successfully developed or tested in the ambulatory female population. The inability to collect urine (due to variations in individual anatomy and adherence of the device) is the major problem. Current external collecting devices are cumbersome and have a low efficacy in the ambulatory population. The development of a product for the external collection of urine in women should be identified as an important area for future clinical research.

Devices that support the bladder neck

Support of the bladder neck to improve stress urinary incontinence has been achieved with varying success with (a) tampons, (b) traditional pessaries and contraceptive diaphragms, and (c) intravaginal devices specifically designed to support the bladder neck. Edwards,[102] Bonnar[103] and Cardozo[104] have reported on devices of historical interest that are not currently available. All studies to date have involved relatively small numbers, with the majority being clinical case series[103,105–107] and one a prospective randomized single-blind study.[108] All studies demonstrated an improvement in continence by the methods employed. Studies performed in the acute setting demonstrate better performance than diary-based studies performed over time, regardless of the device. Efficacy is also higher in patients with minimal to moderate urinary leakage. Continence rates were 6/14 cured and 2/14 improved with tampons;[108] 4/10 improved with a diaphragm;[109] 9/12 improved with an oversized contraceptive diaphragm.[105] The bladder-neck support prosthesis provided continence in the laboratory in 25/30 of patients, with an overall significant decrease in average incontinence episodes in the population.[106,107] The authors reported minimal side effects associated with the diaphragms and support prosthesis, specifically the absence of significant urinary retention, urinary tract infection or vaginal irritation.

There thus appears to be some evidence that support of the bladder neck resulting in improved continence is possible with intravaginal devices without causing significant lower urinary tract obstruction or morbidity. Vaginal support devices should be included in the treatment options when counselling women with stress urinary incontinence. However, long-term results are not available and no studies have compared these therapies with other forms of therapy. Further research is recommended.

Occlusive devices

Devices have been developed that block urinary leakage at the external urethral meatus. In addition to a simple barrier effect, compression of the wall of the distal urethra has been hypothesized to contribute to continence. Several devices are currently marketed that utilize an adhesive or mild suction to occlude urinary loss at the urethral meatus, but there is only a single full published report available.

Eckford *et al.*[110] studied an external pad which provided urethral occlusion by an adhesive seal attached over the urethral meatus in 19 women with the symptom of stress incontinence: 17 women reported a cure or improvement, measured by the number of incontinence episodes per week. There was a significant decrease in both the number of episodes and pad-test leakage when using the device. Difficulties were limited to those in placing and removing the device.

Although Eckford *et al.*[110] found that the external urethral device was safe and efficacious, efficacy for different grades of incontinence has not been established, nor are long-term efficacy and safety data available; further research into the role of devices that block urinary leakage at the external urethral meatus is now recommended.

Intra-urethral devices

Devices that are inserted into the urethra to block urinary leakage have been described. Similarities among the devices include a means to (a) prevent intravesical migration (a meatal plate), (b) enhance retention within the urethra (spheres, inflatable balloons or flanges), and (c) accomplish bladder emptying (removal of the device or a pumping mechanism). A primary differentiation can be made between single-use disposable devices (which allow insertion and removal by the patient for voiding) and indwelling devices (which require insertion by the physician).

Neilsen *et al.*[111] studied 40 patients, who utilized a device composed of an oval meatal plate, a soft stalk with a removable semi-rigid guide pin which is removed after insertion, and either one (the original device) or two (the improved device) spheres along the stalk with fixed distances between the meatal plate and the spheres. They studied both the one- and the two-sphere devices in a crossover study for 2 weeks, and then the patients selected the device that they preferred for an additional 2 months of usage. Peschers *et al.*[112] screened 53 patients with GSI and 21 patients accepted treatment with the two-sphere device. During a 4-month study, the investigators analysed subjective improvement and performed pad-weight and cough tests.

Staskin[113] reported on a 4-month study of 135 of 215 patients who utilized a disposable balloon-tipped urethral insert made from thermoplastic elastomer, inflated with an applicator on insertion and deflated by pulling a string at the meatal plate for removal during voiding. Urodynamic studies excluded patients with urge incontinence and classified patients into those with anatomical hypermobility and those with intrinsic sphincter deficiency. The patients reported on diary and quality-of-life questionnaires. Miller and Bavendam[114] reported on 63 of the 135 patients from the above cohort, who utilized the balloon-tipped intra-urethral insert for a year.

Regarding the results, most patients who completed the studies were subjectively and objectively continent or improved. Cure or improvement rates have been reported as 94.4% by Neilsen *et al.*,[111] 66.7% by Peschers,[112] and 96% (based on pad-weighing tests) by Staskin[113] and Miller and Bavendam.[114] However, it is important to emphasize that there was a high drop-out rate of patients completing the above studies: completion rates were reported as 18 of 40 enrolled for Neilsen *et al.*,[111] 14/21 with 53 screened for Peschers *et al.*,[112] 135/215 for Staskin,[113] and 63/135 with 215 screened for Miller and Bavendam.[114] The most common morbidities reported were discomfort,[113] urinary tract infection (31% treated for positive urine cultures with 20% symptomatic and 11% asymptomatic),[113] and one or more episodes of gross haematuria (24%).[114]

In conclusion, intra-urethral inserts have demonstrated efficacy in the control of urinary incontinence. The morbidity associated with the use of these devices varies with the design of the device. The most common morbidities are urinary tract infection, haematuria and discomfort. There are no long-term studies on devices that are not removed following each void.

Conclusions

Advances in the technology of anti-incontinence devices have provided additional options for conservative approaches to treatment; randomized controlled studies are, however, lacking. The main role of these devices would appear to be for patients in whom other conservative therapies have failed, those who would prefer a rapid intervention while performing physical therapies, or those who wish to avoid or who have failed operative intervention. Device efficacy and morbidity are related to the degree of invasiveness of the treatment. Device cost will vary with frequency and duration of use. Studies comparing overall management and treatment cost, patient acceptance, and quality of life are necessary. These studies should compare devices with physical therapies, device with device, and device with surgical intervention, in subsets of patients with varying pathophysiologies and different social requirements.

GENERAL CONCLUSIONS

Conservative treatment (lifestyle interventions, physical therapies, bladder retraining and anti-incontinence devices) should be included in the counselling of incontinent women regarding these treatment options. The evidence for their efficacy is summarized in Table 29.2.

At present, of all the conservative treatments, most evidence is available regarding physical therapies on the basis of three systematic reviews (with qualitative syntheses) of the available RCTs in this area. However, it is important to stress that, to date, no quantitative synthesis (meta-analysis) has been carried out and that qualitative synthesis may be open to errors due to subjective interpretation of trial outcomes. The same deficiency applies to the evidence relating to bladder retraining. Further RCT research is needed to provide additional evidence of efficacy of physical therapies and bladder retraining.

Regarding lifestyle interventions, most studies to date have reported associations only and have not assessed the actual effect of applying or removing the behaviour in question. Similarly, RCTs are lacking in the area of anti-incontinence devices.

Further research on the efficacy of conservative management is necessary and investigators should use well-established methodological criteria when planning and implementing trials. These trials need to include the use of valid and reliable outcome measures (measures of cost, patient satisfaction, clinical morbidity, function and quality of life) that are lacking from much of the existing research. Investigation of factors affecting outcomes (e.g. severity, age, previous surgery and parity) is also urgently needed.

Table 29.2. *Summary of evidence for efficacy of conservative treatments for women with stress, urge and mixed incontinence*

Multiple RCTs with consistent findings

- PFMT better than no treatment
- Bladder retraining better than no treatment
- PFMT with biofeedback or intravaginal resistance no more effective than PFMT alone

Multiple RCTs with inconsistent findings* or single RCTs[†]

- PFMT vs ES, surgery, medication (for stress incontinence)[†]
- High-intensity PFMT vs home treatment[†]
- PFMT with ES or vaginal cones vs PFMT[†]
- ES vs no treatment for (genuine) stress incontinence[†]
- ES vs sham ES for (genuine) stress incontinence*
- ES vs sham ES for urge incontinence[†]
- Bladder retraining vs medication*
- Bladder retraining alone vs PFMT (with biofeedback) vs bladder retraining with PFMT[†]
- Bladder retraining with medication vs bladder retraining alone*
- Hodge pessary vs super tampon vs no device[†]

No RCTs available

- All lifestyle interventions
- All remaining anti-incontinence devices
- PFMT vs vaginal cones (abstracts only)

RCT, randomized controlled trial; PFMT, pelvic floor muscle training; ES, electrical stimulation.

ACKNOWLEDGEMENTS

This chapter is based largely on the work of the Conservative Treatment of Women Group of the 1st International Consultation on Incontinence. Particular thanks are due to Ingrid Nygaard (principal author for Lifestyle Interventions), Jean Wyman (principal author for Bladder Retraining), David Staskin (principal author for Anti-Incontinence Devices) and also Alain Bourcier (for his contribution to the Physical Therapies section).

REFERENCES

1. Elwood JM. *Critical Appraisal of Epidemiological Studies and Clinical Trials*, 2nd edn. Oxford: Oxford University Press, 1998

2. Agency for Health Care Policy and Research. Public Health Service, US Department of Health and Human Services, *Acute Pain Management: Operative or Medical*

Procedures and Trauma. AHCPR Publ. no. 92–0038. Rockville, MD: 1992.

3. Wilson PD, Herbison RM, Herbison GP. Obstetric practice and the prevalence of urinary incontinence three months after delivery. *Br J Obstet Gynaecol* 1996; 103: 154–161

4. Rasmussen KL, Krue S, Johansson LE *et al*. Obesity as a predictor of postpartum urinary symptoms. *Acta Obstet Gynecol Scand* 1997; 76: 359–362

5. Mommsen S, Foldspang A. Body mass index and adult female urinary incontinence. *World J Urol* 1994; 12: 319–322

6. Dwyer PL, Lee ETC, Hay DM. Obesity and urinary incontinence in women. *Br J Obstet Gynaecol* 1988; 95: 91–96

7. Kölbl H, Riss P. Obesity and stress urinary incontinence: significance of indices of relative weight. *Urol Int* 1988; 43: 7–10

8. Yarnell JWG, Voyle GJ, Sweetnam PM, Milbank J. Factors associated with urinary incontinence in women. *J Epidemiol Community Health* 1982; 36: 58–63

9. Brown JS, Seeley DG, Fong J *et al*. Urinary incontinence in older women: who is at risk? *Obstet Gynecol* 1996; 87: 715–721

10. Bump RC, Sugerman JH, Fantl A, McClish DM. Obesity and lower urinary tract function in women: effect of surgically induced weight-loss. *Am J Obstet Gynecol* 1992; 167: 392–398

11. Deitel M, Stone E, Kassam HA *et al*. Gynecologic–obstetric changes after loss of massive excess weight following bariatric surgery. *J Am Coll Nutr* 1988; 7: 147–153

12. Subak L. Weight reduction in moderately obese women and urinary incontinence. Personal communication, 1998

13. Nygaard IE, DeLancey JO, Arnsdorf L, Murphy E. Exercise and incontinence. *Obstet Gynecol* 1990; 75: 848–851

14. Bø K, Mæhlum S, Oseid S, Larsen S. Prevalence of stress urinary incontinence among physically active and sedentary female students. *Scand J Sports Sci* 1989; 11: 113–116

15. Bø K, Stien R, Kulseng-Hanssen S, Kristofferson M. Clinical and urodynamic assessment of nulliparous young women with and without stress incontinence symptoms: a case-control study. *Obstet Gynecol* 1994; 84: 1028–1032

16. Nygaard IE. Does prolonged high-impact activity contribute to later urinary incontinence? A retrospective cohort study of female Olympians. *Obstet Gynecol* 1997; 90: 718–722

17. Davis GD, Goodman M. Stress urinary incontinence in nulliparous female soldiers in airborne infantry training. *J Pelv Surg* 1996; 2: 68–71

18. Jörgensen S, Hein HO, Gyntelberg F. Heavy lifting at work and risk of genital prolapse and herniated lumbar disc in assistant nurses. *Occup Med* 1994; 44: 47–49

19. Tampakoudis P, Tantanassis T, Grimbizis G *et al*. Cigarette smoking and urinary incontinence in women – a new calculative method of estimating the exposure to smoke. *Eur J Obstet Gynecol Reprod Biol* 1995; 63: 17–30

20. Bump RC, McClish DM. Cigarette smoking and pure genuine stress incontinence of urine: a comparison of risk factors and determinants between smokers and non-smokers. *Am J Obstet Gynecol* 1994; 170: 579–582

21. Hisayama T, Shinkai M, Takaynagi I, Toyoda T. Mechanism of action of nicotine in isolated bladder of guinea-pig. *Br J Pharmacol* 1988; 95: 465–472

22. Koley B, Koley J, Saha JK. The effects of nicotine on spontaneous contractions of cat urinary bladder in situ. *Br J Pharmacol* 1984; 83: 347–355

23. Wilson PD, Bø K, Bourcier A *et al*. Conservative management of women (Committee 14). In: Abrams P, Khouri S, Wein A (eds) *Incontinence*. Plymouth: Health Publication Limited, 1999; 579–563

24. Creighton SM, Stanton SL. Caffeine: does it affect your bladder? *Br J Urol* 1990; 66: 613–614

25. Griffiths DJ, McCracken PN, Harrison GM, Gormley EA. Relationship of fluid intake to voluntary micturition and urinary incontinence in geriatric patients. *Neurourol Urodyn* 1993; 12: 1–7

26. Wyman JF, Elswick RK, Wilson MS, Fantl JA. Relationship of fluid intake to voluntary micturitions and urinary incontinence in women. *Neurourol Urodyn* 1991; 10: 463–473

27. Spence-Jones C, Kamm MA, Henry MM, Hudson CN. Bowel dysfunction: a pathogenic factor in uterovaginal prolapse and urinary stress incontinence. *Br J Obstet Gynaecol* 1994; 101: 147–152

28. Diokno AC, Brock BM, Herzog AR, Bromberg J. Medical correlates of urinary incontinence in the elderly. *Urology* 1990; 36: 129–138

29. Lubowski DZ, Swash M, Nicholls RJ, Henry MM. Increase in pudendal nerve terminal motor latency with defaecation straining. *Br J Surg* 1988; 75: 1095–1097

30. Jorge JMN, Wexner SD, Ehrenpreis ED *et al*. Does perineal descent correlate with pudendal neuropathy? *Dis Colon Rectum* 1993; 36: 475–483

31. Norton PA, Baker JE. Postural changes can reduce leakage in women with stress urinary incontinence. *Obstet Gynecol* 1994; 84: 770–774

32. Bø K. Physiotherapy to treat genuine stress incontinence. *Int Continence Surv* 1996; 6(2): 2–8

33. Berghmans LCM, Hendriks HJM, Bø K et al. Conservative treatment of stress urinary incontinence in women. A systematic review of randomized clinical trials. *Br J Urol* 1998; 82: 181–191

34. Bump RC, Hurt G, Fantl A, Wyman J. Assessment of Kegel muscle exercise performance after brief verbal instruction. *Am J Obstet Gynecol* 1991; 165: 322–329

35. American College of Sports Medicine. The recommended quantity and quality of exercise for developing and maintaining cardiorespiratory and muscular fitness in healthy adults. *Med Sci Sports Exerc* 1990; 22: 265–274

36. Åstrand PO, Rodahl K. *Textbook of Work Physiology: Physiological Basis of Exercise.* New York: McGraw-Hill, 1986

37. DiNubile NA. Strength training. *Clin Sports Med* 1991; 10: 33–62

38. Burns PA, Pranikoff K, Nochajksi TH et al. A comparison of effectiveness of biofeedback and pelvic muscle exercise treatment of stress incontinence in older community-dwelling women. *J Gerontol* 1993; 48: M167–M174

39. Bø K, Hagen RH, Kvarstein B et al. Pelvic floor muscle exercise for treatment of female stress urinary incontinence: III. Effects of two different degrees of pelvic floor muscle exercises. *Neurourol Urodyn* 1990; 9: 489–502

40. Wells TJ, Brink DA, Diokno AC et al. Pelvic muscle exercise for stress urinary incontinence in elderly women. *J Am Geriatr Soc* 1991; 39: 785–779

41. Lagro-Janssen ALM, Debruyne FMJ, Smits AJA, Van Weel C. The effects of treatment of urinary incontinence in general practice. *Fam Pract* 1992; 9: 284–289

42. O'Brien J, Austin M, Sethi P, O'Boyle P. Urinary incontinence: prevalence, need for treatment and effectiveness of intervention by nurse. *Br Med J* 1991; 303: 1308–1312

43. Nygaard IE, Kreder KJ, Lepic MM et al. Efficacy of pelvic floor muscle exercises in women with stress, urge and mixed urinary incontinence. *Am J Obstet Gynecol* 1996; 174: 120–125

44. Gallo ML, Staskin DR. Cues to action: pelvic floor muscle exercise compliance in women with stress urinary incontinence. *Neurourol Urodyn* 1997; 16: 167–177

45. Henalla SM, Hutchins CJ, Robinson P, MacVicar J. Non-operative methods in the treatment of female genuine stress incontinence of urine. *J Obstet Gynaecol* 1989; 9: 222–225

46. O'Brien J, Long H. Urinary incontinence: long term effectiveness of nursing intervention in primary care. *Br Med J* 1995; 311: 1208

47. Ramsay IN, Thou M. A randomised, double blind, placebo controlled trial of pelvic floor exercises in the treatment of genuine stress incontinence. Proceedings of the 20th Annual Meeting International Continence Society. *Neurourol Urodyn* 1990; 9: 398–399

48. Bø K, Talseth T. Long-term effect of pelvic floor muscle exercise 5 years after cessation of organized training. *Obstet Gynecol* 1996; 87: 261–265

49. Wilson PD, Herbison GP, Glazener CMA et al. Postnatal incontinence: a multicentre, randomised controlled trial of conservative treatment. Proceedings of the 27th Annual Meeting, International Continence Society. *Neurourol Urodyn* 1997; 16: 349–350

50. Ramsay IN, Ali HM, Hunter M et al. A prospective, randomized controlled trial of inpatient versus outpatient continence programs in the treatment of urinary incontinence in the female. *Int Urogynecol J* 1996; 7: 260–263

51. Hofbauer VJ, Preisinger F, Nürnberger N. Der stellenwert der physiokotherapie bei der weiblichen genuinen streß-inkontinenz. *Z Urol Nephrol* 1990; 83: 249–254

52. Laycock J, Jerwood D. Does pre-modulated interferential therapy cure genuine stress incontinence? *Physiotherapy* 1993; 79: 553–560

53. Smith JJ. Intravaginal stimulation randomized trial. *J Urol* 1996; 155: 127–130

54. Hahn I, Sommar S, Fall M. A comparative study of pelvic floor training and electrical stimulation for the treatment of genuine female stress urinary incontinence. *Neurourol Urodyn* 1991; 10: 545–554

55. Hahn I, Nauclér J, Sommar S, Fall M. Urodynamic assessment of pelvic floor training. *World J Urol* 1991; 9: 162–166

56. Laycock J. Interferential therapy in the treatment of genuine stress incontinence. Proceedings of the 18th Annual Meeting International Continence Society. *Neurourol Urodyn* 1988; 7: 268–269

57. Wise BG, Haken J, Cardozo LD, Plevnik S. A comparative study of vaginal cone therapy, cones + Kegel exercises, and maximal electrical stimulation in the treatment of female genuine stress incontinence. Proceedings of the International Continence Society 23rd Annual Meeting. *Neurourol Urodyn* 1993; 12: 436–437

58. Laycock J, Knight S, Naylor D. Prospective, randomised, controlled clinical trial to compare acute and chronic electrical stimulation in combination therapy for GSI. Proceedings of the International Continence Society 25th Annual Meeting. *Neurourol Urodyn* 1995; 14: 425–426

59. Klarskov P, Belving D, Bischoff N et al. Pelvic floor exercise versus surgery for female urinary stress incontinence. *Urol Int* 1986; 41: 129–132

60. Tapp AJS, Hills B, Cardozo LD. Randomised study comparing pelvic floor physiotherapy with the Burch colpo-

suspension. Proceedings of the International Continence Society 19th Annual Meeting. *Neurourol Urodyn* 1989; 8: 356–357

61. Peattie AB, Plevnik S. Cones versus physiotherapy as conservative management of genuine stress incontinence. Proceedings of the International Continence Society 18th Annual Meeting. *Neurourol Urodyn* 1988; 7: 265–266

62. Haken J, Benness C, Cardozo L, Cutner A. A randomised trial of vaginal cones and pelvic floor exercises in the management of genuine stress incontinence. Proceedings of the International Continence Society 21st Annual Meeting. *Neurourol Urodyn* 1991; 10: 393–394

63. Castleden CM, Duffin HM, Mitchell EP. The effect of physiotherapy on stress incontinence. *Age Ageing* 1984; 13: 235–237

64. Berghmans LCM, de Bie Frederiks RA, Weil EHJ *et al.* Efficacy of biofeedback, when included with pelvic floor muscle exercise treatment, for genuine stress incontinence. *Neurourol Urodyn* 1996; 15: 37–52

65. Glavind K, Nøhr SB, Walter S. Biofeedback and physiotherapy versus physiotherapy alone in the treatment of genuine stress incontinence. *Int Urogynecol J* 1996; 7: 339–343

66. Shepherd AM, Montgomery E. Treatment of genuine stress incontinence with a new perineometer. *Physiotherapy* 1983; 69: 113

67. Ferguson KL PL McKey, Bishop KR, Kloen P *et al.* Stress urinary incontinence: effect of pelvic muscle exercise. *Obstet Gynecol* 1990; 75: 671–675

68. Pieber D, Zivkovic F, Tamussino G *et al.* Pelvic floor exercise alone or with vaginal cones for the treatment of mild to moderate stress urinary incontinence in premenopausal women. *Int Urogynecol J* 1995; 6: 14–17

69. Sand PK, Richardson DA, Staskin DR *et al.* Pelvic floor electrical stimulation in the treatment of genuine stress incontinence: a multicenter, placebo-controlled trial. *Am J Obstet Gynecol* 1995; 173: 72–79

70. Blowman C, Pickles C, Emery S *et al.* Prospective double blind controlled trial of intensive physiotherapy with and without stimulation of the pelvic floor in the treatment of genuine stress incontinence. *Physiotherapy* 1991; 77: 661–664

71. Brubaker L, Benson T, Bent A *et al.* Transvaginal electrical stimulation for female urinary incontinence. *Am J Obstet Gynecol* 1997; 177: 536–540

72. Luber KM, Wolde-Tsadik G. Efficacy of functional electrical stimulation in treating genuine stress incontinence: a randomized clinical trial. *Neurourol Urodyn* 1997; 16: 543–551

73. Abel I, Ottesen B, Fischer-Rasmussen W, Lose G. Maximal electrical stimulation of the pelvic floor in the treatment of urge incontinence: a placebo controlled study. Proceedings of the International Continence Society 26th Annual Meeting. *Neurourol Urodyn* 1996; 15: 283–284

74. The Coronary Drug Project Research Group. Influence of adherence to treatment and response of cholesterol on mortality in the Coronary Drug Project. *N Engl J Med* 1980; 303: 1038–1041

75. Ramsay I, Hassan A, Hunter M, Donaldson K. A randomised controlled trial of urodynamic investigations prior to conservative treatment of urinary incontinence in the female. Proceedings of the International Continence Society 24th Annual Meeting. *Neurourol Urodyn* 1994; 13: 455–456

76. Wyman JF, Fantl JA. Bladder training in the ambulatory care management of urinary incontinence. *Urol Nurs* 1991; 11(3): 11–17

77. Jarvis GJ, Millar DR. Controlled trial of bladder drill for detrusor instability. *Br Med J* 1980; 281: 1322–1323

78. Fantl JA, Wyman JF, McClish DK *et al.* Efficacy of bladder training in older women with urinary incontinence. *J Am Med Assoc* 1991; 265: 609–613

79. Wyman JF, Fantl JA, McClish DK *et al.* Effect of bladder training on quality of life of older women with urinary incontinence. *Int Urogynecol J* 1997; 8: 223–229

80. McClish DK, Fantl JA, Wyman JF *et al.* Bladder training in older women with urinary incontinence: relationships in urodynamic observations. *Obstet Gynecol* 1991; 77: 281–286

81. Svigos JM, Matthews DC. Assessment and treatment of female urinary incontinence by cystometrogram and bladder retraining programmes. *Obstet Gynecol* 1977; 50: 9–12

82. Frewen WK. The management of urgency and frequency of micturition. *Br J Urol* 1980; 52: 367–369

83. Frewen WK. A reassessment of bladder training in detrusor dysfunction in the female. *Br J Urol* 1982; 54: 372–373

84. Pengelly AW, Booth CM. A prospective trial of bladder training as treatment of detrusor instability. *Br J Urol* 1980; 52: 463–466

85. Jarvis GJ. The management of urinary incontinence due to primary vesical sensory urgency by bladder drill. *Br J Urol* 1982; 54: 374–376

86. Publicover C, Bear M. The effect of bladder training on urinary incontinence in community-dwelling older women. *J Wound Ostomy Continence Nurs* 1997; 24: 319–324

87. Wyman JF, Fantl JA, McClish DK *et al.* Bladder training in older women with urinary incontinence: relationship between outcome and changes in urodynamic observations. *Obstet Gynecol* 1991; 77: 281–286

88. Jarvis GJ. A controlled trial of bladder drill and drug therapy in the management of detrusor instability. *Br J Urol* 1981; 53: 565–566

89. Columbo M, Zanetta G, Scalambrino S *et al.* Oxybutynin and bladder training in the management of female urinary urge incontinence: a randomized study. *Int Urogynecol J* 1995; 6: 63–67

90. Wyman JF, Fantl JA, McClish DK *et al.* Comparative efficacy of behavioral interventions in the management of female urinary incontinence. *Am J Obstet Gynecol* 1998; 179: 999–1007

91. Macauley AJ, Stern RS, Homes DM *et al.* Micturition and the mind: psychological factors in the aetiology and treatment of urinary symptoms in women. *Br Med J* 1987; 294: 540–543

92. Frewen W. Role of bladder training in the treatment of the unstable bladder in the female. *Urol Clin North Am* 1979; 6: 273–277

93. Elder DD, Stephenson TP. An assessment of the Frewen regime in the treatment of detrusor dysfunction in females. *Br J Urol* 1980; 52: 467–471

94. Fantl JA, Hurt WG, Dunn LJ. Detrusor instability syndrome: the use of bladder retraining drills with and without anticholinergics. *Am J Obstet Gynecol* 1981; 140: 885–890

95. Holmes DM, Stone AR, Bary PR *et al.* Bladder retraining – 3 years on. *Br J Urol* 1983; 55: 660–664

96. Szonyi G, Collas DM, Ding YY *et al.* Oxybutynin with bladder retraining for detrusor instability in elderly people: a randomized controlled trial. *Age Ageing* 1995; 24: 287–291

97. Wiseman PA, Malone-Lee J, Rai GSA. Terodiline with bladder retraining for treating detrusor instability in elderly people. *Br Med J* 1991; 302: 994–996

98. Klarskov P, Gerstenberg TC, Hald T. Bladder training and terodiline in females with idopathic urge incontinence and stable detrusor function. *Scand J Urol Nephrol* 1986; 20: 41–46

99. Ferrie BG, Smith JS, Logan D *et al.* Experience with bladder training in 65 patients. *Br J Urol* 1984; 55: 482–484

100. Castleden CM, Duffin HW, Asher MJ *et al.* Factors influencing outcome in elderly patients with urinary incontinence and detrusor instability. *Age Ageing* 1985; 14: 303–307

101. Nativ O, Moskowitz B, Issaq E *et al.* A new intraurethral sphincter prosthesis with a self contained urinary pump. *ASAIO J* 1997; 43: 197–203

102. Edwards L. The control of incontinence of urine in women with a pubo-vaginal spring device. Objective and subjective results. *Br J Urol* 1971; 43: 211–225

103. Bonnar J. Silicone vaginal applicance for control of stress incontinence. *Lancet* 1977; 2: 1161

104. Cardozo L. Evaluation of female urinary incontinence device. *Urology* 1979; 13: 398–401

105. Suarez G. Use of a standard contraceptive diaphragm in management of stress urinary incontinence. *Urology* 1991; 37: 119–122

106. Davila GW. Introl bladder neck support prosthesis: a nonsurgical urethropexy. *J Endourol* 1996; 10: 293–296

107. Bernier F. Harris L. Treating stress incontinence with the bladder neck support prosthesis. *Urol Nurs* 1995; 15: 5–9

108. Nygaard I. Prevention of exercise incontinence with mechanical devices. *J Reprod Med* 1995; 40: 89–94

109. Realini JP, Walters MD. Vaginal diaphragm rings in the treatment of stress incontinence. *J Am Board Fam Pract* 1990; 3: 99–103

110. Eckford SD, Jackson SR, Lewis PA, Abrams P. The continence control pad – a new external urethral occlusion device in the management of stress incontinence. *Br J Urol* 1996; 77: 538–540

111. Neilsen KK, Walter S, Maeffaard E, Kromann-Andersen B. The urethral plug II: an alternative treatment in women with genuine urinary stress incontinence. *Br J Urol* 1993; 72: 428–432

112. Peschers U, Zen Ruffinen F, Schaer GN, Schussler B. The VIVA urethal plug: a sensible expansion of the spectrum for conservative therapy of urinary stress incontinence? *Geburtshilfe Frauenheilkd* 1996; 56: 118–123

113. Staskin DR, Bavendam T, Miller J *et al.* Effectiveness of a urinary control insert in the management of stress urinary incontinence: early results of a multicenter study. *Urology* 1996; 47: 629–636

114. Miller JL, Bavendam T. Treatment with the Reliance urinary control insert: one-year experience. *J Endourol* 1996; 10: 287–292

30

Behavioural therapies in the management of urinary incontinence in women

J. A. Fantl

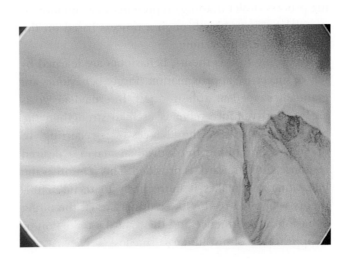

INTRODUCTION

Urinary continence represents the capability of collecting urine in the bladder, not allowing it to exit until it is voluntarily emptied in an appropriate place – the toilet. Although simplistically described, this represents a complex function.

There is clinical as well as experimental evidence that a significant interplay exists between sympathetic and parasympathetic autonomic innervations, both at peripheral and central levels. Somatic innervation through the pelvic and pudendal nerves also influences sphincteric function, primarily through its effect on striated musculature of the pelvic floor.

Bladder and urethral function are coordinated through specific cortical, brain stem and spinal centres. Complex reflex arcs involving both autonomic and somatic nerves are modulated centrally through facilitation and inhibition. Specific loops and circuits have been described and can be identified experimentally as well as clinically.

The appropriate function of the lower urinary tract depends on the harmonic interaction of anatomical and neuromuscular mechanisms. However, the ultimate accomplishment of continence includes the appropriate incorporation of a learned behaviour.

BEHAVIOURAL BASIS OF URINARY CONTINENCE

Newborn babies empty the bladder automatically because of a bladder contraction triggered by critical volume. During early childhood and after a period of somato/neural growth and maturation, the child 'learns' to inhibit bladder contractions, thus avoiding bladder emptying at inappropriate times. Such a learning process (toilet training) represents an adaptation to a social norm taught through a process based on the theory of operant learning.

According to this theory, behaviours are learned by way of successive approximation. Target behaviours are gradually shaped in a desired way. Intermediate goals are set and reinforcement is used to strengthen the behaviour, increasing the chances of it recurring. In operant conditioning the individual makes a desired response and a 'reward' is provided. This reinforces the behaviour and makes it more likely to recur. If this theory is applied to the lower urinary tract, the target behaviour is continence and the reward a reduction or disappearance of involuntary urine loss.

In summary, continence represents the ability to control the lower urinary tract to fulfil a social norm. It requires normal anatomy and function of the lower urinary tract, as well as appropriate learning of a behaviour (Fig. 30.1).

BEHAVIOURAL TREATMENT OF URINARY INCONTINENCE

Several management strategies used to treat urinary incontinence are incorporated under the category of: 'behavioural treatments.'[1] In general, these strategies tend to reduce the frequency of incontinence episodes with almost no reported side effects. In addition, there is no limitation regarding the use of additional interventions such as surgery or drugs.

Behavioural treatments are usually divided into those useful in individuals with cognitive or functional

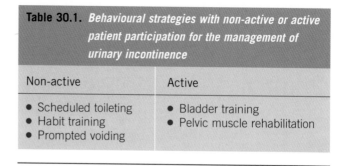

Table 30.1. *Behavioural strategies with non-active or active patient participation for the management of urinary incontinence*

Non-active	Active
• Scheduled toileting • Habit training • Prompted voiding	• Bladder training • Pelvic muscle rehabilitation

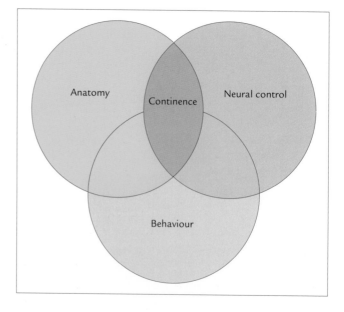

Figure 30.1. *Urinary continence: conceptual model.*

deficits, or both, and those where active patient participation is needed (Table 30.1). It must be emphasized, however, that this distinction is, to some extent, arbitrary. Some patients with functional disabilities but intact cognitive function may benefit from strategies where active participation is needed; therefore treatment should be carefully tailored to the individual.

Non-active patient participation

Scheduled toileting

The technique of scheduled toileting is usually offered to individuals who are institutionalized, suffer cognitive impairment and cannot participate in independent activities. No efforts are made toward motivation and the intervention basically establishes a strict voiding schedule to keep the patient as dry as possible. Usually, the schedule indicates toileting every 2–4 hours around the clock.

Overall success rates have been reported to be as high as 79%.

Habit training

Habit training attempts to match the individual's voiding habits to a 'preventative' toileting schedule. An initial period of monitoring is used to determine the specific profile of the patient's incontinence and a schedule is then individualized. A significant reduction in incontinence has been found in 85% of subjects. Because of the need for significant disruption of nursing routines, the technique can be difficult to establish in nursing homes and is best suited to patients receiving individual care.

Prompted voiding

Prompted voiding requires the patient to be able to recognize the need to void and to respond by requesting toileting or responding when prompted. The three basic elements of the technique are (1) monitoring, (2) prompting and (3) praise or reward.

Reduction of an average of 1–2 episodes of urinary incontinence in patient's having otherwise 8–9 episodes in 24 hours was found when studied under controlled circumstances. The technique was found to be effective in cognitively impaired institutionalized patients. Characterists of the patient's voiding or incontinence episode profile may identify good from poor responders.

Active patient participation

Bladder training (bladder drill)

Originally described by Jeffcoate[2] in 1966, the technique of bladder training was then popularized in Europe by Frewen.[3] It was primarily prescribed for what were originally described as 'functional disorders' and then became known as 'urge incontinence' or 'detrusor instability'. The technique relies on three basic concepts: (1) education, (2) voiding schedule and (3) positive reinforcements.

The education includes description of the basic anatomy and function of the lower urinary tract, with emphasis on the voluntary control over motor and sensory impulses. For this purpose, a slide tape programme using simple drawings and utilizing very basic explanations has been found to be extremely effective in educating patients on micturition and continence physiology. Distractive techniques to control urinary urgency are also incorporated: these techniques include the use of tasks to be performed in order to distract the mind from the sensation of urgency such as reviewing personal accounts, making up the weekly menu, or drawing up the weekly food shopping list etc.

The voiding schedule includes mandatory voidings at specific intervals. These intervals are extended through the training period until a reasonable spacing is reached (usually of 2–3 hours).

Positive reinforcements are an integral part of the management strategies and should emphasize the achievements as well as the efforts. This is best achieved during diary review and it provides compliance check at the same time.

Approximately 75% of patients are likely to reduce the number of incontinence episodes by at least 50%. Twelve per cent may become completely continent. Individuals with sphincteric problems seem to respond similarly to those with pure detrusor dysfunction.

A summary of trials using bladder training in the management of urinary incontinence is presented in Table 30.2.

Pelvic muscle rehabilitation

Pelvic muscle rehabilitation has been known to be effective in managing genuine stress incontinence (GSI) since Arnold Kegel's work in the late 1940s.[16,17] Although primarily used in women with GSI, it has proved beneficial in men after prostatectomy and also

Table 30.2. *Bladder training in women with urinary incontinence*

Investigators/ref. no.	Study design	'Cure rate' (%)
Svigos and Matthews[4]	Series	50
Frewen[5]	Series	82
Pengelly and Booth[6]	Series	44
Elder and Stephenson[7]	Series	52–86
Mahady and Begg[8]	Series	75–90
Jarvis and Millar[9]	Randomized	86–90
Fantl et al.[10]	Series	72
Jarvis[11]	Randomized	46–64
Jarvis[12]	Series	61–65
Frewen[13]	Series	66–97
Fantl et al.[14]	Randomized	12 'cured'/64 improved

Modified from ref. 15.

in women with urge incontinence or mixed syndromes. Pelvic rehabilitation can be enhanced with biofeedback techniques, vaginal weights and/or electrical stimulation. Although techniques have varied, the major elements of the therapy are (a) awareness of pelvic muscle function, (b) identification and utilization of appropriate muscle groups and avoidance of contraction of antagonist groups(abdomen and buttocks) and (c) exercise routine of successive contractions (usually 30–80 times a day for 8 weeks).

Biofeedback aims at using electrical or mechanical instruments to relay back to patients information about their lower urinary tract function, particularly their pelvic muscular activity.

Vaginal weight training uses specifically designed weights which can be inserted and used in the vagina while the patient is ambulatory. The attempt to avoid the loss of the weight through continued pelvic muscle contraction underlies the effectiveness of this technique.

Electrical stimulation of the perineal muscles induces striated muscle contraction as well as inhibition of detrusor activity. A presacral reflex arc must be intact for the latter to be effective. This treatment has been shown to be effective, either alone or in combination with a pelvic floor muscle rehabilitation programme. It is most effective in patients with GSI; however, good

results have also been noted in patients with urge incontinence alone or in cases of mixed syndrome.

Success rates of these different forms of pelvic muscle rehabilitation have varied, depending on the outcome variable used as well as the population studied. It is, however, reasonable to assume that more than 50% of those treated have reduced their incontinence significantly (by 50–80% of their baseline). Complete continence is usually seen in only 15–20% of the cases studied. A summary of trials using a form of pelvic muscle rehabilitation is presented in Table 30.3.

POSSIBLE TREATMENT EFFECT MECHANISMS

The correlation between clinical success and changes in urodynamic variables has been discouraging. The mechanisms by which these interventions affect lower urinary tract functioning are obscure. Pelvic floor rehabilitation acts on striated musculature, possibly improving sphincteric function; bladder training is believed to act by increasing cortical inhibition over the sacral micturition reflex centre. However, none of these theories has yet been proved by objective evidence. Only a few mechanisms could theoretically be influenced by these behavioural techniques, namely voluntary striated muscle contractility, reflex striated muscle contractility,

Table 30.3. *Pelvic floor rehabilitation in women with urinary incontinence*

Investigators/ref. no.	Design	Results (%)
Kegel[17]	Series	84 'cure'
Hendrickson[18]	Series	85 reduction
Kujansuu[19]	Series	56 'successful'
Burgio et al.[20]	Randomized	50–73 reduction
Benvenuti et al.[21]	Series	32 'cured'
Hanalla et al.[22]	Series	37 'cured'
Bø[8] et al.[23]	Randomized	17 'cured'
Burns et al.[24]	Randomized	54–61 reduction
Lagro-Jansen et al.[25]	Randomized	72 reduction
Cammau et al.[26]	Series	25 'cured'/81 improved
Hahn et al.[27]	Series	23 'cured'/48 improved
Dougherty et al.[28]	Series	61 reduction
Elia and Bergman[29]	Series	56 reduction or 'cured

Modified from ref. 15.

cortical inhibition and cortical facilitation. These variables are not easy to quantify, and their modification as the result of a behavioural intervention remains unproven.

Because of the lack of a specific known response and the fact that different interventions appear to have similar therapeutic effects overall, a prospective, randomized trial was conducted using various behavioural protocols – bladder training, pelvic floor muscle rehabilitation, or a combination of these two techniques. The results indicate similar responses in all treatment groups and across all diagnostic strata at 12 weeks of follow-up.[30]

Behavioural techniques in themselves may not be responsible for the treatment effect; rather, the effect may result from the structure and implementation of the programme itself. Education and bladder-control strategies are likely to reduce the condition of incontinence through mechanisms unique to each case. Hypothetically, the lower urinary tract, like other organ systems, has a reserve or compensatory function (Fig. 30.2), which can be implemented either subconsciously or consciously. Individual education, coaching and

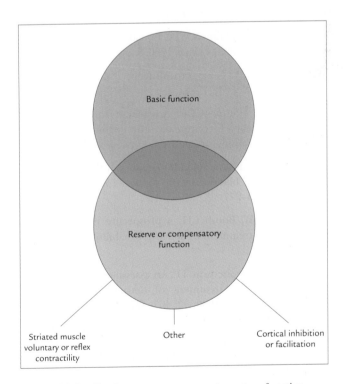

Figure 30.2. *Continence: reserve or compensatory function*

prompting will stimulate these compensatory mechanisms to increase continence.

Behavioural interventions have a place in the management of urinary incontinence. A basic evaluation to demonstrate the clinical condition and to rule out important co-morbidity is mandatory. The therapy appears to depend chiefly on the degree of education, bladder-control strategies and overall structure of the intervention rather than on the actual type of technique used. Interventions will, in most cases, reduce rather than abolish incontinence but can also be used in conjunction with other forms of interventions, such as drugs or surgery. However, a reduction in incontinence may be all that is needed to improve an individual's quality of life. The effect of behavioural therapy may be independent of whether the incontinence is primarily a consequence of sphincter or of detrusor dysfunction.

REFERENCES

1. Fantl JA, Newman DK, Colling J *et al. Urinary Incontinence in Adults: Acute and Chronic Management. Clinical Practice Guideline, No. 2, 1996 Update.* AHCPR Publication No. 96-0682.Rockville, MD: U.S. Department of Health and Human Services. Public Health Service, Agency for Health Care Policy and Research. March 1996

2. Jeffcoate TNA, Francis WJA. Urinary incontinence in the female. *Am J Obstet Gynecol* 1996; 94: 604–618

3. Frewen WK. Urgency incontinence. *J Obstet Gynaecol Br Commonw* 1972; 79: 77–81

4. Svigos JM, Matthews DC. Assessment and treatment of female urinary incontinence by cystometrogram and bladder retraining programs. *Obstet Gynecol* 1977; 50: 9–12

5. Frewen WK. Role of bladder training in the treatment of the unstable bladder in the female. *Urol Clin North Am* 1980; 5: 273–277

6. Pengelly AW, Booth CH. A prospective trial of bladder training as treatment of detrusor instability. *Br J Urol* 1980; 5: 463–466

7. Elder DD, Stephenson TP. An assessment of the Frewen regime in the treatment of detrusor dysfunction in females. *Br J Urol* 1980; 52: 467–471

8. Mahady IW, Begg BM. Long term symptomatic and cystometric cure of the urge incontinence syndrome using a technique of bladder re-education. *Br J Obstet Gynaecol* 1981; 322–333

9. Jarvis GJ, Miller DR. Controlled trial of bladder drill for detrusor instability. *Br Med J* 1980; 281: 322–333

10. Fantl JA, Hurt WG, Dunn LJ. Detrusor instability syndrome: the use of bladder retraining drills with and without anticholinergics. *Am J Obstet Gynecol* 1981; 140: 885–890

11. Jarvis GJ. A controlled trial of bladder drill and drug therapy in the management of detrusor instability. *Br J Urol* 1982; 54: 374–376

12. Jarvis GJ. The management of urinary incontinence due to primary vesical sensory urgency by bladder drill. *Br J Urol* 1981; 53: 565–566

13. Frewen WK. A reassessment of bladder training in detrusor dysfunction in the female. *Br J Urol* 1982; 54: 372–373

14. Fantl JA, Wyman JF, McClish DK *et al.* Efficacy of bladder training in older women with urinary incontinence. *J Am Med Assoc* 1991; 265: 609–613

15. Fantl JA. Bahavioral intervention in community dwelling women with urinary incontinence. *Urology* 1998; Suppl 2: 30–34

16. Kegel AH. Progressive resistance exercise in the functional restoration of the perineal muscles. *Am J Obstet Gynecol* 1948; 56: 238–249

17. Kegel AH. Physiologic therapy for urinary incontinence. *J Am Med Assoc* 1951; 146: 915–917

18. Hendrickson LS. The frequency of stress incontinence in women before and after the implementation of an exercise program. *Issues Health Care Women* 1981; 3: 81–92

19. Kujansuu E. The effect of pelvic floor exercises on urethral function in female stress urinary incontinence: a urodynamic study. *Ann Chir Gynaecol* 1983; 72: 28–32

20. Burgio KL, Robinson JC, Engel BT. The role of biofeedback in Kegel exercise training for stress urinary incontinence. *Am J Obstet Gynecol* 1986; 154: 58–64

21. Benvenuti F, Caputo GM, Bandinelli S *et al.* Reeducative treatment of female genuine stress incontinence. *Am J Phys Med Rehabil* 1987; 66: 155–168

22. Hanalla SM, Kirwan P, Castleden DM *et al.* The effect of pelvic floor muscle exercises in the treatment of genuine stress incontinence in women at two hospitals. *Br J Obstet Gynaecol* 1988; 98: 81–92

23. Bø K, Hagen RH, Kvarstein B *et al.* Pelvic floor muscle exercise for the treatment of female stress urinary incontinence: III. Effects of two different degrees of pelvic floor muscle exercises. *Neurourol Urodyn* 1990; 9: 489–502

24. Burns PA, Pranikoff K, Nochajski T *et al.* Treatment of stress urinary incontinence with pelvic floor exercises and feedback. *J Am Geriatr Soc* 1990; 38: 341–344

25. Largo-Jansen TLM, Debruyne FMJ, Smits AJA, Van Weel

C. Controlled trial of pelvic exercises in the treatment of urinary stress incontinence in general practice. *Br J Gen Pract* 1991; 41: 445–449

26. Cammau H, Van Hylen M, Derde MP *et al.* Pelvic physiotherapy in genuine stress incontinence. *Urology* 1991; 38: 322–337

27. Hahn I, Milson J, Fall M, Eklund P. Long term results of pelvic floor training in female stress urinary incontinence. *J Reprod Med* 1993; 38: 684–691

28. Dougherty M, Bishop K, Mooney R *et al.* Graded pelvic muscle exercise. Effect on stress urinary incontinence. *J Reprod Med* 1993; 38: 684–691

29. Elia G, Bergman A. Pelvic muscle exercises: when do they work? *Obstet Gynecol* 1993; 81: 283–286

30. Wyman JF, Fantl JA, McClish DK *et al.* Comparative efficacy of behavioral interventions in the management of female urinary incontinence. *Am J Obstet Gynecol* 1998; 179: 999–1007

31

Physiotherapy for incontinence

J. Mantle

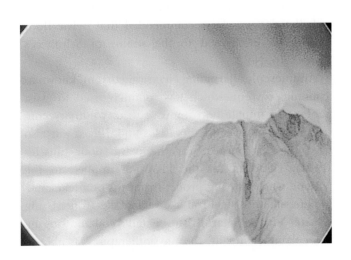

INTRODUCTION

The physiotherapy profession considers urogynaecology to be a specialist field requiring additional post-registration training. Such training is available through specific courses, or by working with experienced colleagues, or both. Physiotherapists have been working for more than 50 years in this field,[1] and bring to it a particularly holistic approach to promoting continence, and with regard to assessment and treatment. The woman's whole physical and mental state, other health problems, lifestyle and responsibilities are considered.

HISTORY

Since the late 1940s, voluntary contractions of the pelvic floor musculature (sometimes called Kegel exercises) have been at the heart of physiotherapy treatment of urinary incontinence. It is often said that Kegel was the first to describe this therapy.[2] However it is of interest to note that in the 1920s and 1930s, Minnie Randell, Sister-in-Charge of the Conjoint Massage and Remedial Exercise Training course at St Thomas's Hospital, London, was training students (the precursors of chartered physiotherapists) to encourage women in the puerperium to practise repeated 'pelvic floor tensing', trying 'to invert the sphincters' … 'until it becomes habitual'.[3] The purpose of this was to prevent and treat symptoms of urine leakage and prolapse.[4] This therapy possibly had some roots in Swedish gymnastics and was disseminated by Randell's ex-students, and also as a result of the formation in 1948 of the Obstetric Physiotherapists' Association (now called the Association of Chartered Physiotherapists in Women's Health), of which Randell was a founder member. Margaret Morris was one of Randell's students and an ex-ballet dancer; she recommended that pelvic floor tensing be performed to the strains of Schubert's Waltzes 16, No 2.[3]

An unevenly alternating electrical current, known as a faradic current, which was routinely used to assist patients to initiate and improve weak voluntary contraction of muscles in the 1940s and 1950s, was also used for this purpose for the pelvic floor muscles (PFM). Faradism for the PFM was applied to the patient, who was lying prone, by means of a fearsome-looking stainless steel rod-like vaginal electrode. Using a battery-driven Smart Bristow Faradic coil and surging the current manually, the physiotherapist was able to produce muscle contractions. With improving techniques, surgery became an increasingly popular solution for stress incontinence through the 1960s and 1970s, partially displacing physical therapies. Surgery appealed to women as a 'quick fix'. However, a number of recent retrospective appraisals[5,6] have shown possible overestimation of cure rates from surgery, some morbidity, and also that relieved symptoms may recur. Thus, there is renewed interest in conservative alternatives.

CURRENT PRACTICE

Currently, a trial of physiotherapy is generally considered appropriate for women with mild-to-moderate genuine stress incontinence (GSI), urge incontinence or mixed incontinence. Treatment should always be preceded by a thorough assessment. Where specific physiotherapy is considered appropriate, the basic treatment options are as follows:

1. For GSI: voluntary pelvic floor muscle contraction (VPFMC) with or without adjuncts such as biofeedback (e.g. pressure perineometry, electromyography [EMG], cones and neuromuscular electrical stimulation), together with education concerning the functioning of the urinary tract and individualized continence-promoting advice.
2. For urge incontinence: bladder training with deferment and control strategies using VPFMC, and the option of electrical stimulation, together with education concerning the functioning of the urinary tract and individualized continence-promoting advice.
3. For mixed incontinence: a combination of the two above options.

ASSESSMENT

Assessment by a physiotherapist has much in common with that by other relevant professionals, but includes consideration of general mobility, strength, coordination and mental acuity which are so crucial to independent safe toileting. Following a carefully elicited description of the current problem and its exact effects on lifestyle, history-taking includes body mass index, obstetric history, previous surgery and other pathologies, menstrual status, family and childhood history of continence problems.

All women should be offered a digital assessment *per vaginam* of the vagina and pelvic floor musculature, after informed consent has been obtained. The procedure has been described in detail elsewhere.[7,8] Briefly, physiotherapists use a modification of the Oxford 0–5 Classification Scale of muscle strength, as follows:

0 = no contraction
1 = flicker
2 = weak contraction
3 = moderate contraction
4 = good contraction
5 = strong contraction.

The patient is examined while lying down with hips and knees flexed and abducted, and is asked to contract the PFM maximally several times; the physiotherapist grades what she feels. Many other aspects can be palpated and recorded, including whether a voluntary contraction can be produced; the speed at which the muscle can be contracted; the speed of relaxation; how long a sub-maximal contraction can be sustained in seconds (static endurance) and how many such contractions can be completed in a series, with equal length rests between, before fatigue occurs (dynamic endur-ance); how many short maximal contractions can be completed in a series before fatigue occurs; whether there is a reflex contraction with a cough. Sensation may be checked, and the sensation and muscle strength of the left and right sides can be compared.

For objective pre- and post-treatment outcome measures, physiotherapists use frequency/volume charts and pad tests, together with the results of the digital assessment, validated quality-of-life questionnaires and analogue scales as subjective measures.

TREATMENT

Pelvic floor exercises

A systemic review of the literature by Berghmans *et al.*[9] (an international group of highly respected physiotherapists), confirms expert opinion that PFM training is of value for patients with GSI. However, as yet there is little hard, scientific, objective evidence as to exactly what changes produce this improvement – but the understanding of incontinence is far from complete.

Uses

Logic and clinical experience support the use of VPFMC for three purposes, and it is motivating for a woman to understand what she is trying to achieve by her efforts.

First, a progressive and intensive programme of voluntary contractions may be used to attempt to strengthen and improve the endurance of the PFM. This may decrease any tendency for the pelvic floor to sag, and by the muscle-training effect, the muscle fibres should hypertrophy, optimizing their ability to support the bladder base and the urethra and to increase urethral closure pressure. The so-called training effect requires at least 3 months of intensive exercise to produce and is achievable only if the muscle tissue has the capability to respond. These points must be clearly explained to the patient at the outset.

Recent research[10] suggests that the volume of the external urethral sphincter is reduced in those with GSI compared with continent women. To date, no one has claimed the ability to contract the external urethral sphincter selectively, either voluntarily or electrically, in the therapeutic setting. Indeed, there is controversy as to whether the nerve supply of the sphincter is autonomic or somatic (or both). However, it has been suggested that intensive voluntary contraction of the PFM also recruits the musculature of the external urinary sphincter and would, over time, increase its strength and bulk – provided, again, that the relevant muscle fibres are capable of responding.

Secondly, strong, precisely timed VPFMCs may be utilized by those with stress urinary incontinence to give added urethral support and control against leakage in stress situations such as coughing, sneezing and lifting. This would be particularly appropriate for women who, on digital assessment, are found to have an absence of (or a very weak) reflex contraction of the PFM, for example on coughing. Obviously, voluntary reinforcing contractions should start just ahead of the stress event and continue through it. In the past, physiotherapists termed this 'counterbracing'; in 1996 it was renamed 'the knack'.[11] This can be taught to a woman at her first visit and often brings some immediate improvement in control. However, clinicians must be aware of the possible effect on repeat stress and pad test results of habitually using 'the knack'.

The use of 'the knack' may be extended, as a means of protection, to conditions where raised intra-abdominal pressure in stress situations, such as lifting, could cause undesirable stretching of vulnerable pelvic floor tissue arising from prolapse, forceps delivery or vaginal repair, for example.

Thirdly, there is reciprocal innervation between the bladder and the urethral sphincter mechanism/PFM,[12] and this can be used to advantage by patients with detrusor overactivity to attempt to inhibit the detrusor, reduce sensations of urgency, defer micturition and give a little more time to reach a convenient toileting place. On experiencing urgency, rather than immediately rushing to reach the toilet, the woman is encouraged to stop, to relax in a sitting or standing position and to perform three or four strong VPFMCs. This is often sufficient to defer micturition for a useful length of time. Perineal pressure may be a useful adjunct. The physiotherapist combines these concepts with the other aspects of bladder training or timed voiding described elsewhere (see chapter 30) for patients experiencing urgency or urge incontinence.

Much of the success of VPFMC as a treatment lies in three factors:

1. The accuracy of the professional judgement on the basis of assessment that VPFMC will be efficacious;
2. Success in teaching the patient how to accomplish the contraction;
3. A woman's understanding of, and compliance with, the proposed usage, and her motivation and diligence to continue long enough for its effectiveness to become evident. Obviously, the length of time required will vary according to the purpose of the VPFMCs.

Teaching VPFMC is difficult, and demands skill and time.[13] Some women become aware of what is required and achieve a contraction easily; others are uncertain; a few are unable to contract voluntarily – this variation may well be a measure of sensory or motor dysfunction, or both. It is crucial that the ability to contract is checked, if only to guard against patients who contract incorrectly (i.e. produce a Valsalva manoeuvre) Although it is appreciated that, in the course of normal activities, healthy PFM normally coordinate with a range of other muscles, in the therapeutic situation, not only has it been found wise initially to discourage co-contraction of accessory muscles, such as the gluteal or abdominal muscles, but also the patient should not

hold her breath. There is one possible exception – that of teaching the patient to contract the transversus abdominis muscles selectively and to become aware of the reflex contraction of the PFM that occurs.

The healthy PFM contain a range of type 1 (slow – i.e. lower strength but fatigue resistant) and type 2 (fast – i.e. greater strength but poor endurance) striated muscle fibres which recruit in an orderly fashion from slow to fast on demand. The slow fibres are designed for more-or-less continuous postural activity, whereas fast fibres are for intermittent bursts of high-intensity activity to give additional support and control in stress situations such as when coughing or lifting. Both Gosling *et al.*[14] and Gilpin *et al.*[15] have investigated the proportion of type 1 to type 2 fibres at various points in the pelvic floor. Following trauma to muscle, nerve and/or connective tissue, and with age, these proportions are likely to alter and this may account for some of the symptoms of incontinence and prolapse. However, there is no precise and validated way for a physiotherapist to gauge such changes accurately. Thus, current practice is for women to be taught to contract in two ways: maximal short (1-second) contractions encourage activation of the type 2 (fast) fibres; submaximal 'held' contractions (which in reality may last from 1 to 20 or more seconds) activate the type 1 (slow) fibres. In other words, the objective is to gain the maximum possible contribution from every fibre. The concept, suggested by Jozwik and Jozwik[16] for patients with stress incontinence, of using knowledge of the plasticity of muscle fibres and of how specific activity or electrical stimulation (or both) can be used to change fibre type to favour the proportion of slow or fast fibres within a given muscle, needs very cautious consideration. As yet, there is no non-invasive validated clinic-based means of measuring type proportions in a patient's PFM on which to base the necessary clinical judgements.

Assuming that the objective is to strengthen the PFM, no study has yet been carried out to quantify the most appropriate number of VPFMCs required daily to be successful – and to be successful most quickly. Indeed, it is probable that this number varies with each patient and over time; however, Kegel[2] has recommended 300, Millard[17] 400, and Bø *et al.*[18] 24–36/day. This last figure was based on general strength-training recommendations.[19] Bø and colleagues[18] asked women with stress incontinence to perform near-maximum intensity contractions three times a day and to attend a weekly group where contractions were performed for 45 minutes in a variety of positions (lying, sitting, standing). The women's motivation was thereby maintained and it seems probable that they performed more contractions than instructed. It is a matter of regret that reports of research using PFM training as an intervention rarely give enough (or any!) detail as to the programme of exercise recommended to participants. Harder still to obtain is an accurate measure of actually how much specific PFM exercise is performed by a patient over a given period.

Although VPFMC is a therapy without side effects, it has one major drawback: it seems to be agreed that, to be effective in improving strength and/or endurance, VPFMC has to be performed almost every day and several times a day. To practise VPFMC efficiently, patients must be free from distractions and able to focus on their exercise efforts. VPFMC is a boring and repetitive exercise requiring considerable discipline. Such are the demands currently being placed on many women by society – to earn, to run the home and to care for family and others – that it is not surprising that women apologize for non-compliance and complain of forgetting, of not having time, or of being too tired to do their exercises – or even of falling asleep when practising.

The pragmatic approach, currently being used by many physiotherapists, is to construct an individualized home practice programme from the findings on digital assessment and in consultation with the patient. The author has found, in south-east London with a high-density multiracial population, that the majority of women will consider trying to exercise for 5–10 minutes three times a day. They rarely achieve this goal, but most do some exercise each day, and the majority, given the option, choose to attend a clinic about once a month over a 4–6-month period for support and guidance in progression. Progression options include increasing the length of 'held' contractions, increasing the number of contractions, reducing the length of intervening rest periods, changing the position in which exercises are performed (e.g. from lying to sitting, to standing, to walking), and adding functional activities, such as coughing.

Biofeedback

Biofeedback can be used to aid the teaching of VPFMC and intensive PFM exercise programmes can be augmented by biofeedback. There are several ways of doing this. Digital assessment has the potential for sensory and verbal biofeedback to the woman but, in this technological age, visual feedback is highly rated. At its most simple this can be obtained from a small perineometer with a pressure probe and a digital display. The equipment most favoured is clinic based and records vaginal squeeze pressure from vaginal probes or pelvic floor EMG activity (sometimes called myofeedback) gathered from surface or vaginal electrodes. These are unreliable in terms of reproducibility because of the many variable factors (such as the time of day, point in the menstrual cycle, overflow from accessory muscles, exact position of the patient, or the contents of the rectum), so are, at best, motivators. However, it seems that a few minutes practice, often on one occasion only, particularly with equipment that gives a graph readout response to a PFM contraction, may greatly assist some women to grasp how to improve their contraction ability. In the future, with the increasing availability of ultrasonography, this could become a further simple and valuable teaching and motivating aid.

Cones

Weighted vaginal cones were first described in 1985 by Plevnik[20] as 'a new method for testing and strengthening of pelvic floor muscles'. Vaginal cones were first marketed in sets of nine, then five, having a common size but in a range of weights from 20 to 100 g. The patient inserted the lightest cone into the vagina and then tried to retain it while walking around. The heaviest cone that could be retained for a minute without voluntarily contracting the PFM was equated with so-called 'passive strength'. The heaviest cone that could be retained for a minute with VPFMC was equated with so-called 'active strength'. As treatment, women tried increasing cone weights, starting with the heaviest that could be retained for a minute with a contraction and twice a day attempting to increase the holding time while moving about. Once the cone could be retained for 15 minutes, progression to the next-heaviest cone was allowed. The theory was that the cone would be used at home by patients, while standing and walking, to give sensory biofeedback, to discourage unwanted abdominal muscle contraction that would push the cone out, and to concentrate effort into contracting the PFM to prevent the cone from slipping out. However, vaginal diameters vary and work by Olah *et al.*[21] underlined the need for cones to be available in several diameters.

The original sets of cones were expensive and proved difficult to sterilize for multiple-user use. More recently, much cheaper but similarly shaped, single-user, hollow shells have been produced (Aquaflex supplied by Thackerycare, UK). The shell is made in two diameters and of two halves that screw firmly together. Any reasonable weighted material (e.g. specifically designed weights, small coins) can safely be progressively introduced into the hollow shell.

The advantages of cones were seen to be chiefly that patients rapidly learnt to use them, so there was a saving in physiotherapist time compared with that necessary to teach VPFMC. However Hahn *et al.*[22] proved radiographically that 'many incontinent women had a flaccid vaginal canal which adapted to the weight of the cone, and the cone took a horizontal position and was thus more easily retained despite poor pelvic floor function'. Conversely, it seems logical that if the distance between the two medial borders of the pubococcygeus is wide, even the larger-size cone on the retail market may not be contained, regardless of weight or the strength of the PFM. Women who elect to use cones must be warned that there may well be a difference in their ability to retain the cone between morning and evening, at certain stages in their menstrual cycle, before and after emptying their rectum, and following intercourse.

However, in their systematic review, Berghmans *et al.*[9] reported that they could find no evidence that PFM exercises with biofeedback are more effective than PFM exercises alone. Indeed, regarding the use of cones, the benefit of encouraging prolonged isometric contractions of the PFM is being challenged and the possibility of producing the overuse injuries that this causes in other muscles has been raised.[23]

Electrical stimulation

Electrical stimulation has been used for more than 50 years by physiotherapists for patients with continence problems. However, there is little agreement as to its value. Berghmans *et al.*,[9] considering stress incontinence, report no consistency between trials in the type of stimulation or parameters used.

Physiotherapists commonly discriminate between parameters that are appropriate for stress incontinence and those for urge incontinence; in either case, electrostimulation is usually combined with VPFMC and continence-promoting advice. Currently, conventional

wisdom is that electrical stimulation for a patient with stress incontinence is most usually given to mimic a normal contraction and is a treatment option particularly for patients who are unable to produce a VPFMC or only a very weak contraction (i.e. grade 0–2). Such electrical stimulation recruits muscle fibres in a less predictable order than that of a voluntary contraction (i.e. type 2 fibres may be recruited before type 1). Having been made aware of the specific PFM activity by means of electrical stimulation, the patient then tries to join in and reproduce the contraction. It has been found that good contractions can usually be produced at a pulse rate of 35–50 Hz and at a phased intensity, which the patient can reasonably tolerate for up to half an hour. Currently, single-user vaginal electrodes are commonly used and the patient is gradually introduced to increased intensity of stimulation. The more complex clinic-based equipment allows the physiotherapist to set a number of parameters, such as the ramping of intensity increase, the length of the contraction, the length of the rest period and the number of contractions. The clinic-based treatment is usually administered by a physiotherapist; it has been suggested that clinic attendance for stimulation increases contact between patient and physiotherapist and that this enables further encouragement, motivation and reminders to do the exercises. However, a patient is unlikely to be willing to attend more than three times a week. The alternative is for the patient to use a battery-operated home stimulator; those commonly available have fewer adjustable parameters but can be used daily. In either case, many patients do not tolerate sufficent current intensity to produce artificial contractions, yet seem to gain benefit; often, patients are also following an intensive programme of VPFMC but Fall and Lindstrom[24] have other hypotheses for this phenomenon. Where there has been muscle denervation, no voluntary contraction is possible and currently available stimulators will not activate the degenerated muscle fibres. However, low-frequency (10 Hz), phased stimulation used daily for several hours over several months has apparently been successful in the treatment of patients in whom VPFMC cannot be obtained initially, or is weak:[25] such treatment places considerable demands on the patient.

For urge incontinence, continuous low-frequency (5–10 Hz) alternating current is recommended,[26] with the objective of inhibiting the bladder overactivity. Here, a home stimulator with a single-user vaginal electrode enables patients to give themselves stimulation for 20–30 min daily at a comfortable current intensity. In his study Fall[26] asked patients to use the stimulator all day or all night. His numbers were small (27) and improvement (18) or rehabilitation/cure (9) took anything up to 23 months to achieve; however, there was a claim that the improvement was more permanent than that obtained by other types of therapy.

The practical issues are that, in general, women are wary of electrical devices and dislike the prickly sensation that accompanies the stimulation of muscles. It is probable that many women, using home stimulators, do not tolerate current of sufficient intensity for an electrically produced contraction to be achieved. Generally, women find it difficult to have time to come to a clinic, especially two or three times a week, for treatment. In towns and cities, travelling time is increasing, so a stimulator for use at home would seem to be a logical solution. However, finding privacy and peace to apply stimulation at home, even for as little as 20 minutes a day, seems very difficult for many. It is usual practice not to apply stimulation during menstruation and stimulation should not be employed if there is any possibility of pregnancy.

NORMAL FUNCTION OF THE URINARY TRACT AND CONTINENCE-PROMOTING ADVICE

Few women have even a rudimentary understanding of how the urinary tract functions: indeed, many who present with continence problems have mistaken ideas concerning normality. For example, some think that to be able to void a little more, 15 minutes after an initial void, is abnormal. Some also are of the opinion that the normal person never, ever, leaks under any circumstances. Is this realistic? This state of affairs may be due to overzealous efforts to raise public awareness that incontinence can be treated.

Physiotherapists are good communicators and have the neuromuscular knowledge and skills to assess and, where appropriate, to treat and advise patients with continence problems. They are also equipped to promote continence – for example to check that women are drinking enough and not too much, what they are drinking and that they are not crouching to void when away from home; to show them the optimum position for defecation and to explain the results of straining; to assess whether the patient is capable of independent toileting or could be enabled to be so; to discuss lifestyle and personal circumstances in terms of activities that put strain on the pelvic floor, such as lifting and handling of frail or heavily disabled relatives or patients, or inappropriately designed fitness training. In addition, physiotherapists are trained to promote health in its widest sense, so they will encourage general fitness and social interaction, both of which may have been lost by patients with continence problems.

REFERENCES

1. Gardiner MD. *Principles of Exercise Therapy*. London: Bell and Sons, 1953

2. Kegel AH. Progressive resistance exercises in the functional restoration of perineal muscles. *Am J Obstet Gynecol* 1948; 56: 238–249

3. Morris M. *Maternity and Post-operative Exercises*. London: Heinemann, 1936; 111

4. Randall M. *Fearless Childbirth*. London: Churchill, 1948

5. Kjolhede P, Ryden G. Prognostic factors and long-term results of the Burch colposuspension. *Acta Obstet Gynecol Scand* 1994; 73: 642–647

6. Black NA, Downs SH. The effectiveness of surgery for stress incontinence in women: a systematic review. *Br J Urol* 1996; 78: 497–510

7. Laycock J. Clinical evaluation of the pelvic floor. In: Schussler J, Laycock J Norton P, Stanton S (eds) *Pelvic Floor Re-education*. London: Springer-Verlag, 1994; 42–48

8. Haslam J. The physical assessment of the pelvic floor. *J Assoc Chartered Physiother Women's Health* 1995; 77: 8–9

9. Berghmans LCM, Hendriks HJM, Bø K *et al*. Conservative treatment of stress urinary incontinence in women: a systematic review of randomized clinical trials. *Br J Urol* 1995; 82: 181–191

10. Martan A, Masata M, Halaska M, Voigt R. Ultrasound of the urethral sphincter. *Neurourol Urodyn* 1997; 16: 389–390

11. Miller J, Ashton-Miller J, DeLancey JOL. The knack: use of precisely timed pelvic muscle contraction can reduce leakage in SUI. *Neurourol Urodyn* 1996; 15: 392–394

12. Mahoney D, Laferte R, Blais D. Integral storage and voiding reflexes. *Urology* 1977; 9: 95–106

13. Mantle J. Essential education: re-educating the pelvic floor muscles. *J Community Nurs* 1994; 8: 14–20

14. Gosling JA, Dixon JS, Caitchley HOD, Thompson S. A

comparative study of the human external sphincter and periurethral levator ani muscles. *Br J Urol* 1981; 53: 35–41

15. Gilpin SA, Gosling JA, Smith ARB, Warrell DW. The pathogenesis of genitourinary prolapse and stress incontinence of urine. *J Obstet Gynaecol* 1989; 96: 15–23

16. Jozwik M, Jozwik M. The physiological basis of pelvic floor exercises in the treatment of stress urinary incontinence. *Br J Obstet Gynaecol* 1998; 105: 1046–1051

17. Millard RJ. *Bladder Control: a Simple Self-help Guide.* Sydney: McLennon & Petty, 1987; 21

18. Bø K, Hagen R, Kvarstein B *et al.* Pelvic floor muscle exercise for the treatment of female stress urinary incontinence: III. Effects of two different degrees of pelvic floor muscle exercises. *Neururol Urodyn* 1990; 9: 489–502

19. American College of Sports Medicine. The recommended quantity and quality of exercise for developing and maintaining cardio-respiratory and muscular fitness in healthy adults. *Med Sci Sports Exerc* 1990; 22: 265–274

20. Plevnik S. New method for testing and strengthening of pelvic floor muscles. Proceedings of the 15th Annual Meeting, International Continence Society 1985; 247: 8

21. Olah KS, Bridges N. Denning J *et al.* The conservative management of patients with symptoms of stress incontinence: a randomised prospective study comparing vaginal cones and interferential therapy. *Am J Obstet Gynecol* 1990; 162: 87–92

22. Hahn I, Milson I, Ohlsson B *et al.* Comparative assessment of pelvic floor function using vaginal cones, vaginal digital palpation and vaginal pressure measurements. *Gynecol Obstet Invest* 1996; 41: 269–274

23. Bø K. Vaginal weighted cones. Theoretical framework, effect on pelvic floor muscle strength and female stress urinary incontinence. *Acta Obstet Gynecol Scand* 1995; 74: 87–92

24. Fall M, Lindstrom S. Electrical stimulation. *Urol Clin North Am* 1991; 18: 393–407

25. Farragher DJ. Trophic electrical stimulation: home treatment for women with urinary incontinence. Proceedings of the World Confederation of Physical Therapy. Private Practitioners' International Meeting, Hong Kong. London, WCPT, 1992

26. Fall M. Does electrical stimulation cure urinary incontinence? *J Urol* 1984;131: 664–667

32

Drug treatment of voiding dysfunction in women

E. S. Rovner, A. J. Wein

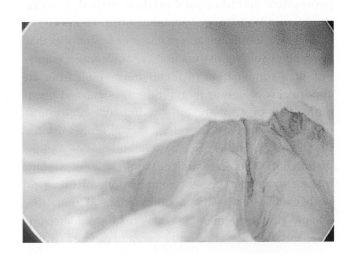

Introduction

The lower urinary tract performs two basic functions – storage of urine and emptying of urine. The physiology and pharmacology of micturition have been described by many qualified authors, each of whom has reported his or her own particular concept of the neuroanatomy, neurophysiology and neuropharmacology of the smooth and striated muscle structures involved; of the peripheral, autonomic and somatic neural factors; and of the spinal and supraspinal influences that are necessary for normal function.[1–5] Although there are significant disagreements about the finer details, it is important to realize that exact agreement about neuromorphology, neurophysiology and neuropharmacology is not necessary for an understanding of the pharmacological principles and applications involved in drug-induced alteration of voiding function and dysfunction. Despite such disagreements, all 'experts' would doubtless agree that, for the purposes of description and teaching, one can succinctly summarize the two phases of micturition from a conceptual point of view. Bladder filling and urine storage require: (1) accommodation of increasing volumes of urine at a low intravesical pressure and with appropriate sensation; (2) a bladder outlet that is closed at rest and remains so during increases in intra-abdominal pressure; and (3) absence of involuntary bladder contractions (detrusor instability [DI] or hyperreflexia). Bladder emptying requires: (1) a coordinated contraction by the bladder smooth musculature of adequate magnitude and duration; (2) concomitant lowering of resistance at the level of the smooth sphincter (the smooth muscle of the bladder neck and proximal urethra) and of the striated sphincter (the periurethral and intramural urethral striated musculature); and (3) absence of anatomic obstruction.

This very simple but acceptable overview implies that any type of voiding dysfunction (i.e. of storage, emptying, or a combination of these) must result from an abnormality of one or more of the factors listed previously. This description, with its implied subdivisions under each category, provides a logical framework for the discussion and classification of all types of voiding dysfunction. There are, indeed, some types of voiding dysfunction that represent combinations of filling or storage and emptying abnormalities. Within this scheme, however, these become readily understandable, and their detection and treatment can be logically described. In addition, all aspects of urodynamic, radiological and videourodynamic evaluation can be conceptualized within this scheme in regard to exactly what they evaluate in terms of either bladder or outlet activity during filling or storage or emptying. Likewise, one can easily classify all known treatments for voiding dysfunction under the broad categories of facilitating either filling–storage or emptying, and achieving this by acting primarily on the bladder or one or more of the components of the bladder outlet.

As a result of advances in the knowledge of the neuropharmacology and neurophysiology of the lower urinary tract, effective pharmacological therapy now exists for the management of many types of voiding dysfunction. This chapter summarizes the treatments available for female voiding dysfunction within this functional classification (Tables 32.1, 32.2). As an apology to others in the field whose works have not been specifically cited in this chapter, it should be noted that citations have generally been chosen primarily because of their review or informational content or sometimes their controversial nature, and not because of their originality or initial publication on a particular subject.

Clinical uropharmacology of the lower urinary tract: some ufseful concepts

Clinical uropharmacology of the lower urinary tract is based primarily on an appreciation of the innervation and receptor content of the bladder and its related anatomical structures. The drugs or classes of drugs used were, in general, developed originally for their actions on other organ systems, the functions of which are controlled or affected by innervation or drug–receptor interaction. The targets of pharmacological intervention in the bladder body, base or outlet include nerve terminals that alter the release of specific neurotransmitters, receptor subtypes, cellular second-messenger systems and ion channels identified in the bladder and urethra. Peripheral nerves and ganglia, spinal cord and supraspinal areas are also sites of action of some agents discussed. Because autonomic innervation and receptor content are ubiquitous throughout the human body's organ systems, there are no agents in clinical use that are purely selective for action on the lower urinary tract. The majority of side effects attributed to drugs facilitating bladder storage or emptying

Table 32.1. *Therapy used to facilitate bladder emptying*

A. Increasing intravesical pressure or bladder contractility
 1. External compression, Valsalva manoeuvre
 2. Promotion or initiation of reflex contractions
  a. Trigger zones or manoeuvres
  b. Bladder training, tidal drainage
 3. Pharmacological therapy
  a. Parasympathomimetic agents
  b. Prostaglandins
  c. Blockers of inhibition
   (1) α-Adrenergic antagonists
   (2) Opioid antagonist
 4. Electrical stimulation
  a. Directly to the bladder or spinal cord
  b. To the nerve roots
  c. Transurethral intravesical electrotherapy
 5. Reduction cystoplasty

B. Decreasing outlet resistance
 1. At a site of anatomical obstruction
  a. Prostatectomy, otomy (diathermy, laser, heat)
  b. Balloon dilatation
  c. Intra-urethral stent
  d. Pharmacological decrease in prostate size or tone
   (1) Luteinizing hormone-releasing hormone agonists
   (2) Antiandrogens
   (3) 5α-Reductase inhibitors
   (4) α-Adrenergic antagonists
  (e) Urethral stricture repair or dilatation
 2. At the level of the smooth sphincter
  a. Pharmacological therapy
   (1) α-Adrenergic antagonists
   (2) β-Adrenergic agonists
  b. Transurethral resection or incision of the bladder neck
  c. Y-V plasty of the bladder neck
 3. At the level of the striated sphincter
  a. Pharmacological therapy
   (1) Skeletal muscle relaxants
    (a) Benzodiazepines
    (b) Baclofen
    (c) Dantrolene
   (2) α-Adrenergic antagonists
  b. Urethral overdilatation
  c. Surgical sphincterotomy, botulinum A toxin
  d. Urethral stent
  e. Pudendal nerve interruption
  f. Psychotherapy, biofeedback

C. Circumventing the problem
 1. Intermittent catheterization
 2. Continuous catheterization
 3. Urinary diversion

Table 32.2. *Therapy used to facilitate urine storage*

A. Inhibiting bladder contractility, decreasing sensory input, or increasing bladder capacity
 1. Habit training (timed voiding); prompted voiding
 2. Bladder training (± biofeedback)
 3. Pharmacological therapy
  a. Anticholinergic agents
  b. Musculotropic relaxants
  c. Calcium antagonists
  d. Potassium-channel openers
  e. Prostaglandin inhibitors
  f. β-Adrenergic agonists
  g. Tricyclic antidepressants
  h. Dimethyl sulphoxide (DMSO)
 4. Bladder overdistension
 5. Electrical stimulation (reflex inhibition)
 6. Acupuncture
 7. Interruption of innervation
  a. Central (subarachnoid block)
  b. Peripheral (sacral rhizotomy, selective sacral rhizotomy)
  c. Dorsal
  d. Perivesical (peripheral bladder denervation)
 8. Augmentation cystoplasty

B. Increasing outlet resistance
 1. Physiotherapy (± biofeedback)
 2. Electrical stimulation of the pelvic floor
 3. Pharmacological therapy
  a. α-Adrenergic agonists
  b. Tricyclic antidepressants
  c. β-Adrenergic antagonists
  d. Oestrogens
  e. β-Adrenergic agonists
 4. Vesicourethral suspension (SUI)*
  a. Transvaginal
  b. Transabdominal
 5. Bladder outlet reconstruction
 6. Surgical mechanical compression
  a. Sling procedures
  a. Artificial urinary sphincter
 7. Non-surgical mechanical compression
  a. Periurethral collagen, Polytef, fat injection
  b. Occlusive devices (hydrophilic urethral patch/suction cup/urethral insert)
  c. Compressive devices (pessaries)

C. Circumventing the problem
 1. Antidiuretic-hormone-like agents
 2. Intermittent catheterization
 3. Continuous catheterization
 4. Urinary diversion
 5. External collecting devices
 6. Absorbent product

* SUI, stress urinary incontinence.

are collateral effects on organ systems that share some of the same neurophysiological or neuropharmacological characteristics as the bladder.

Generally speaking, the simplest and least hazardous form of treatment should always be tried first. A combination of therapeutic manoeuvres or pharmacological agents can sometimes be used to achieve a particular effect, especially if their mechanisms of actions are different and their side effects are not synergistic. At the outset it should be noted that, in our experience, although great improvement often occurs with rational pharmacological therapy, a perfect result (restoration to 'normal' status) is seldom, if ever, achieved.

SPECIAL CONSIDERATIONS IN THE ELDERLY PATIENT

In the ageing patient many non-urinary pathological, anatomical and physiological factors serve as co-morbidities in the development of acute incontinence or the aggravation of chronic incontinence. Potentially reversible pathologies (such as infection, atrophic vaginitis and urethritis, faecal impaction, limited mobility, delirium and hyperglycaemia) should be appreciated by the treating physician. Elderly patients are frequently taking many drugs, and iatrogenic (physician-induced) incontinence may result from the pharmacological side effects of well-intentioned therapy. Sedative hypnotics and alcohol depress general behaviour and sensorium; they may also depress bladder contractility and reduce attention to bladder cues. Diuretics produce polyuria and may be the source of complaints of urgency, frequency and nocturia. Agents with anticholinergic properties may significantly decrease detrusor contractility: these include antihistamines, antidepressants, antipsychotics, opiates, gastrointestinal antispasmodics and antiparkinsonian drugs. α-Adrenergic agonists (contained in many decongestants or cold remedies) can increase bladder-neck tone and may promote urinary retention; α-adrenergic antagonists may predispose to sphincteric incontinence. Calcium-channel blockers for hypertension or coronary artery disease are smooth muscle relaxants, can facilitate bladder storage and may cause urinary retention and overflow incontinence.

Specific methods of pharmacological treatment

FACILITATION OF BLADDER EMPTYING

Absolute or relative failure to empty results from decreased bladder contractility, increased outlet resistance, or both.[6] Absolute or relative failure of adequate bladder contractility may result from temporary or permanent alteration in any one of the neuromuscular mechanisms necessary for initiating and maintaining a normal detrusor contraction. In a neurologically normal individual, inhibition of the micturition reflex may also be secondary to painful stimuli, especially stimuli from the pelvic and perineal areas, or it may be psychogenic. Some types of drug therapy may also inhibit bladder contractility through either neurological or myogenic mechanisms. Non-neurogenic causes include intrinsic impairment of bladder smooth muscle function, which may result from overdistension, severe infection or fibrosis. Increased outlet resistance is generally secondary to anatomical obstruction but may be secondary to a failure of coordination of the smooth or striated sphincter during bladder contraction. Treatment of failure to empty generally consists of attempts to increase intravesical pressure, to facilitate the micturition reflex or to decrease outlet resistance – or some combination of the above.

Increasing intravesical pressure or facilitating bladder contraction

Parasympathomimetic agents

Because a major portion of the final common pathway in physiological bladder contraction is the stimulation of parasympathetic postganglionic muscarinic cholinergic receptor sites, agents that imitate the actions of acetylcholine (ACh) might be expected to be effective in treating patients who cannot empty because of inadequate bladder contractility. ACh itself cannot be used for therapeutic purposes because of its actions at central and ganglionic levels and because of its rapid hydrolysis by acetylcholinesterase and butyrylcholinesterase.[7] Many ACh-like drugs exist, but only bethanechol chloride (BC) has a relatively selective action *in vitro* on the urinary bladder and gut, with little or no nicotinic action.[7] BC is cholinesterase resistant and *in vitro* causes a contraction of smooth muscle from all areas of the bladder.[8,9]

Agents similar to BC have long been recommended[10] for the treatment of postoperative or post-partum urinary retention. In such cases, BC should be used only if the patient is awake and alert and if there is no outlet obstruction. The dose is 5–10 mg given subcutaneously. For more than 30 years BC has been recommended for the treatment of the atonic or hypotonic bladder,[11] and it has been reported to be effective in achieving 'rehabilitation' of the chronically atonic or hypotonic detrusor.[12] When so used, it is recommended that the drug be initially administered subcutaneously in a dose of 5–10 mg (usually 7.5 mg) every 4–6 hours. This is done preferably with an intermittent bladder-decompression regimen. The patient is asked to try to void 20–30 minutes after each dose. When the residual urine volume has decreased to an acceptable level, the dose is gradually decreased and ultimately changed to an oral dose of 50 mg four times daily. In cases of partial bladder emptying, a therapeutic trial with an oral dose of 25–100 mg four times daily may be utilized in conjunction with attempted voiding every 4 hours. BC has also been used to stimulate or facilitate the development of reflex bladder contractions in patients with spinal shock secondary to suprasacral spinal cord injury.[13]

Although BC has been reported to increase gastrointestinal motility and has been used in the treatment of gastro–oesophageal reflux, and although anecdotal success in specific patients with voiding dysfunction seems to occur, there is little or no evidence to support its success in facilitating bladder emptying in series of patients in which the drug (BC) was the only variable.[14] In one set of trials, a pharmacologically active subcutaneous dose (5 mg) did not result in significant changes in flow parameters or residual urine volume in (1) a group of women with a residual urine volume equal to or greater than 20% of bladder capacity but no evidence of neurological disease or outlet obstruction, (2) a group of 27 'normal' women of approximately the same age, or (3) a group of patients with a positive reaction to a BC supersensitivity test.[15,16] This dose did increase cystometric filling pressure and also reduced the bladder capacity threshold, findings previously described by others.[12] Short-term studies in which the drug was the only variable have generally failed to demonstrate significant efficacy in terms of flow and residual urine volume data.[17] Farrell and colleagues conducted a double-blind randomized trial that looked at the effects of two catheter-management protocols and the effect of BC on postoperative urinary retention following gynaecological incontinence surgery:[18] they concluded that BC was not at all helpful in this setting. Although BC is capable of eliciting an increase in bladder smooth muscle tension, as would be expected from studies *in vitro*, its ability to stimulate or facilitate a coordinated and sustained physiological bladder contraction in patients with voiding dysfunction has been unimpressive.[14] Similar sentiments have been expressed by others.[9]

With regard to the bladder outlet, there is no agreement about whether cholinergic stimulation produces an increase in urethral resistance.[15,16] It appears that pharmacologically active doses do, in fact, increase urethral closure pressure, at least in patients with detrusor hyperreflexia;[17] this would, of course, tend to inhibit bladder emptying. It is unclear whether cholinergic agonists can be combined with agents to decrease outlet resistance, to facilitate emptying and achieve an additive or synergistic effect. Our own experience with such therapy, using even as much as 200 mg oral BC daily, has been extremely disappointing. Certainly, most clinicians would agree that a total divided daily dose of 50–100 mg rarely affects any urodynamic parameter at all.

The potential side effects of cholinomimetic drugs include flushing, nausea, vomiting, diarrhoea, gastrointestinal cramps, bronchospasm, headache, salivation, sweating and difficulty with visual accommodation.[7] Intramuscular and intravenous use can precipitate acute and severe side effects, resulting in acute circulatory failure and cardiac arrest, and is therefore prohibited. Contraindications to the use of this general category of drug include bronchial asthma, peptic ulcer, bowel obstruction, enteritis, recent gastrointestinal surgery, cardiac arrhythmia, hyperthyroidism and any type of bladder outlet obstruction.

One potential avenue of increasing bladder contractility is cholinergic enhancement or augmentation. Such an action might be useful as above or in combination with a parasympathomimetic agent. Metoclopramide is a dopamine antagonist with cholinergic properties. It has a central antiemetic effect in the chemoreceptor trigger zone and peripherally increases the tone of the lower oesophageal sphincter, promoting gastric emptying. Its effects seem to be related to its ability to antagonize the inhibitory action of dopamine, to augment ACh release and to sensitize the muscarinic receptors of gastrointestinal smooth muscle.[19] Experiments on dogs suggest that this agent can increase detrusor contractility,[20] and there is one anecdotal case report of improved bladder function in a diabetic patient treated originally with this agent for gastroparesis.[21] Cisapride is a substituted synthetic benzamide that enhances the release of ACh in Auerbach's plexus (in the gastrointestinal tract). In 15 patients with complete spinal cord injury treated with 10 mg cisapride three times a day for 3 days, Carone and associates noted earlier and higher amplitude reflex contractions in those with hyperactive bladders; in those with hypoactive bladders there was a significant decrease in compliance.[22] There was also increased activity and decreased compliance of the anorectal ampulla, with no alteration in striated sphincter activity. In another study in paraplegic patients, cisapride was found to decrease colonic transit time and maximal rectal capacity; an incidental decrease in residual urine was also noted (although only from 51.5 to 27.7 ml).[23] Conversely, in a double-blind placebo-controlled study, Wyndaele and Van Kerrebroeck looked at the effects of 40 mg cisapride daily in 21 patients with clinically complete spinal cord injuries. After 4 weeks of therapy, the authors noted a trend towards a 'stimulating effect' of cisapride on the bladder; however, no statistically significant differences were noted between the treated and placebo groups in any urodynamic parameter measured.[24]

Prostaglandins

The reported use of prostaglandins (PGs) to facilitate emptying is based on the hypothesis that these substances contribute to the maintenance of bladder tone and bladder contractile activity.[1,5] PGE_2 and $PGF_{2\alpha}$ cause bladder contractile responses *in vitro* and *in vivo*. PGE_2 seems to cause a net decrease in urethral smooth muscle tone; $PGF_{2\alpha}$ causes an increase. Bultitude and colleagues reported that instillation of 0.5 mg PGE_2 into the bladders of women with varying degrees of urinary retention resulted in acute emptying and in improvement of longer-term emptying (several months) in two-thirds of the patients studied (n = 22).[25] In general, they reported a decrease in the volume at which voiding was initiated, an increase in bladder pressure and a decrease in residual urine. Desmond and co-workers reported the results of intravesical use of 1.5 mg of PGE_2 (diluted with 20 ml 0.2% neomycin solution) in

patients whose bladders exhibited no contractile activity or in whom bladder contractility was relatively impaired.[26] Of 36 patients, 20 showed a strongly positive response, and six showed a weakly positive immediate response; 14 patients were reported to show prolonged beneficial effects, all but one of whom had shown a strongly positive immediate response. The authors noted additionally that the effects of PGE_2 appeared to be additive or synergistic with cholinergic stimulation in some patients.

Vaidyanathan and colleagues reported that intravesical instillation of 7.5 mg $PGF_{2\alpha}$ produced reflex voiding in some patients with incomplete suprasacral spinal cord lesions.[27] The favourable response to a single dose of drug, when present, lasted from 1.0 to 2.5 months. Tammela and associates reported that one intravesical administration of 10 mg $PGF_{2\alpha}$ facilitated voiding in women who were in retention 3 days after surgery for stress urinary incontinence (SUI).[28] The drug was administered in 50 ml saline as a single dose and retained for 2 hours. It should be noted, however, that in these 'successfully' treated patients, the average maximum flow rate was 10.6 ml/s with a mean residual urine volume of 107 ml; furthermore, the authors state that 'bladder emptying deteriorated in most patients on the day after treatment'. Jaschevatsky and colleagues reported that 16 mg $PGF_{2\alpha}$ in 40 ml saline given intravesically reduced the frequency of urinary retention in a group of women undergoing gynaecological surgery but, inexplicably, only in women undergoing vaginal hysterectomy with vaginal repair – not in those undergoing vaginal repair with urethral plication or vaginal repair alone.[29] Koonings and colleagues reported that daily intravesical doses of $PGF_{2\alpha}$ and intravaginal PGE_2 reduced the number of days required for catheterization after stress incontinence surgery compared with a control group receiving intravesical saline.[30] Other investigators, however, have reported conflicting (negative) results. Stanton and associates[31] and Delaere and co-workers reported no success using intravesical PGE_2 at doses similar to those reported earlier; Delaere and co-workers[32] similarly reported no success using $PGF_{2\alpha}$ in a group of women with emptying difficulties of various causes, although it should be noted that they used lower doses than those reported earlier. Wagner and colleagues[33] used PGE_2 at doses of 0.75–2.25 mg and reported no effect on urinary retention in a group of patients who had undergone anterior colporrhaphy.

Schubler[34] reported that both intravesical PGE_2 and sulprostone (a derivative) caused a strong sensation of urgency in normal female volunteers, resulting in reduced bladder capacity and instability. Both agents also decreased resting urethral closure pressure. PGE_2 increased detrusor pressure at opening and during maximum flow; sulprostone slightly decreased these two parameters. All effects had disappeared 24 hours after administration. PGs have a relatively short half-life, and it is difficult to understand how any effects after a single application can last as long as several months. If such an effect does occur, it must be the result of a 'triggering effect' on some as yet unknown physiological or metabolic mechanism. Because of the number of conflicting positive and negative reports with various intravesical preparations, double-blind placebo-controlled studies would obviously be helpful to determine whether there are circumstances in which PG usage can reproducibly facilitate emptying or treat postoperative retention.

Potential side effects of PG usage include vomiting, diarrhoea, pyrexia, hypertension and hypotension.[35]

Blockers of inhibition

De Groat and co-workers[1,4,36] have demonstrated a sympathetic reflex during bladder filling that, at least in the cat, promotes urine storage partly by exerting an α-adrenergic inhibitory effect on pelvic parasympathetic ganglionic transmission. Some investigators have suggested that α-adrenergic blockage, in addition to decreasing outlet resistance, may in fact facilitate transmission through these ganglia and thereby enhance bladder contractility. Although such an effect may be due solely to an α-adrenergic effect on the outlet (see Decreasing Outlet Resistance, page 369), it may be that α-adrenergic blockade can, under certain circumstances, facilitate the detrusor reflex, through either a direct effect on parasympathetic ganglia or an indirect one (a mechanism associated with a decrease in urethral resistance).

Opioid antagonists

Recent advances in neuropeptide physiology and pharmacology have provided new insights into lower urinary tract function and its potential pharmacological alteration. It has been hypothesized that endogenous opioids may exert a tonic inhibitory effect on the micturition reflex at various levels,[1,3] and agents such as narcotic antagonists may, therefore, offer possibilities for stimulating reflex bladder activity. Wheeler and colleagues,[37] however, noted no significant cystometric changes in a group of 15 patients with spinal cord injury following intravenous naloxone, and 11 of these patients showed decreased perineal electromyographic (EMG) activity. Although this issue is intriguing, it is of little practical use at present.

Decreasing outlet resistance at the level of the smooth sphincter

α-Adrenergic antagonists

Whether or not one believes that there is significant innervation of the bladder and proximal urethral smooth musculature by postganglionic fibres of the sympathetic nervous system, one must acknowledge the existence of α- and β-adrenergic receptor sites in these areas.[1,5] The smooth muscle of the bladder base and proximal urethra contains predominantly α-adrenoceptors. The bladder body contains both types of adrenoceptors, the β type being more common. The implication that α-adrenergic blockade could be useful in certain patients who cannot empty the bladder was first made by Kleeman in 1970.[38] Krane and Olsson[39,40] were among the first to endorse the concept of a physiological internal sphincter that is partially controlled by tonic sympathetic stimulation of contractile α-adrenoceptors in the smooth musculature of the bladder neck and proximal urethra. Furthermore, they hypothesized that some obstructions that occur at this level during detrusor contraction result from an inadequate opening of the bladder neck or an inadequate decrease in resistance in the area of the proximal urethra. They also theorized and presented evidence that α-adrenergic blockade could be useful in promoting bladder emptying in such a patient – one with an adequate detrusor contraction but without anatomical obstruction or detrusor striated sphincter dyssynergia. Abel and colleagues[41] called attention to the fact that such a functional obstruction (which they, too, assumed to be mediated by the sympathetic nervous system) could be maximal at a urethral rather than bladder-neck level, and coined the term 'neuropathic urethra.' Many others have subsequently confirmed the utility of α-blockade in the treatment of what is now usually referred to as smooth sphincter or bladder-neck dyssynergia or dysfunction (see reference 9 for other references).

Successful results – usually defined as an increase in flow rate, a decrease in residual urine and an improvement in upper tract appearance (when that is pathological) – can often be correlated with an objective decrease in urethral profile closure pressures.

One would expect such success with α-adrenergic blockade in treating emptying failure to be least evident in patients with detrusor striated sphincter dyssynergia, as reported by Hachen.[42] Although most would agree that α-blockers exert their favourable effects on voiding dysfunction primarily by affecting the smooth muscle of the bladder neck and proximal urethra, some information suggests that they may affect (decrease) striated sphincter tone as well. Other data suggest that they may exert some effects on the symptoms of voiding dysfunction in certain circumstances by decreasing bladder contractility (see later discussion: Decreasing Bladder Contractility, page 373 *et sec.*). Much of the confusion about whether α-blockers have a direct (as opposed to an indirect) inhibitory effect on the striated sphincter relates to the interpretation of observations of their effect on urethral pressure and periurethral striated muscle EMG activity in the region of the urogenital diaphragm. It is impossible to tell from pressure tracings alone whether a decrease in resistance in one area of the urethra is secondary to a decrease in smooth or striated muscle activity. Nannings and colleagues[43] found that EMG activity of the external sphincter decreased after administration of phentolamine in three paraplegic patients; they attributed this to direct inhibition of a sympathetic action on the striated sphincter. Nordling and colleagues[44] demonstrated that clonidine and phenoxybenzamine (POB), both of which pass the blood–brain barrier, also decreased urethral pressure in this area but had no effect on EMG activity. They concluded (1) that the effect of phentolamine was due to smooth muscle relaxation alone; (2) that the effect of clonidine and possibly of POB was elicited mostly through centrally induced changes in striated urethral sphincter tonus; and (3) that these agents also had an effect on the smooth muscle component of urethral pressure. None of the three drugs, however, affected the reflex rise in either urethral pressure or EMG activity that was seen during bladder filling, and none decreased the urethral pressure or EMG activity response to voluntary contraction of the pelvic floor striated musculature.

Pedersen and associates[45] showed that thymoxamine (an α–adrenergic antagonist that crosses the blood–brain barrier) decreased peak urethral pressure and striated sphincter EMG activity in patients with spastic paraplegia; they speculated that the drug acted on the striated sphincter via a central mechanism. Gajewski and colleagues[46] concluded that α-blockers do not influence the pudendal nerve-dependent urethral response in the cat through a peripheral action, but that prazosin, at least, can significantly inhibit this response at a central level. Thind and co-workers[47] reported on the effects of prazosin on static urethral sphincter function in 10 healthy women: they found that function was diminished, predominantly in the midurethral area, and hypothesized that this response was due to a decrease in both smooth and striated sphincter muscle tone, the latter as a result of a reduced somatomotor output from the central nervous system (CNS).

α-Adrenergic blocking agents have also been used to treat both bladder and outlet abnormalities in patients with so-called autonomous bladders.[48] These include those with myelodysplasia, sacral or infrasacral spinal cord neural injury, and voiding dysfunction following radical pelvic surgery. Parasympathetic decentralization has been reported to lead to a marked increase in adrenergic innervation of the bladder, resulting in conversion of the usual β (relaxant) bladder response to sympathetic stimulation to an α (contractile) response.[49] Although the alterations in innervation have been disputed, the alterations in receptor function have not. Koyanagi[50] demonstrated urethral supersensitivity to α-adrenergic stimulation in a group of patients with autonomous neurogenic bladders, implying that a change had occurred in adrenergic receptor function in the urethra following parasympathetic decentralization. Parsons and Turton[51] observed the same phenomenon but ascribed the cause to adrenergic supersensitivity of the urethral smooth muscle caused by sympathetic decentralization. Nordling and colleagues[52] described a similar phenomenon in women who had undergone radical hysterectomy and ascribed this change to damage to the sympathetic innervation. Decreased bladder compliance is often a clinical problem in such patients, and this, together with a fixed urethral sphincter tone, results in the paradoxical occurrence of both storage and emptying failure. Norlen[48] has summarized the supporting evidence for the success of α-adrenolytic treatment in these patients. POB is capable of increasing bladder compliance (increasing storage) and decreasing urethral resistance (facilitating emptying). Andersson and co-workers[53] used prazosin in such patients and found that maximum urethral pressure (MUP) during filling was decreased, whereas 'autonomous waves' were reduced. McGuire and Savastano[54] reported that POB decreased filling cystometric pressure in the decentralized primate bladder.

α-Adrenergic blockade can decrease bladder contractility in patients with voiding dysfunction by another mechanism as well. Jensen[55-57] reported an increase in the 'α-adrenergic effect' in bladders characterized as 'uninhibited'. Short- and long-term prazosin administration increased bladder capacity and decreased the amplitude of contractions. Thomas and colleagues[58] found that intravenous phentolamine produced a significant reduction in maximum voiding detrusor pressure, voiding volumes and peak flow rates in patients with suprasacral spinal cord injury with no reduction of outflow obstruction. Rohner and associates[59] found that the normal β response of canine bladder-body smooth musculature was changed to an α response after bladder outlet obstruction. Swierzewski and colleagues[60] prospectively studied the effects of terazosin on 12 patients with spinal cord injuries and decreased compliance. All patients were refractory to medical therapy and intermittent catheterization. Urodynamic studies were conducted before, during and at the conclusion of 4 weeks of therapy with 5 mg terazosin daily. The authors found statistically significant improvements in bladder compliance, 'safe bladder volume' and bladder pressure in all patients, with the additional benefits of decreased episodes of both urinary incontinence and autonomic dysreflexia. They speculated that the improvement was due either to a direct effect on the α-receptors of the detrusor or to a central effect, but not to any effects on outlet resistance.

POB was the α-adrenolytic agent originally used for the treatment of voiding dysfunction; like phentolamine, it has blocking properties at both α_1- and α_2-receptor sites. The initial adult dosage of this agent is 10 mg/day, and the usual daily dose for voiding dysfunction is 10–20 mg. Daily doses larger than 10 mg are generally divided and given every 8–12 hours. After the drug has been discontinued, the effects of administration may persist for days because the drug irreversibly inactivates α-receptors, and the duration of effect depends on the rate of receptor resynthesis.[61] Potential side effects include orthostatic hypotension, reflex tachycardia, nasal congestion, diarrhoea, miosis, sedation, nausea and vomiting (secondary to local irritation). Those who still use POB for long-term therapy should be aware that it has mutagenic activity in the Ames test and that repeated administration to animals can cause peritoneal sarcomas and lung tumours.[61] Furthermore, the manufacturer has reported a dose-related incidence in rats of gastrointestinal tumours,[62] the majority of which were in the non-glandular portion of the stomach. Although this agent has been in clinical use for some 30 years without clinically apparent oncological associations, one must now consider the potential medicolegal ramifications of long-term therapy, especially in younger persons.

Prazosin hydrochloride is a potent selective α_1-antagonist,[61] and its clinical use to lower outlet resistance has already been mentioned. The duration of action is 4–6 hours; therapy is generally begun in daily divided doses of 2–3 mg. The dose may be gradually increased to a maximum of 20 mg daily, although seldom is more than 9–10 mg daily used for voiding dysfunction. The potential side effects of prazosin are a consequence of its α_1-blockade. Occasionally, a 'first-dose' phenomenon occurs, a symptom complex of faintness, dizziness, palpitations and (infrequently) syncope, thought to be due to acute postural hypotension. The incidence of this phenomenon can be minimized by restricting the initial dose of the drug to 1 mg and administering this at bedtime. Other side effects associated with chronic prazosin therapy are generally mild and rarely necessitate withdrawal of the drug. The use of prazosin and other α-blockers for the control of hypertension has been reported to precipitate unwanted SUI in some patients, presumably because of its effects on urethral resistance.[63] Changing the class of antihypertensive agent in these patients is usually effective in reversing the urinary incontinence when it is due to the effects of the α-blocker.

Terazosin and doxazosin are two of the latest in a series of highly selective postsynaptic α_1-blocking drugs. They are readily absorbed and have a high bioavailability and a long plasma half-life, enabling their activity to be maintained over 24 hours following a single dose.[64,65] Their use has been recently promoted for the treatment of voiding dysfunction secondary to benign prostatic hyperplasia (BPH) consequent on the α_1-receptor content of the prostatic stroma and capsule. Their side effects are similar to those of prazosin.[66] Daily doses range from 1 to 10 mg, given generally at bedtime, a convenient advantage over the three-times-daily dosage schedule necessary for prazosin. Terazosin is said to have the same affinity for α_1-receptors in genitourinary as in vascular tissue and a fourfold greater selectivity for α_1-receptors than doxazosin. Alfuzosin is a new agent that is reported to be a selective and competitive antagonist of α_1-mediated contraction of the prostate capsule, bladder base and proximal urethral smooth muscle, with efficacy similar to that of prazosin.[67] It is said to be more specific for such receptors in the genitourinary tract than in the vasculature, raising the possibility that voiding may be facilitated by doses that have minimal vasodilatory effects, thus minimizing postural hypotension.[68] The drug requires three-times-daily dosing (7.5–10 mg total). A sustained-release form of the drug, which allows convenient once-daily dosing, is also now available. In a placebo-controlled study,[69] sustained-release alfuzosin was shown to have no significant incidence of adverse effects above that due to placebo. In addition, effects on blood pressure (orthostatic hypotension) were minimal, supporting its selectivity of the lower urinary tract over the vasculature.

Finally, recent molecular characterization of the α_1-receptor has led to the recognition, classification and cloning of a number of α_1-receptor subtypes. Although at present it is unclear whether these receptor subtypes will lead to clinically significant alterations in the pharmacological management of voiding dysfunction (ideally, the development of superselective, receptor-specific and tissue-specific drugs), in the human prostate at least there appears to be some tissue specificity in that the majority of the stromal α_1-receptors are of the α_{1a} subtype.[70] A drug that is selective for the α_{1a}-receptor subtype would be expected to cause fewer undesired (and dose-limiting) effects than the less-selective drugs while maintaining clinical efficacy. Tamsulosin is an α_1-blocking agent that is selective for the α_{1a}- and α_{1d}-receptor subtypes over the α_{1b} subtype.[71] It appears to have no statistically significant drug-related adverse effects over placebo[72] and has less effect on blood-pressure parameters than alfuzosin.[73] It is unclear whether highly selective α_{1a}-antagonists will have similar effects in women, as virtually all of the studies reported in the peer-reviewed literature have studied the effects of these agents on benign prostatic obstruction in men.

Thus, agents with α-adrenergic blocking properties at various levels of the neural organization have been used in patients with very varied types of voiding dysfunction – functional outlet obstruction, urinary retention, decreased compliance and DI or hyper-reflexia. Our own experience suggests that a trial of such an agent is certainly worthwhile, because its effect or non-effect will become obvious in a matter of days and the pharmacological side effects are, of course, reversible. However, our results with such therapy for non-BPH-related voiding dysfunction have been somewhat less spectacular than those of (at least some) other investigators.

Other potential non-specific therapy

β-Adrenergic stimulation has been shown experimentally to decrease the urethral pressure profile and, by inference, urethral resistance.[74] Vaidyanathan *et al.*[75] reported a decrease in urethral closure pressure after administration of terbutaline, a relatively specific β_2-agonist. Other investigators (see Increasing Outlet Resistance, page 389) have reported that β_2-agonists potentiate periurethral striated muscle contraction *in vitro*. It seems doubtful that a β-agonist will prove clinically useful in facilitating bladder emptying by decreasing outlet resistance.

Progesterone has been suggested as a possible treatment for emptying abnormalities in women. In a study of normal women looking at the effects of oestrogen alone vs oestrogen plus progesterone, maximum flow in the oestrogen-only group increased from 26 to 38 ml/s. A sphincteric effect was hypothesized.[76]

Finally, nitric oxide (NO) has been suggested to be a mediator of non-adrenergic, non-cholinergic (NANC) relaxation of the smooth muscle of the bladder outlet that occurs with bladder contraction.[5] Whether this means that analogues or substances that release NO *in vivo* will prove useful in decreasing smooth-muscle-related outlet resistance in humans remains to be seen. If so, one could envisage a role for NO synthetase inhibitors to stabilize urethral pressure or increase outlet resistance as well. NO is a ubiquitous molecule, however, and also exerts inhibitor effects on the detrusor body *in vitro* (see Decreasing Bladder Contractility, page 373). Opposite functional effects on the bladder and outlet (on contractility and resistance) could well frustrate any clinical application.

Decreasing outlet resistance at the level of the striated sphincter

There is no class of pharmacological agents that selectively relaxes the striated musculature of the pelvic floor. Three different types of drugs have been used to treat voiding dysfunction secondary to outlet obstruction at the level of the striated sphincter – the benzodiazepines (diazepam), dantrolene and baclofen. All are characterized generally as antispasticity drugs.[77] Baclofen and diazepam act predominantly within the CNS, whereas dantrolene acts directly on skeletal muscle. Unfortunately, there is no completely satisfactory form of therapy for alleviation of skeletal muscle spasticity. Although these drugs are capable of providing variable relief in specific circumstances, their efficacy is far from complete and troublesome muscle weakness, adverse effects on gait and a variety of other side effects minimize their overall usefulness as a treatment for spasticity.

Benzodiazepines and baclofen are both thought to exert their effects on the lower urinary tract through interactions with inhibitory neurotransmitters. γ-Aminobutyric acid (GABA) and glycine have been identified as major inhibitory neurotransmitters in the CNS.[78] Evidence favours glycine as the mediator of intraspinal postsynaptic inhibition and the most likely inhibitory transmitter in the reticular formation. GABA appears to mediate presynaptic inhibition in the spinal cord and the inhibitory action of local interneurons in the brain. The specific substrate for spinal cord inhibition consists of the synapses located on the terminals of the primary afferent fibres. GABA is the transmitter secreted by these synapses and activates specific receptors, resulting in a decrease in the amount of excitatory transmitter released by impulses from primary afferent fibres, consequently reducing the amplitude of the excitatory postsynaptic potentials. The inhibitory action of GABA in the brain occurs through an increase in chloride conductance with hyperpolarization of the neuronal membrane.

Benzodiazepines

The benzodiazepines potentiate the action of GABA at both presynaptic and postsynaptic sites in the brain and spinal cord.[79,80] When GABA recognition sites are activated, increased chloride conductance across the neuronal membrane produces inhibitory effects. The benzodiazepines increase the affinity of the GABA receptor sites on CNS membranes, and the increased binding increases the frequency with which the chloride channels open in response to a given amount of GABA. Presynaptic inhibition is augmented, and it is thought that this reduces the release of excitatory transmitters from afferent fibres, thereby reducing the gain of the stretch and flexor reflexes in patients with bladder spasticity. This is a postulated mechanism of action of the muscle relaxant properties of diazepam at least.[79] Another benzodiazepine-binding site exists that is not linked to the GABA receptor: this is a peripheral receptor with different pharmacological characteristics. The organ-specific densities and physiological functions of this second class of benzodiazepine receptor remain incompletely clarified and have unknown relevance, if any, for the lower urinary tract.[81]

Benzodiazepines are used extensively for the treatment of anxiety and related disorders,[82] although pharmacologically they can also be classified as centrally acting muscle relaxants. The generalized anxiety disorder responsive to pharmacotherapy by these agents is characterized by unrealistic or excessive anxiety and worry about life circumstances. Specific symptoms can be related to motor tension, autonomic hyperactivity (frequent urination can be a manifestation of this, as well as nausea, vomiting, diarrhoea and abdominal distress) and excessive vigilance. Other common uses include treatment of insomnia, stress-related disorders, muscle spasm, epilepsy and preoperative sedation.[80]

Side effects of benzodiazepines include non-specific CNS depression, manifested as sedation, lethargy, drowsiness, slowing of thought processes, ataxia and decreased ability to acquire or store information.[82]

Some authors believe that any muscle relaxant effect in clinically used doses is due to the CNS depressant effects and cite a lack of clinical studies showing any advantages of these agents over placebo or aspirin in this regard.[83] Effective total daily doses of diazepam, the most widely used agent of this group, range from 4 to 40 mg. Other benzodiazepine anxiolytic agents include chlordiazepoxide, clorazepate, prazepam, halazepam, clonazepam, lorazepam, oxazepam and alprazolam.

There are few available published papers that provide valuable data on the use of any of the benzodiazepines for treatment of functional obstruction at the level of the striated sphincter. Opinions, however, are commonly expressed, at least in regard to diazepam. In view of the information previously cited on the use of α-adrenergic blocking agents for treating or preventing postoperative urinary retention, it is interesting to note that one of the few articles that specifically mentions diazepam reports that it is more effective than oral POB, intravesical PGE or oral BC in promoting spontaneous voiding after colposuspension surgery.[84] We have not found the recommended oral doses of diazepam effective in controlling the classic type of detrusor striated sphincter dyssynergia secondary to neurological disease. If the cause of incomplete emptying in a neurologically normal patient is obscure, and the patient has what appears urodynamically to be inadequate relaxation of the pelvic floor striated musculature (e.g. occult neuropathic bladder, the Hinman syndrome), a trial of such an agent may be worthwhile. The rationale for its use is either relaxation of the pelvic floor striated musculature during bladder contraction, or that such relaxation removes an inhibitory stimulus to reflex bladder activity. However, improvement under such circumstances may simply be due to the anti-anxiety effect of the drug or to the intensive explanation, encouragement and modified biofeedback therapy that usually accompanies such treatment in these patients.

Finally, diazepam may also have effects on the smooth muscle of the detrusor. Peripheral benzodiazepine receptors have been demonstrated in the rabbit detrusor,[85] although the clinical significance is, at present, unknown. In addition, administration of diazepam resulted in smooth muscle relaxation in the rat detrusor in a GABA-independent fashion through interference with calcium transport.[86] It is unclear whether this effect occurs at physiological doses of diazepam or whether this action has any clinical relevance in humans.

Baclofen

Baclofen depresses monosynaptic and polysynaptic excitation of motor neurons and interneurons in the spinal cord and was originally thought to function as a GABA agonist.[77,79] However, its electrophysiological and pharmacological profiles differ radically from those of GABA. Although its effects superficially resemble those of GABA, some specific GABA inhibitors (e.g. bicucculine) do not antagonize the actions of baclofen. Baclofen does not cause depolarization of primary afferent nerve terminals, and there is no evidence that baclofen increases chloride conduction, the most prominent action of GABA. Because both GABA and baclofen can produce some effects that are insensitive to blockade by classic GABA antagonists, two classes of GABA receptors have been proposed – the $GABA_A$ receptor (the classic receptor) and the $GABA_B$ receptor. Baclofen does not bind strongly or specifically to classic $GABA_A$ receptors but does to $GABA_B$ receptors in brain and spinal membranes. Currently, it is thought that activation of the GABA receptors by baclofen causes a decrease in the release of excitatory transmitters onto motor neurons by increasing potassium conductance or by inhibiting calcium influx. Baclofen's primary site of action is in the spinal cord, but it is also reported to be active at more rostral sites in the CNS. Milanov[87] states that, like a $GABA_B$ agonist, baclofen suppresses excitatory neurotransmitter release but also has direct GABA-ergic activity. Its effect in reducing spasticity is caused primarily by normalizing interneuron activity and decreasing motor neuron activity (perhaps secondary to normalizing interneuron activity).[87]

Baclofen has been found useful for the treatment of skeletal spasticity due to a variety of causes (especially multiple sclerosis and traumatic spinal cord lesions).[77] Determination of the optimal dose in individual patients requires careful titration. Treatment is started at an initial dose of 5 mg twice a day and increased every 3 days up to a maximum daily dose of 20 mg four times a day. With reference to voiding dysfunction, Hachen and Krucker[88] found that a daily oral dose of 75 mg was ineffective in patients with striated sphincter dyssynergia and traumatic paraplegia, whereas a daily intravenous dose of 20 mg was highly effective. Florante and associates[89] reported that 73% of their patients with voiding dysfunction secondary to acute and chronic spinal cord injury had lower striated sphincter responses and decreased residual urine volume following baclofen treatment, but only with an average daily oral dose of 120 mg.

Potential side effects of baclofen include drowsiness, insomnia, rash, pruritus, dizziness and weakness. It may impair the ability to walk or stand and is not recommended for the management of spasticity due to cerebral lesions or disease. Sudden withdrawal has been shown to provoke hallucinations, anxiety and tachycardia; hallucinations due to reductions in dosage during treatment have also been reported.[90]

Drug delivery often frustrates adequate pharmacological treatment, and baclofen is a good example of this. GABA's hydrophilic properties prevent its crossing the blood–brain barrier in sufficient amounts to make it therapeutically useful. For oral use a more lipophilic analogue, baclofen, was developed. However, its passage through the barrier is likewise limited, and it has proved to be a generally insufficient drug when given orally to treat severe somatic spasticity and micturition disorders secondary to neurogenic dysfunction.[91] Intrathecal infusion bypasses the blood–brain barrier: cerebrospinal fluid levels 10 times higher than those reached with oral administration are achieved with infusion amounts 100 times less than those taken orally.[92] Direct administration into the subarachnoid space by an implanted infusion pump has shown promising results, not only for skeletal spasticity but also for striated sphincter dyssynergia and bladder hyperactivity. Nannings and colleagues[93] reported on such administration to seven patients with intractable bladder spasticity: all patients experienced a general decrease in spasticity and the amount of striated sphincter activity during bladder contraction decreased; six showed an increase in bladder capacity. Four previously incontinent patients were able to stay dry with clean intermittent catheterization (CIC). The action of baclofen on bladder hyperactivity is not unexpected, given its spinal cord mechanism of action, and this inhibition of bladder contractility when the drug is administered intrathecally may, in fact, prove to be its most important benefit. Loubser and colleagues[94] studied nine patients with spinal cord injury and refractory spasticity, using an external pump to test the initial response: eight showed objective improvement in functional ability; three of seven studied urodynamically showed an increase in bladder capacity. Kums and Delhaas[91] reported on nine men who were paraplegic or quadriplegic secondary to trauma or multiple sclerosis and also had intractable muscle spasticity; they were treated with intrathecal baclofen. After a successful test period during which the drug was administered through an external catheter, a drug-delivery system was implanted and connected to a spinal catheter. Doses ranged from 74 to 840 mg/24 h. Patients were studied before and 4–6 weeks after initiation of therapy. Mean residual urine volume fell from 224 to 110 ml ($p = 0.01$), mean urodynamic bladder capacity rose from 162 to 263 ml ($p < 0.005$), and pelvic floor spasm decreased at both baseline and maximum bladder capacity ($p < 0.005$ and 0.025, respectively). Three subjects became continent. Additionally, CIC was no longer complicated by adductor spasm.

Development of tolerance to intrathecal baclofen with a consequent requirement for increasing doses may prove to be a problem with long-term chronic usage. Mertens and colleagues[95] reported on the long-term use of intrathecal baclofen in a series of 17 patients with mixed spinal cord lesions and severe refractory limb spasticity. Average follow-up was 37.5 months (range 5–69 months). Intrathecal dose was adjusted every 3 months as needed to maintain 'good clinical and functional condition' with regard to limb spasticity, hypertonia, pain and functional disability, and not necessarily for its effects on the lower urinary tract. The authors noted that the dosage necessary to gain an initial 'satisfactory effect' varied considerably between patients, with dosage titration increasing over the first few months in the majority of patients but 'usually' stabilizing after the first year. Unfortunately, quantitative data (actual dosage adjustment, number of patients requiring adjustment, etc.) were not provided. Only 12 of the 17 patients had an associated neurogenic bladder and underwent urodynamic study. Long-term effects on the lower urinary tract were inconsistent: five of nine patients with decreased functional bladder capacity had significant improvement, and uninhibited contractions were reduced or suppressed in 50% of those with detrusor hyperreflexia at presentation. The authors attribute these inconsistent results as potentially due to inadequate dose titration for effects on the lower urinary tract. They speculated that the 'effective dose' to improve lower-extremity hypertonia (the endpoint in this study) was perhaps not sufficient to improve the lower urinary tract parameters in the majority of patients. Further studies on the long-term efficacy of intrathecal baclofen specifically on the lower urinary tract in patients with neurogenic bladder are anticipated.

Dantrolene

Dantrolene exerts its effects by direct peripheral action on skeletal muscle.[77,79] It is thought to inhibit the excitation-induced release of calcium ions from the sarcoplasmic reticulum of striated muscle fibres, thereby inhibiting excitation–contraction coupling and diminishing the mechanical force of contraction. The blockade of calcium release is not complete, however, and contraction is not completely abolished. It reduces reflex more than voluntary contractions, probably because of a preferential action on fast-twitch rather than slow-twitch skeletal muscle fibres. It has been shown to have therapeutic benefits for chronic spasticity associated with CNS disorders. The drug improves voiding function in some patients with classic detrusor striated sphincter dyssynergia and was initially reported to be very successful in doing so.[96] In adults, the recommended starting dose is 25 mg daily, gradually increasing by increments of 25 mg every 4–7 days to a maximum oral dose of 400 mg given in four divided doses. Hackler and colleagues[97] reported improvement in voiding function in approximately half of their patients treated with dantrolene but found that such improvement required oral doses of 600 mg daily. Although no inhibitory effect on bladder smooth muscle seems to occur,[98] the generalized weakness that dantrolene can induce is often sufficiently significant to compromise its therapeutic effects.

Potential side effects other than severe muscle weakness include euphoria, dizziness, diarrhoea and hepatotoxicity. Fatal hepatitis has been reported in 0.1–0.2% of patients treated with the drug for 60 days or longer, and symptomatic hepatitis may occur in 0.5% of patients treated for more than 60 days; chemical abnormalities of liver function are noted in up to 1%. The risk of hepatic injury is twofold greater in women.[99] One use of dantrolene for which agreement exists is the acute management of malignant hyperthermia, a rare hereditary syndrome characterized by vigorous contraction of skeletal muscle precipitated by excess release of calcium from the sarcoplasmic reticulum, generally in response to neuromuscular blocking agents or inhalational anaesthetics. Virtually all hospital pharmacies stock parenteral dantrolene for this purpose.

Other agents

β-Adrenergic agonists, especially those with prominent β_2 characteristics, are able to produce relaxation of some skeletal muscles of the slow-twitch type.[100,101] This action could be significant in view of the fact that the portion of the external urethral sphincter comprising the outermost urethral wall is said to consist exclusively of slow-twitch fibres,[102] whereas the striated muscle fibres of the levator ani contain both fast- and slow-twitch fibres, although the majority are of the slow-

twitch type. This type of action may account at least in part for the decrease in urethral profile parameters seen with terbutaline (see Decreasing Outlet Resistance at the Level of the Smooth Sphincter, page 365). This area of pharmacology and its clinical relevance is somewhat confusing at the moment because β_2-adrenergic drugs have been reported to potentiate periurethral striated muscle contraction, albeit in a different *in vitro* system (see Increasing Outlet Resistance, page 389).

Botulinum toxin (an inhibitor of ACh release at the neuromuscular junction of striated muscle) has been injected directly into the striated sphincter to treat dyssynergia.[103] Injection carried out weekly for 3 weeks can achieve a duration of effect averaging 2 months. The number of patients tested seems thus far to be small, and more information is needed about criteria for success and side effects. Fowler and colleagues[104] used botulinum toxin injections in six women with difficult voiding or urinary retention secondary to abnormal myotonus-like EMG activity in the striated urethral sphincter. Although voiding did not improve in any patient (attributed to the type of repetitive discharge activity present), three patients developed transient stress incontinence, indicating that the sphincter muscle had, indeed, been weakened.

Clonidine is the prototypical α_2-adrenergic receptor agonist. It is considered to be a centrally acting agent with a variety of associated systemic effects including antihypertensive, antinociceptive and antispasmodic effects. Potential effects on relaxation of the external urethral sphincter have been reported previously.[105,106] Herman and Wainberg[107] administered oral clonidine (400 µg) in three divided doses over a 16 h period under monitored inpatient conditions to five spinal cord injury patients with detrusor hyperreflexia and quantified the effects on the external urethral sphincter (EUS) via needle electrodes. They found that clonidine had a profound suppressive effect on volume-induced EMG activity in the EUS in four of five patients. The one patient in whom there were only minimal effects on the EUS had received an intrathecal dose of morphine 2 days before, which the authors feel may have confounded the effects of clonidine in this patient. Although the possible effects of clonidine throughout the neuraxis are legion, the authors speculate that the somewhat selective effect of clonidine on the EUS is attributable to postsynaptic suppression of excitatory spinal interneurons (unmasked by the spinal lesion) via the α_2-agonist activity of clonidine. Adverse effects included significant reductions in systolic and diastolic blood pressure as well as sedative effects. Further clinical studies on the effects of clonidine on the lower urinary tract and striated sphincter (as well as its clinical utility) may be limited owing to its significant effects on blood pressure.

FACILITATION OF URINE STORAGE

The pathophysiology of failure of the lower urinary tract to fill with or to store urine adequately may be secondary to problems related to the bladder, the outlet or both.[6] Hyperactivity of the bladder during filling can be expressed as discrete involuntary contractions (IVCs) or as reduced compliance with or without phasic contractions. IVCs are most commonly associated with inflammatory or irritating processes in the bladder wall or with bladder outlet obstruction, or they may be idiopathic. Decreased compliance during filling may be secondary to the sequelae of neurological injury or disease but may also result from any process that destroys the elastic or viscoelastic properties of the bladder wall. Purely sensory urgency may also account for storage failure; such urgency may result from inflammatory, infectious, neurological or psychological factors, or it may be idiopathic. A fixed decrease in outlet resistance may result from degeneration of or damage to innervation of the structural elements of the smooth or striated sphincter or from neurological disease or injury, surgical or other mechanical trauma, or ageing. Classic SUI (also termed genuine stress incontinence) in women implies a failure of the normal transmission of increases in intra-abdominal pressure to the area of the bladder neck and proximal urethra. This failure is acknowledged to be associated mainly with changes in the anatomical position of the vesicourethral junction and proximal urethra during increases in intra-abdominal pressure (hypermobility), and this in turn is thought to accompany pelvic floor weakness or relaxation, which may be secondary to a number of causes. The pathophysiology of SUI may also involve a decrease in the reflex striated sphincter contraction, which occurs with a number of manoeuvres that increase intra-abdominal pressure. Treatment of abnormalities related to the filling or storage phase of micturition are directed towards inhibiting bladder contractility, increasing bladder capacity, decreasing sensory input during filling or increasing outlet resistance, either continuously or only during abdominal straining (see Table 32.2).

Decreasing bladder contractility

Anticholinergic agents

The major portion of the neurohumoral stimulus for physiological bladder contraction is ACh-induced stimulation of postganglionic parasympathetic muscarinic cholinergic receptor sites on bladder smooth muscle.[1,5] Atropine and atropine-like agents therefore depress normal bladder contractions and IVC of any cause.[55,108,109] In such patients, the volume to the first IVC is generally increased, the amplitude of the IVC decreased and maximum bladder capacity increased. However, although the volume and pressure thresholds at which an IVC is elicited may increase, the 'warning time' (the time between the perception of an IVC about to occur and its occurrence) and the ability to suppress an IVC are not increased. Thus, urgency and incontinence still occur unless such therapy is combined with a regimen of timed voiding or toileting. Bladder compliance in normal individuals and in those with detrusor hyperreflexia in whom the initial slope of the filling curve on cystometry is normal prior to the involuntary contraction does not seem to be significantly altered.[55] McGuire and Savastano[54] reported that atropine increased both the compliance and the capacity of the neurologically decentralized primate bladder, and that both of these effects were additive to those produced by POB[53] (see previous discussion on inhibition of bladder contractility by α-adrenergic blocking agents). However, the effect of pure antimuscarinics in those who exhibit only decreased compliance has not been well studied. Outlet resistance, at least as reflected by urethral pressure measurements, does not seem to be clinically affected by anticholinergic therapy.

Although antimuscarinic agents usually produce significant clinical improvement in patients with IVCs and associated symptoms, generally only partial inhibition results. In many animal models, atropine only partially antagonizes the response of the whole bladder to pelvic nerve stimulation and of bladder strips to field stimulation, although it does completely inhibit the response of bladder smooth muscle to exogenous cholinergic stimulation. Of the theories proposed to explain this phenomenon, termed 'atropine resistance', the most attractive and most commonly cited is the idea that a major portion of the neurotransmission involved in the final common pathway of bladder contraction is NANC – that is, secondary to a release of a transmitter other than ACh or noradrenaline.[1,2,5] Although the existence of atropine resistance in human bladder muscle is by no means agreed on, this concept is the most common hypothesis invoked to explain clinical difficulty in abolishing IVCs with anticholinergic agents alone, and it is also used to support the rationale of treatment of such types of bladder activity with agents that have different mechanisms of action. Brading[110,111] and Andersson[5] both discuss the difficulty of evaluating apparently conflicting data in the literature with respect to atropine resistance. Brading[111] states that the size of the atropine-resistant component varies markedly among different species and, in a given preparation, also depends on the frequency of nerve stimulation. Brading cites studies showing that, at frequencies producing maximum contractile responses, approximately 76% of the response is atropine resistant in the guinea pig and cat, 56% in the rabbit, 15% in the pig, and zero in strips from normal human detrusor. Andersson[5] states that 'most probably normal human detrusor muscle exhibits little atropine resistance', but does not exclude its existence in morphologically or functionally abnormal bladders.

Receptor subtyping is a particularly relevant concept for drug development in general and for antimuscarinic compounds in particular. Subtyping can be based on functional assays, on radioligand-binding affinity and on receptor cloning and expression. At least five different genetically established (by cloning) muscarinic subtypes exist (muscarinic receptor genes designated m_1–m_5).[112] The nomenclature M_1–M_4 describes the protein products of the m_1–m_5 coding regions (the actual muscarinic receptor subtypes) which are each defined pharmacologically using receptor subtype agonists and antagonists.[5,113,114] A physiological role for the product of the m_5 coding region remains undefined.[114] Pirenzepine (a selective muscarinic blocker) was originally used to subdivide muscarinic receptors into M_1 and M_2 categories; using this subclassification, detrusor muscarinic receptors were classified as the M_2 type.[5,115,116] On further analysis of the M_2 receptor population, a small proportion of glandular M_2 receptors were found which could represent the pharmacological type responsible for muscarinic agonist-induced contractions. This subtype is now called the M_3 receptor.[5,113] Although it appears that the majority of the muscarinic receptors in human smooth muscle including bladder are of the M_2 subtype,[117] *in vitro* data indicate that most smooth muscle contraction, including that of the urinary bladder, is mediated by the M_3 receptor subtype.[117,118] Muscarinic receptor subtyping becomes important when considering the possibility of pharmacologically selecting (and blocking) those receptors responsible for urinary bladder smooth muscle contraction while minimally affecting other muscarinic receptor sites throughout the body. Ideally, this approach would effectively treat the underlying problem (detrusor overactivity) while eliminating the unpleasant systemic side effects of most non-specific antimuscarinic agents (dry mouth, constipation, blurred vision, etc.) which, in many cases, are worse than the problem they are treating and result in patient non-compliance.

During treatment, some patients appear to become relatively refractory to anticholinergic drugs after a while. Such an effect could have many causes, but one pharmacological fact that could contribute to such a phenomenon is a change in receptor density in response to certain stimuli (up- or downregulation). Experimentally, at least, Levin and colleagues have shown that an increase in peripheral muscarinic receptor density occurs with chronic atropine administration (in the rat).[116] On the other hand, certain pathological states may be associated with changes in receptor density, which may in turn affect the response to anticholinergic (and other) agents. Restorick and Mundy[119] described a decrease in density of muscarinic cholinergic receptors and an increase in density of α-adrenoceptors in bladder-dome samples from humans with detrusor hyperreflexia; β-adrenoceptor density remained unchanged. Lepor and associates[120] described a similar decrease in cholinergic receptor density in bladder specimens from children and adults with voiding dysfunction due to myelomeningocele, spinal cord injury or multiple sclerosis, all of whom had IVCs. Proposed mechanisms include downregulation due to hyperactivity, smooth muscle hypertrophy and bladder wall fibrosis.

Specific drugs

Propantheline bromide is the classically described oral agent for producing an antimuscarinic effect in the lower urinary tract. The usual adult oral dose is 15–30 mg every 4–6 hours, although higher doses are often necessary. Propantheline is a quaternary ammonium compound that is poorly absorbed after oral administration.[121] Oral administration in the fasting state rather than with or after meals is preferable from the standpoint of drug bioavailability.[122] There seems to be little difference between the antimuscarinic effects of propantheline on bladder smooth muscle and those of other antimuscarinic agents such as glycopyrrolate, isopropamide, anisotropine methylbromide, methscopolamine and homatropine. Some of these agents, such as glycopyrrolate, have a more convenient dosage schedule (two or three times daily), but their clinical effects on the lower urinary tract are indistinguishable. Although there are obviously many other considerations in accounting for the activity of a given dose of drug at this site of action, no available oral drug has a direct *in vitro* antimuscarinic binding potential that is closer to that of atropine than the long-available and relatively inexpensive propantheline bromide.[123,124] There is a surprising lack of valuable data on the effectiveness of propantheline for the treatment of bladder hyperactivity. As Andersson points out,[109] anticholinergic drugs in general have been reported to have both great and poor efficacy for this indication. To show the range of variation, Zorzitto and colleagues[125] concluded that propantheline bromide administered orally in doses of 30 mg four times a day to a group of institutionalized incontinent geriatric patients had marginal benefits that were outweighed by the side effects. Blaivas and colleagues,[108] on the other hand, by increasing the dose of propantheline (up to 60 mg four times a day) until incontinence was eliminated or side effects precluded further use, obtained a complete response in 25 of 26 patients with IVCs. Differences in bioavailability, selective drug delivery, receptor selectivity, receptor density, atropine resistance, pathophysiology, susceptibility to dose-limiting side effects and mental status are all potential factors that could explain such disparate results. The Agency for Health Care Policy and Research (AHCPR) Clinical Practice Guidelines[126] list five randomized controlled trials for propantheline, in which 82% of the patients were women. Percentage cures (all figures refer to percentage minus percentage on placebo) are listed as 0–5, percentage reduction in urge incontinence as 0–53, percentage side effects 0–50, and percentage dropouts 0–9.

Atropine is reported to be available in a 0.5 mg tablet, although we have yet to find it. Atropine and all related belladonna alkaloids are well absorbed from the gastrointestinal tract. Atropine is said to have almost no detectable CNS effects at clinically used doses.[121] It has a half-life of about 4 hours.

Scopolamine is another belladonna alkaloid marketed as a soluble salt. It has prominent central depressive effects at low doses, probably because of its greater penetration (compared with atropine) through the blood–brain barrier. Transdermal scopolamine has been used for treating IVCs.[127] The 'patch' provides continuous delivery of 0.5 mg daily to the circulation for 3 days. Cornella and associates,[128] however, reported poor results with this form of drug in treating 10 patients with DI: only two patients showed a positive response; an additional one showed a slight improvement, the drug had to be discontinued in eight patients because of side effects. Side effects were related to the CNS (ataxia, dizziness) and included blurred vision and dry mouth. A double-blind placebo-controlled study using transdermal scopolamine was performed on 20 patients with DI: after a 14-day treatment period, the 10 patients randomized to transdermal scopolamine treatment showed statistically significant improvements in frequency, nocturia, urgency and urge incontinence over the placebo group; no adverse effects of the therapy were reported.[129] A double-blind placebo study on the effects of transdermal scopolamine in patients who had undergone suprapubic prostatectomy was performed to investigate its use in the treatment or prevention of pain, IVCs, urgency and bladder pressure rises of 15 cmH$_2$O. No statistical differences were found,[130] although the occurrence of IVCs was 33% in the treated group vs 54% in the placebo group. The percentage of patients requiring injectable analgesia on day 1 was similar in treated and control patients, but on day 2 it was statistically lower in the scopolamine group (4% vs 31%). In our experience of treating patients with IVCs with this method, results were very erratic and skin irritation with the patch was a problem for some patients. Caution should be exercised in the use of the patch in the elderly and young, because of the fixed dose.

Hyoscyamine and hyoscyamine sulphate are reported to have approximately the same general anticholinergic actions and side effects as the other belladonna alkaloids. Hyoscyamine sulphate is available as a sublingual formulation, a theoretical advantage, but controlled studies of its effects on bladder hyperactivity are lacking. Glycopyrrolate is a synthetic quaternary ammonium compound that is a potent inhibitor of both M_1 and M_2 receptors but has a preference for the M_2 subtype.[131] It is available in both oral and parenteral preparations; the latter is commonly used as an antisialogogue during anaesthesia. An anticholinergic agent with a significant ganglionic-blocking action as well as such action at the peripheral receptor level might be more effective in suppressing bladder contractility. Although methantheline has a higher ratio of ganglionic-blocking to antimuscarinic activity than does propantheline, the latter drug seems to be at least as potent in each respect, clinical dose for dose. Methantheline does have similar effects on the lower urinary tract, and some clinicians still prefer it over other anticholinergic agents. Few real data are available regarding its efficacy.

The potential side effects of all antimuscarinic agents include inhibition of salivary secretion (dry mouth), blockade of the ciliary muscle of the lens to cholinergic stimulation (blurred vision for near objects), tachycardia, drowsiness and inhibition of gut motility. Those agents that possess some ganglionic-blocking activity may also cause orthostatic hypotension and erectile dysfunction at high doses (at which nicotinic activity becomes manifest). Antimuscarinic agents are generally contraindicated in patients with narrow-angle glaucoma and should be used with caution in patients with significant bladder outlet obstruction because complete urinary retention may be precipitated.

A lack of selectivity is a major problem with all antimuscarinic compounds as they tend to affect parasympathetically innervated organs in the same order; generally, larger doses are required to inhibit bladder activity than to affect salivary, bronchial, nasopharyngeal and sweat secretions. Physicians who have prescribed antimuscarinic (anticholinergic) preparations of any type would agree that 'dry mouth' is one of the most troublesome side effects and probably causes many patients to discontinue therapy. Several new receptor antagonists with varying degrees of specificity for the lower urinary tract show some promise in improving the undesirable side-effect profiles of this class of medications without compromisng efficacy. Tolterodine and its primary metabolite PNU-200577[132] show some selectivity for bladder tissue over salivary tissue *in vitro* and *in vivo* in the anaesthetized cat.[133,134] These tissue-selective effects do not appear to

be due to muscarinic receptor subtype selectivity[132,133] but may be related to differential affinities of the receptors in the salivary gland and detrusor muscle for tolterodine compared with oxybutynin. Although it appears that the binding affinity of tolterodine and oxybutynin to muscarinic receptors in the urinary bladder (in the guinea pig) are very similar, the affinity of tolterodine for muscarinic receptors in the parotid gland is eight times *lower* than that of oxybutynin.[135] In a pilot study in 12 healthy males, tolterodine was shown to have a greater objective and subjective effect on bladder function than on salivation.[136] Jonas and colleagues[137] looked at the urodynamic effects of tolterodine in a multicentre randomized double-blind placebo-controlled study: 242 patients were enrolled and treated over a 4-week period with 1 or 2 mg tolterodine or placebo twice daily. Compared with placebo, 2 mg tolterodine (but not 1 mg) showed statistically significant improvements in mean volume to first IVC (141 to 230 ml, 142 to 210 ml and 140 to 181 ml in the 2 mg, 1 mg and placebo groups, respectively), mean maximal strength of IVC (52 to 37 cmH_2O, 41 to 35 cmH_2O and 47 to 40 cmH_2O in the 2 mg, 1 mg and placebo groups, respectively) and maximal cystometric capacity (272 to 316 ml, 276 to 294 ml and 264 to 268 ml in the 2 mg, 1 mg and placebo groups, respectively). The proportion of adverse effects between the treated groups and placebo was not statistically significant; however, dry mouth was the most commonly reported event (reported in 9% of treated patients) – significantly less than the 50% incidence reported in the literature for other commonly used anticholinergic preparations.[138] Furthermore, the dry mouth was classified as 'severe' by only 1% of patients. At higher doses, the incidence of side effects of tolterodine may be more significant and approach that of other commonly used anticholinergic drugs. Rentzhog and colleagues[139] noted that, at a dose of 2 mg or less, the incidence of adverse effects (including dry mouth) due to tolterodine was comparable to that of placebo (2/13 patients in the placebo group vs 9/51 patients in the tolterodine group reported dry mouth); however, when the dose of tolterodine was increased to 4 mg, a substantial increase in the incidence of dry mouth occurred (9/16 patients). Overall, it appears that tolterodine and PNU-200577 are safe and efficacious for the treatment of detrusor overactivity. A favourable side-effect profile exists at lower doses (less effect on salivary glands), which may diminish in a dose-dependent fashion. Further studies are needed to compare the efficacy and apparently favourable side-effect profile of tolterodine directly with those of other readily available anticholinergic preparations.

Darifenacin[140,141] and vamicamide[142,143] are reported to be novel antimuscarinic agents with potential applications in the lower urinary tract in that they have demonstrated pharmacological specificity for the M_3 receptor, the probable major contributor to volume induced bladder contractility. Unfortunately, no clinical trials have been reported on the use of either of these compounds in the lower urinary tract in humans.

Musculotropic relaxants

Musculotropic relaxants fall under the general heading of direct-acting smooth muscle depressants, the 'antispasmodic' activity of which is reported to affect smooth muscle directly at a site that is metabolically distal to the cholinergic or other contractile receptor mechanism. Although all of the agents discussed in this section do relax smooth muscle *in vitro* by papavarine-like (direct) action, all have been found to possess variable anticholinergic and local-anaesthetic properties in addition. There is still some uncertainty about how much of their clinical efficacy is due only to their atropine-like effect. If, in fact, any of these agents do exert a clinically significant inhibitory effect that is independent of antimuscarinic action, a therapeutic rationale exists for combining them with a relatively pure anticholinergic agent.

Oxybutynin chloride is a moderately potent anticholinergic agent that has strong independent musculotropic relaxant activity as well as local-anaesthetic activity. Comparatively higher concentrations *in vitro* are necessary to produce direct spasmolytic effects, which may be due to calcium-channel blockade.[144,145] The recommended oral adult dose is 5 mg three or four times a day; side effects are antimuscarinic and dose related. Initial reports documented success in depressing detrusor hyperreflexia in patients with neurogenic bladder dysfunction,[145] and subsequent reports documented success in inhibiting other types of bladder hyperactivity as well.[109] A randomized double-blind placebo-controlled study comparing 5 mg oxybutynin three times a day with placebo in 30 patients with DI was carried out by Moisey and colleagues:[146] 17 of 23 patients who completed the study with oxybutynin had

symptomatic improvement and nine showed evidence of urodynamic improvement, mainly an increase in maximum bladder capacity. Hehir and Fitzpatrick[147] reported that 16 of 24 patients with neuropathic voiding dysfunction secondary to myelomeningocele were cured or improved (17% dry, 50% improved) with oxybutynin treatment: average bladder capacity increased from 197 to 299 ml (with drug) vs 218 ml (with placebo); maximum bladder filling pressure decreased from 47 to 37 cmH$_2$O (with drug) vs 45 cmH$_2$O (with placebo). In a prospective randomized study of 34 patients with voiding dysfunction secondary to multiple sclerosis, Gajewski and Awad[148] found that 5 mg oral oxybutynin three times a day produced a good response more frequently than 15 mg propantheline three times a day; they concluded that oxybutynin was more effective in the treatment of detrusor hyperreflexia secondary to multiple sclerosis. Holmes and associates[149] compared the results of oxybutynin and propantheline in a small group of women with DI. The experimental design was a randomized crossover trial with a patient-regulated variable dose regimen. This kind of dose-titration study allows the patient to increase the drug dose to whatever he or she perceives to be the optimum ratio between clinical improvement and side effects – an interesting way of comparing two drugs while minimizing differences in oral absorption. Of the 23 women in the trial, 14 reported subjective improvement with oxybutynin as opposed to 11 with propantheline. Both drugs significantly increased the maximum cystometric capacity and reduced the maximum detrusor pressure on filling. The only significant objective difference was a greater increase in the maximum cystometric capacity with oxybutynin. The mean total daily dose of oxybutynin tolerated was 15 mg (range 7.5–30) and that of propantheline was 90 mg (range 45–145).

Thuroff and colleagues[150] compared oxybutynin with propantheline and placebo in a group of patients with symptoms of instability and either DI or hyperreflexia. Oxybutynin (5 mg three times a day) performed best, but propantheline was used at a relatively low dose – 15 mg three times a day. The incidence of side effects was higher for oxybutynin at just about the level of clinical and urodynamic improvement. The mean grade of improvement on a visual analogue scale was higher for oxybutynin (58.2%) than for propantheline (44.7%) or placebo (43.4%). Urodynamic volume at the first IVC increased more with oxybutynin (51 vs 11.2 vs 9.7 ml), as did the change in maximum cystometric capacity (80.1 vs 48.9 vs 22.5 ml). Residual urine volume also increased more (27.0 vs 2.2 vs 1.9 ml). The authors further subdivided their overall results into excellent (> 75% improvement), good (50–74%), fair (25–49%) and poor (< 25%). Percentages for treatment with oxybutynin were, respectively, 42, 25, 15 and 18%. The authors compared their 67% rate of good or excellent results with those reported in seven other oxybutynin series in the literature (some admittedly poorer studies included) and concluded that their results compared favourably with the range of results calculated from these studies (61–86%). The results of propantheline treatment generally ranked between those of oxybutynin and placebo but did not reach significant levels over placebo in any variable. Subdivision of propantheline results into excellent, good, fair and poor categories yielded percentages of 20, 30, 14 and 36%, respectively. The authors compared their 50% ratio of good or excellent results with those achieved in six other propantheline studies reported in the literature (30–57%) and concluded that their results were consistent with these. Although this study is better than most in the literature, it does have drawbacks, and anyone using it in a meta-analysis would be well advised to read it and the other cited studies very carefully.

Zeegers and colleagues[151] reported on a double-blind prospective crossover study comparing oxybutynin, flavoxate (see page 380), emepronium and placebo. Although there was a high dropout rate (19 of 60 patients) and the entry criteria were vague (frequency, urgency, urge incontinence), the results were scored as 5 (excellent overall effect) to 1 (no improvement) by both patient and physician, and the results were combined into a single number. The percentages of results in categories 3–5 for the agents used were oxybutynin 61%, placebo 41%, emepronium 34%, and flavoxate 31%. The results of the first treatment gave corresponding percentages of only 63, 29, 18 (probably reflecting eight dropouts due to side effects) and 44% respectively.

Ambulatory urodynamic monitoring and pad weighing were used to assess the effects of oxybutynin on detrusor hyperactivity by Von Doorn and Zwiers.[152] The 24-hour average frequency of IVCs decreased from 8.7 to 3.4; the maximum contraction amplitude decreased from 32 to 22 cmH_2O, and the duration of the average IVC decreased from 90 to 60 seconds. However, the daily micturition frequency did not change (11–10), nor did the amount of urine lost – findings the authors try to minimize by pointing out that some patients also had sphincteric incontinence and that, during treatment, there may have been a higher fluid intake.

The AHCPR guidelines[126] list six randomized controlled trials for oxybutynin; 90% of patients were women. The percentage of cures (all figures refer to percentage minus percentage on placebo) is listed as 28–44%; percentage of reduction in urge incontinence is 9–56%, and the percentages of side effects and dropouts are 2–66% and 3–45%, respectively. There are some negative reports on the efficacy of oxybutynin. Zorzitto and colleagues[153] came to conclusions similar to those resulting from their study of propantheline (see page 375) in a double-blind placebo-controlled trial conducted in 24 incontinent geriatric institutionalized patients: oxybutynin 5 mg twice a day was no more effective than placebo with scheduled toileting in treating incontinence in this type of population with detrusor hyperactivity. An incontinence profile was used to assess results: the only significant difference noted was an increase in residual urine volume (159 vs 92 ml). Ouslander and colleagues[154] reported similar conclusions in a smaller study of geriatric patients, and in an accompanying article they concluded simply that the drug is safe for use in the elderly at doses of 2.5–5 mg three times a day.[154,155]

A controlled-release (CR) form of oxybutynin has recently been released. This once-daily formulation uses a patented drug-delivery system to release the active compound over a period of 24 hours. This eliminates the serum peaks and troughs that are associated with the three- or four-times-daily dosage regimen of immediate-release (IR) oxybutynin.[156] Aside from the ease of once-daily administration, the potential benefit of the CR formulation is that stabilization of serum levels throughout the day should lower the incidence of side effects. Another theoretical advantage may be that less absorption occurs in the proximal portion of the gastrointestinal tract draining into the portal system so that there is less first-pass metabolism.

IR and CR oxybutynin have been compared in a multicentre randomized double-blind trial of 106 patients, all of whom had previously responded to IR oxybutynin.[157] For patients currently on anticholinergic therapy, after a 1-week washout period, a dose-titration schedule was used to reach the maximum allowable dose (20 mg IR or 30 mg CR daily), or to the dose at which no urge urinary incontinence (UUI) episodes occurred over the course of 2 days (as measured from a diary) or until a dose was reached with intolerable side effects (at which point the final dose was decreased by 5 mg). The primary efficacy parameter was the mean number of UUI episodes as recorded from a 7-day diary while receiving drug therapy. Secondary endpoints included the proportion of patients achieving elimination of UUI episodes, the number of incontinence episodes, the proportion achieving continence, and voiding frequency. Endpoints were compared with baseline parameters obtained at the start of the study after the washout period. Thirteen patients discontinued therapy during the trial, four because of anticholinergic events. Overall, similar efficacy was noted for both formulations of oxybutynin in the overall number of episodes (27.4 to 4.8 for CR and 23.4 to 3.1 for IR), the percentage decrease in weekly UUI episodes (84% [CR] and 88% [IR]), and overall incontinence episodes (urge, stress and mixed). The number and proportion of patients achieving continence was also similar between the groups (41% [CR] and 40% [IR]). Curiously, voiding frequency increased in both groups, with a statistically significant percentage increase of voiding frequency in patients receiving the CR compared with those receiving the IR formulation (54% vs 17%; $p < 0.001$). Anticholinergic side effects were noted in both groups. Dry mouth was the most frequent, occurring in 68% of patients receiving CR oxybutynin and 87% of patients receiving IR oxybutynin ($p = 0.04$). Dry mouth was reported as moderate or severe by 25% and 46% of patients receiving the CR and IR formulations, respectively ($p = 0.03$). Other anticholinergic side effects were reported with similar frequency in the CR and IR groups: somnolence (38% vs 40%), blurred vision (28% vs 17%), constipation (30% vs 31%), dizziness (28% vs 38%), impaired urination (25% vs 29%), nervousness (25% vs 23 %) and nausea (19% vs 17%).

In an open-label trial[158] with 256 patients (23.4 % of whom were on anti-incontinence medication at baseline and switched over to CR oxybutynin for the study), CR oxybutynin reduced the number of incontinence episodes per week from 18.8 at baseline to 2.8 at the end of the study (83.1% reduction); 31% of patients remained free of UUI throughout the study. A 14.7% reduction in voiding frequency was noted on therapy compared with baseline, as measured from the voiding diary. Dry mouth was reported by 58.6% of patients; 23.0% reporting moderate or severe dry mouth. Only 1.6% of patients discontinued therapy because of dry mouth. Overall, 7.8% of patients discontinued therapy because of adverse events of which nausea, dry mouth and somnolence were most frequent.

Topical application of oxybutynin and other agents to normal or intestinal bladders has been suggested and implemented.[159] This conceptually attractive form of alternative drug administration, delivered by periodic intravesical instillation of either liquid or timed-released pellets, awaits further clinical trials and the development of preparations specifically formulated for this purpose. Several non-randomized, unblinded and non-placebo-controlled studies have demonstrated the efficacy of this therapy in a variety of patients with neurogenic bladders, showing statistically significant improvements in cystometric capacity, volume at first IVC, bladder compliance and overall continence.[160–162]

Madersbacher and Jilg reviewed the intravesical usage of oxybutynin and presented data on 13 patients with complete suprasacral cord lesions who were on CIC.[163] One 5 mg tablet was dissolved in 30 ml distilled water and the solution was instilled intravesically. Of the 10 patients who were incontinent, nine remained dry for 6 hours. For the group, the changes in bladder capacity and maximum detrusor pressure were statistically significant. Some of the more interesting data were given in a figure showing plasma oxybutynin levels in a group of patients in whom administration was intravesical or oral. The level following an oral dose rose to 7.3 mg/ml within 2 hours and then precipitously dropped to slightly less than 2 mg/ml at 4 hours. Following intravesical administration, the level rose gradually to a peak of about 6.2 mg/ml at 3.5 hours, but at 6 hours it was still greater than 4 mg/ml and at 9 hours it was still between 3 and 4 mg/ml. From these data it is unclear whether the intravesically applied drug acted locally or systemically.

In a later study, Madersbacher and Knoll[164] administered oxybutynin intravesically and then, one week later, orally in six patients with neurogenic bladders in order to study the pharmacokinetics of the drug and investigate the pharmacological properties responsible for its clinical effects; serum drug levels were correlated with urodynamic effects 20 minutes and 2 hours after administration of the drug. The authors concluded that the main effect of intravesical oxybutynin is due to systemic absorption; however, a secondary direct local effect (smooth muscle relaxation or topical anaesthetic effect) could not be excluded.

Weese and colleagues[165] reported on a similar dose of oxybutynin (5 mg in 30 ml sterile water) to treat 42 patients with IVCs in whom oral anticholinergic therapy had failed (11 patients) or who had intolerable side effects (31 patients): 20 had hyperreflexia, 19 had instability, and three had bowel or bladder hyperactivity after augmentation. The drug was instilled two or three times each day for 10 minutes by catheter. Nine patients (21%) withdrew from the study because they were unable to tolerate CIC or retain the solution properly, but there were no reported side effects. Of the patients (33) who were able to follow the protocol, 18 (55%) reported at least a moderate subjective improvement in incontinence and urgency. Nine patients became totally continent and experienced complete resolution of their symptoms; 18 patients improved and experienced a decrease of 2.5 pads per day. There were no urodynamic data. Follow-up ranged from 5 to 35 months (mean 18.4 months).

The lack of side effects prompted some speculation about the mechanism of drug action: one possibility suggested was simply a more prolonged rate of absorption; another (and more intriguing) one was a decreased pass through the liver and therefore a decrease in metabolites, the hypothesis being that perhaps the metabolites and not the primary compound are responsible for the side effects.

Enzelsberger *et al.*[166] reported on the use of intravesical oxybutynin in the treatment of idiopathic DI in 52 women. In the only randomized double-blind placebo-controlled study published on the use of intravesical oxybutynin, patients received once-daily intravesical oxybutynin (20 mg in 40 ml sterile water) or placebo for 12 days. The results revealed statistically significant differences in first desire to void (from 95 ml [pre-treatment] to 150 ml [post-treatment]), cystometric capacity (205 to 310 ml), maximal pressure during filling (16 to 9 cmH_2O), daytime frequency (7.5 to 4) and nocturia (5.1 to 1.8). Side effects were similar in the treated and placebo groups (17 vs 10%, respectively). For unexplained reasons, 19/23 patients in the treated group continued to have symptomatic relief after termination of the study.

Glickman and colleagues[167] reported on the acute systemic and urodynamic effects of a single instillation of intravesical atropine (6 mg atropine sulphate in 20 ml of normal saline indwelling for 2–4 h) in 12 patients with neurogenic bladder and refractory detrusor hyperreflexia. In the seven patients who did not expel the solution shortly after instillation, statistically significant increases in volume to first IVC (from 199 to 389 ml), cystometric bladder capacity (256 to 587 ml) and bladder compliance (36 to 78 ml/cmH_2O) were noted, with a statistically significant fall in the maximum pressure recorded during IVCs (from 50 to 26 cmH_2O). No systemic effects were noted as a result of intravesical atropine, including no changes in pupillary reactions, blood pressure or pulse. Since atropine sulphate is readily available in a liquid form, it may lend itself to easier administration than intravesical oxybutynin. The mechanism of action, ideal dose, duration of action, long-term efficacy, effects on the non-neurogenic bladder or efficacy of intravesical atropine when diluted with urine are, as yet, unknown.

With regard to the subject of hyperactivity in augmented or intestinal neobladders, for which there is no separate section in this chapter, Andersson and colleagues[168] recently reviewed this phenomenon and its pharmacological treatment, and noted few instances of positive results with agents given systemically. Locally applied agents were thought to offer more promise. A list of possibilities and their assessments was included. Pure anticholinergics have not produced good results, either locally or systemically. Oxybutynin has shown poor results with systemic therapy but some good results with local therapy. α-Agonists have produced no effect; β-agonists have shown no local effects and equivocal effects when administered subcutaneously, but the comment was made that such use will probably be limited by side effects. Other possibilities mentioned for future use included opioid agonists (diphenoxylate – a component of Lomotil – and loperamide), calcium antagonists, potassium-channel openers and NO donors.

Dicyclomine hydrochloride is also reported to exert a direct relaxant effect on smooth muscle in addition to an antimuscarinic action.[169] An oral dose of 20 mg three times a day in adults has been reported to increase bladder capacity in patients with detrusor hyperreflexia.[170] Beck and co-workers[171] compared the use of 10 mg dicyclomine, 15 mg propantheline and placebo three times a day in patients with detrusor hyperactivity:[167] the cure or improved rates, respectively, were 62, 73 and

20%. Awad and associates[172] reported that 20 mg dicyclomine three times a day caused resolution or significant improvement in 24 of 27 patients with IVCs.

Flavoxate hydrochloride has a direct inhibitory action on smooth muscle but very weak anticholinergic properties.[109,173] In cats, at least, there is some evidence that flavoxate may also have central effects on the inhibition of the micturition reflex in addition to its effects on the relaxation of smooth muscle.[174] Overall favourable clinical effects have been noted in some series of patients with frequency, urgency and incontinence and in patients with urodynamically documented detrusor hyperreflexia.[175,176] However, Briggs and colleagues[177] reported that this drug had essentially no effect on detrusor hyperreflexia in an elderly population, an experience that coincides with the laboratory effects obtained by Benson and associates.[178] The recommended adult dosage is 100–200 mg three or four times a day. As with all agents in this group, a short clinical trial may be worthwhile. Reported side effects are few.

Trospium and propiverine are classified as predominantly antispasmodic agents (smooth muscle relaxants) with some anticholinergic effects as well. Both drugs have been used in Europe for several years, but are not currently available in the United States. In a randomized placebo-controlled study, Stohrer and associates[179] looked at the effects of 20 mg trospium twice daily on 61 patients with detrusor hyperreflexia over a 3-week period. Only six patients withdrew from the study – four in the placebo group and two in the treated group, neither of which was treatment related (according to the authors). Statistically significant improvements in maximum cystometric capacity (increased capacity of 138.1 vs 2.5 ml, treated vs placebo group, respectively), maximum detrusor pressure (decreased 37.8 vs 1.9 cmH₂O, treated vs placebo group, respectively) and compliance (increased 12.1 vs 2.7 ml/cmH₂O treated vs placebo group, respectively) were noted. Only one patient in the study spontaneously reported dry mouth as an adverse effect, and this was in the placebo group! Other adverse effects reported included constipation (three patients, two in the placebo group), reduced exercise tolerance, nausea and tiredness (one event each, all in the placebo group). Madersbacher and colleagues[180] compared trospium with oxybutynin in a randomized double-blind (but not placebo-controlled) study of 95 patients with detrusor hyperreflexia: there were improvements in maximum bladder capacity, max-

imum voiding pressure and compliance, but there were no significant differences between the two drugs with regard to any of the outcome parameters. The proportion of patients reporting dry mouth, when asked specifically about this adverse effect, was similar (54% in both groups). The most common reason cited for withdrawal from the study (a total of 10 patients withdrew, three in the trospium arm) were 'typical' anticholinergic side effects.

Propiverine is a musculotropic smooth muscle relaxant with anticholinergic activity. Propiverine has been described by Haruno[181] as inhibiting spontaneous or agonist-induced bladder contractility in various preparations by either an anticholinergic or a calcium-channel blocking effect; it has relative selectivity (10–100 times) for bladder and ileum. There is a single clinical study in the English-language literature using propiverine which was neither double blind nor placebo controlled:[182] 185 patients were divided into four groups and received the medication at divided daily doses of 15, 30, 45 or 60 mg for a total of 21 days. Bladder capacity and compliance improved in a dose-dependent fashion, with the most favourable ratio of efficacy to tolerability occurring at the 15 and 30 mg dosages. Adverse reactions were primarily anticholinergic in nature and similar to those with other drugs of this type.

Calcium antagonists

The role of calcium as a messenger in linking extracellular stimuli to the intracellular environment is well established, including its involvement in excitation–contraction coupling in striated, cardiac and smooth muscle.[1,5] The dependence of contractile activity on changes in cytosolic calcium varies from tissue to tissue, as do the characteristics of the calcium channels involved, but interference with calcium inflow or intracellular release is a very potent potential mechanism for bladder smooth muscle relaxation.

Nifedipine has been shown to be an effective inhibitor of contraction induced by several mechanisms in human and guinea pig bladder muscle.[109,183] It has also been shown to block completely the non-cholinergic portion of the contraction produced by electrical field stimulation in rabbit bladder.[184] Nifedipine more effectively inhibited those contractions induced by potassium than those by carbachol in rabbit bladder strips, whereas terodiline, an agent with both calcium-antagonistic and anticholinergic properties, had the opposite effect. However, terodiline did cause complete inhibition of the response of rabbit bladder to electrical field stimulation. At low concentrations, terodiline has mainly an antimuscarinic action, whereas at higher concentration a calcium-antagonistic effect becomes evident. Experiments *in vitro* appeared to show that these two effects were at least additive with regard to bladder contractility. Other experimental studies have confirmed the inhibitory effect of the calcium antagonists nifedipine, verapamil and diltiazem on a variety of experimental models of the activity of spontaneous and induced bladder muscle strips and whole bladder preparations.[185,186] Andersson and colleagues[187] showed that nifedipine effectively (and with some selectivity) inhibited the non-muscarinic portion of the contraction of rabbit detrusor strips, whereas verapamil, diltiazem, flunarizine and lidoflazine caused a marked depression of both the total and the non-muscarinic parts of contraction, suggesting that differences exist between various calcium-channel blockers with respect to their effects on at least electrically induced bladder muscle contraction. These results were used as support for the view that, even if 'atropine-resistant' contractions in rabbit and human bladder had different causes, combined muscarinic-receptor and calcium-channel blockade might offer a more effective way of treating bladder hyperactivity than the single-mechanism therapies currently available. Bodner and colleagues[188] treated 14 spinal cord injury patients with detrusor hyperreflexia who complained of intolerable side effects of oxybutynin alone with oxybutynin and sustained-release verapamil. Although the study was neither blinded nor placebo controlled, 13/14 patients were improved (outcome parameters included volume to first IVC and episodes of urinary leakage) with the combination of oxybutynin and verapamil over oxybutynin alone; the statistical significance of the results was not provided; five patients were able to lower their dose of oxybutynin while on combination therapy, with sustained clinical improvement. Episodes of autonomic dysreflexia were improved in three patients on combined therapy. The authors reported that the combination therapy was better tolerated than oxybutynin alone (including dry mouth), although quantitative data were not included.

A number of clinical studies on the inhibitory action of terodiline on bladder hyperactivity have shown clinical effectiveness.[189] In a double-blind crossover study of 12 women with motor urge incontinence, Ekman and colleagues[190] reported increases in bladder capacity and the volume at which sensation of urgency was experienced in all but one of the patients treated with terodiline, whereas placebo treatment had no objective or subjective effect. Peters and associates[191] reported the results of a multicentre study that ultimately included data from 89 patients (from an original 128) and compared terodiline and placebo in women with motor urge incontinence. The daily dose in this study was 12.5 mg in the morning and 25 mg at night. The authors concluded that terodiline was more effective than placebo, but noted that this improvement was much more apparent on subjective than on objective assessment of cystometric and micturition data; 63% of patients preferred terodiline, regardless of treatment sequence; although statistically significant objective differences between terodiline and placebo were recorded, they were not very impressive. Tapp and colleagues[192] reported on a double-blind placebo study, using a dose-titration technique, that included 70 women with urodynamically proven DI and bladder capacities of less than 400 ml. Of the 34 women in the terodiline group. 62% considered themselves improved, and 38% were unchanged; of the 36 women in the placebo group, 42% considered themselves improved, 47% unchanged and 11% worse – a statistically significant response in favour of terodiline with regard to the improvement percentage. Micturition variables of daytime frequency, daytime incontinence episodes, number of pads used and average voided volumes were statistically changed in favour of terodiline, but the absolute changes were relatively small (for instance, a change in daytime incontinence episodes in patients on placebo from 2.5 to 1.9 per day as opposed to 3.7–1.6 for those taking terodiline). Urodynamic data, although showing a trend in favour of terodiline in each parameter, showed no statistically significant differences in any category. Side effects were noted in a large number and with equal frequency in both groups after the dose-titration phase. However, the incidence of anticholinergic side effects was higher in the drug group: 29% of the terodiline patients vs 11% of the placebo patients spontaneously complained of a dry mouth, and 20% of the terodiline patients but none of the placebo patients complained of blurred vision. The AHCPR guidelines[126] list seven randomized controlled trials for terodiline; 94% of patients were women. The percentage of cures (all figures refer to percentage minus percentage on placebo) is listed as 18–33%, percentage of reduction in urge incontinence as 14–83%, and the percentages of side effects and dropouts are 14–40% and 2–8%, respectively.

Terodiline also exhibits an inhibitory effect on experimental hyperreflexia in the rabbit whole-bladder model, suggesting a possible role for local administration as well.[193] Terodiline is almost completely absorbed from the gastrointestinal tract and has a low serum clearance. The recommended dosage in adults is 25 mg twice a day, reduced to an initial dose of 12 mg twice a day in geriatric patients. The half-life is around 60 hours and Abrams[197] logically proposes, on this basis, a once-daily dose but emphasizes the necessity of dose titration for each patient. The common side effects seen with calcium antagonists (hypotension, facial flushing, headache, dizziness, abdominal discomfort, constipation, nausea, rash, weakness and palpitations) have not been reported in larger initial clinical studies with terodiline, side effects consisting primarily of those consequent on its anticholinergic action. However, questions have been raised about the occurrence of a rare arrhythmia (torsade de pointes) in patients taking terodiline simultaneously with antidepressants or antiarrhythmic drugs.[194,195] Stewart and colleagues[196] reported a prolongation of QT and QTC intervals and a reduction in heart rate in elderly patients taking 12.5 mg terodiline twice a day; these effects were apparent after 1 week but not after 1 day of therapy. These investigators also reported polymorphic ventricular tachycardia in four patients (three over age 80) receiving the drug. They advised avoidance of the drug in patients with cardiac disease requiring cardioactive drugs or those with hypokalaemia, or in combination with other drugs that can prolong the QT interval, such as tricyclic antidepressants or antipsychotics. After other reports of apparent cardiac toxicity, the drug was voluntarily withdrawn by the manufacturer pending the results of further safety studies. The studies conducted for approval by the Food and Drug Administration (FDA) were likewise voluntarily halted by the manufacturer; current activity is directed towards their reinstitution.

Other calcium-antagonist drugs have not been widely used to treat voiding dysfunction. Palmer and colleagues[197] reported a double-blind placebo trial with a single daily dose of 20 mg flunarizine in 14 women with DI and consequent symptoms. A statistically signif-

icant decrease in urgency was produced in the drug-treated group, but there was no change in the frequency of micturition. Although a trend toward improvement of cystometric parameters occurred, it was not statistically significant ($p > 0.05$). Nifedipine is useful as prophylaxis against the development of autonomic hyperreflexia during endoscopic examination in patients with high spinal injury: a 10 mg dose given 30 minutes prior to the examination or a sublingual dose of 10 mg has been effective in relieving an episode.[198]

Potassium-channel openers

Potassium-channel openers efficiently relax various types of smooth muscle by increasing potassium efflux, resulting in membrane hyperpolarization.[109] Hyperpolarization reduces the opening probability of ion channels involved in membrane depolarization, and excitation is reduced. Andersson[199] summarized studies showing that, in isolated human and animal detrusor muscle, potassium-channel openers reduce spontaneous contractions and contractions occurring in response to electrical stimulation, carbachol and low (but not high) external potassium concentrations. There are some suggestions that bladder instability – at least that associated with intravesical obstruction and detrusor hypertrophy – may be secondary to supersensitivity to depolarizing stimuli. Theoretically, then, potassium-channel openers might be an attractive alternative for the treatment of DI in such circumstances without inhibiting the normal voluntary contractions necessary for bladder emptying.[200] Pinacidil is a compound that, in a concentration-dependent fashion, inhibits not only spontaneous myogenic contractions but also contractile responses induced by electrical field stimulation and carbachol in isolated human detrusor[201] and in normal and hypertrophied rat detrusor mucle. Unfortunately, a preliminary study of this agent in a double-blind crossover format produced no effects on symptoms in nine patients with DI and bladder outlet obstruction.[202] Nurse and associates[203] reported on the use of cromakalim, another potassium-channel opener, in 17 patients who had refractory DI or hyperreflexia or had stopped other drug therapy because of intolerable side effects. Six of 16 (37.5%) patients who completed the study showed a decrease in frequency and an increase in voided volume. Long-term observation was not possible because the drug was withdrawn owing to reported adverse effects of high doses in animal toxicology studies. Levcromakalim (the pharmacologically active enantiomer of cromakalim) was administered intravenously to six patients with high spinal cord lesions and reflex micturition:[204] other than an increase in the duration of the detrusor contraction, no other urodynamic parameters associated with the detrusor hyperreflexia were significantly affected. Levcromakalim resulted in a rapid and significant drop in blood pressure which precluded studies at a higher dose. Overall, potassium-channel openers are not at present very specific for the bladder and are more potent in relaxing other tissues – hence their potential utility in the treatment of hypertension, asthma and angina. If tissue-selective potassium-activator drugs can be developed, they may prove very useful for the treatment of DI, irritable bowel syndrome and epilepsy.[205] Intravesical use has also been suggested[204,205] as a method of potentially eliminating some of the intolerable systemic side effects that limit the clinical utility of these agents.

Side effects of pinacidil have been studied best: they include headache, peripheral oedema (in 25–50% of patients and dose related), weight gain, palpitations, dizziness and rhinitis. Hypertrichosis and symptomatic T-wave changes have also been reported (30%). Fewer data are available on cromakalim, which can produce dose-related headache but rarely oedema.[199]

Prostaglandin inhibitors

PGs are ubiquitous compounds that have a potential role in the excitatory neurotransmission to the bladder, the development of bladder contractility or tension occurring during filling, the emptying contractile response of bladder smooth muscle to neural stimulation, and even the maintenance of urethral tone during the storage phase of micturition, as well as the release of this tone during the emptying phase (see references 1 and 5 for discussion and references). Downie and Karmazyn[207] suggest a different type of contractile influence of PGs on detrusor muscle. They found that mechanical irritation of the epithelium of rabbit bladder increased basal tension and spontaneous activity in response to electrical stimulation and that these responses, related to the intensity of the irritative trauma, were mimicked by PGs. The effect was significantly reduced by pretreatment of the epithelium, but not the muscle, with PG synthetase inhibitors. Andersson[109] suggests a possible sensitization of sensory afferent nerves by PGs, increasing afferent input at a given degree of bladder filling and contributing to the triggering of IVCs at a small bladder volume. Thus, there are many mechanisms whereby PG synthesis inhibitors might decrease bladder contractility in response to various stimuli; however, objective evidence that such can occur is scant.

Cardozo and colleagues[208] reported a double-blind placebo study on the effects of 50 mg flurbiprofen (a PG synthetase inhibitor) three times a day on 30 women with DI. They concluded that the drug did not abolish IVCs or abnormal bladder activity but did delay the intravesical pressure rise to a greater degree of distension. Of these patients, 43% experienced side effects – primarily nausea, vomiting, headache, indigestion, gastric distress, constipation and rash. Cardozo and Stanton[209] reported symptomatic improvement in patients with DI who were given indomethacin in doses of 50–200 mg daily, but this was a short-term study with no cystometric data, and the drug was compared only with bromocriptine. The incidence of side effects was high (19 of 32 patients), although no patient had to stop treatment because of them. Numerous PG synthetase inhibitors exist, most of which belong in the category of non-steroidal anti-inflammatory drugs, and every clinician has a favourite. It should be remembered that these drugs can interfere with platelet function and contribute to excess bleeding in surgical patients; some may also have adverse renal effects.[210]

β-Adrenergic agonists

The presence of β-adrenoceptors in human bladder muscle has prompted attempts to increase bladder capacity with β-adrenergic stimulation. Such stimulation can cause significant increases in the capacity of animal bladders, which contain a moderate density of β-adrenoceptors.[1] Studies *in vitro* show a strong dose-related relaxant effect of $β_2$-agonists on the bladder body of rabbits but little effect on the bladder base or proximal urethra. Terbutaline, in oral doses of 5 mg three times a day, has been reported to have a 'good clinical effect' in some patients with urgency and urgency incontinence, but no significant effect on the bladders of neurologically normal humans without voiding difficulty.[211] Although these results are compatible with those seen in other organ systems (β-adrenergic stimulation causes no acute change in total lung capacity in normal humans but does favourably affect patients with bronchial asthma), there are few adequate studies of the effects of β-adrenergic stimulation in patients with detrusor hyperactivity. Lindholm and Lose[212] used 5 mg terbutaline three times a day in eight women with motor and seven with sensory urge incontinence: after 3 months of treatment, 14 patients claimed to have experienced beneficial effects, and 12 became subjectively continent. In six of eight cases, the detrusor became stable on cystometric examination. The volume at first desire to void increased in the patients with originally unstable bladders from a mean of 200 to 302 ml, but the maximum cystometric capacity did not change. Nine patients had transient side effects – including palpitations, tachycardia or hand tremor – and in three of these the side effects continued but were acceptable to the patient. The drug was discontinued in one patient because of severe adverse symptoms. Gruneberger,[213] in a double-blind study, reported that clenbuterol had produced a good therapeutic effect in 15 of 20 patients with motor urge incontinence. Unfavourable results of β-agonist usage for bladder hyperactivity were published by Castleden and Morgan[214] and Naglo and associates.[215]

Tricyclic antidepressants

Many clinicians have found that tricyclic antidepressants, particularly imipramine hydrochloride, are especially useful for facilitating urine storage, both by decreasing bladder contractility and by increasing outlet resistance.[9] These agents have been the subject of extensive and highly sophisticated pharmacological investigation to determine the mechanisms of action responsible for their varied effects.[83,216,217] Most data have been accumulated as a result of trying to explain the antidepressant properties of these agents and consequently involve primarily CNS tissue. Although the results, conclusions and speculations based on the data are extremely interesting, it should be emphasized that it is essentially unknown whether they apply to, or have relevance for, the lower urinary tract. In varying degrees, all of these agents have at least three major pharmacological actions: they have central and peripheral anticholinergic effects at some (but not all) sites; they block the active transport system in the presynaptic nerve ending that is responsible for the reuptake of the released amine neurotransmitters noradrenaline and serotonin; and they are sedatives, an action that occurs presumably on a central basis but is perhaps related to

antihistaminic properties (at H_1 receptors, although they also antagonize H_2 receptors to some extent). There is also evidence that these agents desensitize at least some α_2- and some β_2-adrenoceptors. Paradoxically, they also have been shown to block some α- and serotonin-1 receptors. Imipramine has prominent systemic anticholinergic effects but only a weak antimuscarinic effect on bladder smooth muscle.[218,219] It does have a strong direct inhibitory effect on bladder smooth muscle, however, that is neither anticholinergic nor adrenergic.[175,216,220] This may be due to a local-anaesthetic-like action at the nerve terminals in the adjacent effector membrane – an effect that seems to occur also in cardiac muscle,[221] – or it may be due to an inhibition of the participation of calcium in the excitation–contraction coupling process.[218,220] Akah[223] has provided supportive evidence in the rat bladder that desipramine, the active metabolite of imipramine, depresses the response to electrical field stimulation by interfering with calcium movement (perhaps not only extracellular calcium movement but also internal translocation and binding). Direct evidence suggesting that the effect of imipramine on noradrenaline reuptake occurs in lower urinary tract tissue as well as brain tissue has been provided by Foreman and McNulty[224] in the rabbit. In addition, they describe a significantly greater but similar effect of tomoxetine in the bladder and urethra in this model. Tomoxetine inhibits noradrenaline reuptake selectively, whereas imipramine has a non-selective effect. This fact suggests a potential new clinical approach to the use of more selective and potent reuptake inhibitors for the treatment of incontinence. In attempting to correlate clinical effects with mechanisms of action, one might also postulate a β-receptor-induced decrease in bladder body contractility if peripheral blockade of noradrenaline reuptake does occur there owing to the increased concentration of β-receptors compared with α-adrenoceptors in that area. An enhanced α-adrenergic effect in the smooth muscle of the bladder base and proximal urethra, where α-receptors outnumber β-receptors, is generally considered the mechanism whereby imipramine increases outlet resistance.

Clinically, imipramine seems to be effective in decreasing bladder contractility and increasing outlet resistance.[225–228] Castleden and colleagues[228] began therapy in elderly patients with DI with a single 25 mg night-time dose of imipramine, which was increased every third day by 25 mg until the patient either was continent or had side effects, or a dose of 150 mg was reached. Six of 10 patients became continent and, in those who underwent repeated cystometry, bladder capacity increased by a mean of 105 ml and bladder pressure at capacity decreased by a mean of 18 cmH$_2$O. MUP increased by a mean of 30 cmH$_2$O. Although our subjective impression[226] was that the bladder effects became evident only after days of treatment, some patients in the Castleden series became continent after only 3–5 days of therapy. Our usual adult dose for treatment of voiding dysfunction is 25 mg four times a day; less-frequent administration is possible because of the drug's long half-life. Half that dose is given in elderly patients, in whom the drug half-life may be prolonged. In our experience, the effects of imipramine on the lower urinary tract are often additive to those of atropine-like agents; consequently, a combination of imipramine and an antimuscarinic or an antispasmodic is sometimes especially useful for decreasing bladder contractility.[226] If imipramine is used in conjunction with an atropine-like agent, it should be noted that the anticholinergic side effects of the drugs may be additive.

It has been known for many years that imipramine is relatively effective for the treatment of nocturnal enuresis in children. Doses for this condition range from 10 to 50 mg daily. It is not known whether the mechanisms of drug action in this situation are the same as those for decreasing bladder contractility. Korczyn and Kish[229] have presented evidence that the mechanism of the antienuretic effect differs from that of the peripheral anticholinergic effect and the drug's antidepressant effect. The antienuretic effect occurs soon after initial administration, whereas the antidepressant effects generally take 2–4 weeks to develop.

Doxepin is another tricyclic antidepressant that has been found (using rabbit-bladder strips *in vitro*) to be more potent than other tricyclic compounds with respect to antimuscarinic and musculotropic relaxant activity.[220] Lose and colleagues,[230] in a randomized double-blind crossover study of women with IVCs and frequency, urgency or urge incontinence, found that this agent caused a significant decrease in control over night-time frequency and incontinence episodes and a near-significant decrease in urine loss (by the pad-weighing test) and in the cystometric parameters of first sensation and maximum bladder capacity. The dose of doxepin used was either a single 50 mg bedtime dose or this dose plus an additional 25 mg in the morning. The number of daytime incontinence episodes decreased in both doxepin and placebo groups, and the difference was not statistically significant. Doxepin treatment was preferred by 14 patients, whereas two preferred placebo; three patients had no preference. Of the 14 patients who stated a preference for doxepin, 12 claimed that they became continent during treatment and two claimed improvement; the two patients who preferred placebo also claimed improvement. The AHCPR guidelines[126] combine results for imipramine and doxepin, citing only three randomized controlled trials, with an unknown percentage of women patients. The percentage of cures (all figures refer to percentage minus the percentage on placebo) are listed as 31%, percentage of reduction in urge incontinence as 20–88%, and percentage of side effects as 0–70%.

Duloxetine, a combined serotonin- and noradrenaline-reuptake inhibitor, may enhance the storage ability of the lower urinary tract. This relatively new pharmacological agent has been used clinically as an antidepressant.[231] In a study of its effects on the lower urinary tract in the cat, Thor and Katofiasc[232] noted that duloxetine significantly increased bladder capacity (probably through a CNS effect), as well as enhanced external urethral sphincter activity. At present, no human clinical trials have been reported.

When the tricyclic antidepressants are used in the generally larger doses employed for antidepressant effects, their most frequent side effects are those attributable to their systemic anticholinergic activity.[83,217] Allergic phenomena – including rash, hepatic dysfunction, obstructive jaundice, and agranulocytosis – may also occur but are rare. CNS side effects may include weakness, fatigue, parkinsonian effects, fine tremors (noted mostly in the upper extremities) a manic or schizophrenic picture and sedation, probably from an antihistaminic effect. Postural hypotension may also be seen, presumably due to selective blockade (a paradoxical effect) of α$_1$-adrenoceptors in some vascular smooth muscle. Tricyclic antidepressants may also cause excess sweating of obscure origin and a delay in orgasm or orgasmic impotence, the cause of which is likewise unclear. They may also produce arrhythmias and can interact in deleterious ways with other drugs; thus, caution must be observed in using these drugs in patients with cardiac disease.[83] Whether cardiotoxicity will prove to be a legitimate concern in patients receiving smaller doses (smaller than those used for treatment of depression) for lower urinary tract dysfunction remains to be seen, but is a matter of potential concern. Consultation with a patient's physician or cardiologist is always helpful before such therapy is instituted in questionable situations. The use of imipramine is contraindicated in patients receiving monoamine oxidase inhibitors because severe CNS toxicity can be precipitated, including hyperpyrexia, seizures and coma. Some potential side effects of antidepressants may be especially significant in the elderly – specifically weakness, fatigue and postural hypotension. If imipramine or any of the tricyclic antidepressants is to be prescribed for the treatment of voiding dysfunction, the patient should be thoroughly informed about the fact that this is *not* the usual indication for this drug and that potential side effects exist. Reports of significant side effects (severe abdominal distress, nausea, vomiting, headache, lethargy and irritability) following abrupt cessation of high doses of imipramine in children suggest that the drug should be discontinued gradually, especially in patients receiving high doses.

Dimethyl sulphoxide (DMSO)

DMSO is a relatively simple, naturally occurring organic compound that has been used as an industrial solvent for many years. It has multiple pharmacological actions (membrane penetration, anti-inflammatory, local analgesic, bacteriostatic, diuretic, cholinesterase inhibitor, collagen solvent, vasodilator) and has been used for the treatment of arthritis and other musculoskeletal disorders, generally in a 70% solution. The formulation for human intravesical use is a 50% solution. Sant[233] has summarized the pharmacology and clinical usage of DMSO and has tabulated good-to-excellent results in 50–90% of collected series of patients treated with intravesical instillations for interstitial cystitis. However, DMSO has not been shown to be useful in the treatment of detrusor hyperreflexia or DI, or in any patient with urgency or frequency but without interstitial cystitis.

Polysynaptic inhibitors

Baclofen has been discussed previously with agents that decrease outlet resistance secondary to striated sphincter dyssynergia (page 370). It is also capable of

depressing detrusor hyperreflexia due to spinal cord injury.[234] Taylor and Bates[235], in a double-blind crossover study, reported that it was very effective in decreasing both day and night urinary frequency and incontinence in patients with idiopathic instability. Cystometric changes were not recorded, however, and considerable improvement was also obtained in the placebo group. The intrathecal use of baclofen for treatment of detrusor hyperactivity is a potentially exciting area (see prior discussion), and further reports are awaited.

Other potential agents

NO is hypothesized to be a mediator of the NANC relaxation of the outlet smooth muscle that occurs with bladder contraction.[5] Evidence exists that it is also involved in relaxation of bladder body smooth muscle,[236] and this provides interesting fodder for speculation – is relaxation impaired in some types of hyperactivity and can NO analogues or synthetase stimulators be developed as agents to inhibit detrusor contractility? Glyceryl trinitrate releases NO *in vivo* and achieves its cardiovascular effects by relaxing vascular smooth muscle. A pilot study of 10 patients with instability given transdermal NO showed significant decreases in episodes (per 24 hours) of frequency (from 9.7 to 6.7), nocturia (from 1.84 to 1.09), and incontinence (from 0.6 to 0.36).[234] Although the ubiquity of NO might seem to mitigate its potential use in treating bladder hyperactivity (unless more organ-specific substrates or receptors are found), randomized controlled trials should be conducted.

Soulard and colleagues[238] have described the effects of JO 1870 on bladder activity in the rat. This non-anticholinergic probable opioid agonist increased bladder capacity and threshold pressure responsible for micturition in a dose-dependent fashion, raising the possibility of the use or development of opioid agonists with selectivity for receptors involved in the micturition reflex.

Constantinou[239,240] described the effects of thiphenamil hydrochloride on the lower urinary tract of healthy female volunteers and those with detrusor incontinence. This drug was said to be a 'synthetic antispasmodic'. In a randomized controlled trial, based on diary records from 14 patients with instability, it was reported that voiding frequency per day decreased significantly (from 10.3 to 8.0 times), but placebo values were not given. Daily incontinence episodes decreased in nine analysable patients from 2.3 to 1.6 (not significant, placebo values not given), with pad dryness (rated on a 0–4 scale) improving from 1.6 to 1.2 (significant, but no placebo data given). Objective urodynamic results (in 16 patients) showed no flowmetry changes, no changes in bladder capacity, some increase in first sensation of fullness, and a significant decrease in detrusor voiding pressure (from 46.1 to 31.9 cmH$_2$O) over placebo. The data and interpretation in this article are confusing, especially because the study of healthy volunteers showed no urodynamic differences except an *increase* in maximum flow rate (from 16.9 to 27.7 ml/s) at a drug dose of 800 mg. The most that can be said about the clinical use of thiphenamil is that, now a question has been raised, it needs to be addressed by further 'cleaner' studies with internally consistent results.

Increasing bladder capacity by decreasing sensory (afferent) input

Capsaicin

Decreasing afferent input peripherally is the ideal treatment for both sensory urgency and instability or hyperreflexia in a bladder with relatively normal elastic or viscoelastic properties in which the sensory afferents constitute the first limb in the abnormal micturition reflex. Maggi has written extensively about this type of treatment, specifically with reference to the properties of capsaicin.[241–243] This drug is an irritant and algogenic compound obtained from hot red peppers that has highly selective effects on a subset of mammalian sensory neurons, including polymodal receptors and warm thermoreceptors.[244] Capsaicin produces pain by selectively activating polymodal nociceptive neurons by membrane depolarization and opening a cation-selective ion channel, which can be blocked by ruthenium red. Repeated administration induces desensitization and inactivation of sensory neurons by several mechanisms. Systemic and topical capsaicin produce a reversible antinociceptive and anti-inflammatory action after an initially undesirable algesic effect. Local or topical application blocks C-fibre conduction and inactivates neuropeptide release from peripheral nerve endings, accounting for local antinociception and reduction of neurogenic inflammation. Systemic capsaicin produces antinociception by activating specific receptors on afferent nerve terminals in the spinal cord; spinal neurotransmission is subsequently blocked by a prolonged inactivation of sensory neurotransmitter release. With local administration (intravesical), the potential advantage of capsaicin is a lack of systemic side effects. The actions are highly specific when the drug is applied locally – the compound affects primarily small-diameter nociceptive afferents, leaving the sensations of touch and pressure unchanged, although heat (not cold) perception may be reduced; motor fibres are not affected.[245] The effects are reversible, although it is not known whether initial levels of sensitivity are regained. Craft and Porreca[245] list intravesical doses in the rat as 0.03–10.0 µM for 15–30 minutes and in humans a maximum of 1–2 mM.

Maggi[243] reviewed the therapeutic potential of capsaicin-like molecules. Capsaicin-sensitive primary afferents (CSPAs) innervate the human bladder, and intravesical instillation of capsaicin into human bladder produces a concentration-dependent decrease in first desire to void, decreased bladder capacity and a warm burning sensation. Maggi[241] used doses of 0.01, 1.0 and 10 µM, administered in ascending order at intervals of 10–15 minutes as constant infusions of 20 ml/min until micturition occurred. Five capsaicin-treated patients with 'hypersensitive disorder' reported either a complete disappearance of symptoms (four patients) or marked attenuation of symptoms (one patient), beginning 2–3 days after administration and lasting for 4–16 days; after that time the symptoms gradually reappeared but were no worse. Fowler and colleagues[104] found that considerably higher doses (up to 1–2 mM for 30 min) were necessary to produce an effect in humans;[103] however, these investigators reported that bladder control improved within 2 days, and the improvement lasted for 3–6 months. Lower doses (0.1–100 µM) produced 'no long lasting benefit'. In a later study, Fowler and colleagues[246] administered intravesical capsaicin to 14 patients with detrusor overactivity and intractable urinary incontinence, 12 of whom had known spinal cord disease. A single intravesical instillation of 1 or 2 mmol capsaicin revealed a response in nine patients (all of whom had spinal cord disease), with four of these patients having only a 'partial' response and five patients having complete and durable (3 weeks to 6 months) responses, defined as complete continence on intermittent catheterization. In the nine patients who responded to treatment, mean bladder capacity increased from 106 to 302 ml and maximum detrusor pressure decreased from 54 to

36 cmH$_2$O. There were no long-term adverse effects from the therapy. Similar results were noted by Das and colleagues,[247] who treated seven patients with neurogenic bladders with four increasing doses of intravesical capsaicin over a period of several weeks (100 µmol, 500 µmol, 1 mmol and 2 mmol). Only five of seven patients were able to complete the therapy, owing to the discomfort induced by the instillation. Of these five patients, three had symptomatic and urodynamic improvement. Geirsson and associates[248] treated 10 patients with traumatic spinal cord injury and neurogenic bladder with 2 mmol intravesical capsaicin; urodynamic improvement (decreased voiding pressure and increased bladder capacity) was noted in 9/10 patients at 6 weeks. Subjective improvement was noted in 4/10 patients at 2–7 months after therapy, two of whom became continent. All 10 patients had no improvement or a worsening of symptoms during the first 1–2 weeks after instillation. Adverse reactions included severe burning on instillation in those patients with partial spinal lesions, precipitation of autonomic dysreflexia in several other patients and gross haematuria in four patients. Chandiramani and colleagues[249] were able to reduce significantly the short-term toxicity (triggering of involuntary detrusor contractions) and discomfort of intravesical capsaicin therapy by pretreatment with an instillation of 2% topical lignocaine. Pretreatment with lignocaine did not alter the therapeutic efficacy of the capsaicin.

An *efferent* function of CSPAs is the release of neurotransmitters from the peripheral endings of these sensory neurons, such as tachykinins and calcitonin gene-related peptide.[243] These neurotransmitters can produce events collectively known as neurogenic inflammation, which can include smooth muscle contractions, increased plasma protein extravasation, vasodilatation, mast cell degranulation, facilitation of transmitter release from nerve terminals, and recruitment of inflammatory cells. This is another reason why intravesical capsaicin could theoretically be useful in treating the pain and related problems of interstitial cystitis and certain types of bladder hyperactivity that originate in primary afferents.

The peripheral terminals of CSPAs form a dense plexus just below the bladder urothelium, and fibres penetrating the urothelium come into contact with the lumen. This location, combined with their peculiar chemosensitivity permits CSPAs to detect 'backflow' of chemicals across the urothelium, which is thought to occur during conditions leading to breakdown of the 'barrier function' of the urothelium.[243] If the 'barrier' theory or 'leaky urothelium' theory of the pathogenesis of the interstitial cystitis is true, for some or many of the patients with this condition, the CSPAs in such patients may be stimulated by urine constituents leaking back across the urothelium, and, under these circumstances, a local release of neuropeptides may well contribute to the production of neurogenic inflammation. If this is so, as Maggi suggests,[243] a local treatment leading to desensitization of CSPAs would be doubly advantageous. With capsaicin, however, excitation precedes desensitization, somewhat limiting the potential for therapy in humans. A preferable analogue would produce the latter action while reducing or eliminating the former. Last, Maggi[243] discusses the possible long-term disadvantages of such therapy as related to the potential physiological roles – trophic or protective – of CSPAs and their secretions in response to stimulation.

Overall, intravesical capsaicin treatment may be a promising therapy for detrusor overactivity, and possibly sensory dysfunction of the lower urinary tract; however, many problems exist. Optimal dosage, method and timing of delivery as well as delivery vehicle (diluent) remain unclear. The patients likely to respond to this therapy are not yet defined, and randomized placebo-controlled studies to determine overall efficacy have not yet been performed. Finally, discomfort and triggering of involuntary bladder activity with instillation and post-instillation gross haematuria may be problematic.

Increasing outlet resistance

α-Adrenergic agonists

The bladder neck and proximal urethra contain a preponderance of α-adrenergic receptor sites, which, when stimulated, produce smooth muscle contraction.[1,2,5] The static infusion urethral pressure profile is altered by such stimulation, producing an increase in MUP and maximum urethral closure pressure (MUCP). Various orally administered pharmacological agents producing α-adrenergic stimulation are available. Generally, outlet resistance is increased to a variable degree by such an action. The potential side effects of all these agents include blood pressure elevation, anxiety and insomnia due to stimulation of the CNS, headache, tremor, weakness, palpitations, cardiac arrhythmia and respiratory difficulties. All such agents should be used with caution in patients with hypertension, cardiovascular disease or hyperthyroidism.[251]

The use of ephedrine to treat SUI was mentioned as early as 1948.[251] This is a non-catecholamine sympathomimetic agent that enhances release of noradrenaline from sympathetic neurons and directly stimulates both α- and β-adrenoceptors.[250] The oral adult dosage is 25–50 mg four times a day. Some tachyphylaxis develops in response to its peripheral actions, probably as a result of depletion of noradrenaline stores. Pseudoephedrine, a stereoisomer of ephedrine, is used for similar indications and carries similar precautions. The adult dosage is 30–60 mg four times a day, and the 30 mg dose form is available in the United States without prescription. Diokno and Taub[252] reported a 'good-to-excellent' result in 27–38 patients with sphincteric incontinence treated with ephedrine sulphate. Beneficial effects were most often achieved in those with minimal-to-moderate wetting; little benefit was achieved in patients with severe stress incontinence. A dose of 75–100 mg of norephedrine chloride has been shown to increase MUP and MUCP in women with SUI.[253] At a bladder volume of 300 ml, MUP rose from 82 to 110 cmH$_2$O, and MUCP rose from 63 to 93 cmH$_2$O. The functional profile length did not change significantly. Obrink and Bunne,[254] however, noted that 100 mg norephedrine chloride given twice a day did not improve severe stress incontinence sufficiently to offer it as an alternative to surgical treatment. They further noted in their group of 10 such patients that the MUCP was not influenced at rest or with stress at low or moderate bladder volumes. Lose and Lindholm[255] treated 20 women with stress incontinence with norfenefrine, an α-agonist, given as a slow-release tablet: 19 patients reported reduced urinary leakage; 10 reported no further stress incontinence. MUCP increased in 16 patients during treatment, the mean rise being 53–64 cmH$_2$O. It is interesting and perplexing that most patients reported an effect only after 4 days of treatment. This delay is difficult to explain on the basis of drug action, unless one postulates a change in the number or sensitivity of α-adrenoceptors.

The group at Kolding Hospital in Denmark has published three other articles of note on the use of norfenefrine for sphincteric incontinence, with interesting results. Forty-four patients with SUI were randomized to treatment with norfenefrine (15–30 mg three times a day) vs placebo for 6 weeks.[256] Subjectively, 12 of 23 (52%) of the norfenefrine group reported improvement as opposed to 7/21 (33%) of the placebo group – a difference that was not significant. Continence was reported by six (26%) norfenefrine patients and three (14%) placebo patients (not significant). Judged by a stress test, seven patients in each group became continent; 11 of 23 (48%) improved both subjectively and objectively in the norfenefrine group as opposed to 5/21 (24%) in the placebo group ($p = 0.09$). MUCP increased significantly (from 50 to 55 cmH$_2$O in the norfenefrine group, and from 55 to 65 cmH$_2$O in the placebo group!). Although the patients were said to have 'genuine stress incontinence', 5/12 with 'urge incontinence' were reported cured with norfenefrine, and 4/7 with placebo!

Table 32.3. *Norfenefrine and placebo in 44 women scheduled for surgery for SUI**

Results	Placebo not crossed over (n = 11)	Placebo crossed over to norfenefrine (n = 10)	Norfenefrine not crossed over (n = 13)	Norfenefrine crossed over to placebo (n = 10)
Cured or improved	6	2	3	3
Surgery	2	3	2	3
Wanted medical therapy reinstituted	0	3	7	1
Uncertain	2	0	1	3
Pad or pelvic floor exercises	1	2	0	0

* SUI, stress urinary incontinence.
Data from ref. 258.

Diernoes and associates[257] reported on the results of a 1-hour pad test in 33 women with either SUI or combined stress incontinence and urgency treated with 30 mg norfenefrine three times a day. Leakage of more than 10 g was required for entry into the study. Subjective improvement was reported by 10 patients (30%). Continence as shown by pad test was found in six patients (18%). Pad tests were graded on a scale of 1–4. At 12 weeks, 20 patients (61%) had improved by at least one grade ($p < 0.05$), but at 3 weeks the number was 13 (39%; not significant).

Lose and colleagues[258] studied 44 women scheduled for operation for SUI who were treated with 15–30 mg norfenefrine three times a day vs placebo for 3–4.5 months and were then evaluated for outcome after a median observation period of 30 months. The description and categorization of results were somewhat confusing, but the results were interesting. Originally 23 patients were allocated to the norfenefrine group and 21 to placebo. Results were categorized as follows: cured or much improved with no further treatment wanted; underwent surgery for relief; wanted medical therapy reinstituted; uncertain about what kind of treatment they wanted; used pads or pelvic floor exercises. At the end of a 6-week initial treatment period and re-evaluation, patients whose initial treatment had had no effect at all were crossed over to the other group. Categorization of results is shown in Table 32.3. It is obvious that a powerful placebo effect occurred, for reasons unknown, and therefore caution must be exercised in the evaluation of *all* modalities of therapy for sphincteric (and detrusor) incontinence.

Phenylpropanolamine (PPA) hydrochloride shares the pharmacological properties of ephedrine and is approximately equal in peripheral potency while causing less central stimulation.[250] It is available in tablets of 25 or 50 mg, and 75 mg timed-release capsules, and is a component of numerous proprietary mixtures marketed for the treatment of nasal and sinus congestion (usually in combination with an H_1 antihistamine) and as appetite suppressants. Using doses of 50 mg three times a day, Awad and associates[259] found that 11/13 women and 6/7 men with stress incontinence were significantly improved after 4 weeks of therapy. MUCP increased from a mean of 47 to 72 cmH$_2$O in patients with an empty bladder and from 43 to 58 cmH$_2$O in patients with a full bladder. Using a capsule containing 50 mg PPA, 8 mg chlorpheniramine (an antihistamine)

and 2 mg isopropamide (an antimuscarinic), Stewart and colleagues[260] found that, of 77 women with SUI, 18 were 'completely cured' with one sustained-release capsule; 28 patients were 'much better', six were 'slightly better' and 25 were 'no better'. In 11 men with stress incontinence after prostatectomy, the numbers in the corresponding categories were one, two, one and seven. The formulation of Ornade has now been changed, and each capsule of drug contains 75 mg PPA and 12 mg chlorpheniramine. Collste and Lindskog[261] reported on a group of 24 women with SUI treated with PPA or placebo with a crossover after 2 weeks. Severity of SUI was graded 1 (slight) or 2 (moderate). Average MUCP overall increased significantly with PPA compared with placebo (48–55 vs 48–49 cmH$_2$O). This was a significant difference in grade 2 but not in grade 1 patients. The average number of leakage episodes per 48 hours was reduced significantly overall for PPA patients but not in placebo patients (five to two vs five to six). This was significant for grade 1 but not for grade 2 patients. Subjectively, six of 24 patients thought that both PPA and placebo were ineffective. Among the 18 patients (of 24) who reported a subjective preference, 14 preferred PPA and four placebo. Improvements were rated subjectively as good, moderately good and slight. Improvements obtained with PPA were significant compared with those for placebo for the entire population and for both groups separately. The AHCPR guidelines[126] reported eight randomized controlled trials with PPA 50 mg twice a day for SUI in women. Percentage cures (all figures refer to percentages minus percentages on placebo) are listed as 0–14, percentage reduction in incontinence as 19–60, and percentage side effects and percentage dropouts as 5–33 and 0–4.3, respectively.

Some authors have emphasized the potential complications of PPA. Mueller[262] reported on a group of 11 patients who had significant neurological symptoms (acute headache, psychiatric symptoms or seizures) after taking 'look-alike pills' thought to contain amphetamines but actually containing PPA. Baggioni *et al.*[263] emphasized the possibility of blood pressure elevation, especially in patients with autonomic impairment. Lasagna[264] pointed out that previously reported blood pressure elevations occurred with a product that differed from American PPA and probably contained a different and much more potent isomer. He noted that although a huge volume of PPA has been consumed in the form of decongestants and anorectic medications, the world literature has reported only a minimum number of possible toxic reactions, most of which involved excessively high doses in combination medications. Liebson and colleagues[265] found no cardiovascular or subjective adverse effects with doses of 25 mg three times a day or a 75 mg sustained-release preparation in a population of 150 healthy normal volunteers. Blackburn and colleagues,[266] in a larger series of healthy subjects using many over-the-counter formulations, concluded that a statistically significant but clinically unimportant pressor effect existed during the first 6 hours after administration of PPA and that this was greater with sustained-release preparations. Caution should still be exercised in individuals known to be significantly hypertensive and in elderly patients, in whom pharmacokinetic function may be altered.

Midodrine is a long-acting α-adrenergic agonist reported to be useful in the treatment of seminal emission and ejaculation disorders following retroperitoneal lymphadenectomy. Treatment with 5 mg twice a day for 4 weeks in 20 patients with stress incontinence produced a cure in one and improvement in 14.[267] The MUCP rose by 8.3%, and the planometric index of the continence area on profilometry increased by 9%. The actions of imipramine have already been discussed. On a theoretical basis, an increase in urethral resistance might be expected if, indeed, an enhanced α-adrenergic effect at this level resulted from an inhibition of noradrenaline reuptake. However, as mentioned previously, imipramine also causes α-adrenergic blocking effects, at least in vascular smooth muscle. Many clinicians have noted improvement in patients treated with imipramine primarily for bladder hyperactivity but who had in addition some component of sphincteric incontinence. Gilja and colleagues[268] reported a study of 30 women with stress incontinence who were treated with 75 mg imipramine daily for 4 weeks: 21 women subjectively reported continence; the mean MUCP for the group increased from 34.06 to 48.23 mmH$_2$O.

Although some clinicians have reported spectacular cure and improvement rates with α-adrenergic agonists and agents that produce an α-adrenergic effect in the outlet of patients with sphincteric urinary incontinence, our own experience coincides with those who report that such treatment often produces satisfactory or some improvement in mild cases but rarely total dryness in patients with severe or even moderate stress incontinence. Nevertheless, a clinical trial, when possible, is certainly worthwhile, especially in conjunction with pelvic floor physiotherapy or biofeedback.

β-Adrenergic antagonists and agonists

Theoretically, β-adrenergic blocking agents might be expected to 'unmask' or potentiate an α-adrenergic effect, thereby increasing urethral resistance. Gleason and colleagues[269] reported success in treating certain patients with SUI with propranolol, using oral doses of 10 mg four times a day: the beneficial effect became manifest only after 4–10 weeks of treatment. Cardiac effects occur rather promptly after administration of this drug, but hypotensive effects do not usually appear as rapidly, although it is difficult to explain such a long delay in onset of the therapeutic effect on incontinence on this basis. Kaisary[270] also reported success with propranolol in the treatment of stress incontinence. Although such treatment has been suggested as an alternative to α-agonists in patients with sphincteric incontinence and hypertension, few, if any, subsequent reports of such efficacy have appeared. Others have reported no significant changes in urethral profile pressures in normal women after β-adrenergic blockade.[271] Although 10 mg four times a day is a relatively small dose of propranolol, it should be recalled that the major potential side effects of the drug are related to the therapeutic β-blocking effects. Heart failure may develop, as well as an increase in airway resistance, and asthma is a contraindication to its use. Abrupt discontinuation may precipitate an exacerbation of anginal attacks and rebound hypertension.[250]

β-Adrenergic stimulation is generally conceded to decrease urethral pressure (see reference 5 for references), but β$_2$-agonists have been reported to *increase* the contractility of fast-contracting striated muscle fibres (extensor digitorum longus) from guinea pigs and suppress that of slow-contracting fibres (soleus).[272] Clenbuterol, a selective β$_2$-agonist, has been reported to potentiate, in a dose-dependent fashion, the field stimulation-induced contraction in isolated periurethral muscle preparation in the rabbit. The potentiation is greater that that produced by isoprenaline and is suppressed by propranolol. Kishimoto and colleagues[273] reported an increase in urethral pressure with clinical use of clenbuterol and speculated on its promise in the treatment of sphincteric incontinence. Although the differential effects on the smooth and striated musculature of the outlet and even on different fibre types of the striated sphincter may be functionally antagonistic, one should not ignore the possibility of an augmentative effect on outlet resistance by a drug such as clenbuterol under certain physiological conditions. Other β_2-agonists are salbutamol and terbutaline.

Oestrogens

Although oestrogens were recommended for the treatment of urinary incontinence in women as early as 1941,[271] there is still controversy over their use and benefit–risk ratio for this purpose. This subject is a good example of why it is sometimes difficult to obtain a consensus about the efficacy or non-efficacy of a particular category of drug for the treatment of incontinence. There is an impressive basic science literature on the effects of oestrogen on the lower urinary tract but no strictly appropriate experimental model of either stress incontinence or detrusor hyperactivity or hypersensitivity. There are numerous clinical trials – some controlled and some not, some using oestrogen alone and some using oestrogen plus α-agonists. There is little consistency in methodology, and the manner in which some authors have chosen to express their data and conclusions is confusing at times. In some cases raw data seem to be ignored in favour of statistics; however, as always, there is no lack of opinions.

Much attention has been paid to the innervation, physiology and pharmacology of the smooth muscle of the uterus. Oestrogens have been found to affect many related properties including excitability, neuronal influences on the muscle, receptor density and sensitivity, and transmitter metabolism, especially in adrenergic nerves. The urethra (and trigone) are embryologically related to the uterus, and significant work has also been done on the effects of oestrogenic hormones on the lower urinary tract. Hodgson and associates[275] reported that the sensitivity of the rabbit urethra to α-adrenergic stimulation was oestrogen dependent: castration caused decreased sensitivity, and treatment with low levels of oestrogen reversed this. Levin and co-workers[275,276] showed that parenteral oestrogen administration can change the autonomic receptor content and the innervation of the lower urinary tract of immature female rabbits. A marked increase in response to α-adrenergic, muscarinic and purinergic stimulation occurred in the bladder body but not the base, and there was a significant increase in the number of α-adrenergic and muscarinic receptors in the bladder body but not the base. Other work[5] has shown a decrease in muscarinic receptor density following oestradiol treatment of mature female rabbits, and either no change or a decreased detrusor response to cholinergic and electrical stimulation. Levin and co-workers[278] concluded that pregnancy induced an increase in the purinergic and a decrease in the cholinergic responses of the rabbit bladder to field stimulation, and Tong and colleagues[279] reported a decrease in the α-adrenergic response of the mid-part and base of the bladder of pregnant as opposed to virgin rabbits. Larsson and associates[280] reported that oestrogen treatment of the isolated female rabbit urethra caused an increased sensitivity to noradrenaline. The mechanism was postulated to be related to a more than twofold increase in the α-adrenergic receptor number. Callahan and Creed[281] reported that pretreatment with oestrogen of oophorectomized dogs and wallabies did increase sensitivity of urethral strips to α-adrenergic stimulation, but that this did not occur in the rabbit or guinea pig. Bump and Friedman[282] reported that sex hormone replacement with oestrogen, but not testosterone, enhanced the urethral sphincter mechanism in the castrated female baboon by effects that were unrelated to skeletal muscle. They added that these effects might be related not just to changes in the urethral smooth musculature but to changes in the urethral mucosa, submucosal vascular plexus and connective tissue.

Oestrogen therapy certainly seems to be capable of facilitating urinary storage in some post-menopausal women. Whether this effect is related just to changes in the automonic innervation, receptor content or function of the smooth muscle or to changes in oestrogen-binding sites[283] or changes in the vascular or connective tissue elements of the urethral wall, has not been settled. Batra and colleagues[284] have shown that two doses of oestradiol and oestratriol increased blood perfusion into the urethra (as well as the vagina and uterus) of oophorectomized mature female rabbits. After menopause, urethral pressure parameters normally decrease slightly[285] and, although this change is generally conceded to be related in some way to decreased oestrogen levels, it is still largely a matter of speculation whether the actual changes occur in smooth muscle, blood circulation, supporting tissues or the 'mucosal seal mechanism'. Versi and associates[286] describe a positive correlation between skin collagen content (which does decline with declining oestrogen status) and parameters of the urethral pressure profile, suggesting that the oestrogen effect on the urethra may be predicted, at least in part, by changes in the collagen component. Eika and colleagues[287] reported that bladders from ovariectomized rats weighed less and had a higher collagen content and less atropine resistance than controls, and that oestrogen substitution reversed these parameters.

Raz and co-workers[288] reported that progesterone enhanced the β-adrenergic response of the dog urethra and ureter. Progesterone receptors have been identified in the human urethra,[286] but Rud[290] reported that treatment with oestrogens had no effect on urethral profile parameters.[284] Raz and colleagues[291] reported that oral medroxyprogesterone acetate (20 mg daily) exacerbated stress incontinence in 60% of women so treated, with corresponding changes in urethral pressures.

Raz and associates[291] found that a daily dose of 2.5 mg conjugated oestrogens (Premarin) improved stress incontinence and increased urethral pressure in 65% of post-menopausal patients, effects that the authors attributed to mucosal proliferation with a consequently improved 'mucosal seal effect' and to enhancement of the α-adrenergic contractile response of urethral smooth muscle to endogenous catecholamines. Schreiter and associates[292] reported similar benefits after 10 days of treatment with daily divided doses of 6 mg oestriol.[286] They also presented evidence that the effects of oestrogen and of exogenous α-adrenergic stimulation were additive. In one of the first studies that presented some quantitative data on oestrogen, Rud[290] reported the effects of 4 mg doses of oestradiol and doses of oestriol (8 mg daily) on 30 women with an average age of 61 years, 24 of whom had SUI. Small but statistically significant increases occurred in the MUP (from 59 to 63 cmH$_2$O), functional urethral length (from 25 to 28 mm), and actual urethral length (from 33 to 37 mm). No statistically significant change occurred in urethral closure pressure (from 37 to 39 cmH$_2$O). Eight of the 24 incontinent patients experienced subjective and objective improvement; nine experienced subjective improvement only, and seven experienced neither subjective nor objective improvement. There was no correlation between subjective or objective improvement and urodynamic parameters. However, of 18 patients in whom pressure transmission

to the urethra was recorded during cough, seven improved. All of these reported subjective improvement, and five were shown objectively to be dry. Rud[285] pointed out that it is hard to believe that the small changes in urodynamic measurements that occurred, although statistically significant, were directly related to resumption of continence and noted that the increased pressure transmission ratio might be due to factors outside the urethra – either in the striated musculature of the pelvic floor or in the periurethral vasculature or supporting tissues. Rud also studied profilometry during the menstrual cycle in six women: there was no change in any profilometric value during the menstrual cycle and no correlation between oestrogen levels and MUP. It may be, as suggested, that physiological levels of oestrogens have little influence on urodynamic measurements related to continence and that only pharmacological doses cause urodynamically significant changes. Pharmacological doses may also alter responses to other exogenous autonomic stimulation, particularly α-adrenergic stimulation, as laboratory experiments suggest.

Beisland and colleagues[293] carried out a randomized open comparative crossover trial in 20 post-menopausal women with urethral sphincteric insufficiency: both oral PPA, 50 mg twice a day, and oestriol vaginal suppositories, 1 mg daily, significantly increased the MUCP and the continence area on profilometry. PPA was clinically more effective than oestriol but not sufficiently so to obtain complete continence. However, with combined treatment, eight patients became completely continent, nine were considerably improved, and only one remained unchanged. Two patients dropped out of the study because of side effects. Bhatia and colleagues[294] used 2 g conjugated-oestrogen vaginal cream daily for 6 weeks in 11 post-menopausal women with SUI: six were cured or improved significantly. Favourable response was correlated with increased closure pressure and increased pressure transmission. In an accompanying article, Karram and associates[295] reported that oestrogen administration in six women with premature ovarian failure (but without lower urinary tract problems) did not produce any change in urethral pressure, functional length or cystometric parameters; however, a significant increase in the pressure transmission ratio to the proximal and midurethra (from 89 to 109% and from 86 to 100%, respectively) was noted after vaginal oestrogen but not after oral oestrogen, although serum oestradiol levels and cytological changes were similar in the two modes of administration. Negative effects from oestrogen alone on stress incontinence were reported by Walter and colleagues,[296] Hilton and Stanton[297] and Samsioe and associates;[298] however, in each of these studies urge symptomatology was favourably affected. In a review article, Cardozo[299] concluded that 'there is no conclusive evidence that oestrogen even improves, let alone cures, stress incontinence', although it 'apparently alleviates urgency, urge incontinence, frequency, nocturia and dysuria'.

Kinn and Lindskog[300] described the results of treatment of 36 post-menopausal women with SUI with oral oestriol and PPA, alone and in combination, in a double-blind trial after a 4-week run-in period with PPA. Although some of the data are difficult to interpret, the authors concluded that PPA alone and PPA plus oestriol raised the intra-urethral pressure and reduced urinary loss by 35% (significant) in a standardized physical strain test. Leakage episodes and amounts were significantly reduced by oestriol and PPA given separately (28%) or in combination (40%); the authors found no evidence of a synergistic effect but did indicate that an additive effect was present. Walter and colleagues[301] completed a complicated but logical study of 28 (out of 38 original subjects) post-menopausal women with SUI. After 4 weeks of a placebo run-in, patients were randomized to oral oestriol or PPA alone for 4 weeks and then to combined therapy for 4 weeks. In the group that sequentially received placebo, PPA and PPA/oestriol, the percentages reporting cure or improvement, respectively, were 0 and 13%, 13 and 20%, and 21 and 14%. In the group receiving placebo, oestriol and oestriol/PPA, the corresponding percentages were 0 and 0%, 14 and 29%, and 64 and 7%. Objective parameters showed the following: the number of leak episodes per 24 hours in patients treated with PPA first showed a 31% decrease (~3 to 2) compared with placebo ($p < 0.003$). For those treated with oestriol first, the change was not significant (~1.5 to 0.8). Combined treatment produced a mean decrease of 48% over placebo. There was a greater effect with oestriol/PPA than with PPA/oestriol. Pad weights (in grams in a 1-hour test) decreased significantly with PPA alone (~27 to 6 g), but there was no difference between PPA and PPA/oestriol. Oestriol alone significantly decreased pad weights (~47 to 15 g). Although oestriol/PPA was not significantly different, there was further numerical

loss from ~15 to 3 g. The overall conclusions were that oestriol and PPA are each effective in treating SUI in post-menopausal women, and, on the basis of the subjective data, combined therapy is better than either drug alone. This conclusion was substantiated by a significant decrease in the number of leak episodes in the patients in whom oestriol was given before PPA but was not confirmed statistically by pad-weighing tests.

Hilton and colleagues[302] published the results of a double-blind study of 60 (originally) post-menopausal women with SUI who were treated for 4 weeks with oral and vaginal oestrogen alone and in combination with PPA. There were six groups in this study: 1) vaginal oestrogen (VE) and PPA; 2) VE and oral placebo (OP); 3) oral oestrogen (OE) and PPA; 4) OE and OP; 5) vaginal placebo (VP) and PPA; 6) VP and OP. Subjective symptoms and reported pads per day decreased in all groups: the greatest reduction occurred in those treated with VE, although the reduction in groups 1, 2, 4 and 6 were all significant. Objective pad weight after exercise testing showed a slight decrease in all except the VP/OP group. Reduction was maximal in the VE/PPA group (22 to 8 g), but the pretreatment values for pads per day and pad weight varied greatly (< 0.5 to ~3.5 pads per day; < 5 g to 22 g). There was no change in cystometric or urethral profilometric evaluation, either resting or stress.

Using the number of incontinence episodes, as measured by a voiding diary, as well as a variety of quality-of-life instruments, Fantl and associates[303] looked at the effect of 3 months of cyclic oestrogen-replacement therapy in a randomized placebo-controlled study of 83 women with stress and/or urge incontinence and serologically documented hypo-oestrogenism. The authors noted no significant differences within or between the treated and placebo groups. They concluded that cyclic hormone replacement did not affect either clinical or quality-of-life variables in incontinent, hypo-oestrogenic women. However, the authors did not discount the possibility that oestrogen replacement therapy may be efficacious in patients who maintain normal oestrogen levels from the onset of menopause (i.e. those who never became hypogonadal following menopause).

Sessions and associates[304] reviewed the benefits and risks of oestrogen-replacement therapy. Improvements in vasomotor symptomatology and osteoporosis prevention are well established. There is also substantial evidence of a decreased risk of cardiovascular disease, perhaps because of an effect on the lipid profile. There is little question, however, that unopposed oestrogen use in those with an intact uterus increases the risk of endometrial cancer. Progestogen treatment exerts a protective effect, and daily administration of an oestrogen and a progestogen provides an attractive alternative because of a lack of withdrawal bleeding (with sequential therapy) and consequent increased patient compliance. Whether progestogen administration adversely affects the results of oestrogen treatment of SUI is unknown but must be considered. Progestogens may also cause mastalgia, oedema and bloating. It is concluded, further, that there is no evidence for an increase in thromboembolism or hypertension with oestrogen replacement. Transdermal administration of oestrogen avoids any theoretical problems associated with the first-pass effect through the liver with oral administration (alteration in clotting factors and increase in renin substrate). The evidence does suggest an association between breast cancer and oestrogen replacement therapy, but only for those who have received such therapy for more than 15 years. A preventive role of progestogens in this regard is controversial, as is the dose of oestrogen necessary to produce this effect. Grodstein and colleagues[305] looked at the relationship between long-term post-menopausal hormonal replacement therapy and overall mortality in a cohort of nurses over an 18-year period. Although they noted an overall lower risk of death (relative risk, 0.63) for active oestrogen users as compared to subjects who had never taken hormones, the apparent benefit decreased somewhat (relative risk 0.80) after 10 years of therapy owing to an increased mortality from breast cancer in the hormone-treated group.

As to the type of oestrogen preparation preferred, transdermal seems to be as effective as oral, and subcutaneous implants appear to produce physiological serum levels. Percutaneous and intramuscular oestrogen seem to produce variable serum levels. Vaginal creams are said to produce variable serum levels but physiological oestradiol/oestrone ratios.[304] We agree that 'hands on' application to the 'affected area' may have a psychological benefit as well, as suggested by Murray.[306] None-the-less, many women do not like (or cannot self-administer) the vaginal creams. A unique new method for delivering vaginal oestrogen involves a silicone ring with an oestradiol-loaded core containing 2 mg of 17β-oestradiol. The device is inserted into the vagina, by the patient or the physician. A low, constant dose (5–10 g/24 h) is delivered over a period of 90 days. This mode of administration not only is more acceptable to certain women[307] but also offers a more continuous delivery of oestrogen to the affected tissues.[308]

CIRCUMVENTING THE PROBLEM

Antidiuretic-hormone-like agents

The synthetic antidiuretic hormone (ADH) peptide analogue desmopressin acetate (DDAVP; 1-desamino-8-D-arginine vasopressin) has been used for the symptomatic relief of refractory nocturnal enuresis in both children and adults.[306,309] The drug can be administered conveniently by intranasal spray at bedtime (in a dose of 10–40 μg) and effectively suppresses urine production for 7–10 hours. Its clinical long-term safety has been established by continued use in patients with diabetes insipidus. Normal water-deprivation tests, as described by Rew and Rundle,[310] indicate that long-term use does not cause depression of endogenous ADH secretion, at least in patients with nocturnal enuresis. Changes in diuresis during 2 months of treatment in an elderly group of six men and 12 women with increased nocturia and decreased ADH secretion were reported by Asplund and Oberg:[311] nocturia decreased 20% (in millilitres) in men and 34% in women; however, the number of voids from 20:00 to 08:00 hours decreased from 4.5 to 4.3 in men and from 3.5 to 2.8 in women, but the drug was not given until 20:00 hours. At present, this novel circumventive approach to the treatment of urinary frequency and incontinence has been largely restricted to those with nocturnal enuresis and diabetes insipidus. The fact that the drug seems to be much more effective than simple fluid restriction alone for the former condition is perhaps explained by relatively recent reports suggesting a decreased nocturnal secretion of ADH by such patients.[309] Recently, suggestions have been made that desmopressin might be useful in patients with refractory nocturnal frequency and incontinence who do not belong in the category of primary nocturnal enuresis. Kinn and Larsson[312] reported that micturition frequency 'decreased significantly' in 13 patients with multiple sclerosis and urge incontinence who were treated with oral tablets of desmopressin and that less leakage occurred. The actual approximate average change in the number of voids during the 6 hours after drug intake was from 3.2 to 2.5.

A similar circumventive approach is to give a rapidly acting loop diuretic 4–6 hours before bedtime. This, of course, assumes that the nocturia is not due to obstructive uropathy. A randomized double-blind crossover study of this approach using bumetanide in a group of 14 general practice patients was reported by Pedersen and Johansen.[313] Control nocturia episodes per week averaged 17.5; with placebo, this decreased to 12 (!), and with drug to eight. Bumetanide was preferred to placebo by 11 of 14 patients. It will be interesting to see whether any drug companies pursue this avenue of treatment for the large number of patients with refractory nocturnal bladder storage problems or for 'spot' usage prior to some important event in patients with urgency and frequency with and without incontinence.

REFERENCES

1. Wein AJ, Levin RM, Barrett DM. Voiding function: relevant anatomy, physiology, and pharmacology. In: Duckett JW, Howards ST, Grayhack JT, Gillenwater JY (eds) *Adult and Pediatric Urology*, 2nd edn. St Louis: Mosby Year Book, 1991; 933–999

2. Wein AJ, Van Arsdalen KN, Levin RM. Pharmacologic therapy. In: Krane RJ, Siroky MB (eds) *Clinical Neuro-Urology*. Boston: Little Brown, 1991; 523–558

3. Steers WD. Physiology of the urinary bladder. In: Walsh PC, Retik AB, Stamey TA, Vaughan ED (eds) *Campbell's Urology*, 6th edn. Philadelphia: Saunders, 1992; 142–169

4. de Groat WC. Anatomy and physiology of the lower urinary tract. *Urol Clin North Am* 1993; 20: 383–401

5. Andersson KE. Pharmacology of lower urinary tract smooth muscles and penile erectile tissues. *Pharmacol Rev* 1993; 45: 253

6. Wein AJ. Neuromuscular dysfunction of the lower urinary tract. In: Walsh PC, Retik AB, Stamey TA, Vaughan ED (eds) *Campbell's Urology*, 6th edn. Philadelphia: Saunders, 1992; 573–642

7. Taylor P. Cholinergic agonists. In: Gilman AG, Rall TW, Nies AS, Taylor P (eds) *Goodman and Gilman's The Pharmacological Basis of Therapeutics*, 8th edn. New York: Pergamon Press, 1990; 122–130

8. Raezer DM, Wein AJ, Jacobowitz DM. Autonomic innervation of canine urinary bladder. Cholinergic and adrenergic contributions and interaction of sympathetic and parasympathetic systems in bladder function. *Urology* 1973; 2: 211

9. Barrett DM, Wein AJ. Voiding dysfunction: diagnosis, classification and management. In: Gillenwater JY, Grayhack JT, Howards ST, Duckett JW (eds) *Adult and Pediatric Urology*, 2nd edn. St Louis: Mosby Year Book, 1991; 1001–1099

10. Starr I, Ferguson CK. Beta methylcholine urethane. Its action in various normal and abnormal conditions, especially postoperative urinary retention. *Am J Med Sci* 1940; 200: 372

11. Lee L. The clinical use of urecholine in dysfunctions of the bladder. *J Urol* 1949; 62: 300

12. Sonda L, Gershon C, Diokno A. Further observations on the cystometric and uroflowmetric effects of bethanechol chloride on the human bladder. *J Urol* 1979; 122: 775

13. Perkash I. Intermittent catheterization and bladder rehabilitation in spinal cord injury patients. *J Urol* 1975; 114: 230

14. Finkbeiner AE. Is bethanechol chloride clinically effective in promoting bladder emptying? *J Urol* 1985; 134: 443

15. Wein AJ, Malloy T, Shofar F *et al.* The effects of bethanechol chloride on urodynamic parameters in normal women and in women with significant residual urine volumes. *J Urol* 1980; 124: 397

16. Wein AJ, Raezer DD, Malloy T. Failure of the bethanechol supersensitivity test to predict improved voiding after subcutaneous bethanechol administration. *J Urol* 1980; 123: 202

17. Sporer A, Leyson J, Martin B. Effects of bethanechol chloride on the external urethral sphincter in spinal cord injury patients. *J Urol* 1978; 120: 62

18. Farrell GA, Webster RD, Higgins LM, Steeves RA. Duration of postoperative catheterization: a randomized double-blind trial comparing two catheter management protocols and the effect of bethanechol chloride. *Int Urogynecol J* 1990; 1: 132

19. Albibi R, McCallum RW. Metoclopramide: pharmacology and clinical application. *Ann Intern Med* 1983; 98: 86

20. Mitchell WC, Venable DD. Effects of metoclopramide on detrusor function. *J Urol* 1985; 135: 791

21. Nestler JE, Stratton MA, Hakin CA. Effect of metoclopramide on diabetic neurogenic bladder. *Br J Urol* 1983; 2: 83

22. Carone R, Vercella D, Bertapelli P. Effects of cisapride on anorectal and vesicourethral function in spinal cord injured patients. *Paraplegia* 1993; 31: 125

23. Binnie N, Creasey G, Edmond P *et al.* The action of cisapride on the chronic constipation of paraplegia. *Paraplegia* 1988; 26: 151

24. Wyndaele JJ, Van Kerrebroeck R. The effects of 4 weeks

treatment with cisapride on cystometric parameters in spinal cord injury patients. A double blind, placebo controlled study. *Paraplegia* 1995; 33: 625–627

25. Bultitude M, Hills N, Shuttleworth K. Clinical and experimental studies on the action of prostaglandins and their synthesis inhibitors on detrusor muscle in vitro and in vivo. *Br J Urol* 1976; 48: 631

26. Desmond A, Bultitude M, Hills N *et al.* Clinical experience with intravesical prostaglandin E_2: a prospective study of 36 patients. *Br J Urol* 1980; 53: 357

27. Vaidyanathan S, Rao M, Mapa M. Study of instillation of 15(S)-15–methyl prostaglandin F2a in patients with neurogenic bladder dysfunction. *J Urol* 1981; 126: 81

28. Tammela TL, Kontturi M, Lukkarinen O. Intravesical prostaglandin F2 for promoting bladder emptying after surgery for female stress incontinence. *Br J Urol* 1987; 60: 43

29. Jaschevatsky OE, Anderman S, Shalit A. Prostaglandin F2a for prevention of urinary retention after vaginal hysterectomy. *Obstet Gynecol* 1985; 66: 244

30. Koonings P, Bergman A, Ballard CA. Prostaglandins for enhancing detrusor function after surgery for stress incontinence in women. *J Reprod Med* 1990; 35: 1

31. Stanton DL, Cardozo LD, Ken-Wilson R. Treatment of delayed onset of spontaneous voiding after surgery for incontinence. *Urology* 1979; 13: 494

32. Delaere KJP, Thomas CMG, Moonen WA *et al.* The value of intravesical prostaglandin F2a and E2 in women with abnormalities of bladder emptying. *Br J Urol* 1981; 53: 306

33. Wagner G, Husstein P, Enzelsberger H. Is prostaglandin E2 really of therapeutic value for postoperative urinary retention? Results of a prospectively randomized double-blind study. *Am J Obstet Gynecol* 1985; 151: 375

34. Schubler B. Comparison of the mode of action of PGE2 and sulprostone, a PGE2 derivative, on the lower urinary tract in healthy women. *Urol Res* 1990; 18: 349

35. Rall TW. Oxytocin, prostaglandins, ergot alkaloids and other drugs; tocolytic agents. In: Gilman AG, Rall TW, Nies AS, Taylor P (eds) *Goodman and Gilman's The Pharmacological Basis of Therapeutics*, 8th edn. New York: Pergamon Press, 1990; 933–953

36. de Groat WC, Booth AM. Autonomic systems to the urinary bladder and sexual organs. In: Dyck PJ, Thomas PK, Lambert EH (eds) *Peripheral Neuropathy*. Philadelphia: Saunders; 1984; 285–299

37. Wheeler JS, Jr, Robinson CJ, Culkin DJ *et al.* Naloxone efficacy in bladder rehabilitation of spinal cord injury patients. *J Urol* 1987; 137: 1202

38. Kleeman FJ. The physiology of the internal urinary sphincter. *J Urol* 1970; 104: 549

39. Krane R, Olsson C. Phenoxybenzamine in neurogenic bladder dysfunction: I. Clinical considerations. *J Urol* 1973; 110: 653

40. Krane R, Olsson C. Phenoxybenzamine in neurogenic bladder dysfunction. II. Clinical considerations. *J Urol* 1973; 110: 653

41. Abel B, Gibbon N, Jameson R. The neuropathic urethra. *Lancet* 1974; 2: 1229

42. Hachen H. Clinical and urodynamic assessment of alpha adrenolytic therapy in patients with neurogenic bladder function. *Paraplegia* 1980; 18: 229

43. Nannings J, Kaplan P, Lal S. Effect of phentolamine on peripheral muscle EMG activity in paraplegia. *Br J Urol* 1977; 49: 537

44. Nordling J, Meyhoff H, Hald T. Sympatholytic effect on striated urethral sphincter. A peripheral or central nervous system effect? *Scand J Urol Nephrol* 1981; 15: 173

45. Pederson E, Torring J, Kleman B. Effect of the alpha-adrenergic blocking agent thymoxamine on the neurogenic bladder and urethra. *Acta Neurol Scand* 1980; 61: 107

46. Gajewski J, Downie J, Awad SA. Experimental evidence for a central nervous system site of action in the effect of alpha adrenergic blockers on the external urethra sphincter. *J Urol* 1984; 133: 403

47. Thind P, Lose G, Colatrue H *et al.* The effect of alpha adrenoceptor stimulation and blockade on the static urethral sphincter function in healthy females. *Scand J Urol Nephrol* 1992; 26: 219

48. Norlen L. Influence of the sympathetic nervous system on the lower urinary tract and its clincal implications. *Neurourol Urodyn* 1982; 1: 129

49. Sundin T, Dahlstom A, Norlen L *et al.* The sympathetic innervation and adrenoreceptor function of the human lower urinary tract in the normal state and after parasympathetic denervation. *Invest Urol* 1977; 14: 322

50. Koyanagi T. Further observation on the denervation supersensitivity of the urethra in patients with chronic neurogenic bladders. *J Urol* 1979; 122: 348

51. Parsons K, Turton M. Urethral supersensitivity and occult urethral neuropathy. *Br J Urol* 1980; 52: 131

52. Nordling J, Meyhoff H, Hald T. Urethral denervation supersensitivity to noradrenaline after radical hysterectomy. *Scand J Urol Nephrol* 1981; 15: 21

53. Andersson KE, Ek A, Hedlund H. Effects of prazosin in isolated human urethra and in patients with lower neuron lesions. *Invest Urol* 1981; 19: 39

54. McGuire E, Savastano J. Effect of alpha adrenergic blockade and anticholinergic agents on the decentralized primate bladder. *Neurourol Urodyn* 1985; 4: 139

55. Jensen D, Jr. Pharmacological studies of the uninhibited neurogenic bladder. *Acta Neurol Scand* 1981; 64: 145–174

56. Jensen D, Jr. Altered adrenergic innervation in the uninhibited neurogenic neurogenic bladder. *Scand J Urol Nephrol* 1981; 60: 61

57. Jensen D, Jr. Uninhibited neurogenic bladder treated with prazosin. *Scand J Urol Nephrol* 1981; 15: 229–233

58. Thomas DG, Philp NH, McDermott TE. The use of urodynamic studies to assess the effect of pharmacological agents with particular references to alpha blockade. *Paraplegia* 1984; 22: 162

59. Rohner T, Hannigan J, Sanford E. Altered in vitro adrenergic responses of dog detrusor muscle after chronic bladder outlet obstruction. *Urology* 1978; 11: 357

60. Swierzewski SJ, 3rd, Gormley EA, Belville WD *et al.* The effect of terazosin on bladder function in the spinal cord injured patient. *J Urol* 1994; 151: 951–954

61. Hoffman BB, Lefkowitz RJ. Adrenergic receptor agonists. In: Gilman AG, Rall TW, Nies AS, Taylor P (eds) *Goodman and Gilman's The Pharmacological Basis of Therapeutics*, 8th edn. New York: Pergamon Press, 1990; 221–243

62. *Physicians Desk Reference.* Oradell, NJ: Medical Economics Co., 1992

63. Marshall HL, Beevers DG. Alpha-adrenoceptor blocking drugs and female urinary incontinence: prevalence and reversibility. *Br J Clin Pharmacol* 1996; 42: 507–509

64. Taylor SH. Clinical pharmacotherapeutics of doxazosin. *Am J Med* 1989; 87 (Suppl 2A): 25

65. Lepor H. Role of long acting selective alpha-1 blockers in the treatment of benign prostatic hyperplasia. *Urol Clin North Am* 1990; 17: 651

66. Wilde M, Fitton A, Sorkin E. Terazosin: a review of its pharmacodynamic and pharmacokinetic properties and therapeutic potential in BPH. *Drugs Aging* 1993; 3: 258

67. Buzelin JM, Herbert M, Blondin P. Alpha-blocking treatment with alfuzosin in symptomatic benign prostatic hyperplasia: comparative study with prazosin. The PRAZALF Group. *Br J Urol* 1993; 72: 922–927

68. Wilde M, Fitton A, McTavish D. Alfuzosin – a review of its pharmacodynamic and pharmacokinetic properties and its therapeutic potential in BPH. *Drugs* 1993; 45: 410

69. Buzelin JM, Roth S, Geffriaud-Ricouard C *et al.* Efficacy and safety of sustained-release alfuzosin 5 mg in patients with benign prostatic hyperplasia. ALGEBI Study Group. *Eur Urol* 1997; 31: 190–198

70. Lepor H, Tang R, Kobayashi S *et al.* Localization of the alpha-1A-adrenoreceptor in the human prostate. *J Urol* 1995; 154: 2096–2099

71. Noble AJ, Williams-Chess R, Couldwell C *et al.* The effects of tamsulosin, a high affinity antagonist at functional [a]1A- and [a]1D-adrenoceptor subtypes. *Br J Pharmacol* 1997; 120: 231–238

72. Chapple C, Wyndaele JJ, Nordling J *et al.* Tamsulosin, the first prostate-selective alpha 1A-adrenoceptor antagonist. A meta-analysis of two randomized placebo-controlled, multicentre studies in patients with benign prostatic obstruction (symptomatic BPH). European Tamsulosin Study Group. *Eur Urol* 1996; 29: 155–167

73. Wilde M, McTavish D. Tamsulosin. A review of its pharmacological properties and therapeutic potential in the management of symptomatic benign prostatic hyperplasia. *Drugs* 1996; 52: 883–898

74. Raz S, Caine M. Adrenergic receptors in the female canine urethra. *Invest Urol* 1971; 9: 319

75. Vaidyanathan S, Rao M, Bapna B. Beta adrenergic activity in human proximal urethra. *J Urol* 1980; 124: 869

76. Burton G, Dobson C. Progesterone increases flow rates. A new treatment for voiding abnormalities? *Neurourol Urodyn* 1993; 12: 398

77. Cedarbaum JM, Schleifer LS. Drugs for Parkinson's disease spasticity, and acute muscle spasms. In: Gilman AG, Rall TW, Nies AS, Taylor P (eds) *Goodman and Gilman's The Pharmacological Basis of Therapeutics*, 8th edn. New York: Pergamon Press, 1990; 463–484

78. Bloom FE. Neurohumoral transmission and the central nervous system. In: Gilman AG, Rall TW, Nies AS, Taylor P (eds) *Goodman and Gilman's The Pharmacological Basis of Therapeutics*, 8th edn. New York: Pergamon Press; 1990; 244–268

79. Davidoff RA. Antispasticity drugs: mechanisms of action. *Ann Neurol* 1985; 17: 107

80. Lader M. Clinical pharmacology of benzodiazepines. *Annu Rev Med* 1987; 38: 19

81. Rampe D, Triggle DJ. Benzodiazepines and calcium channel function. *Trends Pharmacol Sci* 1986; November: 461

82. Shader RI, Greenblatt DJ. Use of benzodiazepines in anxiety disorders. *N Engl J Med* 1993; 328: 1398

83. Baldesarini RJ. Drugs and the treatment of psychiatric disorders. In: Gilman AG, Rall TW, Nies AS, Taylor P (eds) *Goodman and Gilman's The Pharmacological Basis of Therapeutics*, 8th edn. New York: Pergamon Press; 1990; 383–435

84. Stanton SL, Cardozo LD, Ken-Wilson R. Treatment of delayed onset of spontaneous voiding after surgery for incontinence. *Urology* 1979; 13: 494

85. Smyth RJ, Uhlman EJ, Ruggieri MR. Identification and characterization of a high-affinity peripheral-type benzodiazepine receptor in rabbit urinary bladder. *J Urol* 1994; 151: 1102–1106

86. Ha H, Lee KY, Kim WJ. The action of diazepam in the isolated rat detrusor muscle. *J Urol* 1993; 150: 229–234

87. Milanov IG. Mechanisms of baclofen action on spasticity. *Acta Neurol Scand* 1991; 85: 304

88. Hachen H, Krucker V. Clinical and laboratory assessment of the efficacy of baclofen on urethral sphincter spasticity in patients with traumatic paraplegia. *Eur Urol* 1977; 3: 327

89. Florante J, Leyson J, Martin B *et al*. Baclofen in the treatment of detrusor sphincter dyssynergy in spinal cord injury patients. *J Urol* 1980; 124: 82

90. Roy CW, Wakefield IR. Baclofen pseudopsychosis: case report. *Paraplegia* 1986; 24: 318

91. Kums JJM, Delhaas EM. Intrathecal baclofen infusion in patients with spasticity and neurogenic bladder disease. *World J Urol* 1991; 9: 99

92. Penn RD, Savoy SM, Corcos DE. Intrathecal baclofen for severe spinal spasticity. *N Engl J Med* 1989; 320: 1517

93. Nannings J, Frost F, Penn R. Effect of intrathecal baclofen on bladder and sphincter function. *J Urol* 1989; 142: 101

94. Loubser PG, Narayan RK, Sadin KJ. Continuous infusion of intrathecal baclofen: long term effects on spasticity in spinal cord injury. *Paraplegia* 1991; 29: 48

95. Mertens P, Parise M, Garcia-Larrea L *et al*. Long-term clinical, electrophysiological and urodynamic effects of chronic intrathecal baclofen infusion for treatment of spinal spasticity. *Acta Neurochir Suppl (Wien)* 1995; 64: 17–25

96. Murdock M, Sax D, Krane R. Use of dantrolene sodium in external sphincter spasm. *Urology* 1976; 8: 133

97. Hackler R, Broecker B, Klein F *et al*. A clinical experience with dantrolene sodium for external urinary sphincter hypertonicity in spinal cord injured patients. *J Urol* 1980; 124: 78

98. Harris JD, Benson GS. Effect of dantrolene on canine bladder contractility. *Urology* 1980; 16: 229

99. Ward AK, Chaffman MO, Sorkin EM. Dantrolene. A review of its pharmacodynamic and pharmacokinetic properties and therapeutic use in malignant hyperthermia, the neuroleptic syndrome and an update of its use in muscle spasticity. *Drugs* 1986; 32: 130

100. Olsson A, Swanberg E, Scedinger I. Effects of beta adrenoceptor agonists on airway smooth muscle and on slow contracting skeletal muscle: in vitro and in vivo results compared. *Acta Pharmacol Toxicol* 1979; 44: 272

101. Holmberg E, Waldeck B. On the possible role of potassium ions on the action of terbutaline on skeletal muscle contractions. *Acta Pharmacol Toxicol* 1980; 46: 141

102. Gosling JA, Dixon JS, Critchley HOD. A comparative study of the human external sphincter and periurethral levator ani muscles. *Br J Urol* 1981; 53: 35

103. Dykstra DD, Sidi AA. Treatment of detrusor–striated sphincter dyssynergia with botulinum A toxin. *Arch Phys Med Rehabil* 1990; 71: 24

104. Fowler CJ, Betts C, Christmas T *et al*. Botulinum toxin in the treatment of chronic urinary retention in women. *Br J Urol* 1992; 70: 387

105. Nordling J, Meyhoff H, Hald T. Sympatholytic effect on striated urethral sphincter. *Scand J Urol Nephrol* 1981; 15: 173–180

106. Rao M, Bapna B, Vaidyanathan *et al*. Use of clonidine in the management of patients with neurogenic bladder dysfunction. *Eur Urol* 1980; 6: 261–264

107. Herman RM, Wainberg MC. Clonidine inhibits vesicosphincter reflexes in patients with chronic spinal lesions. *Arch Phys Med Rehabil* 1991; 72: 539–545

108. Blaivas J, Labib K, Michalik S *et al*. Cystometric response to propantheline in detrusor hyperreflexia: therapeutic implications. *J Urol* 1980; 124: 259

109. Andersson KE. Current concepts in the treatment of disorders of micturition. *Drugs* 1988; 35: 477

110. Brading A. Physiology of bladder smooth muscle. In: Torrens M, Morrison JFB (eds) *The Physiology of the Lower Urinary Tract*. New York: Springer Verlag, 1987; 161–192

111. Brading AF. Physiology of the urinary tract smooth muscle. In: Webster G, Kirby R, King L, Goldwasser B (eds) *Reconstructive Urology*. Boston: Blackwell Scientific, 1987; 15–26

112. Bonner TI. The molecular basis of muscarinic receptor diversity. *Trends Neurosci* 1989; 12: 148

113. Poli E, Monica B, Zappia L *et al*. Antimuscarinic activity of telemyepine on isolated human urinary bladder: no role for M-1 receptors. *Gen Pharmacol* 1992; 23: 659

114. Eglen RM, Watson N. Selective muscarinic receptor agonists and antagonists. *Pharmacol Toxicol* 1996; 78: 59–68

115. Levin RM, Ruggieri MR, Wein AJ. Identification of receptor subtypes in the rabbit and human urinary bladder by selective radio-ligand binding. *J Urol* 1988; 139: 844

116. Levin RM, Ruggieri MR, Lee W *et al*. Effect of chronic atropine administration on the rat urinary bladder. *J Urol* 1988; 139: 1347

117. Nilvebrant L, Andersson KE, Gillberg PG *et al*. Tolterodine – a new bladder-selective antimuscarinic agent. *Eur J Pharmacol* 1997; 327: 195–207

118. Tobin G, Sjögren C. In vivo and in vitro effects of muscarinic receptor antagonists on contractions and release of [^{3}H] acetylcholine release in the rabbit urinary bladder. *Eur J Pharmacol* 1995; 281: 1–8

119. Restorick JM, Mundy AR. The density of cholinergic and alpha and beta adrenergic receptors in the normal and hyper-reflexic human detrusor. *Br J Urol* 1989; 63: 32

120. Lepor H, Gup D, Shapiro E *et al*. Muscarinic cholinergic receptors in the normal and neurogenic human bladder. *J Urol* 1989; 142: 869

121. Brown JH. Atropine, scopolamine and related antimuscarinic drugs. In: Gilman AG, Rall TW, Nies AS, Taylor P (eds) *Goodman and Gilman's The Pharmacological Basis of Therapeutics*, 8th edn. New York: Pergamon Press; 1990; 150–165

122. Gibaldi M, Grundhofer B. Biopharmaceutic influences on the anticholinergic effects of propantheline. *Clin Pharmacol Ther* 1975; 18: 457

123. Levin RM, Staskin D, Wein AJ. The muscarinic cholinergic binding kinetics of the human urinary bladder. *Neurourol Urodyn* 1982; 1: 221

124. Peterson JS, Patton AJ, Noronha-Blob L. Mini-pig urinary bladder function: comparisons of in vitro anticholinergic responses and in vivo cystometry with drugs indicated for urinary incontinence. *J Auton Pharmacol* 1990; 10: 65–73

125. Zorzitto ML, Jewett MA, Fernie GR *et al*. Effectiveness of propantheline bromide in the treatment of geriatric patients with detrusor instability. *Neurourol Urodyn* 1986; 5: 133

126. Urinary incontinence guideline panel: *Urinary Incontinence in Adults: Clinical Practice Guidelines*. AHCPR Pub. No. 92–0038. Rockville, MD: Agency for Health Care Policy and Research, Public Health Service, U.S. Department of Health and Human Services, March, 1992

127. Weiner LB, Baum NH, Suarez GM. New method for management of detrusor instability: transdermal scopolamine. *Urology* 1986; 28: 208

128. Cornella JL, Bent AE, Ostergard DR *et al*. Prospective study utilizing transdermal scopolamine in detrusor instability. *Urology* 1990; 35: 96

129. Muskat Y, Bukovsky I, Schneider D *et al*. The use of scopolamine in the treatment of detrusor instability. *J Urology* 1996; 156: 1989–1990

130. Greenstein A, Chen J, Matzkin H. Transdermal scopolamine in prevention of post open prostatectomy bladder contractions *Urology* 1992; 39: 215

131. Lau W, Szilagyi M. A pharmacological profile of glycopyrrolate: interactions at the muscarinic acetylcholine receptor. *Gen Pharmacol* 1992; 23: 1165

132. Nilvebrant L, Gillberg PG, Sparf B. Antimuscarinic potency and bladder selectivitiy of PNU-200577, a major metabolite of tolterodine. *Pharmacol Toxicol* 1997; 81: 169–172

133. Nilvebrant L, Hallen B, Larsson G. A new bladder selective muscarinic receptor antagonist: preclinical pharmacological and clinical data. *Life Sci* 1997; 60: 1129–1136

134. Nilvebrant L, Sundquist S, Gillberg PG. Tolterodine is not subtype (m1–m5) selective but exhibits functional bladder selectivity in vivo. *Neurourol Urodyn* 1996; 15: 310–311

135. Nilvebrant L, Glas G, Jonsson A *et al*. The in vitro pharmacological profile of tolterodine – a new agent for the treatment of urinary urge incontinence. *Neurourol Urodyn* 1994; 13: 433–435

136. Stahl MM, Ekstrom B, Sparf B *et al*. Urodynamic and other effects of tolterodine: a novel antimuscarinic drug for the treatment of detrusor overactivity. *Neurourol Urodyn* 1995; 14: 647–665

137. Jonas U, Hofner K, Madersbacher H *et al*. Efficacy and safety of two doses of tolterodine versus placebo in patients with detrusor overactivity and symptoms of frequency, urge incontinence, and urgency: urodynamic evaluation. The International Study Group. *World J Urol* 1997; 15: 144–151

138. Yarker YE, Goa KL, Fitton A. Oxybutynin. A review of its pharmacodynamic and pharmacokinetic properties, and its therapeutic use in detrusor instability. *Drugs Aging* 1995; 6: 243–262

139. Rentzhog L, Stanton SL, Cardozo L *et al*. Efficacy and safety of tolterodine in patients with detrusor instablity: a dose-ranging study. *Br J Urol* 1998; 81: 42–48

140. Smith CM, Wallis RM. Characterisation of [3H]-darifenacin as a novel radioligand for the study of muscarinic M3 receptors. *J Recept Signal Transduction Res* 1997; 17: 177–184

141. Alabaster VA. Discovery and development of selective M3 antagonists for clinical use. *Life Sci* 197; 60: 1053–1060

142. Oyasu H, Yamamoto T, Sato N *et al*. Urinary bladder-selective action of the new antimuscarinic compound vamicamide. *Drug Res* 1994 ; 44: 1242–1249

143. Yamamoto T, Koibuchi Y, Miura S *et al*. Effects of vamicamide on urinary bladder functions in conscious dog and rat models of urinary frequency. *J Urol* 1995; 154: 2174–2178

144. Kachur JF, Peterson JS, Carter JP *et al*. R and S

enantiomers of oxybutynin: pharmacological effects in guinea pig bladder and intestine. *J Pharmacol Exp Ther* 1988; 247: 867–872

145. Thompson I, Lauvetz R. Oxybutynin in bladder spasm, neurogenic bladder and enuresis. *Urology* 1976; 8: 452

146. Moisey C, Stephenson T, Brendler C. The urodynamic and subjective results of treatment of detrusor instability with oxybutynin chloride. *Br J Urol* 1980; 52: 472

147. Hehir M, Fitzpatrick JM. Oxybutynin and the prevention of urinary incontinence in spinal bifida. *Eur Urol* 1985; 11: 254

148. Gajewski J, Awad JA. Oxybutynin versus propantheline in patients with multiple sclerosis and detrusor hyperreflexia. *J Urol* 1986; 135: 966

149. Holmes DM, Montz FJ, Stanton SL. Oxybutynin versus propantheline in the management of detrusor instability. A patient-regulated variable dose trial. *Br J Obstet Gynaecol* 1989; 96: 607–612

150. Thuroff J, Bunke B, Ebner A *et al.* Randomized double-blind multicenter trial on treatment of frequency, urgency and incontinence related to detrusor hyperactivity: oxybutynin vs. propantheline vs. placebo. *J Urol* 1991; 145: 813

151. Zeegers A, Kiesswetter H, Kramer A *et al.* Conservative therapy of frequency, urgency and urge incontinence: a double-blind clinical trial of flavoxate, oxybutynin, emepronium and placebo. *World J Urol* 1987; 5: 57

152. Van Doorn ESC, Zweirs W. Ambulant monitoring to assess the efficacy of oxybutynin chloride in patients with mixed incontinence. *Eur Urol* 1990; 18: 49

153. Zorzitto ML, Holliday PJ, Jewett MA. Oxybutynin chloride for geriatric urinary dysfunction: a double-blind placebo controlled study. *Age Ageing* 1989; 18: 195

154. Ouslander JG, Blaustein J, Connor H. Habit training and oxybutynin for incontinence in nursing home patients: a placebo-controlled trial. *J Am Geriatr Soc* 1988; 36: 40

155. Ouslander JG, Blaustein J, Connor H. Pharmacokinetics and clinical effects of oxybutynin in geriatric patients. *J Urol* 1988; 140: 47

156. Gupta SK, Sathyan G. Pharmacokinetics of an oral once-a-day controlled-release oxybutynin formulation compared with immediate-release oxybutynin. *J Clin Pharmacol* 1999; 39: 289–296

157. Anderson R, Mobley D, Blank B *et al.* Once daily controlled versus immediate release oxybutynin chloride for urge urinary incontinence. *J Urol* 1999; 161: 1809–1812

158. Gleason DM, Susset J, White C *et al.* and the Ditropan XL study group. Evaluation of a new once daily formulation of oxybutynin for the treatment of urinary urge incontinence. *Urology* 1999; 54: 420–423

159. Kato K, Kitada S, Chun A *et al.* In vitro intravesical instillation of anticholinergic, antispasmodic and calcium blocking agents (rabbit whole bladder model). *J Urol* 1989; 141: 1471–1475

160. Mizunaga M, Miyata M, Kaneko S *et al.* Intravesical instillation of oxybutynin hydrochloride therapy for patients with a neuropathic bladder. *Paraplegia* 1994; 32: 25–29

161. Connor JP, Betrus G, Fleming P *et al.* Early cystometrograms can predict the response to intravesical instillation of oxybutynin chloride in myelomeningocele patients. *J Urol* 1994; 151: 1045–1047

162. Szollar SM, Lee SM. Intravesical oxybutynin for spinal cord injury patients. *Spinal Cord* 1996; 34: 284–287

163. Madersbacher H, Jilg G. Control of detrusor hyperreflexia by the intravesical instillation of oxybutynin hydrochloride. *Paraplegia* 1991; 19: 84

164. Madersbacher H, Knoll M. Intravesical application of oxybutynin: mode of action in controlling detrusor hyperreflexia. *Eur Urol* 1995; 8: 340–344

165. Weese DL, Roskamp DA, Leach GE *et al.* Intravesical oxybutynin chloride: experience with 42 patients. *Urology* 1993; 41: 527

166. Enzelsberger H, Helmer H, Kurz C. Intravesical instillation of oxybutynin in women with idiopathic detrusor instability: a randomised trial. *Br J Obstet Gynaecol* 1995; 102: 929–930

167. Glickman S, Tsokkos N, Shah PJ. Intravesical atropine and suppression of detrusor hypercontractility in the neuropathic bladder. A preliminary study. *Paraplegia* 1995; 33: 36–39

168. Andersson KE, Hedlund H, Mansson W. Pharmacologic treatment of bladder hyperactivity after augmentation and substitution enterocystoplasty. *Scand J Urol Nephrol* 1992; 142: 42–46

169. Downie J, Twiddy D, Awad SA. Antimuscarininc and non-competitive antagonist properties of dicyclomine hydrochloride in isolated human and rabbit bladder muscle. *J Pharmacol Exp Ther* 1977; 201: 662

170. Fischer C, Diokno A, Lapides J. The anticholinergic effects of dicyclomine hydrochloride in inhibited neurogenic bladder dysfunction. *J Urol* 1978; 120: 328

171. Beck RP, Anausch T, King C. Results in testing 210 patients with detrusor overactivity incontinence of urine. *Am J Obstet Gynecol* 1976; 125: 593

172. Awad SA, Bryniak S, Downie JW *et al.* The treatment of the uninhibited bladder with dicyclomine. *J Urol* 1977; 114: 161

173. Ruffman R. A review of flavoxate hydrochloride in the treatment of urge incontinence. *J Int Med Res* 1988; 16: 317

174. Kimura Y, Sasaki Y, Hamada K *et al.* Mechanisms of suppression of the bladder activity by flavoxate. *Int J Urol* 1996; 3: 218–227

175. Delaere KJP, Michiels HGE, Debruyne FMJ *et al.* Flavoxate hydrochloride in the treatment of detrusor instability. *Urol Int* 1977; 32: 377

176. Jonas U, Petri E, Kissal J. The effect of flavoxate on hyperactive detrusor muscle. *Eur Urol* 1979; 5: 106

177. Briggs RS, Castleden CM, Asher MJ. The effect of flavoxate on uninhibited detrusor contractions and urinary incontinence in the elderly. *J Urol* 1980; 123: 656

178. Benson GS, Sarshik SA, Raezer DM *et al.* Bladder muscle contractility: comparative effects and mechanisms of action of atropine, propantheline, flavoxate and imipramine. *Urology* 1977; 9: 31

179. Stohrer M, Bauer P, Giannetti BM *et al.* Effect of trospium chloride on urodynamic parameters in patients with detrusor hyperreflexia due to spinal cord injuries. *Urol Int* 1991; 47: 138–143

180. Madersbacher H, Stohrer M, Richter R *et al.* Trospium chloride versus oxybutynin: a randomized, double blind, multicentre trial in the treatment of detrusor hyperreflexia. *Br J Urol* 1995; 75: 452–456

181. Haruno A. Inhibitory effects of propiverine hydrochloride on the agonist-induced or spontaneous contractions of various isolated muscle preparations. *Drug Res* 1992; 42: 815

182. Mazur D, Wehnert J, Dorschner W *et al.* Clinical and urodynamic effects of propiverine in patients suffering from urgency and urge incontinence. A multicentre dose-optimizing study. *Scand J Urol Nephrol* 1995; 29: 289–294

183. Forman A, Andersson K, Henriksson L *et al.* Effects of nifedipine on the smooth muscle of the human urinary tract in vitro and in vivo. *Acta Pharmacol Toxicol* 1978; 43: 111–118

184. Husted S, Andersson KE, Sommer L. Anticholinergic and calcium antagonistic effects of terodiline in rabbit urinary bladder. *Acta Pharmacol Toxicol* 1980; 46: 20

185. Finkbeiner AE. Effect of extracellular calcium and calcium-blocking agents on detrusor contractility: an in vitro study. *Neurourol Urodyn* 1983; 2: 245

186. Malkowicz SB, Wein AJ, Brendler K *et al.* Effect of diltiazem on in vitro rabbit bladder function. *Pharmacology* 1985; 31: 24–33

187. Andersson KE, Fovaeus M, Morgan E *et al.* Comparative effects of five different calcium channel blockers on the atropine-resistant contraction in electrically stimulated rabbit urinary bladder. *Neurourol Urodyn* 1986; 5: 579

188. Bodner DR, Lindan R, Leffler E *et al.* The effect of verapamil on the treatment of detrusor hyperreflexia in the spinal cord injured population. *Paraplegia* 1989; 27: 364–369

189. Abrams P. Terodiline in clinical practice. *Urology* 1990; 36(Suppl): 60

190. Ekman G, Andersson KE, Rud T *et al.* A double-blind crossover study of the effects of terodiline in women with unstable bladder. *Acta Pharmacol Toxicol* 1980; 46(Suppl): 39

191. Peters D. Multicentre Study Group: Terodiline in the treatment of urinary frequency and motor urge incontinence: a controlled multicentre trial. *Scand J Urol Nephrol* 1984; 87(Suppl): 21

192. Tapp A, Fall M, Norgaard J *et al.* Terodiline: a dose titrated, multicenter study of the treatment of idiopathic detrusor instability in women. *J Urol* 1989; 142: 1027–1031

193. Levin RM, Scheiner S, Zhao Y *et al.* The effect of terodiline on hyperreflexia (in vitro) and the in vitro response of isolated strips of rabbit bladder to field stimulation, bethanechol and KCl. *Pharmacology* 1993; 46: 346

194. Veldhuis G, Inman J. Terodiline and torsade de pointes (Letter to the Editor). *Br Med J* 1991; 303: 519

195. Connolly MJ, Astridge PS, White EG *et al.* Torsade de pointes ventricular tachycardia and terodiline. *Lancet* 1991; 338: 344

196. Stewart DA, Taylor J, Ghosh S *et al.* Terodiline causes polymorphic ventricular tachycardia due to reduced heart rate and prolongation of QT interval. *Eur J Clin Pharmacol* 1992; 42: 577–580

197. Palmer J, Worth P, Exton-Smith A. Flunarizine: a once daily therapy for urinary incontinence. *Lancet* 1981; 2: 279

198. Dykstra DD, Sidi AA, Anderson L. The effect of nifedipine on cystoscopy-induced autonomic hyperreflexia in patients with high spinal cord injuries. *J Urol* 1987; 138: 1155

199. Andersson KE. Clinical pharmacology of potassium channel openers. *Pharmacol Toxicol* 1992; 70: 244

200. Malmgren A, Andersson K, Andersson PO *et al.* Effects of cromakalim (BRL 34915) and pinacidil on normal and hypertrophied rat detrusor in vitro. *J Urol* 1990; 143: 828

201. Fovaeus M, Andersson KE, Hedlund H. The action of pinacidil in isolated human bladder. *J Urol* 1989; 141: 637

202. Hedlund H, Mattiasson A, Andersson KE. Lack of effect of pinacidil on detrusor instability in men with bladder outlet obstruction. *J Urol* 1990; 143: 369A

203. Nurse DE, Restorick JM, Mundy AR. The effect of cromakalim on the normal and hyper-reflexic human detrusor muscle. *Br J Urol* 1991; 68: 27–31

204. Komersova K, Rogerson JW, Conway EL *et al.* The effect of Levcromokalim (BRL 38227) on bladder function in patients with high spinal cord lesions. *Br J Clin Pharmacol* 1995; 39: 207–209

205. Longman SD, Hamilton TC. Potassium channel activator drugs – mechanism of action, pharmacological properties, and therapeutic potential. *Med Res Rev* 1992; 12: 73–148

206. Levin RM, Hayes L, Zhao Y *et al.* Effect of pinacidil on spontaneous and evoked contractile activity. *Pharmacology* 1992; 45: 1–8

207. Downie JW, Karmazyn M. Mechanical trauma to bladder epithelium liberates prostanoids which modulate neurotransmission in rabbit detrusor muscle. *J Pharmacol Exp Ther* 1984; 230: 445–449

208. Cardozo LD, Stanton SL, Robinson H *et al.* Evaluation of flurbiprofen in detrusor instability. *Br Med J* 1980; 2: 281–282

209. Cardozo L, Stanton SL. An objective comparison of the effects of parenterally administered drugs in patients suffering from detrusor instability. *J Urol* 1979; 122: 58

210. Brooks PM, Day RO. Non-steroidal anti-inflammatory drugs – differences and similarities. *N Engl J Med* 1991; 324: 1716

211. Norlen L, Sundin T, Waagstein F. Beta-adrenoceptor stimulation of the human urinary bladder in vivo. *Acta Pharmacol Toxicol* 1978; 43: 5

212. Lindholm P, Lose G. Terbutaline (Bricanyl) in the treatment of female urge incontinence. *Urol Int* 1986; 41: 158

213. Gruneberger A. Treatment of motor urge incontinence with clenbuterol and flavoxate hydrochloride. *Br J Obstet Gynaecol* 1984; 91: 275

214. Castleden CM, Morgan B. The effect of beta adrenoceptor agonists on urinary incontinence in the elderly. *Br J Clin Pharmacol* 1980; 10: 619

215. Naglo AS, Nergardh A, Boreus LO. Influence of atropine and isoprenoline on detrusor hyperactivity in children with neurogenic bladder. *Scand J Urol Nephrol* 1989; 15: 97

216. Hollister LE. Current antidepressants. *Annu Rev Pharmacol Toxicol* 1986; 26: 23

217. Richelson E. Antidepressants and brain neurochemistry. *Mayo Clin Proc* 1990; 65: 1227

218. Olubadewo J. The effect of imipramine on rat detrusor muscle contractility. *Arch Int Pharmacodyn Ther* 1980; 145: 84

219. Levin RM, Staskin D, Wein AJ. Analysis of the anticholinergic and musculotropic effects of desmethylimipramine on the rabbit urinary bladder. *Urol Res* 1983; 11: 259

220. Levin RM, Wein AJ. Comparative effects of five tricyclic compounds on the rabbit urinary bladder. *Neurourol Urodyn* 1984; 3: 127

221. Bigger J, Giardino E, Perel JE. Cardiac antiarrhythmic effect of imipramine hydrochloride. *N Engl J Med* 1977; 296: 206

222. Malkowicz SB, Wein AJ, Ruggieri MR *et al.* Comparison of calcium antagonist properties of antispasmodic agents. *J Urol* 1987; 138: 667

223. Akah PA. Tricyclic antidepressant inhibition of the electrical evoked responses of the rat urinary bladder strip – effect of variation in extracellular Ca concentration. *Arch Int Pharmacodyn* 1986; 284: 231

224. Foreman MM, McNulty AM. Alterations in K(+)-evoked release of 3-H-norepinephrine and contractile responses in urethral and bladder tissues induced by norepinephrine reuptake inhibition. *Life Sci* 1993; 53: 193

225. Cole A, Fried F. Favorable experiences with imipramine in the treatment of neurogenic bladder. *J Urol* 1972; 107: 44

226. Raezer DM, Benson GS, Wein AJ. The functional approach to the management of the pediatric neuropathic bladder: a clinical study. *J Urol* 1977; 117: 649

227. Tulloch AGS, Creed KE. A comparison between propantheline and imipramine on bladder and salivary gland function. *Br J Urol* 1981; 125: 218

228. Castleden CM, George CF, Renwick AG *et al.* Imipramine – a possible alternative to current therapy for urinary incontinence in elderly. *J Urol* 1981; 125: 218

229. Korczyn AD, Kish I. The mechanism of imipramine in enuresis nocturna. *Clin Exp Pharmacol Physiol* 1979; 6: 31

230. Lose G, Jorgensen L, Thunedborg P. Doxepin in the treatment of female detrusor overactivity: A randomized double-blind crossover study. *J Urol* 1989; 142: 1024

231. Berk M, du Plessis AD, Birkett M *et al.* An open-label study of duloxetine hydrochloride, a mixed serotonin and noradrenaline reuptake inhibitor, in patients with DSM-III-R major depressive disorder. *Int Clin Psychopharmacol* 1997; 12: 137–140

232. Thor KB, Katofiasc MA. Effects of duloxetine, a combined serotonin and norepinephrine reuptake inhibitor, on central neural control of lower urinary

tract function in the chloralose-anesthetized female cat. *J Pharmacol Exp Ther* 1995; 274: 1014–1024

233. Sant GR. Intravesical 50% dimethyl sulfoxide (Rimso-50) in treatment of interstitial cystitis. *Urology* 1987; 4(Suppl): 17

234. Kiesswetter H, Schober W. Lioresal in the treatment of neurogenic bladder dysfunction. *Urol Int* 1975; 30: 63

235. Taylor MC, Bates CP. A double-blind crossover trial of baclofen: a new treatment for the unstable bladder syndrome. *Br J Urol* 1979; 51: 505

236. James MJ, Birmingham AT, Hill SJ. Partial mediation by nitric oxide of the relaxation of human isolated detrusor strips in response to electrical field stimulation. *Br J Clin Pharmacol* 1993; 35: 366

237. James MJ, Iacovou JW. The case of GTN patches in detrusor instability: a pilot study. *Neurourol Urodyn* 1993; 12: 399

238. Soulard C, Pascaud X, Roman FJ *et al.* Pharmacological evaluation of JO-1870 – relation to the potential treatment of urinary bladder incontinence. *J Pharmacol Exp Ther* 1992; 260: 1152

239. Constantinou CE. Pharmacologic treatment of detrusor incontinence with thiphenamil HCl. *Urol Int* 1992; 48: 42

240. Constantinou CE. Pharmacologic effect of thiphenamil HCl on lower urinary tract function of healthy asymptomatic volunteers. *Urol Int* 1992; 48: 293

241. Maggi CA, Barbanti G, Santicioli P *et al.* Cystometric evidence that capsaicin-sensitive nerves modulate the afferent branch of micturition reflex in humans. *J Urol* 1989; 142: 150–154

242. Maggi CA. Capsaicin and primary afferent neurons: from basic science to human therapy? *J Auton Nerv Syst* 1991; 33: 1–14

243. Maggi CA. Therapeutic potential of capsaicin-like molecules – studies in animals and humans. *Life Sci* 1992; 51: 1777–1781

244. Dray A. Mechanism of action of capsaicin-like molecules on sensory neurons. *Life Sci* 1993; 51: 1759

245. Craft RM, Porreca F. Treatment parameters of desensitization to capsaicin. *Life Sci* 1992; 51: 1767

246. Fowler CJ, Beck RO, Gerrard S *et al.* Intravesical capsaicin for treatment of detrusor hyperreflexia. *J Neurol Neurosurg Psychiatry* 1994; 57: 169–173

247. Das A, Chancellor M, Watanabe T *et al.* Intravesical capsaicin in neurologic impaired patients with detrusor hyperreflexia. *J Spinal Cord Med* 1996; 19: 190–193

248. Geirsson G, Fall M, Sullivan L. Clinical and urodynamic effects of intravesical capsaicin treatment in patients with chronic traumatic spinal detrusor hyperreflexia. *J Urol* 1995; 154: 1825–1829

249. Chandiramani VA, Peterson T, Duthie GS *et al.* Urodynamic changes during therapeutic intravesical instillations of capsaicin. *Br J Urol* 1996; 77: 792–797

250. Hoffman BB, Lefkowitz RJ. Catecholamines and sympathomimetic drugs. In: Gilman AG, Rall TW, Nies AS, Taylor P (eds) *Goodman and Gilman's The Pharmacological Basis of Therapeutics*, 8th edn. New York: Pergamon Press, 1990; 187–220

251. Rashbaum M, Mandelbaum CC. Non-operative treatment of urinary incontinence in women. *Am J Obstet Gynecol* 1948; 56: 777

252. Diokno A, Taub M. Ephedrine in treatment of urinary incontinence. *Urology* 1975; 5: 624

253. Ek A, Andersson KE, Gullberg B *et al.* The effects of long-term treatment with norephedrine on stress incontinence and urethral closure pressure profile. *Scand J Urol Nephrol* 1978; 12: 105

254. O'Brink A, Bunne G. The effect of alpha adrenergic stimulation in stress incontinence. *Urol Int* 1978; 12: 205

255. Lose G, Lindholm D. Clinical and urodynamic effects of nofenefrine in women with stress incontinence. *Urol Int* 1994; 39: 298

256. Lose G, Rix P, Diernoes E *et al.* Norfenefrine in the treatment of female stress incontinence. *Urol Int* 1988; 43: 11

257. Diernoes E, Rix P, Sorenson T *et al.* Norfenefrine in the treatment of female urinary stress incontinence assessed by one hour pad weighing test. *Urol Int* 1989; 44: 28

258. Lose G, Diernoes E, Rix P. Does medical therapy cure female stress incontinence. *Urol Int* 1989; 44: 25

259. Awad SA, Downie J, Kirulita J. Alpha adrenergic agents in urinary disorders of the proximal urethra: I. Stress incontinence. *Br J Urol* 1978; 50: 332

260. Stewart B, Borowsky L, Montague D. Stress incontinence: conservative therapy with synpathomimetic drugs. *J Urol* 1976; 115: 558

261. Collste L, Lindskog M. Phenylpropanolamine in treatment of female stress incontinence. Double blind placebo controlled study in 24 patients. *Urology* 1987; 30: 398–403

262. Mueller S. Neurological complications of phenylpropanolamine use. *Neurology* 1983; 33: 650

263. Baggioni I, Onrot J, Stewart CK *et al.* The potent pressor effect of phenylpropanolamine in patients with autonomic impairment. *J Am Med Assoc* 1987; 258: 236

264. Lasagna L. Phenylpropanolamine and blood pressure. *J Am Med Assoc* 1985; 253: 2491

265. Liebson I, Bigelow G, Griffiths RR *et al.* Phenyl-propanolamine: effects on subjective and cardiovascular variables at recommended over-the-counter dose levels. *J Clin Pharmacol* 1987; 27: 685

266. Blackburn GL, Morgan JP, Lavin PT *et al.* Determinants of the pressor effect of phenylpropanolamine in healthy subjects. *J Am Med Assoc* 1989; 261: 3267

267. Kiesswetter H, Hennrich F, Englisch M. Clinical and pharmacologic therapy of stress incontinence. *Urol Int* 1983; 38: 58

268. Gilja I, Radej M, Kovacic M *et al.* Conservative treatment of female stress incontinence with imipramine. *J Urol* 1984; 132: 909

269. Gleason D, Reilly R, Bottaccinin M *et al.* The urethral continence zone and its relation to stress incontinence. *J Urol* 1974; 112: 81

270. Kaisary AU. Beta adrenoceptor blaockade in the treatment of female stress urinary incontinence. *J Urol (Paris)* 1984; 90: 351

271. Donker P, Van Der Sluis C. Action of beta adrenergic blocking agents on the urethral pressure profile. *Urol Int* 1976; 31: 6

272. Fellenius E, Hedberg R, Holmberg E *et al.* Functional and metabolic effects of terbutaline and propranolol in fast and slow contracting skeletal muscle in vitro. *Acta Physiol Scand* 1980; 109: 89

273. Kishimoto T, Morita T, Okamiyo Y. Effect of clenbuterol on contractile response in periurethral striated muscle of rabbits. *Tohoku J Exp Med* 1991; 165: 243

274. Salmon UJ, Walter RI, Geist SH. The use of oestrogens in the treatment of dysuria and incontinence in post-menopausal women. *Am J Obstet Gynecol* 1941; 42: 845

275. Hodgson BJ, Dumas S, Bolling DR *et al.* Effect of oestrogen on sensitivity of rabbit bladder and urethra to phenylephrine. *Invest Urol* 1978; 16: 67

276. Levin RM, Shofer FS, Wein AJ. oestrogen-induced alterations in the autonomic responses of the rabbit urinary bladder. *J Pharmacol Exp Ther* 1980; 215: 614

277. Levin RM, Jacobowitz D, Wein AJ. Autonomic innervation of rabbit urinary bladder following oestrogen administration. *Urology* 1981; 17: 449

278. Levin RM, Zderic SA, Ewalt DH *et al.* Effects of pregnancy on muscarinic receptor density and function in the rabbit urinary bladder. *Pharmacology* 1991; 43: 69

279. Tong Y, Wein AJ, Levin RM. Effects of pregnancy on adrenergic function in the rabbit urinary bladder. *Neurourol Urodyn* 1992; 11: 525

280. Larsson B, Andersson K, Batra S *et al.* Effects of estradiol on norepinephrine-induced contraction, alpha adreno-ceptor number and norepinephrine content in the female rabbit urethra. *J Pharmacol Exp Ther* 1984; 229: 557

281. Callahan SM, Creed KE. The effects of oestrogens on spontaneous activity and responses to phenylephrine of the mammalian urethra. *J Physiol* 1985; 358: 35

282. Bump RC, Friedman CI. Intraluminal urethral pressure measurements in the female baboon: effects of hormonal manipulation. *J Urol* 1986; 136: 508

283. Batra SC, Iosif CS. Female urethra: a target for oestrogen action. *J Urol* 1983; 129: 418

284. Batra S, Byellin L, Sjögren C. Increases in blood flow of the female rabbit urethra following low dose oestrogens. *J Urol* 1986; 136: 1360

285. Rud T. Urethral pressure profile in continent women from childhood to old age. *Acta Obstet Gynecol Scand* 1980; 59: 331

286. Versi E, Cardozo L, Buncat L *et al.* Correlation of urethral physiology and skin collagen in post menopausal women. *Br J Urol Gynaecol* 1988; 95: 147

287. Eika B, Salling LN, Christensen LL *et al.* Long-term observation of the detrusor smooth muscle in rats. Its relationship to ovariectomy and oestrogen treatment. *Urol Res* 1990; 18: 439

288. Raz S, Zeigler M, Caine M. The effect of progesterone on the adrenergic receptors of the urethra. *Br J Urol* 1973; 45: 663–667

289. Batra SC, Iosif CS. Progesterone receptors in the female lower urinary tract. *J Urol* 1987; 138: 1301

290. Rud T. The effects of oestrogens and gestagens on the urethral pressure profile of urinary continent and stress incontinent women. *Acta Obstet Gynecol Scand* 1980; 59: 265

291. Raz S, Ziegler M, Caine M. The role of female hormones in stress incontinence. Proceedings of 16th Congress Society International d'Urologie, volume 1. Paris: 1973; 397–402

292. Schreiter F, Fuchs P, Stockamp K. Estrogenic sensitivity of α-receptors in the urethra musculature. *Urol Int* 1976; 31: 13

293. Beisland HO, Fossberg E, Moer A *et al.* Urethral sphincteric insuffciency in postmenopausal females: treatment with phenylpropanolamine and estriol separately and in combination. *Urol Int* 1984; 39: 211

294. Bhatia NN, Bergman A, Karram MM. Effects of oestrogen on urethral function in women with urinary incontinence. *Am J Obstet Gynecol* 1989; 160: 176

295. Karram MM, Yeko TR, Sauer MV *et al.* Urodynamic changes following hormonal replacement therapy in women with premature ovarian failure. *Obstet Gynecol* 1989; 74: 208

296. Walter S, Wolf H, Barleto H *et al.* Urinary incontinence in post menopausal women treated with oestrogens. *Urol Int* 1978; 33: 135

297. Hilton P, Stanton SL. The use of intravaginal oestrogen cream in genuine stress incontinence. *Br J Obstet Gynaecol* 1983; 90: 940

298. Samsioe G, Jansson I, Mellström D *et al.* Occurrence, nature and treatment of urinary incontinence in a 70-year-old female population. *Maturitas* 1985; 7: 335

299. Cardozo L. Role of oestrogens in the treatment of female urinary incontinence. *J Am Geriatr Soc* 1990; 38: 326

300. Kinn AC, Lindskog M. oestrogens and phenyl-propanolamine in combination for stress urinary incontinence in postmenopausal women. *Urology* 1988; 32: 273

301. Walter S, Kjærgaard B, Lose G *et al.* Stress urinary incontinence in postmenopausal women treated with oral oestrogen (estriol) and an alpha-adrenoceptor-stimulating agent (phenylpropanolamine): a randomized double-blind placebo-controlled study. *Int Urogynecol J* 1990; 1: 74

302. Hilton P, Tweddell AL, Mayne C. Oral and intravaginal oestrogens alone and in combination with alpha-adrenergic stimulation in genuine stress incontinence. *Int Urogynecol J* 1990; 1: 80

303. Fantl JA, Bump RC, Robinson D *et al.* Efficacy of oestrogen supplementation in the treatment of urinary incontinence. *Obstet Gynecol* 1996; 88: 745–749

304. Session DR, Kelly AC, Jewelewicz R. Current concepts in oestrogen replacement therapy in the menopause. *Fertil Steril* 1993; 59: 277

305. Grodstein F, Stampfer MJ, Colditz GA *et al.* Post-menopausal hormone therapy and mortality. *N Engl J Med* 1997; 336: 1769–1775

306. Murray K. Medical and surgical management of female voiding difficulty. In: Drife JO, Hilton P, Stanton SL (eds) *Micturition.* London: Springer-Verlag, 1990; 179

307. Ayton RA, Darling GM, Murkies AI *et al.* A comparative study of safety and efficacy of continuous low dose estradiol released from a vaginal ring compared with conjugated equine oestrogen vaginal cream in the treatment of postmenopausal urogenital atrophy. *Br J Obstet Gynaecol* 1996; 103: 351–358

308. Johnston A. Estrogens: pharmacokinetics and pharmacodynamics with special reference to vaginal administration and the new estradiol formulation – Estring. *Acta Obstet Gynecol Scand* 1996; 165: 16–25

309. Norgaard JP, Rillig S, Djurhuus JC. Nocturnal enuresis: an approach to treatment based on pathogenesis. *J Pediatr* 1989; 114: 705

310. Rew DA, Rundle JSH. Assessment of the safety of regular DDAVP therapy on primary nocturnal enuresis. *Br J Urol* 1989; 63: 352

311. Asplund R, Oberg H. Desmopressin in elderly subjects with increased nocturnal diuresis: a 2 month treatment study. *Scand J Urol Nephrol* 1993; 27: 77

312. Kinn AC, Larsson PO. Desmopressin: a new principle for symptomatic treatment of urgency and incontinence in patients with multiple sclerosis. *Scand J Urol Nephrol* 1990; 24: 109

313. Pederson PA, Johansen PB. Prophylactic treatment of adult nocturia with bumetanide. *Br J Urol* 1988; 62: 145

33

Catheters; pads and pants; appliances

K. Anders, S. Foxley, J. Haken

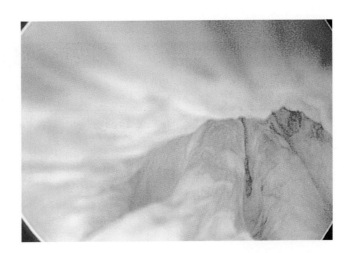

INTRODUCTION

Incontinence is a common and complex condition affecting women of all ages and of all social and cultural backgrounds. Unfortunately, for some, treatment is ineffective, or diagnosis and treatment of the condition can take some time to establish; their incontinence or their inability to micturate normally therefore must be contained or managed. Many products are marketed worldwide, but these must be carefully and appropriately selected for each individual, with consideration to their needs, wishes and social circumstances. Products fall into three main categories – catheters, pads and pants, and aids and appliances. This chapter attempts to provide an overview of what is available and how these can be applied in practice.

CATHETERS

Catheters are used for effective drainage of the bladder, either temporarily or permanently, in the presence of physiological and anatomical defects or obstruction of the lower urinary tract. The word catheter derives from the Greek word *katheter* meaning 'to set down' or 'let down into' and its usage is said to date back to the Sumerian culture in 3000 BC. It was suggested that gold was used as it was easily moulded and was suited to drain urine from the bladder.[1] Today, catheters are an integral part of patient care and the prevalence rate for short-term catheterization[2] among hospitalized patients in the UK is 12.6% (median 4 days) and around 4% in patients in the community.[3] Catheters are used for a variety of reasons, which are summarized below. Catheterization, however, should be undertaken only after full consideration of the implications of the pro-

cedure and with informed consent from the person to be catheterized.

Reasons for catheterization are as follows:

- Prophylaxis; to maintain bladder drainage during and following surgery or epidurals, thus minimizing the risk of distension injury to the bladder
- Investigations; during urodynamic investigations; for accurate urine output measurement (e.g. in intensive care units); measurement of post-micturition residuals
- Treatment; to relieve urinary retention; bladder irrigation; for chemotherapy instillation
- Intractable incontinence; only as a final option for containment.

Catheter insertion falls into two main groups – urethral and suprapubic. Urethral catheterization can be indwelling (or self-retaining) or intermittent/single use (or non-retaining), for example clean intermittent self-catheterization (CISC).

Urethral catheterization

A self-retaining catheter was first described by Reybard in 1853,[4] but it was not until the 1930s that Frederick Foley[5] perfected a method of devising a latex catheter with an integrated balloon that did not disintegrate. With modern techniques and the development of new materials, there is now an extensive range that can be utilized for short-term and long-term use (Table 33.1).

The urethral catheter is still the most commonly used catheter for the drainage of urine as it can be quickly and easily inserted. Female urethral

Table 33.1. *Catheter materials*			
Short-term use (max. 7 days)	Medium use (max. 4 weeks)	Long-term use (max. 12 weeks)	Specialist use
• Latex rubber • Siliconized latex (used to facilitate insertion only) • Plastic/PVC (used when there is extensive debris in the urine, particularly postoperatively)	• Latex coated with Teflon/ PTFE	• Silicone elastomer-encapsulated (coated) latex • Hydrogel-coated latex (hydrogels facilitate insertion and have similar properties to silicone) • 100% silicone	• Roberts (Teflon-coated with one eye below the balloon for drainage) • Three-way irrigation (plastic or latex rubber, usually with reinforcement to prevent collapse with suction) • Whistle-tip catheter

catheterization is an accepted aseptic procedure and should be undertaken under the guidance of strict local hospital or community infection-control policies.

Catheter selection

With different modes of catheterization and the availability of different materials, it is important to make the right choice for each individual's needs. Not surprisingly, a review of hospitals (in the UK)[6] found that many staff had insufficient knowledge of, and inadequate training in, the selection of catheters.

Designs and materials (Table 33.1)

Plastic or PVC and latex rubber should be used for only a very short time and are generally used only in immediate postoperative circumstances. Although cheap, plastic catheters are rigid and uncomfortable, causing bladder spasm and bypassing.[7] Both plastic and latex catheters tend to attract surface deposits, causing encrustation and fractures within the catheter. Following reports that some catheters were associated with cytotoxity,[8] all catheters in the UK must now conform to British Standards. Attempts to improve on the latex catheter include 'siliconizing' the surface of the catheter, producing a lubricant effect to facilitate insertion. Latex has also been coated in Teflon (polytetrafluoroethylene or PTFE) to make it more inert, and giving it a smoother surface in an attempt to reduce urethritis and encrustation.

Silicone elastomer-encapsulated (coated) latex catheters differ from the 'siliconized' catheters described above and are recommended for use in the long term. Silicone is an inert material, reducing the incidence of trauma, urethritis and encrustation, and therefore can be used long term (i.e. up to 3 months). Hydrogel catheters are similar to silicone catheters but they become smoother when hydrated. A comparison of urethral reactions to 100% silicone catheters, hydrogel-coated catheters and siliconized latex catheters demonstrated that 100% silicone catheters had the lowest incidence of urethral inflammation; hydrogel catheters proved to be the most superior in preventing encrustation; the siliconized latex catheters were the least effective in preventing both urethral inflammation and encrustation.[9]

The majority of catheters have a semi-rigid rounded tip with two drainage eyes, placed either laterally or opposed. Opposite drainage eyes generally facilitate better drainage with fewer blockages. There are some variations, including the Tiemann catheter which is curved at the tip, although this is not usually used in women as the curve is designed to facilitate insertion past an enlarged prostate. A whistle-tipped catheter aids drainage of urine containing large amounts of debris because of its open-ended tip (Fig. 33.1).

Other specialist catheters include the Roberts catheter, which has two drainage eyes, either side of the balloon of the catheter. The design allows urine to drain through the distal eye, rather than bypassing the catheter. This is particularly useful in patients with abnormal detrusor activity or when the catheter is susceptible to blockage.

A study in 1984[10] demonstrated that the urethral lumen was not circular and that, therefore, a circular catheter tended to distort the urethra. This finding led to the development of the 'Conformacath', which has a collapsible, flexible urethral section designed to adopt the shape of the female urethra. It is intended to be more comfortable and to reduce the incidence of encrustation and, possibly, of urinary bypassing.[11] A more recent study had mixed results, demonstrating increased blocking and bypassing with the catheter, but concluded that it did offer an alternative for those who were unable to tolerate conventional catheters.[12]

Catheter size and length

To develop a standard measurement, a French instrument maker, J.F.B Charriere, suggested a scale based on the metric system. This measurement is termed as

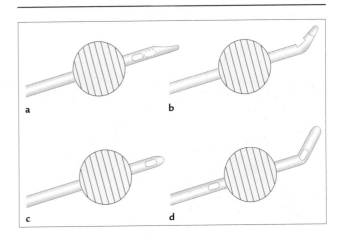

Figure 33.1. *Catheter tips: (a) whistle; (b) Tiemann; (c) round; (d) Roberts.*

either 'French gauge' (Fg) or 'Charriere' (Ch). It is the measurement of the external circumference in millimetres, which is approximately equal to three times the external diameter, depending on the catheter material. Catheters used in women should range from size 12 to 16F, with a small balloon that holds 10 ml sterile water. All 10 ml must be instilled to ensure correct inflation of the balloon, as underinflation may cause distortion of the balloon and deflection of the catheter tip. Many healthcare professionals continue to use larger-diameter catheters even though there is evidence that larger catheters are associated with discomfort and bypassing.[13,14] There is also evidence that too large a catheter will block the para-urethral glands, causing a build-up of secretions which in turn become infected and lead to abscess and stricture[15] (Fig. 33.2). Larger catheters, however, are useful for draining heavy haematuria. The 30 ml balloon associated with a larger catheter was developed to aid homoeostasis and therefore is useful only following prostate surgery in men.

Catheters are available in three lengths: 42 cm (male length); 26 cm (female length); and a shorter paediatric catheter. A female-length catheter is generally unsuitable for a woman who is overweight.

Catheter-associated problems

Infection

The incidence of urinary tract infection (UTI) is high with long-term urinary catheter use and is the most common complication with indwelling catheters. Most users of a catheter will have bacteria in the urine within 3 days[16] and, because of overgrowth of resistant bacteria, prophylactic antibiotics are discouraged[17] unless the patient develops systemic symptoms. Similarly, although irrigation of the bladder with antibiotic and antiseptic agents continues to be used,[18,19] such management is generally of limited value.[20] In particular, the readily available pre-packed chlorhexidine has not been shown to be effective in long-term usage against a number of frequently occurring pathogens: it has been shown to remove sensitive bacteria in the normal urethral flora and thus to allow subsequent colonization by resistant organisms.[21]

One of the main reasons why infections are so difficult to eradicate is the growth of bacterial populations as an adherent biofilm on the catheter surface. Common pathogens, such as *Escherichia coli*, may be eliminated from the urine, but persist in the biofilm and restart the cycle of infection.[22] Laboratory tests have been performed on 'an infection-inhibiting' urinary catheter material with promising results. A silicone rubber elastomer catheter compounded with chlorhexidine gluconate was found to be effective for 4 weeks against *E. coli*, *Proteus mirabilis* and *Staphylococcus epidermidis*.[23] However, a study comparing 18 types of catheter in current use found that none was capable of resisting encrustation by *P. mirabilis* biofilms.[24]

Catheter leakage, bypassing and blockage

Too large a catheter, detrusor spasm, blockage, debris or the presence of bladder calculi are all reasons for catheter failure. Blockage is frequently the result of a urinary tract infection leading to encrustation. The incidence of catheter blockage and bypassing in long-term catheterization is about 48% for blockage and 37% for bypassing,[25] and this may indicate a need for early changing.

The use of a large catheter often irritates the bladder, causing it to contract and squeeze urine out past the catheter. The use of an appropriate smaller catheter will reduce the incidence of abnormal bladder contractions, although some may benefit from the instigation of anticholinergic therapy if there is concomitant detrusor instability or hyperreflexia. In an attempt to avoid any systemic side effects, such therapy can be instilled intravesically.[26]

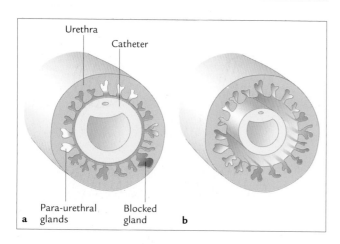

Figure 33.2. *Use of too large a catheter, leading to blockage of para-urethral glands; (b) use of appropriate-sized catheter.*

Urinary catheters also tend to become blocked when biofilm from urease-producing organisms builds up on the catheter surface. This will be indicated by an alkaline urine which precipitates crystals, encrusts the catheter and reduces the catheter lumen, eventually resulting in blockage. Approximately 50% of patients suffer from recurrent encrustation of their urinary catheters,[14,27-29] and regular bladder washouts are advocated in the prevention and treatment of blockage (see Table 33.2 for types of solutions used). Nevertheless, if a patient's catheter repeatedly becomes blocked, excessive bladder washouts are not always the answer and the catheter should, perhaps, be changed more frequently in an effort to pre-empt blockage.

To protect against blockage it is vital to increase the fluid intake. A reduction in acidic fluids (e.g. fruit juice), calcium-rich foods and supplements, and a reduction in alcohol (which may lead to dehydration), is recommended.[30] Debris in the urine is almost inevitable in any woman who has a long-term catheter. General mobilization can protect against debris accumulating and subsequently blocking the drainage eyes of the catheter. In women who are immobile, assisted regular change of position will reduce the incidence of this accumulation. Constipation should be avoided as this can cause leakage and bypassing. Straining on defecation can also contribute to the expulsion of the catheter.

Urethral catheter care

For both short-term and long-term catheterized patients, advice is needed on careful meatal cleansing. A mild unscented soap with water is sufficient, as antiseptic solutions for long-term catheter care have no proven advantage and can lead to the development of resistant organisms.[31] Women certainly need to be instructed in correct perineal cleaning after bowel motions (i.e. to wipe toilet paper away from the urethral opening [front to back] and talcum powder should be avoided as it can become clogged around the catheter.

Care and maintenance of the drainage system is discussed in the section on drainage bags and valves (pages 414-416).

Suprapubic catheterization

Suprapubic catheterization is the insertion, under a general or local anaesthetic, of a catheter into the bladder wall just above the symphysis pubis (Fig. 33.3), for a variety of reasons (Table 33.3). Suprapubic catheters are particularly useful following urogynaecological or urological procedures. They allow safe drainage of the bladder during attempts at postoperative voiding, without the trauma of reinsertion of a urethral catheter each time if attempts are unsuccessful, or if there is a large post-micturition residual. The suprapubic

Table 33.2. *Commonly used bladder washout solutions*	
Type	Indications for use
Citric acid (3.23%)	• To prevent/dissolve crystals forming in the catheter or bladder
Citric acid (6%)	• Dissolves persistent crystals in the catheter or bladder • Minimizes trauma on catheter removal • Unblocks an encrusted catheter
Mandelic acid (1%)	• Prevents growth of urease-producing bacteria (e.g. Pseudomonas) through acidification of the bladder
Chlorhexidine (0.2%)	• Reduces growth of bacteria especially *E. coli* and *Klebsiella* (short-term use only)
Saline (0.9%)	• Mechanical effect to remove blood clots and debris

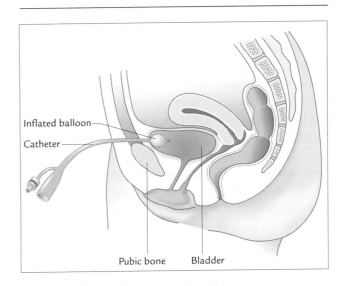

Figure 33.3. *Position of suprapubic catheter.*

413

Table 33.3. *Indications for suprapubic catheterization*

- Urogynaecological/gynaecological (e.g. colposuspension, anterior colporrhaphy, pelvic floor repair, vaginal hysterectomy)
- Urological (e.g. urethral stricture/trauma, ileal augmentation, caecocystoplasty (open prostatectomy)
- Anorectal surgery
- Neurogenic bladder
- Cardiothoracic surgery
- Acute retention
- Inability to self-catheterize
- Need for long-term catheterization
- Intractable incontinence

catheter can be clamped and unclamped according to the patient's progress.[32] This also applies to women in acute retention, as voiding can be tried without removal of the catheter.

Following major abdominal surgery, suprapubic catheters have been found to be the method of choice for urinary drainage, with a lower incidence of bacteriuria and discomfort than with urethral catheterization.[33]

Suprapubic catheterization can be used in women who have intractable incontinence, but this should be a last resort, when all other treatment and forms of containment have failed. For long-term catheterization it is the preferred route, especially in wheelchair users and for those who are sexually active.

A proper explanation of the procedure must be given and informed consent must be obtained.

Unexplained haematuria is perhaps the only real contraindication for suprapubic catheterization, because of the risk of placing a catheter through a bladder tumour.

In women suffering from voiding difficulties or incomplete bladder emptying, every effort should be made to teach them ISC first. Unfortunately, there are some for whom the procedure may be technically difficult and therefore a permanent catheter may be the only answer to maintain adequate bladder drainage.

The choice of suprapubic catheter will depend on whether it is to be used short term (e.g. following surgery) or long term. Suprapubic catheter insertion via an open technique (i.e. cystotomy into the bladder dome under direct vision) can be used following a retropubic procedure. To insert a suprapubic catheter percutaneously or using a 'closed' technique safely, and

without injury to the bowel (as this could lie between the bladder and the anterior abdominal wall), the bladder should be filled to at least 300 ml (transurethrally) with the patient in the Trendelenburg position. When a suprapubic catheter is used as a first line of management in the case of acute retention, it is advisable to use ultrasonography to assess the bladder volume before insertion.

Catheters for short-term use, such as the Bonnano catheter, should be used for only 2–3 weeks. They are commonly held in place by skin sutures, which can pull on the skin, fall out or cause discomfort; the insertion site is, therefore, susceptible to infection if the catheter is used for too long. Suprapubic catheters used long term should be Foley catheters (i.e. held in place with a fluid-filled balloon) made of an inert material like 100% silicone. Medium-sized catheters (14–16 F) can be used. They can be changed every 3 months with little effort once a 'track' or 'fistula' has been formed, although some may need more frequent changes owing to encrustation or blockage. Generally, the first change is still undertaken in the acute-care setting, but subsequent changes are now done routinely within the community. Nevertheless, if there is delay in reinsertion and the catheter fistula is allowed to close, the suprapubic catheter may need to be re-sited. Insertion sites, once healed, should not require a dressing. Other types of self-retaining catheters used in suprapubic catheterization include the Malecot and de Pezzer catheters, which have 'wings' to keep them *in situ*. Suprapubic catheters, as with urethral catheters, drain urine via a 'closed system' into a drainage bag, although valves are being used as an alternative for some women.

Catheter drainage bags

Catheter drainage bags connected directly to a catheter should have a non-return valve to prevent any refluxing of urine once it has entered the bag. Prior to the 1960s, catheters had an open drainage system with the end of the catheter draining into an open non-sterile container. This was the main cause of ascending infection; the introduction of a 'closed drainage system', in which urine drains directly into a sealed sterile drainage bag (Fig. 33.4) has reduced the incidence of bacteriuria dramatically from 97% to 8–15%.[34,35] This system was further developed by replacing the drainage spigot with

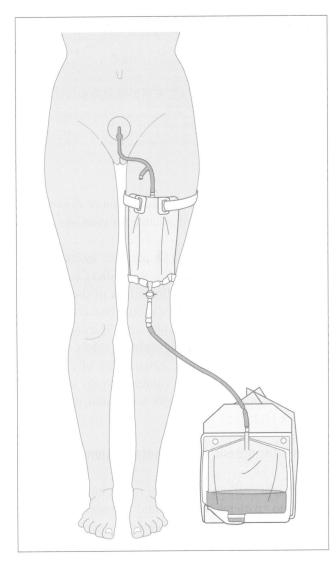

Figure 33.4. *Closed drainage system with a night bag attached to the leg bag; note the short female catheter.*

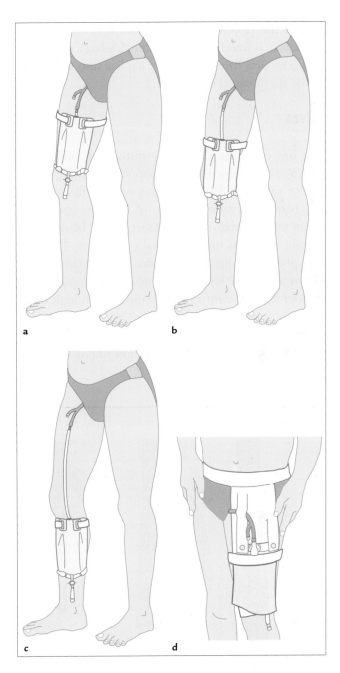

Figure 33.5. *Different lengths of leg bags, ranging from 350 to 750 ml in capacity, and suspensory systems: (a) short-tube bag; (b) medium-tube bag; (c) long-tube bag; (d) alternative method of suspension.*

a non-return outlet tap. It is still possible for bacteria to migrate upwards from the bag, past a non-return valve system, in the form of biofilms;[36] however, if catheter bags are changed once a week, the risk of infection caused by biofilm build-up is minimized.[37] Strict care must be taken when changing bags, with scrupulous attention to hand-washing. Breakage of a closed urinary drainage system should be kept to a minimum; therefore, if a sample of urine is needed, the sampling port must be used, in order to avoid breaking the system.[38]

Women, especially those who are ambulant, should be offered a small body-worn drainage bag (i.e. 'the leg bag'). They come in different sizes (capacity 350, 500 or 750 ml) with long, medium or short tubing (Fig. 33.5). Manufacturers have developed a wide variety of methods to keep the drainage bags in place: these include fabric ties, Velcro straps, 'sporran' belts and integrated pockets or sleeves. Leg bags, however, do not have the capacity for drainage of urine while the user is asleep.

415

So that the closed system is not broken, therefore, a 'night bag' is fitted to the tap of the 'leg bag', so that the urine can flow from the smaller leg bag into the larger, 2-litre, night bag (Fig. 33.4).

Valves

The use of valves (Fig. 33.6) instead of continuous drainage bags is increasing in popularity. The releasing of the valve will be dependent on the fluid intake and bladder capacity. Release of the valve every 3–4 hours will maintain bladder tone, as the bladder will fill and empty as under normal conditions. This may also protect against the erosion of the bladder wall that is associated with the permanent collapse of the bladder in long-term catheterization – although more research is needed in this area. The use of valves is particularly useful for women with voiding difficulties who are unable to perform CISC and who do not wish

Table 33.4. *Contraindications for the use of catheter valves*
• Poor manual dexterity
• Poor mental awareness
• Uncontrolled detrusor instability/hyperreflexia
• Compromised renal function
• Low bladder capacity

to use a drainage bag. It is certainly more discreet for the user, although it is not suitable for everyone (Table 33.4).

A recent multicentre comparative evaluation of catheter valves concluded that prescribers need to be aware of the strengths and limitations of the different types of valves. The ideal valve should be easily manipulated, leak free, comfortable and inconspicuous.[39] Whereas 94% of those using catheter valves preferred this to a standard drainage system, 35% of those who used a bag were happy to continue to do so. In this study, no significant difference was found in the incidence of UTI.[40]

Clean intermittent self-catheterization (CISC)

Intermittent catheterization is a technique mainly taught to patients to facilitate bladder emptying, although it can also be used to enable a patient to instil drugs (e.g. oxybutynin) intravesically, and therefore is appropriate not only for those with voiding difficulties but also for women who have concomitant detrusor instability or hyperreflexia.[26]

CISC (Fig. 33.7) was first introduced by Lapides in 1972.[41] It greatly reduces the incidence of UTI by removing any residual urine and the complications associated with it. It allows women to regain control over their bladders, rather than their bladders controlling them.[42]

CISC should be taught in a relaxed manner by professionals who have an adequate understanding of normal lower urinary tract function and bladder dysfunction. Proper assessment, reassurance and continuing support are vital if women are to be motivated to perform catheterization themselves. Criteria for women performing CISC are summarized in Table 33.5.

CISC can be used in the following voiding disorders and conditions:

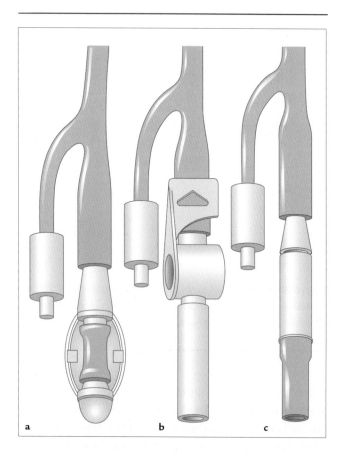

Figure 33.6. *Examples of catheter valves: (a) EMS Medical; (b) Bard Flip-Flo; (c) Sims Portex Uro-Flo.*

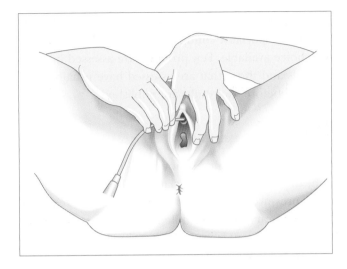

Figure 33.7. *Self-catheterization by a woman.*

Table 33.5. *Criteria for women performing clean intermittent self-catheterization*

- Motivation
- Acceptability
- Adequate manual dexterity
- Adequate mental awareness
- Ability to position themselves to gain access to the urethra
- Sufficient bladder capacity

- Neurogenic bladder
- Hypotonic bladder
- Obstruction
- After surgery.

Neurogenic bladder

CISC is commonly used by women who have urinary dysfunction due to neurological damage from either trauma or a disease such as multiple sclerosis. Recurrent UTIs from persistent residual urine, upper tract damage due to ureteric reflux from high intravesical pressures caused by detrusor hyperreflexia, and subsequent incontinence are prevalent. By the introduction of CISC and thus removal of any persistent urinary residual, all these problems can become greatly reduced. Anticholinergics in addition to CISC are advantageous in this group of women and can be instilled intravesically via the catheter to reduce systemic side effects.

Hypotonic bladder

Women who have little or no sensation of bladder filling or emptying often experience persistent residual urine, giving rise to recurrent UTIs and, in some cases, overflow incontinence. By emptying the bladder at preset times ('by the clock') rather than by desire, they ensure that the bladder capacity is kept within normal limits.

Obstruction

Voiding difficulties caused by urethral stenosis or stricture can be managed temporarily by CISC, which can also be useful for bladder emptying in the presence of an obstructive prolapse or pelvic mass.

After surgery

Many surgical techniques used in an attempt to cure genuine stress incontinence are obstructive in nature.[43] If voiding difficulties do develop, these can easily be managed by CISC. It is important that women are warned of this potential postoperative complication before they consent to such procedures.

There is no set rule as to how long a woman will need to perform CISC, but residuals do tend to decrease with time, unless there was preoperative evidence of voiding difficulties. If women are identified preoperatively (i.e. at urodynamic investigation), it is advisable to teach them CISC before they undergo any surgery. This ensures that they are aware of what is involved should the need to self-catheterize arise.

Catheter types

PVC is frequently used for CISC with a lubricant to facilitate insertion. Plastic catheters can be reused, for up to a week, as long as the user is infection free and has a good technique. Manufacturers have developed self-lubricating (hydrophilic) catheters, with evidence that the higher the osmolality within the catheter the less friction there is on insertion.[44] The disadvantages associated with these catheters are that they are more expensive and can be used only once. Other materials used, although less commonly, include stainless steel and silver. Catheter choice will depend on the individual and what is available. It is quite reasonable for women to use a longer 'male' length catheter if they find it easier. Most women will use a size 10–12 Fg. If women have difficulty in directing the catheter into the urethra there are aids to guide them.

Summary

Careful consideration is necessary before any type of catheterization is used as a long-term form of management. If catheterization is the only feasible solution after appropriate investigation, the choice of catheter should follow comprehensive assessment of the individual.

PADS AND PANTS

Incontinence is frequently accepted as an unavoidable female condition. The use of incontinence pads and pants is, for many women, the first method of control. Women may be unaware of their local continence services and have enormous trouble finding information to help them make a choice,[45] consequently, they buy their own products, usually sanitary towels, which are often unsuitable. The need for appropriate assessment is vital so that the best available treatment or management can be obtained.

In the last 20 years there has been a huge growth in the market of reusable and disposable products. In 1974, Australian Bill Kylie devised an oblong absorbent pad which became the forerunner of the disposable pad industry. Products are continuously changing and developing, with companies endeavouring to ensure that their products suit the users' needs. It is difficult even for a specialist continence nurse to keep up with the choice available. Few products are assessed in quality trials and those that are assessed have usually been changed before the results are published.

Pads

Although incontinence is not a life-threatening condition, the social stigma associated with it can put enormous pressure on the individual. Pads may be required as a temporary measure while investigations are undertaken or treatment is awaited. They should not, however, be used as an alternative to effective continence promotion strategies. Their use should not be considered as the first line of treatment except for the severely incontinent person where containment will be a priority. Accurate assessment of the patient's needs (Table 33.6), should ensure that the correct product to contain incontinence is supplied. For women, absorbent pads are still the most popular form of management and they are manufactured in various shapes and sizes (Fig. 33.8). Pomfret[46] has described the use of an absorbent pad worn (or incorporated) inside a retaining garment as the most common way of managing incontinence.

White[45] stressed that the ideal pad should be 'simple to use, reliable to wear and pleasing in appearance'. The most important point is that the pad should contain the incontinence.

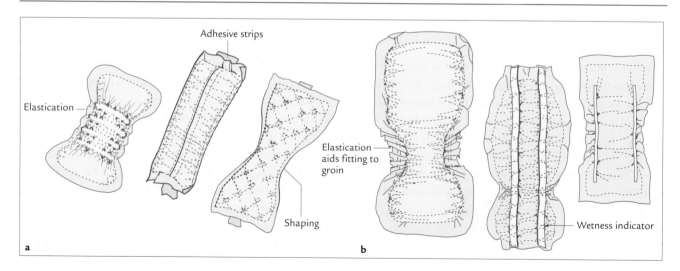

Figure 33.8. *Examples of absorbent pads: (a) insert pads; (b) heavy incontinence pads (used with net pants).*

Table 33.6. *Guidelines when assessing product provision*

Key feature for the 'perfect product'	Individual assessment considerations		
	Requirement	Linked to	Options/variables
Absorbent	Able to receive the loss with no or low leakage	Speed of urine entry and spread Absorbent capacity Core remaining intact	Type of pulp in core, e.g. pulp with super-absorber Reusable
Safe	Able to receive and contain the loss with no or low leakage for a reasonable time period	Absorbent capacity Good fit of pad Pad staying in place Retention of shape Posture of user	Type of pulp in core, e.g. pulp with super-absorber Reusable
Comfort (wet and dry)	Able to be worn dry or wet without being felt unduly and without irritating the skin	Good fit Compliance Retention of shape Low bulk Dry and wet surface texture Core remaining intact	Length, width, thickness Rectangular/shaped Backed/unbacked Method of securing Surface and core materials Disposable/reusable products
Discreet	Won't show Won't rustle Won't smell Won't look different	Low bulk Discreet outline No rustle noise Normal appearance Discreet packaging and delivery Discreet disposal or laundering	With/without super-absorber Rectangular/shaped Reusable pant with integral pad Disposable/reusable system Delivery/mail order
Easy to change	Ease when putting on Ease when taking off Convenient storage immediately before and after use	User disability: mobility; dexterity Facilities	Disposable/reusable system; disposable/reusable materials; pad rectangular, shaped or pants with integral pad; pad pouched, pocketed or loose; adhesive tabs, press-studs or Velcro closures
Secure in position	Won't shift when user moves, walks or transfers	User mobility Pad shape Pad design Method of securing pad	Pad rectangular, shaped or pants with integral pad; pad pouched, pocketed or loose; adhesive tabs, press-studs or Velcro closures
Convenient	Easily used without excessive effort, frustration or anxiety	Availability; storage, temporary and immediate; disposal, immediate and temporary; laundering, ability and facilities; environment, domestic/communal; indoors/out of doors	Disposable/reusable products Disposable/reusable usage cycle
Economical	Able to be used in a cost-effective, non-wasteful manner	Disposables: staying intact to permit reuse if dry Reusables: effect of wash and wear on product life Durability: seam strength; edge-stitching strength; stability of core; stability of dimensions	Disposable: pulp quality; cover-stock strength Reusables: surface, core and backing materials; various qualities of workmanship

From ref. 62.
Reproduced by kind permission of *Nursing Times*, where this table first appeared in the Continence Supplement on 21 April 1993.

Each type of pad has been developed with a particular need in mind (Table 33.7): small pads are used in cases of light incontinence or when a pad can be changed frequently; large pads are used when there is severe incontinence or where toileting is not an option.[47]

Disposable pads

Disposable products are usually made up of two or three layers. The top layer, which is worn next to the skin, is made of a hydrophobic cover which allows urine to pass through to a second absorbent layer composed of a mixture of chemicals and mechanically made pulps, often with added super-absorbent. The third layer, when used, is a waterproof backing to prevent leakage.

The product can also contain a deodorizer. Some pads have elasticated sides, especially around the gusset area, thus ensuring a good fit. A peel-off sticky strip is often integrated into the backing of smaller pads, which attaches to the pants and enables use with normal underclothes or with specially designed net knickers.

One of the major disadvantages with pads is that they can 'bulk up'; in addition, the outside covering comes apart if the pads are not changed often enough.[48]

Disposable pad-and-pants system

Plastic-backed pads used with net pants come in many sizes and shapes (Fig. 33.8) and are recommended for patients who are able to undertake toileting.

Disposable all-in-one pads

All-in-one pads (Fig. 33.9) are worn without additional pants. Some have side fastenings and the size required is determined by the hip size of the patient. They are not necessarily more absorbent than a pad with separate pants but, if well fitted, can be particularly effective in containing urine and poorly formed faeces. They are often used for the severely disabled, bed fast patient, or when toileting is difficult or not appropriate.

Disposable pouch pads

Pouch pads have no waterproof backing; they are designed to be placed in the pouch of a washable pair of pants. The outside of the pouch is lined with a waterproof gusset. The size of the pad required is dependent upon the size of pouch and the degree of absorbency required (Fig. 33.10).

Table 33.7. *Selection of a product*

Type of incontinence	Loss	Recommended product
Urinary	Light (0–50 ml)	Small slim waterproof-backed disposable/reusable liner
		Washable pad built into normal pants
		Male dribble pouch, disposable/reusable
	Moderate (200 ml)	Rectangular or shaped
		Waterproof-backed disposable/reusable liner
	Severe (> 300 ml)	Shaped waterproof-backed disposable pad
		Booster pad with above
		All-in-one disposable/reusable pad
		Female urinary pouch
		Male retracted urinary pouch
Faecal	Staining	Panty liner
		Disposable pants
		Cotton-top reusable slim pad
	Light	Shaped disposable waterproof-backed pad
	Severe	All-in-one disposable pad
		Faecal pouch

From ref. 63.

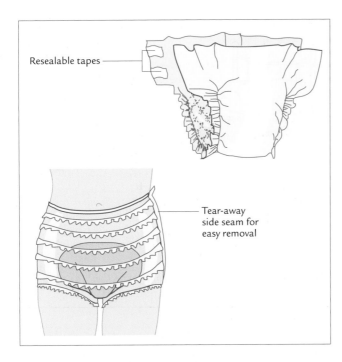

Figure 33.9. *All-in-one pads.*

Disposable absorbent roll

Like the pouch pad, the absorbent roll has no waterproof backing and therefore needs to be used with pants with a waterproof lining. It has the advantage that it can be cut to suit individual requirements, but it is useful only for light incontinence.

Disposable bed pads

Disposable bed pads are available in a range of sizes and absorbencies. They have a liquid-permeable top cover, a cellulose wadding or a fluffy pulp middle layer and a waterproof backing. They are designed as bed protection when there is the added risk of soiling or when a body-worn pad is not suitable (Fig. 33.11).

Reusable pads

The decision whether to use reusable incontinence products rather than disposables is a complex one that will depend on individual needs and preferences. The availability of suitable laundry facilities is also an important factor.[48]

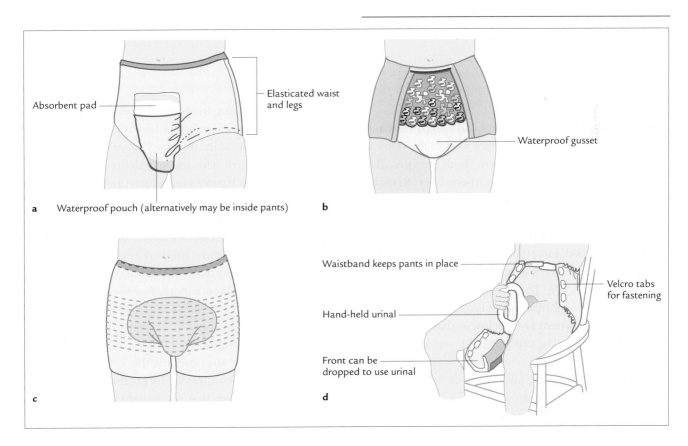

Figure 33.10. *Pouch pads and pants: (a) pouch pants; (b) stretch pants with waterproof gusset; (c) stretch pants for use with plastic-backed pad; (d) drop-front pants.*

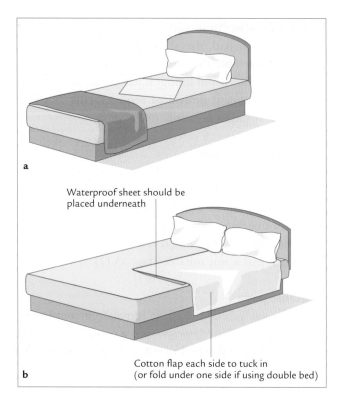

Waterproof sheet should be placed underneath

Cotton flap each side to tuck in (or fold under one side if using double bed)

Figure 33.11. *Disposable and washable types of bed protection: (a) disposable bed pad; (b) washable bed sheet.*

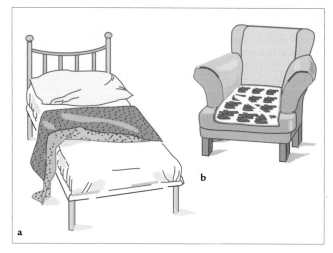

Figure 33.12. *Reusable bed and chair protection: (a) reusable bed pad; (b) reusable chair pad.*

Reusable body-worn pads

Reusable body-worn pads can be a pad-and-pants system or an all-in-one system. The surface next to the skin can be a smooth or a quilted fabric. Both systems allow urine to pass through to an absorbent layer. Reusable pads are available with or without a waterproof backing.

Reusable bed and chair pads

Most reusable bed and chair pads are available with or without 'tuck-in' flaps or waterproof backings; some are non-slip (Fig. 33.12). These pads, like the disposable pads, have a hydrophobic upper layer allowing urine to pass into the absorbent layer below so that the patient's skin stays dry; her skin can therefore remain in direct contact with the pad.

The use of disposable underpads or bed protection (Fig. 33.11) has diminished over the years with the advent of washable bed protectors and more sophisticated disposable and reusable body-worn pads. The advantages and limitations of reusable and disposable products are outlined in Table 33.8.

Pants

Many designs are available to suit varying degrees of incontinence. Most have an integrated waterproof gusset and can be used with or without a pouch pad (Fig. 33.10).

Skin care

The prevention and treatment of any skin condition caused by incontinence is very important. If urine is in contact with the skin the area should be regularly cleaned and dried. The use of talcum powder is not advocated. Thick barrier creams are not recommended for use with pads as this affects the absorption.[49] Urinary incontinence in people with poor skin condition and pressure sores needs careful management. Collier[50] describes how 'moisture predisposes skin to pressure sores because of the effects of skin maceration, which in turn leads to excoriation, increasing the risk of abrasion by friction'. Skin problems associated with incontinence can vary, and need treatment according to the severity of the condition.[51]

Holistic patient assessment is the key to achieving a containment of incontinence by product use, with regular review to ensure that the patient's needs are met. No one product suits everyone, some products are more susceptible to misuse than others, but all work best if the wearers and carers receive proper instruction and ongoing support.[52]

Table 33.8. *Advantages and limitations of reusable and disposable products*

Type of product	Advantages	Limitations
Reusable	• Cannot be torn apart • Retain better shape • Do not break up • Potential for more design options • Facilitate independence from supply system • Eliminate the need for storage • Can be reused if remain dry	• Requires washing • Initial capital outlay • ? Unacceptable to users (especially if menstruating or faecally incontinent)
Disposable	• Flexibility for experimentation to match user's requirements • No need to launder • Materials better suited to faecal incontinence	• Tendency for pulp compression • Tendency for pulp break-up • Can be torn apart

From ref. 45.

AIDS AND APPLIANCES

The female anatomy does not allow easy application of aids and appliances to maintain dryness. For this reason the number of products available for women is far more limited than it is for men. For many women, incontinence will be an ongoing and sometimes intractable problem. It is, therefore, important that women are provided with full information on the range of products available and how to obtain them. The 'range of products and their provision is bewildering to professionals and consumers alike'.[44] The United Kingdom Continence Foundation *Continence Products Directory*[53] lists over a thousand items, ranging from special toilet seats to assist toilet training to odour-control products for use by those with faecal incontinence or who are unable to maintain prompt personal hygiene.

When advising patients or carers about aspects of care on particular aids and appliances, there are several important factors to consider, as shown in Table 33.9.[54] Ideally, the choice of products should be made following full consultation with the user and, where appropriate, with the carers. The opportunity should be given, where possible, for a trial of the aid or appliance prior to purchase. Full explanation of the product's use with supporting written information is needed, together with ongoing support to ensure that the product is meeting the user's needs.

Aids in the toilet

For those with difficulty in bending or managing in the toilet, a raised lavatory seat facilitates sitting down and

Table 33.9. *Implications for the selection of aids and appliances*

• Personal preference	• Hygiene
• Mobility	• Environment
• Manual dexterity	• Financial implications
• Local anatomy	• Laundry or disposal facilities
• Eyesight	• Available helpers (relatives, carers, professionals)
• Mental function	

getting up[55] (Fig. 33.13). Support rails, suitably placed, can also assist elderly or disabled patients to position themselves on the toilet and to manage clothing after voiding. Rails can be positioned on walls or fixed to the floor. Some are designed to swing out of the way to give adequate access for wheelchair users.

Aiding toileting: clothing

The Disabled Living Foundation guidelines for management of incontinence[56] comment that 'the selection of appropriate clothing can make continence so much easier to achieve' (Fig. 33.14). The general recommendations are as follows:

- The fewer the layers of clothing, the easier to manage;
- Loose-fitting clothes are easier to manage than tight ones;
- Light, slippery fabrics cling less and are therefore easier to adjust;

- Short vests, shirts or blouses are less likely to get in the way;
- Fabrics that are easy to launder and do not retain odour should be chosen;
- Thumb or hand loops attached to waistbands may help those who cannot remove trousers or skirts easily;
- Clothes that disguise the chosen method of management (i.e. easy access for toileting or changing pads) are recommended.

Commodes

When the lavatory is not easily accessible, a number of items of equipment can assist in maintaining continence. Commodes and chemical toilets can be used as a substitute to the lavatory (Fig. 33.15).

Commodes can be obtained with a variety of properties, including adjustable-height legs and removable arms and backs.[57] Many look like well-designed chairs and can be kept in a bedroom or living room as part of the ordinary furniture.[58] Chemical toilets have the advantage that they need emptying less often.

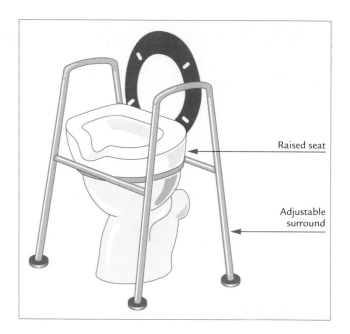

Raised seat

Adjustable surround

Figure 33.13. *Aids in the toilet.*

Female urinals

McIntosh[59] described the major problems that women with incontinence have in managing toileting in the

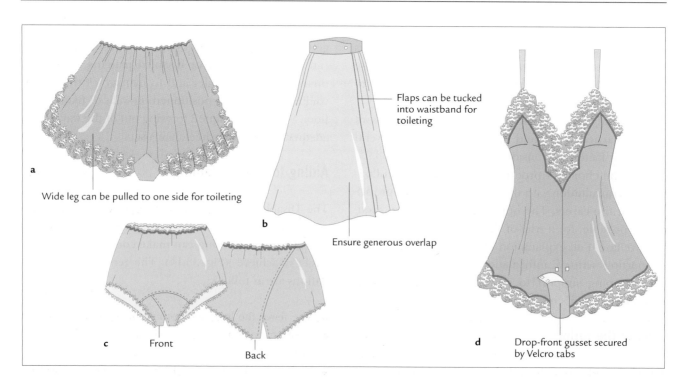

Wide leg can be pulled to one side for toileting

Flaps can be tucked into waistband for toileting

Ensure generous overlap

Front

Back

Drop-front gusset secured by Velcro tabs

Figure 33.14. *Selection of clothing: (a) French knickers: (b) wrap-around skirt; (c) open-crotch knickers; (d) camiknickers.*

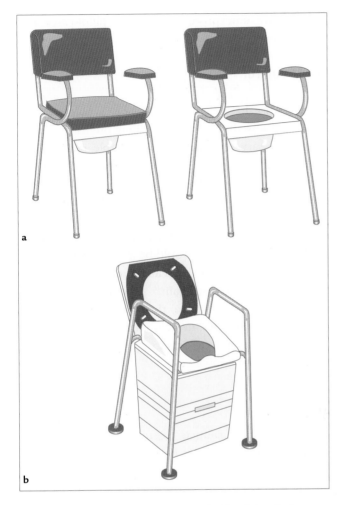

Figure 33.15. *Commode and chemical toilet: (a) typical commode; (b) raised, contoured toilet seat over a chemical commode.*

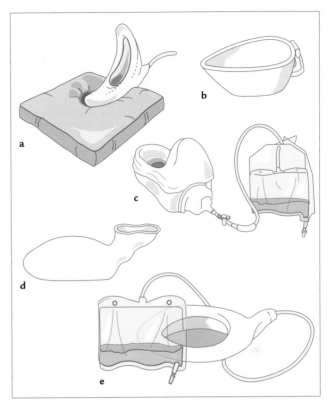

Figure 33.16. *Female urinals: (a) bridge urinal with U-shaped cushion; (b) St Peter's boat; (c) female urinal connected to drainage bag; (d) swan-neck urinal; (e) pan-type urinal connected to drainage bag.*

community, and felt that female urinals could offer a solution for toileting problems and may therefore be the management method of choice. As a viable alternative to commodes, they are particularly helpful for those who cannot get to the toilet in time (Fig. 33.16); this would include women with detrusor instability, frailty due to old age, poor mobility, being without assistance (especially at night), having an inaccessible toilet, and being wheelchair dependent. They also benefit women on social outings and during travel.

A wide range of urinals is available for use in different positions (standing; lying down in bed; lying prone; lying on the side; sitting in bed leaning back or sitting up; sitting up, forwards or backwards in a chair or wheelchair). In addition, small slipper-pan urinals, jug-type urinals (Fig. 33.16) and simple home-made collecting devices can be used. Urinals for women are products that are, however, little used, little known and undervalued.[59]

Body-worn female devices

There are two body-worn female devices: a female urinary pouch with adhesive backing and a device kept in place with straps. These are rarely used and are no longer considered satisfactory appliances for women with urinary incontinence.

Alarms

Three types of alarms are used to promote continence (Fig. 33.17), as follows:

- Body-worn alarm with audible, vibrating or flashing alarm signals;

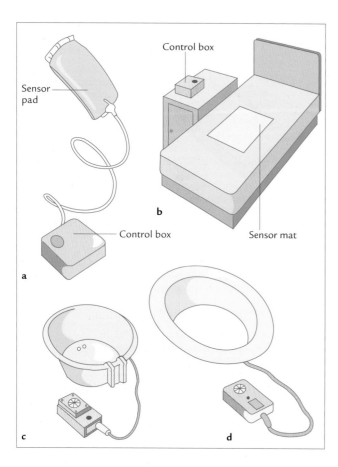

Figure 33.17. *Alarms: (a) mini/personal alarm; (b) bed alarm; (c) potty alarm; (d) toilet bowl alarm.*

- Bed alarm with audible alarm signals;
- Toilet bowl or potty alarms with musical signals.

Body-worn and bed alarms are condition devices used to prompt 'wake up' and 'hold on' to the sensation of a full bladder from sleep. Body-worn alarms can also be used during the day as an aid to bladder retraining or toileting, alerting the patient or her carers to incontinence.

Musical toilet bowls or potty alarms are particularly useful for toilet training for children or for adults with learning difficulties. Every time urine is passed into the toilet or potty, a tune is played; this encourages the recognition of the use of the toilet with the emergence of urine.

Furniture protection

Women with intractable incontinence who have nocturnal enuresis may require waterproof mattress covers to prevent damage to the mattress (Figs 33.11, 33.12). Also

available are waterproof draw-sheets, pillowcases and duvet covers.[60]

Odour control

People who have an incontinence problem often become obsessed by a fear of smelling offensive. This is an unnecessary fear as, with reasonable care, odour need not arise.[61] Good personal hygiene, prompt disposal and storage of products, together with good ventilation, should be all that is needed. Aids and appliances must be cleaned frequently to reduce the risk of crystalline deposits building up and causing a smell. Where possible, it would be an advantage to have two appliances so that one can be cleaned and thoroughly dried before use again.[56] A neutralizing deodorant will help if added to the water when washing appliances, commodes, urinals, chairs and carpets. It is also possible to put a drop or two onto protective padding or onto appliances.

SUMMARY

There are many products to suit a variety of urinary complaints. However, it is crucial that all women with urinary dysfunction are comprehensively assessed and investigated before any form of containment becomes long-term management. For those unfortunate enough to have to rely on catheters, pads and pants or aids and appliances, the right product or mode of containment must be suitable for the individual. The aim with all these products is primarily to improve the individual's quality of life.

REFERENCES

1. Mattelaer JJ, Billet I. Catheters and sounds: the history of bladder catheterization in the early management of traumatic paraplegia and tetraplegia. *Paraplegia* 1995; 33: 429–433

2. Crow RA, Chapman RG, Roe BH, Wilson JH. *Study of Patients with an Indwelling Urinary Catheter and Related Nursing Practice.* Guildford, UK: Nursing Practice Research Unit, University of Surrey, 1986

3. Roe BH. Catheters in the community. *Nurs Times* 1989; 85 (36): 43–44

4. Reybard, JF. *Traité Pratique des Rétrécissements du Canal de l'Urètre.* Paris: Labe, 1853

5. Foley FEB. A self-retaining bag catheter for use as indwelling catheter for constant drainage of the bladder. *J Urol* 1937; 38: 140–143

6. Henry, M. Catheter confusion. *Nurs Times* 1992; 88 (42): 65–72

7. Blannin, J, Hobden J. The catheters of choice. *Nurs Times* 1980; 76 (48): 2092–2093

8. Ruuta M, Alfhan, O, Anderson LC. Cytotoxicity of latex urinary catheters. *Br J Urol* 1985; 57: 82–87

9. Talji M, Korpela A, Jarvi K. Comparison of urethral reactions to full silicone, hydrogel coated and siliconized latex catheters. *Br J Urol* 1990; 66: 652–657

10. Pullan BR, Phillips JI, Hickey DS. Urethral lumen, crossectional shape: its radiological, determination and relationship to function. *Br J Urol* 1982; 54: 399–407

11. Brocklehurst JC, Hickley DS, Davis I *et al*. A new urethral catheter. *Br Med J* 1988; 296: 1691–1693

12. Pomfret I. Comformacath update. *J Community Nurs* 1992; 6: (Nov) 14–16

13. Kennedy AP, Brocklehurst JC, Lye MDW. Factors related to the problems of long-term catheterization. *J Adv Nurs* 1983; 8: 207–212

14. Roe BH, Brocklehurst, JC. Study of patients with indwelling catheters. *J Adv Nurs* 1987; 12: 713–718

15. Blandy JP. How to catheterise the bladder. *Br J Hosp Med* 1981; 26: 58–60

16. Bach D, Hess EA, Prauge CH. Prophylaxis against encrustation and urinary tract infection with indwelling transurethral catheters. *Urol Nephrol* 1990; 2: 25–32

17. Warren JW. Catheter-associated bacteriuria. *Clin Geriat Med* 1992; 8: 805–819

18. Roe BH. Use of bladder washouts: a study of nurse's recommendations. *J Adv Nurs* 1989; 14: 494–500

19. Getliffe KA. The characteristics and management of patients with recurrent blockage of long-term urinary catheters. *J Adv Nurs* 1994; 20: 140–149

20. Gopal Rao G, Elliot TSJ. Bladder irrigation. *Age Ageing* 1988; 17: 373–378

21. Davies AJ, Desai HN, Turton S, Dyas A. Does instillation of chlorhexidine into the bladder of catheterised geriatric patients help reduce bacteriuria? *J Hosp Infect* 1987; 9: 72–75

22. Stickler DI, Chawia IC. The role of antiseptics in the management of patients with long term indwelling bladder catheters. *J Hosp Infect* 1987; 10: 219–228

23. Whalen RL, Cai C, Thompson LM *et al*. An infection-inhibiting urinary catheter material. *ASAIO J* 1997; 43: M842–847

24. Morris NS, Stickler DJ, Winters C. Which indwelling urethral catheters resist encrustation by Proteus mirabilis biofilms? *Br J Urol* 1997; 80: 58–63

25. Kohler-Ockmore J, Feneley RC. Long-term catheterization of the bladder: prevalence and morbidity. *Br J Urol* 1996; 77: 347–351

26. O'Flynn KJ, Thomas DG. Intravesical instillation of oxybutinin hydrochloride for detrusor hyperreflexia. *Br J Urol* 1993; 72: 566–570

27. Brocklehurst J, Brocklehurst S. The management of indwelling catheters. *Br J Urol* 1978; 50: 102–105

28. Kohler-Ockmore J. Urinary catheter complications. *J Dist Nurs* 1992; 10 (8): 18–20

29. Getliffe KA. The characteristics and management of patients with recurrent blockage of long-term urinary catheters. *J Adv Nurs* 1994: 20; 140–149

30. Burr RG, Nuseibeh IM. Urinary catheter blockage depends on urine pH, calcium and rate of flow. *Spinal Cord* 1997; 35: 521–525

31. Stickler DJ. The role of antiseptics in the management of patients undergoing short-term indwelling catheterization. *J Hosp Infect* 1991; 16: 89–108

32. Hilton P, Stanton SL. Suprapubic catheterization. *Br Med J* 1980; 281: 1261–1263

33. O'Kelly JJ, Mathew A, Ross S, Munro A. Optimum method for urinary drainage in major abdominal surgery: a prospective trial of suprapubic versus urethral catheterization. *Br J Surg* 1995; 82: 1367–1368

34. Gillespie WA, Lennon GG, Linton KB, Slacle NN. Prevention of urinary tract infection in gynaecology patients. *Br Med J* 1964; 2: 423–425

35. Thornton GF, Andriole VT. Bacteriuria during indwelling catheter drainage: Effect of a closed sterile drainage system. *J Am Med Assoc* 1970; 214: 339–342

36. Mulhull A. Biofilms and urethral catheter infections. *Nurs Stand* 1991; 5: 26–28

37. Rogers J, Norkett DI, Bracegirdle P *et al*. Examination of biofilm formation and risk of infection associated with the use of urinary catheters with leg bags. *J Hosp Infect* 1996; 32: 105–115

38. Meers P (ed) *Hospital Infection Control for Nurses*. London: Chapman and Hall, 1992

39. Fader M, Pettersson L, Brooks R *et al*. A multi-centre comparative evaluation of catheter valves. *Br J Nurs* 1997; 6: 359, 362–364, 366–367

40. Wison C, Sandhu SS, Kaisory AV. A prospective randomised study comparing a catheter valve with a standard drainage system. *Br J Nurs* 1997; 80: 915–917

41. Lapides J, Dionko AC, Silber SJ, Lowe BS. Clean intermittent catheterization in the treatment of urinary tract disease. *J Urol* 1972; 107: 458–461

42. Moore K. Intermittent self catheterization. Research-based practice. *Br J Nurs* 1995;4: 1057–1062

43. Smith R, Cardozo L. Early voiding difficulties after colposuspension. *Br J Urol* 1997; 80: 911–914

44. Walker L, Telanderm M, Sullivan L. The importance of osmolality in hydrophilic urethral catheters: a crossover study. *Spinal Cord* 1997; 35: 229–233

45. White H. Continence products – the essentials. *J Community Nurs* 1997; 11 (12): 10

46. Pomfret I. The use of continence products. Norton C (ed) In: *Nursing for Continence,* 2nd edn. Beaconsfield, UK: Beaconsfield Publishers, 1996; 335–364

47. Shepherd A, Blannin J. The role of the nurse. In: Mandelstam D (ed) *Incontinence and its Management,* 2nd edn. Beckenham, UK: Croom Helm, 1986; 60–184

48. Norris C, Cottenden A, Ledger D. Underpad overview. *Nurs Times* 1993; 89 (26): 21

49. Le-Leivre S, Addison I. *Incontinence and Skin Care: the Role of the Nurse.* London: Royal College of Nursing, Continence Care Forum, 1996; 5: 16

50. Collier M. Pressure area care. *Nurs Times* 1997; 93 (4): (Suppl): 1–4

51. Watson R. Justifying your practice. *Br J Nurs* 1992; 5: (3) 11–12

52. Cottenden A. In: Roe B (ed) Aids and appliances for incontinence. *Clinical Nursing Practice.* London: Prentice Hall, 1992; 129–152

53. *Continence Products Directory.* 2nd edn. London: The Continence Foundation, 1996

54. Bucknell A. When prevention fails, incontinence must be managed. Geriatric Medicine Supplement. *Community Nurs (Suppl)* 1998; (Sept): 7

55. Disabled Living Foundation. Notes on incontinence. *Information Service Handbook.* Part II, Section 10. London: Disabled Living Foundation, 1989; 13

56. Disabled Living Foundation. Continence. *Hamilton Index.* Part II, Section 10. London: Disabled Living Foundation, 1998; 9

57. Association of Continence Advisers. *Directory of Aids to Toileting.* 1st edn. London: Association of Continence Advisers, April 1985

58. *Disability Equipment Assessment A9: A Comparative Evaluation.* London: Medical Devices Agency, 1994

59. McIntosh J. Realising the potential of urinals for women. *J Community Nurs* 1998; 12: 14

60. Cutner A, Haken J. Aids and appliances. In: Cardozo L (ed) *Urogynaecology: 'The King's Approach'.* London: Churchill Livingstone, 1997; 663–669

61. Norton C. *Nursing for Continence,* 2nd edn. Beaconsfield, UK: Beaconsfield Publishers, 1996

62. Philip J, Cottonden A, Ledger D. Mix and match. *Nurs Times* 1993; 89: 70–74

63. White H. In control with incontinence aids. *Br J Nurs* 1995; 4: 334–338

34

Prevention of incontinence and prolapse

R. M. Freeman

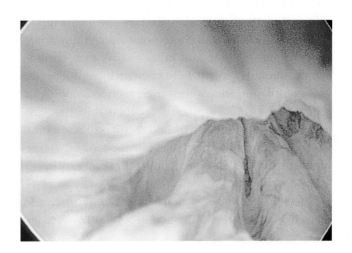

INTRODUCTION

Ideally, the aim of healthcare is prevention rather than cure. Prevention can be classified as *primary* (interventions in asymptomatic individuals to reduce known risk factors for the development of a disease) or *secondary* (to detect symptoms at an early stage and to intervene to stop further development or to improve the prognosis of the condition). To stop recurrence of an illness or preventing it becoming chronic is *tertiary* prevention.

In urogynaecology there is a paucity of large prospective trials to assess the impact of prevention on incontinence and prolapse. Identification of individuals at risk and speculation about methods of prevention is all that can be considered at present.

Predisposing factors for incontinence and prolapse include age, obesity, childbirth, surgery and possibly abnormal voiding habit. How these can produce symptoms and what preventative measures might be adopted is presented in this chapter. In particular, factors associated with age and their prevention are discussed, as is the role of childbirth in pelvic floor dysfunction, irritative symptoms and faecal incontinence after delivery, together with the occurrence and prevention of incontinence and prolapse resulting from gynaecological surgery. Consideration is given to the prevention both of failure of incontinence surgery and detrusor instability (DI).

AGE

Although the prevalence of incontinence is increased in the elderly,[1] the two do not necessarily have a cause-and-effect relationship; other pathological processes associated with ageing might be responsible. Resnick[2] has created the mnemonic DIAPPERS to describe these: **D**elirium, **I**nfection, **A**trophic change, **P**harmacological, **P**sychological, **E**xcess urine output, **R**estricted mobility and **S**tool impaction. Appropriate management of these and other factors (e.g. chronic cough, smoking) might help prevent incontinence as well as prolapse. Simple measures, such as stopping or reducing the dose of diuretics, regular toileting, easy access to toilets, restricting fluids (especially caffeine), and prevention of urinary tract infection (UTI) (possibly by the use of high-dose vitamin C or cranberry juice) might be effective.

There is a known association between constipation and uterovaginal prolapse.[3] Attention to regular bowel habit,

avoiding straining, a high-fibre diet and, if necessary, laxatives should have a positive effect on prevention.

There is a definite ageing process in the lower urinary tract,[4] resulting in atrophic change and poor urethral function. Hormone-replacement therapy should, in theory, prevent lower urinary tract symptoms. However, this has not been proven in patients with genuine stress incontinence (GSI) or DI.[5]

In patients with sensory urgency, oestradiol vaginally (25 µg/day for 3 months) appears to improve the symptom of urgency;[6] this could be important in prevention. Urgency can be distressing for the older patient with restricted mobility, causing panic and anxiety on the sensation of bladder fullness; as a result, the patient voids more frequently to prevent incontinence. This can have the opposite effect, by reducing bladder capacity and resulting in increased urgency and urge incontinence.[7]

In addition to the use of vaginal oestradiol, strategies such as explanation, bladder retraining, pelvic floor exercises, coping strategies, easy access to toilets and the use of bedside commodes may prevent urgency developing into urge incontinence.

OBESITY

Obesity is common in women with urinary incontinence and prolapse. When defined as 'more than 20% above average weight for height and age', obesity has been shown to be more common in patients with GSI and DI than in the normal population.[8] In pregnancy, an increased body mass index has been shown to be an important risk factor for persistent urinary incontinence *post partum*,[9,10] although this is not a consistent finding.[11]

In theory, weight loss should be preventative. One study,[12] in morbidly obese women with incontinence undergoing surgically induced weight loss, showed subjective and objective (urodynamic) improvement in incontinence a year after surgery.

A large prospective study is, therefore, required to see if weight loss (without surgery) can prevent incontinence. Meanwhile, advice on weight loss is probably beneficial.

CHILDBIRTH

There is good evidence that vaginal delivery is associated with pudendal nerve damage through stretch injury.[13,14] This nerve damage is also seen in patients with GSI.[15] It has been assumed, therefore, that damage to the innervation of the pelvic floor with vaginal delivery is responsible for subsequent GSI and prolapse. However, this assumption might not be correct; pregnancy itself may be responsible.[16]

Nulliparous women with GSI do not show evidence of neuromuscular damage; rather, they appear to have weaker pelvic floor collagen.[17] It has been suggested that, in the longer term, connective tissue deficiency might be more important than neuromuscular damage in the aetiology of GSI.[18]

It is possible, therefore, that vaginal delivery might be a risk factor for stress incontinence and prolapse only in those women with defective pelvic floor collagen. For example, primigravidae with excessive bladder-neck mobility antenatally (possibly due to weak pelvic floor collagen) appear to be at higher risk of post-partum stress incontinence.[11] Although intervention in such a group might be preventative, what such intervention might be is a matter of some debate.[19] Although there is evidence that elective caesarean section can prevent neuromuscular damage,[13] this procedure does not always prevent postnatal incontinence.[9] Alternatively, there is some evidence that antenatal pelvic floor exercises might reduce the frequency of urinary incontinence postnatally.[9,20] In addition, post-partum pelvic floor exercises appear to reduce incontinence in 'at-risk' women.[11,21]

The role of obstetric factors is unclear. For example, there is conflicting evidence regarding a prolonged second stage of labour, birth weight, epidural, episiotomy and mode of delivery. Although forceps delivery has been implicated,[13] this is not a consistent finding.[22] The ventouse is arguably less traumatic to the pelvic floor; however, it has not been shown to reduce the incidence of post-partum urinary incontinence or to prevent neuromuscular damage.[14]

It would appear that prevention by changing obstetric practice is not possible with the current state of knowledge. Long-term follow-up studies are required to assess any preventative measures, such as caesarean section or pelvic floor exercises.

Irritative symptoms in pregnancy

Frequency of micturition and nocturia are common in pregnancy.[16] Urge incontinence has been reported to occur in 18% of women in early pregnancy[23] and in 14.8% at 3 months postnatally.[9]

Symptomatic DI has been found in 23% of women during pregnancy and in 15% postnatally.[24] In a larger urodynamic study, rates of 8.4% (antenatally) and 6.8% (postnatally) were reported.[25] A detailed history should identify these women antenatally; bladder retraining might help in secondary prevention. However, follow-up beyond 3 months is necessary to ascertain if the irritative symptoms persist and to assess severity. Prevention might not be necessary if irritative symptoms in pregnancy are shown to subside with time.

Faecal incontinence after delivery

Faecal incontinence, of either liquid or solid stool, has been reported in 4% of women for the first time postnatally.[26] If incontinence of flatus and urgency are added, this figure is increased.[27]

Although pudendal nerve injury in labour may be responsible,[13,14] with the advent of endo-anal ultrasonography, occult anal sphincter defects have been identified in 35% of primiparae and 44% of multiparae after vaginal delivery.[28] In 13 and 23%, respectively, defecatory symptoms (urgency and/or faecal incontinence) have been noted. The main obstetric factor associated with these symptoms was forceps delivery; caesarean section was protective.[27]

In women with recognized third-degree tears, 85% have residual sphincter damage. Symptoms are seen in 50% despite repair at delivery.[28] It is here that obstetric practice can be preventative. For example, prevention of third- and fourth-degree tears is seen with mediolateral episiotomy,[29] whereas the risk is increased by midline episiotomy.[30] Identification of sphincter tears, suturing by an experienced operator, and further assessment of the ventouse rather than forceps delivery might be practical; however, one study has shown both forceps and ventouse deliveries to be risk factors.[26]

Macrosmoia[29] and occiput posterior positions[31] have been shown to be risk factors for pelvic floor damage. These are not under the obstetrician's control; none the less, awareness of those factors might be important in prevention.

It is possible that sphincter tears can occur with delivery of the posterior shoulder as well as with the fetal head. Supporting the perineum at delivery is important to prevent extension of the episiotomy or tear into the anus.

In multiparae with symptomatic anal sphincter defects, secondary prevention can probably be achieved by elective caesarean section, although evidence for this is lacking.

These findings have focused the attention of obstetricians and midwives to the potential risks of anal sphincter tears. This should result in improved training and, it is hoped, prevention.

INCONTINENCE AND PROLAPSE FOLLOWING GYNAECOLOGICAL SURGERY

Hysterectomy

Urinary tract fistulae are (fortunately) rare, but are not always preventable. Between 0.5 and 3% of lower urinary tract injuries have been reported at hysterectomy. Many of these are due to congenital abnormalities and distortion of structures caused by disease.[32] Preoperative intravenous urography and the use of ureteric catheters in potentially difficult cases might help prevent trauma to the urinary tract.

An increased risk of urinary incontinence after hysterectomy has been reported.[33] When assessed 6 years later, women who had had preoperative incontinence had a 36% increased risk of worsening incontinence after hysterectomy. For those patients without incontinence before hysterectomy, the risk of developing incontinence was 15%; however, other short-term studies have failed to confirm these findings.[34] It has been suggested that subtotal hysterectomy might prevent urinary incontinence,[35] but the rationale for this is unclear.

It is possible that the cervix can act as a posterior support for the bladder neck. In addition, it is thought that division of the cardinal ligaments can result in denervation of the pelvic floor.[36] This could result in increased bladder-neck mobility and stress incontinence. It is, therefore, useful to advise those patients with mild stress incontinence preoperatively of the potential risk of worsening incontinence after hysterectomy. Supervised pelvic floor exercises pre- and postoperatively might prevent this exacerbation.

Colposuspension

Following colposuspension for GSI, DI with urge incontinence can occur *de novo* in 15–18.5% of cases.[37,38] Long-term follow-up suggests that this persists.[39] The causes are unclear, but neuropathy, and outlet obstruction as a result of bladder neck overelevation, are possible factors. Of these, bladder-neck elevation of more than 2–6 cm (measured by magnetic resonance imaging) has been shown to correlate with the development of postoperative DI.[40]

Preoperative urodynamic studies would not appear to prevent postoperative DI as in GSI the detrusor is stable. Because of the low specificity and sensitivity of cystometry it is possible that some patients with urgency but a stable bladder might have DI. Other investigations, such as bladder wall thickness[41] and ambulatory monitoring[42] might increase the detection of DI preoperatively and avoid unnecessary surgery in these patients, thus preventing postoperative urgency and urge incontinence. This hypothesis needs to be tested.

Nevertheless, there are many patients with preoperative urgency and urge incontinence who are helped by colposuspension.[43] It is difficult to predict which patients will be helped and which will be made worse by colposuspension. The history might be helpful: for example, it has been suggested that, where the symptom of stress incontinence has preceded the urge incontinence, both are helped by colposuspension; where the urge incontinence has preceded the stress incontinence, the outcome appears to be worse.[44] It is usually recommended that, if the GSI is the main component, symptomatically and urodynamically, then colposuspension can be performed. The patient should be warned of possible postoperative DI.

Despite history and assessment, there will be some patients who develop *de novo* DI without any obvious preoperative risk factors. Further research is required to see how this can be prevented.

Vaginal prolapse surgery

Incontinence is one particularly worrying complication of prolapse surgery. It has been shown that up to 22% of patients developed incontinence *de novo* following vaginal prolapse surgery.[45] A lower figure of 7–14% has also been reported.[46]

A trial of ring pessary preoperatively has attempted to prevent this complication. In an uncontrolled series,[47] 67 patients undergoing anterior repair for large cystocele (without urinary incontinence) had a preoperative ring pessary test. Urodynamic studies were carried out with the ring *in situ*: there was a drop in the pressure transmission ratio on the urethral pressure profile in 24 patients; there was demonstrable stress incontinence in 17; all 24 patients underwent an anti-incontinence procedure (needle suspension) together with the anterior repair, and this resulted in an increase in the pressure transmission ratio, with all patients being dry postoperatively. It is possible that these patients would have been rendered incontinent by the anterior repair alone; however, a small, randomized trial has failed to confirm that an anti-incontinence procedure is preventative in such cases.[46]

Until a larger randomized controlled trial is completed, it seems reasonable to try to detect 'potential' stress incontinence preoperatively, either clinically or by reducing the prolapse with a ring pessary. Whether an anti-incontinence procedure is indicated or will prevent postoperative incontinence is unclear. At least, the patient should be warned of the potential risk of incontinence and the possible need for treatment in the future.

Prolapse after gynaecological surgery

Following hysterectomy, the risk of prolapse of the vaginal vault and enterocele has been reported as 3.6/1000 person-years. The risk increases from 1% at 3 years to 5% 15 years after hysterectomy.[48] Following colposuspension, enterocele has been reported to be between 18 and 30%.[49,38]

Possible causes include reduced and weakened collagen,[50,51] failure to support the vault at hysterectomy or 'anteversion' of the anterior vaginal wall following colposuspension (thus exposing the middle and posterior vaginal compartments to the effects of intra-abdominal pressure).

Prevention will depend on the surgical procedure, the technique and the strength of the supporting structures. Numerous procedures to prevent enterocele (e.g. closure of the pouch of Douglas with a Moscowitz procedure) or vault prolapse (by attaching the round ligaments to the vaginal vault) have been tried. However, long-term follow-up studies are required to see if these measures are effective in preventing prolapse.

Recurrence of stress incontinence after vault suspension

When an enterocele or vault prolapse occurs after successful colposuspension for GSI, some case reports have suggested that repair of the prolapse can result in recurrence of the stress incontinence.[52] The cause is probably related to removal of the pressure effects exerted by the posterior structures (i.e. bowel and vault) on the bladder neck during stress. This can occur as a result of excessive elevation of the anterior vaginal wall at vault suspension. These posterior pressure effects are important in successful colposuspension.[53]

It is important to identify 'potential' incontinence in these cases (see Vaginal prolapse surgery, page 432). Limited vault elevation at sacrocolpopexy or performing a sacrospinous fixation under spinal anaesthesia might be helpful. With the patient awake and able to cough and so to demonstrate stress incontinence, alterations in the placement of the sacrospinous fixation sutures might prevent incontinence.[52]

How often this complication arises is unclear. However, these reports highlight the need to be aware of the possible risk of rendering a patient incontinent again despite a previously successful colposuspension.

Faecal incontinence following surgery

Faecal incontinence is not uncommon following anal stretching for anal fissure. Avoidance of muscle damage during haemorrhoidectomy and surgery for fistula in ano should prevent incontinence.

Following obstetric third-degree tears (see Faecal incontinence after delivery, page 431) an experienced obstetrician or surgeon should repair sphincter defects. Use of a primary overlap technique might be beneficial.[54] It has been shown that 50% of patients have symptoms despite repair at delivery (method not specified).[28] One reason for this might be failure to recognize the defect and to repair it adequately. Unfortunately, it has been shown that knowledge of the anatomy and identification of defects and appropriate repair is poor among many doctors and midwives.[55] Further education, training in identification and improved surgical technique (including avoidance of rapidly absorbing sutures, e.g. catgut), may help to prevent faecal incontinence following obstetric anal sphincter trauma.

PREVENTION OF FAILED SURGERY FOR GSI

The commonly quoted success rates for surgery for GSI are 80–90%;[38] however, this figure has been called into question.[43] Possible reasons for failure include incorrect diagnosis, inadequate preoperative investigation (i.e. urodynamic studies), poor patient selection, an inappropriate operation and an inexperienced surgeon. Previous suprapubic bladder-neck surgery[56] and intrinsic sphincter deficiency (ISD) may be risk factors. A 54% failure rate has been reported in patients with ISD ('low-pressure urethra'),[57] although other studies have failed to confirm these findings.[58]

A study is required to compare the various surgical procedures for the 'low-pressure urethra/ISD', such as slings, colposuspension or injectables. It is only through such a study that the correct procedure for these patients can be identified and failure prevented.

The surgical 'gold standard' for GSI due to excessive bladder-neck mobility appears to be the Burch colposuspension.[59,60] Prevention of failed surgery might be achieved by avoiding procedures with a poor success rate (such as the anterior vaginal repair) or procedures that have not yet been fully evaluated or have failed to show benefit over colposuspension.

Attention to the above should lead to reduced failure rates with surgery. The old adages are still apt: 'The first operation must be the best one' and 'We should choose the right operation for the right patient and the right patient for the right operation'.

PREVENTION OF DETRUSOR INSTABILITY

As the aetiology of DI is unclear, prevention is difficult. Accurate diagnosis by urodynamic studies might prevent unnecessary bladder-neck surgery in patients who have DI.

It is possible that DI may have its origins in childhood. For example, patients with persistent primary nocturnal enuresis have a high incidence of DI;[61] mothers who themselves have symptoms of frequency and urgency often 'toilet' their children more often;[62,63] this could lead to an abnormal voiding habit, resulting in urgency and urge incontinence.[7] Although none of the studies cited here is large, or the findings conclusive, none the less they highlight the need for further investigation in this area. Should symptoms in childhood be relevant to the aetiology of DI then education of parents and of schoolteachers regarding bladder drill and pelvic floor exercises might be preventative.

Psychological factors have been implicated in the aetiology of DI.[64,65] Identification of psychological problems and their possible relationship to the DI, together with appropriate psychotherapy, have produced encouraging results;[59] this might also prove valuable in prevention.

Anecdotal evidence suggests that a high fluid intake is associated with symptoms of frequency and urgency. Restricting bladder stimulants (e.g. caffeine and alcohol) might prevent the development of urge incontinence.

There is also a theory that bladder-neck opening (due to a weak pelvic floor or weak vaginal wall) might lead to the development of DI. It is here that pelvic floor exercises might have a role in prevention by closing the bladder neck. However, long-term studies are needed to test this hypothesis.

Further research is needed into the aetiology of DI, which may be multifactorial. In the meantime, prevention can only be speculative.

CONCLUSIONS

Effective prevention of urinary incontinence and prolapse will be achieved only by long-term prospective studies of interventions; meanwhile, identification of 'at-risk' groups is recommended.

Treatment of coexisting conditions likely to increase the risk of incontinence (such as obesity, chronic cough, or constipation) might help in both the primary and secondary prevention of urinary incontinence and prolapse.

Long-term follow-up of patients with incontinence as a result of pregnancy and vaginal delivery is required before elective caesarean section can be recommended as a preventative measure.

Attention to the potential risk of incontinence following hysterectomy or vaginal prolapse surgery is recommended. For a patient to be rendered incontinent following surgery is distressing; measures to identify this risk preoperatively and to prevent this outcome, possibly by an additional anti-incontinence procedure, should be considered. With attention to the above, appropriate preventative measures should be found to protect women from incontinence and prolapse .

REFERENCES

1. Thomas TM, Plymat KR, Blannin J, Meade TW. Prevalence of urinary incontinence. *Br Med J* 1980; 280: 1243–1245

2. Resnick NM. Geriatric incontinence. *Urol Clin North Am* 1996; 23: 55–74

3. Spence-Jones C, Kamm MA, Henry MM, Hudson CN. Bowel dysfunction: pathogenic factor in utero-vaginal

prolapse and urinary stress incontinence. *Br J Obstet Gynaecol* 1994; 101: 147–152

4. Smith P. Age changes in the female urethra. *Br J Urol* 1972; 44: 667–676

5. Fantl JA, Cardozo LD, McClish D *et al.* Estrogen therapy in the management of urinary incontinence in post-menopausal women – a meta-analysis. *Obstet Gynecol* 1994; 83: 12–18

6. Wise B, Cardozo LD. Unpublished data.

7. Frewen WK. The management of urgency and frequency of micturition. *Br J Urol* 1980; 52: 367–369

8. Dwyer PL, Lee ETC, Hay DM. Obesity and urinary incontinence in women. *Br J Obstet Gynaecol* 1988; 95: 91–96

9. Wilson PD, Herbison GP. Obstetric practice and the prevalence of urinary incontinence three months after delivery. *Br J Obstet Gynaecol* 1996; 103: 154–161

10. Rasmussen KL, Krue ES, Johansson LE *et al.* Pre-pregnancy obesity – a potent risk factor for urinary symptoms post-partum persisting up to 6–8 months after delivery. *Acta Obstet Gynecol Scand* 1997; 76: 359–362

11. King JK, Freeman RM. Can we predict ante-natally those patients at risk of post-partum stress incontinence? *Neurourol Urodyn* 1996; 15: 330–331

12. Bump RC, Sugerman HJ, Fantl JA, McClish DK. Obesity and lower urinary tract function: effect of surgically induced weight loss. *Am J Obstet Gynecol* 1992; 167: 392–399

13. Snooks SJ, Swash M, Setchell M, Henry MM. Injury to innervation of pelvic floor sphincter musculature in childbirth. *Lancet* 1984; 2: 546–550

14. Sultan AH, Kamm A, Hudson CN. Pudendal nerve damage during labour: a prospective study before and after childbirth. *Br J Obstet Gynaecol* 1994; 101: 22–28

15. Smith ARB, Hosker GL, Warrell DW. The role of pudendal nerve damage in the aetiology of genuine stress incontinence in women. *Br J Obstet Gynaecol* 1989; 96: 29–32

16. Stanton SL, Kerr-Wilson R, Harris GV. The incidence of urological symptoms in normal pregnancy. *Br J Obstet Gynaecol* 1980; 87: 897–900

17. Keane DP, Sims J, Abrams P, Bailey J. Analysis of collagen status in pre-menopausal nulliparous women with genuine stress incontinence. *Br J Obstet Gynaecol* 1997; 104: 994–998

18. Peschars UM, Schar GN, Anthuber C, Schussler B. Post-partal pelvic floor damage – is connective tissue impairment more important than neuromuscular change? *Neurourol Urodyn* 1994; 13: 376–377

19. Sultan AH, Stanton SL. Preserving the pelvic floor and perineum during childbirth. Elective caesarean section? *Br J Obstet Gynaecol* 1996; 103: 731–734

20. Henderson JS. Effects of prenatal teaching program on post-partum regeneration of the pubococcygeal muscle. *J Obstet Gynecol Neonatal Nurs* 1983; 8: 403–408

21. Morkved S, Bø K. The effect of post-partum pelvic floor muscle exercise in the prevention and treatment of urinary incontinence. *Int Urogynaecol J* 1997; 8: 217–222

22. Allen RE, Hosker GL, Smith ARB, Warrell DW. Pelvic floor damage and childbirth: a neurophysiological study. *Br J Obstet Gynaecol* 1990; 97: 770–779

23. Cutner A, Cardozo LD, Benness CJ. Assessment of urinary symptoms in early pregnancy. *Br J Obstet Gynaecol* 1991; 98: 1283–1286

24. Nell JT, Diedericks A. A prospective clinical and urodynamic study of bladder function during and after pregnancy (abstract). *Int Urogynaecol J*, 1997; 8: S45

25. Chaliha C, Kaha V, Stanton SL *et al.* What does pregnancy and delivery do to bladder function? A urodynamic viewpoint (abstract). *Neurourol Neurodyn* 1998; 17: 415–416

26. MacArthur C, Bick DE, Keighley MR. Faecal incontinence after childbirth. *Br J Obstet Gynaecol* 1997; 104: 46–50

27. Sultan AH, Kamm MA, Hudson CN. Anal sphincter disruption during vaginal delivery. *N Engl J Med* 1993; 329: 1905–1911

28. Sultan AH, Kamm MA, Bartram I, Hudson CN. Third degree obstetric anal sphincter tears: risk factors and outcome of primary repair. *Br Med J* 1994; 308: 887–891

29. Poen AC, Felt-Bersma RJF, Dekker GA *et al.* Third degree obstetric perineal tears: risk factors and the preventative role of mediolateral episiotomy. *Br J Obstet Gynaecol* 1997; 104: 563–566

30. Helwig JT, Thorp JM, Bowes WA. Does midline episiotomy increase the risk of third and fourth-degree lacerations in operative vaginal deliveries? *Obstet Gynecol* 1993; 82: 276–279

31. Combs CA, Robertson PA, Laros RK. Risk factors for third degree and fourth degree perineal lacerations in forceps and vacuum deliveries. *Am J Obstet Gynecol* 1990; 163: 100–104

32. Hendry WF. Urinary tract injuries during gynaecological surgery. In: Studd J (ed) *Progress in Obstetrics and Gynaecology*, Volume 5. Edinburgh: Churchill Livingstone, 1985; 362–377

33. Brown J, Seeley D, Grady K *et al.* Hysterectomy: the effect on prevalence of urinary incontinence (abstract). *Int Urogynaecol J* 1994; 5: 370

34. Griffith-Jones MD, Jarvis GJ, MacNamara HM. Adverse urinary symptoms after total abdominal hysterectomy – fact or fiction? *Br J Urol* 1991; 67: 295–297

35. Kikku P. Supravaginal uterine amputation v hysterectomy with reference to subjective bladder symptoms and incontinence. *Acta Obstet Gynecol Scand* 1985; 64: 375–379

36. Parys BT, Haylen BT, Hutton JL, Parsons KF. The effects of simple hysterectomy on vesicourethral function. *Br J Urol* 1989; 64: 594–599

37. Cardozo LD, Stanton SL, Williams JE. Detrusor instability following surgery for genuine stress incontinence. *Br J Urol* 1979; 51: 205–297

38. Jarvis GJ. Surgery for genuine stress incontinence. *Br J Obstet Gynaecol* 1994; 101: 371–374

39. Steel SA, Cox C, Stanton SL. Long term follow-up of detrusor instability following the colposuspension operation. *Br J Urol* 1985; 58: 138–142

40. Bombieri L, Freeman R M. Why do women have detrusor instability after colposuspension? (abstract). *Int Urogynecol J* 1998; 9: 326

41. Khullar V, Salvatore S, Cardozo LD et al. Prediction of the development of detrusor instability after colposuspension (abstract). *Neurourol Urodyn* 1995; 14: 486

42. Eckford ESD, Bailey RA, Jackson SR et al. Occult pre-operative detrusor instability – an adverse prognostic feature in genuine stress incontinence surgery (abstract). *Neurourol Urodyn* 1995; 14: 487

43. Black N, Griffiths J, Pope C et al. Impact of surgery for stress incontinence: cohort study. *Br Med J* 1997; 315: 1493–1498

44. Scotti RJ, Angell G, Flora R, Greston WM. Burch colposuspension cure for detrusor instability: predictive value of pre-operative history. *Neurourol Urodyn* 1996; 15: 286

45. Borstad E, Rud T. The risk of developing urinary stress incontinence after vaginal repair in continent women: a clinical and urodynamic follow-up study. *Acta Obstet Gynecol Scand* 1989; 68: 545–54.

46. Bump RC, Hurt WG Theofrastous JP et al. Randomised prospective comparison of needle colposuspension v endopelvic fascia plication for potential stress incontinence, prophylaxis in women undergoing vaginal reconstruction for Stage III or IV pelvic organ prolapse. *Am J Obstet Gynecol* 1996; 175: 326–335

47. Bergman A, Koonings PP, Ballard CA. Predicting post-operative urinary incontinence development in women undergoing operations for genito-urinary prolapse. *Am J Obstet Gynecol* 1988; 158: 1171–1175

48. Mant J, Painter R, Vassey M. Epidemiology of genital prolapse: observations from the Oxford Family Planning Association study. *Br J Obstet Gynaecol* 1997; 104: 579–585

49. Wiskind AK, Crighton SM, Stanton SL. The incidence of genital prolapse after the Burch colposuspension. *Am J Obstet Gynecol* 1992; 167: 399–405

50. Norton PA, Baker JE, Sharp HC, Warenski JC. Genital urinary prolapse and joint hypermobility in women. *Obstet Gynecol* 1995; 85: 225–228

51. Jackson SR, Avery NC, Tarlton JF et al. Changes in metabolism of collagen in genitourinary prolapse. *Lancet* 1996; 347: 1658–1661

52. Bombieri LB, Freeman RM. Recurrence of stress incontinence after vault suspension: can it be prevented? *Int Urogynaecol J* 1998; 9: 58–60

53. Hertogs SK, Stanton SL. Mechanism of urinary continence after colposuspension: barrier studies. *Br J Obstet Gynaecol* 1985; 92: 1184–1188

54. Sultan AH, Monga AK, Kumar D, Stanton SL. Primary repair of obstetric and sphincter rupture using the overlap technique. *Br J Obstet Gynaecol* 1999; 106: 318–323

55. Sultan AH, Kamm MA, Hudson CN. Obstetric perineal trauma. An audit of training. *J Obstet Gynaecol* 1995; 15: 19–23

56. Francis LN, Sand PK, Hamrang K, Ostergard DR. Urodynamic appraisal of success and failure after retropubic urethropexy. *J Reprod Med* 1987; 32: 693–696

57. Sand PK, Bowen LW, Panganiban R, Ostergard DR. The low pressure urethra as a factor in failed retropubic urethropexy. *Obstet Gynecol* 1987; 69: 399–402

58. Richardson DA, Ramahi A, Chalas E. Surgical management of stress incontinence in patients with low urethral pressures. *Gynecol Obstet Invest* 1991; 31: 106–109

59. Burch JC. Urethrovaginal fixation to Cooper's ligament for correction of stress incontinence, cystocele and prolapse. *Am J Obstet Gynecol* 1961; 81: 281–290

60. Stanton SL, Cardozo LD. Results of the colposuspension operation for incontinence and prolapse. *Br J Obstet Gynaecol* 1979; 86: 693–69.

61. Whiteside CG, Arnold EP. Persistent primary enuresis: a urodynamic assessment. *Br Med J* 1975; 1: 364–367

62. De Jonge JA. The urge syndrome. In: Kolvin I, MacKeith RC, Meadow R (eds) *Bladder Control and Enuresis. Clinics in Developmental Medicine* 1973; 48/49: 66–69

63. Foote AJ, Moore KH. Bladder training: should you listen to what your mother says? (abstract) In: Proceedings of the 26th Annual Meeting, International Continence Society, Athens. *Neurourol Neurodyn* 1996; 15: 137–138

64. Freeman RM, McPherson FM, Baxby K. Psychological features of women with idiopathic detrusor instability. *Urol Int* 1985; 40: 257–25.

65. Macauley AJ, Stanton SL, Stern RS, Holmes DM. Micturition and the mind: psychological factors in the aetiology and treatment of urinary disorders in women. *Br Med J* 1987; 294: 540–543.

66. Petros PEP, Ulmsten U. Rule of the pelvic floor in bladder neck opening and closure II: Vagina. *Int Urogynecol J* 1997; 8: 69–73

35

Modern devices for the non-surgical treatment of pelvic organ prolapse and genuine stress incontinence

R. Gardner, D. R. Staskin

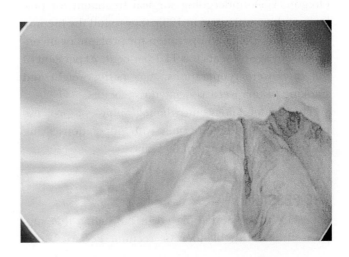

Modern devices to treat pelvic organ prolapse

INTRODUCTION

The pessary is the most common non-surgical method employed to correct pelvic organ prolapse. Pelvic organ prolapse is the descent of one or more of the bladder, rectum, uterus or vaginal apex down the long axis of the vagina. Severe cases of this are marked by protrusion of one or more of these structures at or past the introitus. Prolapse of the genital organs occurs more frequently in women who are multiparous and of advancing age, or both. Additional factors that may predispose to prolapse include obesity, history of heavy smoking or coexisting chronic respiratory disorders. Precise information is lacking about the epidemiology, incidence and prevalence of prolapse. Mant *et al.*[1] prospectively followed women for a total of 292 000 person-years (an average of 17 years per person) who had enrolled in family planning clinics in Scotland and England. They found the incidence of hospital admission with prolapse was 2.04/1000 person-years risk. The incidence of prolapse that required surgical repair after hysterectomy was 3.6/1000 person-years risk. The observed risk of prolapse after hysterectomy was 5.5 times higher in women whose original indication for hysterectomy was prolapse. Parity was the most significant variable related to increased risk for prolapse. The risk for prolapse increased with each child, but the greatest increase in risk occurred after the second child; thereafter, the increase in risk was less dramatic. Olsen *et al.*[2] reported on a retrospective cohort of patients in a managed-care organization in Portland, Oregon, USA undergoing surgical treatment for prolapse and incontinence in 1995: they found the lifetime risk of undergoing an operation for prolapse or incontinence by age 80 years was 11.1 per cent; 29 per cent of the cases were reoperations. Age, parity, weight and smoking history were associated risk factors.

The epidemiology and demographics of prolapse need further study, especially with populations living longer and past the age of 80 years.

THE PESSARY

A pessary is any device placed in the vagina that supports the uterus, bladder or rectum. Pessaries have been used as early as the 5th century BC for the treatment of uterine prolapse. Various materials such as wood, wax, cork, ivory, rubber, metal, fabric, sea sponges, whale bone, and even edible materials such as pomegranates have been used to form and/or serve as pessaries.[3] Modern-day pessaries are made of latex rubber, silicone or acrylic. There were over 100 different types of pessaries available in the late 1800s. Availability was without prescription by mail order or over the counter throughout the 1930s. They are currently available by prescription after office evaluation and fitting performed by a certified healthcare provider.

Commonly used pessaries include the following types:

- Lever: Hodge, Smith–Hodge, and Risser
- Ring
- Shaatz
- Gellhorn
- Gehrung
- Inflato-ball
- Cube
- Donut.

Pessaries are most commonly used for the management of uterine prolapse and to provide vaginal support of the bladder or rectum. There is little information in the literature to prove that one type of pessary is superior to another, but some are favoured for correction of certain types of prolapse.

Uterine prolapse or malposition of the uterus has been observed in the neonatal period. It can occur at any time during the reproductive years, even during pregnancy, but is most commonly seen in the post-reproductive years. Pessaries can be used in the preoperative evaluation of urinary incontinence or to help identify potential problems with postoperative bladder control. Temporary use of pessaries can help delay surgery to a more convenient time. They can be used for longer periods when surgery is either not an option or contraindicated. Pessaries have also been used to deliver medications, to provide support for an incompetent cervix during pregnancy, to correct prolapse of a gravid uterus, or to maintain uterine position after repositioning of an incarcerated uterus. They have been used in years past for the treatment of dysmenorrhoea and menstrual irregularity.[4]

MODERN PESSARIES

Lever pessaries

Lever pessaries include the Hodge (with or without support), the Smith and the Risser devices. The most commonly used pessary in the late 1800s and early 1900s was the Hodge, developed in the 1860s by Dr Hugh Lenox Hodge from the University of Pennsylvania. These pessaries were utilized to correct uterine retrodisplacement or retroversion. They continue to be used to correct uterine prolapse with retroversion, but they are more commonly used to support an incompetent cervix during pregnancy. They are also used in the evaluation of larger cystoceles and stress urinary incontinence (SUI). Initially they were made of rubber but are now made of silicone.

Hodge

The Hodge lever pessary (Fig. 35.1) is an oblong ring with long axis beams that are curved to match the curvature of the vagina; the top beam is squared and wide for those patients with minimal pubic support and a narrow symphysis. The top beam also has a slightly concave notch which prevents urethral obstruction. This modification makes the Hodge a useful choice when prolapse is accompanied by genuine stress incontinence (GSI). The Hodge lever pessary can also be found with a modification of the top beam which forms a shelf to provide support and elevation of a cystocele. The squared-off top beam keeps the device properly positioned in the vagina.

Smith

The Smith lever pessary is a modification of the Hodge lever pessary, by Dr Albert Smith of Philadelphia. It has a more rounded, narrow anterior top beam and a broadly curved posterior beam for a patient with a deep symphysis and well-defined pubic notch.

Risser

The Risser lever pessary is another modification of the Hodge lever pessary, with a wider top beam and a deeper concave notch to provide greater weight-bearing capacity but less soft-tissue pressure necrosis to the urethra. This device is designed for the patient with a flattened pubic arch.

Fitting and insertion of the lever pessaries

The bladder and rectum should be empty. The vaginal depth is estimated by measuring the depth of the vagina with the length of the index or middle finger of the examiner's hand; width is estimated by the distance between the middle and index fingers opposed against each vaginal wall, with care taken to avoid undue stretching of the orifice. Once the proper size pessary is chosen, the pessary must be folded along its long axis, with the broadly curved posterior beam pointed towards the introitus. With the folded pessary held between the thumb and the first two fingers of one hand, the free hand is used to manipulate the cervix to achieve a more anteflexed position of the uterus. Next, the folded pessary is gently advanced into the long axis of the vagina so that the posterior beam of the unfolded pessary lies in the posterior vaginal fornix, behind the cervix. The anterior bar should lie in position behind the pubic symphysis. The uterus is manually held in place until the pessary is completely inserted, then the anterior bar is properly positioned behind the pubis.

A tenaculum applied to the anterior lip of the cervix of the more acutely retroverted uterus can maintain the uterus in an anteverted position during insertion; however, this significantly increases the patient's discomfort during the fitting procedure. Alternatively, the patient can assume a knee–chest position for insertion of the

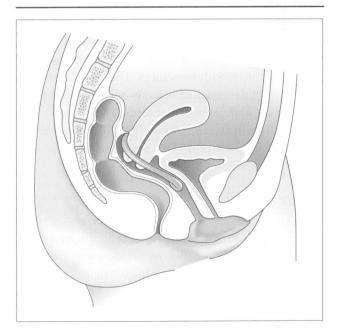

Figure 35.1. *The Hodge lever pessary (courtesy of Milex Products Inc., Chicago, IL, USA).*

device. Once the pessary is in place, the patient should be asked to stand and bear down slightly while being examined. The properly fitted pessary lies behind the pubis anteriorly and the posterior beam is behind the cervix. The patient should walk around the examination room. A successful fitting is one in which the device is not apparent to the patient and remains in position. If the pessary falls out, it is too small. If the pessary feels uncomfortable or painful, or causes urinary obstruction, it is too large.

These pessaries can remain in place during intercourse, and allow for vaginal administration of medications with vaginal applicators. They are available in ten sizes, from 0 to the largest, 9; the most commonly chosen sizes range from 2 to 4.

Ring pessaries

Ring pessaries are commonly used in a patient with first- or second-degree uterine prolapse. The rings are available with or without a porous diaphragm for additional support of a coexisting cystocele. A folding ring without support may remain in place during intercourse. Ring pessaries are commonly made of silicone.

Insertion is accomplished by folding the pessary with the arc concave down and sliding it into the vagina, back to the posterior fornix. Once opened, it should be given a quarter turn to secure its positon. The leading edge of the rim should fit behind the pubic symphysis, but not too snugly. Removal is accomplished by palpating the rim and rotating it slightly to refold and withdraw it in one smooth movement. The ring should take up the redundant vaginal tissue by forming a sling that will support and elevate the uterus. There are 11 sizes ranging from 0 to the largest, 10, which correlate to diameters of 5–10.5 cm. The most commonly chosen sizes range from 3 to 5.

Shaatz pessary

The Shaatz pessary is a disc with a central round opening surrounded by smaller round openings to aid in drainage of vaginal secretions. It was originally made of hard rubber but is now made of flexible silicone. It is used for the support of mild-to-moderate prolapse with a mild cystocele. It is available in sizes 1.5 to 3.5 inches, but the most common sizes chosen are between 2.25 and 2.75 inches.

Gellhorn pessary

The shape of the Gellhorn pessary (Fig. 35.2) resembles a doorknob, with a concave disc-like surface on one side and a short-length handle or knob emanating from the other side. Formerly made of a rigid acrylic material that was non-malleable, the devices are now made of a more flexible silicone material that allows for easier insertion. Regardless of the model chosen, both the rigid acrylic and the flexible silicone pessaries provide excellent support for the patient with third-degree procidentia. The rigid Gellhorn pessary is usually a solid piece of material; the flexible silicone model has perforations in the disc and a channel lengthwise through the handle, which allows for natural drainage of vaginal secretions.

Insertion can be difficult in the patient with a narrow vaginal introitus, as is typical of a woman of advanced age who is neither sexually active nor using oestrogen-replacement therapy. Insertion is accomplished with the patient in the dorsal lithotomy position; the labia are spread with one hand and the other hand holds the handle of the pessary so that the disc lies parallel to the introitus. The disc is gently eased into the vagina into the correct position with the disc flat against the vaginal apex or the cervix, the handle extending down the long axis of the vagina but not protruding from the introitus.

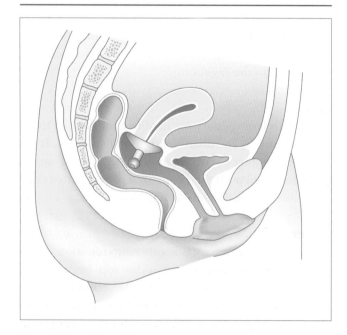

Figure 35.2. *The Gellhorn rigid pessary (courtesy of Milex Products Inc., Chicago, IL, USA)*

The flexible silicone Gellhorn pessaries are malleable enough to conform to some extent to the introitus and vagina as they are being inserted. Atrophic mucosal surfaces can be a source of great discomfort to the patient during insertion and removal, even if a silicone device is chosen. It is wise to caution the patient to expect a certain degree of discomfort from stretching and distension of the introitus and lower end of the vagina. Sometimes superficial abrasion of the introitus can occur during insertion but this should heal quickly.

These pessaries must be removed, cleansed and reinserted on a regular basis. Usually the interval is every 3 months, and is accompanied by general inspection of the vagina and cervix for abrasions or infection. The rigid Gellhorn pessaries can be a challenge to remove without causing discomfort to the patient. The modern silicone model can easily be removed if stuck: a small syringe filled with water or saline should be attached to the opening at the distal end of the handle, then the water is gently injected , thereby breaking the suction of the disc. Gentle traction on the handle will then allow easy removal.

Choosing the proper size of the Gellhorn pessary can be a source of confusion to the examiner. The pessary is available in nine sizes, the diameter of the disc varying from 1.5 to 3.5 inches. The most commonly chosen sizes are 2.25–3 inches. Selecting the best size can be a matter of trial and error, but it is best to begin with a disc of diameter corresponding to the anterior–posterior length of the introitus.

Gehrung pessary

The Gehrung pessary (Fig. 35.3) is useful to support a cystocele and/or rectocele at the same time as a third-degree uterine prolapse. The device has an oblong, ring-like shape but is arched and flexible. The unique shape of the device helps to support the levator sling laterally, avoiding direct pressure on the rectum, but supporting the bladder anteriorly to correct the descensus. The anterior support also aids with micturition. This pessary does not interfere with douching and coitus because of its ring-like shape and relatively slim width. Insertion is accomplished by folding it with the arched-side convex up, keeping both 'heels' parallel to the pelvic floor as the pessary is inserted sideways. Thereafter, one heel is pushed back and the other forward to complete a 90-degree

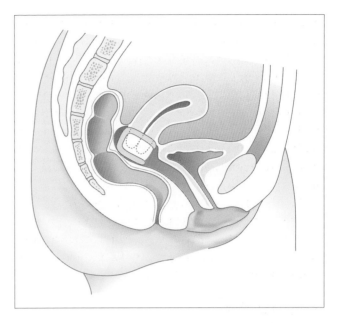

Figure 35.3. *The Gehrung pessary (Courtesy of Milex Products Inc., Chicago, IL, USA).*

rotation so that the back arch is situated in the anterior fornix and the front arch is situated behind the pubic symphysis. The rotation of the pessary as it is being inserted is such that the lateral bars curve convex towards the anterior wall of the vagina. This position creates a 'bladder bridge' to provide support for the cystocele, enabling normal micturition. The device is available in nine sizes but sizes most commonly chosen range from 3 to 5.

Inflato-ball pessary

Inflato-ball pessaries (Fig. 35.4) work by distributing the weight of the prolapsing tissue across this space-occupying device. The size of the Inflato-ball varies according to the amount of air inflated into the device via a two-way valve, so that it adjusts easily to each individual patient's needs. There are four sizes, from small to extra large (diameters of 2–2.75 inches). The medium or large sizes are most commonly chosen.

Cube

The cube pessary (Fig. 35.5) is six-sided with each side concave, one side of which has a string affixed to aid in identification and removal. It is specifically designed for use in third-degree prolapse, with complete procidentia or cystorectocele.

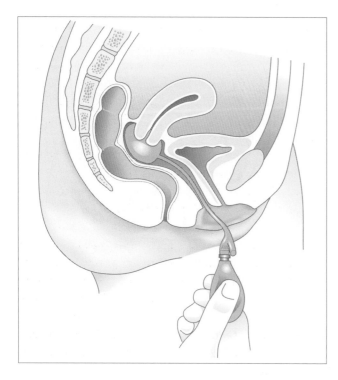

Figure 35.4. *The inflato-ball pessary (courtesy of Milex Products Inc., Chicago, IL, USA).*

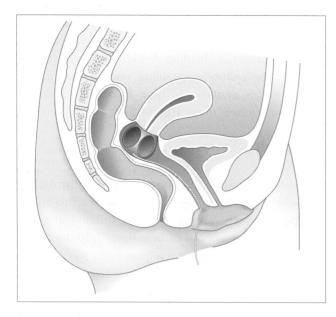

Figure 35.5. *The silicon cube pessary (courtesy of Milex Products Inc., Chicago, IL, USA).*

Insertion is accomplished by compressing the cube's concavities with the fingers of one hand, spreading the labia with the other hand, then gently pushing the cube into the vagina so that the entire cube sits above the introitus. The string should extend out of the vagina. The six concave surfaces provide suction on the vaginal wall. Removal can be difficult because of the suction-vacuum created by the concavities.

The cube is very easy to insert and maintains the prolapsed structures in the correct position; however, proper patient selection is essential for continued use, patient satisfaction and patient compliance. This device must be cleansed daily (or, at least, every other day) because there is no mechanism to allow for drainage of vaginal secretions: bacteria can easily accumulate, causing vaginal infection and malodour. The patient must possess manual dexterity and flexibility sufficient to reach her own genitals and pull down on the string, then to insert her fingers into the vagina to grasp the device and manoeuvre her fingers around the sidewalls of the cube to break the suction and remove it. If the patient cannot do this, she will need someone to help remove, cleanse and replace the device on a daily basis.

The cube pessary is available in seven sizes (1–7) corresponding to 1–2 inches or 25–50 mm. The most commonly chosen sizes are 3–5.

Tandem cube

The tandem cube was designed for the rare patient with third-degree prolapse who is unable to retain even the largest single-cube pessary within the vagina. The tandem cube has 10 concave sides, which provide more surface area for suction. This device demands a great degree of manual dexterity on the part of the patient, or a willing assistant who is able to remove, cleanse and re-position the device daily (or at least every other day). The tandem cube is available in six sizes from a total length of $2\frac{3}{8}$ to 4 inches. The most commonly chosen sizes are from 3 to $3\frac{5}{8}$ inches.

Donut pessary

The Donut pessary (Fig. 35.6) is useful for correction of third-degree prolapse. Formerly made of red rubber but now made of silicone, this pessary is available in six sizes. The diameter ranges from 2 to 3.5 inches. Insertion is simple because it is similar to inserting a diaphragm. Once properly inserted, the Donut pessary can reveal a patient's coexisting SUI because it does not

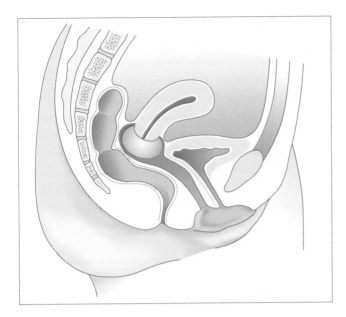

Figure 35.6. *The Donut pessary (courtesy of Milex Products Inc., Chicago, IL, USA).*

provide support to the proximal urethra. The most commonly used sizes range from 2.25 to 3 inches.

GENERAL COMMENTS ON FITTING AND CARE OF THE PESSARY AND THE PATIENT

Fitting is usually done by trial and error but one approach would be to use the index finger as a measure of the length and depth of the vagina. A properly fitted pessary should allow a finger to fit beween the pessary and the vaginal wall, thus aiding and ensuring easy removal. Wood[5] advises starting with the largest pessary that can be comfortably admitted into the introitus but not protrude out of the orifice. A vaginal lubricant is usually applied to the pessary surface to minimize the discomfort of fitting. A low-percentage anaesthetic cream or ointment, especially in the setting of vaginal atrophy, can be used instead of a lubricant. Pretreatment with vaginal oestrogen for 2–3 weeks prior to the insertion appointment is the best way to enhance vaginal lubrication, to decrease atrophy and thereby minimize discomfort at the time of fitting.

Selection of the proper pessary can be very difficult in view of the number of choices and sizes. Davila[6] constructed a table to help identify which pessaries were useful for various degrees of prolapse. In his classification, virtually all pessaries are useful for mild prolapse

and/or enterocele. The lever devices were not considered useful to correct large cystocele, any rectoceles, or any degree of vaginal vault prolapse. The ring pessary was not useful for correction of any degree of rectocele. Sexual activity is another important matter to consider when selecting the type of pessary. Miller[3] states, 'Coitus is possible with the ring, lever and Gehrung pessaries'.

Brubaker[7] states that there are no scientific data to identify optimal care of the pessary. Davila[6] and, more recently, Wu *et al.*[8] offered protocols for pessary management. The patient should be asked to walk around, bear down and void prior to leaving the office to ensure there is no urethral obstruction and that the pessary does not cause discomfort. Once the pessary is deemed appropriate and properly fitted, the patient's return appointment should be scheduled within 1–3 days, depending on the pessary and the patient. The less dexterous the patient, and the fewer family, friends or caretakers she possesses, then the sooner she should return for follow-up. Follow-up for pessary removal, cleansing, inspection of the vagina, and reinsertion of the pessary should occur on a regular basis. Some protocols advise every 3–4 months, some every 6–12 months, but the frequency of return visits depends greatly on the patient and type of pessary chosen.

Intermittent use of oestrogen cream is helpful when the vagina is atrophic. If oestrogen is contraindicated or not an option then Trimo-San (Milex Products Inc., Chicago, IL, USA) vaginal gel can be used to maintain a proper vaginal pH and normal acidity to prevent bacterial overgrowth. It is imperative to remember that the cube pessary is 'unforgiving' because there are no ports to allow for spontaneous drainage of vaginal secretions. The cube is the one pessary that must be removed daily or (at least) every other day for cleansing. Douching may help cleanse the vagina of bacteria while any of the pessaries are in place, apart from the cube. There is little scientific proof that douching is useful or necessary, but the effects of a neglected or forgotten pessary are well documented and are reviewed below.[9]

COMPLICATIONS OF PESSARIES

Complications of pessaries include the following:

- Vaginal discharge, odour, bleeding
- Vaginal infection

- Vaginal abrasions or erosions
- Cytological atypia of the cervix or vagina, usually inflammatory changes
- Incarceration with or without fistula to adjacent organs
- Symptoms of urinary tract infection
- Urinary retention and/or obstruction
- Urinary incontinence

Zeitlin and Lebherz[10] reviewed pessary use in the geriatric population and reported inflammation and infection as the most frequent problems associated with pessaries. They avoided using pessaries made of latex because of the increased frequency of latex sensitivity. Sulak *et al.*[11] reported no major complications associated with use of pessaries in a retrospective study of 107 patients fitted with pessaries for pelvic relaxation. More recently, Myers *et al.*[12] reported on the use of two pessaries, 'a double pessary' – in 5 women who had long-standing vaginal vault prolapse. They observed no problems with infection, erosion or urinary retention.

Vaginal bleeding may be due to infection or erosion of the vaginal mucosa. It is a symptom that warrants immediate office evaluation, removal of the pessary and careful inspection of the vagina and cervix. Most pessary-related vaginal infections, discharge and odour resolve with a more frequent schedule of removal and cleansing of the device and the vagina. Usually, soap and water are sufficient to cleanse the pessary. Douching may be useful to eradicate, prevent or minimize vaginal discharge and odour, but this depends on the patient and her medical provider. Minor infections can be treated with topical antibiotics. Oral broad-spectrum antibiotics are usually not necessary but may be used for severe infections that involve adjacent organs.

Minor ulcerations or granulation tissue may resolve by temporarily discontinuing use of the pessary, or by restricting use to short periods during the day. Brubaker[7] advises a 'pessary free interval' and topical oestrogens for recurrent ulcerations. Frequent recurrence or persistent erosions are common reasons to discontinue the pessary. When Wu *et al.*[8] prospectively followed 81 women successfully fitted with a pessary, they found that the highest rate of discontinuation occurred within the first 12 months, mostly within the first month. Brubaker[7] also noted that one-third of women fitted with a pessary would discontinue use within the first 6 months. Common reasons for discontinuing use included failure to

support the prolapsed organs, persistent vaginal discharge, recurrent erosions, vaginal or rectal pain, urinary incontinence, or desire for surgical repair.

Cytological atypia of the cervix or vagina is usually a result of foreign-body inflammation and irritation of mucosal surfaces. Schraub *et al.*[13] in France reported an association of cervical–vaginal cancer within 18 years of last-time pessary use. Miller[3] in 1995 provided reassurance about the lack of causation of pessary use and the development of vaginal or cervical cancer, although the actual material formerly used to make pessaries may have contributed to isolated cases of 'pessary cancer'.

Incarceration occurs infrequently but it is usually the result of neglect, the so-called 'forgotten' pessary. Poma[14] reported on three cases of pessary incarceration treated with serial application of topical oestrogen to allow for successful removal of the pessary. Rigid pessaries such as the Gellhorn provide some interesting challenges for removal, but usually this can be accomplished with a schedule of topical oestrogen. Difficulty in removal may require regional or general anaesthesia in the operating room to facilitate maximal pelvic relaxation. It is even more unusual to accomplish removal by piecemeal destruction of the pessary. A pessary, on rare occasion, can induce fistula formation to adjacent organs. This is usually seen in long-standing neglect of a rigid pessary, leading to severe local inflammation and invasion of aggressive bacteria through the mucosal surfaces.

Urinary frequency, urgency or incontinence (or all of these) are symptoms that require prompt evaluation and treatment. Urinary tract infections usually respond to oral antibiotics. Suppressive, daily low-dose oral antibiotics can be used in cases of recurrent infection; however, successful treatment may require removal of the device. Refitting with a different type or smaller device may lead to success. Incontinence may not respond to refitting of the pessary, but it may indicate that surgical intervention is warranted. Pessaries can be used to reveal coexisting incontinence after the genital organs are repositioned. Bergman and Bhatia[15] reported that the pessary is a valuable tool in predicting successful outcome of incontinence surgery.

Urinary retention or obstruction is usually due to an incorrectly fitted device and requires immediate removal. Meinhardt *et al.*[16] reported an unusual case of a woman who presented with anuria, urosepsis and bilateral hydronephrosis. However, most situations have not progressed to this unusual degree of severity and resolve after the device is removed.

CONTRAINDICATIONS

Acute vaginal, urinary or pelvic infection; unexplained vaginal or cervical lesions; and unexplained vaginal bleeding are all contraindications to fitting and use of a pessary. The option to use a pessary depends on factors such as the patient's vision, manual dexterity and ability to provide adequate hygiene. If the patient cannot care adequately for herself, then the living arrangement must include competent caretakers – whether they be family, friends or professionals – who will not neglect the proper care of the patient and pessary.

SUMMARY

Pessaries have been used for a variety of reasons since the 5th century BC. They will continue to be used in the non-surgical management of pelvic organ prolapse, perhaps more frequently given the demographic shift towards an ageing population. Demographics of an ageing population, combined with managed healthcare industries worldwide seeking to contain cost and minimize frequency of surgical interventions, may serve to promote the use of pessaries for the management of genital prolapse. There is little in the medical literature about the epidemiology and demographics of urogenital prolapse, although Brett *et al.*[17] commented on uterine prolapse as it relates to the epidemiology of hysterectomy in the USA. Their study was published just after the epidemiological reports of Mant *et al.*[1] and Olsen *et al.*[2] Menotti[18] explored the problems of ageing and quality of life in a population of Italian women over 40 years of age but did not specifically examine the problem of urogenital prolapse. The effects on quality of life, or cost–benefit analysis of surgical versus non-surgical intervention in urogenital prolapse, are areas for further study. This concern is shared by Toozs-Hobson *et al.*[19] of the UK in their review on management of vaginal vault prolapse. There are no prospective, randomized studies to identify which pessary works best, under what conditions and what is the best method of management for the patient fitted with a pessary. This information

would help to increase patient satisfaction and compliance, especially for those patients who are medically or otherwise unable to have surgical correction of their prolapse.

Modern devices to treat genuine stress incontinence

INTRODUCTION

GSI is the result of underactivity of the bladder outlet in the absence of true bladder activity. The bladder outlet or sphincteric mechanism is composed of the bladder neck, the proximal urethra, the region of the external sphincter supported by the vaginal wall and vaginal attachments, and the levator ani complex. The pathophysiology of GSI may be secondary to either abnormal bladder-neck support or low urethral closure pressure associated with intrinsic sphincter deficiency (ISD). The coexistence of GSI in combination with detrusor overactivity (urge incontinence) or underactivity (urinary retention) is clinically important when using devices that increase urinary outlet resistance. Recent technological advances, and the adaptation of products that traditionally have been utilized for other purposes, have provided interesting options for the non-surgical management of urinary loss in the female patient. Devices used to treat this condition include those that provide for external urinary collection, intravaginal support of the bladder neck, or blockage of urinary leakage by occluding egress either at the external meatus or within the urethra. These devices attempt to correct, compensate for, or circumvent the pathophysiology of the bladder outlet in order to improve urinary storage.

Modern devices (apart from biofeedback or physiotherapy devices) for the direct treatment of GSI are reviewed in this chapter. A review of the literature (Medline 1970–1998) for data on device efficacy and safety reveals that many devices currently in use have not been studied objectively, especially those devices traditionally used for other purposes. Many published reports describe devices not currently marketed. There is little, if any, clinical research for many of those recently developed and used specifically to treat incontinence.

EXTERNAL COLLECTION DEVICES

External collection devices are placed over the urethral meatus or within or around the introitus. They are secured with adhesives or special straps, or by suction. The most common of these devices are diapers (nappies), pads and incontinence pants. Some devices collect the urine in a drainage bag. Most published articles are small descriptive studies of patients in rehabilitation centres or nursing homes, not an ambulatory population.[20-24] The major difficulties with these devices are related to method of adherence to the periurethral area and potential skin irritation, and anatomical positioning of the device and how that affects or is affected by activities of daily living or by variation in patient anatomy. Degree of mobility and activity of the patient and duration of use are factors that must be considered. This is an area for future clinical research, especially in an ambulatory population, since most devices currently available are cumbersome to use.

OCCLUSIVE DEVICES

Occlusive devices block urinary leakage at the external urethral meatus. Several devices are currently marketed but peer-reviewed literature is limited. Only one peer-reviewed study, by Eckford *et al.*,[25] was published in 1996. Those authors studied 19 women with symptoms of stress incontinence who used an external urethral occlusive pad, which adhered by an adhesive seal over the urethral meatus. The median age of the 19 women was 45 years, range 36–72 years. Continence data were collected using pad tests, urinary diaries and symptom review. Seventeen women reported a cure or improvement measured by the number of incontinent episodes per week. There was a significant decrease in both the number of episodes ($p < 0.001$) and pad-test leakage ($p < 0.002$) when using the device. Ability to place and remove the device were the major difficulties encountered (Fig. 35.7).

Several products exist to occlude urinary loss at the meatus by simple barrier effect, but compression of the distal urethra has been hypothesized as a contributor to continence. Long-term efficacy and safety data are not currently available. Studies of larger populations, especially of ambulatory patients, are required to obtain data on device efficacy and local effects of adhesives and suction on the periurethral area.

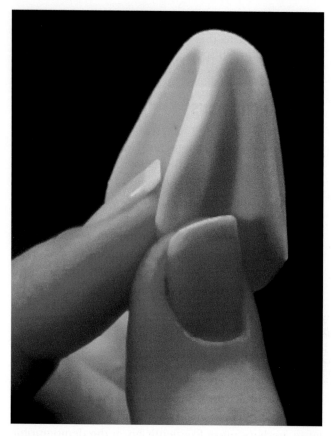

Figure 35.7. *The Impress device (Uromed Corporation, Needham, MA, USA).*

INTRAVAGINAL DEVICES TO SUPPORT THE BLADDER NECK

Support of the bladder neck to improve SUI has been achieved with varying success with tampons, pessaries, contraceptive diaphragms and intravaginal devices specifically designed to support the bladder neck. The quality of the data varies depending on the individual device studied. Many abstracts have been presented at national and international meetings, but the data are limited by short-term or laboratory-only use. Nygaard[26] performed a prospective, randomized laboratory-based study of 18 patients using a Hodge pessary with support, a super tampon, or no device. All patients performed three standardized aerobics sessions of 40 minutes each: both devices decreased the amount of urine loss; however, half of the tampon users were either continent or had only mild leakage (< 4 g).

Pessaries to correct prolapse have been used to identify those women with coexisting but unsuspected stress incontinence in studies conducted by Bhatia *et al.*[27,28] Bhatia reported on the use of a Smith–Hodge pessary in

12 women who underwent urodynamic testing (uroflowmetry, post-void residual, functional urethral length, urethral closure pressure, urethral closure pressure profile and cough pressure profile) as well as Q-tip testing. Ten of these 12 patients[10] became continent in the laboratory. Long-term clinical data were not obtained. Later, 30 women were evaluated with a pessary in hopes of identifying a more clinically useful test than the Bonney test. The pessary equalized pressure transmission in 26/30 women, 21/30 of whom were continent in the standing position. Long-term treatment data were not reported.

The contraceptive diaphragm has been studied for use in support of the bladder neck, providing continence without urethral obstruction or vaginal wall ulceration. Realini and Walters[29] analysed the benefit of a coil-type diaphragm ring, softer than a pessary, in 10 women with incontinence. The women used the diaphragm for a week and recorded events in a urinary diary. A 2-hour pad test was performed. Six patients reported subjective improvement, four experienced no change in symptoms and no patients were worse. Objectively, 40% of the women responded with a 50% reduction on the pad test and 50% reduction in leakage episodes per week.

Suarez[30] studied the efficacy of using a 60–70 mm contraceptive diaphragm in 12 patients. Urodynamic studies were performed with and without the device in place. Flow decreased (29 ml/s to 24 ml/s) and resting maximal urethral pressures increased (37.5 to 81.0 cmH$_2$O) consistent with the investigator's desire to place a size large enough to cause compression of the urethra against the posterior aspect of the symphysis pubis. One woman was not continent; two women discontinued the device because of discomfort; nine women were continent and had no complaints of either obstruction or urinary tract infection.

DEVICES DESIGNED SPECIFICALLY FOR BLADDER-NECK SUPPORT

The use of a pubovaginal spring device was described and studied by Edwards[31] in 1971. The device is not now commercially available but was then inserted into the vagina to apply pressure on the urethra through the vaginal wall and removed for voiding. It was somewhat cumbersome to use and 1/43 women developed vaginal ulceration.

Bonnar[32] and Cardozo[33] described results in separate reports studying different populations using a single-sized, inflatable device of flexible silicone. The device had two horns which projected laterally and which, when inserted into the vagina, would be positioned in the lateral fornices, and an inflatable balloon positioned at the midline anteriorly to support the upper urethra and bladder neck when inflated. Deflating the device allowed for voiding. Bonnar[32] reported a 40% success rate in the 60 women he studied. Cardozo[33] studied 33 patients for one month, 20 of whom finished the study. Two of the 20 women chose to continue with the device when the study had finished. Four patients who were cured of incontinence considered that the device was too cumbersome to use because of sizing, discomfort and difficulties with insertion and inflation. The 14 women who were not cured also considered that the problems with using the device outweighed its usefulness.

Davila and Osterman[34,35] and Bernier and Harris[36] reported on the same patient group in separate publications. Thirty-two physically active women were enrolled, 30 of whom completed the protocol. The majority of these women were dry with the device (Fig. 35.8) in place during stress testing. Urodynamic testing performed with and without the device demonstrated significant changes in functional urethral length, pressure transmission ratio and Q-tip angle, with no evidence of urethral obstruction. There was a documented decrease in the number of weekly incontinence episodes from 10 to 3 ($p < 0.05$) over a 4-week period of observation. The device was acceptable, convenient and comfortable for most women.

Thyssen[37] reported on the use of a disposable polyurethane vaginal device in 22 of 26 patients between the ages of 27 and 69 years. Patients completed a 3-day diary, 24-hour home pad test and urodynamic testing (uroflowmetry and post-void residuals). Urine and vaginal cultures were also obtained over a one-month study period. The diaries showed that 41% of patients were subjectively cured, 45% improved, and 14% unchanged. All patients showed an objective improvement, with a decrease in urinary leakage, but only 1 of the 19 improved patients was dry. Three of four patients with urine loss greater than 100 ml without the device showed a 50% reduction of leakage. There were no urinary tract infections and no problems with bladder emptying.

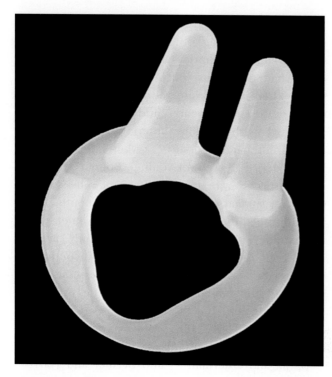

Figure 35.8. *The Introl bladder-neck-support prosthesis (Uromed Corporation, Needham, MA, USA): a flexible, ring-shaped, vaginal device with two ridges at one end. When the device has been placed in the vagina, the ridges raise the urethrovesical junction and bladder neck in the same way as an urethropexy.*

INTRA-URETHRAL DEVICES

Intra-urethral devices to block urinary leakage are inserted into the urethra. These devices must have a means to prevent intravesical migration (usually with a meatal plate). They must physically enhance urine retention in the urethra, usually with an inflatable balloon, spheres or flanges. They require a means by which to accomplish bladder emptying, such as by removal of the device or with a pumping mechanism. Some devices are indwelling, with insertion by a physician for 28 days or longer; others are single-use disposable devices which are inserted and removed by the patient.

Single-use devices with spheres have been studied by Neilsen *et al.*[38–40] and the results published between 1990 and 1995. The urethral plug device had an oval meatal plate, a soft stalk with a removable semi-rigid guide pin (removed after insertion) and either one or two spheres along the stalk with fixed distances between the meatal plate and the spheres. The one-sphere (original) and two-sphere (improved) devices were studied.

Of 40 patients, 18 completed the study. Most of these patients (17/18, or 94.4%) were subjectively and objectively continent or improved. Most preferred the two-sphere device. Urinary tract infections in 6/18 and migration of the device into the bladder in 2/18, necessitating cystoscopic removal, were the major complications experienced with the device.

Peschers *et al.*[41] screened 53 patients with GSI and 21 patients agreed to participate in their study of a two-sphere urethral plug device. Of these 21 patients, 14 completed the 4-month study, and 7/14 experienced no improvement in their symptoms. Urinary tract infection and device migration were the major complications with this device.

SINGLE-USE INFLATABLE DEVICE

Staskin *et al.*[42] reported on 135/215 patients observed in a 4-month multicentre study of a disposable balloon-tipped urethral insert made of a thermoplastic elastomer (Fig. 35.9). The balloon was inflated with an applicator after insertion and deflated by pulling a string at the meatal plate for removal and to allow for voiding. Urodynamic studies excluded patients with urge incontinence and classified patients into those with anatomical hypermobility or ISD. The patients reported 72% complete dryness with 17% improvement on diary, and demonstrated 80% complete dryness and 15% improvement (decrease of 80% in measured loss) on pad weight testing. There was a decrease from 43.2 ml without the device to 2.3 ml with the device. Treatment for positive urine cultures was undertaken in 20% of symptomatic and 11% asymptomatic patients: 39% of patients had positive cultures but were not treated, and 30% had negative cultures at all monthly intervals during the 4-month study. The main reason for dropout was discomfort with the device.

Miller and Bavendam[43] reported on 63 of the 135 patients from the cohort just mentioned who used the balloon-tipped intra-urethral device for a year. Of these 63 patients, 79% reported complete dryness and 16% significant improvement on objective pad-weight testing. These findings were consistent with improvement in subjective diaries ($p < 0.0001$). The patients reported improved comfort and ease of use over time, with sensation of device presence decreasing from 35% at week 1 to 7% at 12 months. One or more episodes of gross haematuria (24%), cystoscopic findings of mucosal irri-

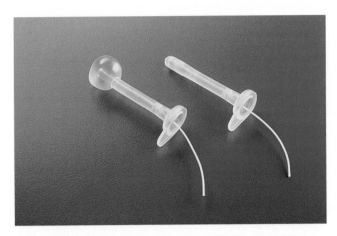

Figure 35.9. *The Reliance device (Uromed Corporation, Needham, MA, USA).*

tation at 4 or at 12 months (9%) and symptomatic bacteriuria on monthly cultures (30%) over the year were the most common morbidities. This device is no longer commercially available.

Intra-urethral inserts have demonstrated efficacy in the control of urinary incontinence. The morbidity associated with the use of these devices will vary with design of the device. There are no long-term studies on those devices that are not removed at each void. The morbidity associated with device usage should be considered when the patient is interested in their efficacy.

SUMMARY

Technological advances will continue to supply workable alternatives in the non-surgical treatment of the underactive bladder outlet. More long-term outcome research is needed to identify which device or devices provide optimal convenience and efficacy and the lowest morbidity in non-surgical treatment of GSI.

REFERENCES

1. Mant J, Painter R, Vessey M. Epidemiology of genital prolapse: observations from the Oxford Family Planning Association Study. *Br J Obstet Gynaecol* 1997;104: 579–585

2. Olsen AL, Smith VJ, Bergstrom JO *et al.* Epidemiology of surgically managed pelvic organ prolapse and urinary incontinence. *Obstet Gynecol* 1997; 89: 501–506

3. Miller DS. Contemporary use of the pessary. In: Sciarra JJ (ed) *Gynecology and Obstetrics*, Volume 1. Philadelphia: JB Lippincott, 1995; 39: 1–12

4. Deger R, Menzin A, Mikuta J. The vaginal pessary: past and present. *Postgrad Obstet Gynecol* 1993; 13: 1–7

5. Wood N. The use of vaginal pessaries for uterine prolapse. *Nurse Pract* 1992; 17: 31–38

6. Davila GW. Vaginal prolapse: management with nonsurgical techniques. *Postgrad Med* 1996; 99: 171–185

7. Brubaker L. The pessary: an important gynecological option. *Menopausal Management* 1994; 2: 1–4

8. Wu V, Farrell SA, Baskett TF, Flowerdew G. A simplified protocol for pessary management. *Obstet Gynecol* 1997; 90: 990–994

9. Friedman AJ. The vaginal pessary. *AUGS Q Rep* 1991; 9: 1–2

10. Zeitlin M, Lebherz TB. Pessaries in the geriatric patient. *J Am Geriatr Soc* 1992; 40: 635–639

11. Sulak PJ, Kuehl TJ, Shull BL. Vaginal pessaries and their use in pelvic relaxation. *J Reprod Med* 1993; 38: 919–923

12. Meyers DL, LaSala CA, Murphy JA. Double pessary use in grade 4 uterine and vaginal prolapse. *Obstet Gynecol* 1998; 91: 1019–1020

13. Schraub S, Sun XS, Maingon P *et al.* Cervical and vaginal cancer associated with pessary use. *Cancer* 1992; 69: 2505–2509

14. Poma PA. Management of incarcerated vaginal pessaries. *J Am Geriatr Soc* 1981; 29: 325–327

15. Bergman A, Bhatia NN. Pessary test: simple prognostic test in women with stress urinary incontinence. *Urology* 1984; 24: 109–110

16. Meinhardt W, Schuitemaker NW, Smeets MJ, Venma PL. Bilateral hydronephrosis with urosepsis due to neglected pessary. *Scand J Urol Nephrol* 1993; 27: 419–420

17. Brett KM, Marsh JV, Madans JH. Epidemiology of hysterectomy in the United States: demographics and reproductive factors in a nationally representative sample. *J Womens Health* 1997; 6: 309–316

18. Menotti A. Demography and public health: the complexity of interventions in women. *Ann Ist Super Sanita* 1992; 28: 329–333 (in Italian)

19. Toozs-Hobson P, Boos K, Cardozo L. Management of vaginal vault prolapse. *Br J Obstet Gynaecol* 1998; 105: 13–17

20. Crowley IP, Cardozo LJ, Lawrence LC. Female incontinence: a new approach. *Br J Urol* 1997; 34: 492–498

21. Johnson DE, Muncie HL, O'Reilly JL, Warren JW. An external urine collection device for incontinent women: evaluation of long-term use. *J Am Geriatr Soc* 1990; 38: 1016–1022

22. Johnson DE, O'Reilly JL, Warren JW. Clinical evaluation

of an external urine collection device for non-ambulatory incontinent women. *J Urol* 1989; 141: 535–537

23. Pieper B, Cleland V, Johnson DE, O'Reilly JL. Inventing urine incontinence devices for women. *Image – Journal of Nursing Scholarship* 1989; 21: 205–209

24. Pieper B, Cleland V. An external urine-collection device for women: a clinical trial. *J ET Nurs* 1993; 20: 51–55

25. Eckford SD, Jackson SR, Lewis PA, Abrams P. The continence control pad – a new external urethral occlusion device in the management of stress incontinence. *Br J Urol* 1996; 77: 538–540

26. Nygaard I. Prevention of exercise incontinence with mechanical devices. *J Reprod Med* 1995; 40: 89–94

27. Bhatia NN, Bergman A, Gunning JE. Urodynamic effects of a vaginal pessary in women with stress urinary incontinence. *Am J Obstet Gynecol* 1983; 147: 876–884

28. Bhatia NN, Bergman A. Pessary test in women with urinary incontinence. *Obstet Gynecol* 1985; 65: 220–226

29. Realini JP, Walters MD. Vaginal diaphragm rings in the treatment of stress incontinence. *J Am Board Fam Pract* 1990; 3: 99–103

30. Suarez G. Use of a standard contraceptive diaphragm in management of stress urinary incontinence. *Urology* 1991; 37: 119–122

31. Edwards L. The control of incontinence of urine in women with a pubo-vaginal spring device. Objective and subjective results. *Br J Urol* 1971; 43: 211–225

32. Bonnar J. Silicone vaginal appliance for control of stress incontinence. *Lancet* 1977; 2: 1161

33. Cardozo L. Evaluation of female urinary incontinence device. *Urology* 1979; 13: 398–401

34. Davila GW, Osterman KV. The bladder neck support prosthesis: a non-surgical approach to stress incontinence in adult women. *Am J Obstet Gynecol* 1991; 171: 206–211

35. Davila GW. Introl bladder neck support prosthesis: a non-surgical urethropexy. *J Endourol* 1996; 10: 293–296

36. Bernier F, Harris L. Treating stress incontinence with the bladder neck support prosthesis. *Urol Nurs* 1995; 15: 5–9

37. Thyssen H. New disposable vaginal device (continence guard) in the treatment of female stress incontinence: design, efficacy and short term safety. *Acta Obstet Gynecol Scand* 1996; 75: 170–173

38. Neilsen KK, Kromann-Andersen B, Jacobsen H *et al.* The urethral plug: a new treatment modality for genuine urinary stress incontinence in women. *J Urol* 1990; 144: 1199–1202

39. Neilsen KK, Walter S, Maeffaard E, Kromann-Andersen B. The urethral plug II: an alternative treatment in women with genuine urinary stress incontinence. *Br J Urol* 1993; 72: 428–432

40. Neilsen KK, Walter S, Maeffaard E, Kromann-Andersen B. The urethral plug – an alternative treatment of women with urinary stress incontinence. *Ugeskr Laeger* 1995; 157: 3194–3197

41. Peschers U, Zen Ruffinen F, Schaer GN, Schussler B. The VIVA urethral plug: a sensible expansion of the spectrum for conservative therapy of urinary stress incontinence? *Geburtshilfe Frauenheilkd* 1996; 56: 118–123

42. Staskin DR, Bavendam T, Miller J *et al.* Effectiveness of a urinary control insert in the management of stress urinary incontinence: early results of a multi-center study. *Urology* 1996; 47: 629–636

43. Miller JL, Bavendam T. Treatment with the Reliance urinary control insert: one-year experience. *J Endourol* 1996; 10: 287–292

36

Outcomes and incontinence: current status of results reporting and the future

R. R. Dmochowski

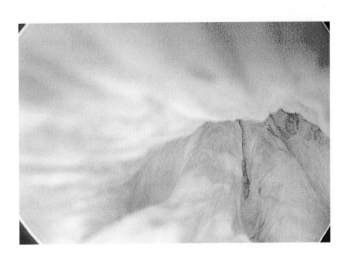

INTRODUCTION

Urinary incontinence is a common condition. In the USA 13–15 million individuals are estimated to be incontinent.

Increased public awareness regarding voiding dysfunction and incontinence has produced heightened interest in the effects of incontinence on the quality of the individual's life. Furthermore, a marked increase in the options for incontinence treatment has produced the need to assess not only symptomatic change, morbidity and mortality, but also the impact on the individual's quality of life resulting from these interventions.

Hitherto, outcomes assessment for incontinence has been founded on physician-reported results, often established on the basis of patient interview, physician opinion, non-standardized surveys and a variable combination of physical examination, voiding diaries, non-validated symptom scores, and urodynamic evaluation. Non-standardized results reporting has prevented critical analysis not only of the influence of incontinence on the individual, but also of the assessment of treatment interventions for voiding dysfunction.

This chapter reviews the assessment of outcomes and the utilization of these outcomes to establish diagnostic and treatment options and guidelines for the behavioural, medical and surgical management of urinary incontinence.

SYMPTOMATIC ANALYSIS

The demographics of female voiding dysfunction continue to evolve on the basis of emerging population-based data as extracted from questionnaire-type instruments. Depending on age, 10–40% of women will develop urinary incontinence.[1]

Incontinence is a symptom complex rather than a pure condition. Associated aspects of voiding dysfunction include irritative (urgency, frequency) and obstructive symptoms (hesitancy, intermittency, incomplete bladder emptying), and the complicated component of nocturnal voiding dysfunction. Further confounding the delineation of incontinence is the relatively minor degree of morbidity associated with urinary incontinence (except in those women with concomitant recurrent urinary tract infection and related sequelae or in those patients who have some aspect of bladder storage failure that compromises renal function).

The major impact of incontinence, therefore, is on the sufferer's quality of life and the related physical activity limitations, plus the social, emotional and psychological implications. Standard results reporting and prevalence testing have been founded on subjective observer data (surgical results reporting), questionnaire data – which, in many cases, lack general validation (prevalence data) – or on patient self-reported tools (voiding diaries). Each of these methods provides a partial definition of incontinence; however, none, when taken incrementally, provides a global perspective of incontinence. Additionally, the individual's perception of level of self functionality is often ignored by these instruments.

Global assessment of the impact of incontinence implies the necessity for health-related quality-of-life (HRQOL) measures which reflect the broader impact of this symptomatic complex. HRQOL measures can be classified into two broad types – generic and condition specific. Generic measures allow assessment and comparison of quality of life across populations. However, these measures may not reflect all the specifics of the disease or symptom being studied and may not be as specific as those measures that are focused on the specific condition under study. Specific measures provide more critical analysis of the condition under evaluation but lack the capability for cross-population or group comparison.

Previously, investigators relied on generic measures[2] for urinary incontinence, given the absence of disease-specific measures. However, recent development of disease-specific, validated instruments has provided investigators with improved tools with which to analyse better the impact of incontinence, including subjective bother and objective interference with life activities.[3] These performance-scale instruments provide information additional to that obtained by objective historical and physical assessment and urodynamic testing.

The Urogenital Distress Inventory (UDI) and Incontinence Impact Questionnaire (IIQ) provide a multiple-component quantification of the effects of the symptoms associated with incontinence and bother on the individual's daily activities.[4] Shortened versions of this questionnaire can easily be administered over minimal time intervals and can be used for cross-comparison of results of intervention.[5]

Different investigators have addressed bladder-symptom questionnaires that assess symptomatic urge and stress incontinence, pad usage and incontinence amount (volume), as well as bothersomeness of symptomatic incontinence, using visual analogue scales.[6] Reproducibility and accuracy have also been validated for these instruments. Other testing methods have relied on the assessment of incontinence severity judged by caregivers in chronic settings (using third-party assessment).[7]

Other measures that have been used to measure the severity of incontinence include standardized diaries as well as pad-weighing tests. Voiding diaries assess several parameters, including volume voided, micturition frequency, number and degree of incontinent episodes, mean and largest voided volumes and time of voiding.[8] The International Continence Society utilizes the largest voided volume recorded in the patient's diary as the definition of functional bladder capacity.[9] Diaries are routinely kept for discrete 24 h periods, and repeated for 48–72 h periods.[10]

Pad tests provide a semi-objective method for assessing the degree (volume) of urine loss over a specified time interval. Several time periods and testing modalities have been described for pad testing, including 1, 6 and 24 h intervals.[9,11,12] Pad testing is often supplemented by the ingestion of phenazopyridine hydrochloride, which provides a visual corollary to the actual change in weight of the used pad. Pad-testing is subject to significant variability between and within individuals. This modality is best correlated with the patient's own assessment of urinary loss. Pad-testing types have previously been validated and subjected to testing reliability; however, poor test–retest validation and variability in performance of testing limit widespread usage.[13]

Despite the presence and proven validity of the aforementioned instruments, they have not been routinely and globally used in outcomes reporting for incontinence. Results reporting across literature sources may comprise any or none of the above and may be complicated further by author opinion and subjective interpretation. Variability is also encountered when assessing the impact of incontinence interventions: some authors interpret successful intervention as any degree of symptomatic improvement; others strictly use cure (complete continence) as the standard definition of success. The criteria for the assessment of success may utilize any or none of the techniques listed previously.

Two major efforts have recently attempted to assess the success of interventions for urinary incontinence. Both have been hindered by the relative lack of standardized results reporting, the absence of homogeneity in the type of results assessed and the impact of the interventions on the patient's symptomatic bother. Despite these shortcomings, the guidelines generated by the Agency for Health Care Policy Research (AHCPR) and the American Urologic Association (AUA) have synthesized extensive literature reviews and distilled useful and complementary documents for the purposes of standardizing the interventions for urinary incontinence.

AHCPR guidelines

Initially presented in 1992 and updated in 1996, the AHCPR guidelines encompassed a broad-based literature-founded review concerning the diagnosis and therapy of incontinence in both sexes.[14] Urinary incontinence was considered to be a global diagnosis and all types (stress, urge, mixed, overflow and functional) were considered. A main focus of these guidelines was the diagnosis and therapy of incontinence from the primary-care standpoint. Literature review (approximately 1200 articles) derived evidential data. Data were evaluated and recommendations formulated on the basis of the supporting evidence. A grading system was used to assess the quality of the evidence, which was used to formulate the individual recommendations. The grading system was as follows:

A Adequate evidence from properly formulated clinical trials with *statistical substantiation* supporting the recommendation statement;
B Adequate evidence from properly formulated clinical trials supporting the recommendation statement.
C Expert opinion (consensus) supporting the recommendation.

The panel concluded initially that incontinence was an under-reported condition with poor documentation of services, and that major variations existed in diagnostic modalities and therapeutic treatments. They concluded that evidence did exist to support the treatment of incontinence in most individuals. Subsequently (1996), the panel reviewed more recent pertinent medical literature and derived some changes in the previously reported algorithm for diagnosis and management of urinary incontinence in primary care. The emphasis of this algorithm was accurate diagnosis and exclusion of confounding conditions. Basic evaluation was recommended to include history (with assessment of bother, bladder record, mental status and patient expectations for treatment outcomes), physical examination, post-void residual determination and urinalysis. The guidelines concluded that further testing with urodynamic studies, cystoscopy and upper urinary tract imaging was indicated only in those individuals who were not candidates for therapy based upon presumptive diagnosis, or in whom such therapy had failed.

Treatment was categorized into three broad types – behavourial, pharmacological and surgical. Behavioural therapies (toileting assistance; voiding retraining; pelvic muscle rehabilitation exercises, biofeedback and pelvic floor electrical stimulation) were considered generally efficacious in both stress and mixed incontinence. However, variability in reporting of outcomes criteria (definition of success and length of follow-up), non-standardized behavioural techniques and application thereof, and use of concurrent interventions, confounded interpretation of the merits of any individual behavioural intervention. Chronic catheters, supportive devices and intermittent catheterization were presented as optional in highly selected individuals with concomitant anatomical or functional abnormalities.

Pharmacological therapy for stress incontinence was identified as providing few cures, but improvement in variable percentages of patients. Drug therapy for detrusor instability was identified as being somewhat more efficacious, and this benefit was augmented by the combination of anticholinergic agents with behavioural therapies.

Surgery was evaluated for urethral, bladder and combined dysfunction. The guidelines concluded that surgical intervention was a recommended treatment for stress incontinence, and could be considered as first-line therapy in patients 'unable to comply with other nonsurgical therapies'. The panel considered procedures for hypermobility of the proximal urethra and intrinsic sphincteric deficiency (ISD) separately: they concluded that retropubic and needle suspension procedures were superior to anterior repairs for patients with hypermobility as the aetiology of their incontinence. Sling procedures and periurethral bulking agents were recommended as first-line treatment for ISD without hypermobility. Slings were also recommended as treatment for ISD with coexistent hypermobility. Artificial urinary sphincters were recommended as an option in those patients with severe ISD, those who are unable to perform intermittent catheterization and those who are unresponsive to other surgical interventions.

In discussing these options with the patient, the panel concluded that a comprehensive discussion of risks, benefits and outcomes should be undertaken with the patient. In general, least-invasive treatments were advocated as first-line therapies, although combinations of therapeutic types may offer optimum interventions for 'specific patient groups'. The panel recognized the limitation in outcomes reporting, and the relative non-exclusivity and non-discrete nature of the reporting modalities (diaries, pad tests, urodynamics and quality-of-life instruments).

Criticism of the AHCPR guidelines has centred on the general nature of the document and a perceived lack of focus on specific diagnostic and treatment entities. The inclusion of all types of incontinence prohibited detailed analysis of interventions for any specific subtype. Specifically, surgical intervention techniques were superficially examined and considered as a secondary intervention.

These criticisms do not consider the primary-care nature of the guidelines nor the requirement to evaluate incontinence broadly as a symptom and not as a specific condition.

AUA guidelines

The goal of the AUA guidelines was to examine specifically the existing medical literature regarding the surgical treatment of stress urinary incontinence (SUI) in women.[15] The index (typical) patient was defined as the otherwise healthy woman, without significant pelvic organ prolapse, who had decided to have surgical correction for SUI as either primary or secondary therapy. The panel evaluated the medical literature pertaining to the surgical treatment of SUI from 1950 to 1993: over 5000 articles were identified, of which 457 were selected for data retrieval. Articles were excluded if there was insufficient follow-up (less than 12 months' postsurgical outcome data), if more than 50% of the initial cohort of treated patients was lost to follow-up, or if specific outcome data (number cured or failed) were unstated. The explicit data analysis method was utilized to evaluate abstracted results.

Owing to the large number of individual procedure types reviewed and the lack of significant difference in outcome data between these types, the panel grouped the surgical approaches into four broad categories – retropubic suspensions, slings, transvaginal suspensions and anterior repairs. The procedural types were analysed for surgical success (cure of incontinence – dry, improved, failed) as well as outcomes such as postoperative urgency/urge incontinence, urinary retention, urinary outflow obstruction and pelvic prolapse, and complications. Given variations in reporting of surgical complications, six general categories were defined by the panel: general medical complications, intraoperative complications, perioperative complications, subjective complications, complications requiring surgery, and transfusions.

Detailed data tables were constructed after analysis of these data. Table 36.1 represents detailed outcomes data for efficacy of the four types of suspension. The actual percentages are weighted means, reflecting the varying numbers of individual patients that constituted each group. Table 36.2 summarizes complication data of the five broad complication categories. Table 36.3 lists more specific data on discrete types of surgical procedures (e.g. Burch, Raz). These data were pooled to provide the broad results that were seen for the four main procedural categories. Tables 36.4–36.7 list detailed complications data for the broad procedural categories (retropubic, transvaginal, anterior repair and sling procedures) by category and specific complication type. Again, these tables reflect pooled data, with percentages determined from the number of patients reported with that complication. If no specific complication was reported, it was assumed that the incidence of that complication was nil.

On the basis of data in the articles, three time frames were established for reporting of results: these were 12–23 months (short term), 24–27 months (intermediate) and 48 months or longer (long term). Comparison of the short-term data revealed similar outcomes between all categories of procedures (80–85% cured or improved) except for anterior repairs (68%). Retropubic suspensions and sling procedures maintained this level of efficacy at the

intermediate and long-term periods. Cure/dry rates for transvaginal suspensions decreased to 70% at long-term follow-up. Anterior repairs demonstrated an increase in cure/dry rates to 85% at the intermediate time frame but then a decrease to 61% at long-term follow-up. The panel considered that this anomaly was due to aberrant data reporting rather than being a true representation of outcome.

The panel also attempted to analyse the effect of confounding variables such as prior incontinence surgery, subjective urgency, urodynamically proven detrusor instability, age, prior hysterectomy, parity and menopausal status on outcomes of surgery. No definite effect of any of the above variables on surgical success was noted, owing to incomplete data reporting.

In evaluating other surgical outcomes, retropubic suspensions showed a higher persistence of preoperative urgency after surgery. However, with all procedure types, if urgency and detrusor instability were present on preoperative evaluation there was a significant risk of these symptoms persisting after surgery. Sling procedures demonstrated an increased rate of new-onset urgency after surgery compared with the other types of operations.

No significant differences in either short-term (less than 4 weeks) or long-term (greater than 4 weeks) postoperative urinary retention were noted between the various procedure types. Additionally, no difference in postoperative urinary obstructive symptoms was identifiable. No difference between procedure types for transfusion rates (3–5%) was noted, nor were any major differences found between procedure types for the various complication categories.

In the opinion of the panel, certain aspects of the preoperative work-up were crucial to appropriate diagnosis and surgical outcome. The panel agreed that the following are essential components of the preoperative evaluation:

- History, including impact of incontinence on the patient's quality of life;
- Physical examination, with demonstration of incontinence;
- Urinalysis;
- Diagnostic studies to assess relative contributions of detrusor dysfunction, hypermobility and ISD to overall symptomatic presentation;

- Estimation of the severity and frequency of incontinence;
- Assessment of the patient's expectations for therapeutic outcome.

The panel considered that determination of the patients' quality of life comprised a significant component of preoperative and postoperative evaluation. Although semi-objective, the quality-of-life determination quantifies subjective bother and disruption of daily activities that symptomatic incontinence causes to the patient.

Implicit to a discussion of therapeutic intervention for female SUI is consideration of the patient's understanding of, and expectations for, treatment results. In order for appropriate decision-making by both patient and physician, extensive counselling and communication are necessary during the informed-consent process. Counselling should include a discussion of reasonable options for treatment, the risks and benefits of each of the options, and any particular aspect of the patient's presentation that may modify treatment results. Additionally, the physician's experience with the interventions being considered affects the final choice. The panel concluded that, although all four types of procedure represented options for the patient, the patient should be made aware of important differences in outcomes between the procedural types.

Criticisms of the AUA guidelines were based on the lack of any definitive recommendations for choice of surgical procedure. Unfortunately, owing to inadequate results reporting in the literature, no specific procedural type was found to be optimal or to cause less morbidity. However, the trend for sling and retropubic procedures to demonstrate better long term-results has resulted in a shift towards these procedures in general practice. Another strident criticism of these guidelines was the lack of analysis of coexistent pelvic organ prolapse as an outcome variable: this analytical decision was made early in data retrieval to simplify data extraction and data reporting

CONCLUSIONS

Comprehensive evaluation of urinary incontinence includes objective, semi-objective and subjective data. The composite of all components provides the most complete and critical baseline analysis of the individual's urinary incontinence. Results reporting should include sufficient testing components to establish the initial degree of incontinence and to interpret the impact of reported interventions for urinary incontinence. Although investigator opinion can be valuable when expressed, this opinion should be clearly segregated from objective and subjective results reporting. Continued evolution of modalities to assess the degree of incontinence and standardization of reporting practices will improve outcomes analysis for urinary incontinence. The patient, however, remains the final arbiter of the success (or lack thereof) for incontinence interventions. Appraisal of subjective impact on the patient's quality of life must be included in therapeutic decision-making and results analysis. Both the AHCPR and AUA guidelines similarly concluded that assessment of patient expectations is essential for creating reasonable outcome expectations, as these expectations have a crucial role in the patient's perception of intervention success.

Each guideline provided a unique viewpoint of current results reporting for incontinence intervention. Both demonstrated the fragmented and incomplete nature of symptomatic appraisal and specified the need to continue the development and inclusion of methodologies (such as the UDI/IIQ) that allow the inclusion of the patient's perception of incontinence and incontinence interventions into overall assessment. Perhaps the inclusion of the patient's subjective perception is the single most important result of the guidelines efforts to date.

Table 36.1. *Comparative outcomes for procedure categories*

Outcomes	Retropubic suspension			Transvaginal suspension			Anterior repair			Sling procedure		
	G/P	Median	CI (2.5–97.5)%	G/P	Median	CI(2.5–97.5)%	G/P	Median	CI (2.5–97.5)%	G/P	Median	CI (2.5–9.7)%
Cure/dry												
12–23 months	15/943	84	(77–89)	13/700	79	(71–86)	6/310	68	(55–80)	5/135	82	(73–89)
24–47 months	23/1870	84	(80–88)	8/424	65	(50–77)	3/113	85	(69–95)	7/34	82	(73–89)
48 months and longer	17/2196	84	(79–88)	4/292	67	(53–79)	5/1088	61	(47–72)	7/473	83	(75–88)
Cure/dry/improved												
12–23 months	16/961	86	(80–90)	13/700	82	(74–87)	6/310	78	(65–88)	5/135	91	(84–96)
24–47 months	24/1941	88	(85–91)	8/424	78	(71–83)	3/113	95	(89–98)	7/344	85	(77–91)
48 months and longer	18/2204	90	(87–92)	4/292	82	(73–89)	6/1101	73	(70–76)	7/473	87	(80–92)
Postoperative urgency												
For patients with urgency and DI preoperatively	6/78	66	(50–79)	6/33	54	(35–73)				4/45	46	(24–68)
For patients with urgency and no DI preoperatively	6/319	36	(22–52)							5/110	34	(13–61)
For patients with no urgency but with DI preoperatively	1/6	4	(0–33)	1/3	7	(0–54)				4/36	20	(5–45)
For patients with no urgency and no DI preoperatively	8/241	11	(8–16)	6/150	5	(3–10)				7/140	7	(3–11)
Retention												
Longer than 4 weeks	5/340	5	(3–7)	6/479	5	(4–8)				7/578	8	(6–11)
Permanent	Less than 5%											
Days in the hospital (panel survey)	From 0 to 5 days											

cont.

457

Table 36.1. *Comparative outcomes for procedure categories (cont.)*

Outcomes	Retropubic suspension			Transvaginal suspension			Anterior repair			Sling procedure		
	G/P	Median	CI (2.5–97.5)%	G/P	Median	CI (2.5–97.5)%	G/P	Median	CI (2.5–97.5)%	G/P	Median	CI (2.5–97.5)%
Resumption of normal activities	Typically 6 weeks for all treatment modalities											
Death	Death rate for all procedures presumed to be no different than for other types of elective vaginal/abdominal surgery: approximately 5 out of 10000											
Transfusion	9/1131	5	(3–8)	10/1083	3	(1–6)	3/857	3	(1–9)	6/279	4	(2–7)
General medical complications												
Significant	21/3136	2	(2–3)	10/805	2	(1–3)	5/1005	2	(1–3)	14/1127	4	(2–5)
Not significant	7/1549	2	(1–4)	7/646	4	(1–9)	3/650	8	(2–17)	2/258	6	(3–10)
Intraoperative complications												
Significant	13/1992	2	(1–3)	5/532	2	(1–5)	1/294	1	(0–2)	6/326	3	(1–6)
Not significant	16/2284	3	(1–4)	25/1835	5	(4–8)	1/313	0	(0–1)	19/1077	8	(5–12)
Perioperative complications												
Significant	40/3598	4	(3–5)	40/2814	7	(5–9)	5/970	2	(1–5)	20/1723	7	(5–10)
Not significant	64/6044	14	(14–15)	54/3330	12	(9–15)	13/2322	16	(10–23)	26/1916	12	(8–17)
Subjective complications	13/1001	9	(5–15)	24/1412	11	(8–15)	3/341	2	(1–6)	4/301	6	(2–13)
Complications requiring surgery	15/2718	2	(1–3)	15/1575	2	(1–4)	2/1074	0	(0–1)	11/1119	3	(2–5)

DI, detrusor instability; G, number of groups/treatment arms extracted; P, number of patients in these groups; CI, confidence interval.
Reprinted with permission of the American Urological Association.

Table 36.2. *Comparative outcomes for procedure categories*

Outcomes	Retropubic suspension			Transvaginal suspension			Anterior repair			Sling procedure		
	G/P	Median	CI (2.5–97.5)%	G/P	Median	CI (2.5–97.5)%	G/P	Median	CI (2.5–97.5)%	G/P	Median	CI (2.5–97.5)%
General medical complications												
Abdominal complication	1/19	6	(1–22)				1/519	0	(0–1)	1/88	1	(0–5)
Cardiovascular	21/3136	3	(2–3)	10/805	2	(1–3)	5/1005	2	(1–3)	14/1127	4	(2–5)
Pulmonary	6/1000	2	(1–3)	5/516	4	(1–11)	3/650	8	(2–17)	2/258	6	(3–10)
Intraoperative complications												
Bladder complication	16/2284	3	(2–4)	25/1835	5	(4–8)	1/313	0	(0–1)	19/1077	8	(5–12)
Ureteral complication	6/730	2	(1–4)	1/255	1	(0–2)						
Urethral complication	5/1003	1	(0–3)	2/128	3	(1–8)				6/326	3	(1–6)
Perioperative complications												
Bleeding	19/1608	5	(3–7)	21/1392	4	(3–5)	3/889	3	(1–6)	4/500	3	(1–6)
UTI	46/4141	13	(12–14)	33/1598	10	(7–13)	11/1743	9	(5–16)	14/984	12	(7–19)
Wound complication	57/5633	7	(5–8)	61/4096	7	(6–8)	7/1806	10	(6–17)	30/2499	9	(6–12)
Subjective complications												
Dysuria	3/175	13	(6–24)	4/119	16	(6–32)				2/178	8	(1–25)
Pain	5/349	6	(3–10)	16/1151	10	(7–14)				1/54	4	(1–11)
Sexual dysfunction	9/766	6	(3–12)	10/609	8	(6–11)	3/341	2	(1–6)	1/69	2	(0–7)
Complications requiring surgery												
Fistula	15/2718	1	(1–2)	14/1568	2	(1–3)	2/1074	1	(0–1)	10/829	3	(1–5)
Stone formation	4/744	2	(1–4)	1/7	16	(2–50)				2/417	3	(1–7)

G, number of groups/treatment arms extracted; P, number of patients in these groups; CI, confidence interval; UTI, urinary tract infection.
Reprinted with permission of the American Urological Association.

Table 36.3. Comparative outcomes for individual procedures – cure/dry detail

	G/P	Median	CI (2.5–97.5)%	G/P	Median	CI (2.5–97.5)%	G/P	Median	CI (2.5–97.5)%
Retropubic suspension									
	Burch			MMK			Lapides		
12–23 months	8/644	85	(78–91)	3/107	72	(55–85)			
24–47 months	9/756	84	(79–88)	10/718	83	(75–89)	2/98	86	(60–98)
48 months and longer	6/529	83	(75–90)	6/1156	83	(76–88)	1/41	44	(30–59)
	Paravaginal			Other					
12–23 months				4/192	85	(70–95)			
24–47 months				5/298	83	(69–93)			
48 months and longer	1/213	88	(83–92)	3/258	90	(83–96)			
Transvaginal suspension									
	Pereyra			Pereyra – modified			Stamey		
12–23 months	1/99	79	(70–86)	5/205	75	(62–86)	2/66	67	(48–83)
24–47 months				2/168	76	(40–97)	3/87	52	(33–70)
48 months and longer				2/196	69	(40–90)	2/96	65	(47–80)
	Raz			Gittes			Other		
12–23 months				2/49	73	(33–96)	3/281	93	(88–96)
24–47	1/41	34	(21–49)	1/108	81	(73–88)	1/20	75	(54–90)
48 months and longer									

cont.

Table 36.3. *Comparative outcomes for individual procedures – cure/dry detail (cont.)*

	G/P	Median	CI (2.5–97.5)%	G/P	Median	CI (2.5–97.5)%	G/P	Median	CI (2.5–97.5)%
Anterior repair	Kelly plication			Other					
12–23 months	4/270	71	(54–84)	2/40	61	(31–86)			
24–47 months	2/51	94	(83–99)	1/62	74	(62–84)			
48 months and longer	3/1006	60	(41–77)	2/82	62	(38–83)			
Sling procedure	Abdominal fascia			Fascia lata			Vaginal wall		
12–23 months				1/10	69	(39–91)			
24–47 months	1/67	82	(72–90)	1/52	98	(91–100)			
48 months and longer	2/98	82	(68–92)				1/82	95	(89–98)
	Homologous			Synthetic			Other		
12–23 months	1/6	96	(67–100)	2/35	86	(68–96)	1/84	82	(73–89)
24–47 months	2/17	61	(18–94)	3/208	82	(70–91)			
48 months and longer				2/91	71	(59–81)	3/202	85	(71–93)

MMK, Marshall–Marchetti–Krantz procedure; G, number of groups/treatment arms extracted; P, number of patients in these groups; CI, confidence interval. Reprinted with permission of the American Urological Association.

Table 36.4. *Comparative outcomes for retropubic suspension procedures: complications details*

Outcomes	Retropubic suspension						Lapides			Paravaginal			Other		
	Burch			MMK											
	G/P	Median	CI (2.5–97.5)%	G/P	Median	CI (2.5–97.5)%	G/P	Median	CI (2.5–97.5)%	G/P	Median	CI (2.5–97.5)%	G/P	Median	CI (2.5–97.5)%
Death	Death rate for all procedures presumed to be no different than for other types of elective vaginal/abdominal surgery: approximately 5 out of 10000														
Transfusion	2/214	3	(1–7)	2/231	8	(4–14)				2/359	2	(0–9)	3/327	5	(1–13)
General medical complications															
Abdominal complication													1/19	6	(1–22)
Cardiovascular	8/916	2	(1–4)	8/1557	3	(1–4)				1/146	2	(1–5)	4/517	3	(1–6)
Pulmonary	1/77	3	(1–8)	3/535	1	(0–3)				1/213	1	(0–2)	1/175	3	(1–6)
Intraoperative complications															
Bladder complication	6/519	5	(2–10)	8/1613	2	(1–3)							2/152	1	(0–4)
Ureteral complication	4/454	2	(1–5)	1/239	0	(0–2)							1/37	3	(0–12)
Urethral complication	1/156	0	(0–2)	4/847	1	(0–4)									
Perioperative complications															
Bleeding	6/702	7	(3–12)	8/400	4	(2–7)							5/506	3	(1–6)
UTI	17/1341	24	(17–33)	19/2036	7	(5–10)	1/63	2	(0–7)	1/146	11	(7–17)	8/555	10	(5–17)
Wound complication	17/1667	6	(4–9)	23/2604	8	(6–11)	2/75	4	(1–12)	2/359	2	(0–5)	13/928	7	(4–11)
Subjective complications															
Dysuria				2/75	18	(6–39)							1/100	6	(3–12)
Pain	3/189	6	(2–14)	1/60	2	(0–8)									
Sexual dysfunction	7/639	5	(2–10)	2/217	10	(0–49)							1/100	6	(3–12)
Complications requiring surgery															
Fistula	3/468	2	(0–5)	9/1867	1	(1–2)							3/383	1	(0–3)
Stone formation	1/117	3	(1–7)	1/270	0	(0–2)							2/357	2	(1–4)

MMK, Marshall–Marchetti–Krantz procedure; G, number of groups/treatment arms extracted; P, number of patients in those groups; CI, confidence interval; UTI, urinary tract infection.
Reprinted with permission of the American Urological Association (AUA).

Analysis of individual procedures complications (Tables 36.4–36.7)

Subgroupings of complications for the various individual procedures under each of the four major procedure groupings are displayed in Tables 36.4–36.7. Under the retropubic suspension grouping (Table 36.4), the individual procedures are: Burch, MMK, Lapides, Paravaginal and Other. For transvaginal suspensions (Table 36.5), the individual procedures are Pereyra, Modified Pereyra, Stamey, Raz, Gittes and Other. For the anterior repair grouping (Table 36.6), the Kelly plication and Other are the only procedures listed (because of considerable variability in types of procedures in the Other category). Finally Table 36.7 summarizes sling procedures: Abdominal fascia, Fascia lata, Vaginal wall, Homologous materials, Synthetic materials and Other.

The Other category in each of these tables contains combined procedures as well as a variety of additional procedure modifications. A technical supplement to this report, *Evidence Working Papers* (available from the AUA) contains a full listing of procedures in the Other category.

Rates of complications are generally similar between the types of retropubic suspensions (Table 36.4), with some exceptions. For example, the Burch procedure appears to have a higher UTI rate (median 24%) than other retropubic procedures. In the panel's opinion, such differences are due to reporting variances between studies and to small overall sample sizes.

For transvaginal suspension procedures (Table 36.5), complication rates are also generally similar. Inconsistencies are due to small numbers of patient groups and/or patients. This is true of the transfusion rate of Pereyra (17%) and of the dysuria rate for Stamey (41%).

Complication rates for anterior repairs (Table 36.6) are generally low and reflect differences in reporting and older literature references rather than real differences from the other procedure groupings. Table 36.7 displays complication rates for sling procedures. Differences in data reported are due to small sample size and older literature.

Table 36.5. *Comparative outcomes for transvaginal suspension procedures: complications details*

Outcomes	Transvaginal suspensions								
	Pereyra			Pereyra – modified			Stamey		
Death	Death rate for all procedures presumed to be no different than for other types of elective vaginal/abdominal surgery: approximately 5 out of 10 000								
	G/P	Median	CI (2.5–97.5)%	G/P	Median	CI (2.5–97.5)%	G/P	Median	CI (2.5–97.5)%
Transfusion	1/95	17	(10–25)	1/93	7	(3–13)	4/457	1	(0–3)
General medical complications									
Abdominal complication									
Cardiovascular	2/285	1	(0–4)	1/30	7	(1–20)	6/465	2	(1–4)
Pulmonary	1/186	1	(0–2)	1/225	1	(0–2)	2/85	5	(0–18)
Intraoperative complications									
Bladder complication	6/565	4	(2–8)	7/539	4	(2–9)	5/189	12	(6–19)
Ureteral complication				1/225	1	(0–2)			
Urethral complication	1/46	3	(0–10)	1/82	1	(0–6)			
Perioperative complications									
Bleeding	3/310	5	(2–9)	3/177	3	(1–7)	7/386	4	(2–6)
UTI	3/306	11	(7–17)	6/216	14	(6–26)	14/684	7	(4–11)
Wound complication	5/614	6	(3–11)	9/611	8	(5–12)	25/1481	12	(8–16)
Subjective complications									
Dysuria				1/30	4	(0–15)	1/44	41	(27–56)
Pain	1/99	27	(19–37)	1/114	2	(0–6)	11/584	12	(9–15)
Sexual dysfunction				1/114	16	(10–23)	2/62	8	(1–23)
Complications requiring surgery									
Fistula	3/420	1	(0–2)	3/393	1	(0–3)	3/147	9	(3–19)
Stone formation							1/7	16	(2–50)

cont.

Table 36.5. *Comparative outcomes for transvaginal suspension procedures: complications details (cont.)*

Outcomes	Transvaginal suspensions Raz			Gittes			Other		
Death	Death rate for all procedures presumed to be no different than for other types of elective vaginal/abdominal surgery: approximately 5 out of 10 000								
	G/P	Median	CI(2.5–97.5)%	G/P	Median	CI (2.5–97.5)%	G/P	Median	CI (2.5–97.5)%
Transfusion	2/306	1	(0–4)				2/132	6	(1–20)
General medical complications									
Abdominal complication									
Cardiovascular							1/25	1	(0–9)
Pulmonary				1/20	35	(17–57)			
Intraoperative complications									
Bladder complications	2/142	6	(1–16)	2/54	8	(2–19)	3/346	1	(0–3)
Urethral complications									
Urethral complications									
Perioperative complications									
Bleeding	1/17	13	(3–33)	3/177	4	(1–8)	4/325	3	(1–7)
UTI	2/61	15	(4–36)	2/106	6	(1–19)	6/225	4	(7–23)
Wound complication	5/384	7	(3–14)	5/286	6	(3–11)	12/720	9	(6–13)
Subjective complications									
Dysuria							2/45	9	(2–22)
Pain	2/247	5	(2–12)				1/107	3	(1–7)
Sexual dysfunction	2/247	4	(1–12)	2/72	3	(0–12)	3/114	4	(1–10)
Complications requiring surgery									
Fistula	1/206	0	(0–1)				4/402	1	(0–2)
Stone formation									

G, number of groups/treatment arms extracted; P, number of patients in those groups; CI, confidence interval; UTI, urinary tract infection. Reprinted with permission of the American Urological Association.

Table 36.6. *Comparative outcomes for anterior repair procedures: complications details*

Outcomes	Anterior repairs Kelly plication			Other		
	G/P	Median	CI (2.5–97.5)%	G/P	Median	CI (2.5–97.5)%
Death	Death rate for all procedures presumed to be no different than for other types of elective vaginal/abdominal surgery: approximately 5 out of 10000					
Transfusion	3/857	3	(1–9)			
General medical complications						
Abdominal complication	1/519	0	(0–1)			
Cardiovascular	4/965	1	(0–3)	1/40	3	(0–11)
Pulmonary	2/610	7	(1–23)	1/40	5	(1–15)
Intraoperative complications						
Bladder complication	1/313	0	(0–1)			
Ureteral complication						
Urethral complication						
Perioperative complications						
Bleeding	2/849	2	(0–7)	1/40	3	(0–11)
UTI	9/1689	8	(3–15)	2/54	22	(4–55)
Wound complication	5/1706	13	(7–20)	2/100	3	(1–9)
Subjective complications						
Dysuria						
Pain						
Sexual dysfunction	2/319	1	(0–4)	1/22	5	(0–19)
Complications requiring surgery						
Fistula	2/1074	0	(0–1)			
Stone formation						

G, number of groups/treatment arms extracted; P, number of patients in those groups; CI, confidence interval; UTI, urinary tract infection.
Reprinted with permission of the American Urological Association.

Table 36.7. *Comparative outcomes for sling procedures: complications details*

Outcomes	Sling procedures								
	Abdominal fascia			Fascia lata			Vaginal wall		
Death	Death rate for all procedures presumed to be no different than for other types of elective vaginal/abdominal surgery: approximately 5 out of 10 000								
	G/P	Median	CI (2.5–97.5)%	G/P	Median	CI (2.5–97.5)%	G/P	Median	CI (2.5–97.5)%
Transfusion				1/10	2	(0–22)	1/54	0	(0–5)
General medical complications									
Abdominal complication				1/88	1	(0–5)			
Cardiovascular	2/114	3	(1–9)	4/405	2	(1–5)	1/54	2	(0–8)
Pulmonary				2/258	5	(3–10)			
Intraoperative complications									
Bladder complication	2/77	21	(2–64)	2/147	12	(5–23)	1/82	3	(1–8)
Ureteral complication									
Urethral complication	3/171	3	(1–7)						
Perioperative complications									
Bleeding				1/170	1	(0–3)			
UTI	2/77	18	(1–67)	2/258	9	(5–14)	1/54	4	(1–11)
Wound complication	3/157	7	(2–17)	4/421	8	(4–14)	1/82	3	(1–8)
Subjective complications									
Dysuria	1/80	1	(0–6)						
Pain							1/54	4	(1–11)
Sexual dysfunction									
Complications requiring surgery									
Fistula				2/93	6	(1–16)			
Stone formation									

cont.

Table 36.7. *Comparative outcomes for sling procedures: complications details (cont.)*

Outcomes	Sling procedures								
	Homologous			Synthetic			Other		
Death	Death rate for all procedures presumed to be no different than for other types of elective vaginal/abdominal surgery: approximately 5 out of 10 000								
	G/P	Median	CI (2.5–97.5)%	G/P	Median	CI (2.5–97.5)%	G/P	Median	CI (2.5–97.5)%
Transfusion				2/80	5	(1–13)			
General medical complications									
Abdominal complication									
Cardiovascular	1/10	11	(1–38)	4/399	2	(1–5)	2/145	7	(1–21)
Pulmonary									
Intraoperative complications									
Bladder complication	1/10	11	(1–38)	8/339	8	(4–14)	5/422	5	(2–10)
Ureteral complication									
Urethral complication				1/20	6	(1–21)	2/135	2	(0–6)
Perioperative complications									
Bleeding				2/125	7	(1–20)	1/205	1	(0–3)
UTI	1/10	40	(15–70)	7/564	11	(5–19)	1/21	6	(1–20)
Wound complication	1/10	31	(9–61)	13/1038	10	(6–15)	8/791	9	(4–16)
Subjective complications									
Dysuria				1/98	15	(9–23)			
Pain									
Sexual dysfunction				1/69	2	(0–7)			
Complications requiring surgery									
Fistula				7/576	3	(1–5)	1/160	0	(0–2)
Stone formation				2/417	3	(1–7)			

G, number of groups/treatment arms extracted; P, number of patients in those groups; CI, confidence interval; UTI, urinary tract infection.
Reprinted with permission of the American Urological Association.

REFERENCES

1. Herzog AR, Fultz NH. Prevalence and incidence of urinary incontinence in community dwelling populations. *J Am Geriatr Soc* 1990; 34: 273–281

2. Grimby A, Milsom I, Molander U *et al.* The influence of urinary incontinence on the quality of life of elderly women. *Age Ageing* 1993; 22: 82–89

3. Shumaker SA, Wyman JF, Uebersax JS *et al.* Health related quality of life measures for women with urinary incontinence: the Incontinence Impact Questionnaire and the Urogenital Distress Inventory. *Qual Life Res* 1994; 3: 291–306

4. Wyman JF, Harkins SC, Choi SC *et al.* Psychosocial impact of urinary incontinence in women. *Obstet Gynecol* 1987; 70: 378–381

5. Uebersax JS, Wyman JF, Shumaker SA *et al.* Short forms to assess life quality and symptom distress for urinary incontinence in women: the Incontinence Impact Questionnaire and the Urogenital Distress Inventory. *Neurourol Urodyn* 1995; 14: 131–139

6. Romanzi L, Blaivas JG. Office evaluation of incontinence. In: O'Donnell PD (ed) *Urinary Incontinence.* St Louis: Mosby, 1997; 475–479

7. O'Donnell PD, Sutton LE, Beck CE. Urinary incontinence detection in elderly inpatient men. *Neurourol Urodyn* 1987; 6: 101–108

8. Larsson G, Victor A. Micturition patterns in a healthy female population studied with a frequency/volume chart. *Scand J Urol Nephrol* 1988; 114: 53–57

9. Abrams P, Blaivas JG, Stanton SL, Anderson JT. The standardization of terminology of lower urinary tract function. *Scand J Urol Nephrol* 1988; 114(Suppl): 5–19

10. Hahn I, Fall M. Objective quantification of stress urinary incontinence: a short, reproducible, provocative pad weighing test. *Neurourol Urodyn* 1991; 10: 475–481

11. Lose G, Gammelgard J, Jorgensen TJ. The one hour pad weighing test: reproducibility and the correlation between the test result, start volume in the bladder and the diuresis. *Neurourol Urodyn* 1986; 5: 17–21

12. Fantl JA, Harkins SW, Wyman JF *et al.* Fluid loss quantitation test in women with urinary incontinence: a test–retest analysis. *Obstet Gynecol* 1987; 70: 739–743

13. Christensen SJ, Golstrup H, Hertz JB *et al.* Inter and intradepartmental variations of the perineal pad weighing test. *Neurourol Urodyn* 1986; 5: 23–28

14. Fantl JA, Newman D, Colling J *et al. Urinary Incontinence in Adults: Acute and Chronic Management. Clinical Practice Guideline.* Rockville, MD: US Dept of Health and Human Services, 1996 (2) 1–65

15. Leach GE, Dmochowski RR, Appell RA *et al.* Female stress urinary incontinence clinical guidelines panel. Summary report on the surgical management of female stress urinary incontinence. *J Urol* 1997; 158: 875–879

37

Preparation for surgery

J. Bidmead, L. Cardozo

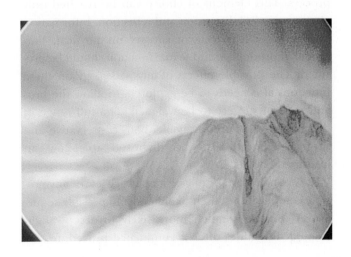

INTRODUCTION

A great deal of a surgeon's attention is naturally focused on the technical performance of an operation. Although surgical technique is a major factor influencing outcome, other factors such as appropriate patient selection, preoperative investigation and preparation also have a major influence on the results of surgery.

Most urogynaecological surgery is elective. Urinary incontinence and urogenital prolapse, although undeniably distressing, are rarely life threatening. Urogynaecological surgery can therefore be planned in advance and time is available for preparation, which can be used to improve the outcome of surgery.

The elective nature of most urogynaecological surgery means that operative morbidity must be kept to a minimum. Adequate preparation and intervention to reduce surgical and anaesthetic complications is mandatory, as is the provision of preoperative counselling.

PROCEDURE SELECTION

One of the most important factors governing the success of any gynaecological surgery is patient selection. This applies as much to the selection of procedure by the woman herself as it does to the selection of an operation for a patient by the surgeon. In the past the phrase 'patient selection' has applied more often to the latter.

In gynaecology, the type of surgery performed may have a profound influence on the emotional, psychological and sexual well-being of a woman. It is, therefore, vital that, before proceeding to an irreversible surgical procedure, a woman should feel that she has had the opportunity to take part in the decision-making process. This element of choice can be reached only after a period of discussion and reflection. Information on the possible effects of surgery on physical, hormonal, reproductive and sexual function should be provided. The possible effects of any pathology on these functions also needs to be explored, to allow the pros and cons of surgery to be weighed. The full range of therapeutic measures available, both conservative and surgical, should also be discussed to allow an informed choice.

It is also important to give a realistic view of any possible complications, their likelihood and possible sequelae. A woman is much more likely to accept slight voiding difficulties after a continence procedure, for example, if this has been explained in advance. Explaining unanticipated difficulties 'after the event' can be fraught and is much more likely to lead to medicolegal action, often with unsatisfactory outcomes for both parties.

PATIENT SELECTION

It has often been said that the key to successful surgery lies not only with the technical skills of the surgeon but with his or her ability to select cases appropriately. This means that the skill and experience of the surgeon should be used during consultation to help guide a woman in making choices about treatment.

USE OF ALTERNATIVE THERAPIES

Time is also available to permit a number of alternative therapies to be tried before surgical intervention is undertaken.

Recently, alternative conservative treatments for incontinence have become available that offer increased choice for those women unsuitable or unwilling to undergo surgery.

Pelvic floor physiotherapy, with or without electrical stimulation, remains the mainstay of conservative management of genuine stress incontinence (GSI). Many studies have shown excellent results, although it is clear that closely monitored therapy by a physiotherapist interested and experienced in this area is necessary. Vague instructions to perform pelvic floor exercises (PFE) are ineffective and may even be counterproductive: fewer than 70% of women are able to perform these exercises correctly without tuition.[1] The use of PFE was first described by Kegel in 1948.[2] In a series of studies Kegel was able to demonstrate an impressive success rate of 84% in women with stress incontinence. More recent studies have confirmed good long-term results.[3,4] Although there are no published data to suggest that prior effective pelvic floor physiotherapy improves the eventual outcome of surgery, this is the impression of many urogynaecologists. As the success rate of physiotherapy is good and its influence on surgical outcome may be beneficial, it is recommended that surgical intervention is not resorted to until a woman has had an adequate course of physiotherapy.

A number of mechanical devices have also become available recently. These may be useful in a number of situations: they may be helpful in the short term, allowing women to regain continence while undergoing physiotherapy or while awaiting surgery.[5] Some women, particularly those with mild GSI only on exercise, may choose to use them as an alternative to surgery (for example during aerobics classes or tennis). Lastly, there remains a group of women for whom surgery has failed and where further surgery is inadvisable; women in this group are able to use devices to regain control or manage their incontinence.

Devices vary, as do the women who use them, and so it is often worth trying more than one.

Prosthetic devices for the control of prolapse are also available. Those most commonly used today are a silicon ring pessary which can control vaginal prolapse very effectively if pelvic floor tone is good. Uterovaginal prolapse may be more effectively controlled with a shelf pessary. Although these pessaries may not be suitable for younger women they can be useful for older women wishing to avoid surgery.

Use of such devices while awaiting surgery can improve a woman's quality of life in the short term; they may also be advantageously employed while a woman is undergoing a course of physiotherapy and while coming to a final decision regarding surgery.

PSYCHOLOGICAL PREPARATION FOR SURGERY

Whereas it may be considered desirable to bring any intervention to a satisfactory conclusion as rapidly as possible, the very nature of this surgery allows time for both surgeon and patient to consider all the available options and select the most appropriate. Time is also available to consider factors that may improve the likelihood of a satisfactory outcome and to take measures to reduce the possibility of adverse outcomes. Finally, the effect of surgery on lifestyle can be considered and any period of convalescence planned for.

It is well documented that only 10% of verbal information given during a consultation is remembered by the patient afterwards. This can be substantially increased by the use of written information given to patients during a consultation.[6] Patient information leaflets can be particularly useful if they have been written locally to reflect practice in a particular unit.

Written information leaflets can also be re-read at leisure by women and allow time to consider treatment options and think of any questions that may

addressed at subsequent consultations. Although the primary objective of patient information leaflets is not to save the surgeon's time, it would be impractical to discuss all aspects of all the treatment options at a single consultation.

Although not a primary objective, the use of such written information and documentation of this may be particularly useful medicolegally. Many medicolegal disputes arise when patients complain of sequelae about which they feel they were not warned. Often, the case may be that such problems were discussed but that this was not among the 10% of the consultation remembered by the patient. The documentation of written information being given may be useful in such circumstances.

Use of a nurse counsellor

Involvement of nursing staff may be particularly beneficial. Increasingly, a number of units are offering a preoperative counselling service. This is often provided by suitably experienced and trained nursing staff and allows discussion of any anxieties in a more relaxed and leisurely fashion than is possible on a traditional preoperative ward round. It is particularly helpful if a woman has the opportunity to discuss a procedure with an experienced member of the nursing team preoperatively, so that she can discuss aspects of surgery that she may have felt unable to discuss with the surgical staff. Nursing staff are also appropriately placed to give information about preoperative and postoperative care, catheter regimens, drains, dressings and ward routine. Ideally, the nurse should be one of the team providing care on the ward; this is currently the practice in our unit and has proved most useful.

As previously stated, because most urogynaecological surgery is elective, any investigations can be carried out in advance of any proposed intervention and plans can be modified as a result. There should be no need for a procedure to be performed under conditions of undue stress and there should be no hesitation in deferring an operation until a more appropriate time – when there may be more time available on a theatre list, for example. If a procedure is felt to be inappropriate, further investigations necessary or the patient's condition not optimal, then surgery should be deferred.

Finally, the surgeon has the ultimate sanction and, if it is felt that an intervention is inappropriate or not in a patient's best interest, then (after appropriate explanation) it may be wise to refer back to the general practitioner or suggest a further opinion. Although this may seem to be an extreme measure, it is preferable to continuing on a course of action that may have untoward results for both patient and doctor!

PHYSICAL PREPARATION FOR SURGERY

Fitness

Before undergoing any surgical procedure it is essential that a woman is as fit, physically, as possible. The elective nature of most urogynaecological procedures allows surgery to be deferred if any intercurrent illness has reduced a woman's fitness. In addition to exercising the pelvic floor muscles, a programme of exercise may be beneficial in reducing morbidity and speeding up postoperative recovery. Preoperative exercise will also enhance weight loss if this is a concern. The physiotherapist is in an ideal position to advise a woman on preoperative exercise.

Smoking

In addition to its well-known effects on general health smoking increases the risk of postoperative problems, such as thromboembolism. The issue of thromboprophylaxis is covered elsewhere (page 475). Pulmonary atelectasis and subsequent pneumonia is a particular risk following general anaesthesia and this is substantially increased by smoking.

In addition, chronic cough is a factor in development or recurrence of urogenital prolapse. For these reasons it is worth impressing on women the importance of stopping smoking preoperatively.

Weight

It comes as a surprise to many women that obesity is a major cause of surgical difficulty. In addition to the technical difficulties faced by the surgeon, obesity also increases virtually all perioperative risks. For the anaesthetist, intravenous access, induction of anaesthesia and intubation are all more difficult. Postoperatively, obesity increases the risk of thromboembolism, wound infection, haematoma and respiratory infection.

Although there is little published evidence, it appears that obesity, by raising intra-abdominal pressure, increases the risk of failure of incontinence procedures and increases the recurrence of urogenital prolapse.

For these reasons the obese woman should be encouraged to lose weight prior to surgery. Rather than giving a general instruction to 'lose some weight', it is more effective to set a reasonable target for weight loss and offer surgery once that target has been achieved. Referral to a dietician is often helpful and appetite suppressants may be useful in the short term.

Anaemia

Anaemia may well be a problem in women presenting for urogynaecological surgery with concomitant menorrhagia. As well as reducing the safe margin for intraoperative blood loss, anaemia increases the risk of postoperative wound infection and delays full recovery. Mild-to-moderate anaemia may respond to simple oral iron replacement in the form of ferrous sulphate (200 mg daily). Other measures to reduce menstrual loss and allow replenishment of iron stores include the use of mefanamic acid (500 mg three times daily) alone or in combination with tranexamic acid (1 g four times daily).[7] Gonadotropin releasing hormone (GnRH) analogues may be useful, with or without 'add-back' hormone-replacement therapy (HRT), in extreme cases to suppress menstruation prior to surgery.[8] GnRH analogues have also been shown to be useful in reducing the volume of uterine fibroids prior to hysterectomy or myomectomy and in reducing blood loss at myomectomy or hysterectomy.[9]

Bowel preparation

It is worth paying attention to preoperative bowel preparation. In women with normal bowel habit undergoing routine surgery, complicated preoperative regimens are unnecessary. However, it is worth ensuring an empty rectum prior to surgery as this may avoid postoperative discomfort and constipation. A single mild aperient such as a sodium lauryl sulphoacetate enema given the evening before surgery should suffice.

Women undergoing pelvic reconstructive surgery, such as colposuspension or vaginal repair, may benefit from more thorough bowel preparation (to prevent a loaded rectum interfering with surgery) and a regimen of postoperative laxatives (to reduce postoperative straining that may compromise the repair). A sachet of sodium picosulphate taken the afternoon before surgery will ensure an empty rectum; postoperatively, a stool softener such as lactulose will prevent discomfort and straining due to constipation.

Prior to undertaking operations which require complete access to the sacral promontory and where mobilization of the rectum may be required, more thorough bowel preparation is necessary. A full rectum may make the performance of sacrocolpopexy difficult or impossible. A low-residue low-fibre diet for 48 hours prior to surgery, together with a half sachet of sodium picosulphate daily, will help to ensure an empty rectum. A disposable phosphate enema can be given preoperatively to women with a history of marked constipation.

PREOPERATIVE INVESTIGATIONS

The majority of preoperative investigations should be performed on an outpatient basis with the results available for review prior to admission to allow time for any remedial action to be taken.

An exhaustive list of preoperative investigations is beyond the scope of this chapter and should be tailored to an individual woman's general health and any existing medical problems. Basic preoperative investigations may include haematological and biochemical investigations, urinalysis, electrocardiography (ECG) and imaging.

Haematological investigations

Every woman should have a full blood screen performed to include haemoglobin, haematocrit, white cell count and differential and haemoglobinopathy screen where appropriate. For all procedures where there is significant risk of transfusion, typing should be performed and serum retained for cross-matching at short notice.

Biochemical investigations

For the majority of women, no particular biochemical investigations are necessary. However, in women with pre-existing disease such as hypertension or diabetes, biochemical screening may be necessary. Renal function tests should be performed if there is any suspicion of renal failure or ureteric obstruction.

Urinalysis

Simple ward urinalysis is useful to exclude glycosuria and infection. Urine should be tested for beta human chorionic gonadotropin if there is any possibility of pregnancy.

ECG

ECG traces are not required for most fit women undergoing surgery, but may be required if there is a history of hypertension or cardiac disease. Most departments of anaesthesia now have guidelines for preoperative ECG testing.

Imaging

The roles of plain and contrast radiology, computed tomography, ultrasonography and magnetic resonance imaging are discussed in the relevant sections of this book.

Routine preoperative chest radiography is now rarely required except in women with cardiac or pulmonary disease. Most departments of anaesthesia now have guidelines for preoperative chest radiography. An intravenous urogram should be performed if an anatomical abnormality suggests that the course of the ureters may be aberrant, if malignancy is suspected or in major prolapse where ureteric obstruction is a possibility.

ANAESTHETIC PRE-ASSESSMENT

Preoperative assessment by the anaesthetist is essential to ensure the safe and smooth running of the list. It is good practice for the patient to be seen the evening before surgery with the notes and results of investigations available. Where major medical problems exist, or if there have been previous anaesthetic problems such as difficult intubation, anaesthetic consultation may be carried out prior to admission. The most appropriate type of anaesthetic (general, regional or local) should also be selected.

The advice of the relevant specialist should also be sought in the case of significant existing medical conditions. The specialist team will be able to give advice on preoperative preparation and therapy in the immediate postoperative phase.

INFORMED CONSENT

Before embarking upon any surgical procedure it is imperative that adequate informed consent has been obtained and documented. Increasingly, medicolegal claims involving the issue of consent are being pursued and, as an aspect of good practice as well as risk management, it is important to understand the ethical and legal issues surrounding the concept of informed consent. When considering the issue of informed consent, the British courts use what is known as the Bolam principle. This was developed in the case *Bolam* v *Friern Hospital Management Committee*, [1957] 1 Wlr 582. This states that 'a Doctor is not negligent when he acts in accordance with a practice accepted as proper by a responsible body of medical men skilled in that particular art'.

Consent is difficult to define succinctly but requires three elements – volition, capacity and knowledge.

Volition

Volition is based on the principles of self-determination and a respect for individual integrity. This requires that a woman is able to make a decision regarding consent without undue pressure from a third party, either a relative or a member of the medical staff. Legally, a spouse or relative cannot give or withhold consent on a woman's behalf, although it is considered good practice to involve the spouse, particularly where the treatment proposed will affect fertility.

Capacity

Capacity to consent requires that a woman has sufficient intellect to appreciate information discussed prior to giving consent, and the mental capacity to appreciate the risks and consequences of the operation proposed. This is a particularly difficult area when dealing with women whose mental capacity is limited as a result of either intellectual handicap or psychiatric illness. In these situations it is important to seek additional professional opinion and to seek legal clarification where time allows.

The situation when dealing with minors (in the UK under 16 years of age) is another delicate area. In general, both the parents and child would be involved in giving informed consent. However, in the UK the circumstances of minors giving consent without parental approval or knowledge has recently been clarified in the case of *Gillick* v *West Norfolk and Wisbech Health Authority*, [1985] 3 All ER 402, in which the House of Lords ruled that parental rights give way to a child's right to make her own decision upon sufficient maturity to understand the nature and consequences of that decision. This has led to the concept of 'Gillick' competency, where a medical practitioner must make a clinical judgement as to whether a minor has sufficient maturity to give informed consent. Although this has clarified the situation in the UK, it is important that practitioners are aware of the law regarding minors in their own country or state.

Knowledge

The third aspect of consent is that of knowledge. This implies that a woman should be given sufficient information concerning the diagnosis and prognosis to make a reasoned decision regarding treatment. A woman must also be given sufficient information about alternative treatments and also any reasonably foreseeable adverse effects of the proposed treatment. This is another difficult area, as women's ability to understand the technicalities of a medical condition and its treatment may vary. Similarly, it would be unreasonable to describe in depth every conceivable complication arising from surgery. This area was clarified in the case of *Sidaway v Board of Governors of Bethlem Royal Hospital*, [1985] 1 ALL ER 643, in which the courts applied the Bolam principle to information about potential risks. In general, the information given should conform to that given by a responsible body of medical opinion. Those risks that are commonly associated with a procedure should certainly be discussed; more uncommon complications need not be. It is left to the medical practitioner to decide on an individual patient's ability or wish to discuss these issues. The need to discuss complications also varies with their potential severity and implications for future health. This means that it is essential to discuss the possibility of a complication that may be relatively remote but which would have a major impact on a woman's life. A good example of this is the need to perform hysterectomy to control haemorrhage at myomectomy; although this is well reported it is, in fact, a relatively uncommon occurrence. However, as myomectomy is primarily performed to preserve fertility and the loss of the uterus has such major implications for a woman wishing to bear further children, the remote possibility of this should always be discussed and recorded beforehand.

Oophorectomy performed without specific consent has been the subject of a number of recent court actions – both civil cases for negligence and criminal cases for assault. It is essential that the possibility of oophorectomy, either as a technical necessity or for an unforeseen indication, is discussed and documented.

The risks of surgical complications such as bladder trauma requiring catheterization, wound infection and urinary tract infection should also be discussed, as appropriate.

The issue of informed consent has become clearer in recent years, with some guidance from the cases cited above. The final decision regarding a woman's capacity to give consent and her ability to understand the information given is left to the professional judgement of the surgeon.

Most practitioners will use a standard consent form and record any particular information on this. However, the concept of informed consent embraces more than just a signature and so it is important that good records are kept of any discussion and information given prior to informed consent.

THROMBOEMBOLISM AND THROMBOPROPHYLAXIS

Thromboembolism accounts for around 20% of perioperative hysterectomy deaths.[10] As prophylaxis has been shown to be effective in reducing the risk of thromboembolism, women undergoing gynaecological surgery should be assessed for clinical risk factors and overall risk of thromboembolism, and should receive prophylaxis according to the degree of risk: this is highest for surgery associated with malignancy, less in abdominal hysterectomy and lowest for vaginal hysterectomy.[11] Other risk factors associated with the disease or surgical procedure include infection, polycythaemia and heart failure. Risk factors associated with the patient are age over 37 years, obesity, previous deep vein thrombosis (DVT), blood group other than O and the presence of congenital or acquired thrombophilias. Assessment of these risk factors allows categorization into low-, medium- or high-risk categories.

The Royal College of Obstetricians and Gynaecologists (RCOG) has issued guidelines on the use of thromboprophylaxis in gynaecological surgery.[12] Patients deemed at low risk require attention to hydration and early mobilization only. Those at moderate risk should receive specific prophylaxis with either low-dose subcutaneous heparin (5000 units 12-hourly) or intermittent pneumatic compression. Patients deemed to be high risk should be given heparin as above and in addition be fitted with graduated compression stockings.

The use of heparin is associated with a small increase in the risk of wound haematoma but no significant fall in postoperative haemoglobin or increase in the need for blood transfusion.

Low molecular weight heparin (e.g. Enoxaparin 20 mg or Tinzaparin once daily) may also be used, as once-daily administration may be more convenient for patients and staff (although these preparations are more expensive).

In many units these guidelines are exceeded and heparin, intermittent compression and compression stockings are used for all but minor day-case procedures.

COMBINED ORAL CONTRACEPTIVE PILL

The combined oral contraceptive (COC) pill has been implicated as a risk factor for postoperative thromboembolism. However, most of the evidence for this has relied on the clinical diagnosis of DVT, which is in itself unreliable. A study by Vessey et al.[13] showed a modest increased risk in users of the COC. The recent RCOG guidelines suggest that the COC need not be stopped but that appropriate prophylaxis should be given. Alternatively, if the COC is to be stopped 4–6 weeks before surgery then appropriate alternative contraceptive measures should be taken.[12]

HORMONE-REPLACEMENT THERAPY (HRT)

Recent studies have suggested an increased risk of venous thrombosis in women taking HRT. There is at present no evidence associating HRT, at physiological levels, with an increase in postoperative DVT.[14] Therefore there seems little to be gained by stopping HRT prior to surgery and exposing the patient to a recurrence of perimenopausal symptoms. However, routine assessment of risk and appropriate prophylaxis should be undertaken, as many patients in this age group will have other, more significant, risk factors for thrombosis.[15]

Atrophic changes in the vaginal skin can cause difficulty during vaginal reconstructive surgery and compromise postoperative wound healing. Preoperative treatment with topical oestrogen for 6 weeks is worthwhile and carries little risk.

ANTIBIOTIC PROPHYLAXIS

Prophylactic antibiotics have been clearly shown to reduce the risk of postoperative wound infection. The use of perioperative antibiotic prophylaxis has been shown, in a systematic review, to reduce markedly the risks of febrile morbidity after elective and emergency caesarean section.[16] A similar reduction in infectious morbidity has been shown with the use of broad-spectrum antibiotic prophylaxis in both abdominal and vaginal hysterectomy.[17,18] This reduction was also seen in a study of antibiotic prophylaxis in both general and gynaecological surgery.[19]

Adverse reactions to prophylactic antibiotic regimens are reported rarely, with an incidence of less than 1%. The cost of antibiotic cover is outweighed by the considerable economic savings, most notably the reduction in inpatient stay. The clinical and economic evidence clearly demonstrates the effectiveness of routine perioperative antibiotic prophylaxis.

The choice of antibiotic appears to be between a broad-spectrum penicillin or cephalosporins, either alone or in combination with an aminoglycoside or metronidazole. There appears to be little difference between the penicillins and cephalosporins. The studies showing the greatest reduction in postoperative infection are those where an aminoglycoside was used as part of the combination. As the pattern of microbial resistance varies, the most appropriate combination of agents should be selected after consultation with the local microbiology service, and should be reviewed at regular intervals.

The development of microbial resistance is a particular concern. Given the clear advantages of routine chemoprophylaxis, it is sensible to continue this; however, to reduce bacterial resistance, short courses should be used with routine 'first-line' agents. Newer agents should be reserved for treatment of established antibiotic-resistant infections.

As the aim of chemoprophylaxis is the prevention rather than the treatment of established infection, regimens used should aim to achieve a high tissue concentration of the chosen antibiotics at the time of surgery when inoculation of the wound occurs. This would mean the administration of intravenous antibiotics some hours prior to surgery; a more practical compromise is to give the first dose at the time of induction of anaesthesia, with a further two doses in the first 24 hours postoperatively.

ANTICIPATION OF POSTOPERATIVE VOIDING PROBLEMS

Voiding difficulties may occur acutely following any pelvic surgery; after continence procedures in particular, voiding difficulties may persist in the medium or long term. The importance of relieving acute urinary retention cannot be overstated. Acute overdistension of the bladder leads to damage to detrusor syncytium with ischaemic damage to the postsynaptic parasympathetic fibres. This may result in insidious deterioration of detrusor function and, later, the onset of voiding dysfunction.[20] A number of factors that increase the risk of acute postoperative retention have been identified: these include increased age, long operation time, high doses of opiate analgesia and patient-controlled analgesia, together with large amounts of intravenous fluid.[21] In view of the possible long-term sequelae of acute overdistension of the detrusor, it is important that steps are taken to prevent this. Postoperative indwelling urethral catheterization should be used following any pelvic surgery, although some authors prefer intermittent catheterization.[22] In women judged clinically or urodynamically to be at high risk of retention, suprapubic catheterization may be preferable; this may performed easily at the time of surgery and avoids the need for repeated urethral catheterization. Following removal of a catheter, close monitoring of fluid balance should be continued to prevent recurrent retention.

As previously stated, voiding difficulties are particularly common following continence procedures initially and may persist for a variable time following surgery. After colposuspension they are particularly common in women with preoperative flow rates of less than 15 ml/s or maximum voiding detrusor pressure below 15 cmH$_2$O. Between 12 and 25% of women are reported to suffer delayed voiding postoperatively and 11–20% have increased residual volumes and reduced flow rates when measured at 3 months postoperatively.[23] In a recent study by Smith and Cardozo[24] of 100 women undergoing colposuspension, 21% experienced significant voiding difficulties for up to 6 months following their surgery, although this persisted beyond 6 months in only 2%. Hilton and Stanton[25] performed postoperative urodynamic studies on women 3 months after colposuspension and found highly significant reduced flow rates and increased voiding pressure.

Voiding problems are also common following needle suspension procedures, although published figures vary. Ashken *et al.*[26] noted no significant changes in flow rate, voiding pressures or urine residual volume in a study of 60 women after successful Stamey procedure; Hilton and Mayne[27] studied 100 women undergoing Stamey procedure and found increased functional urethral length and improved pressure transmission but no significant changes in resting urethral profile or voiding pressure; Mundy[28] found a higher incidence of voiding difficulties and irritative symptoms compared with colposuspension.

Sling procedures are particularly prone to causing voiding difficulty as their mechanism of action is to increase outflow resistance.[25,29]

Whichever continence procedure is to be performed, it is important that women are counselled adequately. The need for suprapubic catheterization, which may occasionally be prolonged, should be carefully explained preoperatively. The occasional need for clean intermittent self-catheterization (CISC) should be discussed. When voiding difficulty is predicted by urodynamic studies it may be worth teaching CISC prior to surgery. Even though perhaps only a minority of these women will need to self-catheterize, from the psychological standpoint short-term voiding problems are much better dealt with when they have been anticipated.

ENTEROCELE AND RECTOCELE FORMATION

The formation of enteroceles and rectoceles is thought to occur as a result of elevation of the anterior vaginal wall creating a posterior defect and causing intra-abdominal pressure to be transmitted directly to the posterior vaginal wall. The incidence of postoperative posterior compartment defects is estimated to be 7–17%.[30] It is important that this is discussed with women preoperatively, together with the potential need for interval posterior vaginal repair.

DE-NOVO DETRUSOR INSTABILITY

It has been shown that detrusor instability (DI) arises *de novo* in 12–18.5% of women postoperatively,[31] and occurs more commonly following previous continence surgery. It seems likely that a number of cases reflect pre-existing DI not detected at cystometry preoperatively. In addition, it has been suggested that damage to the autonomic nerve supply occurs during lateral displacement of the bladder during surgery.[32] The presence of preoperative DI should be excluded with urodynamic investigations. Where DI is present, a trial of anticholinergic therapy should be carried out. This will ensure that symptoms of frequency and urgency can be controlled and that the woman is able to tolerate the side effects of anticholinergic therapy if it is required postoperatively. Such women should be warned that symptoms of frequency and urgency may persist after surgery for stress incontinence and this should be recorded in the case notes.

CONCLUSIONS

Adequate preparation for surgery has an important role in ensuring an optimal outcome and reducing morbidity.

The elective nature of most urogynaecological surgery allows time to ensure that women are well prepared, both psychologically and physically, before undergoing the chosen operation.

REFERENCES

1. Laycock J. *The Investigation and Management of Urinary Incontinence in Women.* London: RCOG Press 1995

2. Kegel AH. Progressive resistance exercise in the functional restoration of the perineal muscles. *Am J Obstet Gynecol* 1948; 56: 238–248

3. Tapp AJS, Hills B, Cardozo L. Who benefits from physiotherapy? *Neurourol Urodyn* 1988; 7: 259–265

4. Bø K, Talseth T. Five year follow up of pelvic floor exercise for the treatment of stress urinary incontinence. *Neurourol Urodyn* 1994; 13: 374–376

5. Choe JM, Staskin DR. Clinical usefulness of urinary insert devices. *Int Urogynecol J* 1997; 8: 307–313

6. Collings LH, Pike LC, Binder A *et al.* Value of written information in a general practice setting. *Br J Gen Pract* 1991; 41: 466–467

7. Bonnar J, Sheppard BL. Treatment of menorrhagia: a randomised controlled trial of ethamsylate, mefenamic acid and tranexamic acid. *Br Med J* 1996; 313: 579–582

8. Thomas EJ, Okuda M, Thomas NM. The combination of a depot GnRH analogue and cyclical HRT for dysfunctional uterine bleeding. *Br J Obstet Gynaecol* 1991; 98: 1155–1159

9. Sternquist M. Treatment of uterine fibroids with GnRH

analogues prior to hysterectomy. *Acta Obstet Gynecol Scand Suppl* 1997; 194: 94–97

10. Department of Health Report of the National Enquiry Into Perioperative Deaths London: HMSO, 1993

11. Bergquist D. *Postoperative Thromboembolism.* London: Springer-Verlag, 1983; 106–107

12. Royal College of Obstetricians and Gynaecologists. *Report of the RCOG Working Party on Prophylaxis Against Thromboembolism in Gynaecology and Obstetrics.* London: RCOG 1995

13. Vessey MP, Mant D, Smith A, Yeates D. Oral contraceptives and venous thromboembolism. *Br Med J* 1986; 292: 526

14. Carter CJ. Thrombosis in relation to oral contraceptives and hormone replacement therapy. In: Greer IA, Turpie AAG, Forbes CD (eds) *Haemostasis and Thrombosis in Obstetrics and Gynaecology.* London: Chapman and Hall 1992; 371–388

15. Lowe G, Greer I, Cooke T *et al.* Risk and prophylaxis for venous thromboembolism in hospital patients. *Br Med J* 1992; 305: 567–574

16. Smaill F. Propylactic antibiotics in caesarean section (all trials). In: Keirse MJNC, Renfrew MJ, Neilson JP, Crowther C (eds) *The Cochrane Pregnancy and Childbirth Database; Issue 2.* Oxford: Oxford University Press, 1994

17. Hemsall DL, Molly C, Heard RA *et al.* Single dose prophylaxis for vaginal and abdominal hysterectomy. *Am J Obstet Gynecol* 1987; 157: 498–501

18. Duff P, Park RC. Antibiotic prophylaxis in vaginal hysterectomy: a review. *Obstet Gynecol* 1980; 55 (Suppl): 193–202

19. Regiori A, Ravera M, Coccozza E *et al.* Randomised study of antibiotic prophylaxis for general and gynaecological surgery from a single centre in rural Africa. *Br J Surg* 1996; 83: 356–359

20. Osborne JL. *Urodynamics and the Gynaecologist.* Alec Bourne Lecture. London: RCOG Press, 1981

21. Tammela T, Konturri M, Lukkarien O. Postoperative urinary retention 1. Incidence and predisposing factors. *Scand J Urol Nephrol* 1986; 20: 197–201

22. Smith NGK, Murrant JD. Postoperative urinary retention in women management by intermittent catheterisation. *Age Ageing* 1990; 19: 337–340

23. Stanton SL, Cardozo LD, Williams JE *et al.* Clinical and urodynamic features of failed incontinence surgery in the female. *Obstet Gynecol* 1978; 51: 515–520

24. Smith RN, Cardozo L. Early voiding difficulties after colposuspension. *Br J Urol* 1997; 160: 911–914

25. Hilton P, Stanton SL. A clinical and urodynamic assessment of the Burch colposuspension for genuine stress incontinence. *Br J Obstet Gynaecol* 1983; 90: 934–939

26. Ashken MH, Abrams PH, Lawrence WT. Stamey endoscopic bladder neck suspension for stress incontinence. *Br J Urol* 1984; 56: 629–634

27. Hilton P, Mayne C. The Stamey endoscopic bladder neck suspension: a clinical and urodynamic investigation including actuarial follow up over four years. *Br J Obstet Gynaecol* 1991; 98: 1141–1149

28. Mundy AR. A trial comparing the Stamey bladder neck suspension with colposuspension for the treatment of stress incontinence. *Br J Urol* 1983; 55: 687–690

29. Beck RP, McCormack RN. Treatment of urinary stress incontinence with anterior colporrhaphy. *Obstet Gynecol* 1982; 59: 269–274

30. Burch JC. Coopers ligament urethrovesical suspension for urinary stress incontinence. *Am J Obstet Gynecol* 1968; 100: 764–772

31. Alcalay M, Monga A, Stanton SL. Burch colposuspension: a 10–20-year follow up. *Br J Obstet Gynaecol* 1995; 102: 740–745

32. Cardozo LD, Stanton SL, Williams JE. Detrusor instability following surgery for GSI. *Br J Urol* 1979; 58: 138–142

38

Intra-urethral injection therapy

R. A. Appell

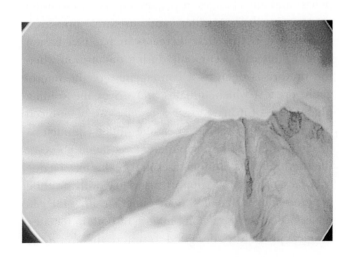

INTRODUCTION

The correction of the problem of failure to store urine may be simplified by considering the location of the cause of the patient's embarrassing situation, at which time treatment may be directed at the dysfunctioning area in the lower urinary tract, either the bladder or its outlet. When the problem originates in the outlet, the difficulty is often related to the competency of the urethral sphincteric mechanism at the neck of the bladder. Although this incompetence of the sphincteric mechanism may be the result of some defect in anatomical support (so-called genuine stress urinary incontinence [SUI] secondary to hypermobility of the vesicourethral junction with resultant unequal transmission of intra-abdominal pressure to the bladder and urethra), it may also be related to a problem in the intrinsic urethral closure mechanism itself as a result of sympathetic neurological injury, surgical trauma or myelodysplasia. Urodynamically, in these cases of intrinsic sphincteric deficiency (ISD), the bladder neck and proximal urethra remain open at rest in the absence of a detrusor contraction. However, it must be recognized that ISD may exist alone or concomitantly with hypermobility of the outlet, and the existence of this variable of hypermobility may very well influence the choice of therapy for the ISD.

The urethra faces two potential expulsive forces: These are (1) detrusor pressure (p_{det}) and (2) abdominal pressure (p_{abd}). Detrusor pressure reflects outlet resistance, as any increase in p_{det} tends to force the urethral sphincter open when the p_{det} and the urethral pressure (p_{ur}) become equalized. Increases in p_{abd} cannot open a normal urethra because the sphincteric portion is positioned within the abdominal cavity (true pelvis) and any changes in p_{abd} are equally transmitted to the intrinsic bladder and urethral pressures. Although it is true that increases in p_{abd} can hasten voiding, this can occur only during micturition when the urethra is open as a consequence of the neurogenic process which initiates and drives the voiding phase. Thus, if urinary loss *per urethram* can be induced by increasing p_{abd} alone, then the outlet (sphincteric mechanism) must be incompetent. As stated above, if the urethra leaks with increases in p_{abd}, this may be due to a lack of urethral support associated with urethral hypermobility in females, poor outlet closure (ISD) in males or females, or a combination of both in females. Surgical procedures designed to restore the urethra to its proper resting position and to keep it there during excursions in p_{abd} do not resolve incontinence related to poor urethral sphincteric function (ISD). To obviate that problem, surgeons have performed slings or implanted artificial sphincters to compress the urethra, but increasing urethral resistance to p_{abd} may result in a parallel increase in p_{det} with untoward effects on bladder compliance leading to upper urinary tract damage. One does not wish to increase resistance to p_{det} just to obviate stress incontinence produced by increases in p_{abd}, and injectable materials can be used successfully in patients with ISD as they markedly improve the ability of the urethra to resist p_{abd} without changing voiding pressure or the p_{det} at the time of leakage.

PATIENT SELECTION

Injectables are not a panacea for all types of incontinence. Strict criteria for their consideration as a treatment modality have been ascertained and injectables are most suitable for patients with sphincter incompetence and normal detrusor muscle function.

It is important to elucidate if previous surgery has been performed or an underlying neurological disorder exists. The activity precipitating the urinary leakage is important. Patients who leak in the supine position, have bedwetting, or leak with a sensation of urinary urgency do not have genuine SUI and need to be investigated for ISD. Urodynamic studies are performed to evaluate possible bladder causes of incontinence and to evaluate urethral function, easily ascertained by abdominal leak-point pressure (ALPP) (i.e. the p_{abd} required to drive urine through the continence mechanism). This corresponds to urethral opening pressure. Low ALPP ($< 100\,cmH_2O$) resulting in urinary leakage implies ISD. ALPP appears to relate to the grading or severity of incontinence reported by the patient and is less variable and measurement is easier to perform than urethral pressure profilometry. Videourodynamic studies demonstrate an open bladder outlet at rest in the absence of a detrusor contraction, the classic definition of ISD. The ideal patient for the use of injectables to treat incontinence is one with poor urethral function (ISD), normal bladder capacity and compliance, and good anatomical support. Contraindications to injectables include active urinary tract infection, untreated detrusor hyperreflexia, or known hypersensitivity to the proposed injectable agent.

Adult female patients

As stated above, stress incontinence in women can be divided into urethral hypermobility and ISD. In my experience, injectables are most suitable for patients with pure ISD. Therefore, the physical examination is essential to ascertain whether associated prolapse and urethral hypermobility are present. A pelvic examination that shows no urethral mobility with straining or coughing in conjunction with a positive 'stress test' where leakage is seen to occur when the patient strains in the upright position with 200 ml in the bladder constitutes presumptive evidence of ISD. The cotton-swab test is employed, with an angle of greater than 30 degrees signifying urethral hypermobility.[1,2] Radiographically, the presence of an open bladder neck and proximal urethra with the bladder at rest in the absence of a detrusor contraction implies the presence of ISD. Urodynamic investigation is performed to rule out possible detrusor causes of incontinence, as well as to obtain ALPP to evaluate urethral function. This measurement of the abdominal pressure required to induce leakage is a confirmatory step. Patients best suited for suspension procedures and, therefore, less suited for injection therapy are those with urethral hypermobility and high ALPP. Patients with combined ISD and hypermobility are better served, in my experience, with alternative surgical endeavours such as the artificial urinary sphincter or a sling procedure.

Paediatric female patients

In paediatric female patients, although the aetiology of the ISD may be differ from that in adults (e.g. myelodysplasia instead of post-surgical ISD), the criteria of adequate bladder capacity, lack of detrusor dysfunction and lack of anatomical abnormality (hypermobility) in the presence of ISD lead to the best candidates.

INJECTABLE MATERIALS

Historical chronology

The technique of periurethral and intra-urethral injection of material to increase outflow resistance in patients with urinary incontinence is not new. The first report[3] involved 20 patients and described the injection of a sclerosing solution (sodium morrhuate or cod-liver oil) into the anterior vaginal wall. An inflammatory response developed with secondary scarring and resultant compression of the incompetent urethra. Cure or improvement was reported in 17 patients; however, the complications included pulmonary infarction and cardiorespiratory arrest. Quackels[4] reported two patients successfully treated with periurethral paraffin injection without complications. Sachse[5] treated 31 patients with another sclerosing agent, Dondren: 12/24 men with post-prostatectomy incontinence and 4/7 women were reported as cured. Again, however, pulmonary complications were the major drawbacks.

Polytetrafluoroethylene (PTFE)

The first report of the use of PTFE paste in a glycerol base (Polytef; Urethrin) by Berg[6] described three women with surgically induced ISD who experienced resolution of symptoms, although two required a repeat injection. The only complication was asymptomatic bacteriuria in one patient. The use of PTFE injection for incontinence was promulgated in the USA by Politano and associates at the University of Miami for many years.[7–10] However, this procedure did not attain universal acceptance, despite reports from various other centres demonstrating its efficacy.[11–16] These and other studies were extensively reviewed for efficacy and safety by the Department of Technology Assessment of the American Medical Association,[17] which concluded that PTFE injection is a reasonably effective treatment for incontinence and technically easy to perform; however, owing to migration of particles[18] and granuloma formation,[19] the safety of the product remains uncertain. Despite these findings there have been no reports of untoward sequelae in humans. Additionally, this product has had so many reports (listed above) of such great success in so many different types of incontinence problems that they have been treated with incredulity by many physicians. A current investigation into the efficacy and safety of PTFE injections for incontinence due to ISD only has begun under monitoring by the United States Food and Drug Administration (US FDA) and it is hoped that this will clarify many of these concerns with respect to efficacy and safety.

Glutaraldehyde cross-linked bovine collagen (GAX-collagen)

Bovine dermal collagen has long been recognized as a biocompatible biomaterial primarily in the form of resorbable sutures and haemostatic agents. Cross-linking with glutaraldehyde results in a fibrillar collagen with resistance to collagenase digestion and significantly enhanced persistence, with stabilization preventing synesis. For this reason, overcorrection is not necessary or desirable with GAX-collagen implants, as the volume does not undergo rapid shrinkage soon after injection; this is due to the formation of this compact fibrous structure which promotes incorporation into surrounding host connective tissue, with additional production and deposition of new host collagen within the implant.[20] This material does not cause granuloma formation, and migration of particles to distant body sites does not appear at autopsy.[20] Shortliffe et al.[21] reported a small series of 16 men and one woman with demonstrable efficacy in nine (53%) with no adverse complications or adverse effects on urodynamic parameters.

GAX-collagen is a highly purified 35% suspension of bovine collagen in a phosphate buffer containing at least 95% type I collagen and 1–5% type III collagen prepared by selective hydrolysis of the non-helicoidal amino-terminal and carboxy-terminal segments (telopeptides) of the collagen molecules, which has the effect of decreasing the antigenicity[22] and increasing the duration of the implant within the human body by increasing its resistance to collagenase.[23] GAX-collagen is biocompatible and biodegradable and elicits only a minimal inflammatory reaction without foreign body reaction.[24] GAX-collagen begins to degrade in 12 weeks and is completely degraded in 19 months, yet the transformation of the injected material into living connective tissue[25] explains its ability to maintain its effectiveness in nearly 80% of those who have attained continence.[26] Despite US FDA approval for the treatment of ISD in males and females in the latter part of 1993, GAX-collagen does have the potential for eliciting an allergic reaction and, although it is more compatible than PTFE in biological systems, it is considerably more expensive and requires more treatment sessions to attain continence, hence the continued search for a better injectable.

Autologous injectables

Concerns over the negative aspects of PTFE and GAX-collagen discussed above have led to attempts to use autologous materials such as blood and fat.

Autologous blood appears to have no lasting quality. In one small study of 14 women,[27] 30 ml of blood from an antecubital vein in a heparinized syringe was used: within two treatment sessions each patient was rendered continent; however, the duration of continence lasted only 10–17 days, with the resultant recommendation that, in questionable cases, the inexpensive injection of autologous blood under local anaesthesia in an office setting can answer the question whether other injectables are worth the expense and effort for that individual patient.

Autologous fat provides the advantages of ready availability and biocompatibility; it is easily obtainable through liposuction. The first report was by Gonzalez de Gariby et al.[28] in 10 women; in a follow-up report a year after a single injection in 15 women and five men, they noted 'good' results in 33% of the women and none of the post-prostatectomy men,[29] an efficacy that does not compare favourably with PFTE or GAX-collagen. The reason for this appears to be that, in the ultimate fate of the injected fat, only a very small proportion remains viable as neovascularity is never adequately achieved at the centre of the graft to maintain its long-term viability. Some fat integrates as a graft, but only 10–20% survives overall, with 60% lost only 3 weeks after injection,[30] owing to destruction of the normal adipocyte architecture.[31] For this reason the potential advantages of autologous fat over other injectables must be tempered against the uncertain outcome.

Silicone polymers

Macroplastique or Bioplastique are textured polydimethyl siloxane macroparticles (> 100 μm) suspended within a bioexcretable carrier hydrogel of polyvinylpyrrolidone (povidone [PVP]) where the solid particle content is 33% of the total volume. Henly et al.[32] compared migratory and histological tendencies of solid silicone macrospheres with those of smaller silicone particles in dogs: nuclear imaging showed that small particles were disseminated throughout the lung, kidney, brain and lymph nodes 4 months after injection, whereas only one episode of large-particle migration to the lung occurred without associated inflammation. Recently, a number of presentations of early results have been favourable,[33–36] with fewer injection treatments than PTFE, GAX-collagen or autologous fat; however, the concerns over migration of particles and the adverse publicity over silicone gel implants will probably limit the use of this material in the USA.

INTRA-URETHRAL INJECTION TECHNIQUES

The techniques used to inject the varying materials are not difficult, even when the substance requires some special instrumentation, such as liposuction prior to autologous fat injection.[37] However, it is essential to place the material (whichever is utilized) precisely in order to ensure an optimal result. The injections[26] can be performed suburothelially through a needle placed directly through a cystourethroscope (transurethral injection) or periurethrally with a spinal needle or special injector used percutaneously and positioned in the urethral tissues in the suburothelial space while observing the manipulation endoscopically *per urethram* or via ultrasound probe *per vaginam* in females[38] or *per rectum* in male patients;[39] thus, regardless of technique used, the implant is placed within the wall of the urethra (i.e. intra-urethrally), optimally in the lamina propria. The cause of the incontinence, the tissue at the injection site and the plane of delivery of the injectable substance will affect the treatment results. Nearly every patient can be injected under local anaesthesia, which has the added advantage of allowing the patient to stand to perform a few provocative manoeuvres immediately after the injection, in an attempt to cause urinary leakage, which can then be addressed before the patient is released from treatment.

The methods of injection should not pose great difficulty to the surgeon comfortable with transurethral surgery. Precise localization of the site of deposition of the collagen material is essential to ensure an optimal response. Male patients are injected through the transurethral approach, and female patients are injected by either approach. I prefer periurethral injections in female patients, as this approach decreases bleeding complications that hamper visualization and extrusion of the injected material.

Female patients may be injected by a transurethral technique,[40] using a spinal needle inserted percuta-neously through the wall of the urethra while observing needle placement directly by cystoscopy,[41] or transvaginally with the needle placed through the biopsy port of an ultrasound probe.[38] Manoeuvres to help in localization of the needle tip are useful, such as preinjecting during the periurethral technique with methylene blue to enable the surgeon to place the implant more accurately.[42] In either case, the patient is placed in the lithotomy position and 'prepped' in the usual sterile fashion. Topical 2% lignocaine (lidocaine) gel is used in the urethra and 20% benzocaine in the vestibule. The periurethral tissues are infiltrated with 2–4 ml 1% plain lignocaine injected at the 3 o'clock and 9 o'clock positions. Use of a female sound to straighten the urethra may be helpful in 'removing' the curve upwards of the urethra at the level of the bladder neck and to guide placement of the periurethral injection of lignocaine. It is most important to emphasize that the material injected should be positioned at the bladder neck and proximal urethra (Fig. 38.1); placement too distally will ultimately be doomed to failure.

Transurethral approach

In the transurethral approach, a zero-degree lens is used. The endoscope is placed at the midurethra and the needle is advanced in the 4 o'clock position. The point of submucosal insertion is immediately beyond midurethra and advanced proximally to the level of the

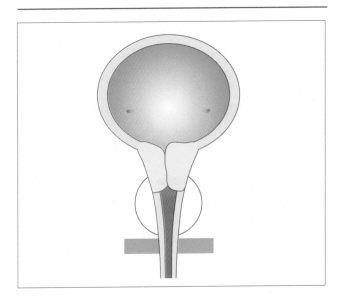

Figure 38.1. *Schematic representation of a cushion of injectable material just below the bladder neck.*

bladder neck. The material is then injected, and the urethral mucosa can be seen to protrude gradually to the midline. It is important to inject slowly, to allow the tissue to accommodate the material adequately. When the mucosal bleb reaches the midline, the needle is withdrawn while the injection is continued slowly. The needle is then repositioned in the 8 o'clock position and the injection is continued until the urethral mucosal blebs again approximate into the midline, creating the appearance of an obstructed prostatic urethra in the male.

Periurethral approach

In the periurethral approach (which I prefer, to minimize intra-urethral bleeding and extravasation of the injectable substance), the goal of creating urethral mucosal coaptation is the same. After infiltration of the periurethral tissues, the appropriately gauged needle (with GAX-collagen this is accomplished with a 20 or 22 gauge standard spinal needle) with the obturator in place is inserted into the periurethral tissue at the 4 o'clock position. The needle should be positioned within the lamina propria; in this plane, the needle advances with minimal resistance. During advancement of the needle, urethroscopy is performed to monitor placement of the needle at the level of the bladder neck. It is quite easy to hold the endoscope with one hand while advancing the needle with the

other hand. Gentle rocking of the needle assists in confirming the proper location and depth of the needle tip. Once this is confirmed, the material is injected, treating a mucosal bleb precisely as in the transurethral technique. Once the mucosal bleb meets the midline, the needle is repositioned in the 8 o'clock position and the injection is carried out on the contralateral side (Fig. 38.2). If extravasation occurs, the needle is repositioned in a more anterior location and the injection is repeated. Once the appearance of obstruction is created by urethral coaptation, the procedure is terminated.[43]

In order to avoid instrumentation of the urethra and running the risk of compressing the freshly placed implant by the endoscope, transvaginal ultrasound-guided injections have been demonstrated to work equally as well.[38] Regardless of the technique of injection chosen, the goal is closure of the bladder outlet in such a way that there is mucosal apposition, as demonstrated endoscopically (Fig. 38.3).

For paediatric patients, the techniques are identical to those for adults. Williams needles as small as 3.7 F are available for the less viscous injectable implants (e.g. GAX-collagen).

POSTOPERATIVE CARE

Perioperative antibiotic coverage is recommended even when the preprocedure urinalysis is normal for 2–3

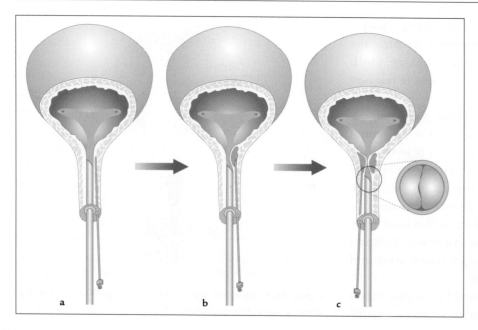

Figure 38.2. *(a) Apperance of the urethra prior to treatment; (b) periurethral needle positioned in the proximal urethra below the bladder neck (note submucosal location within the lamina propria); (c) urethra following injection.*

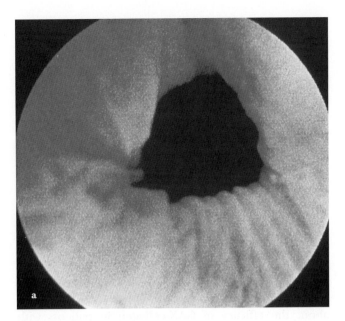
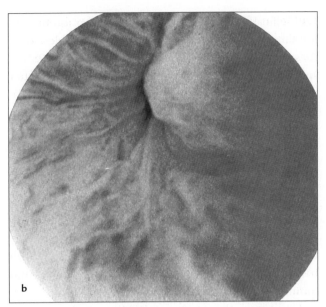

Figure 38.3. *Endoscopic appearance of the bladder neck from midurethra in a female patient with intrinsic sphincter deficiency before (a) and after (b) collagen injection.*

days. Most patients are able to void fairly easily or by Valsalva technique following the procedure. However, if urinary retention should occur, clean intermittent catheterization should be utilized with a 10–14 F catheter. Indwelling catheters should be avoided in patients undergoing implantation, as this promotes moulding of the intra-urethral material around the catheter. Although rarely necessary, if long-term catheterization is needed, I recommend suprapubic cystotomy until voiding has again been initiated.

Scheduled repeat injection treatment sessions for those requiring more implant should be based upon the desired period of time for the substance used: for example, GAX-collagen can be reinjected within a week (however, I prefer to wait 4 weeks), whereas with PTFE a wait of at least 4 months is recommended because syneresis may result in improved coaptation and continence with time.

EFFICACY OF INJECTABLE TREATMENT

No controlled, long-term follow-up reports are available on any injectable substance in male, female or paediatric patients. In fact, it is difficult to glean information as to the aetiology of the incontinence in any of these groups. For example, many groups report their results of the use of injectables in stress incontinence without differentiating between patients with hypermobility, those with ISD and those with both. There has been very little in the way of objective reporting – mostly subjective patient statements of cure, improvement or failure. Additionally, mixed techniques of injection and instrumentation are often intertwined. Regrettably, I am among the investigators who have failed to report the data as cleanly as 'true' science requires. All of this means that results are really a combination of anecdotal reporting mixed with conjecture, speculation and the hope that the truth is involved. In evaluating the results of intra-urethral injections these procedures are compared with slings and the artificial sphincter. Having stated this, it appears that injectables are very helpful for some incontinent patients. Recently, primarily due to the fact that it was used in the North American GAX-collagen Study, a subjective grading of incontinence has been used to evaluate treatment success or failure. Improvement is noted when there appears to be a decrease in the grade of incontinence, as stated by the patient. Cure includes those patients with 'social continence', a term coined by Brantley Scott *et al.*[44] meaning that any perceived wetting by the patient is controlled with the use of tissues or a minipad. Patients rendered dry or socially continent are considered successful in evaluation of these results. If one also includes as cured those dry individuals who must empty their bladders with self-catheterization, results may appear astounding for slings, the artificial sphincter and injectables. With these criteria, sling surgery is successful in 81–98%,[45] sphincter surgery in over 90% (regardless of whether the abdominal[46] or transvaginal[47] approach is utilized), PTFE injections in 70–95%,[16] GAX-collagen in 64–95%,[41] fat in 70–90%,[37] and silicone macrospheres in 70–82%.[33,36] As all of these procedures appear to have comparable success rates, the question arises as to the reasons for lack of universal acceptance of injectables. There are two major disadvantages to the use of injectables:[48] these are (1) the inability to determine the quantity of material needed for an individual patient and (2) the safety of non-autologous products for injection with respect to migration, foreign body reaction and immunological effects.

In women, the results of PTFE paste for incontinence have been relatively good, at least in the short term.[17] A recent report[49] of women followed for 21–72 months (mean 49 months) is less encouraging, with a success rate of only 38% and the occurrence of late local side effects such as fibrosis in the urethra and bladder granuloma balls in 15%, indicating a need for a more inert substance.

Recent reports with autologous fat have had less than impressive results.[50,51] Santarosa and Blaivas[51] reported on 12 women with ISD, where 83% were improved subjectively, but this improvement appeared to drop precipitously at 1 year. Additionally, the role of injectable fat in urethral hypermobility is not reliable or efficacious.[52] Therefore, although autologous fat injections seem to work reasonably well for ISD, the long-term follow-up requires further assessment, as it appears that autologous fat undergoes a rapid rate of reabsorption due to its high water content.

The first report of silicone particles used for incontinence in women appeared in 1992 and was encouraging, with a short-term cure rate of 82% in 84 patients.[33] When the follow-up ran to 14 months the cure rate was 70%.[36] Obviously, more and longer trials are necessary to determine the true efficacy using this injectable agent.

This leads the discussion to the most widely used injectable at present, GAX-collagen. The summary of the North American multicentre clinical investigation was presented in 1994:[53] 127 women with ISD were followed-up for 1 year and 88 were followed-up for 2 years. Of the patients followed-up for 2 years, 46% were dry and

another 34% 'socially continent', meaning significantly improved with management for urinary leakage by a single minipad or tissues. This was accomplished with a rise in ALPP of 40 cmH$_2$O. Continent women received a mean volume of 18.4 ml GAX-collagen implanted over a mean of 2.1 ($\pm$ 1.5) treatment sessions. Once attaining continence, 77% remain dry and do not require a repeat injection. It had previously been reported that 55% of women could regain continence after a single treatment session.[54]

These multicentre results have been supported by other worldwide independent studies[55–62] and compare favourably with results obtained using slings and the artificial sphincter for ISD.[48] Although the success and efficacy of collagen implantation for females with ISD has been reproduced in these series, debate exists about the efficacy of GAX-collagen in patients with type II hypermobility of the vesicourethral junction, genuine anatomical SUI. Eckford and Abrams[60] treated 25 female patients with SUI and reported 80% cured or improved 36 months after injection with GAX-collagen, again with markedly improved ALPP. However, 90% of the women had prior surgery and it is difficult to determine from the paper whether these patients had hypermobility alone or ISD. Furthermore, 72% required re-treatment and it is difficult to accept the 36-month follow-up from the first injection and an 80% cure rate. Herschorn et al.[55] reported equal success rates among patients with hypermobility and patients with ISD; however, the number of injections and the amount of material injected were higher in patients with anatomical urinary incontinence. It has also been documented that elderly female patients with anatomical incontinence do well with the injections of GAX-collagen.[63] This contrasts with the 17 patients from the North American multicentre trial with hypermobility, where the early 82.3% success was short-lived, as all 17 patients required bladder-neck suspension surgery within 2 years of the initial 'dryness'.[64]

Reports of the use of injectables in children are sparse. Vorstman et al.[10] reported on 11 children (nine girls and two boys) injected with PTFE: of the four girls with myelodysplasia or sacral agenesis, 50% were rendered dry and required intermittent catheterization to empty; the other five girls and the two boys had ISD due to previous surgery and the success rate was 85.7%. Appell[48] reported on 14 children treated with GAX-collagen, where 5/6 boys and all of the eight girls were rendered continent; however, the volume of material needed was significant (31.8 ml for the boys and 14.5 ml for the girls). ALPP rose by 56.5 cmH_2O in the boys and 23.6 cmH_2O in the girls. Wan et al.[65] treated eight children with GAX-collagen, with an 7/8 cured at 14 months. More recently, the Cleveland Clinic experience[66] in treating seven children with GAX-collagen for ISD was presented where 4/7 are dry but the other three had no benefit from multiple injections, and it appears that the children who do benefit have large bladder capacities and moderate (as opposed to severe) ISD.

COMPLICATIONS

Perioperative complications associated with periurethral injections are uncommon. The rate of urinary retention in patients undergoing PTFE injections is approximately 20–25%;[67] these patients may require a transient period of catheterization. In the multicentre US clinical trial of GAX-collagen injections, transient urinary retention developed in approximately 15% of patients.[68] Indwelling catheters are avoided in these patients, as this promotes moulding of the GAX-collagen around the catheter, resulting in a failure. Therefore, if intermittent catheterization is not feasible, suprapubic trochar cystotomy should be performed.

Irritative voiding symptoms develop in 20% of patients following injection of PTFE, but resolve after several days[14] and urinary tract infection is stated to be 2%.[13] With GAX-collagen, only 1% of patients experienced irritative voiding symptoms while 5% had a urinary tract infection.[68] After PTFE injection, patients have been noted to develop fever with negative blood and urine cultures at a rate of about 25%, this also resolves after a few days and probably indicates a mild allergic response, especially in the 5% who also report perineal discomfort that spontaneously resolves.[67,69]

During injection, perforation and extravasation of the injected material can occur if the mucosa is disrupted. This may also result in minor urethral bleeding. Whereas the transurethral technique is mandatory in male patients, these complications of bleeding and extrusion of the injectable material are eliminated by injecting by the periurethral approach in female patients. With GAX-collagen, extravasation is generally not a problem as the material is easily flushed away in the urinary stream; however, during injection of PTFE,

any extrusion of material can be problematic as it may be difficult to remove from the lumen.

Regardless of the material, the act of repeated injection into the urethra may result in some other minor complications. A recent report[70] of sterile abscess formation at the injection site after routine transurethral injection of collagen may, again, indicate an advantage in using the periurethral approach.

SAFETY

When PTFE is injected, the acute reaction following injection is a histiocytic and giant cell response with an ingrowth of fibroblasts among the small PTFE particles. This creates a compression of the tissue at the injection site; subsequently, foreign body giant cells and granuloma formation are seen at the site of injection with encapsulation of the material. After injection of PTFE, the particles are found within lymphatics and blood vessels. Particles have also been found 1 year after injection in the pelvic lymph nodes, lungs, brain, kidneys and spleen of animal models.[18,71] In humans, PTFE particle migration to the lungs has been documented in two patients: the first report, by Mittleman and Marraccini,[19] described a PTFE granuloma in the lung of a patient 2 years after injection; another case has been reported with an apparent clinically significant febrile response.[72] A PTFE granuloma has also been reported to mimic a cold thyroid nodule several months after injection.[73] No adverse clinical events were attributable to these findings by Mittelman and Marraccini[19] or Sanfilippo et al.[73] However, the first clinically significant case of migration of PTFE following injection therapy was reported by Claes et al.[72] Their patient had received injections of PTFE for urinary incontinence 3 years prior to presenting with unexplained fevers associated with new lung lesions. A bronchial lavage and lung biopsy revealed PTFE granulomas with surrounding inflammation.

The major concern associated with the use of PTFE particles is that, following particle migration, there is foreign body granuloma formation and this has the potential to be carcinogenic – sarcoma formation has been induced in rats and mice following implantation of material similar to PTFE,[74] and chondrosarcoma of the larynx 6 years after PTFE injections for the treatment of vocal cord paralysis has been reported.[75] It is important to note that no case of carcinogenesis has been identified following widespread use of this material for over 30 years in laryngeal and urethral augmentation procedures. A complete review[76] concluded that PTFE does not have any carcinogenic potential: there have been only three reported cases of malignancy adjacent to PTFE implants, and no cause and effect has been demonstrated.[75,77,78] However, the fear of this potential problem has caused many to reserve the use of PTFE for older patients and, recently, PTFE for injection has been withdrawn from the market by the US FDA, although it has allowed a long-term study to begin comparing PTFE and GAX-collagen for efficacy and safety.

GAX-collagen, as stated, is both biocompatible and biodegradable. The low concentration of glutaraldehyde minimizes the immunoreactivity and cytotoxicity of the implant; therefore, this substance elicits no foreign body reaction as it becomes incorporated into the host tissue.[79] A minimal inflammatory response has been associated with the injection of GAX-collagen, but no granuloma formation was present.[80] GAX-collagen begins to degrade in 12 weeks; however, neovascularization and deposition of fibroblasts with host collagen formation occurs within the implant.[81] The GAX-collagen degrades completely within 10–19 months[24] and there are no reports of particle migration of the collagen material as it is transformed into living connective tissue.[25] Owing to the minimal inflammatory response and no evidence of migration, GAX-collagen is the most widely used bulk-enhancing agent for the treatment of incontinence in adults and children.

Safety of GAX-collagen is further enhanced by the use of a dermal skin test with the more immunogenic non-cross-linked bovine collagen. Although those with a positive skin test could conceivably not suffer from injection with the less immunogenic GAX-collagen, this is not advised. Positive skin tests in the multicentre study amounted to less than 4% of female patients.[53] This is important because there have been legal claims by patients who had collagen injections for soft-tissue augmentation (facial plastic surgery techniques) of signs and symptoms of collagen-vascular disorders such as dermatomyositis. Despite these claims, there has been no evidence to link injections of bovine collagen with any disorder.[48] The patient population has, thus far, actually had a lower incidence of such disorders than would be expected in the general population,[20] and no plaintiffs have been able to glean support during litigation.

THE PRESENT AND FUTURE ROLES OF INJECTABLES FOR INCONTINENCE

In properly selected patients with ISD, periurethral injections offer excellent results. Patients with no anatomical hypermobility and ISD in the presence of a stable bladder of adequate capacity appear to be the most satisfactory candidates for periurethral injections. GAX-collagen is the most widely used injectable, as it has been shown to be both biocompatible and biodegradable. There are no reports of particle migration with this material, and repeat injections can be performed safely under local anaesthesia. Autologous fat has been the alternative in intra-urethral injectables, particularly in patients who have had positive skin tests to the collagen material.

The treatment response in female patients undergoing these procedures is similar to that in those undergoing surgical procedures to correct ISD, and the complications are minimal. Although there are few reports of long-term results (>5 years) for all of these procedures in the literature, injected patients have been followed-up for only short periods and the data available do not take into consideration reinjection rates, which run as high as 22% with collagen at 2 years after attaining dryness[43] and this affects the cost of this therapy. Additionally, in male patients, the success rate of intra-urethral injections does not approach that of the artificial urinary sphincter, to date. On the other hand, minimal perioperative complications are associated with the use of injectables

In selected elderly and less mobile female patients with anatomical incontinence, recent data suggest that collagen may be useful. The use of periurethral injections in the treatment of ISD certainly has a role in the treatment of the correctly selected patient, and allows treatment of incontinence in patients who are poor candidates for surgery and may be denied other forms of therapy.

Injectables must be considered to still be in the developmental stages and their roles in the management of incontinence still need to be defined more precisely; the development of new, non-migrating, safe and technically simple-to-use injectables must also be considered. The optimal substance must be inert and non-degradable; it must become encapsulated and remain where injected, and must neither lose nor gain bulk (syneresis). It must not be too viscous, so that it can be injected with standard cystoscopic equipment used for other purposes under local anaesthesia in an outpatient setting, in order to keep the procedure safe and cost-effective. Additionally, more accurate techniques for determining the quantity of material to inject in an individual must be developed in order to achieve the optimal result in a single treatment session. This 'wish list' for injectable therapy is not beyond our ability to develop.

REFERENCES

1. Crystle CD, Charme LS, Copeland WE. Q-tip test in stress urinary incontinence. *Obstet Gynecol* 1971; 39: 313–315

2. Appell RA, Ostergard D. *Practical Urodynamics. Illustrated Medicine, Female Urology Series, Volume 2.* New York: MP Partners, 1992; 4–9

3. Murless BC. The injection treatment of stress incontinence. *J Obstet Gynaecol Br Emp* 1938; 45: 67–73

4. Quackels R. Deux incontinence après adenonectomie queries par injection de paraffine daris de perinée. *Acta Urol Belg* 1955; 23: 259–262

5. Sachse H. Treatment of urinary incontinence with sclerosing solutions, indications, results, complications. *Urol Int* 1963; 15: 225–244

6. Berg S. Polytef augmentation urethroplasty: correction of surgically incurable urinary incontinence by injection technique. *Arch Surg* 1973; 107: 379–381

7. Politano VA, Small MP, Harper JM, Lynne CM. Periurethral Teflon injection for urinary incontinence. *J Urol* 1974; 111: 180–183

8. Lewis RI, Lockhart JL, Politano VA. Periurethral polytetrafluoroethylene injection in incontinent female subjects with neurogenic bladder disease. *J Urol* 1984; 131: 459–462

9. Kaufman M, Lockhart JL, Silverstein MJ, Politano VA. Transurethral polytetrafluoroethylene injection for post-prostatectomy urinary incontinence. *J Urol* 1984; 132: 463–464

10. Vorstman B, Lockhart JL, Kaufman MR, Politano VA. Polytetrafluoroethylene injections for urinary incontinence in children. *J Urol* 1985; 133: 248–250

11. Heer H. Die behandlung der harnin-kontinenz mit der Teflon-paste. *Urol Int* 1977; 32: 295–302

12. Lampante I, Kaesler FP, Sparwasser H. Endourethrale submuckose tefloninjektion zur erzielung von harninkontinenz. *Aktuel Urol* 1979; 10: 265–272

13. Lim KB, Ball AJ, Feneley RCL. Periurethral Teflon injection: a simple treatment for urinary incontinence. *Br J Urol* 1983; 55: 208–210

14. Schulman CC, Simon J, Wespes F, Germeau F. Endoscopic injection of Teflon for female urinary incontinence. *Eur Urol* 1983; 9: 246–247

15. Deane AM, English P, Hehir M *et al.* Teflon injection in stress incontinence. *Br J Urol* 1985; 57: 78–80

16. Appell RA. Commentary: periurethral polytetrafluoroethylene (Polytef™) injection. In: Whitehead ED (ed) *Current Operative Urology.* Philadelphia: Lippincott, 1990; 63–66

17. Cole HM (ed). Diagnostic and therapeutic technology assessment (DATTA). *J Am Med Assoc* 1993; 269: 2975–2980

18. Malizia AA Jr, Reiman JM, Myers RP *et al.* Migration and granulomatous reaction after periurethral injection of Polytef (Teflon). *J Am Med Assoc* 1984; 251: 3277–3281

19. Mittleman RE, Marraccini JV. Pulmonary Teflon granulomas following periurethral Teflon injection for urinary incontinence. *Arch Pathol Lab Med* 1983; 107: 611–612

20. DeLustro F, Keefe J, Fong AT, Jolivette DM. The biochemistry, biology, and immunology of injectable collagens: Contigen™ Bard collagen implant in treatment of urinary incontinence. *Pediatr Surg Int* 1991; 6: 245–251

21. Shortliffe LM, Freiha FS, Kessler R *et al.* Treatment of urinary incontinence by the periurethral implantation of glutaraldehyde cross-linked collagen. *J Urol* 1989; 141: 538–541

22. DeLustro F, Dasch J, Keefe J, Ellingsworth L. Immune response to allogeneic and xenogeneic implants of collagen and collagen derivatives. *Clin Orthop* 1990; 260: 263–179

23. McPherson J, Sawamura S, Armstrong R. An examination of the biologic response to injectable glutaraldehyde cross-lined collagen implants. *J Biomed Mater Res* 1986; 20: 93–97

24. Canning DA, Peters CA, Gearhart JR, Jeffs RD. Local tissue reaction to glutaraldehyde cross-linked bovine collagen in the rabbit bladder. *J Urol* 1988; 139: 258–259

25. Remacle M, Marbaix E. Collagen implants in the human larynx. *Arch Otorhinolaryngol* 1988; 245: 203–209

26. Appell RA. Collagen injection therapy for urinary incontinence. *Urol Clin North Am* 1994; 21: 177–182

27. Appell RA. Unpublished data. (Presented at the American Urogynecologic Society Annual Meeting, Toronto, 1994.)

28. Gonzalez de Gariby AS, Castro-Morrondo JM, Castro-Jimeno JM. Endoscopic injection of autologous adipose tissue in the treatment of female incontinence. *Arch Esp Urol* 1989; 42: 143–146

29. Gonzalez de Gariby AS, Castillo-Jimeno JM, Villanueva-Perez PI. Treatment of urinary stress incontinence using paraurethral injection of autologous fat. *Arch Esp Urol* 1991; 44: 595–600

30. Bartynski J, Marion MS, Wang TD. Histopathologic evaluation of adipose autografts in a rabbit ear model. *Otolaryngol Head Neck Surg* 1990; 102: 314

31. Nguyen A, Krystyna AP, Bouvier JN. Comparative study of survival of autologous adipose tissue taken and transplanted by different techniques. *Plast Reconstr Surg* 1990; 85: 378

32. Henly DR, Barrett DM, Esiland TL *et al*. Particulate silicone for use in periurethral injections: local tissue effects and search for migration. *J Urol* 1995; 153: 2039–2043

33. Buckley JF, Scott R, Meddings R *et al*. Injectable silicone microparticles: a new treatment for female stress incontinence. *J Urol* (Pt 2) 1992; 147: 280A

34. Patterson PJ, Buckley JF, Smith M, Kirk D. Injectable silicone macroparticles for post-prostatectomy incontinence. *J Urol* (Pt 2) 1993; 149: 235A

35. Iacovou J, Lemberger J, James M, Kockelbergh R. Periurethral silicone microimplants for the treatment of simple stress incontinence: a one year follow-up. *J Urol* (Pt 2) 1993; 149: 402A

36. Buckley JF, Lingham K, Lloyd SN *et al*. Injectable silicone macroparticles for female urinary incontinence. *J Urol* (Pt 2) 1993; 149: 402A

37. Ganabathi K, Leach GE. Periurethral injection techniques. *Atlas Urol Clin North Am* 1994; 2: 101–109

38. Appell RA. Treatment of intrinsic sphincter dysfunction. Collagen injections. In: Raz S (ed) *Female Urology*, 3rd edn. Philadelphia: Saunders, 1996; 399

39. Kageyama S, Kawabe K, Susuki K *et al*. Collagen implantation for post-prostatectomy incontinence: early experience with a transrectal ultrasonographically guided method. *J Urol* 1994; 152: 1473–1475

40. O'Connell HE, McGuire FJ, Aboseifs UA. Transurethral collagen therapy in women. *J Urol* 1995; 154: 1463–1465

41. Appell RA. Injectables for urethral incompetence. *World J Urol* 1990; 8: 208–211

42. Neal ED Jr, Lahaye ME, Lowe DC. Improved needle placement technique in periurethral collagen injection. *Urology* 1995; 45: 865–866

43. Winters JC, Appell RA. Periurethral injection of collagen in the treatment of intrinsic sphincteric deficiency in the female patient. *Urol Clin North Am* 1995; 22: 673–678

44. Scott FB, Bradley WE, Timm GW. Treatment of urinary incontinence by an implantable prosthetic sphincter. *Urology* 1973; 1: 252–259

45. Blaivas JG. Treatment of female incontinence secondary to urethral damage or loss. *Urol Clin North Am* 1991; 18: 355–363

46. Light JK, Scott FB. Management of urinary incontinence in women with the artificial urinary sphincter. *J Urol* 1985; 134: 476–478

47. Appell RA. Technique and results in the implantation of the artificial urinary sphincter in women with type III stress urinary incontinence by a vaginal approach. *Neurourol Urodyn* 1988; 7: 613–619

48. Appell RA. Use of collagen injections for treatment of incontinence and reflux. *Adv Urol* 1992; 5: 145–165

49. Buckley JF, Lingham K, Meddings RN, Scott R. Injectable Teflon paste for female stress incontinence: long-term follow-up and results. *J Urol* (Pt 2) 1993; 149: 418A

50. Cervigni M. Panei M. Periurethral autologous fat injection for type III stress urinary incontinence. *J Urol* (Pt 2) 1993; 149: 403A

51. Santarosa RP, Blaivas JG. Periurethral injections of autologous fat for the treatment of sphincteric incontinence. *J Urol* 1994; 151: 607–611

52. Blaivas JG, Herwitz D, Santarosa RP *et al*. Periurethral fat injection or sphincteric incontinence in women. *J Urol* (Pt 2) 1994; 151: 419A

53. Appell RA, McGuire FJ, DeRidder PA *et al*. Summary of effectiveness and safety in the prospective, open, multi-center investigation of contigen implant for incontinence due to intrinsic sphincteric deficiency in females. *J Urol* (Pt 2) 1994; 151: 418A

54. Appell RA. New developments; injectables for urethral incompetence in women. *Int Urogynecol J* 1990; 1: 117–119

55. Herschorn S, Radomski SB, Steele DJ. Early experience with intraurethral collagen injection for urinary incontinence. *J Urol* 1992; 148: 1797–1800

56. Striker P, Jaylen B. Injectable collagen for type 3 female stress incontinence: the first 50 Australian patients. *Med J Aust* 1993; 158: 89–91

57. Swami SK, Eckford SD, Abrams P. Collagen injections for female stress incontinence: conclusions of a multistage analysis and results. *J Urol* (Pt 2) 1994; 151: 479A

58. Goldenberg SL, Warkentin MJ. Periurethral injection for patients with stress urinary incontinence. *J Urol* (Pt 2) 1994; 151: 479A

59. Richardson TD, Kennelly MJ, Faerber GJ. Endoscopic injection of glutaraldehyde cross-linked collagen for the treatment of intrinsic sphincteric deficiency in women. *Urology* 1995; 46: 378–381

60. Eckford SD, Abrams P. Para-urethral collagen implantation for female stress incontinence. *Br J Urol* 1991; 68: 586–589

61. Monga AK, Robinson D, Stanton SL. Periurethral collagen injections for genuine stress incontinence: a 2-year follow-up. *Br J Urol* 1995; 75: 156

62. Smith DN, Appell RA, Winters JC, Rackley RR. Collagen injection therapy for female intrinsic sphincteric deficiency. *J Urol* 1997; 157: 1275–1278

63. Faerber GJ. Endoscopic collagen injection therapy for elderly women with type I stress urinary incontinence. *J Urol* (Pt 2) 1995; 153: 527A

64. Press SM, Badlani GH. Injection therapy for urinary incontinence. *AUA Update Ser* 1995; 14: 14–20

65. Wan J, McGuire EJ, Bloom DA, Ritchey ML. The treatment of urinary incontinence in children using glutaraldehyde cross-linked collagen. *J Urol* 1992; 147: 127–130

66. Ross JR, Kay R, Appell R. Unpublished data. (Presented at the 69th Annual Meeting of the North Central Section, AUA, Minneapolis, 1995.)

67. Politano VA. Periurethral polytetrafluoroethylene injection for urinary incontinence. *J Urol* 1982; 127: 439–442

68. Bard CR Inc. PMAA submission to United States Food and Drug Administration for IDE #G850010, 1990

69. Politano VA. Periurethral Teflon injection or urinary incontinence. *Urol Clin North Am* 1978; 5: 415–422

70. Sweat SD, Lightner DJ. Complications of sterile abscess formation and pulmonary embolism following periurethral bulking agents. *J Urol* 1999; 161: 93–96

71. Vandenbossche M, Delhobe O, Dumortier P *et al.* Endoscopic treatment of reflux: experimental study and review of Teflon and collagen. *Eur Urol* 1994; 23: 386

72. Claes H, Stroobants D, van Meerbeck J *et al.* Pulmonary migration following periurethral polytetrafluoroethylene injection for urinary incontinence. *J Urol* 1989; 142: 821–822

73. Sanfilippo F, Shelburne J, Ingram P. Analysis of a polytef granuloma mimicking a cold thyroid nodule 17 months after laryngeal injection. *Ultrastruct Pathol* 1980; 1: 471–475

74. Oppenheimer BS, Oppenheimer ET, Stout AP *et al.* The latent period in carcinogenesis by plastics in rats and its relation to the presarcomatous stage. *Cancer* 1958; 11: 204–213

75. Hakky M, Kolbusz R, Reyes CV. Chondrosarcoma of the larynx. *Ear Nose Throat J* 1989; 68: 60–62

76. Dewan PA. Is injected polytetrafluoroethylene (Polytef) carcinogenic? *Br J Urol* 1992; 69: 29–33

77. Lewy RB. Experience with vocal cord injection. *Ann Otol Rhinol Laryngol* 1976; 85: 440–450

78. Montgomery WW. Laryngeal paralysis – Teflon injection. *Ann Otol* 1979; 88: 647–657

79. Ford CN, Martin CW, Warren TF. Injectable collagen in laryngeal rehabilitation. *Laryngoscope* 1984; 95: 513–518

80. Delustro F, Condell RA, Nguyen MA, McPherson JM. A comparative study of the biologic and immunologic response to medical devices derived from dermal collagen. *J Biomed Mater Res* 1986; 20: 109–120

81. Stegman S, Chu S, Bensch K, Armstrong R. A light and electron microscopic evaluation of Zyderm and Zyplast implants in aging human facial skin: a pilot study. *Arch Dermatol* 1987; 123: 1644–1649

39

Vaginal approaches for the treatment of stress incontinence

Y. H. Kim, V. W. Nitti

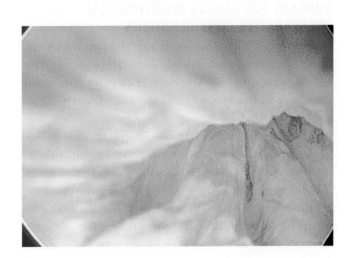

INTRODUCTION

There are a variety of treatments for stress incontinence, including physiotherapy, electrical stimulation, medications, devices, periurethral bulking agents and surgery. The type of treatment chosen by patient and physician will depend upon a multitude of factors, including the type and severity of stress incontinence, patient preference, patient expectations from treatment, co-morbid medical conditions and concomitant genitourinary condition such as prolapse and bladder dysfunction. When surgical treatment is being considered, it is important that the patient is carefully evaluated to determine the aetiology of stress incontinence, the presence of pelvic organ prolapse (which should be corrected at the time of surgery) and the potential for surgery to contribute to prolapse in the future (so that preventative measures can be taken). Similarly, prior to surgical management of vaginal prolapse, the presence of stress incontinence (or potential for it to occur after vaginal prolapse is corrected) should be determined.

A variety of surgical approaches to treat stress incontinence have been introduced during the past century. These include a multitude of retropubic, transvaginal and sling procedures, each having advantages and disadvantages for a given patient. This chapter outlines the various transvaginal surgical options. When evaluating the published literature on such treatments it is critical to look at how success is defined (cured vs 'improved') and the length of follow-up. Most procedures reported in the literature have excellent results in the short term (1–2 years), but may not have durable results in the longer term.

SURGERY FOR STRESS INCONTINENCE: PREOPERATIVE CONSIDERATIONS

Stress urinary incontinence is the involuntary loss of urine with increased intra-abdominal pressure. The aetiology of stress incontinence is described in detail elsewhere in this volume. From a surgical perspective, stress incontinence has classically been divided into two types: these are (1) anatomical incontinence due to urethral hypermobility or a support defect, and (2) intrinsic sphincter deficiency (ISD) due to failure of the intrinsic urethral sphincter mechanism to provide adequate resistance, independent of position or support.[1] It has been difficult to determine the presence or degree of ISD in patients with urethral hypermobil-

ity. The problem with such a classification system is that it looks at the condition as a static rather than a dynamic condition. Recently, DeLancey[2] has emphasized the importance of urethral and bladder neck support, intrinsic urethral sphincter function and the contribution of the levator ani muscles to stress continence. This requires adequate connective tissue and muscular support and function, as well as intact neural innervation. Breakdown to various degrees of one or more of these can result in stress incontinence. Failure of certain surgical procedures to treat stress incontinence adequately may be due in part to incomplete understanding of the causes of incontinence in a given patient.

The work of DeLancey has helped us to understand the mechanisms at work in providing stress continence in female patients.[3] Urethral and bladder-neck support is normally provided by the hammock-like structure which is formed by the anterior vaginal wall and its connection to the arcus tendineus fasciae by the endopelvic fascia. In addition to the passive support provided by this structure, there may also be an active component provided by the attachment of the endopelvic fascia to the levator ani muscles. When there is an increase in intra-abdominal pressure, the urethra lies in such a position that it can be compressed against this supporting hammock. In cases where the supporting structure has been weakened or damaged (e.g. after childbirth), it may no longer be able to provide an adequate backboard upon which the urethra may be compressed. Although many operations to treat stress incontinence were originally based upon the concept of restoring the bladder neck and urethra to a high retropubic position, many in the field of female urology and urogynaecology now believe that such procedures work by restoring support rather than position.

Before surgery is considered for stress incontinence, the following evaluation is recommended by the American Urological Association (AUA) Female Stress Urinary Incontinence Clinical Guidelines Panel:[4]

1. History, including the effect stress incontinence has on the patient's quality of life;
2. Physical examination, including the demonstration of stress incontinence;
3. Urinalysis;
4. 'Other appropriate diagnostic studies' to strengthen the diagnosis of stress incontinence and

evaluate detrusor function, rule out detrusor over-activity and underactivity, and identify ISD and urethral hypermobility.

These components of the patient evaluation, including urodynamic testing, are described in detail elsewhere in this volume.

TRANSVAGINAL PROCEDURES FOR THE TREATMENT OF STRESS URINARY INCONTINENCE

Overview

Most of the transvaginal procedures that have been described were designed to treat anatomical incontinence or urethral hypermobility. Thus, one could predict that if a significant component of ISD were present, patients undergoing such procedures would have a higher incidence of failure.[5] Sling procedures, which can be done transvaginally, treat both a support defect as well as ISD, even if there is no associated urethral hypermobility. Transvaginal procedures, such as the Kelly plication and various needle suspension procedures (see page 496), gained popularity because of surgical ease, relatively low perioperative morbidity and favourable short-term success rates. However, recent reports have suggested that the long-term success rates of such procedures are significantly lower and in some series do not match those of retropubic and sling procedures.

Trockman *et al.*[6] retrospectively reviewed data on 125 women undergoing modified Pereyra bladder-neck suspension with a mean follow-up of 9.8 years: they found only a 51% success rate in treating stress incontinence and a 20% overall dry rate. Kondo *et al.*[7] reported only a 37% rate of continence for women undergoing a Gittes no-incision bladder-neck suspension at 6 years' follow-up. Finally, the AUA Female Stress Urinary Incontinence Clinical Guidelines Panel,[4] in an extensive review of the world literature, found significantly higher long-term (4 years or more) cure rates for retropubic and sling procedures than for transvaginal procedures and anterior repairs, with slightly increased morbidity for the former two procedures (Table 39.1). Therefore, indications for transvaginal procedures appear to have narrowed with the most recent data. It is important to consider factors such as perioperative morbidity, patient's overall medical condition and expectations of treatment in the short and long term. There are select cases where reduced morbidity and/or surgical ease may be opted for in spite of a lower long-term cure or success rate. When there is coexisting genitourinary pathology – such as cystocele, uterine prolapse, enterocele, rectocele, urethral diverticulum, perineal laxity or incompetent anal sphincter – these should be addressed at the same time as a transvaginal incontinence procedure.

BASIC PRINCIPLES

Several basic principles should be adhered to when performing vaginal surgery. The patient should be positioned in a high lithotomy position to allow for adequate exposure. We prefer the use of 'candy cane' stirrups. In addition, the vagina should be carefully scrubbed and 'prepped' with an antimicrobial solution. Broad-spectrum antibiotics are given perioperatively (usually ampicillin and gentamicin or the equivalent)

Table 39.1. *Long-term (48 months and longer) cured/dry and cured/dry/improved rates for various incontinence operations as reported by the American Urological Association Female Stress Urinary Incontinence Clinical Guidelines Panel*

	Cured/dry (%)	Cured/dry/improved (%)
Anterior repairs	61	73
Transvaginal suspensions	67	82
Retropubic suspensions	84	90
Sling procedures	83	87

From ref. 4.

and are continued in an oral form for 7–10 days post-operatively. A weighted speculum maximizes exposure of the operative field. Because of the transient urinary retention that is common after needle suspensions, surgeons have the option of placing a suprapubic catheter at the time of surgery; this can be done percutaneously or by using the Lowsley retractor technique described by Zeidman *et al.*[8] or a similar method. A vaginal packing that can be impregnated with an antimicrobial agent (e.g. povidone solution or bacitracin vaginal ointment) is usually left in the vagina for about 24 hours to prevent bleeding.

Anterior repair with Kelly suburethral plication

The use of anterior vaginal repair or anterior colporrhaphy is still considered by some to be an appropriate treatment for cystourethrocele and associated stress incontinence. Kelly is given much of the early credit in the gynaecological literature for identifying urethral support mechanisms as well as the deficits in these mechanisms that result in stress incontinence (namely musculofascial relaxation of the levator hiatus as a result of childbearing, resulting in a cystourethrocele).[9] The Kelly urethral plication, described in 1914,[10] had been used by gynaecologists as one of the primary ways to repair this condition. In this procedure, a urethral catheter is placed to empty the bladder, thus allowing identification of the urethrovesical junction. Saline may be injected just beneath the vaginal mucosa to 'hydrodissect' the avascular plane just beneath the vaginal mucosa. A midline anterior vaginal wall incision is made from the vaginal apex to the urethral meatus. The avascular plane just beneath the vaginal mucosa is developed sharply laterally to the pubic ramus to dissect the vagina from the bladder, bladder neck and urethra. Two or three non-absorbable vertical mattress sutures are placed at the bladder neck and proximal urethral to plicate and buttress musculofascial tissue bordering the levator hiatus, namely periurethral fascia. Two steps thought to be important in the success of the Kelly plication are (1) elevation of the urethrovesical junction in the retropubic space high above the urogenital diaphragm and (2) restoration of the suburethral fascial support in an effort to 'strengthen' the urethral musculature and

increase intra-urethral pressure.[9] An accompanying cystocele can be repaired by placing absorbable vertical mattress sutures into the mobilized pubocervical or paravesical fascia, also bordering the levator hiatus, to plicate this tissue across midline, elevating and supporting bladder involved in the cystocele. Excess anterior vaginal epithelium is sparingly trimmed to, and then reapproximated across, the midline with absorbable sutures. Aggressive excision of epithelium may result in vaginal stenosis.

Unfortunately, it has been shown that the long-term rates for the cure of stress incontinence using anterior repair (anterior colporrhaphy with Kelly plication) are somewhat disappointing: some reports have cited rates as low as 47%.[4] Specific reports on the use of anterior repair to treat incontinence associated with prolapse have shown continence rates of 48–60%.[11,12] Thus, the procedure may correct central prolapse of a cystourethrocele but has a higher failure rate if used to treat stress incontinence. This is probably because insufficient support is restored in many cases; in addition, anterior colporrhaphy corrects only a central defect and does not address the most common musculofascial defect resulting in cystocele and stress incontinence, which is a defect in the attachment of the paravaginal fascia (urethropelvic ligament and pubocervical fascia) to the arcus tendineus, also described as a lateral defect.[13] In fact, in cases of cystocele repair, this procedure may actually worsen or unmask stress incontinence.[14] Anterior colporrhaphy is appropriate for repair of a cystocele with a central defect, but may result in a recurrent cystocele or *de-novo* stress incontinence if used for a cystocele with lateral defects. However, many experts now feel that anterior colporrhaphy should be discouraged as a primary treatment of stress incontinence.

Needle suspension procedures

The needle bladder-neck suspension procedures all share a similar concept. From the original needle procedure described by Pereyra in 1959 to the newer *in situ* vaginal wall slings and bone anchoring procedures, all attempt to restore urethral support by anchoring native vaginal and paravaginal tissue to the abdominal wall (rectus fascia) or symphysis pubis using special instruments or needles to transfer sutures.

Pereyra

The original needle suspension technique, the first alternative technique to that of the abdominal suspension procedures, was described by Pereyra in 1959.[15] This technique represented a major change in incontinence surgery, attempting to simulate retropubic operations with less morbidity. All transvaginal suspension procedures for the treatment of stress incontinence – including bladder-neck suspensions, suburethral slings and needle suspension cystocele repairs – are based at least in part on the original Pereyra procedure.

Pereyra's original operation used a pair of no. 30 stainless steel wires to suspend para-urethral tissues to the rectus fascia. Special cannulas are passed blindly from a small suprapubic stab incision through the retropubic space to the para-urethral area, about 2–3 cm posterior to the urethral meatus. A trocar component of the cannula is then advanced through the anterior vaginal wall at the level of the bladder neck. The cannula and trocar tips are then threaded with the steel wire and are transferred back to the suprapubic area, disengaged, and the wires clamped. After both sides are completed, the wires' sutures are tied. The para-urethral tissues are cauterized at several points along the proximal urethra roughly 1 cm from the urethra, so that support would be rendered by fibrous tissue after the wires cut through the soft para-urethral tissues.

Modifications of the original Pereyra procedure have resulted in the progressive evolution of the technique. Harer and Gunther[16] modified the technique by introducing a vaginal incision for the purpose of mobilizing the urethra and approximating the para-urethral tissues across the midline. Pereyra and Lebherz[17] introduced the concept of entering the retropubic space by opening the lateral para-urethral tissue, which allowed for fingertip guidance of the passage of the cannula, avoiding blind passage from the suprapubic to the vaginal region. Tauber and Wapner[18] advocated placement of non-absorbable suspension sutures under direct vision into the pubocervical fascia at the level of the bladder neck. The free end of each suture is tied, forming a loop around the encircled portion of the fascia. These sutures are transferred to the suprapubic area via a special needle and tied to each other over the rectus fascia. Winter[19] modified the Pereyra method by passing a straightened 3-inch needle with no. 2 nylon plastic suture from the vagina along the side of the bladder neck to the lower abdominal wall on each side. Cobb and Ragde[20] introduced the double-prong ligature in 1978, which minimized the number of passes necessary for suspension and allowed for a sufficient fascial bridge to support the suspension sutures. These modifications have all been important in the evolution of transvaginal needle suspension surgery for stress incontinence. We now discuss in detail several of the more commonly performed needle suspensions.

Stamey endoscopic bladder-neck suspension

In 1973, Stamey[21] developed several novel concepts to bladder-neck needle suspension. The concept of cystoscopic control was introduced, which allowed for accurate suture placement at the bladder neck and visualization of bladder-neck closure with elevation of the suspension sutures. In addition, bolsters were introduced to support the bladder neck.

In the Stamey endoscopic bladder-neck suspension, two short, transverse suprapubic incisions are made just cephalad to the pubic symphysis. A T-shaped incision is made in the anterior vaginal wall epithelium overlying the proximal urethra and urethrovesical junction, and the vaginal epithelium is dissected off the urethra and urethrovesical junction (Figure 39.1). Special needles, either straight, 15 or 30 degrees, with an eye at the tip large enough to thread a no. 2 nylon suture, are introduced through each suprapubic incision and are directed through the rectus fascia and retropubic space, emerging through periurethral tissue at the level of the urethrovesical junction just lateral to the bladder neck. The needle is guided just alongside the internal vesical neck, which can easily be determined by placing gentle traction on the Foley catheter and palpating the balloon. Cystoscopy confirms movement of the bladder neck with motion of the needle and that there is no penetration of the bladder or urethra. A large permanent suture (no. 2 nylon) is threaded onto the needle, which is drawn back out of the suprapubic incision with the suture. A second pass of the needle is made about 1 cm lateral to the original entry site in the rectus fascia, emerging from the periurethral fascia about 1 cm distal to the nylon suture. Cystoscopy is repeated to determine the needle position; then, the end of the nylon suture is placed through a 1 cm tube of a 5 mm Dacron arterial graft. The suture is then threaded onto the needle, which is again drawn back out of the suprapubic

497

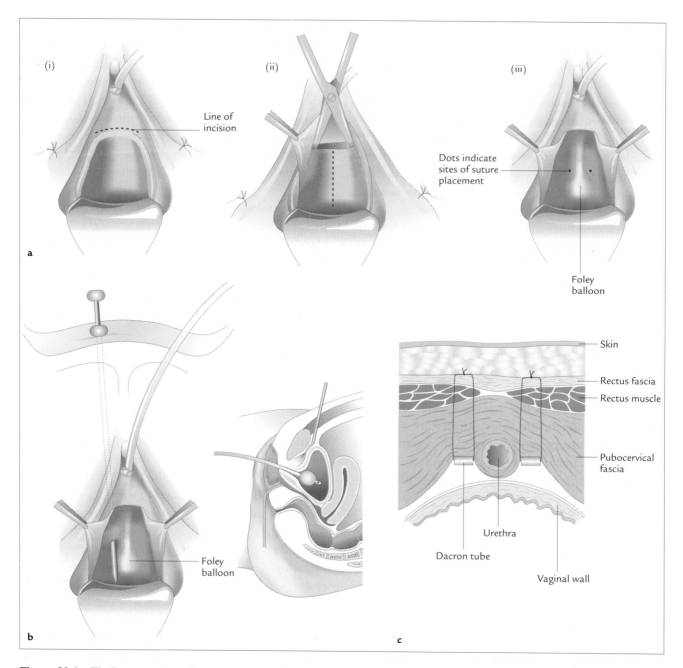

Figure 39.1. *The Stamey endoscopic suspension. (a) 'T'-shaped vaginal incision is performed in three stages to separate the bladder neck from the vaginal epithelium. (b) Passage of Stamey needle during suspension procedure. A vaginal finger palpates the Foley balloon and is used to guide the needle out through the vaginal epithelium. (c) Schematic illustration of the suspending nylon loops on either side of the urethra at the bladder neck.*

incision, creating a suture loop with Dacron bolster that supports a 1 cm bridge of periurethral fascia (Fig. 39.2). The same procedure is repeated on the other side of the bladder neck. Endoscopic examination is performed with traction on the nylon sutures to demonstrate closure of the bladder neck. After place-

ment of a suprapubic catheter, the vaginal wall is closed and the nylon sutures are tied.

In 1980, Stamey[22] reported a 91% cure rate in 203 patients undergoing endoscopic suspension. However, reports by other investigators have shown significantly lower long-term success rates.[23]

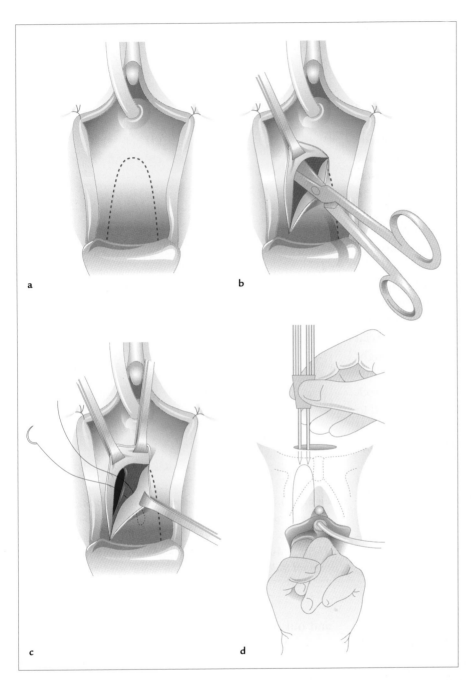

Figure 39.2. *The Raz bladder neck suspension. (a) inverted U incision in the anterior vaginal wall; (b) sharp dissection of the vaginal wall off the glistening surface of the periurethral fascia and sharp perforation of the endopelvic fascia into the retropubic space; (c) no. 1 polypropylene sutures placed in the urethropelvic ligament and vaginal wall minus its epithelium under direct vision; (d) sutures transferred to suprapubic region using a double-pronged ligature carrier passed through the retropubic space under direct finger guidance.*

Raz bladder-neck suspension

Another significant modification of Pereyra's operation is the Raz bladder-neck suspension, described in 1981.[24] This modification incorporated perforation of the endopelvic fascia, placement of sutures into periurethral supporting structures under direct vision, guidance of the needle through the retropubic space under direct finger guidance, the use of polypropylene sutures and endoscopic confirmation of suture placement.

In the Raz bladder-neck suspension, an inverted U (or two parallel oblique incisions) is made in the anterior vaginal wall. The distal extent of the incision is at a point midway between the bladder neck and the external urethral meatus, while proximally the incision extends just proximal to the bladder neck (Fig. 39.2a). Dissection is carried out laterally towards the pubic bone over the glistening surface of the periurethral fascia (Fig. 39.2b). At the level of the bladder neck, the retropubic space is opened sharply with scissors, which should point towards the patient's ipsilateral shoulder upon entering the retropubic space. Once the retropubic space has been opened, the operator's index finger is inserted, and all adhesions along the length of the urethra are bluntly released. Using a long Russian forceps with the jaws separated as a retractor in the retropubic space, no. 1 polypropylene sutures are placed under direct vision into the detached urethropelvic ligament (endopelvic fascia found at the medial edge of the window created in the retropubic space) together with pubocervical fascia and anterior vaginal wall minus the epithelium (Fig. 39.2c). Three or four helical passes through these structures are made, and the strength of the sutures is tested by pulling the patient on the table.

A small transverse lower-abdominal stab incision is made just above the pubic symphysis. A double-pronged needle is passed through the rectus fascial layer under direct finger guidance and is brought through the retropubic space to emerge from the anterior vesicovaginal space at the level of the bladder-neck (Fig. 39.2d). The previously placed suture is attached to the needle and brought through the retropubic space, emerging through the rectus fascia. The anterior vaginal epithelium is closed, and the sutures suspending the periurethral and endopelvic fascia needle are tied over the rectus fascia with minimal tension. Cystoscopy is performed to rule out bladder, urethral or ureteral injury (intravenous indigo carmine, which is administered by the anaesthesiologist, should be seen effluxing from the ureteral orifices) and to ensure that the bladder neck is well supported.

In 1981 Raz reported an initial 96% short-term success rate in the first 100 patients. A subsequent report in 1992 showed a 90% success rate in 206 patients with a mean follow-up of 15 months.[5] The procedure was also reported to have similar results in patients with previous failed surgery.[25] However, studies with longer follow-up reported significantly lower success rates: Trockman et al.[6] reported only a 51% cure rate for stress incontinence and a 20% overall dry rate at a mean follow-up of 9.8 years.

No-incision urethropexy

In 1987, Gittes and Loughlin[26] described a 'no-incision' bladder-neck suspension technique. Without making a vaginal incision, a single-prong needle is passed from a suprapubic stab wound through the retropubic space

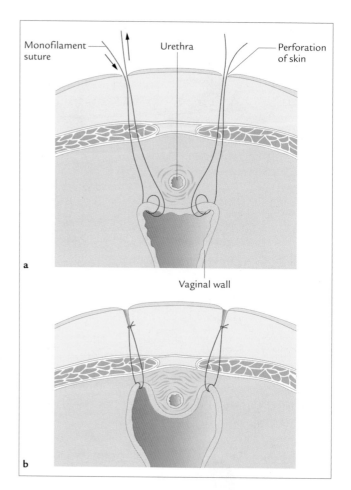

Figure 39.3. *No-incision urethropexy (Gittes procedure). Schematic diagram showing placement of suspension sutures without an incision (a) before, and (b) after, tying sutures. The suspension relies upon a full-thickness helical bite of vaginal wall as shown.*

and out of the vaginal wall at the level of the bladder neck. A heavy nylon or polypropylene suture is threaded into the needle suprapubically and withdrawn to the suprapubic region. A second pass of the needle is made and advanced out of the vaginal wall about 2 cm caudal or cephalad from the first puncture site. Before threading the needle again, a full-thickness helical bite of the vaginal wall is taken between the two vaginal perforations (Fig. 39.3). The suture is threaded and transferred suprapubically; a similar procedure is then performed on the other side. Cystoscopy is performed to confirm elevation of the bladder neck with traction. This procedure relies upon the fact that the suspension sutures will break through the vaginal epithelium and remain buried.

Initially, it was claimed that reduced operative time and hospital stay (as well as the possibility of performance under local anaesthesia) were distinct advantages of the no-incision technique. In their initial report, Gittes and Loughlin reported a continence rate of 87% 2.5 years after surgery.[26] Other authors, however, have questioned the durability of cure using this technique, reporting cure rates of only 37–44% in follow-up to a mean of 6 years.[7,27] Many in the field of female urology and urogynaecology would agree that Gittes modification, although the least invasive of the needle suspensions, is also the least durable.

Bone-anchoring techniques

Leach and Labasky first described anchoring of the suspension sutures to the pubic tubercle in 1989.[28] This technique was advocated to avoid several theoretical disadvantage, such as the risk of suture tearing through fascia, reduction of postoperative pain and 'pulling' (thought to be associated with sutures tied over the abdominal fascia) and proper support of the urethra and bladder neck, regardless of differences in fascia rigidity. In the original procedure, a modified Pereyra or Raz suspension was performed and suspension sutures were passed into the ipsilateral pubic tubercle instead of being anchored to the rectus fascia There was no reported incidence of osteomyelitis or osteitis pubis.

In 1994, Benderev[29] described the use of a metal bone anchor, which was used in conjunction with a special percutaneous kit (Vesica, Boston Scientific, Natick, MA, USA). In this modification of the Gittes procedure, a metal bone anchor with an attached non-absorbable suture is drilled into the pubic bone. A special needle is passed percutaneously several times to incorporate a Z-shaped portion of vaginal wall and paravaginal fascia (Fig. 39.4). Appell *et al.*[30] subsequently reported a 94% cure rate at 12 months. Using the same procedure, Schultheiss and associates reported a 43% cure rate at 11 months mean follow-up.[31]

Nativ and colleagues described another device – the In-Tact bone anchoring system (Influence Inc., San Francisco, CA, USA) – which places bone anchors into the undersurface of the pubic bone directly through the vaginal wall without an incision, using a stapler-like device.[32] A 12-month follow-up in 41 patients showed an 82% cure rate. Again, it must be emphasized that pub-

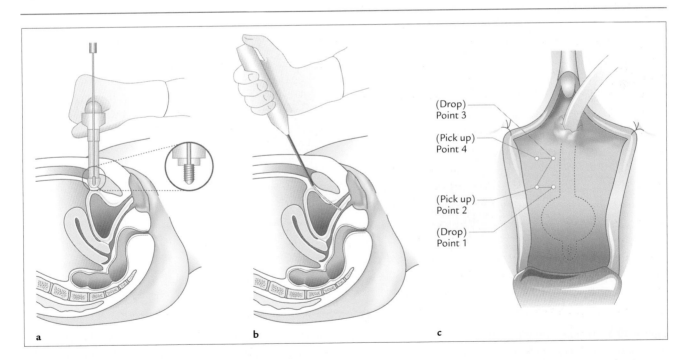

Figure 39.4. *Vesica percutaneous bladder suspension. (a) In this modification of the Gittes no-incision technique, two bone anchors are drilled into the pubic bone on each side of the midline. (b) A special suture passer is used to pass the suture which is attached to the bone anchor through the retropubic space and through the vaginal wall. (c) The suture is then brought back to the suprapubic area and the process is repeated to create a Z-shaped configuration of vaginal wall. The sutures are then tied over a suture spacer to avoid excess tension.*

lished data on this and other similar techniques are based on a relatively short follow-up with respect to success and complications.

Bone-anchoring techniques have recently been applied to a number of anti-incontinence procedures, such as transvaginal bladder-neck suspension, *in situ* vaginal wall sling and pubovaginal sling. It must be emphasized that the theoretical advantages of bone anchoring (more stable point of fixation and less postoperative pain) have not been confirmed in randomized, controlled studies. Furthermore, although initially complications attributable to bone anchors were not described, osteomyelitis has recently been reported.[33]

In situ vaginal wall sling

As an alternative to pubovaginal sling, Raz and associates[34] introduced the *in situ* vaginal wall sling in 1989. The procedure was initially described for the treatment of ISD, but then was also applied to urethral hypermobility. Although described as a sling procedure, the *in situ* vaginal wall sling is conceptually more like a

suspension – re-creating support by reinforcing native structures.

Instead of using a strip of tissue to sling from the rectus fascia to the suburethral area, *in situ* anterior vaginal wall has been used to support and compress the intrinsically damaged urethra. In the original description of the procedure (Fig. 39.5), a rectangular island of anterior vaginal wall is created with the following margins: bladder neck, distal urethra and vaginal fornices. As in the Raz bladder-neck suspension, the periurethral and endopelvic fascia are exposed and penetrated, allowing entrance into the retropubic space, and double-pronged needles are passed from a small suprapubic incision to the vesicovaginal space. Polypropylene sutures (no. 1) are secured to each corner of the sling, including full thickness of the vaginal wall with epithelium and medial edges of periurethral (distal) and endopelvic fascia (proximal), and are threaded through needles and transferred to the abdominal wall. A proximally based vaginal flap covers the 'sling'. In a later modification, an island of vaginal wall was no longer isolated, but two sutures on each side were

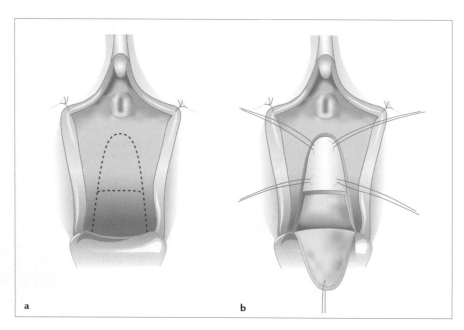

Figure 39.5. *Vaginal wall sling. (a) An inverted U incision is made with the apex of the U just proximal to the urethral meatus. The wings of the U extend about 2 cm proximal to the bladder neck. A transverse incision is made at the level of the bladder neck, creating an island of vaginal wall under the urethra. (b) A proximally based vaginal flap is then created (just below the 'sling'). Four sutures are placed, one in each corner of the sling. The proximal sutures include the urethropelvic ligament (endopelvic fascia) and vaginal wall including the epithelium (as in the Raz bladder-neck suspension). The distal sutures include the periurethral fascia and vaginal wall, including the epithelium. The four sutures are individually transferred to the anterior abdominal wall with a double-pronged needle and the vaginal flap is advanced over the* in situ *sling and suspension sutures are tied.*

simply placed in the aforementioned structures, suspended and tied.[35]

In their initial report, Raz *et al.*[34] reported a 77% cure rate for non-neurogenic stress incontinence secondary to ISD in 26 woman. Length of follow-up was not reported. In a follow-up study using the modified technique in 134 women with all types of stress incontinence, a 96% 'success' rate was reported, with a mean follow-up of 11 months.[36]

Needle suspension and cystocele repair

Needle suspension has been described to treat stress incontinence associated with cystocele and to correct the lateral or paravaginal defect associated with certain cystoceles. The technique is identical to that used for the Raz bladder-neck suspension, either in association with a formal anterior repair of the central defect,[37] or simply by placing an additional pair of sutures more proximally to suspend the base of the bladder in cases of moderate cystocele.[38] The authors reported 88% excellent or good results for the treatment of stress incontinence (mean follow-up 34 months) for the former procedure and 94% excellent or good results for the treatment of stress incontinence (mean follow-up 2 years) for the latter.

Sling procedures

A variety of sling procedures can be performed either partially or totally by a transvaginal technique (see chapters 43 and 44). In many cases the vaginal dissection is similar to that described above for the Raz bladder-neck suspension. These procedures have the advantage of treating both support defects and ISD.

COMPLICATIONS OF VAGINAL SURGERY FOR STRESS INCONTINENCE

A variety of complications following anti-incontinence surgery have been documented and complication rates vary greatly in the literature. Complications may be divided into three types with respect to their temporal occurrence: these are intra-operative, early postoperative and late postoperative (delayed or chronic).[39] In many cases, early postoperative complications will resolve with conservative or no treatment; chronic complications often require more aggressive intervention. Table 39.2 summarizes the complications that may

Table 39.2. *Complications of vaginal procedures for stress incontinence*

Intra-operative complications
  Bleeding
  Bladder and urethral injury
  Ureteral injury
  Bowel injury
  Nerve injury
    Common peroneal nerve (due to positioning)
    Trauma to urethral nerves

Early postoperative complications
  Voiding dysfunction
    Frequency/urgency/urge incontinence
    Obstructive symptoms
    Urinary retention
  Infection
    Urinary tract infection
    Wound infection
    Pelvic abscess

Late postoperative complications (delayed and chronic)
  Pain
  Suture erosion
  Osteitis pubis
  Osteomyelitis (bone anchors)
  Pelvic prolapse
  Chronic voiding dysfunction
    Frequency/urgency/urge incontinence
    Obstructive symptoms
    Urinary retention
  Chronic urinary tract infection

occur, according to type. The reader is referred to chapter 62 for a more detailed description.

REFERENCES

1. Raz S, Little NA, Juma S. Female urology. In: Walsh PC, Retik AB, Stamey TA, Vaughan ED (eds) *Campbell's Urology* (6th edn). Philadelphia: Saunders, 1992; 2782–2828

2. Delancey JOL. The pathophysiology of stress urinary incontinence in women and its implication for surgical treatment. *World J Urol* 1997; 15: 268–274

3. DeLancey JOL. Structural support of the urethra as it relates to stress urinary incontinence: the hammock hypothesis. *Am J Obstet Gynecol* 1994; 170: 1713–1720

4. Leach GE, Dmochowski RR, Appell RA *et al.* Female stress urinary incontinence clinical guidelines panel summary report on surgical management of female stress urinary incontinence. *J Urol* 1997; 158: 875–880

5. Raz S, Sussman EM, Erickson DB *et al.* The Raz bladder neck suspension: results in 206 patients. *J Urol* 1992; 148: 845–850

6. Trockman BA, Leach GE, Hamilton J *et al.* Modified Pereyra bladder neck suspension: 10-year mean followup using outcomes analysis in 125 patients. *J Urol* 1995; 154: 1841–1847

7. Kondo A, Kato K, Gotoh *et al.* The Stamey and Gittes procedures: long-term followup in relation to incontinence type and patient age. *J Urol* 1998; 160: 756–758

8. Zeidman MJ, Chaing H, Larcon A, Raz S. Suprapubic cystotomy using Lowsley retractor. *Urology* 1988; 32: 54–56

9. Thompson JD, Wall LL, Growdon WA, Ridley JH. Urinary stress incontinence. In: Thompson JD, Rock JA (eds) *Te Linde's Operative Gynecology*, 7th edn. Philadelphia: Lippincott, 1992; 887–940

10. Kelly HA, Dumm WM. Urinary incontinence in women, without manifest injury to the bladder. *Surg Gynecol Obstet* 1914; 18: 444–448

11. Low JA. Management of anatomic urinary incontinence by vaginal repair. *Am J Obstet Gynecol* 1967; 82: 1231

12. Ross RA, Singleton HM. Vaginal prolapse and stress urinary incontinence. *W V Med J* 969; 65: 77

13. Richardson AC. Paravaginal repair. In: Gershenson DM, Aronson MP (eds) *Operative Techniques in Gynecologic Surgery: Reconstructive Pelvic Surgery.* Philadelphia: Saunders, 1996; 66–75

14. Raz S, Klutke CG, Golomb J. Four-corner bladder and urethral suspension for moderate cystocele. *J Urol* 1989; 142: 712–715

15. Pereyra AJ. Simplified surgical procedure for the correction of stress incontinence in women. *W J Surg* 1959; 67: 223–226

16. Harer WB, Gunther RE. Simplified urethrovesical suspension and urethroplasty. *Am J Obstet Gynecol* 1965; 91: 1017–1020

17. Pereyra AJ, Lebherz TB. Combined urethrovesical suspension and vaginourethroplasty for correction of urinary stress incontinence. *Obstet Gynecol* 1967; 30: 537–542

18. Tauber R. Wapner P. Surgical repair of severe and recurrent urinary incontinence. *Obstet Gynecol* 1967; 30: 741–745

19. Winter CC. Unilateral and bilateral bladder neck suspension operation for stress urinary incontinence. *J Urol* 1976; 116: 47–51

20. Cobb OE, Ragde H. Simplified correction of female stress incontinence. *J Urol* 1978; 120: 418–420

21. Stamey TA. Endoscopic suspension of the vesical neck for urinary incontinence. *Surg Gynecol Obstet* 1973; 136: 547–554

22. Stamey TA. Endoscopic suspension of the vesical neck for urinary incontinence. *Ann Surg* 1980; 192: 465–471

23. O'Sullivan DC, Chilton CP, Munson KW. Should Stamey colposuspension be our primary surgery for stress incontinence? *Br J Urol* 1995; 75: 457–460

24. Raz S. Modified bladder neck suspension for female stress incontinence. *Urology* 1981; 17: 81–84

25. Leach GE, Raz S. Modified Pereyra bladder neck suspension after previously failed anti-incontinence surgery: surgical technique and results with long-term follow-up. *Urology* 1984; 23: 359–362

26. Gittes RF, Loughlin KR. No-incision pubovaginal suspension for stress incontinence. *J Urol* 1987; 138: 568–570

27. Kil PJM, Hoekstra JW, van der Meijden APM *et al.* Transvaginal ultrasonography and urodynamic evaluation after suspension operations: comparison among the Gittes, Stamey and Burch suspensions. *J Urol* 1991; 146: 132–136

28. Leach GE, Labasky RF. Bone fixation technique for transvaginal needle suspension. *Urol Clin North Am* 1989; 16: 175–182

29. Benderev TV. A modified percutaneous outpatient bladder neck suspension system. *J Urol* 1994; 152: 2316–2320

30. Appell RA, Rackley RA, Dmochowsky RR. Vesica percutaneous bladder neck stabilization. *J Endourol* 1996; 10: 221–225

31. Schultheiss, D, Hofner K, Oelke V *et al.* Does bone anchor fixation improve the outcome of percutaneous bladder neck suspension *J Urol* 1998; 159 (suppl): 215

32. Nativ O, Levine S, Madjar S *et al.* Incisionless per vaginal bone anchor cystourethropexy for the treatment of female stress incontinence. Experience with the first 50 patients. *J Urol* 1997; 158: 1742–1744

33. Matkov TG, Henja MJ, Coogan CL. Osteomyelitis as a complication of Vesica percutaneous bladder neck suspension. *J Urol* 1998; 160: 1427

34. Raz S, Siegel AL, Short JL, Snyder JA. Vaginal wall sling. *J Urol* 1989; 141: 43–46

35. Raz S, Stothers L, Chopra A. Vaginal wall sling (part 1). *Urol Int* 1995; 2: 10–12

36. Stothers L, Chopra A, Raz S. Vaginal wall sling for anatomic incontinence and intrinsic sphincter damage – efficacy and outcome. *J Urol* 1995; 153: 525A

37. Raz S, Klutke CG, Golumb J. Four-corner bladder and urethral suspension for moderate cystoceles. *J Urol* 1989; 142: 712–715

38. Raz S, Little NA, Juma S *et al.* Repair of severe anterior vaginal wall prolapse (grade IV cystourethrocele) *J Urol* 1991; 146: 988–992

39. Ficazzola M, Nitti VW. Complications of incontinence procedures in women. In: Taneja S, Smith RD, Ehrlich R, Taneja S (eds) *Complications of Urologic Surgery*, 3rd edn. 2000, Philadelphia: Saunders.

40

Needle suspensions

G. J. Jarvis

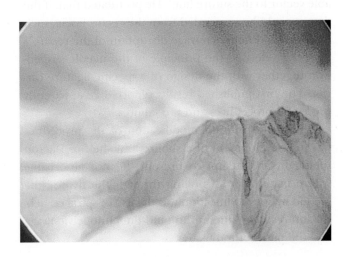

INTRODUCTION

In 1959, Armand Pereyra introduced a novel approach to the surgical treatment of genuine stress incontinence (GSI) in women.[1] Since that first description, needle suspensions have evolved with a series of modifications and with a cycle of popularity. Having been widely embraced as a reasonable balance between the degree of surgical invasion and acceptable success rates, the technique is now no longer considered to be a first-line surgical option in that the promising intermediate-term results have not been sustained in the longer term.

In this chapter, I will discuss the development and modifications of needle suspensions, describe a standard surgical technique, assess results, assess the place of specific modifications, discuss complications and assess the current place of needle suspensions in the surgical repertoire.

DEVELOPMENT OF NEEDLE SUSPENSIONS

In the 1950s, the most popular surgical procedures for GSI were the Marshall–Marchetti–Krantz procedure and anterior colporrhaphy. In 1956, Pereyra left the US Navy and became Chief Medical Officer at the California Institute for Women. Pereyra's duties included being gynaecological surgeon to a local women's prison, which allowed for a unique personal assessment and follow-up of patients on whom he had operated. His preferred operation was the Marshall–Marchetti–Krantz procedure and Pereyra considered that failure 'would often reveal strands of fibrous material between the relaxed tissues and the posterior aspect of the symphysis'. He concluded that 'traction from coughing and Valsalva was an undesirable vector to the suture line'. He postulated that, if the tissues could be suspended from the rectus fascia, such forces should not encourage disruption of the repair.[2]

Pereyra devised the principle of the needle suspension together with the design of a specific ligature carrier. The first published results reported 28 apparently successful procedures and two failures.[1]

The first significant modification of the procedure was the development of a suburethral shelf of Dacron tubing in an attempt to prevent the non-absorbable suture material from pulling through the tissues; the second major modification was the use of spiral or helical sutures in an attempt to bind the endopelvic fascia and the periurethral tissues.[3]

In 1973, Thomas Stamey, also of California, described two major (and several minor) modifications of the needle suspension. Stamey advised the use of a cystoscope in order that the position of the internal bladder neck could be identified with absolute accuracy and the sutures placed in close proximity to this point. The second modification was to insert an endoscope into the urethra during the process of tying the suspension sutures to ensure that 'the approximate amount of suprapubic tension required to close the internal vesical neck, which then serves as a guide as to how tightly to tie the nylon sutures supra pubically'.[4]

Stamey favoured the use of a small transverse incision in the anterior vaginal wall at the level of the bladder neck, whereas Raz reported the modification utilizing a curvilinear incision and including the paravaginal tissues within the helical suture.[5] Other significant modifications have included the advice by Mundy to insert the sutures vaginally rather than suprapubically,[6] while Hilton advocated the use of Silastic rather than Dacron buffers in order to reduce the infection rate;[7] Cobb suggested the use of a double-pronged needle in order to reduce the number of passages of a needle through the tissues while at the same time ensuring optimum width in the loop of nylon.[8]

Whichever of these techniques is favoured by the surgeon, the general principle of the needle suspension remains unchanged – that is, elevation of the bladder neck by use of non-absorbable suture material tied over the rectus sheath. Here, it seemed, was an operation that was relatively easy to perform, was unlikely to compromise the results of any further surgery, had a low complication rate and seemed to be successful.

SURGICAL TECHNIQUE

The general principle of the surgical technique can be seen in Figure 40.1. Given the range of modifications to the original description of a needle suspension, I now describe the surgical technique used in my own practice.

The patient is placed in a modified lithotomy position, cleaned and draped. Two suprapubic incisions are made, each approximately 1 cm in length, with the medial end of each incision being 1 cm above and 1 cm lateral to the pubic tubercle. The incision is oblique, parallel to the inguinal ligament; the fat is opened with a finger. The rectus sheath remains intact. Placing the

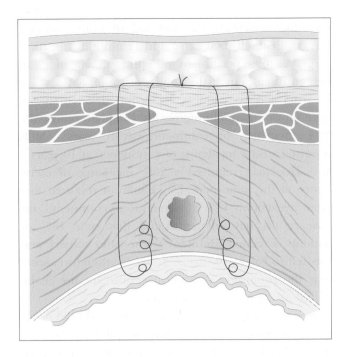

Figure 40.1. *Diagrammatic representation of supporting sutures showing helical modification.*

incision at this point ensures that the loop of nylon will be tied over the rectus sheath.

A cystoscope is passed and the bladder neck identified. An incision is then made into the anterior vaginal wall; I prefer a short (1–2 cm) longitudinal incision. The vaginal wall is then dissected off the bladder neck and proximal urethra. While the operator looks down the cystoscope, a finger may be placed inside the created flap of vagina, the external position of the bladder neck being identified with accuracy.

The supporting sutures are then inserted; I prefer no. 1 nylon. With the patient's bladder relatively empty (50–100 ml fluid) in order to minimize the risk of bladder penetration, and with the surgeon's finger placed just external to the bladder neck, the first loop of the first suture is passed. I favour the Stamey carrier needle with a terminal eye and a 15-degree anterior bend. The needle is inserted initially vertically downwards until the sheath has been pierced, and is then deviated in such a way that the point of the needle can be advanced, keeping as close as possible in contact to the posterior aspect of the pubic bone. The point of the needle should be aimed at the surgeon's own finger, thereby allowing the first loop of nylon to be as close as possible to the bladder neck without traversing the bladder. It is good practice to leave the

cystoscope in place throughout the procedure, supported by an assistant; the surgeon can then look down the cystoscope in order to confirm that the needle has not traversed the bladder and that, when the needle is rocked by an assistant, the bladder neck moves. If the needle has traversed the bladder, the needle is simply removed and insertion repeated minimally more laterally.

Once the surgeon is satisfied that the needle will have placed the first part of the nylon loop in the correct position, the nylon is removed from the eye of the needle; the needle is withdrawn and then reinserted approximately 1 cm lateral to the original insertion. This time, however, the needle should pierce the vaginal skin and be brought out into the vagina. If a paravaginal buffer is to be used (I favour a 1 cm piece of Silastic infant feeding tube size 6), it is inserted over the nylon at this point; this is said to have the advantage of reducing the incidence of 'cheesewiring' through the paravaginal tissues. Cystoscopy again confirms that the bladder has not been traversed and the loop of nylon is then inserted through the eye of the needle, which is withdrawn back into the abdominal incision, thereby placing a U-shaped loop of nylon on one side of the bladder neck. The procedure is repeated on the other side, thereby placing a second U-shaped loop of nylon on the other side of the bladder neck.

The bladder should then be filled to a greater capacity in order to make a final visualization that suture material has not traversed the bladder. The commonest place to find suture material is high up in the bladder, laterally. Once it is confirmed that there is no suture material through the bladder, the cystoscope is withdrawn from the bladder.

It is preferable to close the vaginal incision before tying the loops of nylon, because elevation of the vagina makes closure more difficult. Once the vagina is closed (I prefer to use interlocking polyglycolic acid sutures) and haemostasis is confirmed, the loops of nylon should be tied.

Judging tension is an integral part of the procedure and different authors suggest different techniques. If there is a speculum in the vagina it should be removed at this stage in case it exerts counter-traction. Whereas Stamey used an endoscope in the urethra to judge closure, others judged tension by the minimum required to prevent urethral leakage of fluid when suprapubic pressure is applied; I place a size 14 soft Foley catheter through the urethra and into the bladder and then tie both sutures using tension which is best described as 'more than minimum and less than moderate'. Tension-measurement studies using a spring balance intraoperatively have suggested that there is a wide middle range of tension associated with success but that insufficient tension or excess tension will be associated with failure.[9]

It is customary to give gentamicin intramuscularly during the procedure in order to reduce the possibility of infection of the non-absorbable suture or the buttress, and the bladder is then drained suprapubically. The skin incisions are closed with the material of choice.

RESULTS

The expected chance for cure of incontinence varies greatly throughout the literature, as it does for any surgical procedure. Results depend upon many factors, including initial patient selection, and a range of results for short-term continence (39–97%) can be found in the literature.[10,11] A meta-analysis of such results gives a mean subjective cure rate of 78% and a mean objective cure rate of 70%.[12]

The technique of meta-analysis may be used to assess outcome in different circumstances. Thus, the results for procedures based upon the Pereyra procedure, (where an endoscope is not used to judge suture placement), as opposed to a Stamey procedure (where an endoscope is used to judge suture placement), suggests, perhaps surprisingly, that the use of a cystoscope to judge suture placement with accuracy is not essential for short-term continence. The mean objective continence rate in one study for the Pereyra procedure was 72% with a mean objective continence rate of 71% for the Stamey.[13]

It is a general principle of surgery for GSI that an operation performed in the absence of previous surgery is more likely to render the patient continent than an operation performed when previous surgery has failed. This general principle holds in needle-suspension procedures, one meta-analysis suggesting that the mean objective cure rate for a primary needle suspension was 75% compared with 73% if there was recurrent incontinence.[13]

Unfortunately, much of the surgical literature relating to the management of GSI reports continence rates at a relatively short period of time following surgery, generally between 3 and 12 months. Clearly, if surgery is to be performed to improve quality of life in benign disease, then the results of surgery at 5 years, 10 years and even longer are required. Such studies have shown disappointing results: Bergman reported a 43% incidence of continence at 5 years;[14] Mills reported a 33% incidence of continence at 10 years,[15] and Trockman reported a 20% incidence of continence at the same period;[16] O'Sullivan reported that after 5 years only 18% of women were continent;[17] my own results have demonstrated that only 18% of patients remained continent 4 years after surgery, and this fell to 6% at 10 years.[18] It would, therefore, seem that the promising short-term results are not maintained in the intermediate term.

It is not entirely clear why such failure should occur and it is likely that such failure is multifactorial. The minimally invasive nature of the procedure is associated with minimal fibrosis and this may mitigate against permanent support of the tissues. Suture material may fracture or may cheesewire through the tissues. When patients have had an initially successful needle suspension that has ultimately failed, and further surgery is undergone, the suprapubic knot of nylon over the rectus sheath appears to be in the correct position but the vaginal end of the loop appears to be misplaced (personal observation). This being so, modification such as a bone-anchoring technique (designed to improve poor success rate in the long term), may not achieve this result.[19]

The importance of this intermediate-term failure rate means that specific indications for needle suspension must be identified; these are discussed below.

COMPLICATIONS

Although all surgical procedures carry complications, one of the original advantages advocated for needle suspensions was the relative lack of complications compared with those associated with more formal suprapubic surgery. Stamey described an absence of operative deaths and an absence of need for blood transfusion, but also mentioned that, in 10 of 300 patients, a suprapubic suture had to be removed because of 'pain, infection, or both'.[20] If pain is a feature after the early postoperative stage, then the major causes are either entrapment of a small branch of the ilio-inguinal nerve or erosion of the suture through the bladder wall with the subsequent possibility of stone formation.[21-23]

All surgical procedures for GSI should, logically, be associated with some incidence of *de-novo* detrusor instability and/or a voiding disorder, as all such surgery involves either relocation of the bladder neck or an increase in urethral resistance (or both). The reported incidence of *de-novo* detrusor instability following needle suspensions has varied between zero and 20%, with a mean incidence in the region of 5.8%. Voiding disorders may also follow this procedure, with a mean of 5.8% and a range of 1–24%.[21] A single study has demonstrated a decrease in voiding disorder postoperatively, presumed to relate to the reduction of cystocele without a significant increase in urethral resistance.[7] A recent assessment of the literature concluded: 'compared with a suprapubic procedure the morbidity is low, although not negligible'.[24]

INDICATIONS

The disappointing intermediate- and longer-term results mean that needle suspensions can no longer be considered to be a first-line surgical option for the treatment of GSI in a woman who has not undergone previous surgery, who is relatively fit, and who is wishing for a surgical procedure that is likely to give a significant chance of continence for the subsequent 10 or more years.

Needle suspensions do, nevertheless, have a significant place in the surgical repertoire. They may be particularly indicated in the patient in whom surgical access for a more formal suprapubic procedure is anticipated to be limited (or even dangerous), or in patients who are considered to be medically frail by virtue of coexisting medical pathology, age, limited mobility or limited longevity. In such a group of patients, the only realistic surgical options may be either a needle suspension or the use of a substance injected into the proximal urethra; given the present state of knowledge, it cannot be stated which of these two general treatment options will give the lower long-term morbidity but higher success.

CONCLUSIONS

Needle suspensions initially seemed to be a most attractive surgical option, with the combination of minimal invasive technique and minimal complication; however, the results have not been encouraging in the longer term. Nevertheless, specific indications remain in contemporary practice.

If there is to be a wider indication for such techniques in the future, one or more modifications that increase the intermediate-term chance of continence without increasing morbidity will be necessary. Such techniques are likely to depend upon the development of alternative material for support rather than upon modifications of surgical technique. In the absence of such development, needle suspensions will remain a valuable technique in highly specific circumstances.

REFERENCES

1. Pereyra AJ. A simplified surgical procedure for the correction of stress urinary incontinence in women. *West J Obstet Gynecol* 1959; 67: 223–226

2. Cornella JL, Pereyra AJ. Historical vignette of Armand J Pereyra. *Int Urogynaecol J* 1990; 1: 25–30

3. Pereyra AJ, Lebherz TB, Growdon WA *et al.* Pubourethral supports in perspective. *Obstet Gynecol* 1982; 59: 643–648

4. Stamey TA. Cystoscopic suspension of the vesical neck for urinary incontinence. *Surg Gynecol Obstet* 1973; 136: 547–554

5. Raz S, Modified bladder neck suspension for female stress incontinence. *Urology* 1981; 17: 82–85

6. Mundy AR. A trial comparing Stamey bladder neck suspension with colposuspension for the treatment of stress incontinence. *Br J Urol* 1983; 55: 687–690

7. Hilton P, Mayne C. The Stamey endoscopic bladder neck suspension – a clinical and urodynamic investigation including actuarial follow-up over 4 years. *Br J Obstet Gynaecol* 1991; 98: 1141–1149

8. Cobb OE, Ragde H. Simplified correction of female stress incontinence. *J Urol* 1978; 120: 418–420

9. Condo A, Kato K, Goto HM *et al.* Quantifying thread tension is of clinical use in Stamey bladder neck suspension. *J Urol* 1989; 141: 38–42

10. Peattie AB, Stanton SL. The Stamey operation for correction of genuine stress incontinence in the elderly woman. *Br J Obstet Gynaecol* 1989; 96: 983–986

11. Roberts JA, Angel JR, Thomas R *et al.* Modified Pereyra procedure for stress incontinence. *J Urol* 1981; 125: 787–789

12. Jarvis GJ. Stress incontinence. In: Mundy AR, Stephenson TP, Wein AJ (eds) *Urodynamics: Principles, Practice and Application,* 2nd edn. New York: Churchill Livingstone, 1994; 299–326

13. Jarvis GJ. Long needle bladder neck suspension for genuine stress incontinence – does endoscopy influence results? *Br J Urol* 1995; 76: 467–469

14. Bergman A, Elia G. Three surgical procedures for genuine stress incontinence – a 5 year follow-up of a prospective randomised study. *Am J Obstet Gynecol* 1995; 173: 66–71

15. Mills R, Persad R, Ashken MH. Long-term follow-up results for the Stamey operation for stress incontinence of urine. *Br J Urol* 1996; 77: 86–88

16. Trockman BA, Leach GE, Hamilton J *et al*. Long-term results for needle suspension. *J Urol* 1995; 154: 1841–1847

17. O'Sullivan DC, Chilton CP, Munson KW. Should Stamey colposuspension be our primary surgery for stress incontinence? *Br J Urol* 1995; 75: 457–460

18. Kevelighan EH, Jarvis GJ, Aagaard J *et al*. The Stamey endoscopic bladder neck suspension – a 10 year follow-up study. *Br J Obstet Gynaecol* 1998; 105: (Suppl 17): 47

19. Schultheiss D, Hofner K, Oelke M *et al*. Does bone anchor fixation improve the outcome of percutaneous bladder neck suspension in female urinary stress incontinence? *Br J Urol* 1998; 82: 192–195

20. Stamey TA. Endoscopic suspension of the vesical neck. In: Stanton SL, Tenagho EA (eds) *Surgery of Female Incontinence*. Berlin: Springer-Verlag, 1998; 77–91

21. Jarvis GJ. Surgery for genuine stress incontinence. *Br J Obstet Gynaecol* 1994; 101: 371–374

22. Weiss RE, Cohen E. Erosion of buttress following bladder neck suspension. *Br J Urol* 1992; 69: 656–657

23. Jarvis GJ. Erosion of buttress following bladder neck suspension. *Br J Urol* 1992; 70: 695

24. Bidmead J, Cardozo L. Four decades of needle bladder neck suspension. *Br J Urol* 1998; 82: 171–173

41

Retropubic cystourethropexies

E. Petri

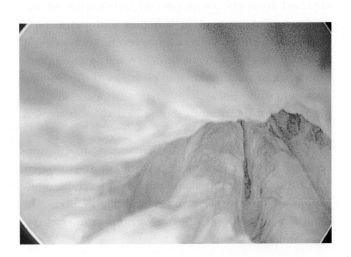

INTRODUCTION

There is still considerable debate about the best surgical approach for the treatment of genuine stress incontinence. However, retropubic urethropexy is considered by most to be the 'gold standard' for surgical correction of sphincter incompetence .

The earliest documented surgical approach to stress incontinence was in 1864 by Baker Brown;[1] since his description, over the decades more than 200 different surgical procedures have been designed to correct female genuine urinary stress incontinence (USI).[2] Unfortunately, it is often difficult to compare the results published in the literature because of important differences in the surgical techniques and in the selection of the patients. Another confusing factor is that most authors generally report only short-term results, whereas it would be meaningful to analyse long-term cure at 5 years (preferably, 10 years) after surgery.[3] In addition, randomized studies with objective control of success rates are rare.

In 1949, two urologists and a gynaecologist (Marshall, Marchetti and Krantz) described vesicourethral suspension in a 54–year-old man who had developed USI following abdominoperineal resection.[4] This urethropexy constituted the first step in the history of the surgical management of female sphincter incompetence with an abdominal approach.

TECHNIQUES

Marshall *et al.* performed colposuspension by suturing the periurethral tissue to the back of the pubic bone. Krantz, the gynaecologist (and anatomist) of the three authors, stated that the control of incontinence was obtained from the elevation and stabilization of the urethrovesical junction in a higher endopelvic position. In fact, in the light of more recent knowledge, it is known that all anti-incontinence retropubic operations work by stabilization and elevation of the bladder neck and the vesical base to prevent excessive displacement of the urethra during periods of increased physical stress.[3,4]

Subsequently, Marshall *et al.*[5] reported an 82% success rate for their procedure performed on 44 women with USI. These authors have published several modifications of their procedure, even though 'success in approximately 95% of primary and repeat operations' was claimed.

In 1972, Symmonds[6] described a modification of this procedure, which consisted essentially of the opening of the bladder dome for a more accurate positioning of the sutures. Using this modification, Lee and co-authors[7] obtained an excellent cure rate of 91% in 227 patients with primary stress incontinence.

In 1976, Richardson and colleagues[8] described a new concept – that urethrocystocele and stress incontinence may be the result of an isolated paravaginal defect in the pubocervical segment of the endopelvic fascia. This defect was found lateral to the vagina, in the connective tissue attachment of the pubocervical fascia to the aponeurosis overlying the obturator internus muscle at the level of the tendineous arch of the endopelvic fascia (white line). An abdominal surgical approach with closure of the paravaginal defect produced high cure rates without significant complications. In the series of Shull and Baden,[9] the middle two sutures were placed through Cooper's ligament, so this was not strictly a paravaginal repair. To date there are only a few studies of the objective outcome of this procedure.

The cornerstone of today's technique of cystourethropexy was laid by Burch,[10] who first used the term 'urethrovaginal fixation' and then later 'urethrovesical suspension'.[11]

In 1958, John C. Burch , during a Marshall–Marchetti–Krantz (MMK) procedure, experienced the common problem whereby the sutures in the periostium continued to pull out and it became necessary to attach the sutures to another point. The 'white line' of the pelvic fascia overlying the levator ani muscles was initially used for this purpose. The vaginal wall was found to be very mobile and Burch sutured the paravaginal fascia instead of the periurethral tissue to the white line. Soon, Burch realized that in some patients the white line was too weak to hold the sutures; he used Cooper's ligament instead as the point of fixation. This ligament, also designated the ileopectineal ligament, which is located at the posterior and superior border of the superior ramus of the pubic bone, is a strong thick fibrous band that is eminently suitable for passing and holding the sutures. He used three chromic catgut sutures on each side of the urethra.[10,12]

'Colposuspension' was first used by Turner-Warwick and Whiteside,[13] Since then, numerous modifications of this concept and different terminologies have been published, e.g. colpocystourethropexy,[14] retropubic urethropexy,[15] and obturator shelf procedure (Turner-

Warwick, unpublished work cited by Stanton).[16] In 1976, Tanagho[14] described a modification of this technique in which he recommended that dissection should be avoided in the midline over the urethra. He also recommended placement of the sutures far lateral to the urethra, and tying of sutures so that two fingers could easily be inserted between the fascia and the symphysis, thus preserving mobility and motility of the proximal urethra.[16,17] Such factors as different techniques of placement of sutures, suture materials used and height of elevation make colposuspension a procedure that may have as many modifications as 'vaginal repair'.

INDICATIONS AND CONTRAINDICATIONS

Taking into account the very different socio-economic situations and healthcare systems in different countries, as well as the objective success rates of different forms of treatment of female urinary incontinence, together with the medicolegal burdens for the physicians in large parts of Europe and the North American continent, I would always recommend a conservative treatment in primary cases. Conservative treatment has few complications, does not compromise future surgery and should be available as an option to all incontinent women. I am averse to the use of drugs and of long-term compliance to mechanical devices in many patients, preferring such physiotherapeutic regimens as intravaginal cones or spheres, pelvic floor exercises, perineometry and various forms of electrostimulation. If this treatment is not acceptable to the patient or has failed over a period of more than 6 months, a urogynaecological clinical investigation (described elsewhere in this book) is performed, with complete urinalysis, urethrocystoscopy, urodynamic study and perineal/introital ultrasonography. Urodynamic investigation allows classification of the disease and rules out such risk factors as hypotonic urethra and concomitant neurogenic disorders. Identification of a low-pressure urethra by preoperative urethral profilometry suggests a greatly increased risk for operative failure and should be explained to the patient.

The morphological investigation allows correct selection of the procedure, giving information about additional pelvic floor defects such as enterocele, rectocele, different types of vesical descent and additional pathology of the small pelvis. In primary cases of sphincter incompetence, a modified colposuspension is treatment of first choice; a prospective study of the value of a tension-free vaginal tape (TVT), which is inserted under local anaesthesia, reducing duration in hospital (thus reducing costs), might change this strategy in the future.[18] Where there is additional **symptomatic** pathology, colposuspension is combined with vaginal or abdominal reconstruction of the pelvic floor. In case of recurrence, it is important to ensure that the vagina has adequate capacity and mobility, so that the lateral fornices can be elevated towards each ipsilateral ileopectineal ligament (Fig. 41.1). If this is not the case, I either treat with local oestrogens for 6–8 weeks in post-menopausal women, or combine a soft silicone pessary with local oestrogens, which effectively softens scars from previous vaginal surgery. No special preparation is necessary, apart from a suprapubic shave and heparin prophylaxis. I do not use perioperative antibiotics routinely.

AIM OF SURGERY

Proper urethral function and maintenance of continence requires that the proximal urethra is positioned (and well supported) within the abdominal cavity. The anatomical fault in the majority of cases of sphincter incompetence is a weakening of the extrinsic support of the proximal urethra, resulting in downwards and backwards movement of the bladder neck during stress (so-called rotational descent of the bladder neck and proximal urethra or hypermobility of the urethrovesical junction). Rising intra-abdominal pressure does not force the urethra against the well-supported vagina, and the pressure cannot be transmitted to the proximal urethra, resulting in stress incontinence.[3,19] The dynamic urethral pressure changes during stress will be modified by surgery, owing to the intra-abdominalization of the urethra which will allow better transmission of the abdominal pressure to the urethra.[20,21] The goal of anti-incontinence procedures is to re-establish the correct intra-abdominal location of the proximal urethra. The success of surgery is determined by (a) suburethral support, (b) height of elevation and (c) stability of fixation. However, crucial to the success of these procedures is the avoidance of excessive elevation of the urethrovesical junction. Urinary retention and detrusor instability (DI) can occur as a result of urethral obstruction because of overcorrection of the anatomical defect.[17]

PERSONAL TECHNIQUE

A low Pfannenstiel incision is made approximately two fingers above the symphysis at a length of 7–10 cm. If there has been previous abdominal surgery (46% in my patients), parts of the old scar are used. The rectus muscles are carefully separated from the underlying transversalis fascia, taking care to avoid injury to the inferior epigastric vessels. The pelvic side walls are opened by blunt finger dissection, avoiding the space of Retzius with its delicate neural and vascular supply. Pulling aside the rectus muscle with retractors, the surgeon places his first and second fingers in the vagina to elevate the lateral vaginal fornix (Fig. 41.1). From above, the balloon of the transurethral catheter is seen or palpated and the hand in the abdomen dissects carefully the para-urethral tissue and the bladder base medially off the paravaginal fascia until the upward pressure cone of the finger in the vagina is identifiable (Fig. 41.2).

Where there has been previous surgery it may be necessary to dissect scars or fibrous tissue by electrocautery or scissors; frequently I have had to dissect or excise alloplastic materials from previous alloplastic slings or needle suspensions together with granulomas around the knots.

The paravaginal fascia is recognized as a white tissue, the veins being compressible by the vaginal finger (impossible if only the bladder wall is visualized!).

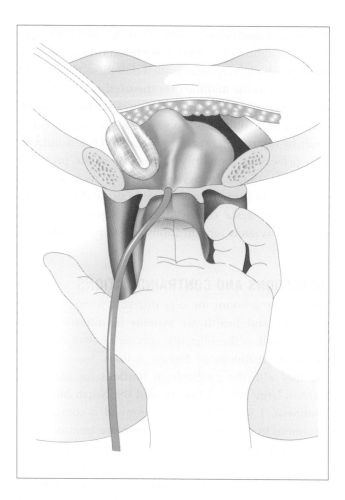

Figure 41.2. *Elevation of the lateral vaginal fornix, careful dissection of the para-urethral tissue and the bladder base medially off the paravaginal fascia.*

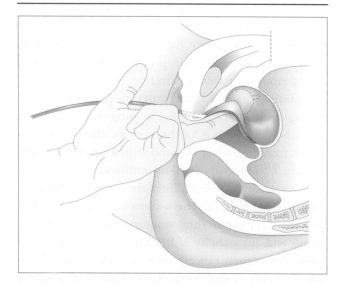

Figure 41.1. *Ensure that the vagina has adequate capacity and mobility, so that the lateral fornices can be elevated towards each ipsilateral ileopectineal ligament.*

Whereas Burch applied three sutures on each side, I use only two sutures through all layers of tissue except the vaginal epithelium as far laterally in the vaginal wall as possible – the first at the level of the lower pole of the catheter balloon and the second at the level of the maximal circumference of the balloon and then to the nearest point on the ipsilateral ileopectineal ligament (Cooper's ligament) (Fig. 41.3). Some surgeons use a sterilized thimble; others even introduce an amnioscopic tube instead of their fingers in order to prevent lacerations of their fingers. This happens rarely during the first 15–20 procedures; I prefer to slip into a second glove before inserting the fingers into the vagina.

The vagina is then elevated by the surgeon without any pressure or tension, the assistant tying the knots (Fig. 41.4). I have never tried a complete apposition of vaginal fascia and ligament, as described by Burch; in

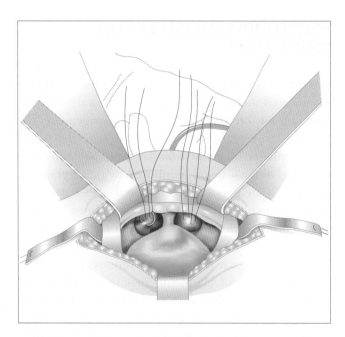

Figure 41.3. *Two sutures through all layers of tissue except the vaginal epithelium as far laterally in the vaginal wall as possible and then to the nearest point on the ipsilateral ileopectineal ligament.*

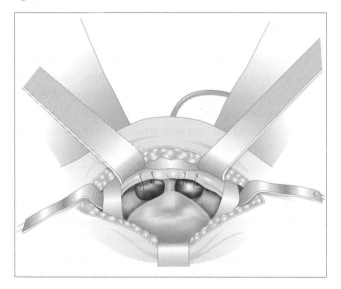

Figure 41.4. *Elevation of the vagina by the surgeon without any pressure or tension, the assistant tying the knots.*

my opinion this is not feasible in most post-menopausal women and will result in unnecessary overcorrection, with consequent urgency symptoms and obstructive micturition (Fig. 41.5). In most cases there is at least 1.5–2 cm between the tissues, which is why permanent sutures (Ethibond 0 with a strong MOX needle or, alternatively, Gore-tex or Cardiofil) are preferred. There has

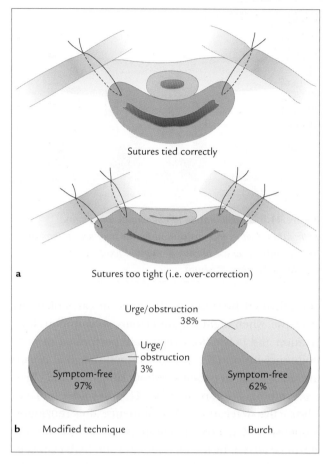

Figure 41.5. *(a) Original Burch procedure with complete apposition of vaginal fascia and ligament and loose approximation of the tissues. (b) Incidence of micturition problems following overcorrection during colposuspension.*

been no randomized controlled study of the optimal type of suture material.[22] In my experience with more than 2500 cases, no complications have been ascribed to the suture material.

The sutures should not be placed higher at a more proximal level beyond the urethrovesical junction because of the risk of injuring or obstructing the juxtavesical parts of the ureter. Obstruction can be caused by kinking of scar tissue left by previous needle suspension procedures when pulling the sutures upwards.

After completion of the sutures on the other side I check for haemostasis, using soft drains only in diffuse bleeding or where the bladder has been opened. A suprapubic catheter is inserted. In case of additional procedures, in 15 years' experience I have had no problems in going from above to below and vice versa. In rare cases of large central cystoceles with residual or recurrent urinary tract infection (UTI), the vaginal

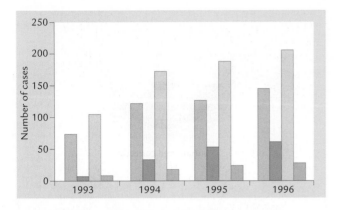

Figure 41.6. *Combination of abdominal and vaginal approaches used in this institution for the treatment of prolapse and incontinence.* (■ *plastic;* ■ *vaginal fixation;* ■ *colposuspension;* ■ *sling*)

route is used first; this is also done in cases of severe prolapse, when vaginal hysterectomy, sacrospinous vault fixation and pelvic floor repair are performed prior to colposuspension (Fig. 41.6). 'Cosmetic' vaginal repairs are inadvisable in patients without subjective and objective symptoms (e.g. recurrent UTI, post-void residual or obstructive defecation). As continence after retropubic suspension depends on compression of the urethra during exertion by the bladder base and high cystocele, a surgical technique that re-positions and supports the bladder neck but leaves the bladder base free should give the best results.[23] In cases of relaxation of the posterior vaginal wall and lack of perineum I start with the colposuspension, subsequently changing to the vaginal posterior repair. Even though enterocele formation is a possibility, I no longer routinely obliterate the cul-de-sac, as described by Burch and others; neither a Moschowitz or a McCall-type culdoplasty nor high peritonealization via the vaginal route has proved satisfactory, as not only has mechanical ileus occurred twice but also long-term follow-up has shown that, in cases of wide small pelvis, enteroceles have recurred after 6–12 months.

Suturing of the peritoneum, no matter what technique is used, will not suffice to prevent recurrence because of the lack of strength of this tissue. As described, I prefer to perform sacrospinous fixation (from below or above) together with reconstruction of the perineum (good plication of the levator ani muscle); in my opinion, this is the only structure of strength that can be found in nearly all patients.

POSTOPERATIVE MANAGEMENT AND COMPLICATIONS

Patients are mobilized on the evening of the day of surgery, receiving 2–2.5 litres of parenteral fluids. Continuous mobilization together with oral fluids are commenced on day 1. Catheter management has become more aggressive from year to year: the suprapubic catheter is clamped on day 2 to enable micturition, the residual being monitored by the suprapubic drainage. Catheters can be removed at 3.7 days (on average) when residuals have repeatedly been less than 100 ml urine. Perioperative antibiotics are given only to those women with pre-existing UTI or intra-operative complications such as major lacerations of the bladder, extirpation of alloplastic materials with several approaches or additional hysterectomy. The final catheter specimen of urine is sent for culture and sensitivity tests, allowing specific treatment if needed. The rate of hospital-borne infection in my department was between 0.6 and 1.6% over the last few years. In rare cases of longer-lasting obstruction of micturition (<1%), electrostimulation is used initially in cooperation with the physiotherapist (possibly a psychosomatic approach?).

Voiding difficulties after abdominal colpourethropexy are described as a frequent problem, often combined with symptoms of frequency and urgency, and can be persistent. In my own recent series, 18.1% of women after MMK needed drainage for more than 10 days. Immobile fixation of the urethra – urethral rigidity secondary to periurethral fibrosis – may be the reason for this complication.

A rate of postoperative obstructive micturition[24,25] of 22–52% encouraged a change in our surgical technique (see above), reducing the symptoms to 3%. Nevertheless, in a 10-year follow-up study of 434 women, of a group of 159 women who considered themselves to be only 'improved', 82% were completely dry but complained of impaired flow without marked residual; as they had become used to emptying the bladder by straining, now having to relax the pelvic floor and wait for detrusor contraction seemed to be a reduction in quality of life for them. No relationship can be found between postoperative voiding difficulties and perioperative finding of bladder-neck elevation or approximation of paravaginal tissue to the ileopectineal ligament.[16]

Whereas Stanton[16] did not see any relationship between the cure of stress incontinence and presence of voiding difficulties, my experience is in accordance with that of Aagaard *et al.*[26] who found voiding difficulties in 60% of those women in whom surgery later failed, but in only 26% of those with subsequent surgical success. This corresponds to my experience with sling procedures, where 23% of those patients with postoperative retention, but only 9% of those without obstructive micturition, had a recurrence in a 12-year follow-up.[27]

Elderly, post-menopausal women are more likely to require prolonged catheterization after colposuspension. Such patients should be warned about this risk during the preoperative consultation. For every 10 years of age, a patient is 77% more likely to require catheterization on any given day. This fact seems to be related to age rather than to oestrogen status.[28] In increasing age, elevation of the bladder neck by more than 25 mm was a risk factor for postoperative voiding difficulties in a study by Bombieri and Freeman,[29] together with a higher degree of anxiety and depression, pain and preoperative voiding by abdominal straining.

Other postoperative complications are infrequent. Minor complications are correlated with bladder trauma and venous bleeding during surgery. No vesical or ureteral fistula was seen, but it was necessary to revise three major haematomas at the pelvic side wall (in all cases a drain had thrombosed) and one case of arterial bleeding of the bladder wall, induced by the trocar for the suprapubic drainage. If there is macrohaematuria caused by bladder sutures or by puncturing the bladder, the transurethral catheter is left in place and the bladder is rinsed until the urine becomes clear.

A rarely described complication is ureteral kinking, which tends to occur in patients with previous pelvic surgery (Fig. 41.7). Three cases have been encountered, all after several previous incontinence procedures, all having undergone needle suspension with broad scars in the para-urethral and trigonal area. Placing the sutures far lateral at the area of the bladder neck with good visualization of the anterior vaginal wall should prevent this serious complication.[30–32]

DI following colposuspension was first reported by Cardozo *et al.*[33] Definitions of DI vary greatly, and incidence rates of 5% (own data) and in the literature of 5%,[16,33] 14.7%,[24] 27%,[34] 35%[35] and 41% in patients with success and 81% in those with failure[26] have been

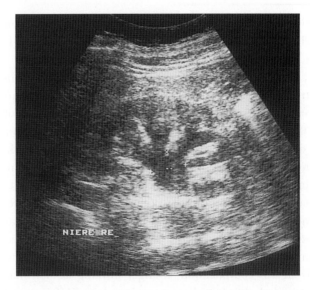

Figure 41.7. *Ureteral obstruction after colposuspension: four previous procedures that had failed, including two different types of needle suspension. During relaparotomy there was no direct laceration but kinking occurred within the elevated scar tissue.*

reported. It may be that there is a difference in patient material (such as previous surgery or age) but possibly also in surgical modifications. The highest rates of DI are found in patients who underwent an original Burch procedure; with a modified technique I have found an incidence of 3% in the last 10 years, with reliance on fewer sutures and a smaller shelf of supporting tissue, without having encountered a reduction in durability of postoperative result as anticipated by Hertogs and Stanton.[23]

Colposuspension with its high anterior elevation seems to aggravate posterior wall weakness. The incidence of enterorectoceles ranges from 5 to 60%, requiring reoperation in up to 15%.[36] Nevertheless, even in the more 'anatomical' paravaginal repair, Shull[9] reported a rate of enterocele formation of about 6%. Again, Aagaard *et al.*[26] reported a marked difference between successful (26% enteroceles) and unsuccessful (60%) procedures, presumably caused by surgical errors and technical problems. With stable fixation of the bladder neck, progressive relaxation of the tissue with ageing seems to increase the problem at follow-up: Alcalay *et al.*[24] demonstrated an increase in incidence of enteroceles from 9.2% after 3 months and 17.8% after 5 years up to 19.2% after 10–20 years.

As previously mentioned, rather than relying on the stability of peritoneum in closing the cul-de-sac, I prefer to perform a sacrospinous fixation of the vaginal vault or at least to correct the pelvic floor herniation when the levator muscles are lateralized and there is no perineum.

Little has been published on the Burch pain syndrome, which has attracted my attention in recent years. Aagaard et al.[26] have described an incidence of 20% in successfully treated patients and of 37% after failed procedures. In long-term follow-up studies, working women have reported to me that pain in the 'inguinal area' (point of fixation at Cooper's ligament) has bothered them to the point of permanent disablement. Information about this possible complication has now been included in the informed-consent form used in my institution; in the future, as there seems no way to avoid this complication, younger working women may be excluded from colposuspension and a TVT inserted instead.

RESULTS

Even though the original MMK procedure showed objective success rates of 71–89.2% in a follow-up of at least 12 months,[37] most European studies have had difficulty in reproducing this, showing rates of 52–85%;[38–40] in my own series, continence was achieved in 62.5%

after 1 year, with a gradual decrease from year to year. Even with additional use of fibrin sealing, Stolz et al.[41] had a cure rate of only 52.5% with MMK. The complication rate is higher, including voiding difficulties (in my experience these improved after dissolution of the resorbable sutures) and its unique complication of osteitis ossis pubis in up to 5%.[42]

The Burch urethropexy and its modifications are the best-studied procedures, with good objective and long-term follow-up. There are marked differences between subjective and objective data, as well as between primary and recurrent cases (Tables 41.1, 41.2). I do not accept the universal tendency to include 'improved' cases in the category of successful treatment, as urodynamically improved patients demonstrate the same unchanged pressure transmission and, morphologically, incorrect repositioning of the bladder neck, as found in those designated as surgical failures.

In my own patients (n = 2500 up to 1999), with 47% having undergone up to 19 previous anti-incontinence procedures, the success rate with a follow-up of at least 24 months was 89% for primary procedures but only 72% for cases of recurrence.

Fairly good results were achieved by my team in patients with mixed incontinence, when urgency was

Table 41.1. *Results of colposuspension*

Source	No. of patients	Percentage continent	Follow-up (months)
Jarvis meta-analysis, 1994*	2300	84.3	>12
Stanton and Cardozo, 1979*	25	84	> 4
Mundy, 1983*	26	73	>12
Stanton, 1984*	60	83	>12
Milani, 1985*	44	79	>12
Galloway, 1987*	50	84	> 6
Larsson et al.[45]	99	94	>24
Schürmann and Ralph[25]	31	82	>12
Cardozo and Cutner, 1992*	100	80	6–12
Herbertssen, 1993*	72	90.3	84–144
Feyereisl et al.[46]	87	81.6	>12
Petri, 1997*	1500	81	>24

*Cited in ref. 37.

Table 41.2. *Results of colposuspension in patients with previously unsuccessful surgery*

Source	Percentage continent	Follow-up (months)
Jarvis meta-analysis*	82.5 (?)	>12
Stanton, 1984*	65	60
Galloway, 1987*	63	54
Stanton and Cardozo, 1979	77	>24
Wolf and Noesselt[47]	73	6–12
Petri, 1997*	72	>24
Cardozo et al. 1999[43]	78	9
Maher et al. 1999[44]	72	9

*Cited in ref. 37.

Table 41.3. *Long-term results of colposuspension*

Source	No. of patients	Percentage continent			
		1 year	2–5 years	5–10 years	>10 years
van Geelen et al.[50]	90	85.3	–	79.2	
Larsson et al.[47]	99	99	94	–	
Herbertsson and Iosif[51]	47	–	–	89.4	
Kjoelhede and Ryden[36]	243	–	–	63	
Aagaard et al.[26]	960 (!)	–	–	54	
Alcalay et al.[24]	109	93.6	79.8	72.5	69
Petri, 1997*	732	89	81	72	
Borstad[35]	78	80	–	73	

*Cited in ref. 37.

caused by funnelling of the proximal urethra because of a lack of anatomical fixation. Colombo described a 75% success rate in mixed incontinence,[3] whereas Jorgensen et al.[45] had a cure rate of only 26% in a group of patients with urge incontinence.

An increasing number of long-term follow-up studies up to 20 years demonstrate a wide range of results; even so, the poorest of these are better than any results known for other procedures (Table 41.3). All randomized studies comparing colposuspension with other methods demonstrate the superiority of colposuspension (Table 40.4).

CONCLUSIONS

With the reduced resources of healthcare systems in many countries, it is necessary to consider the expense and cost-effectiveness of surgical procedures. Urinary incontinence affects an estimated 13 million men and women in the USA, and 3.5 million in Germany, at an

Table 41.4. *Randomized studies comparing colposuspension with other techniques*

| | Percentage success | | | |
Source	Anterior repair	Pereyra	MMK	Colposuspension
Weil *et al.*[52]	57	50	–	91
vanGeelen *et al.*[50]	44.6	–	–	85.3
Bergman *et al.*[53]	63	65	–	89
Penttinen *et al.*[54]	–	79	–	100
Colombo *et al.*[55]	–	–	65	80

MMK, Marshall–Marchetti–Krantz procedure.
*Cited in ref. 37.

Table 41.5. *Cost and effectiveness of three surgical procedures for stress incontinence*

| | | No. of patients continent | | Cost/cure (US$) | |
Procedure	Cost (US$)	1 year*	5 years*	1 year	5 years
Colposuspension	6460	890	820	7258	7878
Pereyra	5653	650	430	8697	13 147
Anterior colporrhaphy	4978	630	370	7902	13 454

*Per 1000 incontinent women, 1 and 5 years after operation.
Modified from ref. 46.

annual cost (conservatively estimated), of US$15 billion and DM 3 billion, respectively. In many countries (e.g. Germany) budgets are associated with diagnoses: for example, the payment is the same for an intra-urethral injection on an outpatient basis as for a complex abdominovaginal correction of a pelvic floor defect and incontinence surgery; this is because, for the insurance company or the healthcare system, both comprise 'surgical treatment of urinary incontinence'. There is a need for larger prospective studies comparing the effectiveness of different procedures, taking in account recurrence rates and complications.

In view of the major economic and psychological burdens imposed on society by urinary incontinence, pelvic surgeons should use treatments for this condition that are most cost-effective and should re-examine those treatments that effect cures at a higher cost. Retropubic urethropexy is the most cost-effective pro-cedure compared with the modified Pereyra technique and anterior colporrhaphy, as shown by reimbursable costs for the region and effectiveness data at 1 and 5 years after operation from prospective, randomized studies[46] (Table 41.5).

Colposuspension in its different modifications has emerged in most centres as the procedure of choice for patients with uncomplicated sphincter incompetence. Cure rates of about 85% have been reported and the outcome of any new technique is expected to be compared with this figure. The MMK procedure does not achieve the cure rates of colposuspension and has more serious complications; it should, therefore, be consigned to history. The paravaginal repair was originally described for correction of cystourethrocele; those demonstrating good results for the cure of stress incontinence placed Burch stitches bilaterally in addition to the paravaginal stitches.

REFERENCES

1. Baker Brown I. On diseases of women remediable by operation. *Lancet* 1864; i: 263–266

2. Hilton P, Stanton SL. A clinical and urodynamic assessment of the Burch colposuspension for genuine stress incontinence. *Br J Obstet Gynaecol* 1983; 90: 934–939

3. Colombo M. Diagnosis and surgical management of female urinary stress incontinence. *Chir Int* 1998; February–March: 9–12

4. Marshall VF, Marchetti AA, Krantz KE. The correction of stress incontinence by simple vesicourethral suspension. *Surg Gynecol Obstet* 1949; 88: 509–518

5. Krantz KE. The Marshall–Marchetti–Krantz procedure. In: Stanton SL, Tanagho EA (eds) *Surgery of Female Incontinence.* 2nd edn. Berlin: Springer, 1986; 87–91

6. Symmonds RE. The suprapubic approach to anterior vaginal relaxation and urinary stress incontinence. *Clin Obstet Gynecol* 1972; 15: 1107–1121

7. Lee RA, Symmonds RE, Goldstein RA. Surgical complications and results of modified Marshall–Marchetti–Krantz procedure for urinary incontinence. *Obstet Gynecol* 1979; 53: 447–450

8. Richardson AC, Lyon JB, Williams NL. A new look at pelvic relaxation. *Am J Obstet Gynecol* 1976; 126: 568–577

9. Shull BL, Baden WF. A six-year experience with paravaginal defect repair for stress urinary incontinence *Am J Obstet Gynecol* 1989; 160: 1432–1440

10. Burch JC. Urethrovaginal fixation to Cooper's ligament for correction of stress incontinence, cystocele and prolapse *Am J Obstet Gynecol* 1961; 81: 281–290

11. Burch JC. Cooper's ligament urethrovesical suspension for stress incontinence *Am J Obstet Gynecol* 1968; 100: 764–774

12. Kjoelhede PK. *Burch Colposuspension and the Pelvic Floor.* Linköping Univ Med Dissertations Linköping 1996

13. Turner-Warwick R, Whiteside G. Investigations and management of bladder neck dysfunction. In: Riches E (ed) *Modern Trends in Urology.* 3rd edn. London: Butterworths, 1970; 295–311

14. Tanagho EA. Colpocystourethropexy: the way we do it. *J Urol* 1976; 116: 751–753

15. Cowan W, Morgan HR. A simplified retropubic urethropexy in the treatment of primary and recurrent urinary stress incontinence in the female. *Am J Obstet Gynecol* 1979; 133: 295–301

16. Stanton SL. Colposuspension. In: Stanton SL, Tanagho EA (eds) *Surgery of Female Incontinence*, 2nd edn. Berlin: Springer, 1986; 95–103

17. Germain MM, Ostergard DR. Retropubic surgical approach for correction of genuine stress incontinence. In: Ostergard DR, Bent AE (eds) *Urogynecology and Urodynamics.* 4th edn. Baltimore: Williams and Wilkins, 1996; 527–532

18. Ulmsten U, Henriksson L, Johnson P, Varhos G. An ambulatory surgical procedure under local anaesthesia for treatment of female urinary incontinence *Int Urogynaecol J* 1996; 7: 81–86

19. Wall LL, Wiskind AK, Taylor PA. Simple bladder filling with a cough stress test compared with subtracted cystometry for the diagnosis of urinary incontinence. *Am J Obstet Gynecol* 1994; 171: 1472–1479

20. Edwards L, Malvern J. The urethral pressure profile: theoretical considerations and clinical application. *Br J Urol* 1974; 46: 325–331

21. Tenaillon M, Toppercer A, Elhilali M. Clinical and urodynamic evaluation of urethrocystopexy for stress urinary incontinence. *Urology* 1981; 18: 527–530

22. Smits-Braat M, Vierhout ME. Permanent or absorbable sutures for Burch colposuspension? *Int Urogynaecol J* 1995; 6: 350–352

23. Hertogs K, Stanton SL. Mechanism of urinary continence after colposuspension: barrier studies. *Br J Obstet Gynaecol* 1985; 92: 1184–1188

24. Alcalay M, Monga A, Stanton SL. Burch colposuspension: a 10–20 year follow-up. *Br J Obstet Gynaecol* 1995; 102: 740–745

25. Schürmann R, Ralph G. Urodynamic results following colposuspension according to Burch. *Zentralbl Gynakol* 1990; 112: 577–581

26. Aagaard J, Ferlie R, Byrjalsen C *et al.* Colposuspension am Burch – an 18–year follow-up story. *Int Urogynecol J* 1994; 5: 334

27. Petri E, Beckhaus I, Frohneberg D, Thüroff JW. Inguinovaginal sling according to Narik and Palmrich – indication, problems, long-term results. *Aktuel Urol* 1983; 14: 286–290

28. Heit M, Vogt V, Brubaker L. Predicting prolonged catheterization after Burch colposuspension: a new statistical approach. *Int Urogynaecol J* 1994; 5: 385

29. Bombieri L, Freeman RM. Why do women have voiding difficulty after colposuspension? *Int Urogynecol J* 1997; 8: S38

30. Applegate GB, Bass KM, Kubik CJ. Ureteral obstruction as a complication of the Burch colposuspension procedure: case report. *Am J Obstet Gynecol* 1987; 156: 445

31. Ferriani RA, Silva de Sá MF, Moura MD *et al.* Ureteral blockage as a complication of Burch colposuspension: report of 6 cases. *Gynecol Obstet Invest* 1990; 29: 239–240

32. Virtanen HS, Kiilholma PJA, Mäkinen JI *et al.* Ureteral injuries in conjunction with Burch colposuspension. *Int Urogynaecol J* 1995; 6: 114–118

33. Cardozo, L, Stanton SL, Williams J. Detrusor instability following surgery for genuine stress incontinence. *Br J Urol* 1979; 51: 204–207

34. Langer R, Ron-El R, Neuman M *et al.* The value of simultaneous hysterectomy during Burch colposuspension for urinary stress incontinence. *Obstet Gynecol* 1988; 72: 866–869

35. Borstad E. Long-term results after Burch colposuspension: a 11–14 years follow-up. *Int Urogynaecol J* 1997; 8: S28

36. Kjoelhede P, Rydén G. Prognostic factors and long-term results of the Burch colposuspension. *Acta Obstet Gynecol Scand* 1994; 73: 642–647

37. Hill S. Genuine stress incontinence. In: Cardozo L (ed) *Urogynecology.* New York: Churchill Livingstone, 1997; 231–285

38. Behr J, Winkler M, Schwiersch U. Urodynamische Betrachtungen zur Marshall–Marchetti–Krantz-Operation. *Geburtshilfe Frauenheilkd* 1986; 46: 649–653

39. Hochuli E, Lüscher KP, Spinelli A. Results of the operative treatment of severe second degree stress incontinence in 425 cases. *Geburtshilfe Frauenheilkd* 1981; 41: 469–473

40. Milani R, Maggioni A, Colombo M *et al.* Burch colposuspension versus modified Marshall–Marchetti–Krantz for stress urinary incontinence: a controlled clinical study. *Neurourol Urodyn* 1991; 10: 454–455

41. Stolz W, Brandner P, Dory F, Bastert G. The Marshall–Marchetti–Krantz-operation using fibrin sealing – results after 2 years. *Geburtshilfe Frauenheilkd* 1989; 49: 564–567

42. McLennan MT, Bent AE, Richardson DA. Evaluation of different surgical procedures. In: Ostergard DR, Bent AE (eds) *Urogynecology and Urodynamics*, 4th edn. Baltimore: Williams and Wilkins, 1996; 517–526

43. Cardozo L, Hextall A, Bailey J, Boos K. Colposuspension after previous failed incontinence surgery: a prospective observational study. *Br J Obstet Gynaecol* 1999; 106: 340–344.

44. Maher C, Dwyer P, Carey M, Gilmour D. The Burch colposuspension for recurrent urinary stress incontinence following retropubic continence surgery. *Br J Obstet Gynaecol* 1999; 106: 719–724.

45. Jorgensen L, Lose G, Mortensen SO *et al.* The Burch colposuspension for urinary incontinence in patients with stable and unstable detrusor function. *Neurourol Urodyn* 1988; 7: 435–439

46. Holley RL, Rouse DJ, Howard BC *et al.* The cost-effectiveness of three surgical procedures for genuine stress incontinence. *J Pelvic Surg* 1997; 3: 246–250

47. Larsson B, Jonasson A, Fianu S. Retropubic urethrocystopexy with fibrin sealant: a long-term follow-up. *Gynecol Obstet Invest* 1988; 26: 257–261

48. Feyereisl J, Dreher E, Haengi W *et al.* Long-term results after Burch colposuspension. *Am J Obstet Gynecol* 1994; 171: 647–652

49. Wolf H, Noesselt T. Ergebnisse nach modifizierter Kolposuspensionsplastik nach Burch bei Patientinnen mit hypotoner Urethra oder Rezidivinkontinenz. *Arch Gynecol* 1991; 250: 340–341

50. VanGeelen JM, Theeuwes AGM, Eskes TKAB, Martin CB. The clinical and urodynamic effects of anterior vaginal repair and Burch colposuspension. *Am J Obstet Gynecol* 1988; 159: 137–144

51. Herbertsson G, Iosif CS. Surgical results and urodynamic studies 10 years after retropubic colpourethrocystopexy. *Acta Obstet Gynecol Scand* 1993; 72: 298–301

52. Weil A, Reyes H, Bischoff P *et al.* Modifications of the urethral rest and stress profiles after different types of surgery for urinary stress incontinence. *Br J Obstet Gynaecol* 1984; 91: 46–55

53. Bergman A, Ballard CA, Koonings PP. Comparison of three different surgical procedures for genuine stress incontinence: prospective randomized study. *Am J Obstet Gynecol* 1989; 160: 1102–1106

54. Penttinen J, Kaar K, Kauppila A. Colposuspension and transvaginal bladder neck suspension in the treatment of stress incontinence. *Gynecol Obstet Invest* 1989; 28: 101–105

55. Colombo M, Scalambrino S, Maggioni A *et al.* Burch colposuspension versus modified Marshall–Marchetti–Krantz urethropexy for primary genuine stress incontinence: a propective randomized trial. *Am J Obstet Gynecol* 1994; 171: 1573–1579

42

Laparoscopic colposuspension

J. M. Lavin, A. R. B. Smith

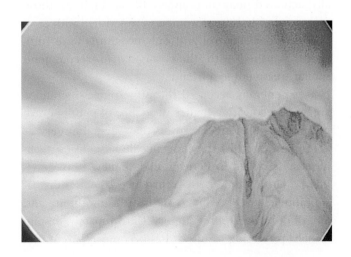

INTRODUCTION

Technological advances in imaging and instrument design have enabled surgeons to perform surgery through a minimal-access approach, with the aim of minimizing perioperative morbidity while maintaining the success rates achieved by conventional surgery. Some operations, such as cholecystectomy, are now widely performed using the laparoscopic approach. Publications have illustrated that it is technically possible to perform a colposuspension with laparoscopic assistance, but the efficacy of this approach is not yet clear.

The description of the Marshall–Marchetti–Krantz procedure,[1] in 1949, and the Burch colposuspension,[2] in 1961, led to the acceptance of the suprapubic approach for surgery for the correction of stress incontinence as being most successful. The Burch colposuspension is the operation that is most widely practised currently, and has been studied most extensively. Published series suggest that an 80–95% success rate can be expected with the Burch procedure.[3] There is a time-dependent decline in efficacy, but this has been shown to plateau at 69% cure of stress incontinence at 10–12 years after surgery.[4] Along with these success rates, it must be remembered that 15% of women may be troubled by new detrusor instability and that 7% may have voiding dysfunction.[3] More recently there has been a greater awareness of the risk of prolapse and dyspareunia following colposuspension: it has been reported that there is a 10% incidence of vaginal prolapse within 12 months of surgery and this figure rises to 25% of women having a vaginal prolapse within 5 years;[5] there is also a 10% incidence of post-colposuspension dyspareunia. A recent cohort study shows that the success rates generally achieved may not always be as high as those reported:[6] only 10% of women were satisfied with postoperative pain control and only two-thirds were sufficiently satisfied with their surgery to recommend similar treatment to a friend.

It is generally accepted that suprapubic operations are associated with a higher incidence of perioperative morbidity and a longer recovery than vaginal surgery; as a response to this, the long needle suspension techniques, described by Pereyra[7] and Stamey,[8] were developed. These aimed to reproduce the results of suprapubic surgery, but to reduce the morbidity and length of recovery after surgery. Unfortunately, despite initially promising results, it has become apparent that the long-term results are disappointing, with 10-year success rates as low as 10%.[9]

Laparoscopic colposuspension was first described by Vancaillie, in 1991.[10] This was designed to reproduce the Burch procedure and its good results, with the advantages of minimal-access surgery. Further published series of laparoscopic colposuspension mainly comprise reports from small retrospective series with short-term follow-up and a lack of standardization of preoperative assessment, surgical technique and follow-up, making meaningful critical analysis difficult. There are, to date, only two published, prospective randomized studies that compare laparoscopic with open Burch colposuspension.[11,12] These studies are highlighted throughout this chapter.

PREOPERATIVE ASSESSMENT

Few papers define the incontinence that was present preoperatively; urodynamic studies were not always carried out prior to surgery to exclude detrusor instability. In some, the diagnosis of stress incontinence was made from the patient's history or from a standing stress test. Objective quantification of the degree of incontinence, such as by pad testing, was rarely performed. Despite the now-recognized risk of new prolapse development following stress incontinence surgery, there was no standardized assessment of prolapse in any of the reports.

TECHNIQUE

Three approaches to access the retropubic space are described, namely transperitoneal, extraperitoneal and 'Retziusscopy'.

1. The transperitoneal approach has the advantage of allowing inspection of the abdomen and pelvis. It provides a wide access and allows other intraperitoneal procedures to be performed. In our own series we found that 30% of women underwent an associated procedure at the same time as the colposuspension. However, this technique requires blind entry into the peritoneal cavity and therefore carries a risk of visceral damage. There is also a risk of herniation of intra-abdominal organs through the port wounds postoperatively.

2. The extraperitoneal approach avoids the peritoneal space and as such removes the risk of injury to the

intra-abdominal viscera. Preperitoneal scarring from previous surgery may interfere with access to the retropubic space. There is a smaller operating field and it is not possible to perform intraperitoneal concomitant surgery. It is generally thought that this approach is faster than the transperitoneal approach and, because the peritoneum is not opened, this technique causes less pain. Neither of these claims has been proven by a controlled study.

3. In the Retziusscopy technique the main trocar is placed suprapubically, rather than at the umbilicus. The risk of bladder perforation is increased and it is therefore less popular.

Various techniques have been described for the fixation of the endopelvic fascia, often bearing little resemblance to the procedure described by Burch.

A range of different sutures has been used, both absorbable and permanent. Burch, in his original description, used catgut, without apparent problems of suspension failure. However, as one of the advantages of laparoscopic surgery is the reduction in tissue damage and subsequent scar formation, it is possible that laparoscopic colposuspension requires permanent sutures.

The size of the needle used also varies between papers. If smaller needles are used than at open colposuspension, too small a 'bite' may be obtained, causing the suture to cut out of the vagina, or leading to only a small area of the paravaginal fascia being apposed to the pelvic side wall. In his prospective study, Burton[11] used Dexon in both series; however, a 12 mm needle was used, in the laparoscopic group, limiting the amount of tissue gathered. This may have influenced the poorer outcome achieved in this group.

The number of sutures placed also varies in different series. Most commonly only two sutures are placed on each side, although it is more usual for three sutures to be sited at the open procedure. There is little description about the position of the sutures. In our own experience the distance between the sutures is less when placed laparoscopically.

Other authors describe the use of mesh, staples, bone anchors and fibrin sealant to elevate the bladder neck. These techniques reduce the operating time by eliminating the requirement of suturing, which is a difficult laparoscopic technique to master. The use of mesh is also aimed at improving the durability of the colposuspension.[13,14] However, mesh has been used in gynaecology for many years and its popularity has waned with increasing recognition of mesh erosion. It may be that, with the improvements in the materials available today, this risk has been reduced, or it might be that, with the resurgence of its popularity, we have yet to see more cases of erosion.

The use of fibrin sealant has been reported.[15] In this technique, the sealant was placed in the retropubic space and the bladder neck was pressed against the retropubic periostium for 5 minutes. This shortened the procedure considerably to an average of 20 minutes. However, as only a single retrospective series of 17 patients has been reported, it is difficult to assess its value.

Laparoscopically assisted needle suspensions using Stamey needles have also been reported.[16] It is not surprising that the long-term results of these operations seem to be similar to those of the Stamey procedure

Learning curve

It is well recognized that there is a learning curve associated with laparoscopic colposuspension, although its length has yet to be established. It is probable that it was longer for the pioneers of this type of surgery, as they had to learn solely by their own experiences. A large prospective study, which began in March 1999, has the stipulation that participating surgeons must have already carried out 50 laparoscopic colposuspensions. Most of the papers do not give information about the number of procedures a surgeon had carried out prior to the published series; however, with some reporting mean operating times in excess of 180 minutes, it is likely that cases carried out during the surgeon's learning curve are being reported and may therefore be unfairly compared with series of open colposuspensions from units carrying out large numbers of these operations. Burton[11] had performed only 10 laparoscopic colposuspensions before embarking on his prospective study in which the success rate in the laparoscopic group was lower. In a prospective study carried out by Ramsay and Hawthorne,[17] the patients undergoing laparoscopic colposuspension were operated upon by an experienced endoscopic surgeon and those undergoing open colposuspension were treated by a urogynaecologist; this study revealed no significant difference in the success rates at 2 years.

We found a clear demonstration of the learning curve in our first 139 cases.[18] Four women required conversion to an open procedure, but all four occurred within our first 42 cases. We also found that the mean operating time halved over the first 50 cases.

Operating time

The operating time for laparoscopic colposuspension is consistently longer than for the open procedure, but with experience (of both the surgeon and theatre staff), this may be a difference of only 15 minutes. The use of mesh and staples may further reduce the duration of the laparoscopic procedure and may lead to similar operating times.

INTRA-OPERATIVE COMPLICATIONS

The reported incidence of urinary tract injury sustained at laparoscopic surgery is higher than that published for open colposuspension. The incidence of bladder injuries in the laparoscopic series is reported as 1–10%. Some of these bladder injuries are small and are noted only on filling the bladder prior to insertion of a suprapubic catheter; these require only drainage or are amenable to laparoscopic repair. The incidence of ureteric injury or kinking is reported as less than 0.1%.

Accepting that the published series of open colposuspensions are generally from reputed centres of urogynaecology, it may be that it is unfair to compare these with the published laparoscopic series which often include the laparoscopic surgeon's learning curve and are not all from gynaecologists with formal training in urogynaecology. A large prospective study is required to compare intra-operative morbidity.

PERIOPERATIVE MORBIDITY AND EARLY RECOVERY

Most series do not comment on pyrexia, need for transfusion and analgesic requirements. In a retrospective study of case records that compared laparoscopic with open colposuspension, we found[18] that the incidence of postoperative pyrexia was decreased from 31 to 11%, wound infection from 8 to 1% and the transfusion rate from 8 to 2%.

We also found that the number of doses of narcotic analgesia required was halved following laparoscopic surgery; however, this and the duration of stay are both open to bias due to both our own and the patient's expectations following surgery. This type of bias was demonstrated by Mackenzie,[19] who showed that the pre-operative information given to patients undergoing hysterectomy had a major influence on time for recovery. The Sheffield cholecystectomy study[20] also illustrated that, when patients are blinded to the method of gall-bladder removal, their recovery rates are the same for open and laparoscopic techniques.

Differing catheter regimens and the (now routine) use of intermittent self-catheterization are influencing time of discharge. The length of postoperative stay, although open to bias, is also difficult to compare between Europe and North America, where financial imperatives dictate early hospital discharge. It is possible that earlier mobilization and voiding may accelerate the return to normal activity. Hawthorne and Ramsay[17] reported that postoperative stay for laparoscopic colposuspension was 2.8 days compared with 6.6 days for open colposuspension. The women in the endoscopic group returned to normal activity faster (3.3 vs 4.9 weeks).

SUCCESS RATES

There is no universal definition of surgical cure of stress incontinence and this lack of clarity is evident in reports on laparoscopic colposuspension. Descriptions such as '100% satisfactory relief' have been used. Some apply very strict criteria based on both subjective and objective data, so the success rates cannot be compared between series. Many reports refer to success rates at 3 months, but it has long been recognized that follow-up should be for a minimum of 2 years. Open colposuspension success rates fall by approximately 10% per 10 years so it is too early to assess the long-term success of laparoscopic colposuspension. The poor long-term results from the Stamey procedure should warn against optimism and it is possible that early mobilization influences long-term results.

Burton, who performed the first randomized controlled trial of laparoscopic and open colposuspension,[11] reported a cure rate of 60% from the laparoscopic cases at 3 years compared with 93% for the open procedure using objective measurement. There was a further deterioration in the results in the laparoscopic group at 5 years.[21] Hawthorne and Ramsay,[17] in a 2-year follow-up of a prospective randomized study of similar size, demonstrated no objective difference in outcome. A further prospective study by Su[12] reported a lower success rate with the laparoscopic colposuspension at 3 months (80.4 vs 95.6%). A prospective randomized trial involving 200 women was reported by Carey *et al.* in 2000.[22] Follow-up at 6 months showed that the laparoscopic approach was as effective as the traditional Burch procedure.

Postoperative detrusor instability, voiding dysfunction, new prolapse development and dyspareunia are all recognized sequelae to open colposuspension. These are rarely reported in the laparoscopic series, so it is difficult to determine an overall incidence from the literature. We found a 10% incidence of *de-novo* detrusor instability, a 5% incidence of short-term voiding difficulty and a 1% incidence of long-term problems, requiring intermittent self-catheterization. We also found that 10% of women developed a new prolapse, similar to the rate reported for the open Burch procedure. Data regarding sexual function following laparoscopic surgery are absent.

RECOVERY

One of the main advantages cited in favour of minimal-access surgery is that there is a quicker postoperative recovery, which confers obvious quality-of-life benefits to the patient. However, two issues need to be examined: (a) does laparoscopic colposuspension lead to an earlier return to normal activities, and (b) is a swift recovery beneficial?

The return to normal activities can be strongly influenced by both the surgeon's and the patient's expectations. Those patients who underwent laparoscopic surgery in our retrospective series reported that they returned to work and normal activities in less than half the time it took for those convalescing after an open Burch colposuspension. Ramsay and Hawthorne[17] found, in their prospective study, that those women who had undergone laparoscopic colposuspension returned to work after 3.1 weeks, whereas those who had undergone open colposuspension took 4.1 weeks off work.

The optimum period of convalescence is not known. It has been argued that one of the reasons why the bladder-neck suspension procedures have high failure rates is that women resume normal activities too soon, before adequate fibrosis has occurred. If this is so, it is possible that with time we will see a similar decline in efficacy of the laparoscopic colposuspension, as witnessed with the Stamey procedure. However, the evidence available for hernia repair operations would suggest that early mobilization is not detrimental to the success of the procedure.

COST

Laparoscopic surgery is associated with high initial capital costs, due to equipment purchase. The surgeon's learning curve also increases the cost of the procedure, reflected in the increased operating time required for the initial cases. However, weighed against this must be the shorter postoperative hospitalization and the faster return to work.

A cost analysis in the United States[23] showed that laparoscopic colposuspension was more expensive than a Burch operation (US$4960 vs US$4079), even though it reduced hospital stay. However, the length of stay was much shorter than would be usual in Europe. Another analysis from Australia concluded that the laparoscopic colposuspension was cost-effective.[24] The different conclusions reached by these authors is probably related to the duration of postoperative stay.

These cost analyses refer only to the hospital costs. If women are returning to work sooner, it can be argued that the overall costs may be less. However, it must be borne in mind that, if recurrence of stress incontinence is found to be higher following laparoscopic colposuspension, the ultimate costs of treating that patient will include any further surgery that she requires. Whereas repeat surgery after a failed Stamey procedure is generally not complicated, surgery following a laparoscopic colposuspension may be complicated by scarring in the retropubic space.

PATIENT EXPECTATIONS

The published series of Burch colposuspensions are generally from centres of urological/gynaecological excellence. However, are these indicative of the results that are generally obtained for this procedure, or do they reflect the expertise of specialists in urogynaecology?

Black and colleagues[6] carried out a prospective cohort study, aimed at assessing the impact of surgery for stress incontinence on morbidity, and questioned 442 women who underwent surgery for stress incontinence in 18 different hospitals. Although most women reported an improvement in their symptoms, only 28%

described themselves as being completely cured. Their surgeons were more optimistic and reported a satisfactory outcome in 85% of the women, whereas only two-thirds of the women considered that their surgery had met their expectations and would recommend it to a friend. Laparoscopic colposuspension series generally report a higher degree of patient satisfaction than this. However, as with so many other parameters, this is open to bias. In our series, 94% said they would recommend laparoscopic colposuspension to a friend; the reasons for this difference need clarification.

CONCLUSIONS

The evidence available to date is not sufficient to determine whether laparoscopic colposuspension is an advance over open colposuspension. The retrospective series are open to so much bias that the information that they provide must be viewed with great caution. The prospective randomized studies provide better-quality data, but are small series and therefore do not have the power to demonstrate a significant difference. A large prospective randomized trial is required to evaluate this procedure fully.

REFERENCES

1. Marshall VF, Marchetti AA, Krantz KE. The correction of stress incontinence by simple vesicourethral suspension. *Surg Gynaecol Obstet* 1949; 88: 509–518

2. Burch JC. Urethrovesical fixation to Cooper's ligament for correction of stress incontinence, cystocele and prolapse. *Am J Obstet Gynecol* 1961; 81: 281–290

3. Jarvis GJ. Surgery for genuine stress incontinence. *Br J Obstet Gynaecol* 1994; 101: 371–374

4. Alcalay M, Monga A, Stanton SL. Burch colposuspension: a 10–20 year follow up. *Br J Obstet Gynaecol* 1995; 102: 740–745

5. Wiskind AK, Creighton SM, Stanton SL. The incidence of prolapse after Burch colposuspension. *Am J Obstet Gynecol* 1992; 167: 399–405

6. Black N, Griffiths J, Pope C *et al.* Impact of surgery for stress incontinence on morbidity: cohort study. *Br Med J* 1997; 315: 1493–1498

7. Pereyra AJ. A simplified surgical procedure for the correction of stress urinary incontinence in women. *West J Surg Obstet Gynecol* 1959; 67: 223–226

8. Stamey TA. Endoscopic suspension of the vesical neck for urinary incontinence. *Surg Gynecol Obstet* 1973; 136: 547–554

9. Kevelighan E, Aagaard J, Jarvis GJ. The Stamey endoscopic bladder neck suspension – a 10 year follow up study (abstr. 142) *Proceedings of the 27th Annual Meeting of the International Continence Society, Yokohama,* 1997, 74–75

10. Vancaillie TG, Schuessler WW. Laparoscopic bladder neck suspension. *J Laparoendosc Surg* 1991; 1: 169–173

11. Burton G. A three year prospective randomised urodynamic study comparing open and laparoscopic colposuspension. *Neurourol Urodyn* 1997; 16: 353–354

12. Su TH, Wang KG, Hsu CY *et al.* Prospective comparison of laparoscopic and traditional colposuspensions in the treatment of genuine stress incontinence. *Acta Obstet Gynecol Scand* 1997; 76: 576–582

13. Seitzinger MR. Laparoscopic modified MMK using direct stapling method. *J Am Assoc Gynecol Laparosc* 1995; 2: S50

14. Birken RA, Legget PL. Laparoscopic colposuspension using mesh reinforcement. *Surg Endosc* 1997; 11: 1111–1114

15. Kiilhoma P, Haarala M, Polvi H *et al.* Sutureless endoscopic colposuspension with fibrin sealant. *Tech Urol* 1995; 1: 81–83

16. Pelosi MA 3rd, Pelosi MA. Laparoscopic-assisted transpectineal needle suspension of the bladder neck. *J Am Assoc Gynecol Laparosc* 1998; 5: 39–46

17. Ramsay IN, Hawthorne R. Personal communication, 1998

18. Lavin JM, Lewis CJ, Foote AJ *et al.* Laparoscopic Burch colposuspension: a minimum of 2 year's follow up and comparison with open colposuspension. *Gynaecol Endosc* 1998; 7: 251–258

19. Mackenzie IZ. Reducing hospital stay after abdominal hysterectomy. *Br J Obstet Gynaecol* 1996; 103: 175–178

20. Majeed AW, Troy G, Nicholl JP *et al.* Randomised, prospective, single-blind comparison of laparoscopic versus small-incision cholecystectomy. *Lancet* 1996; 347: 989–994

21. Burton G. A five-year prospective randomized urodynamic study comparing open and laparoscopic colposuspension. *Neurourol Urodyn* 1996; 18: 295–296

22. Carey M, Rosamilia A, Maher C *et al.* Laparoscopic versus open colposuspension: a prospective multicentre randomized single-blind comparison. *Neurourol Urodyn* 2000: 19; 389–391

23. Kohli N, Jacobs PA, Sze EH *et al.* Open compared with laparoscopic approach to Burch colposuspension: a cost analysis. *Obstet Gynecol* 1997; 90: 411–415

24. Loveridge K, Malouf A, Kennedy C et al. Laparoscopic colposuspension. Is it cost-effective? *Surg Endosc* 1997; 11: 762–765

43

Sling procedures – organic

D. C. Chaikin, J. G. Blaivas

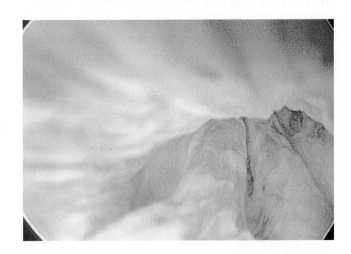

INTRODUCTION

Sling procedures with many different modifications have been used for almost 100 years in the treatment of female incontinence. A variety of techniques have been described, together with a wide range of sling materials. The common feature of sling-type operations is the use of a strip of material, which is passed completely beneath the urethra or bladder neck and anchored anteriorly, usually to some point on the abdominal wall. Throughout the 20th century, the popularity of sling operations has varied, with periods of enthusiasm as new methods have been used and periods of disillusionment as complications have become apparent.

In the early part of the century, sling-type procedures were devised to act by compressing the urethra and producing partial obstruction, leading to a high incidence of voiding problems. It would appear that urethral obstruction is not necessary for successful sling surgery and it is probable that optimal sling tension is much less than was previously thought. A successful sling does not need to increase resting urethral pressure, but acts as a backboard of support for the urethra during stress and allows more effective pressure transmission. The trend has been to reduce sling tension, decreasing the obstructive nature of the procedure and leading to a lower incidence of postoperative voiding difficulties and detrusor instability (DI).

Currently, there is renewed interest in the use of sling techniques as greater understanding of their mechanism of action has developed and means of avoiding some of the pitfalls have been discovered.

HISTORY OF SUBURETHRAL SLING PROCEDURES

Vaginal plastic procedures, the forebears of the modern anterior colporrhaphy, were first described by Schultze[1] in 1888, and modified by a number of authors, most notably Kelly.[2] Kelly described the excision of a portion of anterior vaginal wall and plication of the paravesical tissue (at the bladder neck) and paravaginal fascia. The success of this type of anterior vaginal repair was known to be limited and the need for repeated surgery and the lack of success led to the search for alternative approaches.

From the beginning of the 20th century, a number of operations utilizing a variety of materials to form a suburethral sling were reported. That described by Goebell[3] and Stockell[4] utilized the pyramidalis to form a muscular sling beneath the urethra, and Frangheim[5] suggested the addition of strips of rectus fascia left attached to the pyramidalis. A combination of the Goebell–Stockell–Frangheim[6] procedure became popular for some time.

The use of muscle flaps was also proposed by Giordano,[7] who described the transposition of the gracilis wrapped around the urethra; Martius[8] developed the use of the bulbocavernosus and its associated fat pad to provide bulk around the urethra. The technique described by Martius is, of course, still used today to provide a pedicled flap in fistula repair and radical vulval surgery. These techniques all relied on the provision of bulky tissue to compress the urethra, thereby increasing the urethral closure pressure. Unfortunately, owing to extensive dissection and denervation, this tissue bulk was often short-lived.

Miller,[9] in 1932, described the use of thin strips of rectus fascia to lift and elevate the bladder neck; however, it was not until 1942 that Aldridge[10] described his sling procedure, which can be recognized as the predecessor of modern sling techniques.

Aldridge used thin horizontal strips of rectus fascia raised by a Pfannenstiel incision. These are left attached at their medial border. Through a vaginal incision, a tunnel is created on either side of the urethra at the bladder neck, between the layers of the endopelvic fascia, and developed through the space of Retzius retropubically to reach the insertion of the abdominal muscles. The endopelvic fascia is plicated in the midline to give additional support to the bladder neck. Finally, the fascial strips are brought through the rectus and sutured in the midline at the bladder neck and the vaginal and abdominal incisions are closed.

Aldridge proposed that this technique should be used as a primary technique in women where previous surgery had failed and, particularly, where sphincter function was compromised as a result of either previous surgery or birth trauma and neurological injury.[11] Since Aldridge's description, a number of modifications have been described: sling insertion, utilizing a combined vaginal and abdominal approach, a vaginal approach alone, or a suprapubic technique alone, with blind dissection beneath the urethra and bladder base, have all been described. The use of an abdominal approach alone is claimed to reduce bacterial contamination of the sling, although the incidence of bladder and urethral injury may be slightly higher.[12] However, there is no definitive evidence to suggest which surgical approach is superior, and this appears to be related to the preference and experience of the surgeon. It is the choice of sling material and final sling tension that appear to have most influence on the outcome of sling surgery.

MECHANISM OF ACTION OF PUBOURETHRAL SLINGS

In Aldridge's original description, the mechanism of a sling was proposed to be active. Because the abdominal end of the sling is attached to the abdominal aponeurosis, it moves with the abdominal wall during periods of raised intra-abdominal pressure. During a cough or sneeze, the abdominal wall moves outward and the sling is drawn upward, effectively increasing intra-urethral pressure. A number of authors have described a visible elevation of the bladder neck during a Valsalva manoeuvre following a sling procedure.

DeLancey[13] and Zacharin[14] have proposed that the pubourethral ligaments and endopelvic fascia provide support to the urethra, thereby allowing effective transmission of increases in intra-abdominal pressure. It may be that a suburethral sling, rather than elevating and compressing the urethra during stress, provides passive resistance and support, allowing effective transmission of intra-abdominal pressure to the urethra.

It is not clear whether a passive or an active mechanism (or both) is most important in restoring continence.

PATIENT SELECTION FOR SLING PROCEDURES

Considerable debate surrounds the selection of women for whom sling surgery is the most appropriate. Traditionally, slings have been used for women who have had one or more previously failed incontinence operations and have poor urethral sphincter function as assessed by urethral pressure profilometry.[15] This represents a group of women who are extremely difficult to treat successfully, and cure rates of 82% demonstrate the efficacy of this technique.[16,17] Some experts argue that, owing to the potential for denervation of the urethral sphincter and a higher complication rate than suprapubic surgery, slings should be reserved as secondary procedures.[18] However, protagonists of sling surgery consider that these are appropriate as a primary operation in all cases of stress incontinence.[19] A number of

reports of success rates of over 90% demonstrate that sling surgery may certainly be appropriate as a first-line operation.[20]

EFFECT OF VAGINAL DISSECTION ON THE URETHRAL NERVE SUPPLY

The innervation of the female urethra has been the subject of much controversy. Recent studies by Ball *et al.*[21] and Borirakchanyavat *et al.*[22] have clarified the somatic and autonomic innervation of the urethra. It appears that the somatic component travels in an extrapelvic course via the pudendal nerve, whereas the autonomic nerve supply to the urethra and bladder neck is carried via the pelvic plexus. As a result of detailed anatomical and histological studies, the autonomic nerves of the urethra have been found to travel in close association with the inferior vascular pedicle of the bladder and close to the anterolateral vaginal wall at 4 and 8 o'clock positions to reach the urethral sphincter. This finding offers one potential explanation for the relatively poor results of anterior colporrhaphy, as the wide dissection of the anterior vaginal wall may result in denervation of the urethral sphincter.

Intrinsic sphincter deficiency is most commonly seen after previous incontinence surgery and is one of the most difficult aspects of stress incontinence to treat successfully. It follows that during surgery for stress incontinence, every attempt should be made to avoid damaging the urethral nerve supply during vaginal dissection.

USE OF SLING PROCEDURES IN OLDER WOMEN

Treatment of stress incontinence in older women is complicated by the increased incidence of DI and voiding difficulties in this age group. In addition, the need for a procedure with lower morbidity has led to a reluctance to utilize sling procedures in older women. However, a study by Carr *et al.*[15] found a subjective cure rate of 100% in a group of women over 70 with an incidence of *de-novo* DI of 10%, which was comparable with that in a younger group of women, and no appreciable difference in the incidence of voiding difficulties. Sling surgery was well tolerated in the elderly women, with no significant difference in surgical morbidity. It would appear that age is no bar to successful sling surgery in a carefully selected group of older women.

SLINGS AND UROGENITAL PROLAPSE

The sling technique originally described by Aldridge included an anterior colporrhaphy as a preliminary stage of sling insertion. Cross *et al.*[16] studied the results of sling insertion and anterior repair in a group of women with large cystoceles and stress incontinence: they reported an 89% cure of stress incontinence and 92% cure of prolapse at a mean of 20 months. The successful use of a Marlex mesh patch to reinforce an anterior repair with 'side arms' to act as a sling has also been reported.[17] Recently there have been reports of the use of cadaveric fascia lata as a patch to reinforce an anterior repair.[23]

SLING INSERTION FOLLOWING URETHRAL TRAUMA OR RECONSTRUCTION AND IN MYELODYSPLASIA

Slings have also been utilized to produce continence in women with neuropathic bladders and complete sphincter dysfunction due to myelodysplasia,[18] and following urethral reconstruction and trauma.[19,20] In this situation, the technique differs somewhat from that used in less-complicated stress incontinence. The aim is to produce high elevation of the bladder neck with a greater degree of urethral obstruction and is usually performed after bladder augmentation. This results in a continent low-pressure urine reservoir and allows clean intermittent catheterization.

NATURAL SLING MATERIALS

The Aldridge sling has two disadvantages in the choice of sling material: the harvesting of rectus fascia requires a large abdominal incision and creation of a defect in the rectus fascia, which increases the surgical morbidity; in addition, women with stress incontinence may have connective tissue that is inherently weak,[24,25] leading to poorer long-term results. Women presenting with stress incontinence may also have had previous abdominal surgery, which may cause difficulty in obtaining a sufficient length of good-quality undamaged fascia from this site.

Vaginal wall sling

A number of modifications of a technique for elevating the bladder neck using *in situ* sections of vaginal wall have been described. In these techniques, a patch of freely dissected or *in situ* vaginal skin is secured to the abdominal wall with the use of long sutures, passed using Stamey-type needles, elevating the bladder neck. In the *in situ* method, the defect in the vaginal wall is then closed using an advancement flap. It is claimed that vaginal skin provides more flexible support than a fascial or synthetic sling and good results are reported with this technique. However, although termed the 'vaginal sling', the technique has more in common with the needle-suspension techniques described by Peyrera, Stamey and Raz; it is not, therefore, considered further in this chapter.

Autologous fascia lata

To circumvent the problems of using abdominal wall fascia, the use of a strip of autologous fascia lata was proposed by Price in 1933.[26] Fascia lata has been used extensively in a number of studies.[27–30] It can be obtained in a strip 18–20 cm long, with the use of a fascial stripper, through a small incision just above the lateral femoral condyle. Fascia lata is thicker and stronger than abdominal aponeurosis and there is a reduced risk of an incisional hernia developing subsequently. The technique of fascial stripping, although straightforward, is not without complications: a second operative site is created with a concomitant increase in the risk of haematoma formation, wound infection and postoperative pain. Damage to branches of the lateral cutaneous nerve of the thigh is also a possibility, with subsequent neuralgia. The operative time is increased, as fascia must be harvested and prepared before proceeding with colporrhaphy and sling insertion.[31] It is not clear whether the fascial flap serves merely as a framework for fibrosis or survives intact. Early failure of fascial slings has been ascribed to partial necrosis of the fascia.

Fokaefs *et al.*[32] carried out a histological and biomechanical study of free and pedicled fascial slings in rabbits. In this model, free fascial slings remained viable, presumably as a free graft obtaining nutrients initially by diffusion until neovascularization took place. How these results apply to human tissue is not certain, although shrinkage of the fascia by up to one-third reinforces the fact that excess tension in the sling should be avoided to reduce subsequent voiding difficulties.[33]

Cadaveric fascia lata

Allogenic grafts of fascia lata usually harvested from cadavers have been used for many years, mainly in orthopaedics. Many studies have demonstrated their safety, stability and lack of antigenicity.[34] After implantation, the local response to allogenic fascia[35] does not differ from that with autologous fascia, providing a framework for fibrosis.

Allogenic fascia should therefore provide similar results to autologous grafts without the donor-site morbidity and potential complications associated with intra-operative harvesting of the graft; good results have been reported using these materials.[36,37]

The implantation of allogenic materials raises concerns regarding the antigenicity of the foreign material and the transmission of infectious diseases, such as hepatitis B and C, and the HIV virus. Allografts are fresh-frozen, freeze-dried or solvent dehydrated, all of which effectively destroy their antigenicity. No graft rejection has been noted after the use of such implants.[38] To minimize the risk of viral infection, graft material is sterilized and processed by a multistep process that effectively reduces the graft to an acellular fibrous mesh and which should inactivate any viral agents. The risk of HIV transmission from soft-tissue allografts has been estimated at one in 8 million.[39]

Porcine dermis

Porcine dermis has also been described as an alternative allogenic sling material.[40,41] As with human fascia lata, the process of preservation and sterilization renders the tissue non-immunogenic and should destroy any viral particles. Human dermis processed by a patented technique to preserve and sterilize it has been utilized for vaginal reconstruction and for sling surgery. There are no published reports of long-term complications or durability.

Lyodura

Lyodura (homologous lyophilized dura mater) has been used by Rottenburg *et al.*[42] and Faber *et al.*,[41] again with results comparable to those with other natural sling materials.

OPERATIVE TECHNIQUE FOR PUBOVAGINAL SLING (BLAIVAS–CHAIKIN)

Regional (epidural or spinal anaesthesia) is used unless there is a contraindication or if it proves technically unsatisfactory. The surgery is performed in the dorsal lithotomy position with a weighted speculum in the vagina. A Foley catheter is inserted into the urethra and the balloon inflated with enough saline to facilitate palpation of the vesical neck. In order to minimize blood loss, the abdominal portion of the procedure is completed first. The fascial strip to be used for the sling is harvested and stored in sterile saline while the vaginal portion of the operation is completed.

A short transverse incision is made just beneath the pubic hairline and carried down to the rectus fascia (Fig. 43.1). The surface of the rectus fascia is dissected free of subcutaneous tissue and a suitable site is selected for excision of the fascial strip (Fig. 43.2). If the patient has undergone previous surgery, there may be considerable scarring. It is not necessary to find 'scar-free' fascia – even the most scarred tissue, not even recognizable as fascia, may be used. We have always been able to find a suitable strip to harvest. Two parallel horizontal incisions, 2–3 cm apart, are made near the midline in the rectus fascia. The incisions are extended superolaterally for the entire width of the wound, following the direction of the fascial fibres. If a longer strip is needed, the incisions may be extended superiorly in a vertical direction at the most lateral aspect of the wound. The undersurface of the fascia is freed from muscle and scar. Prior to exercising the strip, each end of the fascia is secured with a long 2/0 non-absorbable suture using a running horizontal mattress which is placed at right angles to the direction of the fascial fibres (Figs 43.3, 43.4). No attempt is made to enter the retropubic space. It is not necessary to mobilize or expose the bladder or vesical neck from above, as this is accomplished through the vaginal dissection. The fascial defect is closed with a continuous 2/0 non-absorbable suture. The wound is temporarily packed with saline-soaked sponges and attention is turned to the vagina.

If donor tissue is to be used, we prefer to use a strip (15 cm × 2 cm) of solvent-dehydrated donor fascia lata. After tissue preparation, we soak the tissue in an antibiotic solution until the vaginal dissection has been completed. A long 2/0 non-absorbable suture using a running horizontal mattress which is placed at right

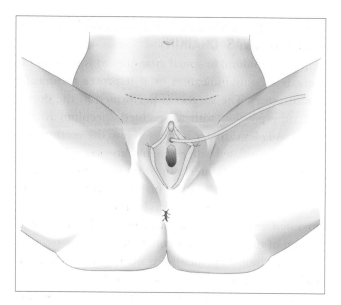

Figure 43.1. *Pfannensteil skin incision.*

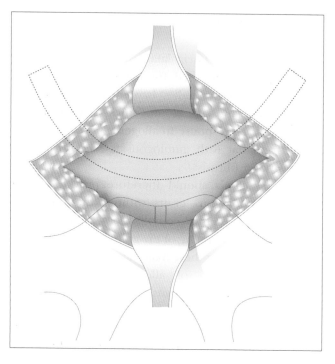

Figure 43.2. *A graft 2–3 cm wide is outlined keeping the incision parallel to the direction of the fascial fibres. The incision is extended laterally to the point where the rectus fascia divides and passes to the internal and external oblique muscles.*

angles to the direction of the fascial fibres is placed at either end of the tissue strip.

The bladder neck is identified by placing gentle traction on the Foley catheter and palpating the balloon. In most patients, the actual position of the vesical neck is about 2 cm proximal to the palpable distal edge of the balloon. A gently curved incision is made over the vesical neck (Fig. 43.5). It is very important that this incision is made in the right plane – just beneath the

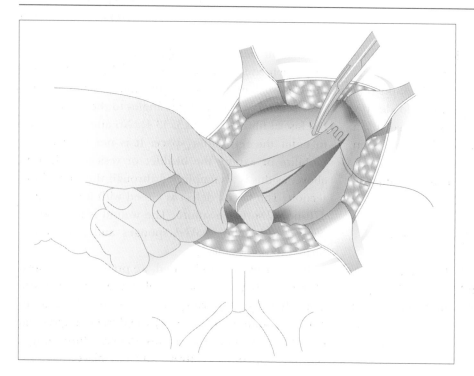

Figure 43.3. *A 2/0 non-absorbable running horizontal mattress suture is placed across the most lateral portion of the graft and the ends are left long. The sling is transected approximately 1 cm lateral to the mattress suture.*

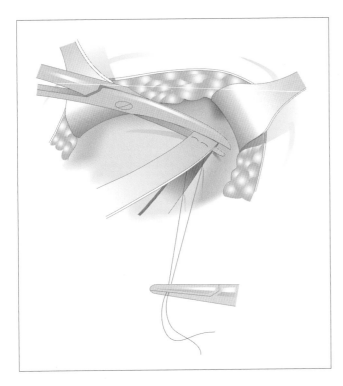

Figure 43.4. *After placing a 2/0 non-absorbable running horizonal mattress suture the sling is transected.*

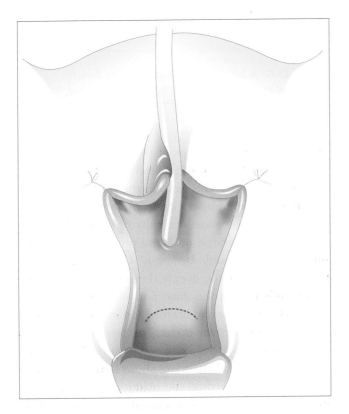

Figure 43.5. *Vaginal incision. A gently curved transverse incision is made 1 cm proximal to the bladder neck.*

vaginal epithelium and superficial to the endopelvic fascia. The proper plane is identified by noting the characteristic shiny white appearance of the undersurface of the anterior vaginal wall. Although the plane is usually described as being bloodless, this is not always the case, but it usually provides the least blood loss. Even more importantly, this plan ensures that the dissection will proceed lateral to the bladder and urethra. If the initial vaginal incision is even a few millimetres too deep, these structures may be injured.

The dissection continues laterally just beneath the vaginal epithelium with Metzenbaum scissors pointed toward the patient's ipsilateral shoulder. The endopelvic fascia is perforated at its most lateral insertion into the ischiopubic ramus with either the Metzenbaum scissors or the surgeon's finger (Fig. 43.6). During this part of the dissection it is important to stay as far lateral as pos-

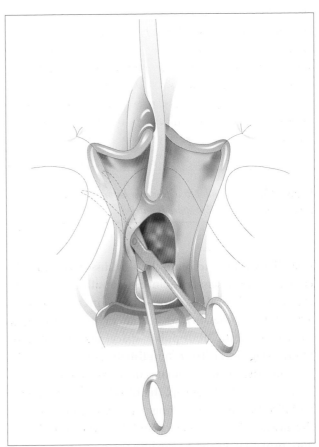

Figure 43.6. *Dissection is begun with Metzenbaum scissors in the avascular plane just beneath the vaginal epithelium. The tips of the scissors are directed toward the patient's ipsilateral shoulder.*

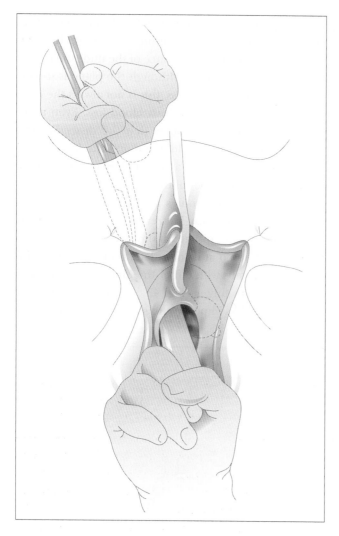

Figure 43.7. *The endopelvic fascia is perforated with the index finger and the retropubic space is entered.*

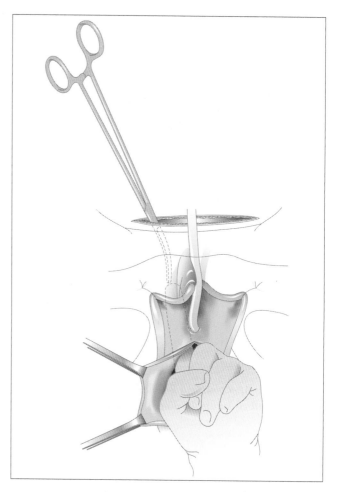

Figure 43.8. *A long DeBakey clamp is passed from the abdominal to the vaginal wound lateral to the urethra.*

sible. This is best accomplished by dissecting with the concavity of the scissors pointing laterally and by exerting constant lateral pressure with the tips of the scissors against the undersurface of the vaginal epithelium. Alternatively, the retropubic space may be entered bluntly (Fig. 43.7). To accomplish this, the tip of the finger, opposite the nail, palpates the periosteum. With the back edge of the fingertip, the bladder and urethra are mobilized medially as the finger advances and perforates the fascia. This completely mobilizes the vesical neck and proximal urethra, freeing these structures from their vaginal attachments. If the dissection does not proceed easily, it may be necessary to complete it sharply with Metzenbaum scissors. The scissors are introduced into the proper plane until the undersurface of the

pubis is palpated. The tips of the scissors are pressed firmly against the bone and spread until they open for a distance of 2–3 cm. This exposes the proper plane and the index finger is reinserted to complete the dissection. Sometimes, this manoeuvre must be repeated several times before the vesical neck and proximal urethra are sufficiently mobilized. However, if the initial vaginal incision was made too deeply (beneath the endopelvic fascia), this part of the dissection will be dangerously close to the bladder and urethra and inadvertent injury to either structure may occur. The retropubic space is entered and the lateral edge of the fascia is separated from the bone for a distance of about 4–6 cm. In cases of obvious vaginal scarring, the bladder base and vesical neck are freed from their vaginal attachments. After completion of the dissection, the surgeon's left index finger is reinserted into the vaginal wound, retracting

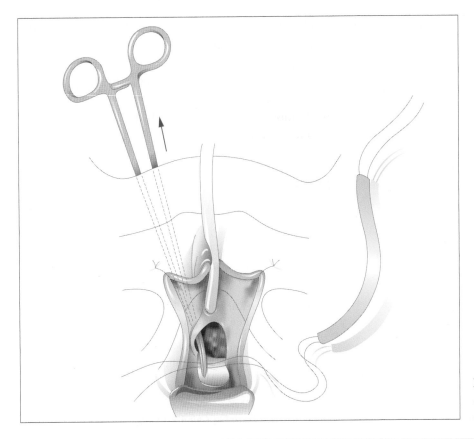

Figure 43.9. *The fascial graft is passed around the urethra and brought to the abdominal wound on either side.*

the vesical neck and bladder medially. A Kocher clamp is placed on the inferior leaf of the rectus fascia and the surgeon's right index finger is placed beneath the fascia and palpates the index finger on the left in the vaginal wound. A long, curved DeBakey clamp is guided beneath the fascia, directed to the undersurface of the pubis. The tip of the clamp is pressed against the periosteum and directed towards the index finger, which palpates the periosteum through the vaginal incision. The index finger is used to guide the clamp into the vaginal wound (Fig. 43.8). When the tip of the clamp is visible, one end of the long suture, which is attached to the fascial graft, is grasped and pulled into the abdominal wound. The procedure is repeated on the other side (Fig. 43.9). The fascial sling is now positioned from the abdominal wall on one side around the undersurface of the urethra at the junction of the bladder neck and back to the abdominal wall on the other side.

If donor fascia lata is to be used, we make a small (2 cm) suprapubic incision and clean the rectus fascia bluntly. We then pass a DeBakey clamp through the fascia in the manner described above (Figs 43.8, 43.9). When the tip of the clamp is visible, one end of the long suture, which is attached to the fascial graft, is grasped

and pulled into the abdominal wound. The procedure is repeated on the other side. The fascial sling is now positioned from the abdominal wall on one side around the undersurface of the urethra at the junction of the bladder neck and back to the abdominal wall on the other side.

Cystoscopy is performed to ensure that there has been no damage to the urethra or bladder neck. A trocar 12F suprapubic tube is inserted percutaneously into the bladder and its position is visually inspected to be sure that is well away from the trigone. The vaginal incision is closed prior to securing the sling in place. The long sutures attached to the sling are tied loosely together over the rectus fascia in the midline without tension and a vaginal pack is left in place. We no longer suture the fascial sling to the rectus fascia (Fig. 43.10). The only exception to this is when the goal of surgery is to create urinary retention and maintain the patient on intermittent catheterization. We have found no precise technique for estimating the tension to be exerted on the fascial strip, but, through experience, have decided that it is far better to err on the side of too little tension.

539

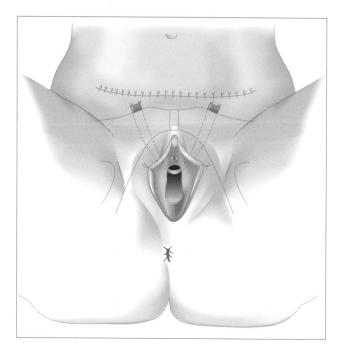

Figure 43.10. *The sling is tied without tension.*

Postoperative care

The vaginal pack is removed the day after surgery. Voiding trials are begun as soon as the patient is ambulating comfortably. If the patient is able to void well, the suprapubic tube is removed; if not, she is taught intermittent catheterization, but, occasionally, patients are discharged with the suprapubic tube in place. One day prior to the return visit, she again has a voiding trial at home.

Conclusion

In our opinion, the recent success of the pubovaginal sling is primarily related to improvements in surgical technique. The most important aspects of surgical technique include the following:

1. Thorough familiarity with vaginal and retropubic anatomy;
2. Confining the vaginal dissection to the 'glistening white surface' just beneath the vaginal epithelium and superficial to the endopelvic fascia;
3. Mobilization of the vesical neck from the vaginal approach, freeing it from tethering to the vagina;

4. Use of a gently curved inverted 'U' incision over the vesical neck to ensure that the sling cannot slip too far proximally or distally;
5. The use of free grafts of fascia for the sling instead of pedicle grafts;
6. Positioning the graft beneath the vesiclal neck without tension.

REFERENCES

1. Schultze BS. *Cor-Bl Allg Artzl Ver Thuringen* (Weimar) 1888; 17: 289

2. Kelly HA, Dumm W. Urinary incontinence in women, without manifest injury to the bladder. *Surg Gynecol Obstet* 1914; 444–450

3. Goebell RG. Zür operativen Behandlung der incontinenz der mannlichen harnrohre *Gynakol Urol* 1910; 2: 187

4. Stockel W. Uber di verwendung der musculi pyramidales bei der operativen behandlung der incontinentia urinae. *Gynakol Urol* 1917; 41: 11

5. Frangheim P. Z.r operativen behandlung der incontinenz. *Verh Dtsch Ges Chir* 43rd Congress: 419.

6. Wheeless CR, Wharton L, Dorsey J, TeLinde R. The Goebell–Stockel operation for universal cases of urinary incontinence. *Am J Obstet Gynecol* 1997; 128: 546.

7. Giordano D. *Twentieth Congress, Français Chir* 1907; 506

8. Martius H. *Chirurg* 1929; 1: 769

9. Miller N. The surgical treatment of stress incontinence in the female. *JAMA* 1932; 98: 628

10. Aldridge AH. Transplantation of fascia for relief of urinary incontinence. *Am J Obstet Gynecol* 1942; 398–411

11. Jeffcoate TNA. Results of Aldridge sling operation for stress incontinence. *J Obstet Gynaecol Br Emp* 1956; 63: 36–39

12. Mason R, Roach M. Modified pubovaginal sling for the treatment of intrinsic sphincter deficiency. *J Urol* 1996; 156: 1991–1994

13. DeLancey J. Structural support of the urethra as it relates to stress urinary incontinence: the hammock hypothesis. *Am J Obstet Gynecol* 1994; 170: 1713–1723

14. Zacharin RF. Abdomino-perineal suspension in the management of recurrent stress incontinence of urine – a 15 year experience. *Obstet Gynecol* 1983; 62: 644–654

15. Carr L, Walsh P, Abraham V, Webster G. Favourable outcome of pubovaginal slings for geriatric women with stress incontinence. *J Urol* 1997; 157: 125–128

16. Cross C, Crepedes D, McGuire E. Treatment results using pubovaginal slings in patients with large cystoceles and stress incontinence. *J Urol* 1997; 158: 431–434

17. Drutz H. Suburethral duplication and anterior colporrhaphy reinforced with a sub-urethral Marlex mesh for the treatment of cystocele and stress urinary incontinence (Abstract). 23rd meeting, IUGA, 1998

18. Elder J. Periurethral and puboprostatic sling repair for incontinence in patients with myelodysplasia. *J Urol* 1990; 144: 434–437

19. Gormeley A, Bloom D, McGuire E, Ritchey M. Pubovaginal slings for the management of urinary incontinence in adolescents. *J Urol* 1994; 152: 822–825

20. Woodside J. Pubovaginal sling procedure for the management of urinary incontinence after urethral trauma in women. *J Urol* 1987; 138: 537–578

21. Ball T, Teichman J, Sharkey F *et al.* Terminal nerve distribution to the urethra and bladder neck: considerations in the management of stress incontinence. *J Urol* 1997; 158: 827–829

22. Borirakchanyavat S, Aboseif S, Carroll P *et al.* Continence mechanism of the isolated female urethra: an anatomical study of the intra-pelvic somatic nerves. *J Urol* 1997; 158: 822–826

23. Groutz *et al.* Personal communication, 2000

24. Ulmsten U, Ekman G, Giertz G, Malstrom A. Different biochemical composition of connective tissue in continent and stress incontinent women. *Acta Obstet Gynecol Scand* 1987; 66: 455–457

25. Landon CR, Smith ARB, Crofts CE, Trowbridge EA. Biomechanical properties of connective tissue in women with stress incontinence of urine. *Neurourol Urodyn* 1989; 8: 369–370

26. Price PB. Plastic operations for incontinence of urine and of faeces. *Arch Surg* 1933; 26: 1043–1048

27. Beck RP, Grove B, Arnusch D, Harvey I. Recurrent urinary stress incontinence treated by the fascia lata sling procedure. *Am J Obstet Gynecol* 1974; 120: 613

28. McLaren C. Late results from sling operations. *J Obstet Gynaecol Br Commonw* 1968; 63: 36

29. Parker TR, Addison AA, Wilson J. Fascia lata urethrovesical suspension for recurrent stress urinary incontinence. *Am J Obstet Gynecol* 1979; 135: 843–852

30. Govier F, Gibbons R, Correa R *et al.* Pubovaginal slings using fascia lata for the treatment of intrinsic sphincter deficiency. *J Urol* 1997; 157: 117–121

31. Kaplan SA, Santarosa RP, Te AE. Comparison of fascial and vaginal wall slings in the management of intrinsic sphincter deficiency. *Urology* 1996; 47: 885–889

32. Fokaefs E, Lampel A, Hoenfellner M *et al.* Experimental evaluation of free versus pedicled fascial flaps for sling surgery of urinary stress incontinence. *J Urol* 1997; 157: 1039–1043

33. McGuire E, Lytton B. Pubovaginal sling procedure for stress incontinence. *J Urol* 1978; 139: 82

34. Cooper JL, Beck RP. History of soft tissue allografts in orthopaedics. *Sports Med Arthrosc Rev* 1993; 1: 2–16

35. Merrit W, Peacock EE, Chvapil M. Comparison of biology of fascial authografts and allografts. *Surg Forum* 1974; 25: 524–526

36. Wright EJ, Iselin CE, Carr LK. Pubovaginal sling using cadaveric allograft. *J Urol* 1998; 169: 1312–1316

37. Handa V, Jensen J, Germain M, Ostergard D. Banked human fascia lata for the suburethral sling procedure: a preliminary report. *Obstet Gynecol* 1996; 88: 1045–1049

38. Buck BE, Malinin TI. Human bone and tissue allografts: preparation and safety. *Clin Orthop* 1994; 303: 8–17

39. Buck BE, Resnick L, Shah SM, Malinin TI. Human immunodeficiency virus cultured from bone: implications for transplantation. *Clin Orthop* 1990; 251: 249–253

40. Iosif CS. Porcine corium sling in the treatment of urinary stress incontinence. *Arch Gynecol* 1987; 240: 131

41. Faber P, Beck L, Heindreich J. Treatment of urinary stress incontinence with the lyodura sling. *Urol Int* 1978; 33: L117

42. Rottenburg R, Weil A, Brioschi P *et al.* Urodynamic and clinical assessment of the Lyodura sling operation for urinary stress incontinence. *Br J Obstet Gynaecol* 1985; 92: 829–834

44

Sling procedures – artificial

J. K. Jensen, H. J. Rufford

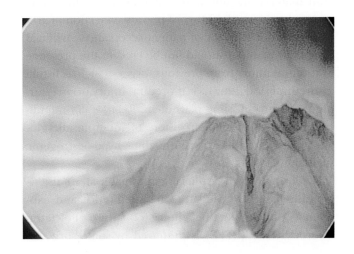

INDICATIONS FOR THE USE OF ARTIFICIAL SLING MATERIAL

Surgeons now have several options of sling material to consider and present to the patient. The major decision to be made involves the use of organic versus inorganic material. The choice of artificial sling material simplifies the operative procedure in that the graft is readily available and does not require harvesting from a second operative site. This readiness and ease of preparation decreases operative time, discomfort and potential postoperative complications. A second operative site is always another potential site of seroma or infection. When harvesting rectus fascia or fascia lata, there is always the potential that the strip obtained will be too short; in these instances, the surgeon must rely on suture to bridge the gap, instead of having tissue-to-tissue apposition and healing. The strength of any patient's fascia is also an unknown variable until obtained and can be found to be suboptimal for a procedure that has, as its goal, support for the urethrovesical junction and maintenance of intra-urethral pressure during stress activities of the body. The use of man-made material bypasses these potential problems of inadequate autologous graft length or strength.

With these facts in mind, the use of artificial sling graft material should be considered in patients with obviously decreased tissue strength, as shown by the presence of significant pelvic prolapse or a history of multiple abdominal procedures where fascial strength may be decreased as a result of repeated healing and scarification. The age of the patient and presence of medical conditions known to attenuate connective tis graft material.

Conversely, contraindications to the use of artificial graft material include known allergy to the inorganic material to be used, history of previous rejection of artificial material and lack of patient acceptance. Artificial sling graft material should not be used in the presence of urethral injury from previous surgery (such as fistula or urethral sloughing), or if urethral injury occurs during the course of sling placement. Relative contraindications include a patient history of multiple allergies and patients with excessively thin hypo-oestrogenic vaginal mucosa.

Choosing which artificial graft material to use is typically based on the surgeon's preference and experience, much like the choice of suture. Polytetrafluoroethylene (PTFE) is preferred by some surgeons over the other available materials, owing to the ease in removing the graft if so needed. Other artificial graft materials which exist in gauze or mesh form result in increased scarification where the fibrous tissue embeds into the mesh. Such material may be extremely difficult to remove from the operative site, putting the adjacent urethra and bladder at increased risk of injury. Removal of PTFE, owing to its lack of bonding to surrounding tissues, is generally atraumatic, with entry into the surrounding sheath of scar tissue and removal of the graft simply by placing tension on one end of the transected graft. The evolution of the patch sling, with reduction of the amount of artificial material used in fashioning the sling, has been successful in decreasing, but not completely eliminating, the risks associated with synthetic slings.

ARTIFICIAL GRAFT MATERIAL OPTIONS

In using synthetic material in surgery, specific material properties are sought that make the graft biocompatible, as well as long lasting. Specifically, the ideal graft material should be chemically and physically inert, permanent and non-degradable, and non-carcinogenic. The material must be mechanically strong to give support over time. The material should be easily fabricated and sterilized for availability and use.

Few reports of the use of absorbable synthetic sling materials are available. An absorbable sling would share the advantages of easy availability without the long-term risks of sling erosion of the permanent synthetic materials. However, durability of the sling would be a concern. Short-term results of the use of polyglactin mesh reported by Fianu and Soderburg[1] appeared promising, but no further information is available.

The non-absorbable artificial materials that have been used for suburethral sling procedures include nylon, Perlon (polycaprolactam), polyethylene terephthalate (Mersilene ribbons or mesh), polypropylene (Marlex mesh), PTFE (Teflon, Gore-tex) and Silastic (Table 44.1). Of these artificial materials, only polyglactin mesh is absorbable; the other synthetic materials used to date are non-absorbable, permanent materials that are non-toxic and have high tensile strength. These materials do differ, however, in composition, weave, porosity and flexibility, which alters their individual propensities to scarification, injury to surrounding tissues, infection and rejection (Fig. 44.1).

Table 44.1. *Artificial materials used for suburethral slings*

Trade name	Composition
Mersilene	Polyethylene terephthalate
Marlex, Prolene	Polypropylene
Teflon	PTFE
Gore-tex	Expanded PTFE
Silastic	Silicone rubber reinforced with polyethylene terephthalate
Vicryl	Polyglactin mesh

PTFE, polytetrafluoroethylene.

Mersilene mesh is a polyester mesh composed of multifilament fibres of polyethylene terephthalate. Marlex mesh is a monofilament mesh composed of polypropylene. Gore-tex is expanded Teflon, a multifilament mesh of PTFE, the production of which is a trade secret. Silastic sheet consists of medical-grade silicone rubber reinforced with woven polyethylene terephthalate.

Theoretically, monofilament mesh withstands infection better than multifilament mesh. The propensity to infection with multifilament fibres is related to the differential entry of small bacteria (compared with larger macrophages and polymorphonuclear leucocytes) into small interstices between filaments; this does not occur with monofilament mesh.

The size, shape and number of pores, or mesh porosity, influences the development of fibrous scarification to adjacent tissue. Tissue bonding is a double-edged sword – bonding is beneficial to the healing process and

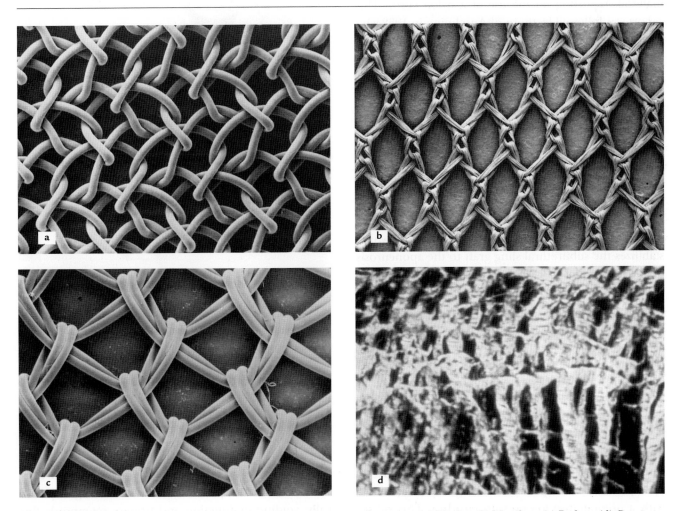

Figure 44.1. *Artificial mesh used for suburethral sling graft; pore configuration: (a) Marlex; (b) Mersilene; (c) Prolene; (d) Gore-tex. (Reprinted from ref. 6, with permission.)*

in rendering support, the goal of incontinence procedures. On the other hand, intense scarification between the implanted mesh and surrounding tissue can make mesh removal technically difficult. Pourdeyhimi has shown that Mersilene has the greatest porosity and, therefore, becomes embedded in fibrous scarification, bonding the mesh firmly to adjacent structures.[2] Likewise, Marlex mesh has been found to act as a scaffold on which connective tissue can grow.[3] On the other hand, PTFE mesh bonds poorly to surrounding tissue owing to its large pore size and chemical composition. Mesh flexibility is greatest with Gore-tex and least with Marlex, a fact that may relate to the propensity of Marlex to erode into adjacent tissue.[4]

Historically, surgeons have looked to alternative, inorganic materials from which to fashion the suburethral sling and give support to the urethrovesical junction. In 1951, Bracht was the first to describe the use of inorganic material, reporting on the use of a nylon cord.[5] This report was followed by those of Anselmino in 1952 who used Perlon, and in 1961 by Zoedler who used nylon.[5] Williams and Telinde, as well as Ridley, fashioned slings from Mersilene ribbon.[6] These early artificial slings caused problems with urethral obstruction, retention and even urethral transection due to their cord-like configuration, which placed direct pressure on the urethra at a narrow location along its length.

Mersilene

In 1968, Moir[7] adapted the use of a wider strip of Mersilene mesh to the Aldridge sling procedure which stabilizes the suburethral sling graft to the aponeurosis of the abdominal wall (Fig. 44.2). The initial series by Moir reported an 83% cure or substantial improvement in incontinence, but did not specifically mention postoperative complications.

Surgeons have continued to use the Mersilene gauze-hammock sling operation over the ensuing 30 years with continued success. Investigators have reported a 73–96% subjective cure rate (Table 44.2).[8–13] Young et al.[8] performed objective evaluation of the Mersilene gauze hammock procedure with pre- and postoperative urodynamic evaluation, showing a 93% objective cure rate. The study found no significant change in MUCP postoperatively except in the subgroup of patients with a preoperative low-pressure urethra. This subset of patients with a mean preoperative MUCP of

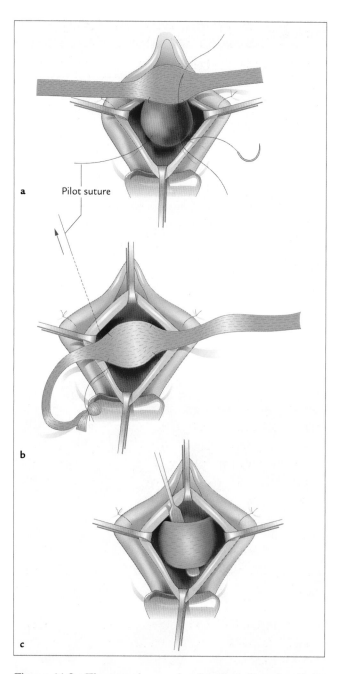

Figure 44.2. *The gauze hammock suburethral sling, described by Moir (ref. 7).*

15 cmH$_2$O showed a mean increase of 8.6 cmH$_2$O (57%) postoperatively. A significant increase in PTR from a mean of 75% preoperatively to 112% ($p < 0.0001$) postoperatively was also found.

A lower incidence of complications was noted than was seen with the previously used cord slings (specifically, voiding dysfunction and urinary retention); this was attributed to the greater width of the sling graft

Table 44.2. *Surgical outcome of the polyethylene terephthalate suburethral sling*

Author (ref. no)	No. of patients	Length of follow-up	Cure rate (%)	Complications
Moir[7]	71	2–24 months	83 (subjective)	Not reported
Nichols[9]	22	1–2 years	95 (subjective)	Not reported
Kersey[10]	105	6 months–5 years	84 (subjective)	Vesicovaginal fistula (2) Vaginal erosions with partial removal (3)
Iosif[11]	44	3–11 years	73 (subjective)	Sling divisions for retention (7) Abscesses (2)
Kersey[12]	100	6 months–5 years	78 (subjective)	Prolene suture exposure (2) Persistent detrusor instability (23%)
Guner[13]	24	24 months	96 (subjective)	Persistent urge incontinence (4.2%)
Young[8]	110	13 months	95 (subjective) 93 (objective)	Voiding dysfunction (3) Vaginal erosions with partial removal (2) Groin sinus (1) Midvaginal band (1)

Adapted from ref. 6.

underlying the bladder neck. However, problems with erosion of the artificial graft into adjacent structures, and abscess and sinus formation at the vaginal and abdominal sites, continued to occur. Patients also experienced urinary retention and voiding dysfunction due to excessive tension on the graft during placement.

Marlex mesh

Following this example of a broader bladder-neck support, Morgan and colleagues[14–16] described the use of a wide band of Marlex mesh, placed by a two-team approach from both abdominal and vaginal routes, and attached to the iliopectineal ligament bilaterally (Fig. 44.3). Marlex was chosen as the graft material owing to its inert properties and monofilament composition, which were thought to bypass the extensive scarring and infection associated with polyethylene terephthalate.

The Marlex mesh suburethral sling has been used by teams in different centres around the world, with subjective cure rates ranging from 79 to 100%.[14–19] One small study performed postoperative urodynamic testing and reported a 70% objective cure at 3 months. Long-term objective cure rates are unknown.

In the initial series of 20 patients, Morgan[14] reported two cases requiring sling removal because of urinary retention in one case and the development of

a vesicovaginal fistula in the other. Further experience by Morgan and other investigators continued to demonstrate an increased incidence of infection, sinus formation, urethral obstruction and vaginal or urethral

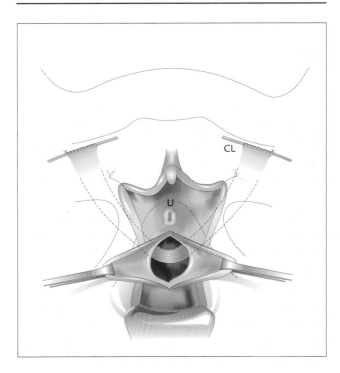

Figure 44.3. *Marlex mesh sling suspending the urethrovesical junction (U) from Cooper's ligaments (CL).*

erosion requiring sling revision or removal. Of most concern has been the propensity for Marlex mesh to cause trauma to the urethra[14–19] (Table 44.3).

Polytetrafluoroethylene (Teflon)

The use of Teflon tape to suspend the urethrovesical junction was described in 1981 by Cato but the procedure is not considered to be a sling as no graft was placed suburethrally.[20] The use of expanded Teflon – Gore-tex – was first reported in 1988 by Horbach, who used a combined vaginal and abdominal approach for placement of a full-circle 'standard' strip sling attached to the aponeurosis of the rectus fascia[21] (Fig. 44.4). The investigators used the suburethral sling specifically for patients with urodynamically diagnosed genuine stress incontinence (GSI) with a low-pressure urethra ($<20\,cmH_2O$): 85% of patients were subjectively cured at 3 months, with 11/13 (84.6%) cured objectively (Table 43.4). At the 1-year subjective follow-up, 12/13 (92%) were continent. Postoperative urodynamic testing revealed an improvement in urodynamic parameters – specifically, a significant increase in MUCP from a mean of 11.4 to $36.1\,cmH_2O$ ($p<0.02$).

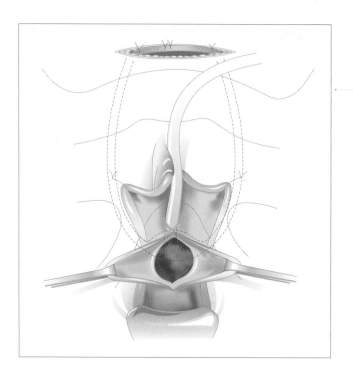

Figure 44.4. *Gore-tex standard strip sling suspending urethrovesical junction from anterior rectus fascia.*

Table 44.3. *Surgical outcome of the polypropylene suburethral sling*

Author (ref. no)	No. of patients	Length of follow-up	Cure rate (%)	Complications
Morgan[14]	20	3–23 months	100 (subjective)	Obstruction (1) Vesicovaginal fistula (1)
Bryans[17]	69	5–8 years	79 (subjective)	Voiding dysfunction (15) Vaginal erosion (4) with vaginal removal (2) Sinus tract (2)
Hilton and Stanton[18]	10	3 months	80 (subjective) 70 (objective)	Not reported
Morgan[15]	208	5 years	77 (subjective)	Urethral erosions (12) with partial transurethral removal Prolonged retention (14) with transurethral resection of the bladder neck (12)
Drutz[19]	65	5 years	95 (subjective)	Vaginal erosion with partial removal (4) Urethral erosion with transurethral resection (1)
Morgan[16]	88		85 (subjective)	Prolonged retention (2) Persistent DI (16.7%); *de-novo* DI

DI, detrusor instability.
Adapted from ref. 6.

Patients with a hypermobile urethrovesical junction preoperatively had restoration of normal urethrovesical junction support, as shown by normalization of their Q-tip test.

Summitt *et al.*[22] followed a larger cohort of patients (48) for 10 months and found an 82% objective cure rate with a suburethral Gore-tex sling. The major postoperative complication experienced was that of delayed return to normal voiding, with a mean time to suprapubic catheter removal of 21.6 days. Two (4.2%) patients required sling revision to relieve outlet obstruction. Delayed complications of vaginal erosion (five or 10.4%) and sinus tract formation (one or 2.1%) also resulted in removal of the Gore-tex sling. All patients remained continent following sling removal.

In another study designed to evaluate the long-term clinical and urodynamic outcomes of the Gore-tex suburethral sling, 62 patients were followed-up for 1 year postoperatively and urodynamic testing was repeated.[23] Of these patients, 73% were subjectively cured of stress incontinence and 61% were objectively cured. There was a significant increase in MUCP postoperatively. There was a 33% incidence of *de-novo* DI. The incidence of artificial graft complications requiring partial or complete graft removal was 22% – 10 patients showed sinus tract formation, four had persistent vaginal granulation tissue, three had anterior vaginal wall erosion, and one patient had persistent groin pain (Table 44.4).

In a separate investigation, a team at the same centre histologically evaluated slings that were removed because of abdominal or vaginal rejection of the sling material, with lack of healing at that site or the development of a sinus tract.[24] Sling rejection or removal occurred in 20/115 patients (17%). Histology revealed Gram-positive cocci in all Gore-tex patch interstices, as well as fibrous tissue, fibroblasts and collagen. These findings suggest an infective process that begins at (or follows) graft placement and that prevents healing of the operative site. The fact that 75% of patients remained continent following removal of the sling was attributed to the characteristic fibrous sheath that forms around Gore-tex following placement and is not removed with the graft.

Silastic

Owing to the difficulties in revising slings once placed, Stanton *et al.*[28] suggested the use of medical-grade Silastic sheet for the suburethral sling graft. Tissue reaction to Silastic is minimal, with formation of only a thin fibrous sheath around the graft material. Much like Gore-tex, which exhibits minimal bonding to the surrounding tissue, this characteristic of Silastic allows for easy revision or removal of the sling if needed. In the initial report on the use of the Silastic sling, Stanton reported an 83% objective cure rate at 1 year. Four (13.3%) patients required release or removal of the sling due to voiding difficulties. The procedure described involves an abdominal approach with creation of a suburethral tunnel for passage of the sling graft. The Silastic graft is attached to the iliopectineal ligament. Other complications reported involved intraoperative entry into the bladder, urethra and vagina, all of which are related to the surgical abdominal approach.

Chin and Stanton[29] reported long-term results of the Silastic sling procedure, as described by Stanton, in a larger cohort of 88 patients. There was no postoperative infection requiring sling removal. However, sling erosion into adjacent structures occurred in 10 patients (11.4%), including vaginal (five), bladder (four) and urethra (one) erosion. Four other patients required sling release or removal secondary to voiding difficulties. Other reasons for removal included intractable groin pain (two) and strangulated hernia (one). In two publications, Korda *et al.*[30,31] have also reported experience with the Silastic sling procedure. In spite of an 80.6% subjective cure rate, 24% of patients have required sling revision to establish postoperative voiding; 4.5% underwent sling removal for sinus tract formation and for intractable pain and 3% developed *de-novo* DI (Table 44.5).

TECHNICAL DEVELOPMENTS

The surgical technique of the artificial suburethral sling procedure has used vaginal, abdominal or combined abdominovaginal routes. The abdominal route has been marred by an increased incidence of injury to the urethra, bladder and vagina, which occurs when creating a suburethral tunnel for passage of the sling. Most surgeons now use a combined abdominal and vaginal approach to avoid the difficult suburethral dissection.

The graft material has been suspended to the iliopectineal ligament or to the aponeurosis of the rectus fascia. The standard strip sling procedure involves

Table 44.4. *Reported surgical outcome of the expanded polytetrafluoroethylene suburethral sling*

Sling type	Author (ref. no)	No. of patients	Length of follow-up	Cure rate (%)	Complications
Standard strip	Horbach[21]	13	3–18 months	85 (subjective)	Sling revision for retention (1) Sling removal for sinus tract (1) Persistent DI (50%) *de-novo* DI (73%)
	Summitt[22]	45	6 months	82 (objective)	Removals for vaginal erosion/infection (5) Revisions for obstruction (2) Abdominal sinus tract (1) Persistent DI (71%); *de-novo* DI (12.2%)
	Bent[24]	115	6 months–5 years	Not reported	Sling rejection/ removal (21)
	Weinberger[23]	62	12 months	73 (subjective)	Abdominal/vaginal sinus tract (10) Vaginal erosions Sling removals (22) Persistent DI (48%); *de-novo* DI (33%)
Patch	Ogundipe[25]	8	6 months	100 (subjective)	Stitch abscess (1) Persistent DI (75%); *de-novo* DI (66%)
	Norris[26]	122	6 months	88 (subjective)	Removal of vaginal erosions (5) Revision for voiding dysfunction (6) Persistent DI (49%); *de-novo* DI (32%)
	Yamada[27]	39	2 years	84 (subjective)	Removal for infection (1)

DI, detrusor instability.
Adapted from ref. 6.

placement of a continuous full circle of graft underlying the bladder neck, meeting above the rectus fascia, where the sling arms are approximated and stabilized to the rectus fascia. Other slings are interrupted, with the sling arms attached to a specific site, such as the rectus fascia or Cooper's ligament.

The majority of synthetic materials used for the sling graft have been non-absorbable. To avoid the known complications of permanent sling material, Fianu used absorbable polyglactin mesh, reporting a 95% success rate at 5–14 months.[1] No mesh-related postoperative complications were experienced. There has been no long-term follow-up or further investigation of absorbable artificial slings.

In trying to minimize the problems experienced with artificial slings (namely, the risk of infection and of graft rejection), surgeons have tried to decrease the amount of artificial graft material used in the operation. The result has been the evolution of 'patch' slings rather than the more traditional 'standard' strip sling or interrupted strip sling (Fig. 44.5).

Ogundipe[25] reported on a small series of patients receiving a Gore-tex patch sling in 1992, and found a 100% objective cure rate at 6 months. Postoperative

Table 44.5. *Reported surgical outcome of the Silastic suburethral sling*

Author (ref. no)	No. of patients	Length of follow-up	Cure rate (%)	Complications
Stanton[28]	30	3–12 months	83 (subjective)	Removals for retention (4) Vesicovaginal fistula (1) Persistent DI (100%); *de-novo* DI (67%)
Chin[29]	88	3 months–5 years	71 (subjective)	Slings removed (17); voiding dysfunction (4); sling erosions (10); groin pain (2); insisional hernia (1) Voiding dysfunction (8) Persistent DI (70%); *de-novo* DI (28%)
Korda[30]	54	4–30 months	77 (subjective)	Revisions for retention (15); sinus tract (2) with removal (1)
Korda[31]	67	4–30 months	81 (subjective)	Revisions for retention (16) Sling removals (3): sinus tract (2); groin pain (1) Persistent DI (61.5%); *de-novo* DI (3.7%)

DI, detrusor instability.

urodynamic parameters showed improved urethrovesical junction support, as measured by Q-tip test, and an increase in functional urethral length. There was no significant improvement in MUCP or PTR. Complications experienced by the cohort of seven patients included three cases of delayed urinary retention requiring bladder drainage and training (42.9%), one abdominal Gore-tex stitch abscess treated with surgical excision and drainage (14.3%), and two cases of *de-novo* DI (28.6%).

In 1996, Norris and colleagues[26] reported on a much larger series of patients undergoing a Gore-tex patch sling procedure with a mean follow-up of 24 months: 88% of patients were subjectively cured of GSI. In this series of 122 patients, six (4.9%) underwent sling revision for urinary retention persisting for more than 3 months; five patients (4.1%) underwent sling removal because of vagina erosion and 17 (14%) experienced onset of *de-novo* DI. Yamada *et al.*[27] in 1998 reported a lower removal rate of 2.6% in a series of 32 patients, using a slightly different technique that minimized dissection of the anterior vaginal wall.

This concept of a patch sling has been teamed more recently with the use of bone anchors embedded into the symphysis pubis in an attempt to provide a fixed site of attachment for the sling. Kovac and Cruickshank[32] reported a 100% subjective cure in 25 patients undergoing this procedure with a 4-year follow-up, with no incidence of infection, rejection or erosion. A 91.4% cure rate at 8 months was found among 35 women undergoing a similar polypropylene mesh patch sling with bone anchors to the pubic tubercles;[33] again, no postoperative complications that have required revision or removal of the sling have been experienced.

Collagen-impregnated synthetic sling

Two sling materials utilized recently consist of synthetic mesh impregnated with collagen. These are Meadox and Protegen, both of which have been used previously as vascular prostheses. No published data are available on success rates and it is not clear what advantages such materials would have had over current synthetic sling materials. These materials were recently removed from commercial sale by the manufacturer because of a high rate of vaginal erosion.

Bone anchors

Most reported techniques rely on the attachment of the abdominal ends of the sling to the rectus aponeurosis, either *in situ*, as in Aldridge's original description or, as in more modern descriptions, via small incisions just above the pubic symphysis, and direct suture to the rectus sheath or Cooper's ligament.

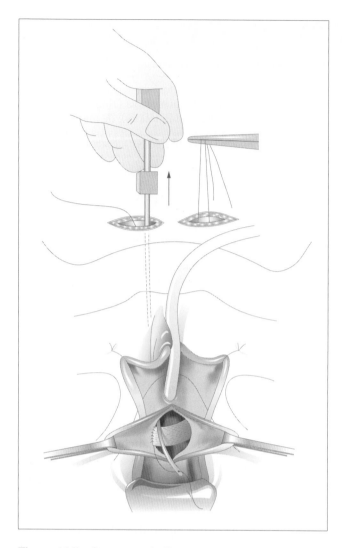

Figure 44.5. *Gore-tex patch sling.*

The technique described by Kovac and Cruikshank[32] and Hom *et al.*[33] relies on the attachment of a Mersilene mesh to the pubic bone with the use of small bone anchors. It is suggested that this more accurately repositions the urethra and provides support at the junction of the proximal urethra.

Bone anchors have also been utilized with other sling procedures, using full strips of artificial or autologous (or homologous) materials. The risk of osteomyelitis from bone anchors has been reported by Maktov and colleagues.[34]

The tension-free vaginal tape

The concept behind the tension-free vaginal tape (TVT) is that stress incontinence results from the failure of the pubourethral ligaments in the mid-urethra.[35,36] This led to the 'integrated theory for the management of female stress incontinence'[37–39] which is based on the model that continence is maintained at the mid-urethra and not at the bladder neck. The aim of the tape is to reinforce the 'functional' pubourethral ligaments and hence secure proper fixation of the mid-urethra to the pubic bone, allowing simultaneous reinforcement of the suburethral vaginal hammock and its connection to the pubococcygeus muscles.[36]

The procedure

The tape is composed of a knitted Prolene mesh. The instrument and sling used for the TVT procedure are shown in Figure 44.6. The aim of the procedure is to place the tape at the mid-urethra.[40] It is inserted via a small vaginal incision using two 5 mm trochars. The procedure can be performed under local, regional or general anaesthesia. The patient is placed in the lithotomy position, and the lower abdomen and the vagina are prepared as a sterile operating field. Two small (1 cm) incisions are made in the abdominal wall, 5 cm apart, just above the superior rim of the pubic bone. A sagittal incision is made in the suburethral vaginal wall starting 1 cm from the external urethral meatus. After minimal bilateral para-urethral dissection of the vaginal wall, the tape, covered by a plastic sheath, is introduced with the help of the trochars. Each trochar perforates the urogenital diaphragm and is then moved through the retropubic space to emerge through the abdominal incision. The tape is therefore lying in a U-shape around the urethra (Fig. 44.7).[41]

Following TVT insertion, a cystoscopy is performed to ensure that there has been no damage to the bladder. If the procedure is being carried out under local or regional anaesthesia, the woman is asked to perform a series of coughs in order to adjust the position of the tape. Obviously, if the procedure is being carried out under general anaesthetic then the patient is unable to cough; the assistant simulates the coughs by applying suprapubic pressure. The aim is to have the tape lying free at rest (hence 'tension-free') whilst exerting sufficient pressure on the urethra during a cough to prevent leakage of urine. When the surgeon is happy with the placement of the tape, the plastic sheath can be removed. Because of the weave, the tape is self-retaining and requires no fixation. The incisions are then sutured with appropriate material.

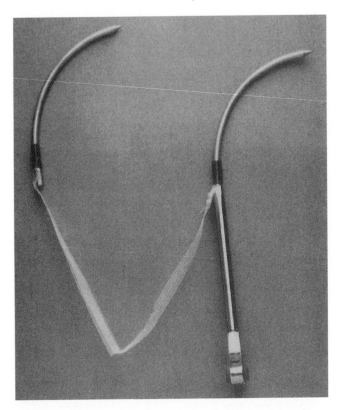

Figure 44.6. *Instrument and sling used for the tension-free vaginal tape procedure. The Prolene sling is covered by a removable plastic sheath connected to two needles which can be attached to a metal handle for placement. (Reproduced from ref. 42, with permission.)*

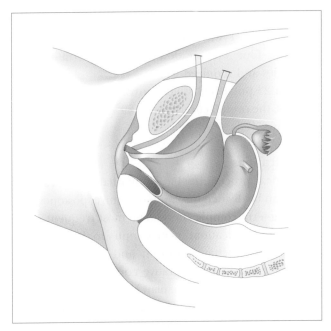

Figure 44.7. *The tension-free vaginal tape in situ.*

Results

The preliminary results came from Ulmsten[42] in Sweden who reported an 84% cure rate with no long-term voiding difficulties or *de-novo* DI. A further study involving 131 women from several centres in Sweden showed a cure rate of 91%.[43] These women had not had any previous surgery and were followed up for at least 12 months.

Long-term follow-up studies are only available from Scandinavia, where the procedure was first performed. The 3-year follow-up data revealed an objective cure rate of 86%.[41] The 5-year data (presented by Nilsson at the International Continence Society, Finland in 2000) come from three centres in Scandinavia.[44] The study involved 62 patients and showed an objective cure rate of 80.6%. A further 14.5% had improved; the procedure had failed in 4.5%. Hence it is concluded that there is no increase in the failure rate over 5 years. However, a lower cure rate associated with increasing age is reported. They were no tape erosions or rejections

in this series and the incidence of *de-novo* DI was less than 5%.

A recent randomized multicentre study carried out in the UK compared the TVT with the current gold standard, the colposuspension.[45] The study involved 14 centres and recruited 344 women. The cure rate was similar in each treatment group, subjectively 66% (TVT) and 71% (colposuspension) and objectively 68% (TVT) and 66% (colposuspension). However, the mean duration of stay was significantly less in the TVT group: 2.2 days compared with 6.5 days in the colposuspension group.[46] Seventy-six per cent of the TVT group and 41% of the colposuspension group had returned to work by 6 weeks post-operatively. At six months all the patients in both groups considered themselves fit for normal activities.

Several small studies have investigated the use of TVT as a secondary procedure after previous failed incontinence surgery. In one series of 25 patients followed up for 3 years the cure rate was 84%; the remainder of the patients had all improved, and the technique did not fail in any patient.[47] However, this study did allow leakage of up to 10 g on a pad test if this was associated with urgency. Hilton and Ward[48] published results from 50 women, of whom 40% had previously undergone at least one incontinence operation. Their results showed an objective cure rate of 75% when TVT was used as a secondary procedure. However, four women developed long-term voiding difficulties and required CISC.

From 23 published studies involving a total of 1392 patients, the overall cure rate was 89% and the improvement rate 5%.[49]

Complications

All surgical procedures have potential complications. These can be divided into intra-operative, postoperative and long-term complications. The most frequent intra-operative complications include injury to the bladder at the time of trochar insertion, and bleeding in the retropubic space. Postoperative complications include voiding difficulties, which may be long term, urinary tract infection, and wound infection. Worrying long-term complications include the risk of tape rejection and tape erosion. A nationwide analysis of complications in Finland[50] (see Table 44.6) found that of 1455 patients from 38 units, all had had a TVT inserted and 40 had had one or more further procedures at the same time.

Other units report similar complications: in a series of 429 women from Italy,[51] bladder perforation occurred in 24 women, a rate of 6%.

Summary

The TVT procedure appears to be a safe and effective surgical procedure for the treatment of female genuine stress incontinence. In the short and medium term the success rates appear to be similar to other procedures already available; long-term data is still awaited. Studies around the world are comparing TVT with colposuspension, both open and laparoscopic, sling procedures, and injectables. Other groups are looking at the feasibility of performing prolapse surgery at the time of inserting a TVT. We await these results with interest.

URODYNAMIC EFFECTS OF SLINGS

The urodynamic changes following sling procedures have been studied by a number of authors.

Hilton[18] studied women undergoing either sling or needle suspension procedures. Maximal urethral closure pressure (MUCP) and functional urethral length were slightly increased in both, but a significant

Table 44.6. *Summary of complications in 1455 patients having had a TVT inserted*

Complication	Number	Percentage
Minor voiding difficulties postoperatively	109	7.5
Complete retention postoperatively	34	2.3
Urinary tract infection	59	4.1
Bladder perforation	56	3.8
Blood loss > 200 ml	27	1.9
Retropubic haematoma	27	1.9
Wound infection	12	0.8
Defective healing of vaginal incision	10	0.7
Injury to major vessel	1	0.1
Obturator nerve injury	1	0.1
Vaginal haematoma	1	0.1
Other	33	2.3

Data from ref. 50.

increase in pressure transmission ratio (PTR) was found in the sling group. The increase in PTR was most marked in the distal urethra in this study, whereas a study by Rottenburg et al.[52] found no changes in resting urethral pressure and a slight decrease in functional urethral length; again, a significant increase in urethral pressure transmission was found. Young et al.[8] followed-up 110 women after Mersilene mesh sling procedures and found an increase in MUCP in women with low MUCP preoperatively, but no change in women with normal-range MUCP preoperatively. Functional urethral length was found to increase slightly in this study, but the most significant change was again in urethral pressure transmission, which increased in 80% of the group. The effect of a Gore-tex sling in women with low MUCP was studied by Horbach et al.,[21] who showed that there was a significant increase in postoperative MUCP, although this increase was not apparent in all women with objective cure of stress incontinence. Pressure transmission was not examined in this study.

RESULTS OF SLING SURGERY

Assessment of the outcomes of sling techniques is complicated, as many series consist of women who have undergone at least one (and, in some cases, many) previous failed incontinence operations. In addition, the majority of publications refer to case series, with few comparative studies available; many results are reported as subjective cure rates only. In the publications reviewed for this chapter, objective cure rates range from 61 to 100% and subjective cure rates from 73 to 93%.

Jarvis,[53] in a meta-analysis of all surgery for stress incontinence, found an objective cure rate of 85.3% and a subjective cure rate of 82.4%. These figures agree closely with the results of the American Urological Association, who report an overall subjective cure rate of 82%.[54]

Few long-term results of sling techniques are available. It appears that the failure of a sling procedure is most likely to become apparent in the first 6 months, and this is probably due to degeneration of fascia or failure of anchoring sutures.

Some long-term studies are available: from these it appears that those sling operations successful after 6 months are likely to remain successful for many years.

General complications

The general surgical complications are no higher with sling surgery than those with other vaginal or suprapubic operations. Wound haematoma rates of about 3% and postoperative urinary infection of 5% have been reported.[55] Pain at the site of sling attachment to the rectus fascia is one specific problem (although it is rarely reported), as is dyspareunia, although this is specifically mentioned in only one of the papers reviewed.

Voiding difficulties following sling procedures

The relatively high incidence of voiding difficulties following sling surgery has been one of the most significant factors preventing more widespread use of this technique.[56] Suburethral slings are reputed to be more obstructive than other incontinence operations, with an incidence of retention varying from 2.2 to 16%, and with 1.5–7.8% of patients requiring long-term CISC.[5]

In a systematic review of surgery for stress incontinence, Jarvis[57] found a mean incidence of postoperative voiding disorders of 12.8% (range 2–37%). However, this figure includes one study by Korda et al.,[30,31] where 28% of women required further surgery to reduce sling tension before voiding could take place. When the figures from this study are removed, the result is a mean of 10.8% (range 2–20%).

Postoperative voiding difficulties may occur as a result of either poor detrusor function or urethral obstruction. Poor detrusor function may be identified preoperatively, using free and pressure–flow studies.[58] Women with suboptimal detrusor function need to be warned of the risk of prolonged postoperative voiding difficulties and the potential need for long-term CISC.[59] Urethral obstruction may occur as a result of excessive sling tension. Hilton[60] found a significant reduction in peak urine flow rate and a small rise in maximum voiding pressure following sling surgery, suggesting that a slight degree of urethral obstruction occurs.

Prolonged catheterization following fascial[61,62] sling placement is 12–60 days, with up to 15% of women performing CISC; following Mersilene sling placement,[9] 11% of women catheterized for longer than 14 days and, after Marlex[63] graft placement, 9% of women catheterized for 3–6 months and 1% developed permanent retention.

Recently, the importance of avoiding excessive sling tension has been recognized and there is a trend for slings to be placed under less tension or even completely loose;[64] this may reduce the incidence of voiding dysfunction. Appell[65] reports that only 2% of women required long-term CISC with fascial slings placed under minimal tension.

Predicting which women are most at risk of developing postoperative voiding difficulties seems difficult. A higher incidence of voiding difficulties has been described following colposuspension in women who void using a Valsalva manoeuvre.[66] This was not found by McLennan et al.[67] in a study of voiding following fascia lata sling procedures. Age over 65 years, low urine flow rate (less than 20 ml/sec) and concomitant surgery appeared to increase the risk of delayed spontaneous voiding. The retention rate of 5% was lower in this study than in previous reports; again, the authors ascribe this to reduced sling tension.

Detrusor instability following sling procedures

Prior to 1970, the concept of DI was not fully recognized and, therefore, data cannot be reliably obtained from studies before this date.[68] In addition, many of the published series relate to a group of women who have undergone numerous previous unsuccessful operations. It has been shown that the incidence of DI in this group is, in any case, higher than in women undergoing a first operation for GSI.[69]

The reported incidence of postoperative symptoms of urge incontinence varies widely, from 3 to 30%. In a review of published series, the American Urological Association found the incidence of *de-novo* DI to be 7% (95% confidence interval 3–11%).[54]

DI arising after bladder-neck surgery appears inevitable in some cases. Whether this is due to pre-existing DI, undiagnosed by preoperative cystometry, or, as has been suggested, is due to denervation following surgical dissection is not clear. Overelevation of the bladder neck, excessive sling tension and irritation of the bladder neck by synthetic sling materials have also been implicated. It may be significant that one of the studies reporting the highest rate of *de-novo* DI (33%) involved the use of a Gore-tex sling.[23] In this study, postoperative urethral pressure measurement showed a significant increase in MUCP. This supports the view that excess tension, combined with the use of an unyielding synthetic material, increases the incidence of *de-novo* DI and voiding difficulties. However, postoperative voiding dysfunction is common to all suburethral sling proce-

dures, and is probably more a reflection of surgical technique than of sling material. Early studies did not investigate the occurrence of urge incontinence symptoms in relation to the sling procedure, so little is known regarding the incidence with the use of Mersilene and Marlex. In more recent studies assessing the success of Gore-tex, preoperative and postoperative urodynamic tests were utilized to indicate clearly the rates of persistent and *de novo* DI.[21–23,70]

These rates are significant, with up to a 77% rate of persistent DI and a 66% rate of *de novo* DI related to the use of standard or patch Gore-tex slings. Subjective rates of persistent and *de novo* DI with the use of Silastic slings have similarly been found to be high, at 61.5–100% and 3.7–66.7%, respectively[28–31] (Table 44.7).

Although it may not be possible to eliminate completely problems from postoperative DI, it seems sensible to attempt to limit them by appropriate preoperative urodynamic investigations, patient selection, a trial of anticholinergic therapy and repeat urodynamics in women with pre-existing DI.

Sling-release techniques

It is clear that overelevation of the urethra and bladder neck is associated with a high incidence of voiding difficulties. A number of techniques for

Table 44.7. *Artificial suburethral slings: reported postoperative complication rates (%) based on type of artificial material*

Complication	Material				
	Mersilene	Marlex	Standard Gore-tex	Patch Gore-tex	Silastic
Fistula	1.9–3.3	0–5	Not reported	Not reported	1.9–3.3
Sinus tract formation	0–3.3	0–2.9	2.2–17.7	0–7.6	3–3.7
Vaginal erosion	1.8–2.8	6.2–7.2	11.1–16.1	2.6–4.0	0–9.3
Urethral erosion	Not reported	1.5–5.8	Not reported	Not reported	0–1.9
Voiding dysfunction	2.7–15.9	2.3–21.7	4.4–7.7	4.9	9.3–23.9
Persistent DI	4.2–23	16.7	48–77	49–75	61.5–100
De-novo DI	Not reported	7.3	11–33	32–66	3.7–67
Sling revision/removal	1.8–15.9	2.9–11.5	15.4–35.5	2.6–9	13.3–31.5

Not reported indicates not reported in published series.
DI, detrusor instability.

avoiding and correcting excessive sling tension have been advocated.

Various intra-operative techniques to gauge correct sling tension have been described, including measurement of Q-tip angle, intra-operative urethral pressure profilometry and cystoscopy. Although these techniques have enthusiastic advocates, there is no convincing evidence that they correctly determine appropriate sling tension. Avoiding excess tension appears to rely on the experience of the surgeon. The TVT procedure uses a novel method of determining sling tension: as the technique is performed under local or regional anaesthesia, sling tension can be adjusted while the patient coughs with a full bladder. How this relates to sling tension in an ambulant woman is not clear, but it may avoid excessive bladder-neck elevation.

When obstruction occurs postoperatively, simple urethral dilatation has been suggested, which may produce temporary relief but also progressive worsening of the obstruction due to periurethral fibrosis.[62,71] Transurethral resection or incision of the bladder neck may fail and is *not* advised, as the cause of the obstruction – the sling – is extraluminal.[72]

Transvaginal urethrolysis[73] has been described, as well as transvaginal division of the sling material. Ghoniem and Elgamasy[74] advanced this by incising the suburethral portion of the sling and then using a patch of vaginal epithelium to reunite the two ends.

A novel approach described by Brubaker[75] is to free the abdominal end of the sling by creating fascial plugs, which can be resutured below the rectus fascia once the sling tension has been adjusted.

Graft erosion

Problems related to erosion of the sling material, through either the vagina or the urethra, appear to be encountered almost exclusively with synthetic sling materials. Although the incidence of such problems is low, graft erosion can pose a formidable management problem with persistent vaginal discharge, vesicovaginal fistula formation and fibrosis and destruction of the urethral sphincter. Assessing the true incidence of such problems is difficult. Many early reports of new sling techniques do not feature sling erosion, even when using materials now well known to cause problems.

Reviewing the available reports, some conclusions can be drawn about the likelihood of such problems and the characteristics of graft materials most likely to lead to erosion.

It is a basic surgical principle that chronic inflammation in or around a foreign body will lead to erosion to an adjacent epithelial surface.[76,77] In the case of a sling, this will usually be either the vagina or urethra. An alternative is abscess and chronic sinus or fistula formation. A chronic inflammatory response occurs, owing to either the inherent tissue reaction of the material itself, or, more probably, chronic infection. Even in an era of easy access to broad-spectrum chemoprophylaxis, caution needs to be exercised when insertion of a foreign body into a potentially contaminated wound is contemplated.

Gore-tex has been associated with a high rate of local infection and sling removal of up to 23% in some studies.[24] It appears that the microporous structure, in fact, inhibits ingrowth of fibrous tissue and, possibly, provides inaccessible areas for bacterial colonization and chronic infection.[78] Infection rates in 'patch' procedures with Gore-tex may relate to graft size and technique and have been reported to be less than 3%.[26]

Marlex has a large open-weave mesh, which may allow free ingrowth of fibrous tissue. However, lack of healing of the vaginal wall appears to be a particular problem with this material and is reported as occurring in 7%[17] and 6.2%[19] of cases. However, in a 16-year review of the Marlex sling operation, Morgan *et al.*[15] report a success rate of 80%, with two cases of urethral transection but no other graft-related complications.

Low rates of erosion and mesh removal of 2.5% have been ascribed to the open weave, flexibility and thinness of Mersilene mesh, although in this study by Young *et al.*, three women (3.6%) had complications related to mesh erosion after a mean follow-up of 16 months.[8]

Urethral transection is another problem that is related to erosion and reported only with synthetic materials. It was a particular problem with Mersilene tape and led to its use being abandoned.[79]

Interestingly, where sling erosion and infection have necessitated resection of division of the sling material, continence is often maintained, reinforcing the view that it is the fibrosis induced by the sling that provides urethral support rather than the material itself.[29]

An ideal synthetic material would provide a framework for tissue ingrowth and vascularization without causing an excessive chronic inflammatory response.[22]

Estimating the true incidence of problems related to synthetic slings is complicated by the fact that many problems related to erosion may not become apparent until relatively late. Erosion of graft material may occur relatively late, at 1–4 years postoperatively.[23] Whereas good early results of surgery are often submitted for publication, late adverse events are less likely to be reported, leading to a bias in the literature and to under-reporting of complications. It appears that, as new techniques become more widely used, complications such as erosion become more widely encountered, but it is often 10 or more years before the true incidence of such problems becomes apparent. From those publications reviewed, the incidence of significant problems associated with synthetic materials (excluding Gore-tex) appears to be low, in the region of 1–6%.

COMPARATIVE COST OF SLING SURGERY

Few comparative studies of the economic aspects of sling techniques are available. However, Berman and Kreder carried out an economic analysis of periurethral injection of collagen in 1997.[80] They found that sling surgery was more expensive, at US$10,382, than periurethral injection of collagen, at US$4996 per case. Despite this, the cure rates of 71.4 and 27.7%, respectively, make sling surgery far more cost-effective.

CONCLUSIONS

The principal difference between natural and synthetic materials is in the complication rate due to chronic infection or tissue reaction. Some synthetic materials appear less likely to cause these problems than others. However, a certain incidence of erosion and related problems is probably inevitable following the insertion of a permanent implant through a potentially contaminated wound. It appears that the main function of the sling material, whether natural or synthetic, is to provide a framework for fibrosis. Once this has taken place, the sling material itself is largely redundant. It would, therefore, seem logical to utilize the newer generation of absorbable materials in sling surgery. These would provide easily available lengths of material, without

increasing surgical morbidity, and would avoid the problems of permanent synthetic grafts, as these materials do not persist beyond the time taken for fibrosis to occur.

Whether sling surgery is more appropriate for complex cases of stress incontinence or should be used as first-line therapy is impossible to determine at present. Randomized comparative trials are needed to assess the suitability of slings as a primary procedure.

Sling procedures are currently enjoying a revival of interest. If we are to advance our understanding of these techniques, thorough evaluation of surgical procedure, objective and subjective outcomes, and complications over at least a 5-year follow-up will be required.

There is little doubt that sling operations, in expert hands, can produce very good results. The type of sling material chosen probably does not affect outcome, in terms of cure rates, provided that the characteristics of the chosen material are considered carefully.

The main drawback of sling surgery has been the relatively high complication rate. However, it appears that the rates of voiding difficulties and *de-novo* DI can be reduced by avoiding excess sling tension, as it does not appear that urethral compression and obstruction is necessary for a successful result.

REFERENCES

1. Fianu S, Soderberg G. Absorbable polyglactin mesh for retropubic sling operations in female urinary stress incontinence. *Gynecol Obstet Invest* 1983; 16: 45–50

2. Pourdeyhimi B. Porosity of surgical mesh fabrics: new technology. *J Biomed Mater Res* 1989; 23: 145–152

3. Usher FC. The repair of incisional and inguinal hernias. *Surg Gynecol Obstet* 1970; 131: 342–344

4. Chu CC, Welch L. Characterization of morphological and mechanical properties of surgical mesh fibers. *J Biomed Mater Res* 1985; 19: 903–916

5. Ghoniem GM, Shaaban A. Sub-urethral slings for treatment of stress urinary incontinence. *Int Urogynecol J* 1994; 5: 228–239

6. Iglesia CB, Fenner DE, Brubaker L. The use of mesh in gynecologic surgery. *Int Urogynecol J* 1997; 8: 105–115

7. Moir JC. The gauze-hammock operation: a modified Aldridge sling procedure. *J Obstet Gynaecol Br Commonw* 1968; 75: 1–9

8. Young SB, Rosenblatt PL, Pingeton DM *et al.* The Mersilene mesh suburethral sling: a clinical and

urodynamic evaluation. *Am J Obstet Gynecol* 1995; 173: 1719–1726.

9. Nichols DH. The Mersilene mesh gauze-hammock for severe urinary stress incontinence. *Obstet Gynecol* 1973; 41: 88–93

10. Kersey J. The gauze hammock sling operation in the treatment of stress incontinence. *Br J Obstet Gynaecol* 1983; 90: 945–949

11. Iosif CS. Sling operation for urinary incontinence. *Acta Obstet Gynecol Scand* 1985; 64: 187–190

12. Kersey J, Martin MR, Mishra P. A further assessment of the gauze hammock sling operation in the treatment of stress incontinence. *Br J Obstet Gynaecol* 1988; 95: 382–385

13. Guner H, Yildiz A, Erdem A *et al.* Surgical treatment of urinary stress incontinence by a suburethral sling procedure using a Mersilene mesh graft. *Gynecol Obstet Invest* 1994; 37: 52–55

14. Morgan JE. A sling operation, using Marlex polypropylene mesh, for treatment of recurrent stress incontinence. *Am J Obstet Gynecol* 1970; 170: 369–377

15. Morgan JE, Farrow GA, Stewart FE. The Marlex sling operation for the treatment of recurrent stress urinary incontinence: a 16–year review. *Am J Obstet Gynecol* 1985; 151: 224–226

16. Morgan JE, Heritz DM, Stewart FE *et al.* The polypropylene pubovaginal sling for the treatment of recurrent stress urinary incontinence. *J Urol* 1995; 154: 1013–1015

17. Bryans FE. Marlex gauze hammock sling operation with Cooper's ligament attachment in the management of recurrent urinary stress incontinence. *Am J Obstet Gynecol* 1979; 133: 292–294

18. Hilton P, Stanton SL. Clinical and urodynamic evaluation of the polypropylene (Marlex) sling for genuine stress incontinence. *Neurourol Urodyn* 1983; 2: 145–153

19. Drutz HP, Buckspan M, Flax S, Mackie L. Clinical and urodynamic reevaluation of combined abdominovaginal Marlex sling operations for recurrent stress urinary incontinence. *Int Urogynecol J* 1990; 1: 70–73

20. Cato RJ. Teflon tape suspension for the control of stress incontinence. *Br J Urol* 1981; 53: 364–367

21. Horbach NS, Blanco JS, Ostergard DR *et al.* A suburethral sling procedure with polytetrafluoroethylene for the treatment of genuine stress incontinence in patients with low urethral closure pressure. *Obstet Gynecol* 1988; 71: 648–652

22. Summitt RL, Bent AE, Ostergard DR, Harris TA. Suburethral sling procedure for genuine stress incontinence and low urethral pressure: a continued experience. *Int Urogynecol J* 1992; 3: 18–21

23. Weinberger MW, Ostergard DR. Long-term clinical and urodynamic evaluation of the polytetrafluoroethylene suburethral sling for treatment of genuine stress incontinence. *Obstet Gynecol* 1995; 86: 92–96

24. Bent AE, Ostergard DR, Zwick-Zaffuto M. Tissue reaction to Gore-tex suburethral sling for incontinence: clinical and histological study. *Am J Obstet Gynecol* 1993; 169: 1198–1204

25. Ogundipe A, Rosenzweig BA, Karram MM *et al.* Modified suburethral sling procedure for the treatment of recurrent or severe stress urinary incontinence. *Surg Gynecol Obstet* 1992; 175: 173–176

26. Norris JP, Breslin DS, Staskin DR. Use of synthetic material in sling surgery: a minimally invasive approach. *J Endourol* 1996; 10: 227–230

27. Yamada T, Arai G, Masuda H *et al.* The correction of type 2 stress incontinence with a polytetrafluoroethylene patch sling: 5-year mean followup. *J Urol* 1998; 160: 746–749

28. Stanton SL, Brindley FS, Holmes DM. Silastic sling for urethral sphincter incompetence in women. *Br J Obstet Gynaecol* 1985; 92: 747–750

29. Chin YK, Stanton SL. A follow-up of Silastic sling for genuine stress incontinence. *Br J Obstet Gynaecol* 1995; 102: 143–147

30. Korda A, Peat B, Hunter P. Experience with Silastic slings for female urinary incontinence. *Aust NZ J Obstet Gynaecol* 1989; 29: 150–154

31. Korda A, Peat B, Hunter P. Silastic slings for female incontinence. *Int Urogynecol J* 1990; 1: 66–69

32. Kovac SR, Cruickshank SH. Pubic bone stabilization sling for recurrent urinary incontinence. *Obstet Gynecol* 1997; 89: 624–627

33. Hom D, Deautel MJ, Lumerman JH *et al.* Pubovaginal sling using polypropylene mesh and Vesica bone anchors. *Urology* 1998; 51: 708–713

34. Maktov TG, Hejna, Coogan CL. Osteomyelitis as a complication of vesica percutaneous bladder neck suspension. *J Urol* 1998; 160: 1427

35. Petros P, Ulmsten U. An integral theory on female urinary incontinence. Experimental and clinical considerations. *Acta Obstet Gynecol Scand* 1990; 69(Suppl): 153

36. Petros P, Ulmsten U. An integral theory and its method for the diagnosis and management of female urinary incontinence. *Scand J Urol Nephrol* 1993; 151: 1–93

37. Petros P, Ulmsten U. Urethral pressure increase on effort originates from within the urethra, and continence from musculovaginal closure. *Neurourol Urodyn* 1995; 14: 337–350

38. Petros P, Ulmsten U. Role of the pelvic floor in bladder neck opening and closure: I Muscle forces. *Int Urogynecol J* 1997; 8: 74–80

39. Petros P, Ulmsten U. Role of the pelvic floor in bladder neck opening and closure: II Vagina. *Int Urogynecol J* 1997; 8: 69–73

40. Petros P, Ulmsten U. Intravaginal slingplasty. An ambulatory surgical procedure for treatment of female urinary stress incontinence. *Scand J Urol Nephrol* 1995; 29: 75–82

41. Ulmsten U, Johnson P, Rezapour M. A three year follow up of TVT for surgical treatment of female stress incontinence. *Br J Obstet Gynaecol* 1999; 106: 345–350

42. Ulmsten U, Henriksson L, Johnson P, Varhos G. An ambulatory surgical procedure under local anaesthesia for treatment of female urinary incontinence. *Int Urogynecol J* 1996; 7: 81–86

43. Ulmsten U, Falconer C, Johnson P *et al.* A multicentre study of tension-free vaginal tape (TVT) for surgical treatment of stress urinary incontinence. *Int Urogynecol J* 1998; 9: 210–213

44. Ulmsten U, Nilsson CG, Upsalla, Sweden. Personal communication. Presented at the International Continence Society meeting, August, 2000: Tampere, Finland.

45. Ward K, Hilton P. A randomised trial of colposuspension and tension free vaginal tape (TVT) for primary genuine stress incontinence. *Neurourol Urodyn* 2000; 19: 386–387

46. Ward K, Hilton P, Browning J. Changes in quality of life following surgery with tension free vaginal tape (TVT) or colposuspension for primary stress incontinence (GSI) (abstract). Presented at the International Continence Society meeting, August 2000, Tampere, Finland.

47. Jomaa M. TVT: tension free vaginal tape for surgical treatment of recurrent stress incontinence in local anaesthesia. A prospective open study at 3 years follow up (abstract). *Int Urogynecol J* 2000; 11(suppl 1): S33

48. Ward K, Hilton P. TVT: early experience. *Int Urogynecol J* (Abstract 20) IUGA Meeting 1998, p319

49. Ethicon; Edinburgh UK: data on file.

50. Kuuva N, Nilsson CG. A nationwide analysis of complications associated with the tension free vaginal tape (TVT) procedure. *Neurourol Urodyn* 2000; 19: 394–395

51. Meschia M, Gattei U, Pifarotti P *et al.* Tension free vaginal tape in the treatment of stress urinary incontinence. *Int Urogynecol J* 2000; 11(Suppl): S1–S21

52. Rottenburg R, Well A, Brioschi P *et al.* Urodynamic and clinical assessment of the Lyodura sling operation for urinary stress incointinence. *Br J Obstet Gynaecol* 1985; 92: 829–834

53. Jarvis GJ. Stress incontinence. In: Mundy AR, Stephenson TP, Wein AJ (eds) *Urodynamics: Principles, Practice and Application,* 2nd edn. New York: Churchill Livingstone, 1994; 299–326

54. Leach G, Dmochowski R, Appell R *et al.* Female stress urinary incontinence clinical guidelines panel summary report on surgical management of female stress urinary incontinence. *J Urol* 1997; 158: 875–880

55. McGuire EJ. Abdominal procedures for stress incontinence. *Urol Clin North Am* 1985; 12: 285–290

56. Horbach NS. Suburethral sling procedures. In: Ostergard DR, Bent AE (eds) *Urogynecology and Urodynamics,* 3rd edn. Philadelphia: Williams and Wilkins, 1991; 413–421

57. Jarvis GJ. Surgery for genuine stress incontinence. *Br J Obstet Gynaecol* 1994; 101: 371–374

58. Webster GD, Kreder KJ. Voiding dysfunction following cystourethropexy: its evaluation and management. *J Urol* 1990; 140: 670–673

59. Carr LX, Webster GD. Bladder outlet obstruction in women. *Urol Clin North Am* 1996; 23: 385–391

60. Hilton P. A clinical and urodynamic study comparing the Stamey bladder neck suspension and suburethral sling procedures in the treatment of genuine stress incontinence. *Br J Obstet Gynaecol* 1989; 96: 213–220

61. McGuire EJ, Bennett CJ, Konnack JA *et al.* Experience with pubovaginal slings for urinary incontinence in the University of Michigan. *J Urol* 1987; 138: 525–526

62. Beck RP, McCormick S, Nordstrom L. The fascia lata sling procedure for treating recurrent genuine stress incontinence of urine. *Obstet Gynecol* 1988; 72: 699–703

63. Bryans FE. Marlex gauze hammock sling operation with Coopers ligament attachment in the management of recurrent stress urinary incontinence. *Am J Obstet Gynecol* 1979; 41: 88–93

64. Blaivas G, Jacobs B. Pubovaginal fascial sling for the treatment of complicated stress urinary incontinence. *J Urol* 1991; 145: 1214–1218

65. Appell R. Primary slings for everyone with genuine stress incontinence: the argument for ... (editorial) *Int Urogynaecol J Pelvic Floor Dysfunct* 1998; 9: 249–251

66. Bahtia NN, Bergman A. Urodynamic predictability of voiding following incontinence surgery. *Obstet Gynecol* 1984; 63: 564–567

67. McLennan M, Melick C, Bent A. Clinical and urodynamic predictors of delayed voiding after fascia lata suburethral sling. *Obstet Gynecol* 1998; 98: 608–612

68. Bates CP, Whiteside CG, Turner-Warwick RT. Synchronous Cine/pressure/flow/cysto-urethrography with special reference to stress and urge incontinence. *Br J Urol* 1970; 42: 714–723

69. Cardozo LD, Stanton SL, Williams JE. Detrusor instability following surgery for GSI. *Br J Urol* 1979; 48: 138–142

70. Sand PK, Utrie J, Summitt RL, Ostergard DR. The effect of a suburethral sling on detrusor instability. *Int Urogynecol J* 1993; 4: 396

71. Zimmern P, Hadley H, Leach G, Raz S. Female urethral obstruction after Marshall–Marchetti–Krantz operation. *J Urol* 1987; 138: 517

72. Moloney P, Fenster H. Bladder neck incision for relief of obstruction after anti-incontinence surgery. *Int J Urogynecol* 1993; 4: 68

73. McGuire E, Leston W, Wang S. Transvaginal urethrolysis after obstructive urethral suspension procedures. *J Urol* 1989; 142: 1037–1039

74. Ghoniem G, Elgamasy A. A simplified surgical approach to bladder outlet obstruction following pubovaginal sling. *J Urol* 1995; 154: 181–183

75. Brubaker L. Suburethral sling release. *Obstet Gynecol* 1995; 86: 686–688

76. Avtan L, Avci C, Bulut T, Fourtanier G. Mesh infections after laparoscopic inguinal hernia repair. *Surg Laparosc Endosc* 1997; 7: 192–195

77. Miller K, Junger W. Ileocutaneous fistula formation following laparoscopic polypropylene mesh hernia repair. *Surg Endosc* 1997; 11: 772–773

78. Bent AE, Ostergard DR, Zwick-Zaffuto M. Tissue reaction to expanded polytetrafluoroethylene suburethral sling for urinary incontinence: clinical and histologic study. *Am J Obstet Gynecol* 1993: 169: 1198–1204

79. Melnick I, Lee R. Delayed transection of the urethra by Mersilene tape. *Urology* 1976; 8: 580–581

80. Berman C, Kreder K. Comparative cost analysis of collagen injection and fascia lata sling cystourethropexy for the treatment of type III incontinence in women. *J Urol*

45

The artificial urinary sphincter in the female patient

H. R. Hadley, M.-O. Bitker

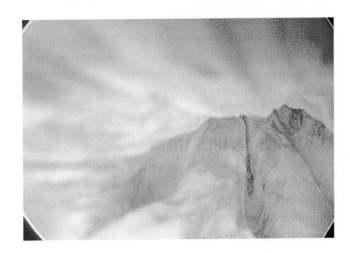

INTRODUCTION

The artificial urinary sphincter (AUS) is an effective alternative to the urethral sling and periurethral injection therapy for the treatment of urinary incontinence due to primary urethral sphincter insufficiency (type III stress urinary incontinence, or intrinsic sphincter deficienc – ISD).[1-3] The placement of the artificial sphincter may be accomplished through a transabdominal incision or the sphinter cuff may be implanted through a transvaginal approach.

ISD is the most common indication for the placement of the AUS in women. ISD may be the result of urethral scarring following multiple prior anti-incontinence operations, neurological disorders (myelomeningocele, sacral cord tumour or peripheral neuropathy), radical pelvic operations (abdominoperineal resection or radical hysterectomy), pelvic radiation therapy and, in certain cases, oestrogen deficiency or senile changes of the vaginal wall. Because the cause of incontinence in women with ISD is inadequate urethral closure, a standard bladder-neck suspension will not alleviate the patient's inadequate urethral resistance. The AUS may be utilized as an alternative to a sling procedure or periurethral injection, especially in cases of severe urethral dysfunction. The AUS is composed of three parts: these are the inflatable cuff, the pressure-regulating balloon and the pump (Fig. 45.1). The cuff is placed circumferentially around the bladder neck, the pressure-regulating balloon is positioned in the prevesical space and the pump is inserted into the labium majus. When the pump is compressed, fluid within the system is transferred from the cuff to the regulating balloon. This decompression of the cuff opens the bladder neck and allows the patient to void. After 1–2 minutes the pressure-regulating balloon promotes cuff filling by transfer of fluid through a resistor in the pump, re-establishing urethral compression, coaptation and continence. The American Medical System AS-800 is the only AUS that is currently implanted.

EVALUATION OF THE PATIENT

Preoperative evaluation of the patient should include a general (as well as a focused urological and neurological) history and physical examination. Radiographic and urodynamic studies of the lower urinary tract to assess detrusor and sphincter function during the stor-

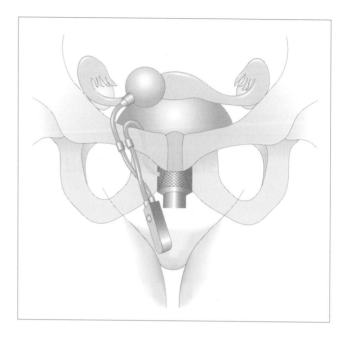

Figure 45.1. *The AS-800 artificial urinary sphincter in a woman. The cuff is placed around the bladder neck, the pressure-regulating balloon in the prevesical space and the pump in the labium majus.*

age and emptying phases should be performed prior to increasing lower urinary tract outlet resistance.

A history of incontinence surgery may affect the vascularity and thickness of the periurethral tissue and anterior wall of the vagina. Major difficulties during the periurethral and bladder-neck dissection can be expected in patients with a history of multiple surgical attempts to treat incontinence, particularly by a transvaginal incision or in the case of previous pelvic radiotherapy. The history should document radical pelvic operations, and orthopaedic or neurological disorders. The ability of the patient to 'pump' the device is dependent on satisfactory upper-extremity mobility and dexterity.

The patient with genuine stress urinary incontinence due to primary urethral insufficiency will typically report a significant loss of urine with abdominal straining. However, a history of significant urinary loss may represent bladder overactivity with or without normal sensation alone, or associated with ISD.

In addition to a focused genitourinary examination, special attention should be paid to the anterior vaginal wall and the lower abdomen for signs of significant scarring, tissue defects or infection.

Objective demonstration of stress urinary incontinence in the supine or upright position is required. A Q-tip test can be utilized to demonstrate urethral mobility, with the understanding that hypermobility of the bladder neck does not establish the presence of ISD and is not a contraindication to AUS implantation. Cystourethroscopy can be performed to assess urethral coaptation and bladder trabeculation, and to rule out the possibility of a fistula.

Urinary storage at low intravesical pressure is critical before increasing urethral resistance with the AUS. High-pressure urinary storage is a contraindication to AUS placement! Urodynamic studies should be utilized to assess detrusor and sphincter function during urinary storage and emptying.

Uroflowmetry and measurement of post-voiding residual urine reflect bladder emptying. Adequate bladder capacity at low intravesical pressure can be confirmed with a filling cystometrogram, which will record bladder capacity, bladder compliance and the absence of uninhibited bladder contractions.

Measurement of urethral leak-point pressure is recommended. Leakage of urine associated with a leak-point pressure of less than $80\,cmH_2O$ in the absence of a detrusor contraction supports the diagnosis of ISD. The urethral pressure profile is utilized, primarily in France, to confirm low urethral closure pressures ($< 25\,cmH_2O$).[4]

Radiographic evaluations should include a voiding cystourethrogram (VCUG) with resting and straining views. A well-supported urethra with an open bladder neck at baseline intravesical pressure is consistent with primary urethral insufficiency. The VCUG will also confirm the absence of vesicoureteric reflux.

INDICATIONS

The AUS is indicated for those patients who suffer from intrinsic urethral insufficiency with low-pressure urinary storage. Some patients with decreased bladder emptying may require intermittent self-catheterization following the procedure, especially if they have significant urinary residuals preoperatively. Urethral sling and periurethral bulking agents are alternative treatments and should be considered when the surgeon and patient are moving towards operative treatment of her incontinence.

Patients who demonstrate elevated intravesical storage pressures are subject to upper tract deterioration if the outlet resistance is increased. A response to anticholinergic drug therapy should be demonstrated prior to AUS implantation. Simultaneous or staged augmentation cystoplasty should be considered as an alternative to lifelong anticholinergic therapy.

As in most patients with urinary incontinence due to primary urethral insufficiency, conservative measures should be considered before operative intervention. These non-operative measures include timed voiding, fluid restriction, pelvic floor exercises, systemic or topical oestrogens, α-receptor agonists and anticholinergic medication. If the patient continues to be incontinent despite conservative treatment, operative intervention may be considered.

Patients who are unable or unwilling to perform intermittent catheterization but can operate the labial pump may be candidates for the AUS. When compared with the urethral sling the AUS is less likely to cause permanent urinary retention. When voiding, the patient with the AUS is capable of temporarily reducing urethral outlet resistance by decompressing the cuff. The bladder may be emptied by abdominal straining or by exploiting gravity with the cuff open. The patient with an AUS has less resistance to bladder emptying than the patient with a urethral sling, which often relies on urethral compression. Patients with poorly contractile or acontractile bladders, therefore, may be less likely to suffer from postoperative urinary retention than may the patients with a urethral sling.

Women of childbearing age are eligible for sphincter implantation. The sphincter should be deactivated during vaginal delivery to permit bladder emptying. There is no contraindication to caesarean section as the components are within the retropubic space.

From a medicolegal point of view, although informed consent is not routinely obtained in some European countries, it is recommended that those patients who are candidates for an AUS should be particularly aware of the existence of alternative procedures and of the possibility of postoperative complications and device failures.

TECHNIQUE

Transvaginal implantation

The advantage inherent in the transvaginal approach for AUS cuff placement, compared with a purely abdominal approach, is the accessibility of the poorly defined urethrovaginal plane. The dissection of this poorly defined plane is even more onerous following one or more anti-incontinence procedures. As opposed to the transabdominal approach, the transvaginal technique allows dissection of this urethrovaginal plane under direct vision. A controlled surgical entrance and optimal closure of the anterior vaginal wall eliminates the need for dissection of this difficult plane from within the retropubic space. An inadvertent and potentially unrecognized entrance through the vaginal wall and into the vagina can be eliminated.[1,5,6]

The patient is admitted to the hospital on the day of the operation. Preoperative parenteral antibiotics (cefazolin, gentamicin and metronidazole) are administered 1 hour prior to the operation. After a regional or general anaesthetic has been given, the patient is placed in the modified dorsal lithotomy position. The lower abdomen and vagina are shaved and prepared with povidone-iodine in the usual manner. The labia majora are sutured to the skin laterally, and a posterior-weighted vaginal retractor is placed for exposure of the anterior vaginal wall. After insertion of a Foley catheter to drain the bladder, saline is injected into the subepithelial tissue of the anterior vaginal wall near the bladder neck to facilitate dissection of the vaginal flap.

A vertical incision is made in the anterior vaginal wall (Fig. 45.2). The incision extends from a point midway between the bladder neck and the external meatus to the proximal bladder neck. A plane under the vaginal wall is created on each side of the incision, using sharp dissection. The dissecting scissors are first pointed laterally to the edge of the inferior pubis ramus and then upwards towards the ipsilateral shoulder of the patient (Fig. 45.3). Sufficiently thick vaginal flaps are created in anticipation of closure of the vagina over the soon-to-be-placed AUS cuff. If the patient has not had a previous bladder-neck operation, blunt finger dissection may be performed to separate the endopelvic fascia from its lateral attachments to the pubic rim. The finger should sweep from lateral to medial, creating a window into

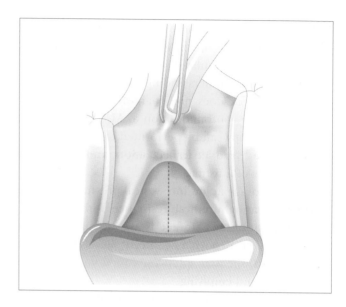

Figure 45.2. *With the patient in the modified dorsolithotomy position, a vertical incision is made in the anterior vaginal wall.*

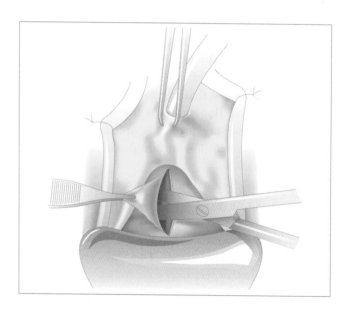

Figure 45.3. *Using a combination of sharp and blunt dissection, the retropubic space is entered lateral to the bladder neck.*

the retropubic space. The urethra and bladder neck can then be separated posteriorly and laterally from the vagina and the pelvic sidewall with sharp and blunt dissection. A similar procedure is followed on the opposite side.

Attention is next directed to the anterior aspect of the proximal urethra and bladder neck to free its attachments from the overlying symphysis pubis. If possible, blunt finger dissection through the vaginal incision should be used to perform this part of the procedure. However, in the patient who has had a previous retropubic operation, dense scarring may be encountered in the anterior portion of the urethra. The dissection on the anterior side of the urethra, therefore, may be particularly difficult because of its relative inaccessibility through the transvaginal approach. Overly aggressive dissection may lead to unintentional bladder opening or urethral tear. If unintentional entry to the bladder occurs, conventional wisdom may dictate that the procedure be abandoned. Salisz and Diokno, however, reported on their success in repairing the injury

and proceeding with implantation of the device.[7] To facilitate exposure of the dorsal surface of the urethra a separate suprameatal incision (1–2 cm) may be used[8] (Fig. 45.4a). Through this incision, sharp dissection is done in the midline below the symphysis pubis (Fig. 45.4b). After the bladder and urethra are allowed to drop away from their attachments to the symphysis, lateral blunt dissection can easily be performed to complete the dissection to the retropubic space previously opened through the vaginal incision. Thus, a circumferential dissection is completed around the bladder neck (Fig. 45.5).

After the proximal urethra has been freed circumferentially, a broken-back small vascular clamp (Dale femoral–popliteal anastomosis clamp, Pilling 353543) is passed around the urethra from left to right. The cuff-measuring tape is grasped and passed around the bladder neck, and the circumference of the bladder neck is measured. If the circumference is equivocal, it is best to err in favour of a slightly larger cuff size. Using a curved clamp, the appropriate-sized cuff of the AUS is placed around the bladder neck (Fig. 45.6). If the pump of the AUS is to be inserted into the right labium majus, the cuff is withdrawn from right to left; if, however, the pump is to be placed in the left labium majus, the cuff should be withdrawn from left to right. The cuff is then locked in place (Fig. 45.6) and rotated 180 degrees so

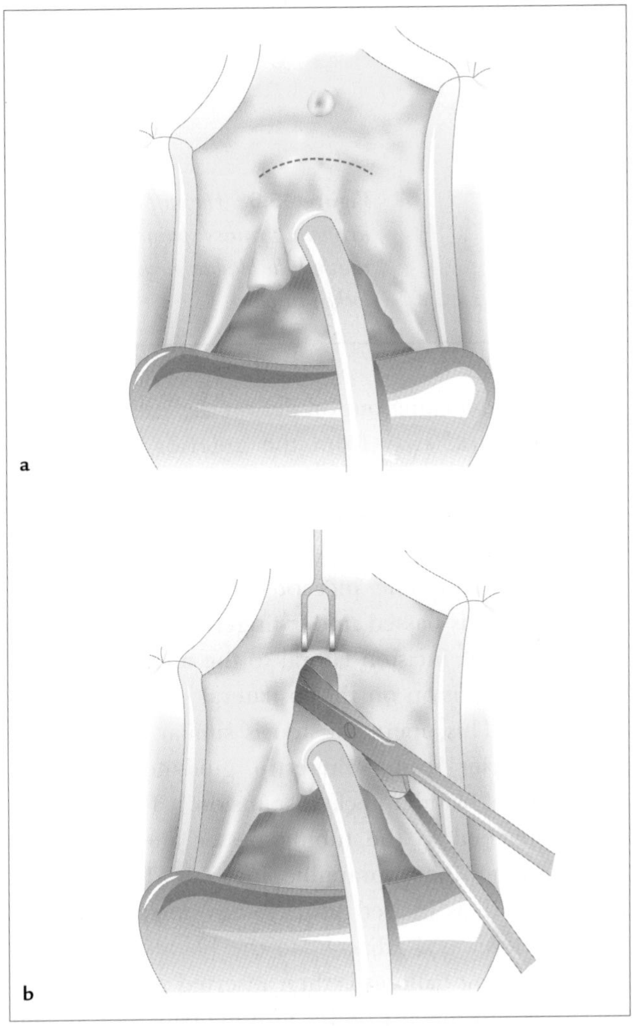

Figure 45.4. *(a) If dense scarring is encountered anterior to the urethra, a separate incision is made above the urethral meatus; (b) The suprameatal dissection is done in the midline just below the symphysis pubis.*

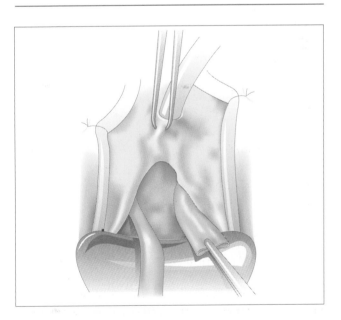

Figure 45.5. *A Penrose drain is placed around the bladder neck to demonstrate the completed circumferential dissection.*

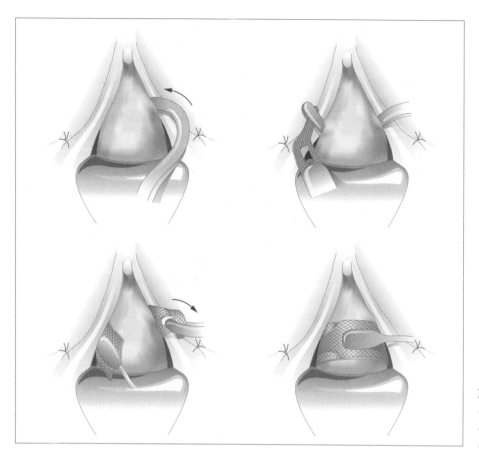

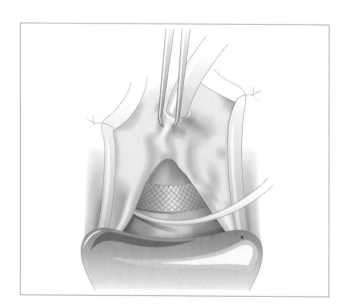

Figure 45.6. *The cuff of the artificial urinary sphincter is passed around the bladder neck and then locked in place.*

Figure 45.7. *The cuff is rotated 180 degrees clockwise so that the hard-locking button lies anterior to the urethra, away from the anterior vaginal wall.*

that the hard-locking button lies on the anterior aspect of the urethra, away from the anterior vaginal wall (Fig 45.7).

On the side on which the pressure-regulating balloon and pump mechanism will be implanted, a transverse suprapubic incision (4 cm) is made. The tubing passer is passed under fingertip guidance from the suprapubic incision lateral to the midline down to the vaginal incision on the ipsilateral side of the bladder neck. (This operative step is similar to passing a needle carrier under fingertip guidance during a Pereyra-type bladder-neck suspension.) The cuff tubing is attached to the tubing passer and then withdrawn up to the suprapubic incision. The anterior rectus sheath is incised transversely, and a prevesical space is developed adjacent to the bladder. The pressure-regulating balloon is then inserted in the prevesical space. In women I prefer to use a balloon reservoir at 51–60 cmH$_2$O pressure.

From the suprapubic incision a subcutaneous tunnel into the labium majus is created through which the pump will be inserted. The pump is passed into the labium majus to the level of the urethral meatus with the deactivation button facing anteriorly. A Babcock clamp is used to secure the pump in position. The tubes are trimmed to the appropriate lengths and then irrigated to remove any air or debris from their ends. A straight connector is placed between the pump and the balloon reservoir. A right-angle connector attaches the pump to the cuff. Monofilament suture ties or Quick Connectors are used to secure these attachments. Preparation of the cuff and reservoir is performed according to the instructions specified by the manufacturer.

The suprapubic and vaginal wounds are irrigated copiously with antibiotic solution. The wounds are then closed in multiple layers with absorbable sutures to ensure good coverage of the prosthesis with healthy overlying tissue. If the integrity of the vaginal wall appears to be compromised, an interposition of a vascularized flap (e.g. Martius flap) should be considered. The pump is left in the deactivated mode for 6 weeks.

A vaginal gauze pack is placed, and is removed on the first postoperative day. The Foley catheter is removed on the third postoperative day.

Transabdominal implantation

In France, the transabdominal approach is most commonly used for implantation of an AUS because it gives easy access to the retropubic extraperitoneal space.[9] A 2–3 day preadmission period is scheduled for learning about the device and for preparation of the skin and vagina with antibacterials. Preoperative skin preparation is also performed for 15 minutes in the operating room.

The patient should be placed in the lithotomy position with her knees at the same level as the abdomen, which provides access to both the abdominal and perineal area. After the patient has been draped, a 14F Foley catheter is introduced into the urethra. It is extremely important to use this catheter size, as measurement of cuff size will be corrected for this diameter during intra-operative measurement of the urethral diameter. The device is prepared and the filling solutions of iso-osmotic saline or radiographic contrast selected for filling of the device.

A midline or a Pfannenstiel incision can accomplish access to the retropubic space. The dissection of the retropubic space may be difficult, especially with patients who have undergone several previous pelvic operations for incontinence. The dissection must

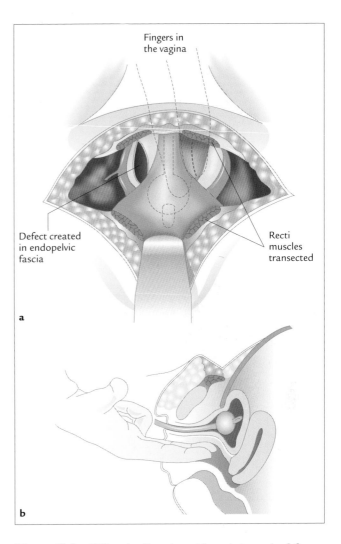

Figure 45.8. *Aiding the dissection with an intravaginal finger: (a) frontal view; (b) lateral view.*

follow the posterior face of the pubic bone, trying not to enter the anterior wall of the bladder. Repair of any cystotomy can be performed with absorbable suture, or the cystotomy may be left open and utilized for the remaining dissection.

As it approaches the bladder neck, the dissection will go laterally and can be aided with an intravaginal finger (Fig. 45.8). The vesicovaginal plane is then dissected alternately from each side of the bladder neck. Extreme care must be taken to avoid perforation into the vagina during sharp and right-angle dissection (Fig. 45.9). In difficult cases an intentional cystotomy of the anterior bladder wall may also aid identification of the bladder neck and facilitate separation within the vesicovaginal plane.

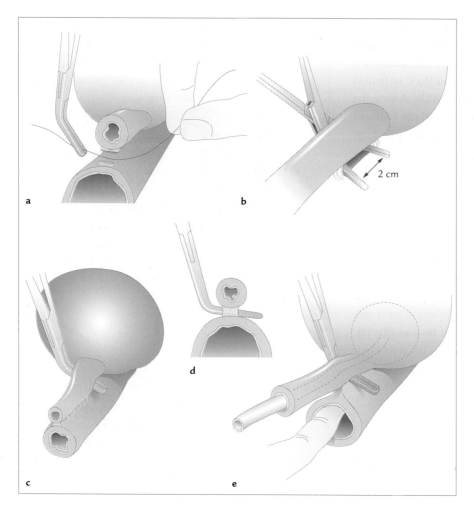

Figure 45.9. *(a, b) Insertion of right-angled clamp; (c, d) right-angled clamp in place; (e) clamp, catheter and finger in position.*

The cuff sizer is used, taking care always to choose the larger size in cases of intermediate measurement. The cuff is placed around the bladder neck so that the hard-locking button lies on the opposite side from the labium majus, where the pump is to be implanted.

Any vesical incision is closed in two layers with absorbable suture. Any bladder perforation is ruled out by filling the bladder intra-operatively through the Foley catheter.

In the case of an accidental perforation of the vaginal wall, especially if unrecognized, there is a high risk of erosion of the cuff through the vaginal wall in the postoperative period. It is advisable, in cases of significant vaginal wall trauma, to consider converting the operation to a sling procedure. If an AUS is the only possibility for cure, it is preferable to implant only the cuff and to close the vaginal wall after the interposition of a Martius flap.

The choice of reservoir balloon is influenced by the quality of the tissue of the bladder neck. If the dissection has been difficult, or in the setting of previous pelvic irradiation, it is more advisable to choose a low-pressure-regulating balloon (51–61 cmH$_2$O). In the majority of cases a balloon of 61–70 cmH$_2$O pressure will be a good choice. The balloon is usually placed on the same side as the labium majus where the pump will be implanted.

The pump is first filled with 22 ml iso-osmotic contrast medium to prime the cuff; subsequently, it will be refilled up to a total volume of 20 ml. After the pump has been filled with contrast medium, it is placed within the labium majus, on the side of hand dominance, and a 3/0 absorbable polyglycolic suture is placed within the tunnel to prevent migration.

The three parts of the device are then connected, usually using a right-angle connector between the cuff and the pump tube and a straight-angle connector between the balloon and the pump tube. Tubes usually run better from the pump to the balloon and the cuff through the abdominal muscles than through the midline incision. The cuff is then deflated and the device deactivated. After careful verification of the haemostasis and irrigation of the operative site, the abdominal wall is closed without drainage.

The Foley catheter is withdrawn on postoperative day 2 or 3 if a cystotomy has not been performed. In the case of incidental or intentional bladder entrance, a 12-day period of catheter drainage is recommended. Prophylactic antibiotics are continued for 3 days and there is careful follow-up of the surgical wound and monitoring of the sterility of the urine until the patient is discharged. The device is activated after a 4–6-week period to allow healing of the periurethral tissues.

DECREASED DEVICE EFFICACY

With improvements in the design and manufacture of the device, fluid loss secondary to tubing fracture at the connector sites, cuff leakage at the stress points created by deflation and kinking of the tubing have decreased significantly. If the device has been filled with iso-osmotic contrast, a plain radiograph of the kidney, ureter and bladder or fluoroscopy are useful to diagnose fluid leak; a urethral pressure profile or cystoscopy can be utilized to observe decreased urethral pressure or an open cuff, respectively.

Urethral atrophy decreases the compressive bulk within the cuff. Urinary leakage may occur without device malfunction. The preferred treatment is replacement with a smaller cuff rather than increasing reservoir pressure. During any revision of the device, the surgeon's judgement concerning replacement of a malfunctioning portion of the device rather than the whole device is critical. Significant indications for complete device replacement include device leakage, which may allow foreign material within the system, or a device that has been in place for more than 2–3 years.

INFECTION AND EROSION

Induration and tenderness of the pump site or suprapubic inflammation or induration usually reflect infection of the device. Erosion of the sphincter cuff into the urethra is commonly associated with the recurrence of urinary incontinence, although urinary tract infection may be the first and only symptom. Erosion of the cuff through the vaginal wall is associated with vaginal bleeding and discharge. Erosion of the reservoir into the bladder is rare, and may present as a urinary tract infection or infection of the device. Pump erosion through the labium majus is diagnosed by direct examination.

Infection of the device, or erosion through the skin or vagina or into the urinary tract, must be treated by explantation of the entire device. Reimplantation can be considered after 4–6 months. In the case of cuff erosion, the placement of an omentum flap between urethra and cuff is recommended.

Experience with the penile prosthesis has revealed the ability to irrigate the wound thoroughly with antibiotic solution and proceed with immediate reimplantation of the device. However, erosion of the cuff into the urinary tract presents unique challenges, which discourage this manoeuvre. In the isolated case of erosion of the sphincter tubing through the abdominal skin, or where there is erosion of the pump through the labium, aggressive irrigation of the wound and debridement of surrounding tissue, wound closure may be successful. The pump should be replaced and moved to the opposite labum majus. The device with cuff erosion through the vaginal wall has been salvaged utilizing a Martius flap and vaginal wall closure. In all cases of infection and erosion, when device salvage is attempted, the patient should be informed of the high risk of additional surgery to perform complete device removal.

DISCUSSION

The few published papers relating to implantation of the AUS through the transvaginal approach report favourable outcomes. Appell reported a series of 34 patients in whom the AUS was placed through simultaneous vaginal and abdominal incisions:[1] 19 patients underwent follow-up of 3 years. The overall continence rate was 100%; three patients, however, required revision operations for inadequate cuff compression and connector leak. Abbassian[8] described the implantation of the AUS utilizing the vaginal incision alone in four patients: at mean follow-up of 14 months, all patients were dry.

The potential advantage of the AUS over the urethral sling is that a known circumferential compressive force can be placed around the entire urethra rather than only on the posterior surface of the urethra. Because the patient with an AUS will not void against outlet obstruction, there is a decreased likelihood of urinary retention and bladder instability than with the urethral sling. The incidence of prolonged postoperative urinary retention after the urethral sling operation has been reported to be up to 10%. Patients with a hypocontractile bladder are especially at risk for permanent urinary retention after the urethral sling.[7]

A disadvantage of the AUS is the risk of erosion by the device. Cuff erosion probably occurs more commonly in patients who previously have undergone pelvic irradiation.[8] With the use of a low-pressure-regulating balloon (51–60 cmH$_2$O pressure), delayed primary activation of the cuff and exclusion of the patient with prior pelvic radiotherapy, the incidence of device erosion may be reduced.[1,8]

In the past, mechanical malfunction of the AUS has been common, with revision necessary in 31–43% of women with the device.[9,10] However, since the introduction of new cuff designs the incidence of mechanical malfunction has decreased.[2]

Long-term follow-up data for the AUS in women are sparse. Fulford *et al.*[3] reported on 61 patients of both sexes who could be followed-up for at least 10 years after implantation of the AUS. There were 18 women (technique of implantation not described) in this series: of the nine women who underwent implantation for neurological reasons, four had erosion and three had either cuff or pump failure. This paper,[3] and a recent look at my own data (men and women) with long-term follow-up, indicate that revision of the AUS is likely to be necessary 10 years after implantation for either mechanical or non-mechanical reasons. I suggest, therefore, that if a mechanical or non-mechanical problem that requires operative intervention is encountered, serious consideration should be given to replacing the entire device if it was implanted more than 2–3 years previously.

SUMMARY

The management of women with stress urinary incontinence associated with a non-mobile well-supported urethra and bladder neck is certainly a challenge to the surgeon. Many of these patients have undergone previous unsuccessful anti-incontinence operations. The AUS is a viable alternative to the urethral sling or periurethral injection therapy for these difficult patients.

The advantage of the transvaginal approach in the placement of the AUS is that it offers the surgeon the ability to dissect through the difficult urethrovaginal plane under direct vision. In the patient with abundant scar tissue, the addition of a suprameatal incision reduces the likelihood of an inadvertent cystotomy or urethral injury during the anterior dissection of the urethra. With familiarization of implantation technique, the use of a low-pressure-regulating balloon reservoir (51–60 cmH$_2$O pressure), delayed primary activation of the cuff and selective patient criteria (e.g. exclusion of patients with prior pelvic irradiation), the AUS can result in reasonable long-term social continence in patients with urinary incontinence due to intrinsic urethral insufficiency. In the subgroup of patients with a combination of hypocontractile bladder and ISD, the AUS may be the initial treatment of choice over the urethral sling because of its lower incidence of prolonged postoperative urinary retention and vesical instability.

REFERENCES

1. Appell RA. Techniques and results in the implantation of the artificial urinary sphincter in women with type III stress urinary incontinence by a vaginal approach. *Neurourol Urodyn* 1988; 7: 613–619

2. Webster GD, Perez LM, Khoury JM *et al.* Management of type III stress urinary incontinence using artificial urinary sphincter. *Urology* 1992; 39: 499–503

3. Fulford SCV, Sutton C, Bales G *et al.* The fate of the 'modern' artificial urinary sphincter with a follow-up of more than 10 years. *Br J Urol* 1997; 79: 713–716

4. Appell RA. Sphincter insufficiency: testing and treatment. *Curr Opin Urol* 1997; 7: 197–204

5. Wang Y, Hadley HR. Artificial sphincter: trans-vaginal approach. In: Raz S (ed) *Female Urology*, 2nd edn, volume 1. Philadelphia: Saunders, 1996; 428–434

6. Hadley R. Transvaginal placement of the artificial urinary sphincter in women. *Neurourol Urodyn* 1988; 7: 292–293

7. Salisz JA, Diokno AC. The management of injuries to the urethra, bladder or vagina encountered during difficult placement of the artificial urinary sphincter in the female patient. *J Urol* 1992; 148: 1528–1530

8. Abbassian A. A new operation for insertion of the artificial urinary sphincter. *J Urol* 1988; 140: 512–513

9. Long RL, Barrett DM: Artificial sphincter: abdominal approach. In: Raz S (ed) *Female Urology*, 2nd edn, volume 1. Philadelphia: Saunders, 1996; 419–427

10. Richard F, Chartier-Kastler E, Lebret T *et al.* Résultats des colposuspensions, des bandelettes sous-uréthrales modifiées et du sphincter artificiel dans l'incontinence grave avec pressions de clôture inférieures à 30 cm d'eau. In: Chatelain C, Jacobs C (eds) *Séminaires d'Uro-Néphrologie de la Pitié-Salpêtrière*, 22nd series. Paris Masson 1996; 400–408

11. Bitker MO, Barrou B, Aranda B *et al.* Résultats du traitement de l'insuffisance urinaire post-opératoire de l'homme par implantation du sphincter artificiel AS800. A propos de 15 observations. *J Urol (Paris)* 1987; 93: 275–278

46

Aetiology and classification of pelvic organ prolapse

S. Swift, J. Theofrastous

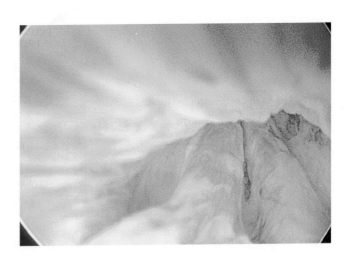

AETIOLOGY

The aetiology of pelvic organ prolapse (POP; Fig. 46.1) is difficult to describe, for several reasons, prominent among which is the problem with defining this condition. The American College of Obstetricians and Gynecologists (ACOG) technical bulletin defines POP as the protrusion of the pelvic organs into or out of the vaginal canal.[1] This is a very loose definition and technically could encompass a range from any woman who has the slightest relaxation of the cervix, such that it descends 1–2 cm into the vagina on Valsalva manouevre, to the woman who has complete vaginal eversion and uterine procidentia. Obviously, as these are two extremes of the degree of support found in adult women, it becomes difficult to determine the transition between normal and pathological POP. Part of this difficulty arises because the degree and stage of POP in the general female population has not been described. Several investigators have documented the presence of specific symptoms in the general population that are often associated with POP, but have not correlated these symptoms with the degree of prolapse as determined by physical examination.[2–6] Others have determined the prevalence and degree of POP in selected populations (i.e. patients attending referral clinics for incontinence and POP), but these data cannot be extrapolated to the general population.[7,8]

Two reports have described the incidence of surgically corrected POP and urinary incontinence in a specific population of patients: one involved patients attending a family-planning clinic and the other described all patients participating in one insurance plan.[9,10] They reported incidences of 2.04–2.63 surgical procedures for prolapse or genuine stress incontinence (GSI) per 1000 women-years, with an increasing incidence as women age, and a lifetime risk of undergoing surgery for prolapse or incontinence of 5–11.1%.

The greatest single causative factor for the development of prolapse is hypothesized to be the result of pregnancy and vaginal delivery of a term infant. This may be secondary to damage to the fascial supports and neurological innervation of the pelvic floor muscles which occur as the fetal vertex passes through the birth canal.[11,12] Other factors, such as poor-quality connective tissue, underlying neurological disease, chronic states that increase intra-abdominal pressure (e.g. chronic obstructive pulmonary disease, chronic constipation or obesity) and lifestyle are commonly noted as risk factors or associated findings in subjects with POP and incontinence.[1] The data on the contributions of these various factors are reviewed and discussed in detail in this chapter in an attempt to describe the current state of knowledge regarding the aetiology of POP.

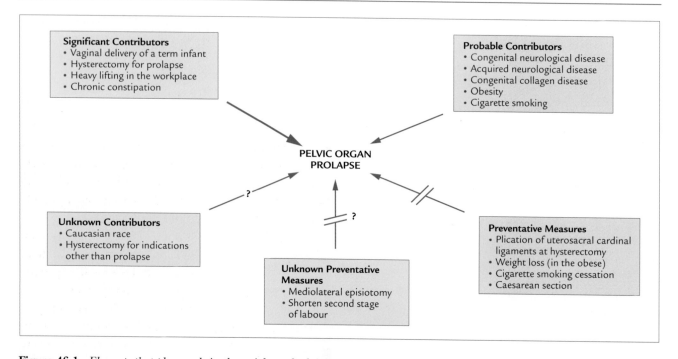

Figure 46.1. *Elements that play a role in the aetiology of pelvic organ prolapse.*

Childbirth

Vaginal delivery of a term infant has been postulated to be the most significant contributor to the subsequent development of POP. It is postulated that, as the fetal vertex passes through the vaginal canal, this stretches the levator ani muscles and the pudendal nerve, leading to damage with permanent neuropathy and muscle weakness. Several studies in the literature describe the effects of vaginal delivery on the innervation of the pelvic floor.[11-13] They demonstrate that there is an increase in the pudendal nerve terminal motor latency following vaginal delivery that is consistent with damage to the nerve. In the majority of these women, recovery from the nerve damage occurs in the first 2–3 months following delivery. However, in a small percentage of women, there is evidence of persistence of the nerve damage; nevertheless, the data regarding which aspects of the delivery process place the woman at risk for persistence of the damage are controversial. In one study, the use of forceps in multiparous women appeared to increase the risk of prolonged nerve damage;[13] in another, the use of forceps did not increase the risk of prolonged nerve damage, but the length of the second stage of labour was the only significant factor associated with persistent nerve damage.[11] There is also evidence that this damage can be avoided by caesarean delivery.[14] It is considered that the damage to the pudendal nerve leads to long-term weakness of the levator ani that eventually is responsible for the POP and GSI seen later in life.

There are also data to suggest that acute damage to the pelvic floor supporting structures may occur at the time of vaginal delivery. This has been documented by ultrasonographic measurements of the descent of the vesical neck shortly before and after vaginal delivery. Women had similiar support during pregnancy, but in those who underwent a vaginal delivery there was greater descent of the vesical neck with straining in the immediate post-partum period than in those who underwent elective caesarean section.[15]

The aforementioned data suggest that some damage occurs to the pudendal nerve and the pelvic support structures with almost all vaginal deliveries, but that, in most cases, there is recovery from this damage in the immediate post-partum period. What part of the birth process leads to prolonged damage is difficult to determine, but both use of forceps and a long second stage may play a role. It should also be noted that there are older studies suggesting that a mediolateral episiotomy versus either a midline episiotomy or delivery over an intact perineum protects against the subsequent development of POP.[16]

Although this provides some clinical information on the acute effects of vaginal delivery, it does not explain how this acute damage affects the long-term support and function of the pelvic viscera. One population-based study demonstrated an 11-fold increase in the risk of prolapse in women with more than four children compared with the risks in nulliparous women, and most of this increased risk occurred in women who had borne two or more children.[9]

Congenital pelvic floor defects

One of the greatest questions concerning the aetiology of POP is that of which patients are at risk. From the above discussion, it appears that, although pudendal neuropathy and pelvic floor damage occur commonly with vaginal delivery, severe POP is relatively uncommon. Therefore, do those patients destined to develop prolapse have a congenital defect – either neurological or structural – that prevents recovery of their pelvic support mechanism from the trauma of vaginal delivery, and might this also account for prolapse that is occasionally seen in the nulliparous woman?

It has been demonstrated in several studies that women who develop POP have an increased prevalence of pudendal neuropathy.[10,17,18] These changes in pudendal nerve function are reminiscent of the nerve damage that is seen following childbirth. However, one of the difficulties in evaluating this information is that pudendal nerve terminal motor latencies are difficult to interpret, and the 95% confidence interval between controls and subjects with stress incontinence overlaps, so that there is not a statistically significant difference; however, there does appear to be a trend toward worsening pudendal neuropathy in subjects with POP and urinary incontinence.[19]

In addition, it has been noted that younger women (average age 30 years) who present with prolapse have a higher incidence of recognized nerve injury from other causes (e.g. cervical spine injury, poliomyelitis and Guillain–Barré syndrome) than older women with prolapse (average age 60 years).[20] Although this is an interesting observation, this study involved very small numbers, making it difficult to draw valid conclusions.

Muscle biopsies from the levator ani of subjects with POP and GSI demonstrate histological evidence of a neuropathic process involving partial denervation and then reinnervation.[18] This suggests pudendal nerve damage with recovery. However, these changes were not present throughout the levator ani muscle (the most significant differences were noted in biopsies taken from the posterior compartment) and were not related to severity of symptoms or the patient's parity.[18] The changes were strongly related to the subject's age and may simply reflect age-related changes as opposed to neuropathic sequelae.[21] One of the questions regarding these studies involves the cause of the pudendal neuropathy and whether it was a result of a difficult vaginal delivery or some other insult. There are currently no long-term studies demonstrating that women with prolonged pudendal neuropathy, as a direct result of childbirth, are at an increased risk of POP and GSI later in life.

There is also evidence that women with POP have defective collagen. It has been shown that women with POP have less total collagen in their pubocervical fascia than do controls, and that the collagen present is of a weaker type than that in controls with normal support.[22,23] There is also the observation that subjects with POP have a greater degree of joint hypermobility, suggesting a collagen defect.[24] If POP is related to collagen defects, then women with congenital connective tissue diseases should have a greater incidence of prolapse. However, when women with Ehlers–Danlos syndrome were evaluated there was no relationship between greater degrees of joint mobility and more prominent POP.[25]

Another congenital defect that is thought to have a role in POP is spina bifida. Although this is often quoted as a cause of prolapse, particularly in the young nulliparous patient, there are only a few case reports describing its relationship to prolapse and most of these were in the newborn.[26,27] The report by Torpin[26] mentioned a group of adult women with prolapse who had a 28% incidence of spina bifida occulta compared with a 10% incidence in their control population without prolapse. Although the relationship may not be straightforward, in the young nulliparous woman with severe prolapse an evaluation to identify spina bifida occulta is warranted.

Is there a congenital predilection for pelvic support dysfunction in some subjects that may be responsible for the more severe degrees of POP? If so, can these women be identified and recommendations made for ways to protect their pelvic floor support structures, particularly during childbirth? Until these questions are answered, no universal recomendations can be made.

Racial differences

One component that may predict those subjects likely to develop prolapse is their genetic background, as reflected in their race. There are a few anecdotal reports that certain populations have a higher or lower incidence of POP, but these tend to be more opinion than fact.[28–30] One study that specifically addressed racial differences showed a similar rate and severity of prolapse between black and white populations.[7] In this study, the population examined was selected for the symptom of prolapse and may be more a reflection of the racial make-up of the local population than a statement on the relative incidence of prolapse in a given race. There is also a study examining the difference in anatomy and collagen content of cadaver specimens between Caucasian and Asian women:[30] there appears to be a greater collagen content in the fascial supports of Asian than in Caucasian women. However, the populations compared were not adequately described to determine what other influences may have explained the results. Furthermore, a recent study on the incidence of urinary incontinence (a condition commonly associated with POP) in Asian women demonstrated similiar rates to those published for predominantly Caucasian populations.[31]

There is much anecdotal evidence that Caucasian women are at greater risk of developing prolapse than either black or Asian women; however, there is little objective evidence to back this up. Although there may be differences in pelvic anatomy between races, how this translates into the risk of developing POP remains speculative.

Pelvic surgery (hysterectomy)

The role of surgery to correct the various aspects of POP and the predisposition for recurrence of (or new) sites of relaxation that occur with specific procedures are discussed in chapter 47 which describes surgical correction of prolapse and incontinence. In this chapter, we limit the discussion to the relationship between hysterectomy and subsequent vaginal-vault prolapse. The incidence of massive vaginal-vault prolapse following hysterectomy is not known but has been estimated to be 2.0–3.6 /1000 women-years.[9,32] There is a general opinion that enterocele formation and prolapse are greater following a vaginal hysterectomy than after abdominal hysterectomy. However, the rates and degree of prolapse appear to be similar, regardless of the type of antecedent hysterectomy.[33] There is a correlation between subsequent prolapse and the initial indication for the hysterectomy, with prolapse rates as high as 15/1000 women-years in patients whose indication for hysterectomy was uterine prolapse.[9]

Disruption of the attachments of the uterosacral-ligament/cardinal-ligament complex to the cuff is considered to be responsible for post-hysterectomy vaginal-vault prolapse. Most authors feel that the incidence of prolapse can be reduced by paying particular attention to reattaching these ligaments to the cuff and obliterating the cul-de-sac. There are a few uncontrolled reports that the incidence of enterocele following a hysterectomy can be reduced by more than 50% if cul-de-sac obliteration is performed at the time of hysterectomy.[33,34] It would seem that, if disruption of the attachments of the uterosacral and cardinal ligaments were the the main reason for subsequent prolapse, then supracervical (sub-total) hysterectomy would provide some degree of protection. In the one report on the prevalence of post-hysterectomy prolapse, the author stated that, in his practice, there were 31 cases of eversion of the vagina and cervical stump and only seven cases of vaginal eversion of the cuff; this was despite the mention that more total than supracervical hysterectomies were performed in that practice.[35] This suggests that preservation of the uterosacral and cardinal ligamentous attachments to the cervix does not prevent subsequent prolapse.

Prolapse following hysterectomy appears to be unrelated to the route of surgery but may be related to the indication, with vaginal-vault prolapse occurring most commonly, following a hysterectomy for prolapse. The cause of subsequent prolapse is still unknown; however, if attention is paid to securing the cardinal and uterosacral ligaments to the cuff and obliterating the cul-de-sac, the incidence may be reduced.

Lifestyle

It is widely believed that women who participate in high-impact activities, whether at work or at play, will have more complications with prolapse and associated symptoms than their sedentary counterparts. Urinary incontinence during high-impact activities – particularly sports – is common, with up to 25% of young physically fit women reporting some urinary incontinence while participating in their sport.[36] However, when elite athletes are followed over time the incidence of incontinence developing later in life is similiar to that in age-matched controls.[37] These reports did not comment on POP, so how this relates to high-impact sports remains unknown.

Although sports do not appear to cause urinary incontinence later in life, there are reports of other activities that predispose to urinary incontinence. Pelvic support defects and stress urinary incontinence in six nulliparous infantry trainees were attributed to airborne training for the military in the form of repeated parachute drops.[38] The cause of their prolapse and incontinence was thought to be related to the repetitive high-impact stress with parachute jump landings or parachute deployment that weakened the pelvic floor, leading to the dysfunction. These were all young, physically fit, nulliparous women with no symptoms prior to their airborne training.

Heavy lifting at work also appears to be related to POP and herniated lumbar disc disease.[39] In one study, the number of prolapse operations performed on over 28 000 nursing assistants was compared with the number performed on the general population. For this study, nursing assistants were identified as a population that performs a lot of heavy lifting and manual labour. A 60% increased risk of operation for prolapse in these women over the general population was noted and it was felt this was secondary to their work-related duties. A similiar increase in the risk of surgery for herniated disc was also noted, validating the selection of this population as one participating in heavy lifting and manual labour.

The question becomes one of why elite athletes have none of the long-term consequences to their high-impact activities that are experienced by the average individual with heavy lifting in the workplace experiences. It may be that trained athletes have greater tone in their pelvic floor musculature that is associated with years of training, whereas individuals who are suddenly exposed to heavy lifting in the work place may be at greater risk because their pelvic floor musculature has not been prepared by any preceding training. Furthermore, the increased incidence of disc and back problems experienced by the women involved in heavy lifting may demonstrate a tendency toward poor technique in performing their lifting, which may also play a role in the development of POP.

Although there does not appear to be an increased risk for the athlete for subsequent development of pelvic floor dysfunction, it does appear that heavy lifting at work may play a role in its development. In addition, extreme insults to the pelvic support (e.g. those that occur with repetitive parachute jumps) probably do have long-term sequelae.

Chronic disease

Chronic illnesses that result in constant stress and strain on the pelvic floor are often quoted as a significant predisposing condition for POP.[1,40] Conditions such as chronic obstructive pulmonary disease or chronic cough, chronic constipation and obesity are the diseases most often implicated, but there are few data in the literature to substantiate this. One study describes an association between chronic constipation and POP:[41] in this study, 61% of subjects with uterovaginal prolapse reported straining with stool as young adults prior to the onset of the prolapse, whereas in a control group, only 4% reported straining with stool as young women. Furthermore, studies of severely constipated women have demonstrated abnormalities in pudendal nerve function similar to those noted in subjects with uterovaginal prolapse.[42]

The relationship between obesity and GSI has been investigated and, although there is some conflicting evidence, most agree that obesity appears to predispose the individual to GSI.[43,44] It has also been demonstrated that surgically induced weight loss will cure over 50% of subjects with GSI.[45,46] The effect of weight-management programmes that do not involve surgery have not been evaluated to date, so conclusive statements regarding weight loss outside of surgery cannot be made. The effects of chronic pulmonary disease have not been studied, but there is a relationship between cigarette smoking and GSI, with smokers having a 2.5-fold increase in the risk of developing GSI, independent of other factors.[47] The more violent coughing by smokers

is considered to promote this; other conditions that result in vigorous coughing would, therefore, be expected to have similar consequences. These studies suggest a relationship between chronic diseases and GSI, a common symptom of prolapse; however, their relationship to POP has not been studied.

Chronic constipation, obesity and cigarette smoking all appear to be related to the development of pelvic floor dysfunction. Other conditions, such as chronic obstructive pulmonary disease, that result in insults to the pelvic floor, also probably have a role in the aetiology of this condition but have not been sufficiently investigated.

Summary

The role of childbirth in the development of pelvic floor dysfunction and prolapse remains central; whether there are congenital conditions that place the individual at risk remains controversial. Furthermore, are there conditions that can be identified and corrected to reduce the individual's risk of subsequently developing POP? These are important considerations that need more investigation before conclusive recommendations can be made.

CLASSIFICATION OF PELVIC ORGAN PROLAPSE

In few areas in medicine does something seem so obvious and intuitive, but is, in fact, replete with obfuscation and confusion, than the clinical evaluation of POP. Over the last few decades, dozens of schemes for evaluating POP have flourished and waned, leaving investigators in 1961 to lament that misleading discrepancies exist with reference to classification of the uterus in disorders involving fascial relaxation.[48] These authors noted that, although Howard Kelly had recognized the need for an accurate method to record the details of the pelvic examination as early as 1898, little progress had been made to codify performance or documentation of the pelvic examination. Kelly and his disciples differentiated only between complete prolapse with total vaginal eversion (procidentia uteri) and incomplete prolapse.[49] Given that hysterectomy was highly morbid in these early days, vaginal-cuff prolapse was a rarity. Friedman and Little concluded: 'Perhaps we have stirred up the proverbial tempest in a teapot without just cause' and went on to propose yet another system.[48]

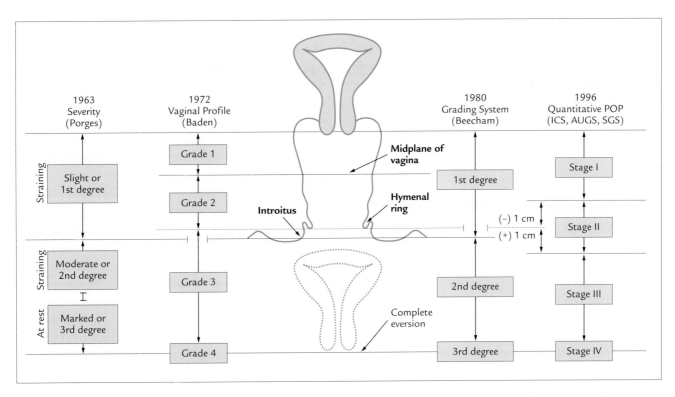

Figure 46.2. *Comparison of the four most commonly used pelvic organ prolapse (POP) grading systems. ICS, International Continence Society; AUGS, American Urogynecologic Society; SGS, Society of Gynecologic Surgeons.*

One of the earliest systems of evaluating prolapse, which gained widespread usage, was that developed by Porges in 1963[50] (Fig. 46.2). Porges recognized the importance of examining the patient during straining in order to reproduce the *in vivo* anatomy and stratified his classification system accordingly. Porges recommended two separate sets of observations – at rest and with straining – sounding the uterus to exclude cervical elongation; he disparaged the then-common practice of placing a tenaculum on the cervix and applying traction, as it in no way simulates a life situation: the reference point for this system was the introitus.

Baden and Walker proposed a method of classifying vaginal support by a site-specific examination during straining, in which six different anatomical reference points were assigned a numerical value between zero and four to generate a vaginal profile.[51] The vaginal profile evaluates urethroceles, cystoceles, prolapse and rectoceles according to a half-way system, with graduations half-way to (grade 2) and half-way through (grade 3) the hymen (Fig. 46.2). Unlike the system for the above structures, Baden proposed the evaluation

of enteroceles using a system in which the vaginal length was divided into quarters and herniation to the hymen was assigned as grade 4. Perineal lacerations were also graded, with involvement of the perineal body equivalent to grade 2, involvement of the anal sphincter grade 3, and laceration to the rectal mucosa grade 4. Baden and Walker were among the first investigators to report specific anatomical findings before and after reconstructive surgery; however, they concluded that 'the pelvic examination is just a pelvic examination' and that gynaecologists should employ additional testing such as cystometry or cystoradiography at their discretion.[52]

One of the most widely used grading systems currently in use was published by Beecham in 1980 in the 'Communications in Brief' section of the *American Journal of Obstetrics and Gynecology*. Beecham decried the morass of various non-standardized systems that were in use and proposed a system in which prolapse was rated in degrees during straining, in order 'to determine what troubles the patient all the time'.[53] The reference point for this scheme was the introitus, with prolapse to or above the introitus considered to be first degree and complete eversion as third degree (Fig. 46.2). Beecham stipulated that prolapse that was only visible at the introitus by depressing the perineum should be considered first degree, and he coined the term 'cystourethrocele' given that it was difficult to discriminate between prolapse of the urethra or of the bladder without surgery.

THE QUANTITATIVE PELVIC EXAMINATION

The most current system of evaluating POP was devised because of the frustration that clinicians felt when attempting to communicate with colleagues using existing non-standardized unvalidated systems. The quantitative POP examination system is the outcome of collaboration between several groups of international investigators and has been adopted by the International Continence Society, the American Urogynecologic Society (AUGS), and the ACOG. The final draft was published in 1996 and, unlike previous systems, has been validated with high reproducibility between and within examiners, and can also be learned and performed rapidly.[54-56]

The quantitative POP examination measures the position of midline vaginal structures in centimetres relative to the hymenal ring. The remnant of the hymenal ring is used as the reference point because it is a fixed and easily identified landmark, as opposed to the introitus which is a non-standardized anatomical structure (it is defined as 'entrance into the vagina'). The examination is performed during straining, which reproduces the patient's complaints. Structures above the hymenal ring are measured in negative centimetres; those which prolapse beyond the hymenal ring are measured in positive centimetres (Fig. 46.2). Any structure that descends to the level of the hymenal ring is measured as zero centimetres. Nine measurements are recorded during the examination, with two taken anteriorly, two apically, two posteriorly, two externally, and vaginal length (Table 46.1; Fig. 46.3a). These points are depicted diagramatically in Figure 46.3b in two profiles demonstrating a large anterior wall defect with some apical decsent (Profile A) and a large posterior defect (Profile B). Although these points may be recorded in any fashion, a convenient method using a three-by-three grid is noted in Figure 46.3. Any rigid measuring device, such as a ruler or engraved instrument may be used. A ring forceps which has been engraved in centimetre increments (e.g. 1, 2, 3, 4, 5, 7.5 and 10 cm) is convenient, in that is readily available and can be used to evaluate midline and paravaginal defects. For descriptive purposes, an ordinal staging system is used whereby the prolapse stage is defined by the structure that demonstrates the greatest degree of prolapse. As with measuring the nine reference points, the staging is defined relative to the hymenal ring (Table 46.2). An easy method of remembering this staging system is that any prolapse where the leading edge is at or between

Table 46.1. *Sites measured in the quantitative pelvic organ prolapse examination*

Point	Description
A anterior (Aa)	A point on the anterior vaginal wall 3 cm above the hymenal ring
B anterior (Ba)	Most dependent or distal point on the anterior vaginal wall segment between A anterior and point C or the cuff if subject is status post hysterectomy
C	Anterior lip of the cervix or the cuff if the subject is status post hysterectomy
A posterior (Ap)	A point on the posterior vaginal wall 3 cm above the hymenal ring
B posterior (Bp)	Most dependent or distal point on the posterior vaginal wall segment between A posterior and point D or the cuff if subject is status post hysterectomy
D	Posterior fornix (this space is left blank in the subject who is status post hysterectomy)
Genital hiatus (gh)	Middle of external urethral meatus to posterior hymenal remnant
Perineal body (pb)	Posterior hymen to middle of anal opening
Total vaginal length (tvl)	Hymenal ring to vaginal apex

From ref. 54.

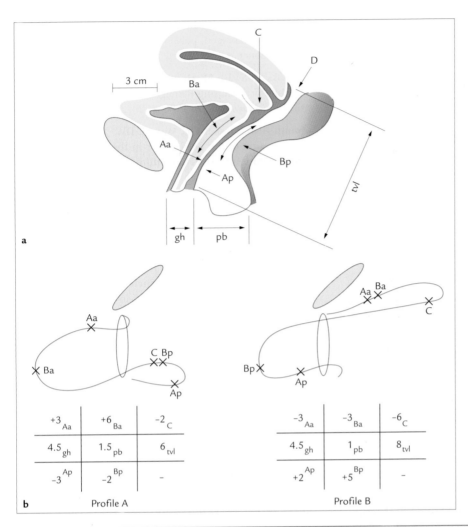

Figure 46.3. *(a) Diagrammatic representation of the nine points recorded for the pelvic organ prolapse classification system. Terms are defined in Table 46.1. (b) Profile A represents a large anterior wall defect with some apical descent; Profile B represents a large posterior defect. Note the grid system used for recording the nine points.*

Stage	Description
Table 46.2. *Staging of pelvic organ prolapse*	
0	No descensus of pelvic structures during straining
I	The leading surface of the prolapse does not descend below 1 cm above the hymenal ring
II	The leading edge of the prolapse extends from 1 cm above the hymen to 1 cm through the hymenal ring
III	The prolapse extends more than 1 cm beyond the hymenal ring, but there is not complete vaginal eversion
IV	The vagina is completely everted

From ref. 55.

1 cm above and 1 cm through the hymenal ring represents stage II; any prolapse above this is stage I, and any beyond is stage III up to complete eversion, which is stage IV.

A comparison of all the evaluation systems discussed above is represented diagrammatically in Figure 46.2, which was inspired by the paper of Friedman and Little.[48] A reproducibility comparison demonstrated that this system had a higher interobserver reproducibility than Baden's vaginal profile (κ 0.79 vs 0.68; $p<0.001$ for both).[56]

At a practical level, an efficient method of performing the examination consists of placing a bivalved speculum in the vagina and measuring apical descent, using the posterior blade of the speculum to measure anterior and then posterior structures and then measuring the perineal structures. Vaginal length is the least-reproducible measurement but can be measured by noting the distance between the end and proximal digit during bimanual examination.[55] Further information regarding the performance of the quantitative pelvic organ examination, including a videotape, is available at the AUGS website (http://www.augs.org).

One aspect of this system that may be awkward (or even anathema) to adherents of previous systems is the strict avoidance of terms such as cystocele, rectocele or enterocele. The rationale behind this seemingly dogmatic practice is to avoid erroneous assumptions regarding the prolapsing organs. It is often difficult even for experienced observers to discriminate between a high rectocele and a pulsion enterocele. Furthermore, patients who have had previous reconstructive pelvic surgery may have gross alterations in their vaginal axis that result in unusual patterns of prolapse (e.g. anterior enterocele after sacrospinous ligament suspension).

REFERENCES

1. American College of Obstetricians and Gynecologists. *Pelivic Organ Prolapse. ACOG Technical Bulletin 214.* Washington, DC: ACOG, 1995

2. Herzog AR, Fultz NH. Prevalence and incidence of urinary incontinence in community-dwelling populations. *J Am Geriatr Soc* 1990; 38: 273–281

3. Mommsen S, Lam GW, Feldspang A, Elwing LB. Descriptive epidemiology and social consequences of urinary incontinence in women age 30–59. *Neurourol Urodyn* 1990; 9: 327–328

4. Burgio KL, Matthews KA, Engel BT. Prevalence, incidence and correlates of urinary incontinence in healthy, middle-aged women. *J Urol* 1991; 146: 1255–1259

5. Rekers H, Drogendijk AC, Valkenburg H, Riphagen F. Urinary incontinence in women from 35–79 years of age; prevalence and consequences. *Eur J Obstet Gynecol Rep Med* 1992; 43: 229–234

6. Brocklehurst JC. Urinary incontinence in the community – analysis of a MORI poll. *Br Med J* 1993; 306: 832–834

7. Bump RC. Racial comparisons and contrasts in urinary incontinence and pelvic organ prolapse. *Obstet Gynecol* 1993; 81: 421–425

8. Peacock LM, Wiskind AK, Wall LL. Clinical features of urinary incontinence and urogenital prolapse in a black inner-city population. *Am J Obstet Gynecol* 1994; 171: 1464–1469

9. Mant J, Painter R, Vessey M. Epidemiology of genital prolapse: observations from the Oxford Family Planning Association study. *Br J Obstet Gynaecol* 1997; 104: 579–585

10. Olsen AL, Smith VJ, Bergstrom JO *et al.* Epidemiology of surgically managed pelvic organ prolapse and urinary incontinence. *Obstet Gynecol* 1997; 89: 501–506

11. Snooks SJ, Swash M, Henry MM, Setchell M. Risk factors in childbirth causing damage to the pelvic floor innervation. *Int J Colorectal Dis* 1986; 1: 20–24

12. Smith ARB, Hosker GL, Warrell DW. The role of partial denervation of the pelvic floor in the aaetiology of genital prolapse and stress incontinence of urine. A neurophysiological approach. *Br J Obstet Gynaecol* 1989; 96: 24–28

13. Allen RE, Hosker GL, Smith ARB, Warrell DW. Pelvic floor damage and childbirth: a neurophysiological study. *Br J Obstet Gynaecol* 1990; 97: 770–779

14. Snooks SJ, Swash M, Setchell M, Henry MM. Injury to innervation of pelvic floor sphincter musculature in childbirth. *Lancet* 1984; September 8: 546–550

15. Peschers U, Schaer G, Anthuber C *et al.* Changes in vesical neck mobility following vaginal delivery. *Obstet Gynecol* 1996; 88: 1001–1006

16. Gainey HL. Postpartum observations of pelvic tissue damage: further studies. *Am J Obstet Gynecol* 1955; 70: 800–807

17. Gilpin SA, Gosling JA, Smith ARB, Warrell DW. The pathogenesis of genitourinary prolapse and stress incontinence of urine: a histological and histochemical approach. *Br J Obstet Gynaecol* 1989; 96: 15–23

18. Smith ARB, Hosker GL, Warrell DW. The role of pudendal nerve damage in the aaetiology of genuine stress urinary incontinence. *Br J Obstet Gynaecol* 1989; 96: 29–32

19. Sultana C, Young P. Comparison of pudendal and perineal nerve terminal motor latencies in women with urinary incontinence and normal controls (Abstract). Presented at the American Urogynecologic Society 18th Annual Meeting, Tucson, Arizona, September 1997

20. Strohbehn K, Jakary JA, DeLancey JOL. Pelvic organ prolapse in young women. *Obstet Gynecol* 1997; 90: 33–36

21. Koelbl H, Strassegger H, Riaa PA, Gruber H. Morphologic and functional aspects of pelvic floor muscles in patients with pelvic organ prolapse and genuine stress incontinence. *Obstet Gynecol* 1989; 74: 789–795

22. Jackson SR, Avery NC, Tarlton JF *et al.* Changes in metabolism of collagen in genitourinary prolapse. *Lancet* 1996; 347: 1658–1661

23. Makinen J Soderstrom KO, Kiilhoma P, Hirvonen T. Histological changes in the vaginal connective tissue of patients with and without uterine prolapse. *Arch Gynecol* 1986; 239: 17–20

24. Norton P, Baker J, Sharp H, Warenski J. Genitourinary prolapse; relationship with joint mobility. *Neurourol Urodyn* 1990; 9: 321–322

25. McIntosh LJ, Stanitski DF, Mallett VT *et al.* Ehlers–Danlos syndrome: relationship between joint hypermobility, urinary incontinence, and pelvic floor prolapse. *Gynecol Obstet Invest* 1996; 41: 135–139

26. Torpin R. Prolapse uteri associated with spina bifida and clubfeet in newborn infants. *Am J Obstet Gynecol* 1942; 43: 892–894.

27. Ajbor LN, Okojie SE. Genital prolapse in the newborn. *Int Surg* 1976; 61: 496–497

28. van Dongen L. The anatomy of genital prolapse. *S Afr Med J* 1981; 60: 357–359

29. Cox PSV, Webster D. Genital prolapse amongst the Pokot. *East Afr Med J* 1975; 52: 694–699

30. Zacharin RF. 'A chinese anatomy' – the pelvic supporting tissues of the chinese and occidental female compared and contrasted. *Aust N Z J Obstet Gynaecol* 1977; 17: 1–11

31. Brieger GM, Yip SK, Hin LY, Chung TKH. The prevalence of urinary dysfunction in Hong Kong chinese women. *Obstet Gynecol* 1996; 88: 1041–1044

32. Richter K. Massive eversion of the vagina; pathogenesis, diagnosis and therapy of the 'true' prolapse of the vaginal stump. *Clin Obstet Gynecol* 1982; 25: 897–899

33. Symmonds RE, Williams TJ, Lee RA, Webb MJ. Posthysterectomy enterocele and vaginal vault prolapse. *Am J Obstet Gynecol* 1981; 140: 852–859

34. Waters EG. Vaginal prolapse: technique for prevention and correction at hysterectomy. *Obstet Gynecol* 1956; 8: 432–436

35. Phaneuf LE. Inversion of the vagina and prolapse of the cervix following supracervical hysterectomy and inversion of the vagina following total hysterectomy. *Am J Obstet Gynecol* 1952; 64: 739–743

36. Nygard IE, Thompson FL, Svengalis SL, Albright JP. Urinary incontinence in elite nulliparous athletes. *Obstet Gynecol* 1994; 84: 183–187

37. Nygard IE. Does prolonged high-impact activity contribute to later urinary incontinence? A retrospective cohortstudy of female olympians. *Obstet Gynecol* 1997; 90: 718–722

38. Davis GD, Goodman M. Stress urinary incontinence in nulliparous female soldiers in airborne infantry training. *J Pelvic Surg* 1996; 2: 68–71

39. Jorgensen S, Hein HO, Gyntelberg F. Heavy lifting at work and risk of genital prolapse and herniated disc in assistant nurses. *Occup Med* 1994; 44: 47–49

40. DeLancey JOL. Pelvic floor dysfunction: causes and prevention. *Contemp Obstet Gynecol* Jan 1993: 68–80

41. Spence-Jones C, Kamm MA, Henery MM, Hudson CN. Bowel dysfunction: a pathogenic factor in uterovaginal prolapse and urinary stress incontinence. *Br J Obstet Gynaecol* 1994; 101: 147–152

42. Snooks SJ, Barnes PRH, Swash M, Henry MM. Damage to the innervation of the pelvic floor musculature in chronic constipation. *Gastroenterology* 1985; 89: 977–981

43. Wingate L, Wingate MB, Hassanein R. The relationship between overweight and urinary incontinence in postmenopausal women: a case control study. *Menopause* 1994; 1: 199–203

44. Dwyer PL, Lee ET, Hay DM. Obesity and urinary incontinence in women. *Br J Obstet Gynaecol* 1988; 95: 91–96

45. Bump RC, Sugerman HJ, Fantl JA, McClish DK. Obesity and lower urinary tract function in women: effect of surgically induced weight loss. *Am J Obstet Gynecol* 1992; 167: 392–399

46. Dietel M, Stone E, Kassam HA *et al.* Gynecological–obstetric changes after loss of massive excess weight following bariatric surgery. *Am J Coll Nutr* 1988; 7: 145–153

47. Bump RC, McClish DK. Cigarette smoking and urinary incontinence in women. *Am J Obstet Gynecol* 1992; 167: 1213–1218

48. Friedman EA, Little WA. The conflict of nomenclature for descensus uteri. *Am J Obstet Gynecol* 1961; 81: 817–820.

49. Kelly HA. *Operative Gynecology.* New York: Appleton, 1898

50. Porges RF. A practical system of diagnosis and classification of pelvic relaxations. *Surg Gynecol Obstet* 1963; 117: 761–773

51. Baden WF, Walker TA. Genesis of the vaginal profile: a correlated classification of vaginal relaxation. *Clin Obstet Gynecol* 1972; 15: 1048–1054

52. Baden WF, Walker TA. Physical diagnosis in the evaluation of vaginal relaxation. *Clin Obstet Gynecol* 1972; 15: 1055–1069

53. Beecham CT. Classification of vaginal relaxation. *Am J Obstet Gynecol* 1980; 136: 957–958

54. Bump RC, Mattiasson A, Bø K *et al.* The standardization of terminology of female pelvic floor dysfunction. *Am J Obstet Gynecol* 1996; 175: 10–17

55. Hall AF, Theofrastous JP, Cundiff GC *et al.* Interobserver and intraobserver reliability of the proposed International Continence Society, Society of Gynecologic Surgeons, and American Urogynecologic Society Pelvic organ prolapse classification system. *Am J Obstet Gynecol* 1996; 175: 1467–1471

56. Kobak WH, Rosenberger K, Walters MD. Interobserver variation in the assessment of pelvic organ prolapse. *Int J Urogynecol Pelvic Floor Dysfunct* 1996; 7: 121–124

47

Anterior vaginal prolapse with and without genuine stress incontinence

M. D. Walters, A. M. Weber

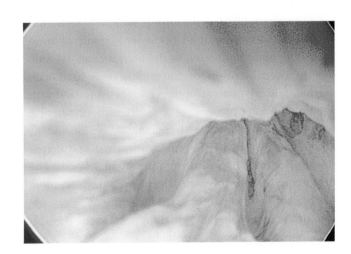

INTRODUCTION

Anterior vaginal prolapse occurs commonly, and may coexist with disorders of micturition. Mild anterior vaginal prolapse frequently occurs in parous women, but usually presents few problems. As prolapse progresses, symptoms may develop and worsen, and treatment becomes indicated. This chapter reviews the anatomy and pathology of anterior vaginal prolapse, with and without genuine stress incontinence (GSI), and describes methods of vaginal repair.

ANATOMY AND PATHOLOGY OF ANTERIOR VAGINAL PROLAPSE

Anterior vaginal prolapse ('cystocele') is defined as pathological descent of the anterior vaginal wall and bladder base. According to the International Continence Society standardized terminology for prolapse grading, the term anterior vaginal prolapse is preferred to 'cystocele,' as information obtained at physical examination does not allow the exact identification of structures behind the vaginal wall.[1] (See chapter 46.)

The aetiology of anterior vaginal prolapse is not completely understood but is probably multifactorial, with different factors implicated in individual patients. Normal support for the vagina and adjacent pelvic organs is provided by interaction between pelvic muscles and connective tissue.[2] The upper vagina rests on the levator plate and is stabilized by superior and lateral connective tissue attachments; the mid-vagina is attached to the arcus tendineus fasciae pelvis (ATFP; 'white line') on each side.[3] Pathological loss of support may occur with damage to the pelvic muscles, connective tissue attachments, or both.

Nichols and Randall described two types of anterior vaginal prolapse – distension and displacement.[4] Distension was thought to occur as a result of overstretching and attenuation of the anterior vaginal wall, due to overdistension of the vagina associated with vaginal delivery or to atrophic changes associated with ageing and menopause. The distinguishing physical feature of this type was described as diminished or absent rugal folds of the anterior vaginal epithelium due to thinning or loss of midline vaginal fascia. The other type of anterior vaginal prolapse – displacement – was attributed to pathological detachment or elongation of the anterolateral vaginal supports to the ATFP. It may occur unilaterally or bilaterally and frequently

coexists with some degree of distension cystocele and with urethral hypermobility. Rugal folds may or may not be preserved.

Another theory attributes most cases of anterior vaginal prolapse to disruption or detachment of the lateral connective tissue attachments at the ATFP, resulting in a paravaginal defect and corresponding to the displacement type discussed above. This was first described by White in 1909[5] and 1912,[6] but was disregarded until reported by Richardson *et al.* in 1976.[7] Richardson also described transverse defects, midline defects and defects involving isolated loss of integrity of 'pubourethral ligaments.' Transverse defects were said to occur when the 'pubocervical fascia' separated from its insertion around the cervix, whereas midline defects represented an anteroposterior separation of the 'fascia' between the bladder and vagina.

There has never been a systematic or comprehensive description of anterior vaginal prolapse based on physical findings and correlated with findings at surgery, to provide objective evidence for any of these theories of pathological anatomy. However, recent improvements in pelvic imaging may lead to a greater understanding of normal pelvic anatomy and the abnormalities associated with prolapse. Magnetic resonance imaging (MRI) holds great promise with its excellent ability to differentiate soft tissues and its capacity for multiplanar imaging. Further work is needed to correlate the different images with anatomy and histology under normal conditions and under conditions of pelvic organ prolapse. The main limitation for imaging related to prolapse has been the inability to image patients in the standing position, to evaluate for the effects of gravity and increased intra-abdominal pressure; eventually, this limitation will be overcome.

The pelvic organs, pelvic muscles and connective tissues can be identified easily with MRI. Various measurements can be made that may be associated with anterior vaginal prolapse or urinary incontinence, such as the urethrovesical angle, bladder-base descent and the relationship between the vagina and its lateral connective tissue attachments. Aronson *et al.* used an endoluminal surface coil placed in the vagina to image pelvic anatomy with MRI, and compared four continent nulliparous women with four incontinent women with anterior vaginal prolapse.[8] Lateral vaginal attachments were identified in all continent women. In Figure 47.1, the 'posterior pubourethral ligaments' (bilateral

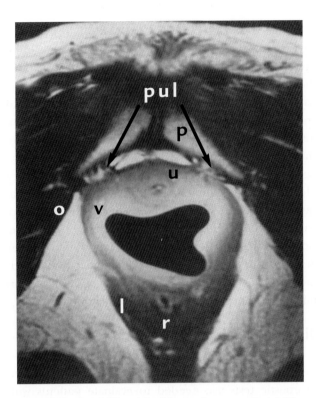

Figure 47.1. *Axial T1-weighted image from a continent 38-year-old nulliparous woman, showing the connection of the anterior vaginal wall (v) to the posterior pubic symphysis (p) by the 'pubourethral ligaments' (pul). The anterior vaginal wall and endopelvic fascia function as a sling or hammock for support of the urethra (u). o, Obturator internus muscle; r, rectum; l, levator ani musculature. (From ref. 8. with permission.)*

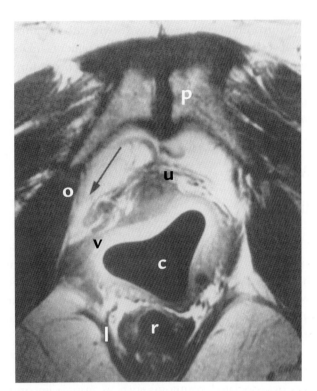

Figure 47.2. *Axial T1-weighted image from a 57-year-old woman, para 5, with genuine stress urinary incontinence. The paravaginal detachment (arrow) is seen at the level of the urethrovesical junction. v, anterior vaginal wall; p, posterior pubic symphysis; u, urethra; o, obturator internus muscle; c, endovaginal coil; r, rectum; l, levator ani musculature. (From ref. 8. with permission.)*

attachment of the ATFP to the posterior aspect of the pubic symphyses) are clearly seen. In the two subjects with clinically apparent paravaginal defects, lateral detachments were evident (Fig. 47.2). Although this study involved only a small number of subjects, it provides the basis for further work in describing anatomical abnormalities that accompany anterior vaginal prolapse and other disorders of pelvic support. This may ultimately guide the choice of surgical repair.

Anterior vaginal prolapse commonly coexists with GSI. Some features of pathophysiology may overlap, such as loss of anterior vaginal support with bladder-base descent and urethral hypermobility; other features, such as sphincteric dysfunction, may occur independent of vaginal and urethral support. The pathophysiology of GSI is covered more fully in chapter 8.

At one time, suburethral (Kelly) plication was the mainstay of surgical treatment for GSI. First described by Kelly and Dumm in 1914, anterior colporrhaphy with suburethral plication corrected anterior vaginal prolapse (distension type of cystocele) while stabilizing the suburethral fascia to prevent urethral descent.[9] The Kelly–Kennedy modification, described by Kennedy in 1937,[10] involved dissection of the urethra from the vaginal wall with plication of the injured sphincter muscle at the urethrovesical junction, to provide preferential support to the proximal urethra and bladder neck and to create posterior urethral angulation compared with the bladder base. Because failure rates are higher with this procedure than with retropubic procedures,[11,12] suburethral plication is, generally, not currently used as a first-line surgical treatment for GSI. Nevertheless, it is a useful procedure in selected clinical situations such as stress incontinence, usually coexistent with advanced prolapse, in elderly or medically fragile patients unable to undergo extensive or lengthy abdominal procedures. If significant stress incontinence persists or develops postoperatively, bulking agents such as collagen injection can be used.

EVALUATION

History

When evaluating women with pelvic organ prolapse and urinary and/or faecal incontinence, attention should be paid to all aspects of pelvic support. The reconstructive surgeon must determine the specific sites of damage for each patient, with the ultimate goal of restoring both anatomy and function.

Patients with anterior vaginal prolapse may complain of either symptoms directly related to vaginal protrusion or associated symptoms such as urinary incontinence or voiding difficulty. Symptoms related to prolapse may include the sensation of a vaginal mass or bulge, pelvic pressure, low back pain and sexual difficulty. Stress urinary incontinence commonly occurs in association with anterior vaginal prolapse. Voiding difficulty may result from advanced prolapse. Women may require vaginal pressure or manual replacement of the prolapse in order to accomplish voiding. They may relate a history of previous urinary incontinence that has since resolved with worsening of their prolapse. This can occur with urethral kinking and obstruction to urinary flow; women in this situation are at risk for incomplete bladder emptying, and recurrent or persistent urinary tract infections.

Physical examination

The physical examination should be conducted with the patient in the lithotomy position, as for a routine pelvic examination. The examination is first performed with the patient supine. If physical findings do not correspond to symptoms, or if the maximum extent of the prolapse cannot be confirmed, the woman is re-examined in the standing position.

The genitalia are inspected and, if no displacement is apparent, the labia are gently spread to expose the vestibule and hymen. The integrity of the perineal body is evaluated and the approximate size of all prolapsed parts is assessed. A retractor or Sims' speculum can be used to depress the posterior vagina to aid in visualizing the anterior vagina. After the resting examination, the patient is instructed to strain down forcefully or to cough vigorously. During this manoeuvre, the order of descent of the pelvic organs is noted, as is the relationship of the pelvic organs at the peak of straining. It may be possible to differentiate between 'lateral' defects, identified as detachment or effacement of the lateral vaginal sulci, and 'central' defects, seen as midline protrusion but with preservation of the lateral sulci. Anterior vaginal wall descent usually represents bladder descent with or without concomitant urethral hypermobility. Less commonly, an anterior enterocele can mimic a 'cystocele' on physical examination.

Diagnostic tests

After a careful history and physical examination, few diagnostic tests are needed to evaluate patients with anterior vaginal prolapse further. Urinalysis for urinary tract infection should be performed if the patient complains of any lower urinary tract dysfunction. If the patient's oestrogen status is unclear, a vaginal cytological smear can be obtained to assess maturation index. Hydronephrosis occurs in a small proportion of women with prolapse; however, even if identified, it does not alter the management in women for whom surgical repair is planned;[13] routine imaging of the kidneys and ureters is, therefore, unnecessary.

If urinary incontinence is present, further diagnostic testing is indicated to determine the cause of the incontinence. Urodynamics (simple or complex), endoscopy, or radiological assessment of filling and voiding function are generally indicated only when symptoms of incontinence or voiding dysfunction are present.[14,15] Even if no urological symptoms are noted, voiding function should be assessed to evaluate for completeness of bladder emptying. This usually involves a timed, measured void, followed by urethral catheterization or ultrasonography to measure residual urine volume.

In women with severe prolapse, it is important to check urethral function after the prolapse is repositioned. As demonstrated by Bump *et al.*,[16] women with severe prolapse may be continent owing to urethral obstruction; when the prolapse is reduced, urethral dysfunction may be unmasked, with occurrence of incontinence.[16] A pessary or vaginal packing can be used to reduce the prolapse before office bladder filling or electronic urodynamic testing.[17] If urinary leaking occurs with coughing or Valsalva manoeuvre after reduction of the prolapse, the urethral sphincter is probably incompetent, even if the patient is normally continent. In this situation, the surgeon can choose an anti-incontinence procedure in conjunction with anterior vaginal prolapse repair. If sphincteric incompetence is not present even after reduction with a pessary, a specific anti-incontinence procedure is not indicated, although the urethra and bladder neck should be supported as part of the anterior vaginal prolapse repair.

SURGICAL REPAIR TECHNIQUES

Anterior colporrhaphy with suburethral plication

The objective of anterior colporrhaphy is to plicate the layers of vaginal muscularis and adventitia overlying the bladder ('pubocervical fascia') or to plicate the paravaginal tissue in such a way as to reduce protrusion of the bladder and vagina.[18] In most cases, regardless of whether the patient suffers from urinary incontinence, plicating sutures at the urethrovesical junction should be placed to augment posterior urethral support and to ensure that stress incontinence, if not present at the time of operation, does not develop postoperatively.[19,20] Modifications of the basic technique depend on how lateral the dissection is carried, where the plicating sutures are placed and whether additional layers (natural or synthetic) are placed in the anterior vagina for extra support.

The operative procedure begins with the patient supine, with the legs elevated and abducted and the buttocks placed just past the edge of the operating table. The chosen anaesthetic has been administered, and one perioperative intravenous dose of an appropriate antibiotic may be given as prophylaxis against infection. The vagina and perineum are sterilely 'prepped' and draped, and a 16F Foley catheter with a 5 ml balloon is inserted for easy identification of the bladder neck. If indicated, a suprapubic catheter is placed into the bladder.

A weighted speculum is placed in the vagina. If a vaginal hysterectomy has been performed, the incised apex of the anterior vaginal wall is grasped transversely with two Allis clamps and elevated; otherwise, a transverse incision is made in the vaginal mucosa near the apex. A third Allis clamp is placed about 1 cm below the posterior margin of the urethral meatus and pulled up. Additional Allis clamps may be placed in the midline between the urethra and apex. Haemostatic solutions (such as 0.5% lignocaine with 1: 200,000 adrenaline) or saline may be injected submucosally, along the midline of the anterior vaginal wall, to decrease bleeding and to aid in dissection. The points of a pair of curved Mayo scissors are inserted between the vaginal epithelium and the vaginal muscularis, or between layers of the vaginal muscularis, and gently forced upward while partially opening and closing the scissors. Countertraction during this manoeuvre is important to minimize the likelihood of bladder perforation. The vagina is then incised in the midline, starting at the apex and continuing to the level of the midurethra. As the vagina is incised, the edges are grasped with Allis or T-clamps and drawn laterally for further mobilization. Dissection of the vaginal flaps is then accomplished by turning the clamps back across the forefinger and incising the vaginal muscularis with a scalpel or Metzenbaum scissors, as shown in Figure 47.3. An assistant maintains constant traction medially on the remaining vaginal muscularis and underlying vesicovaginal adventitia and bladder.

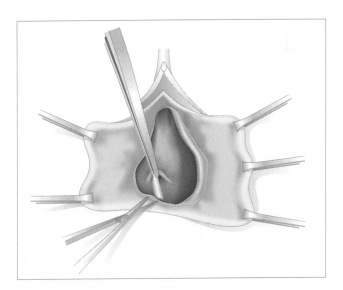

Figure 47.3. *Sharp dissection is used to mobilize the bladder base and overlying vaginal muscularis from the vaginal apex during anterior colporrhaphy.*

This procedure is performed bilaterally until the entire extent of the anterior vaginal prolapse has been dissected; in general, the dissection should be carried further laterally with more advanced prolapse. The spaces lateral to the urethrovesical junction are sharply dissected toward the inferior pubic rami.

Once the vaginal flaps have been completely developed, the urethrovesical junction can be identified visually or by pulling the Foley catheter downwards until the bulb obstructs the vesical neck. Repair should begin at the urethrovesical junction, using a No. 2-0 or 0 delayed absorbable suture. The first plicating stitch is placed into the periurethral endopelvic fascia at the urethrovesical junction on one side and then on the other side (Fig. 47.4a, b). One or two additional stitches are placed to support the length of the urethra and urethrovesical junction. When these sutures are tied, tissue pulled to the midline creates a suburethral shelf that creates or augments posterior urethral support.

After the stitches for vesical neck plication have been placed and tied, attention is turned to the anterior vaginal prolapse repair. In standard anterior colporrhaphy, stitches using No. 2-0 or 0 delayed absorbable sutures are placed in the vaginal tissue (muscularis and adventitia) medial to the vaginal flaps and plicated in the midline without tension. Depending on the severity of the prolapse, one or two rows of plication sutures or a purse-string suture followed by plication sutures are placed (Fig. 47.4c, d). The vaginal epithelium is then trimmed from the flaps bilaterally and the remaining anterior vaginal wall is closed with a running No. 3-0 subcuticular or locking suture.

One modification of the standard repair is to extend the dissection and mobilization of the vaginal flaps laterally to the descending pubic rami on each side. After the vesical neck plication has been performed, stitches are placed laterally in the paravaginal tissue (lateral to the vaginal muscularis and adventitial layers, but not including the epithelium of the vaginal flaps). The paravaginal connective tissue is plicated in the midline under tension using No. 0 delayed absorbable or permanent suture. This produces a firm bridge of tissue across

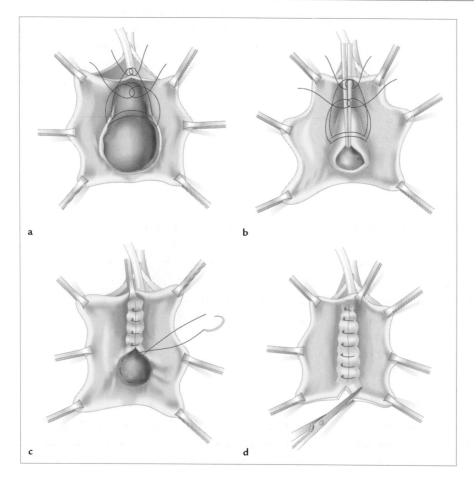

a　　　　　　　　　　　b

c　　　　　　　　　　　d

Figure 47.4. *Technique of anterior colporrhaphy: (a) after dissection of vaginal wall from the bladder and urethra, one to three plication sutures are placed in the periurethral endopelvic fascia at the urethrovesical junction; (b) the plication sutures at the vesical neck are tied; (c) a purse-string suture can be placed in the vaginal muscularis to reduce large cystoceles; (d) the entire cystocele has been repaired with plication sutures and the vaginal epithelium is trimmed before closure.*

the anterior vaginal space, but it also results in narrowing of the anterior vagina, which must be considered when planning concomitant posterior colporrhaphy. The vaginal flaps are trimmed and closed as usual.

Another modification involves the use of an additional layer of support in the anterior vagina. After the plication sutures have been placed and tied, this layer is placed over the stitches and anchored in place at the lateral limit of the previous dissection, using interrupted stitches of No. 3-0 absorbable or permanent suture. Natural materials that have been used include resected segments of vaginal wall,[21] rectus or cadaveric fascia. Permanent or absorbable mesh may be used, although permanent material carries a risk of infection or erosion with need for subsequent removal.[22]

Anti-incontinence operations are frequently performed at the same time as anterior vaginal prolapse repair. Urethral suspension procedures (sling procedures, needle or retropubic urethropexies) may effectively treat mild anterior vaginal prolapse associated with urethral hypermobility. More advanced anterior vaginal prolapse will not be treated adequately and in these cases anterior colporrhaphy should be performed as well. Surgical judgement is required to perform the plication tightly enough to reduce the anterior vaginal prolapse sufficiently, yet preserve enough mobility of the anterior vagina to allow for adequate urethral suspension. If anterior colporrhaphy is combined with a sling procedure, the cystocele should be repaired before the sling sutures are tied.

Vaginal paravaginal defect repair

The objective of paravaginal defect repair for anterior vaginal prolapse is to reattach the detached lateral vagina to its normal place of attachment at the level of the ATFP.[23] This can be accomplished using a vaginal or retropubic approach. Retropubic paravaginal defect repair is discussed in chapter 40, together with other retropubic procedures such as Burch colposuspension.

The preparation for vaginal paravaginal defect repair begins as for an anterior colporrhaphy. Marking sutures are placed on the anterior vaginal wall on each side of the urethrovesical junction, identified by the location of the Foley balloon after placing gentle traction on the catheter (Fig. 47.5a). In patients who have undergone hysterectomy, marking sutures are also placed at the vaginal apex. If a cul-de-plasty is being performed, the stitches are placed but not tied until the completion of the paravaginal repair and closure of the anterior vaginal wall. As for anterior colporrhaphy, vaginal flaps are developed by incising the vagina in the midline and dissecting the vaginal muscularis laterally. The dissection is performed bilaterally until a space is developed between the vaginal wall and retropubic space. Blunt dissection using the surgeon's index finger is used to extend the space anteriorly along the inferior pubic rami, medially to the pubic symphysis, and laterally toward the ischial spine. If a paravaginal defect is present and dissection is occurring in the appropriate plane, the retropubic space should be entered easily, so that retropubic adipose tissue can be seen. The ischial spine can then be palpated on each side. The ATFP can be followed from the ischial spine to the back of the symphysis pubis (Fig. 47.5b). Once dissection is complete, midline plication of vaginal muscularis can be performed, either at this point or after placement and tying of the paravaginal sutures.

On the lateral pelvic sidewall, the obturator internus muscle and the ATFP are identified by palpation and then visualization. Retraction of the bladder and urethra medially is best accomplished with a Briesky–Navratil retractor, and posterior retraction is provided with a lighted right-angle retractor. Using a No. 0 permanent suture, the first stitch is placed around the tissue of the white line just anterior to the ischial spine. If the white line is detached from the pelvic sidewall or is not felt to be durable clinically, then the stitch should be placed in the fascia overlying the obturator internus muscle. The placement of subsequent sutures is facilitated by putting tension on the first suture. A series of four to six stitches is placed and held, working anteriorly along the white line from the ischial spine to the level of the urethrovesical junction (Fig. 47.5c). Starting with the most anterior stitch, the surgeon picks up the edge of the periurethral tissue (vaginal muscularis or pubocervical fascia) at the level of the urethrovesical junction and then tissue from the undersurface of the vaginal flap at the previously marked sites. Subsequent stitches move posteriorly until the last stitch closest to the ischial spine is attached to the vagina nearest the apex, again using the previously placed marking sutures for guidance. Stitches in the vaginal wall must be carefully placed to allow adequate tissue for subsequent midline vaginal closure. After all stitches are placed on one

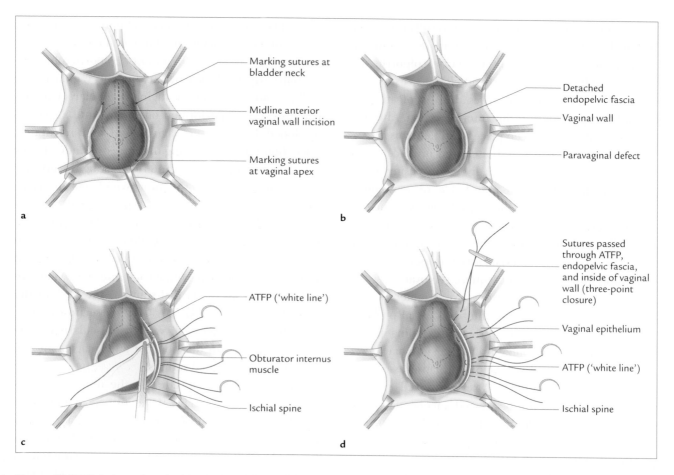

Figure 47.5. *Technique of vaginal paravaginal defect repair. (a) The vagina is opened through a midline incision. Marking sutures are placed at the bladder neck and vaginal apex to ensure correct suture placement on vaginal epithelium. (b) The opened vagina reveals bilateral paravaginal defects. Note the detached endopelvic fascia on the lateral edge of the bladder. (c) Access to the arcus tendineus fasciae pelvis (ATFP) or 'white line' is obtained by retracting the bladder medially. Permanent sutures are passed through the ATFP or fascia over the obturator internus muscle. Four or five sutures are placed, starting at the ischial spine. Tension on sutures facilitates placement of subsequent sutures. (d) Each suture is passed through the ATFP, detached endopelvic fascia and the inside of the vaginal epithelium, forming the three-point closure. Once they have been placed on both sides (if indicated), they are individually tied by alternating right and left sides.*

side, the same procedure is carried out on the other side. The stitches are then tied in order from the urethra to the apex, alternating from one side to the other. This repair is a three-point closure involving the vaginal epithelium, vaginal muscularis and endopelvic fascia ('pubocervical fascia'), and lateral pelvic sidewall at the level of the ATFP (Fig. 47.5d). There must be tissue-to-tissue approximation between these structures. Suture 'bridges' must be avoided by careful planning of suture placement. Vaginal tissue should not be trimmed until all the stitches are tied. As previously stated, vaginal muscularis can then be plicated in the midline (if this

has not already been done) with several interrupted stitches using No. 0 delayed absorbable suture. The vaginal flaps are trimmed and closed with a running subcuticular or interlocking delayed absorbable suture.

Complications

Intra-operative complications are relatively uncommon with anterior vaginal prolapse repair. Excessive blood loss may occur, requiring blood transfusion(s), or a haematoma may develop in the anterior vagina. The lumen of the bladder or urethra may be entered in the course of dissection. Accidental cystotomy should be repaired in layers at the time of the injury. After repair of cystotomy, the bladder is generally drained for 7–14 days to allow for adequate healing. Other rare complications include ureteral damage, intravesical or urethral suture placement (and associated urological problems), and fistula – either urethrovaginal or vesicovaginal. If permanent sutures or mesh material are used in the repair, erosion, draining sinuses or chronic areas of vaginal granulation tissue can result. The actual incidence of these complications is unknown. Urinary tract infections occur commonly but other infections such as pelvic or vaginal abscesses are less common.

Voiding difficulty can occur after anterior vaginal prolapse repair. This problem may occur more frequently in women with subclinical preoperative voiding dysfunction. Treatment is bladder drainage or intermittent self-catheterization until spontaneous voiding resumes, usually within 6 weeks.

Sexual function may be positively or negatively affected by vaginal operations for anterior vaginal prolapse. Haase and Skibsted studied 55 sexually active women who underwent a variety of operations for stress incontinence or genital prolapse.[24] Postoperatively, 24% of the patients experienced improvement in their sexual satisfaction, 67% experienced no change, and 9% experienced deterioration. Improvement often resulted from cessation of urinary incontinence; deterioration was always due to dyspareunia after posterior colporrhaphy. These authors concluded that the prognosis for an improved sex life is good after surgery for stress incontinence, but that posterior colpoperineorrhaphy causes dyspareunia in some patients.

RESULTS

The main indication for surgical repair of anterior vaginal prolapse is to relieve symptoms when they exist, or as part of a comprehensive pelvic reconstructive procedure for multiple sites of pelvic organ prolapse, with or without urinary incontinence. Anterior colporrhaphy with vesical neck plication may also be effective for treatment of mild stress incontinence associated with urethral hypermobility.

Few studies have addressed the long-term success of surgical treatments for anterior vaginal prolapse. All published studies are uncontrolled series. Definitions of recurrence vary and sometimes are not stated, and loss to follow-up often is not stated. In our review of surgical techniques for the correction of anterior vaginal prolapse, reported failure rates ranged from 0% to 20% for anterior colporrhaphy and from 3% to 14% for paravaginal defect repair.[2] No controlled studies have compared different procedures performed primarily for anterior vaginal wall prolapse.

Women with advanced anterior vaginal prolapse, with or without stress incontinence, frequently have other abnormal bladder symptoms such as urgency, urge incontinence and voiding difficulty. In a study by Gardy et al.,[20] of surgical repair of large cystoceles, stress incontinence resolved in 94%, urge incontinence in 87%, and significant residual urine (more than 80 ml) in 92% of patients 3 months after needle-suspension procedures and anterior colporrhaphy. Approximately 5% of patients developed recurrent anterior vaginal prolapse and 8% developed recurrent enterocele after an average of 2 years' follow-up.

Risk factors for failure of anterior vaginal prolapse repair have not been specifically studied. Vaginal prolapse recurs with increasing age, but the actual frequency is unknown. Recurrence may represent a failure to identify and repair all support defects, or weakening, stretching or breaking of patients' tissues, as occurs with advancing age and after menopause. Sacrospinous ligament suspension of the vaginal apex, with exaggerated retrosuspension of the vagina, may predispose patients to recurrence of anterior vaginal prolapse. Other characteristics that may increase the chance of recurrence are genetic predisposition, constipation, subsequent pregnancy, heavy lifting, chronic pulmonary disease, smoking, obesity and absence of oestrogen replacement after menopause.

The literature varies markedly in the reported success of suburethral plication for GSI, from 34% to 91%.[12,25] The extent of preoperative evaluation including diagnostic assessment of incontinence is often poorly described in reports on suburethral plication. In addition, length of follow-up and outcome measures (subjective vs objective) are often highly variable and inconsistent, even within individual studies. In many reports, the main indication for anterior colporrhaphy with suburethral plication is anterior vaginal prolapse repair; the effects on GSI are often incidental and poorly documented.

In a review of 11 studies on anterior repair for GSI, 957 patients had an overall 'cure' rate of 65% (range 31–91%) and a 'cure or improvement' rate of 74% (range 31–98%); the complication rate averaged 14%.[25] The variation in reported success rates may be due to different surgical techniques, including the extent of endopelvic fascial dissection, location and depth of stitch placement, and use of permanent versus absorbable suture. It probably also relates to differences in patient populations and selection bias in study design. As very few studies have used random assignment to treatment, patients undergoing suburethral plication probably differ from patients having retropubic procedures or suburethral slings for incontinence. The poor long-term results of suburethral plication may be explained in part by the nature of periurethral endopelvic fascia that lacks the durability required to adequately support the bladder neck over time. Because of these poor long-term results, in most cases suburethral plication is no longer recommended for surgical correction of GSI.

REFERENCES

1. Bump RC, Mattiasson A, Bø K *et al.* The standardization of terminology of female pelvic organ prolapse and pelvic floor dysfunction. *Am J Obstet Gynecol* 1996; 175: 10–17

2. Weber AM, Walters MD. Anterior vaginal prolapse: review of anatomy and techniques of surgical repair. *Obstet Gynecol* 1997; 89: 311–318

3. DeLancey JOL. Anatomic aspects of vaginal eversion after hysterectomy. *Am J Obstet Gynecol* 1992; 166: 1717–1728

4. Nichols DH, Randall CL (eds). *Vaginal Surgery*, 4th edn. Baltimore: Williams and Wilkins, 1996

5. White GR. A radical cure by suturing lateral sulci of vagina to white line of pelvic fascia. *J Am Med Assoc* 1909; 21: 1707–1710

6. White GR. An anatomical operation for the cure of cystocele. *Am J Obstet Dis Women Child* 1912; 65: 286–290

7. Richardson AC, Lyon JB, Williams NL. A new look at pelvic relaxation. *Am J Obstet Gynecol* 1976; 126: 568–573

8. Aronson MP, Bates SM, Jacoby AF *et al.* Periurethral and paravaginal anatomy: an endovaginal magnetic resonance imaging study. *Am J Obstet Gynecol* 1995; 173: 1702–1710

9. Kelly HA, Dumm WM. Urinary incontinence in women, without manifest injury to the bladder. *Surg Gynecol Obstet* 1914; 18: 444–450

10. Kennedy WT. Incontinence of urine in the female, the urethral sphincter mechanism, damage of function and restoration of control. *Am J Obstet Gynecol* 1937; 34: 576–584

11. Fantl JA, Newman DK, Colling J *et al. Urinary Incontinence in Adults: Acute and Chronic Management. Clinical Practice Guideline, No. 2, 1996 Update.* AHCPR Publication No. 96–0682. Rockville, MD: Agency for Health Care Policy and Research, Public Health Service, U.S. Department of Health and Human Services. March 1996

12. Leach GE, Dmochowski RR, Appell RA *et al.* Female Stress Urinary Incontinence Clinical Guidelines Panel summary report on surgical management of female stress urinary incontinence. *J Urol* 1997; 158: 875–880

13. Beverly CJ, Walters MD, Weber AM *et al.* Prevalence of hydronephrosis in women undergoing surgery for pelvic organ prolapse. *Obstet Gynecol* 1997; 90: 37–41

14. Richardson DA, Bent AE, Ostergard DR. The effect of uterovaginal prolapse on urethrovesical pressure dynamics. *Am J Obstet Gynecol* 1983; 146: 901–905

15. deGregorio G, Hillemanns HG. Urethral closure function in women with prolapse. *Int Urogynecol J* 1990; 1: 143–145

16. Bump RC, Fantl JA, Hurt WG. The mechanism of urinary continence in women with severe uterovaginal prolapse: results of barrier studies. *Obstet Gynecol* 1988; 72: 291–295

17. Bhatia NN, Bergman A. Pessary test in women with urinary incontinence. *Obstet Gynecol* 1985; 65: 220–226

18. Stanton SL, Norton C, Cardozo L. Clinical and urodynamic effects of anterior colporrhaphy and vaginal hysterectomy for prolapse with and without incontinence. *Br J Obstet Gynaecol* 1982; 89: 459–463

19. Beck RP, McCormick S. Treatment of urinary stress incontinence with anterior colporrhaphy. *Obstet Gynecol* 1982; 59: 269–274

20. Gardy M, Kozminski M, DeLancey JOL *et al.* Stress incontinence and cystoceles. *J Urol* 1991; 145: 1211–1213

21. Zacharin RF. Free full-thickness vaginal epithelium graft in correction of recurrent genital prolapse. *Aust N Z J Obstet Gynaecol* 1992; 32: 146–148

22. Julian TM. The efficacy of Marlex mesh in the repair of severe, recurrent vaginal prolapse of the anterior mid-vaginal wall. *Am J Obstet Gynecol* 1996; 175: 1472–1475

23. Shull BL, Benn SJ, Kuehl TJ. Surgical management of prolapse of the anterior vaginal segment: an analysis of support defects, operative morbidity, and anatomic outcome. *Am J Obstet Gynecol* 1994; 171: 1429–1439

24. Haase P, Skibsted L. Influence of operations for stress incontinence and/or genital descensus on sexual life. *Acta Obstet Gynecol Scand* 1988; 67: 659–661

25. Kohli N, Karram MM. Surgery for genuine stress incontinence: vaginal procedures, injections, and the artifical urinary sphincter. In: Walters MD, Karram MM (eds) *Urogynecology and Reconstructive Pelvic Surgery*, 2nd edn. St Louis: Mosby, 1999; 171–196

48

Enterocele

N. Kohli

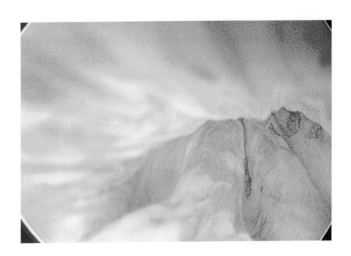

INTRODUCTION

Pelvic organ prolapse is a major healthcare problem, accounting for more than 500,000 gynaecological operations performed annually in the USA alone. Of all the different types of prolapse, the enterocele continues to perplex and challenge the gynaecological surgeon the most, partly owing to our poor understanding of its anatomy as well as difficulty in its diagnosis. First described by Garengeot in 1736,[1] the enterocele has previously been referred to as posterior vaginal hernia, primary and secondary enterocele, cul-de-sac hernia, pouch of Douglas hernia, and rectovaginal hernia, further reinforcing our poor understanding of its anatomy.[2] As late as 1932, enterocele was considered a rare clinical entity and Bueerman noted only 86 recorded cases.[1] Since then, developing knowledge regarding enterocele anatomy and diagnosis has led to increased experience but there are still few large series reported.

The actual incidence of enterocele is difficult to determine, as most women present with a combination of pelvic support defects, and the diagnosis of enterocele can often be difficult. Previous investigators have reported a range from 0.1 to 16% of women undergoing gynaecological surgical procedures.[3-5] The incidence of enterocele following bladder-neck suspension or colposuspension has been reported to be between 3 and 17%.[6-8] It has also been associated with colorectal dysfunction, with enteroceles found in 19% of patients with defecation disorders.[9] Risk factors include advanced age, increased parity, menopause and obesity.[2] Enteroceles are more common in women who previously have undergone hysterectomy, with equal frequency whether the procedure was performed abdominally or vaginally.[10] Some have postulated that this association may be due to poor vault support or failure to reapproximate the anterior and posterior fascial planes at the time of hysterectomy; thus, an enterocele may have an iatrogenic aetiology in many cases. A thorough understanding of the anatomy, pathophysiology and surgical principles of the enterocele are critical in developing strategies to treat and prevent this condition.

ANATOMY

An enterocele has classically been defined as a herniation of the small intestine into the vagina. In contrast to the sliding hernias present in cystoceles or rectoceles, an enterocele is a true hernia with a sac, a neck and contents. According to Kinzel,[2] the neck of the sac is usually located between the uterosacral ligaments in front of the sacrum and behind the cervix, if it is present. The enterocele hernia slips through the endopelvic fascia and down the posterior fornix, presenting as a bulge in the posterior vaginal wall proximally or, in extreme cases, in the lower vagina or even at the perineal body (Fig. 48.1). An anterior enterocele, a rare entity, occurs when the enterocele sac dissects between the bladder and the uterus.[2]

In his review of the functional anatomy of the pelvic floor in relation to pulsion enterocele, Zacharin[12] hypothesized that the development of an enterocele was related to anatomical abnormalities in

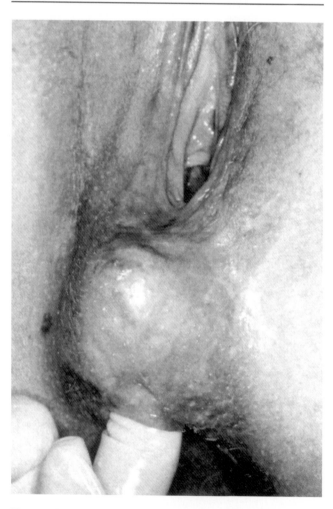

Figure 48.1 *Posterior enterocele along the posterior vaginal wall and extending to the perineal body. (From ref. 11, with permission.)*

the recto-uterine pouch associated with the upper third of the posterior vaginal and anterior rectal walls. These abnormalities include weakness of both the pelvic floor musculature and fascial supports.[12] Nichols *et al.*[13] demonstrated that the normal axis of the upper vagina is nearly horizontal in the standing position, lying on the rectum which, in turn, lies on and is parallel to the levator plate, a fusion of the muscles of the pelvic diaphragm posterior to the rectum. Berglas and Rubin[14] further correlated the degree of inclination of the levator plate with the tendency toward uterovaginal prolapse, concluding that a 'sagging' levator plate results in an increase in the levator hiatus and subsequent propensity to develop pelvic prolapse including enterocele. Although the pelvic organs are supported from below by the levator ani muscle complex in a 'trampoline' fashion, support and strength from the endopelvic fascia and its components is equally important in preventing the development of pelvic hernias.

The endopelvic fascia is composed of parietal and visceral components (Fig. 48.2). As described by Harrison and McDonagh,[15] the parietal endopelvic fascia covers the pelvic surfaces of the muscles lining the pelvic cavity, including the internal obturator, piriformis and levator ani. The visceral endopelvic fascia leaves the lateral pelvic wall where it is inserted along the white line of the pelvic fascia. At this point it is continuous with the

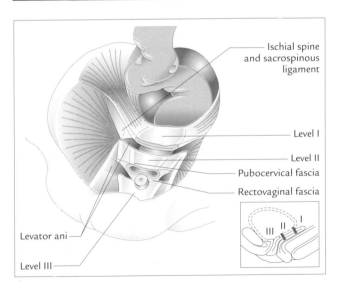

Figure 48.2 *The parietal and visceral components of the endopelvic fascia support the upper and mid vagina through suspension (I) and attachment (II).*

parietal portion of the endopelvic fascia. It stretches medially as a broad sheet of aponeurotic fibrous tissue that splits into three layers to envelop the visceral contents of the pelvis – the bladder, the vagina and cervix and the rectum. The ventral layer ensheathes the bladder, the dorsal layer ensheathes the rectum, and the median layer envelops the vagina, its cranial part being fused centrally to the cervix and laterally to the cardinal ligaments of the uterus.[15] These anatomical relationships have been confirmed by cadaveric dissections performed by Curtis *et al.*[16]

The posterior layer of the fascial sheet encircling the vagina and its lateral extension to the pelvic walls is continuous with the cardinal ligament.[17] The upper posterior vaginal fascia is frequently traumatized during parturition, and this defect may lead to development of an enterocele. The peritoneum of the cul-de-sac normally extends to a point approximately 3 cm caudal to the posterior cervical vaginal junction. Here, it lies between the fascial layers of the vaginal and rectal walls and is bordered laterally by the uterosacral ligaments as they course along the pelvic sidewalls and attach to the sacral promontory at S3–S4 on each side of the rectum.[18] As these fascial boundaries tear and weaken, extension of the cul-de-sac along the posterior vaginal segment results in enterocele formation. Conditions that either alter the integrity or weaken the support of these fascial and muscular structures predispose to enterocele.

Contrary to the traditional belief that enteroceles result from a generalized attenuation or stretching of the fascial supports and extension of the cul-de-sac into the posterior vaginal segment, Richardson's observations implicate site-specific fascial defects in the aetiology of pelvic prolapse resulting in a different description of the anatomical basis of an enterocele.[11] Richardson postulates that an apical enterocele results from a defect in the integrity of the endopelvic fascia at the vaginal apex; he defines an enterocele as a fascial hernia where peritoneum comes into direct contact with vaginal mucosa. The vagina, a fibromuscular tube lined with a superficial epithelial layer, is supported anteriorly by the pubocervical fascia and posteriorly by the rectovaginal fascia. In the patient with an intact uterus, the hiatus between the proximal edges of these fascial layers is bridged by the cervix and uterine fundus. In rare cases, detachment of the rectovaginal fascia from the posterior surface of the uterus occurs, resulting in a posterior enterocele with an intact uterus. More commonly, in the case of the patient who has previously undergone hysterectomy, failure to reapproximate the anterior and posterior fascial layers during vaginal cuff closure, or subsequent detachment of these two layers, results in a fascial defect, generally at the posterior vaginal apex (Fig. 48.3). This break in the integrity of the fibromuscular tube results in an area where the peritoneum comes into direct contact with the vaginal epithelium, eventually stretching and creating an enterocele noted on clinical examination (Fig 48.4). Thus, the enterocele sac, as described by Richardson, is bordered by the detached edge of the pubocervical fascia anteriorly, the detached edge of the rectovaginal fascia posteriorly, the pelvic sidewalls laterally, and the vaginal mucosa inferiorly.[11] Surgical repair of the enterocele is accomplished by reapproximation of these fascial edges (Fig. 48.5).

A complete understanding of the anatomy of an enterocele is critical for proper diagnosis and surgical correction. Traditional techniques for prevention and treatment of an enterocele have focused on plication of the enterocele sac and closure of the cul-de-sac based on the hypothesis that an enterocele results from an extension of the pouch of Douglas. However, newer techniques based on Richardson's site-specific fascial defect theory advocate restoration of fascial integrity without excision of the enterocele sac or obliteration of the cul-de-sac. Further anatomical investigations and studies of surgical outcomes are required to further our understanding of enterocele anatomy.

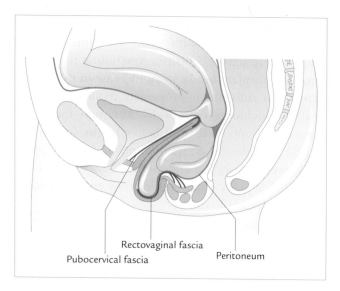

Rectovaginal fascia

Pubocervical fascia   Peritoneum

Figure 48.4 *Stretching of the peritoneal and mucosal components of the enterocele sac results in extension of the prolapse along the posterior vaginal wall to the perineal body.*

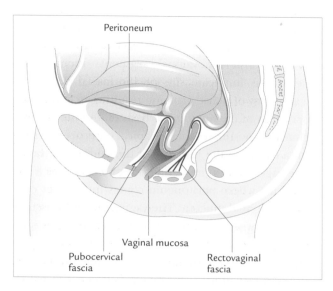

Peritoneum

Vaginal mucosa

Pubocervical fascia   Rectovaginal fascia

Figure 48.3 *Apical enterocele due to a defect in the anterior and posterior fascial planes allowing contact of the peritoneum with the vaginal mucosa.*

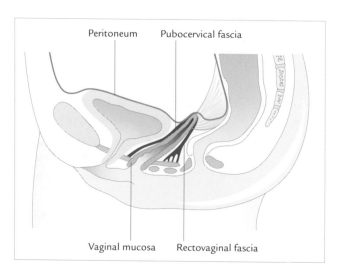

Peritoneum   Pubocervical fascia

Vaginal mucosa   Rectovaginal fascia

Figure 48.5 *Surgical correction of the enterocele sac by reapproximation of the anterior and posterior fascial planes via an abdominal or transvaginal approach.*

PATHOPHYSIOLOGY

Enteroceles can be classified into one of four types – congenital, pulsion, traction or iatrogenic – on the basis of aetiology and anatomy. A *congenital enterocele* is associated with an unusually deep pouch of Douglas due to failure of fusion of the anterior and posterior peritoneum of the cul-de-sac during late fetal development. This type is generally not associated with prolapse of the vaginal vault. *Pulsion enterocele* results from chronically increased abdominal pressure due to such factors as obesity, chronic cough, constipation and heavy lifting, which 'pushes' out the hernia. It is often found in conjunction with uterovaginal prolapse as well as cystocele and rectocele. In contrast, *traction enterocele* is associated with loss of support of the pelvic floor, eversion of the lower vagina and traction upon a poorly supported vaginal vault by structures prolapsing from below. Finally, *iatrogenic enterocele* occurs as a sequel to surgical procedures, such as retropubic urethropexies or uterine suspensions, which alter the normal vaginal axis and expose the cul-de-sac to increased abdominal pressure.[19] According to Richardson's site-specific fascial-defect theory, iatrogenic enteroceles can also be caused by failure to reapproximate the anterior and posterior fascial layers at the apex during vaginal vault closure following hysterectomy. Proper classification of enteroceles is mostly of academic interest as the principles of repair and diagnosis should be identical for all types.

Enteroceles can also be classified according to their location. They most commonly occur either at the vaginal apex or along the proximal posterior vaginal segment. Less frequently, anterior enteroceles may present as a bulge in the anterior vaginal segment, often mimicking a high cystocele (Fig. 48.6). According to Masson, the apical/posterior type of enterocele occurs 16 times more frequently than the anterior type.[20] Lateral hernias, as described by Nichols, are rare and enter the vagina through the lateral fornices either anterior or posterior to the broad ligament.[21]

DIAGNOSIS

An enterocele is often difficult to diagnose and is commonly overlooked or mistaken for a high rectocele or simple vaginal vault descensus. This is partly due to its variable presentation in terms of symptomatology and physical examination findings. The astute clinician

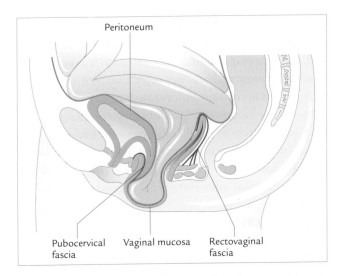

Figure 48.6 *The clinical appearance of an anterior enterocele often mimics that of a high cystocele and is indistinguishable before surgery.*

should be aware of common presenting symptoms, as well as techniques and tests that may aid in accurate preoperative diagnosis. Even the most experienced gynaecological surgeon may fail to make the diagnosis until the time of surgery.

Signs and symptoms

The classic symptoms of an enterocele include pressure or fullness in the rectum, sensation of a bulging mass in the vagina, pelvic pressure and pain, and difficulty during sexual intercourse.[2] In Timmons' study of 163 patients with advanced vault prolapse and enterocele, all patients had symptoms of tissue protrusion and pelvic pressure, while difficulty in walking and impaired coitus were reported by approximately 50% of patients surveyed.[22] Nichols postulated that the subjective 'bearing down' symptoms are often related to mesenteric traction from the presence of bowel, omentum or ovary within the enterocele sac.[21] If the enterocele compresses or pulls the urethra, obstructive voiding symptoms (including incomplete bladder emptying or even urinary retention) may result.[23] Patients may also report symptoms of constipation due to the enterocele obstructing the rectum during increases in intra-abdominal pressure.[24] Defecation disorders are often found to have a greater prevalence in patients with an enterocele. In a study of 69 patients with enterocele undergoing defecography, Mellgren *et al.*[25] reported that 55% had concomitant rectal intussusception, 38% had rectal prolapse and 30% had faecal incontinence. Similarly, Timmons *et al.*[22] reported that 39% of patients with post-hysterectomy enterocele had defecation difficulties. Less commonly, patients may complain of low back pain or report vagal responses with straining. Any or all of these symptoms may be present and worsen with the patient in an upright position or during activities that increase intra-abdominal pressure.

Physical examination

Careful physical examination is the cornerstone for preoperative diagnosis of an enterocele. A detailed pelvic examination with the patient in the dorsal lithotomy position should be performed to identify support defects in all pelvic compartments. This is most easily accomplished using half of a bivalve speculum with sequential visualization of the anterior, posterior and apical vaginal segments. Attention should be given to site-specific analysis, as previously described by Schull *et al.*[26] All concurrent prolapse should be reported quantitatively using standardized grading systems such as those proposed by Baden and Walker or the International Continence Society (pelvic organ prolapse questionnaire).[27,28] The presence of vaginal vault prolapse should be carefully noted. Most commonly, an enterocele will present as a bulge in the upper third of the posterior vaginal wall or as complete vault eversion (Fig. 48.7). In some patients, peristalsis of small bowel may be seen beneath a thin, postmenopausal vagina and is considered pathognomonic for an enterocele sac. Smaller enteroceles are difficult to diagnose and can either be mistaken for a high rectocele or overlooked completely.

Various authors have reported techniques to increase the ability of the physical examination to diagnose accurately an enterocele prior to surgery. Meigs[29] recommended examining the patient in the standing position with the examiner's index finger in the rectum and thumb in the vagina. The patient is asked to strain and any enterocele present is identified by palpation of a bowel-filled sac dissecting between the rectum and the vagina (Fig. 48.8).[29] In 1946, Waters[30] described a manoeuvre using a bivalve speculum in the vagina and the examiner's index finger in the rectum simultaneously, to differentiate between rectocele and enterocele

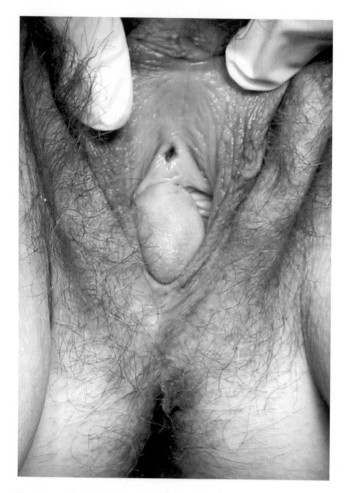

Figure 48.7 *Complete vaginal vault eversion with enterocele following hysterectomy in a post-menopausal woman.*

(Fig. 48.9). Altchek[31] reported transillumination of the rectovaginal septum with a light source in the rectum for diagnosis of enterocele. When the light source intensity was increased, some transillumination of the enterocele was evident, although it was distinctly less bright than at the rectocele.[31] Despite these techniques, clinical examination may still miss a majority of enteroceles preoperatively, so intra-operative assessment of the cul-de-sac and detection of an enterocele should be routinely performed.

Radiological testing

Given the limitations of clinical examination in the accurate preoperative diagnosis of enterocele, recent research has concentrated on radiological testing to

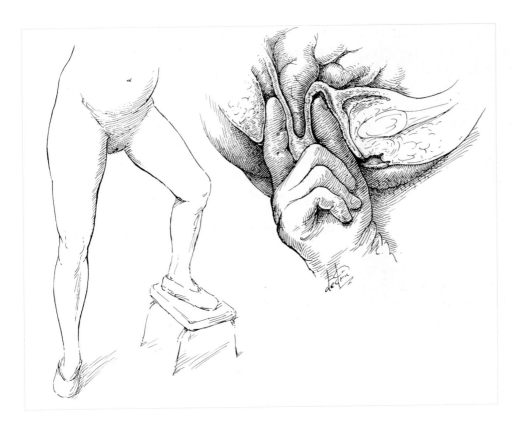

Figure 48.8 *Technique of vaginal examination in the standing position to differentiate between rectocele and enterocele. When the patient strains in the standing position, the enterocele sac will descend between the surgeon's thumb and forefinger. (From ref. 20, with permission.)*

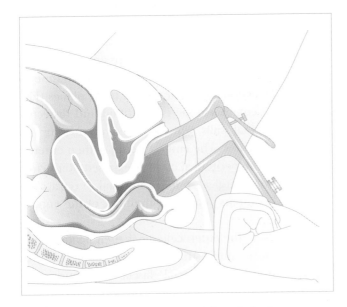

Figure 48.9 *Waters' manoeuvre for differentiation between rectocele and enterocele using a bivalve speculum and digital rectal examination.*

make the diagnosis (Fig. 48.10). Kelvin *et al.*[33] utilized evacuation proctography (defecography) to evaluate 74 patients with pelvic prolapse who had, by description, primarily posterior compartment defects. Enteroceles were detected by defecography in 13 patients, six of whom had not been diagnosed with enterocele on physical exam.[33] In 197 patients with colorectal dysfunction, Mellgren *et al.*[25] found that 69 had an enterocele demonstrated by defecography studies. Tepetes *et al.*[34] reported diagnosis of a perineal enterocele using peritoneography. Under fluoroscopy, contrast dye was infused intraperitoneally by tapping the anterior abdominal wall in the midline just below the umbilicus. Follow-up radiographic evaluation revealed peritoneal invagination of the pouch of Douglas consistent with an enterocele.[34] Fast magnetic resonance imaging was used by Yang *et al.*[35] to diagnose pelvic prolapse accurately during dynamic increases in intra-abdominal pressure. Despite encouraging results, the clinical utility and cost-effectiveness of radiological testing in the diagnosis of enteroceles and other pelvic support defects is still controversial and should be considered investigational pending further data.

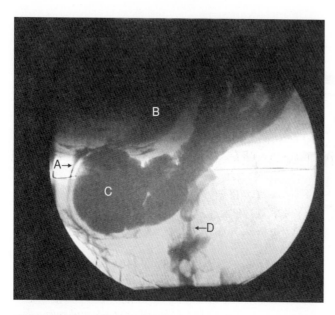

Figure 48.10 *Radiological appearance of a large enterocele on fluoroscopy: A, vagina; B, cystocele; C, enterocele; D, rectocele. (From ref. 32 with permission.)*

PREVENTION AND TREATMENT

Treatment of enterocele with or without concurrent vault prolapse can be either medical or surgical. For patients who are poor surgical candidates secondary to advanced age or coexisting medical conditions, or for women who prefer non-surgical treatment, a medical regimen consisting of oestrogen vaginal cream, Kegel's exercises and pessary placement should be considered. Biofeedback with or without functional electrical stimulation may also be helpful. Medical treatment is most effective in the properly selected patient with mild-to-moderate symptoms and early-stage prolapse on physical examination.

Surgery for treatment or prevention of enterocele should be considered for each patient, on the basis of the severity of prolapse, presence of concurrent support defects and desires of the patient. Although traditional enterocele repair can be performed abdominally, vaginally or laparoscopically, each approach follows the same basic principles: (1) identification and dissection of the enterocele sac; (2) excision or obliteration of the enterocele; (3) high ligation of the sac, and (4) repair of pelvic floor defects to provide horizontal support along the levator plate and reconstruct the normal axis of the vagina. Choice of approach is based on a variety of factors, including the surgeon's experience, the need for concurrent surgery and the presence of a uterus. More recently, site-specific fascial defect repair of an enterocele has been described with reapproximation of the detached fascial edges. This newer technique can also be performed by any of the surgical approaches mentioned for the traditional enterocele repair. There are few comparative data regarding surgical outcomes of the various procedures or approaches in the surgical treatment of enterocele.

Vaginal procedures for enterocele repair

The vaginal approach to enterocele repair has many advantages, including ability to perform concurrent vaginal repairs, decreased morbidity, shortened hospitalization and reduced recovery time. However, it provides limited visualization of the abdominopelvic cavity and requires greater surgical skill and knowledge of pelvic anatomy for an effective repair. Vaginal enterocele repair is routinely performed in conjunction with vaginal hysterectomy, anterior and posterior colporrhaphy and sacrospinous ligament vault suspension. With the recent trend toward increased vaginal surgery, it is probably the most common approach to enterocele repair.

Vaginal enterocele repair

First reported by Ward in 1922, the classic vaginal enterocele repair has undergone little modification since its first description. The vaginal mucosa overlying the enterocele is grasped with Allis clamps and the vaginal wall is infiltrated with normal saline in the midline to facilitate dissection and separation of tissue planes (Fig. 48.11). The enterocele sac is identified and dissected from the vaginal walls, with care to prevent injury to adjacent structures. The enterocele sac is then entered sharply and the peritoneal cavity is exposed. Retractors and moistened surgical sponges are used to retract the peritoneal contents away from the neck of the enterocele sac.

The neck of the enterocele sac is then ligated using one or more purse-string non-absorbable sutures incorporating the prerectal fascia posteriorly, the uterosacral–cardinal ligament complex laterally on each side, and the peritoneal fold overlying the bladder anteriorly (Fig. 48.12). Each individual suture is then tied separately to obliterate the enterocele. The

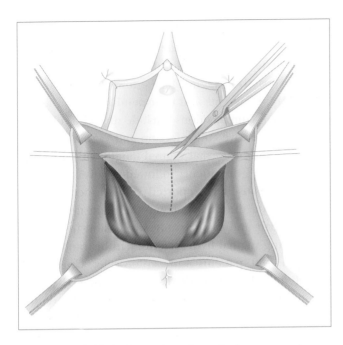

Figure 48.11 *Vaginal entry into the vaginal mucosa and dissection of the enterocele sac.*

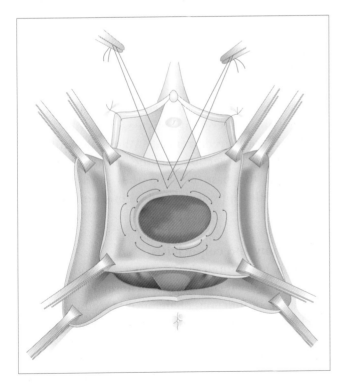

Figure 48.12 *High ligation of the enterocele sac using a series of purse-string sutures.*

enterocele sac distal to the plication sutures is then excised. To provide additional support, a delayed absorbable suture is used to plicate the uterosacral–cardinal ligament complex in the midline distal to the enterocele repair to provide an additional layer of strength and support. In patients with weak attenuated uterosacral ligaments, additional repair such as a 'crown suture' in the musculofascial layers of the upper posterior vagina is required.[15] Finally, excess vaginal wall is excised and closed using a running delayed absorbable suture. Care must be taken not to excise too much vaginal wall, which would cause shortening of vaginal length or narrowing of vaginal calibre. Potential complications include rectal or bowel injury and ureteral kinking.

This basic technique has been endorsed by numerous authors. Although surgical results in most series have been favourable, long-term follow-up has generally been poor.[36–38] In an effort to improve clinical outcomes, various modifications of Ward's original technique have been proposed. Parsons and Ulfelder[39] recommended a combined vaginal and abdominal repair, closing the sac and performing a levator plication from below, then closing the uterosacral ligaments from above, incorporating the neck of the enterocele sac in the closure. Hiller[40] described a vaginal approach, suturing the uterosacral and cardinal ligaments together in the midline and then attaching the sutures to levator ani, obliterating the hernial sac. There are no data comparing the efficacy of these modifications with that of the original technique described by Ward.

Modified McCall cul-de-plasty

First described in 1957, the classic McCall cul-de-plasty obliterates the redundant cul-de-sac of Douglas, using a series of continuous sutures suspended to the uterosacral ligaments which are then plicated in the midline.[41] Current modifications incorporate suspension of the vaginal apex with reattachment to the uterosacral ligaments. The procedure is performed immediately after vaginal hysterectomy but can also be performed separately in the post-hysterectomy patient with enterocele and/or vaginal vault prolapse.

After hysterectomy is completed, a finger is inserted into the posterior cul-de-sac to assess its depth and presence of enterocele. The bowel and omentum are packed out of the surgical field using a moist sponge. A permanent suture is then placed through the left uterosacral ligament (identified by traction on the previously tagged uterosacral ligament particles), through the anterior serosa of the sigmoid colon in a purse-string fashion, and then through the opposite uterosacral ligament. The sutures are held and one to three more identical sutures are placed, progressing toward the posterior vaginal cuff. The number of internal sutures placed depends on the size and depth of the enterocele sac. Tie-down of the sutures will eventually obliterate the dependent portion of the cul-de-sac. After the internal sutures have been placed, one or two delayed absorbable sutures are used to resuspend the vaginal apex to the uterosacral ligament complex. A full-thickness 'bite' incorporating vaginal epithelium and peritoneum is taken approximately 1 cm from the edge of the vaginal apex just lateral to the midline. The needle is then passed through the left uterosacral ligament, the peritoneum of the posterior cul-de-sac in a purse-string fashion, the right uterosacral ligament, and finally full-thickness peritoneum and vaginal epithelium adjacent to the needle entry point previously described (Fig. 48.13). The permanent sutures are then tied in sequence, obliterating the

enterocele sac. The vaginal apex is subsequently closed using interrupted delayed absorbable suture and the external McCall sutures are then tied, pushing the posterior vaginal apex toward the plicated uterosacral ligaments and resuspending the cuff.

Potential complications include ureteral obstruction, postoperative cuff infection and vaginal stenosis. McCall reported normal vaginal length with no surgical failures in 45 patients followed-up over 3 years.[41] Other surgeons have reported similar success rates, and this procedure has become the mainstay of enterocele repair and vaginal vault suspension in patients undergoing vaginal hysterectomy.[42] In his randomized study of 100 patients with enterocele, Cruikshank reported the McCall cul-de-plasty technique to be superior to both a vaginal Moschowitz-type procedure and simple peritoneal closure in preventing subsequent enteroceles on 3-year clinical follow-up.[43] Given the success of this procedure via the vaginal approach, Wall has adapted the technique to be performed via laparotomy following abdominal hysterectomy (Fig. 48.14).[44]

Torpin[45] and Waters[46,47] also advocated culdoplastic techniques for enterocele correction and prevention. Torpin described resection of the cul-de-sac by excising a triangular section of tissue, including excess peritoneum and vaginal vault, after vaginal hysterectomy. The exposed edges were then reapproximated using a continuous spiral suture, the uterosacral ligaments were plicated in the midline and the vaginal cuff was closed. In Torpin's series of 135 patients undergoing cul-de-sac excision, there were no reported recurrences.[45] Waters also utilized a wedge-shaped resection of the posterior vaginal vault, with the base between the uterosacral ligaments and the apex at the mid-vagina, with excellent results.[46,47]

Colpectomy and colpocleisis

Although most surgical techniques for correction of prolapse involve reconstruction of normal anatomy and restoration of function, obliterative procedures should also be considered for the treatment of advanced pelvic prolapse including enterocele. Obliterative procedures are ideally suited for the elderly or medically fragile patient who no longer desires to maintain sexual function and would benefit from a minimally invasive procedure. It can be performed quickly under local or

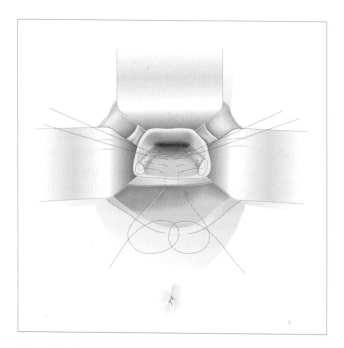

Figure 48.13 *McCall cul-de-plasty technique used to obliterate the cul-de-sac and enterocele by approximating the uterosacral ligaments and posterior peritoneum of the cul-de-sac.*

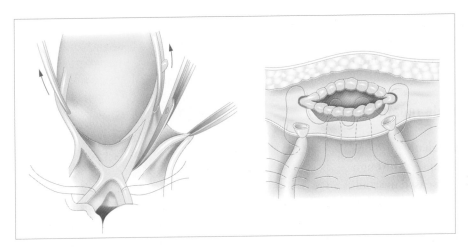

Figure 48.14 *Abdominal cul-de-plasty incorporating the uterosacral ligaments and posterior peritoneum, performed at the time of hysterectomy.*

regional anaesthesia and has been associated with excellent cure rates.

The operation is performed by grasping the prolapsed vaginal mucosa in the midline. Submucosal injection with a haemostatic agent helps to facilitate dissection and minimize bleeding. The midline mucosal incision is extended from the perineal body posteriorly to the bladder neck anteriorly. The vaginal mucosa is dissected off the underlying prolapse and endopelvic fascia. The dissection should extend to the levator ani

muscles on both sides. A series of purse-string sutures is placed, slowly inverting the prolapse and overlying fascia. Tie-down of these sutures results in reduction of the underlying cystocele, enterocele and/or rectocele (Fig. 48.15). A standard Kelly plication is performed to create suburethral support of the bladder neck. The levator ani muscles are then plicated in the midline from the bladder neck to the perineum, creating a strong wall of support to prevent recurrent prolapse. The vaginal mucosa is then completely excised close to the

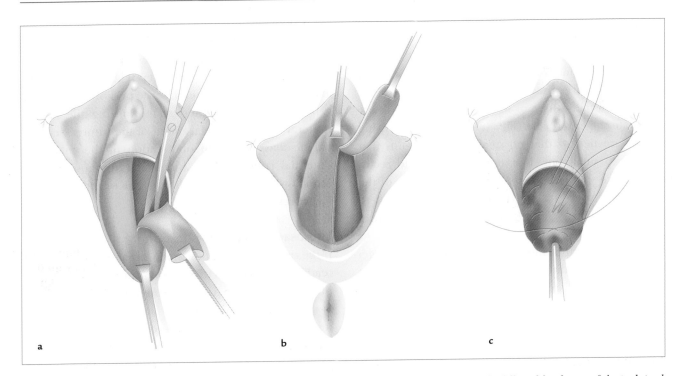

Figure 48.15 *Colpectomy performed by removal of vaginal mucosa anteriorly (a) and posteriorly (b) followed by closure of the prolapsed segment using a series of purse-string sutures (c).*

609

vaginal introitus. A tight perineoplasty is performed and the vaginal mucosa is subsequently closed. After completion of the procedure, the vagina ends in a blind sac with a small introitus.

Abdominal procedures for enterocele repair

The abdominal approach is preferred by many surgeons for the treatment of pelvic organ prolapse. Although this approach may be associated with increased morbidity and mortality, increased length of hospitalization and prolonged recovery, various studies have reported improved results in the surgical treatment of incontinence and prolapse using the abdominal approach rather than the vaginal route.[48] Abdominal repair of enterocele should be considered on the basis of the surgeon's experience, especially when there is coexisting pathology requiring concurrent abdominal procedures.

Moschowitz procedure

Moschowitz,[49] in 1912, first reported his experience in treating prolapse of the rectum by placing concentric, purse-string sutures around the cul-de-sac, including the anterior wall of the rectum. Since then, this technique has formed the cornerstone of abdominal repair of enterocele. The initial suture is placed at the base of the cul-de-sac. Peritoneal sutures should be placed over the posterior vaginal wall, the right pelvic sidewall, the serosa of the sigmoid and the left pelvic sidewall. The number of sutures used depends on the depth of the cul-de-sac: usually, three or four sutures will completely obliterate the enterocele (Fig. 48.16). The purse-string sutures are tied so that no small defect remains that could trap small bowel or lead to enterocele recurrence. Care should be taken, during placement of the purse-string sutures along the pelvic sidewall, not to include or kink the ureter medially when the sutures are tied.

Potential complications include ureteral or large-bowel injury, bleeding and abdominal pain. Dicke[50] has reported a case of small-bowel obstruction secondary to a Moschowitz procedure.[49]

Halban procedure

Nichols and Randall[19] described an alternate means of obliterating the cul-de-sac as suggested by Halban,[51] who proposed that a series of stitches be placed in a

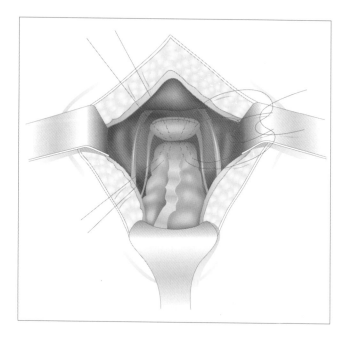

Figure 48.17 *Halban procedure obliterating the cul-de-sac using sagittal sutures through the serosa of the sigmoid, the peritoneum of the cul-de-sac and the back of the vaginal wall.*

sagittal direction. Sutures are placed in a longitudinal fashion incorporating the serosa of the sigmoid, the deep peritoneum of the cul-de-sac and the posterior vaginal wall. Four or five sutures are placed across the pelvis, each adjacent to the next, extending from one uterosacral ligament to the other (Fig. 48.17). Sutures are not placed in the lateral pelvic peritoneum or adjacent to the ureters, thereby minimizing the risk of ureteral injury. After placement of the sutures, sequential tie-down results in obliteration of the cul-de-sac. Potential complications are similar to those for the Moschowitz procedure, although risk of ureteral injury is theoretically decreased.

Uterosacral ligament plication

If the uterus is present or the uterosacral ligaments are readily identifiable, cul-de-plasty can be performed by plicating the uterosacral ligaments in the midline. Sutures are placed into the medial portion of one uterosacral ligament, then into the back wall of the vagina and finally into the medial portion of the contralateral uterosacral ligament. Three to five such sutures are placed from the upper portion of the vagina down towards the rectum. The lowest suture incorpo-

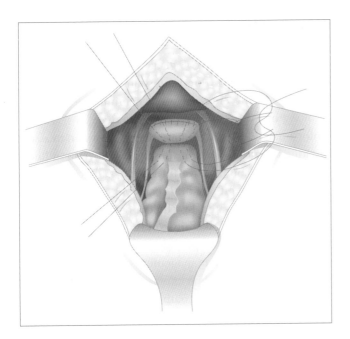

Figure 48.17 *Halban procedure obliterating the cul-de-sac using sagittal sutures through the serosa of the sigmoid, the peritoneum of the cul-de-sac and the back of the vaginal wall.*

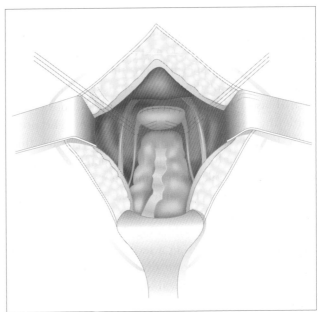

Figure 48.18 *Abdominal uterosacral ligament plication.*

rates the anterior rectal serosa, to bring the rectum adjacent to the uterosacral ligaments and vagina in the midline (Fig. 48.18). After the sutures are tied, the entire length of the uterosacral ligament should be brought together in the midline, thereby obliterating the cul-de-sac. As in the Moschowitz procedure, care should be taken to identify the ureter prior to suture placement to prevent unintentional ureteral obstruction or kinking.[52]

Laparoscopic procedures for enterocele repair

A detailed description of laparoscopic techniques for the treatment of enterocele is beyond the scope of this chapter. However, most of the abdominal repairs outlined, as well as the site-specific fascial-defect repair recently introduced, can be performed laparoscopically. Surgical outcomes and cost-effectiveness of the laparoscopic approach are primarily dependent on operator experience, as laparoscopic reconstructive procedures are often associated with a steep learning curve. If the laparoscopic technique is performed in a manner identical to the open procedure, equivalent results should be expected. We recommend that, before performing enterocele repair laparoscopically, the sur-

geon should have sufficient experience with traditional vaginal and abdominal approaches to gain a complete understanding of the anatomical principles underlying enterocele repair.

Site-specific fascial-defect repair

Recently, site-specific fascial defect has been implicated in the aetiology of pelvic organ prolapse including enterocele. In contrast to traditional enterocele repairs, which emphasize obliteration of the cul-de-sac and high ligation of the enterocele neck, site-specific defect repair advocates identification of the fascial defect and reapproximation of its detached edges. There is currently little information to support these anatomical concepts or surgical techniques, owing to the recent introduction of this theory.

Miklos *et al.*[53] have reported their initial experience with site-specific enterocele repair using a combined laparoscopic–vaginal approach to repair the enterocele and resuspend the vaginal vault. The procedure is begun with open laparoscopy to identify and suture-tag the uterosacral ligaments along the pelvic sidewall. A midline incision is then made along the posterior vaginal mucosa. The vaginal mucosa is then dissected off the underlying rectovaginal septum. As the dissection is continued toward the vaginal apex, a distinct loss of rectovaginal septum with sudden protrusion of peritoneum (enterocele sac) is noted. The enterocele sac is isolated, entered sharply and then resected. The detached edges of the pubocervical fascia and rectovaginal fascia are identified anteriorly and posteriorly bordering the enterocele sac, respectively. The previously tagged uterosacral ligament sutures are then retrieved through the vaginal incision and attached to the vaginal apex bilaterally by incorporating one end of the suture through the anterior fascia and the other end through the posterior fascia. Next, the enterocele is repaired by reapproximating the anterior fascia to the posterior fascia using a series of interrupted permanent sutures. Tie-down of the uterosacral suspension sutures results in apical support of the vaginal cuff (Fig. 48.19). The rectocele is repaired, if indicated, and the vaginal mucosa is then closed. In 17 patients undergoing this procedure with a mean follow-up of 6.3 months (1–17 months), there were only two cases of mild vault descensus and no cases of recurrent enterocele; no significant complications were noted.[51] Although initial results are encouraging, further research is required before this technique can gain widespread acceptance.

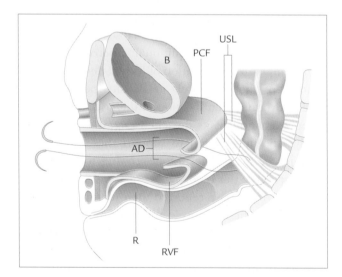

Figure 48.19 *Site-specific defect repair of apical defect (AD) enterocele with reapproximation of the pubocervical fascia (PCF) to the rectovaginal fascia (RVF) with suspension to the uterosacral ligament (USL). (B, bladder; R, rectum.)*

CONCLUSIONS

The diagnosis and anatomy of the enterocele continues to challenge the gynaecological surgeon. Since its first description in 1736, our understanding of the pathophysiology of the enterocele has continued to develop, resulting in a variety of surgical techniques for its repair. Unfortunately, few studies have been performed to assess the long-term outcomes of these procedures in either a descriptive or comparative format. In addition, current strategies to prevent new and recurrent enteroceles have not been substantiated by clinical data. As our understanding of this clinical entity continues to improve, additional data will help to provide a scientific basis for the diagnosis and surgical management of enterocele. Meanwhile, clinicians should be familiar with current concepts regarding the anatomy, pathophysiology and surgical management of enterocele. Regardless of the technique used for enterocele repair, the basic principles of reconstructive pelvic surgery should be followed – accurate diagnosis and correction of all support defects, with the goal of restoring normal anatomy and function.

REFERENCES

1. Bueerman WH. Vaginal enterocele: a report of three cases. *J Am Med Assoc* 1932; 99: 1138

2. Kinzel GE. Enterocele: a study of 265 cases. *Am J Obstet Gynecol* 1961; 81: 1166

3. Austin RC, Damstra EF. New fascia plastic repair of enterocele. *Surg Gynecol Obstet* 1955; 101: 297

4. Weed JC, Tyrone C. Enterocele: an analysis of 52 cases. *Am J Obstet Gynecol* 1950; 60: 324

5. Ranney B. Enterocele, vaginal prolapse, pelvic hernia: recognition and treatment. *Am J Obstet Gynecol* 1981; 140: 53

6. Raz S, Sussman EM, Erickson DB *et al.* The Raz bladder neck suspension: results in 206 patients. *J Urol* 1992; 148: 845

7. Wiskind AK, Creighton SM, Stanton SL. The incidence of general prolapse following the Burch colposuspension operation. *Neurourol Urodyn* 1991; 10: 453

8. Korda A, Ferry J, Hunter P. Colposuspension for the treatment of female urinary incontinence. *Aust N Z J Obstet Gynaecol* 1989; 29: 146

9. Ekberg O, Nylander G, Fork FT. Defecography. *Radiology* 1985; 155: 45

10. Addison WA, Livengodd CH, Sutton GP *et al.* Abdominal sacral colpopexy with Mersilene mesh in the retroperitoneal position in the management of posthysterectomy

vaginal vault prolapse and enterocele. *Am J Obstet Gynecol* 1985; 153: 140

11. Richardson CA. The anatomic defects in rectocele and enterocele. *J Pelvic Surg* 1995; 1: 214

12. Zacharin RF. Pulsion enterocele: review of functional anatomy of the pelvic floor. *Obstet Gynecol* 1980; 50: 135

13. Nichols DH, Milley PS, Randall CL. Significance of restoration of normal vaginal depth and axis. *Obstet Gynecol* 1970; 36: 251

14. Berglas B, Rubin IC. Study of the supportive structures of the uterus by levator myography. *Surg Obstet Gynecol* 1953; 97: 677

15. Harrison JE, McDonagh JE. Hernia of Douglas' pouch and high rectocele. *Am J Obstet Gynecol* 1950; 60: 83

16. Curtis AH, Anson BJ, Beaton LE. The anatomy of the sub-peritoneal tissues and ligamentous structures in relation to surgery of the female pelvic viscera. *Surg Gynecol Obstet* 1939; 68: 161

17. Uhlenhuth E, Day ED, Smith RD *et al.* The visceral endopelvic fascia and hypogastric sheath. *Surg Gynecol Obstet* 1948; 86: 9

18. Uhlenhuth E, Wolfe WM, Smith EM *et al.* The rectogenital septum. *Surg Gynecol Obstet* 1948; 86: 148

19. Nichols DH, Randall CL. *Vaginal Surgery*, 3rd edn. Baltimore: Williams and Wilkins, 1989; 313–327

20. Masson JC. Vaginal hernia. *Surg Gynecol Obstet* 1928; 47: 36

21. Nichols DH. Types of enterocele and principles underlying choice of operation for repair. *Obstet Gynecol* 1972; 40: 257

22. Timmons MC, Addison WA, Addison SB *et al.* Abdominal sacral colpopexy in 163 women with post hysterectomy vaginal vault prolapse and enterocele: evolution of operative techniques. *J Reprod Med* 1992; 37: 323

23. Nitti VW. Variations on enterocele repair. *Contemp Obstet Gynecol* 1995; Dec: 52

24. Wallden L. Defecation block in cases of deep rectogenital pouch. *Acta Chir Scand* 1952; 165: 1

25. Mellgren A, Johansson C, Dolk A *et al.* Enterocele demonstrated by defecography is associated with other pelvic floor disorders. *Int J Colorect Dis* 1994; 9: 121

26. Shull BL, Capen CV, Riggs MV, Kuehl TJ. Preoperative and post operative analysis of site-specific pelvic support defects in 81 women treated with sacrospinous ligament suspension and pelvic reconstruction. *Am J Obstet Gynecol* 1992; 166: 1764

27. Baden WF, Walker T, Lindsey JH. The vaginal profile. *Tex Med* 1968; 64: 56

28. Bump RC, Mattiasson A, Bø K *et al.* The standardization of terminology of female pelvic organ prolapse and pelvic floor dysfunction. *Am J Obstet Gynecol* 1996; 175: 10

29. Meigs JV. Enterocele or posterior vaginal hernia. *Surg Clin North Am* 1947; 1226

30. Waters EG. A diagnostic technique for the detection of enterocele. *Am J Obstet Gynecol* 1946; 52: 810

31. Altchek A. Diagnosis of enterocele by negative intrarectal transillumination. *Obstet Gynecol* 1965; 26: 636

32. Pitkin RM, Scott JR (eds) *Clinical Obstetrics and Gynecology*. Philadelphia: Lippincott, 1993.

33. Kelvin FM, Maglinte DDT, Hornback JA, Benson JT. Pelvic prolapse: assessment with evacuation proctography (defecography). *Radiology* 1992; 184: 547

34. Tepetes K, Petsas T, Siamplis D, Tzoracoleftherakis E. Peritoneographic diagnosis of perineal enterocele after hysterectomy. *ROFO* 1995; 163: 367

35. Yang A, Mostwin JL, Rosenshein NB, Zerhouni EA. Pelvic floor descent in women: dynamic evaluation with fast MR imaging and cinematic display. *Radiology* 1991; 179: 25

36. Reich WJ, Nechtow MJ, Keith L. Diagnosis and modified surgical treatment of posterior direct vaginal hernia (enterocele). *Clin Obstet Gynecol* 1966; 9: 1070

37. Bemis GG. Repair of enterocele (posterior vaginal wall hernia). *Clin Obstet Gynecol* 1975; 18: 3

38. Hiller RI. Repair of enterocele with preservation of the vagina. *Am J Obstet Gynecol* 1952; 64: 409

39. Parsons L, Ulfelder H. *An Atlas of Pelvic Operations*, 2nd edn. Philadelphia: Saunders, 1968

40. Hiller RI. Repair of enterocele with preservation of the vagina. *Am J Obstet Gynecol* 1952; 64: 409

41. McCall MH. Posterior cul-de-plasty. *Obstet Gynecol* 1957; 10: 595

42. Given FT. Posterior cul-de-plasty: revisited. *Am J Obstet Gynecol* 1985; 153: 135

43. Cruikshank SH, Kovac SR. Randomized comparison of three surgical methods used at the time of vaginal hysterectomy to prevent posterior enterocele. *Am J Obstet Gynecol* 1999; 180: 859

44. Wall LL. A technique for modified McCall culdeplasty at the time of abdominal hysterectomy. *J Am Coll Surg* 1994; 178: 507

45. Torpin R. Excision of the cul-de-sac of Douglas. *J Int Coll Surg* 1955; 24: 322

46. Waters EG. Vaginal prolapse: technique for correction and prevention of hysterectomy. *Obstet Gynecol* 1956; 8: 432

47. Waters EG. Culdoplastic technique for prevention and correction of vaginal vault prolapse and enterocele. *Am J Obstet Gynecol* 1961; 81: 291

48. Bergman A, Elia G. Three surgical procedures for genuine stress incontinence: five-year followup of a prospective randomized study. *Am J Obstet Gynecol* 1995; 173: 66

49. Moschowitz AV. The pathogenesis, anatomy and cure of prolapse of the rectum. *Surg Gynecol Obstet* 1912; 15: 7–21

50. Dicke JM. Small bowel obstruction secondary to a prior Moschowitz procedure. *Am J Obstet Gynecol* 1985; 152: 887

51. Halban J. *Gynäkologische Operationslehre*. Berlin: Urban and Schwarzenberg, 1912

52. Karram MM, Walter MD. *Clinical Urogynecology*. St Louis: Mosby-Year Book, 1993

53. Miklos JR, Kohli N, Lucente V, Saye WB. Site-specific fascial defects in the diagnosis and surgical management of enterocele. *Am J Obstet Gynecol* 1998; 179: 1418

49

Pathophysiology, diagnosis and management of rectoceles

M. M. Karram, W. Porter

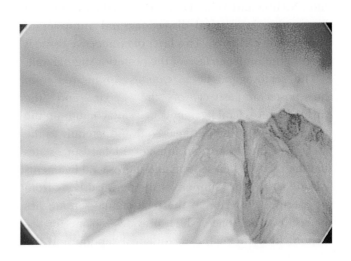

INTRODUCTION

Since the early 19th century, surgeons have performed posterior colporrhaphy to manage complete tears of the perineum. The supports of the genital organs were largely a mystery, and there was little distinction between prolapses of the rectum, bladder and uterus. As anatomical concepts developed, surgeons ascertained that the main support of the uterus was the vagina, which in turn was supported by the insertion of the levator ani muscles into the perineum. This concept was the basis for the incorporation of plication of the levator ani muscles into posterior colpoperineorrhaphy, with the surgical goals of constriction of the vaginal tube, creation of a perineal shelf and partial closure of the genital hiatus. Until recently, very little attention has been given to the functional derangements that are commonly associated with rectoceles.

A rectocele is an outpocketing of the anterior rectal and posterior vaginal wall into the lumen of the vagina.[1] Some rectoceles may be asymptomatic, whereas others may cause such symptoms as incomplete bowel emptying, vaginal mass, pain and pressure. The prevalence of rectoceles ranges from 20 to 80% in the general population.[2] A rectocele is fundamentally a defect of the rectovaginal septum, not of the rectum. The size of the defect does not necessarily correlate with the amount of functional derangement. This chapter reviews the anatomy, pathophysiology, diagnosis and management of rectoceles.

ANATOMY

In 1839, Denonvilliers first described a layer of fascia found in males, which he named the 'rectovesical septum'. Nichols and Milley later recorded the existence of this septum in surgical dissections and autopsies of fresh female cadavers.[3] This layer of connective tissue is fused to the undersurface of the posterior vaginal wall.

The rectovaginal fascia extends downwards from the posterior aspect of the cervix and the cardinal–uterosacral ligaments to its attachment on the upper margin of the perineal body and laterally to the fascia over the levator ani muscles. Richardson[3] states that the rectovaginal septum and uterosacral ligaments provide suspensory support of the perineal body from the sacrum. Posterior to the rectovaginal septum lies the rectovaginal space, which provides a plane for dissection. In between the rectovaginal septum and the rectum is the pararectal fascia; inside this fibromuscular layer lie blood vessels, nerves and lymph nodes, which supply the rectum. The pararectal fascia, originating from the pelvic sidewalls, divides into fibrous anterior and posterior sheaths, which encompass the rectum. These layers provide additional support to the anterior rectal wall.[4]

Further support is provided by the levator ani, which are composed of paired iliococcygeus, puborectalis and pubococcygeus muscles. These muscles function to maintain a constant basal tone and a closed urogenital hiatus. This constant basal tone prevents the urogenital hiatus from widening and the eventual descent of the pelvic viscera. These muscles also provide a contraction reflex to increased intra-abdominal pressures, preventing incontinence and prolapse. The anterior sacral nerve roots S2–S4, which innervate these muscles, cross the pelvic floor and are stretched and compressed during labour, increasing the risk of injury.[4,5]

AETIOLOGY

Rectocele was once thought to be a condition affecting only multiparous females and resulting from obstetric damage or increased tissue laxity with ageing and menopausal atrophy. However, recently, rectoceles and enteroceles have been noted to occur in approximately 40% of asymptomatic parous women.[6] Shorvon *et al.*[7] performed defecography on healthy, young, nulliparous, asymptomatic volunteers, noting that 17/21 women had small or moderately sized rectoceles. Rectoceles may thus have a wider prevalence than previously thought and may not be a result of parity.

The most common causes of rectoceles are obstetric events. Traumatic obstetric events, which usually occur when the presenting part descends quickly in the second stage of labour, can predispose to rectocele formation. The forces of labour may separate, tear or distend the pelvic floor, altering the functional and anatomical position of the muscles, nerves and connective tissues. The rectal fascia may separate from the perineal body, causing a transverse defect and low rectocele. Low rectoceles are isolated defects in the suprasphincteric portion of the rectovaginal fascia. They are usually caused by obstetric trauma that disrupts the attachments of the levator ani fascia and bulbocavernosus muscles. An eversion of the introitus will be noted on physical examination. This will aggravate constipation and will result in inefficient bowel movements and the need for stronger Valsalva manoeuvre.[8–12] If mid or high rectoceles form, they may alter the vaginal axis.[1,4,8,9] Laxity of the levator ani secondary to the levator detaching from the perineal body along the vaginal axis allows the pelvic organs to slide downwards, following the new altered axis. Women with an android pelvis are at increased risk because labour forces are directed towards the posterior vaginal wall and perineum, leaving the anterior vaginal wall relatively protected.

Mid-vaginal rectoceles are most likely caused by obstetric trauma not involving the levator ani. The rectovaginal fascia is damaged by the stretching and laceration of the tissue, which results in the thinning of the fascia, leading to subsequent adhesion formation. This adhesion of the rectovaginal septum, vagina and rectal capsule inhibits independent function. Symptoms may include incomplete bowel emptying, rectal pressure, and pain after bowel movements; they may also coexist with a high rectocele.[12]

High rectoceles often occur from pathological overstretching of the posterior vaginal wall. The cardinal ligaments fuse with the vagina and cervix, causing the cervix to fuse with the anterior vaginal wall. The rectovaginal septum is absent from the posterior vaginal wall, causing loss of the anterior rectal wall support. High rectocele may also coexist with congenital deepness of the pouch of Douglas.[12]

Rectoceles may occur as a result of pathological stretching of the pudendal nerves during descent of the fetal head, causing atrophy and denervation of the pelvic floor muscles. Sultan[13,14] reported that most damage to the pelvic support occurs in the first vaginal delivery. EMG studies demonstrate an 80% incidence of denervation of perineal muscles after vaginal delivery.[5,15,16] Denervation will probably recover after the post-partum period; however, it has been demonstrated that injury may be cumulative with increasing parity.[5] Increased labour duration and weight of the baby directly influence the perineal damage and denervation of the pelvic floor. This neuropathy can lead to the weakening of pelvic floor muscles and development of a rectocele. Thus, shortening of the second stage of labour by episiotomy or forceps may decrease the risk of denervation and subsequent pelvic floor damage.[8]

Defecation disorders may account for a subgroup of rectoceles. They may lead to the weakening of the rectovaginal septum by continuous straining against an obstruction. One disorder, the perineal descent syndrome, is clinically diagnosed when the individual strains and the perineal plane descends past the ischial tuberosities;[15] this disorder may be confused with a rectocele. Other conditions, such as paradoxical sphincter reaction (anismus), cause unconscious contraction of the voluntary striated muscles when attempting to defecate. This constant straining with bowel movements has been shown to cause or worsen a pre-existing rectocele and increasingly to weaken the rectovaginal septum by denervation injury.[17] Anismus eventually leads to the accumulation of stool in the rectum, which may complicate pelvic outlet obstruction and cause a progressive cycle, worsening the rectocele.[18]

Congenital absence of the perineum may mimic a rectocele. This pseudorectocele has its posterior vaginal wall exposed because of lack of inferior support; this may be corrected by surgical reconstruction of the perineum. Congenital absence allows for deepening of the cul-de-sac and weakening of the rectovaginal septum, leading to the development of a high rectocele and enterocele.[6,12]

Some studies have found differences in connective tissue strengths between races, which may contribute to rectoceles. Africans have been noted to have a decreased frequency of laceration after normal spontaneous deliveries and a subsequent decrease of uterine prolapse. This may be related to constitutional factors such as pelvis type, connective tissue and ability to fibrose,[12] whereas Hispanic, Filipino and Chinese women may have an increased risk of laxity of tissue.[19]

CLINICAL PRESENTATION

Clinical symptoms vary from being non-existent to severe bowel symptoms. A common complaint is constipation, which may occur in up to 75% of patients with rectoceles.[2] Patients may also complain of incomplete rectal emptying, a sense of rectal pressure or a vaginal bulge.[1,20,21] Vaginal digitation or perineal support is sometimes necessary to facilitate defecation.[20] Many non-specific symptoms, such as rectal pain, bleeding, faecal or gas incontinence, low back pain worsening throughout the day but relieved by lying down, and dyspareunia may occur, as well as many other defecatory disorders.[6] As previously mentioned, the majority of rectoceles are totally asymptomatic.

PHYSICAL EXAMINATION

Physical examination begins with the patient in the dorsal supine position (for the gynaecologist) or in the left lateral decubitus position (for the colorectal surgeon). Delemarre *et al.*[22] found that examination in the supine position leads to the underscoring of the rectocele, whereas the lateral decubitus position more closely matches the findings of defecography. After the external genitalia, the introitus and vaginal vault have been inspected, the strength, integrity and signs of descent (prolapse) of the perineum are tested. The patient is then asked to forcefully strain down or cough. This manoeuvre allows the pelvic organs to descend to determine the extent of the prolapse. Digital support of the perineum opens the genital hiatus, allowing visualization of the anatomy. Posterior wall prolapse caused by rectocele or enterocele is assessed by using a finger in the rectum to evaluate anterior displacement of the rectovaginal septum and perineal body. This can be differentiated from enterocele by noting bowel in the rectovaginal space: with the patient standing, the rectovaginal examination will reveal small bowel herniating into this space when an enterocele is present. Of women with rectoceles, 80% are asymptomatic and can be diagnosed only on physical examination.[7–18]

Although a good physical examination is the best diagnostic method available to the clinician, the diagnostic tests discussed below have been used for the evaluation of posterior vaginal wall defects and defecatory dysfunction.

DIAGNOSTIC STUDIES

Defecography

Defecography, first described in 1964,[7] is increasingly being used for preoperative evaluation of pelvic organ prolapse. Defecography is considered by some to be useful because it provides objective outcomes and identifies anatomical abnormalities. The technique involves filling the rectum with a barium paste with the consistency of stool and opacifying the vagina. Fluoroscopy is used with the patient at rest, on contracting the pelvic floor muscles, on straining down and during defecation.[18] The fluoroscopic examination grades rectoceles during maximal distension as small (< 2 cm), moderate (2–4 cm), and large (> 4 cm).[1,9,18] Kelvin *et al.*[18] noted

that barium was retained only in moderate-to-large rectoceles. The relevance of the rectocele size as related to symptoms has not been ascertained;[23] however, larger rectoceles are associated with faecal trapping.[9]

Defecography is a good diagnostic tool to help exclude other defecation disorders that may increase the risk of recurrence of symptoms despite anatomical repair. Radiographically, anismus or paradoxical sphincter response is observed as a decrease or less than 5% increase in the anorectal angle during straining.[16,24] The anterior rectal wall infolding 6–8 cm inside the rectum identifies internal intussusception.[18] Lastly, enterocele may be suspected if the distance between the vagina and the rectum is 2 cm or more and there is concurrent herniation of small loops of bowel within the rectovaginal space.[18]

Although defecography has been shown to be reproducible when clinical data are present,[25] the significance of faecal trapping and usefulness of correlating data between faecal trapping and the need for repair is controversial and needs to be studied further.

Scintographic defecography is another tool to evaluate the physiology of rectal emptying. It not only assesses the rate and completeness of emptying but also assesses the anorectal angle and pelvic floor descent. The advantages are less radiation exposure and more precise quantification; however, the disadvantages are its inability to evaluate the anatomical detail or view pelvic floor anatomy.[16]

Ultrasonography

Endosonography of the anus has proved to be valuable in detecting incontinence disorders by imaging the anatomical integrity of the internal and external anal sphincters. In the opinion of Sandridge and Thorp,[26] anatomical defects are best detected by means of an endovaginal probe, by measuring rectal length and diameter, puborectalis thickness and angle, thickness and integrity of the internal and external anal sphincters, and curvature of the anal canal.

Anal manometry

Anal manometry measures rectal pressures by a transducer or balloon. Its measurement of rectal sensation evaluates the first feeling, urge, and discomfort; this information is used to distinguish causes of constipation.

When an individual is able to tolerate increased volumes without signs of increased discomfort or the urge to defecate, overflow incontinence may occur. Careful consideration must be given to this evaluation process because individuals able to tolerate only small volumes in the rectum may have an irritable rectum, causing incontinence or urgency. Overflow incontinence and irritable bowel syndrome may mimic rectocele symptoms such as incontinence or incomplete emptying. If misdiagnosis of a rectocele is made, rectocele repair may exacerbate these disorders by causing worsening of symptoms.[16,17,27]

Electromyography and nerve conduction studies

Electromyography (EMG) and nerve conduction studies also have been used to evaluate defecation disorders. Obstetric trauma denervates and causes atrophy of the pelvic floor muscles and tissue, which may lead to subsequent pelvic floor weakness. This denervation may be detected by EMG studies, and pudendal terminal motor latency can be used as a method to detect the causes of pelvic floor weakness.

Colonic transit studies

For colonic transit studies, the patient ingests radio-opaque markers, which are measured and counted in the right colon, left colon, sigmoid colon and rectum. Clinically slow transit time is defined as less than two bowel movements per week over several years. The utility of this test in individuals with rectoceles is debatable: some have normal transit times whereas others have prolonged times.[24] Patients whose symptoms did not improve after repair were found to have longer transit times preoperatively.[20]

MANAGEMENT

Once the clinical diagnosis has been made and (if necessary) confirmed by ancillary studies, the decision to operate or to treat conservatively must be made. Most non-surgical treatments consist of proper bowel training, following an active lifestyle and eating an appropriate amount of dietary fibre.[28,29] These steps are most important when the main complaint is constipation. The only non-surgical therapy available for the prolapse symptoms is oestrogen-replacement therapy in post-menopausal women and the use of a vaginal pessary. In our experience, pessaries have not been very effective in women with isolated symptomatic rectoceles. Indications for surgery should include being symptomatic, having an anatomical defect, or undergoing other pelvic reconstructive surgery with an asymptomatic rectocele.[9]

Symptoms that respond well to surgery include pelvic pressure and a vaginal bulge, vaginal digitalization or splinting (which occurs in 20–75% of symptomatic patients) and outlet-obstruction constipation. Janssen *et al.*[27] noted that repair increased rectal sensitivity, causing the urge to defecate earlier as a positive predictor of a good outcome. In the colorectal literature it has been noted that defecography showing a rectocele greater than or equal to 2 cm with symptoms is also a good indicator for surgery; however, this finding has not been conclusive in all studies.[2] Sullivan *et al.*[30] reported that anoscopic evidence of the rolling down of the anterior rectal wall will be present before surgical correction;[2] however, this may not be valid for all female patients.[27]

Signs and symptoms that are predictive of a poor surgical outcome include a history of use of potent laxatives, incidence of preoperative pain and, possibly, large rectoceles in women who had previously undergone hysterectomy.[20,21,27,31] A few studies in the colorectal literature have noted that hysterectomy disrupts parasympathetic nerves, causing decreased rectal sensation as well as increased rectal compliance, which may not be improved after anatomical correction.[27,31] The persistence or development of dyspareunia after rectocele repair has been variable and is dependent on the surgical technique: levator plication and overnarrowing of the introitus may lead to increased dyspareunia, whereas defect-specific repair has been associated with disappearance or improvement of dyspareunia.[32]

SURGICAL REPAIR

Three different surgical techniques are currently utilized to repair symptomatic rectoceles. Gynaecological surgeons have traditionally advocated a transvaginal repair involving a levatoroplasty. Owing to the development of dyspareunia in some patients and the relatively poor functional outcome of these repairs, recently some gynaecological surgeons have advocated a defect-specific rectocele repair. Colorectal surgeons continue to repair rectoceles via a transanal approach.

Defect-specific rectocele repair

According to Richardson,[3] rectoceles are caused by a variety of breaks in the fascia. He described the most common break as being a transverse separation above the attachment to the perineal body, resulting in a low rectocele. Another common fascial break was explained to result from an obstetric tear or episiotomy that was incorrectly repaired. This midline vertical defect may involve the lower vagina and extend to the vaginal apex. Less-common separations involving a lateral separation down one side of the fascia were also found to exist (Fig. 49.1). Richardson also stated that a U- or L-shaped tear in the fascia might occur. Since Richardson's observations there has been an increased movement among gynaecologists towards site-specific rectocele repair. Richardson recommends performing the repair with a finger in the rectum, so that defects can be easily identified and fascia can be appropriately approximated with interrupted sutures (Fig. 49.2).

Before starting any rectocele repair, the surgeon should approximate the introitus by using Allis clamps bilaterally to help determine how much perineal and vaginal tissue should be excised to correct a

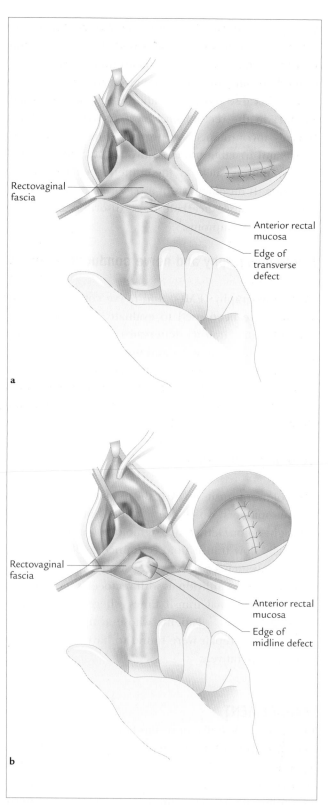

Figure 49.2. *Transverse and midline defect detected on rectal examination. Inset demonstrates a site-specific defect closed with interrupted suture.*

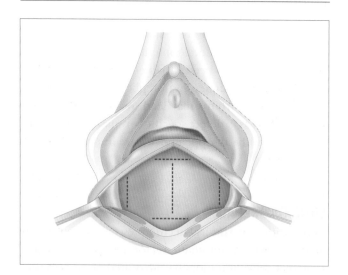

Figure 49.1. *Diagrammatic representation of the various locations where breaks in the rectovaginal septum have been observed in patients with rectocele, as seen through a posterior colporrhaphy incision*

gaping introitus. The repaired opening should accommodate three fingerbreadths, taking into account that the levator ani and perineal muscles are relaxed from general anaesthesia and may further constrict postoperatively and with postmenopausal atrophy. The next step is to place Allis clamps on the posterior perineum; a diamond-shaped perineal incision is made and the overlying skin is removed (Fig. 49.3). The length and width of the perineal incision are dependent on the epithelium needed for restoration of the perineal body. Mayo scissors are used to make a plane in the rectovaginal space. As much fascia is left on the rectum as possible. Sharp dissection is usually required over the perineal body, because of previous scarring from episiotomies. The surgeon performs blunt and sharp dissection to the apex of the vagina. This is continued laterally to the tendinous arch of the levator ani and extends inferiorly to the perineal body.

If perineal lacerations are present, dissections are continued as follows. For grade 3 perineal lacerations, adequate exposure is needed to reapproximate the divided anal sphincter. In complete or grade 4 perineal lacerations, dissection continues to allow enough tissue exposure for the subsequent edge-to-edge anal mucosal suturing to be tension free. Haemostasis is ensured, and irrigation may be used to attain a clean operative field to allow inspection for defects. The rectovaginal fascia is inspected for defects, by the surgeon inserting a finger of the non-dominant hand into the rectum (Fig. 49.4). The rectal wall is brought forwards, distinguishing the uncovered muscularis (fascial

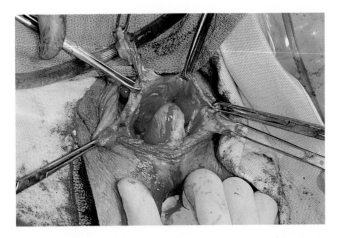

Figure 49.4. *Complete mobilization of the posterior vaginal wall from anterior rectal wall. Rectal examination demonstrates obvious rectocele, with minimal fascia on the anterior rectal wall.*

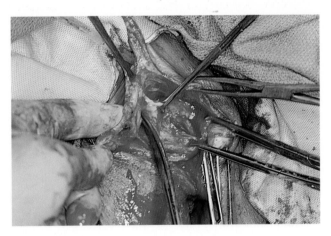

Figure 49.5. *The fascia is being mobilized off the vaginal epithelium.*

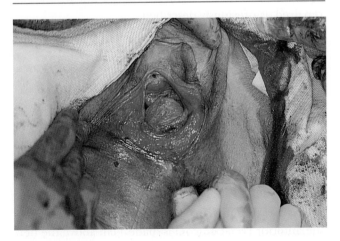

Figure 49.3. *Rectocele demonstrated on rectal examination. Note that perineal skin has been excised.*

defect) from the muscularis covered by the smooth semi-transparent rectovaginal septum. According to the plane of dissection and the location of the defect, frequently the rectovaginal fascia must be mobilized off the lateral vaginal epithelium (Fig. 49.5). After the defect has been identified, Allis clamps are used to grasp the connective tissue (perirectal or rectovaginal fascia), which is pulled over the bare area to facilitate repair (Fig. 49.6). The rectal finger is then used to determine if a defect has been corrected. Next, this area is sewn together with interrupted sutures plicating the fascia over the rectal wall with a no. 2/0 delayed absorbable suture (Fig. 49.7). The surgeons must continuously examine the vaginal calibre to ensure a smooth contour and a diameter of three fingerbreadths.[3,4,6,33,34]

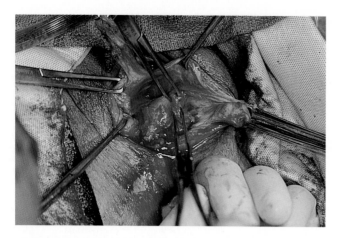

Figure 49.6. *Enough fascia has been mobilized to cover the defect sufficiently.*

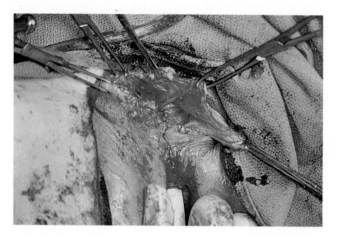

Figure 49.7. *The fascial edges have been sutured together and the defect closed.*

Whereas rectocele repair is accomplished for identification of the fascial defect and re-approximation of the connective tissue, evaluation of the levator hiatus is an entirely different issue. In women who have an enlarged levator hiatus, it may be appropriate to place another set of interrupted sutures horizontally to narrow the levator hiatus. This portion of the operation is not necessary in all patients and is independent of rectocele repair.

Perineorrhaphy is the next step in posterior segment reconstruction. The perineal body consists of the anal sphincter, the superficial and deep transverse perineal muscles, the bulbocavernosus muscles and the junction of the rectovaginal fascia with the anal sphincter. Perineorrhaphy implies identification and reconstruction

of these components. The first step in perineorrhaphy is to remove any old scar tissue to the point that fresh viable tissue is revealed. If a grade 4 laceration is present, the rectal mucosa is completely mobilized off the vaginal wall and reapproximated with interrupted sutures. The external anal sphincter is then reapproximated. After stepwise reapproximation of the transverse perineal muscles, the perineal body is sewn over the sphincter. Finally, the bulbocavernosus muscle ends are attached to the perineal body. This musculofascial complex is covered by suturing the overlying vulvar skin with no. 3/0 suture in a running fashion. Vaginal packing is removed on postoperative day 1 and diet is advanced as tolerated.[33,34]

Traditional transvaginal repair

The traditional rectocele approach has been described and illustrated by Nichols, Wheeless and others.[35,36] The opening of the vagina is as previously described, via a midline incision or by removal of a triangular wedge of vaginal wall. Some surgeons will place an initial row of 2/0 interrupted sutures approximating the rectovaginal fascia. The rectocele is then depressed in the midline with the surgeon's finger to reveal the margin of the puborectalis portion of the levator ani muscle. With the rectocele still depressed, a no. 1/0 absorbable suture is used to suture the margins of the levator ani muscles in an interrupted fashion (Fig.49.2c). After all the sutures have been placed, they are tied.

The posterior vaginal mucosa is appropriately trimmed and closed with either interrupted or continuous 3/0 absorbable suture. The perineal body is repaired as previously described.

Transrectal approach

The transrectal approach was described by Sarles *et al.*[11] In this method, all patients are treated preoperatively with oral laxatives and are given antibiotics: metronidazole (500 mg twice daily for 2 days prior to surgery) and cefuroxime (250 mg i.v. 1 hour before surgery). The anus and vagina are cleansed with povidone-iodine. A Park retractor is inserted into the anal canal to expose the anterior rectal surface. An incision of the anterior rectal mucosa is made 1 cm above the dentate line. The submucosal plane is sharply dissected 8–10 cm from the anal verge. Bleeding is controlled by diathermy. Dissection is performed anteriorly and laterally; the resulting bare areas are plicated using interrupted polyglycolic acid 2/0 sutures 0.5 cm apart; the suture includes the rectal muscle and the rectovaginal septum. If the vaginal mucosa is perforated, the stitch is removed. The mucosal flap at least 6 cm long is excised. A second layer of polyglycolic acid sutures 3/0 close the mucosal defect. Postoperative care includes delaying food by mouth for 48 hours after surgery and slowly advancing the diet over several days.

RESULTS

Few studies have addressed the long-term success of vaginal plastic procedures for treating rectocele. Early recurrence of the rectocele is probably the result of missed and unrepaired support defects. Rectoceles that occur late after repair are usually due to constitutional factors such as weakening of the support tissue as a result of advancing age, chronic straining, post-menopausal atrophy and other factors. These anatomical success rates have ranged from 80[37] to 90%,[4] using any of the three types of repairs. Only a few studies have objectively addressed visceral and sexual function after rectocele repair.[29,32]

COMPLICATIONS

Postoperative complications are reviewed in Table 49.1. These include constipation, incontinence, incomplete rectal emptying, splinting, pain, bleeding and sexual dysfunction.[16] Pain seems to be more persistent and severe after transvaginal surgery.[29,37] Postoperative constipation develops or persists in 44–69% of patients.[1,10,11,37] Rectoceles may cause sexual dysfunction preoperatively and postoperatively. Levator plication will lead to increased dyspareunia due to pressure atrophy of the included muscle and the resulting scarring.[29,35] Vaginal tightness and dyspareunia were also

reported following transanal rectocele repair.[37] Kahn and Stanton[29] suggest that long-term sexual dysfunction may occur after vaginal posterior repair and may be increased with increased age, postmenopausal atrophy and other types of vaginal surgery. However, there is a significant background prevalence of dyspareunia in the general population, which ranges from 17 to 34%.[38] In 1961, a study by Francis and Jeffcoate[39] reported a 50% prevalence of dyspareunia after vaginal surgery, usually from overnarrowing of the introitus. Another study had a dyspareunia rate of 9%, whereas 24% of patients stated there was improvement in their sex life after surgery. The authors concluded that this low rate of dyspareunia was due to early return to sexual intercourse, only 3 weeks after surgery.[40] Kahn and Stanton[29] also reported an increased rate of faecal incontinence, from 4 to 11%, after rectocele repair.

If proctotomy occurs accidentally during repair, the rectum should be repaired in layers. Oral feeding should be delayed until 48 hours after surgery, and is slowly increased from clear liquids, to soft, to low-residue diet over the next 48 hours. Laxatives should be avoided for 4–5 days to keep the terminal rectum and anus free of faecal material. If infection occurs, a rectovaginal fistula may develop.[6]

CONCLUSIONS

The prevalence of surgical repair for urinary incontinence or genital prolapse has exceeded more than 10% of all women who reach the eighth decade of life.[41] With society's gradually ageing population, there will be a large population suffering from rectoceles or defecation disorders. Therefore, it will be important that the clinician is well versed in the proper evaluation of, and the reparative techniques utilized to manage, these defects. More research is needed to understand fully the correlation between anatomical defects and functional derangements that can occur secondary to posterior vaginal wall prolapse.

Table 49.1. *Complications of rectocele repair*

• Bleeding	• Difficulty with bowel emptying
• Constipation	• Faecal incontinence
• Dyspareunia	• Proctotomy
• Pelvic pain/pressure	• Rectovaginal fistula

REFERENCES

1. Mellgren A, Anzen B, Nilsson BY *et al.* Results of rectocele repair: a prospective study. *Dis Colon Rectum* 1995; 38: 7–13

2. Mollen RMHG, van Larrhoven CJHM, Kuijpers JHC. Pathogenesis and management of rectoceles. *Sem Colorectal Surg* 1996; 7: 192–196

3. Richardson AC. The rectovaginal septum revisited: its relationship and its importance in rectocele repair. *Clin Obstet Gynecol* 1993; 36: 976–983

4. Babiarz JW, Raz S. Pelvic floor relaxation. In: Babiarz JW, Raz S (eds) *Female Urology*, 2nd edn. Philadelphia: Saunders, 1996; 445–456

5. Handa VL, Harris TA, Ostergard DR. Protecting the pelvic floor: obstetric management to prevent incontinence and pelvic organ prolapse. *Obstet Gynecol* 1996; 88: 470–478

6. Walters MD. Pelvic floor prolapse: cystocele and rectocele. In: Walters MD, Karram MM (eds) *Clinical Urogynecology*. St Louis: Mosby-Year Book, 1993; 225–236

7. Shorvon PJ, McHugh S, Diamant NE *et al.* Defecography in normal volunteers: results and implications. *Gut* 1989; 30: 1737–1749

8. Nichols DH, Randall CL. Reduction of maternal injuries associated with childbirth. In: Nichols DH, Randall CL (eds) *Vaginal Surgery*, 4th edn. Baltimore: Williams and Wilkins, 1996; 43–57

9. Brubaker L. Rectocele. *Curr Opin Obstet Gynecol* 1996; 8: 376–379

10. Khubchandani IT, Clancy JP III, Rosen L *et al.* Endorectal repair of rectocele revisited. *Br J Surg* 1997; 84: 89–91

11. Sarles JC, Arnaud A, Selezneff I, Olivier S. Endo-rectal repair of rectocele. *Int J Colorectal Dis* 1989; 4: 167–171

12. Nichols DH, Randall CL. Types of prolapse. In: Nichols DH, Randall CL (eds) *Vaginal Surgery*, 4th edn. Baltimore: Williams and Wilkins, 1996; 101–118

13. Sultan AH. Anal incontinence after childbirth. *Curr Opin Obstet Gynecol* 1997; 9: 320–324

14. Sultan AH, Stanton SL. Preserving the pelvic floor and perineum during childbirth – elective caesarean? *Br J Obstet Gynaecol* 1996; 103: 731–734

15. Benson JT. Vaginal approach to posterior vaginal defects: the perineal site. In: Baden WF, Walker T (eds) *Surgical Repair of Vaginal Defects*. New York: Lippincott, 1992; 219–233

16. Kahn MA, Stanton SL. Techniques of rectocele repair and their effects on bowel function. *Int Urogynecol J* 1998; 9: 37–47

17. Johansson C, Nilsson BY, Holmstrom B *et al.* Association between rectocele and paradoxical sphincter response. *Dis Colon Rectum* 1992; 35: 503–509

18. Kelvin FM, Maglinte DDT, Benson JT. Evaluation proctography (defecography): an aid to the investigation of pelvic floor disorders. *Obstet Gynecol* 1994; 83: 307–314

19. Green JR, Soohoo SL. Factors related with rectal injury in spontaneous delivery. *Obstet Gynecol* 1989; 73: 732–736

20. Karlbom U, Graf W, Nilsson S, Pahlman L. Does surgical repair of a rectocele improve rectal emptying? *Dis Colon Rectum* 1996; 39: 1296–1302

21. Murthy VK, Orkin BA, Smith LE, Glassman LM. Excellent outcome using selective criteria for rectocele repair. *Dis Colon Rectum* 1996; 39: 374–378

22. Delemarre JBVM, Kruyt RH, Dorrnbos J *et al.* Anterior rectocele: assessment with radiographic defecography, dynamic magnetic resonance imaging, and physical examination. *Dis Colon Rectum* 1994; 37: 249–259

23. Hutchinson R, Mostafa AB, Kumar D. Rectoceles: are they important? *Int J Colorectal Dis* 1993; 8: 232–233

24. Pucciani F, Rottoli ML, Bologna A *et al.* Anterior rectocele and anorectal dysfunction. *Int J Colorectal Dis* 1996; 11: 1–9

25. Klauser AG, Ting KH, Mangel E *et al.* Interobserver agreement in defecography. *Dis Colon Rectum* 1995; 37: 1310–1316

26. Sandridge DA, Thorp JM. Vaginal endosonography in the assessment of the anorectum. *Obstet Gynecol* 1995; 86: 1007–1009

27. Janssen LWM, van Dijke CF. Selection criteria for anterior rectal wall repair in symptomatic rectocele and anterior rectal wall prolapse. *Dis Colon Rectum* 1994; 37: 1100–1107

28. Infantino A, Masin A, Melega E *et al.* Does surgery resolve outlet obstruction from rectocele? *Int J Colorectal Dis* 1995; 10: 97–100

29. Kahn MA, Stanton SL. Posterior colporrhaphy: its effects on bowel and sexual function. *Br J Obstet Gynaecol* 1997; 104: 82–86

30. Sullivan ES, Leaverton GH, Hardwick CE. Transrectal perineal repair: an adjunct to improved function after anorectal surgery. *Dis Colon Rectum* 1968; 11: 106–114

31. Smith AN, Varma JS, Binnie NR, Papachrysostomou M. Disordered colorectal motility in intractable constipation following hysterectomy. *Br J Surg* 1990; 77: 1361–1366

32. Cundiff GW, Weidner AC, Visco AG *et al.* An anatomic and functional assessment of the discrete defect rectocele repair. *Am J Obstet Gynecol* 1998; 179: 1451–1457

33. Baden WF, Walker T. Evolution of the defect approach. In: Baden WF, Walker T (eds) *Surgical Repair of Vaginal Defects*. New York: Lippincott, 1992; 1–7

34. Baden WF, Walker T. Vaginal approach to posterior vaginal defects: the rectal site. In: Baden WF, Walker T (eds) *Surgical Repair of Vaginal Defects*. New York: Lippincott, 1992; 209–218

35. Nichols DH, Randall CL. Posterior colporrhaphy and perineorrhaphy. In: Nichols DH, Randall CL (eds) *Vaginal Surgery*, 4th edn. Baltimore: Williams and Wilkins, 1996; 257–289

36. Wheeless CR. Posterior repair. In: Wheeless CR (ed) *Atlas of Pelvic Surgery*, 3rd edn. Baltimore: Williams and Wilkins, 1997; 46–49

37. Arnold MW, Stewart WRC, Aguilar PS. Rectocele repair: four years' experience. *Dis Colon Rectum* 1990; 33: 684–687

38. Jamieson DJ, Steege JF. The prevalence of dysmenorrhea, dyspareunia, pelvic pain, and irritable bowel syndrome in primary care practices. *Obstet Gynecol* 1996; 87: 55–58

39. Francis WJA, Jeffcoate TNA. Dyspareunia following vaginal operations. *Br J Obstet Gynaecol* 1961; 68: 1–10

40. Hasses P, Skibsted L. Influence of operations for stress incontinence and/or genital descensus on sexual life. *Acta Obstet Gynecol Scand* 1988; 67: 659–661

41. Olsen AL, Smith VJ, Bergstrom JO *et al.* Epidemiology of surgically managed pelvic organ prolapse and urinary incontinence. *Obstet Gynecol* 1997; 89: 501–506

50

Perineal and primary anal sphincter repairs

A. H. Sultan, M. A. Kahn

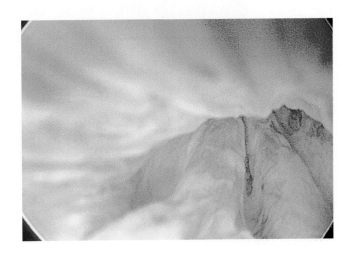

INTRODUCTION

Vaginal delivery – particularly instrumental delivery – is the most frequent cause of perineal and anal sphincter disruption.[1-3] Consequently, vaginal delivery has been directly implicated as a major aetiological factor in urinary/faecal incontinence, dyspareunia and uterovaginal prolapse.[4] Although some symptomatic women may present early, the majority tend to present much later, particularly during the perimenopausal years. This delay may be related to embarrassment or to other aggravating factors associated with pelvic floor weakness, such as ageing, oestrogen deficiency and progression of pelvic neuropathy.[5] It is, therefore, crucial to ensure that obstetric anal sphincter injuries are recognized and repaired appropriately. It is now a widely recognized tenet in pelvic floor and incontinence surgery that the best chance of sustained success follows the first repair. Unfortunately, the majority of perineal and secondary anal sphincter repairs are the sequelae of unrecognized trauma or inadequate primary repair.

ANATOMY

Anatomists regard the perineum as a diamond-shaped area of the pelvic outlet caudal to the pelvic diaphragm (levator ani); the triangular fibromuscular area between the vagina and anal canal is regarded as the perineal body.[6] The borders of the perineum are formed by the inferior pubic rami anteriorly and the sacrotuberous ligaments posteriorly. A transverse line joining the anterior aspect of the ischial tuberosities into an anterior urogenital triangle and a posterior anal triangle (Fig. 50.1) divides the pelvic outlet. The perineal body is made up of interlacing muscle fibres from the bulbospongiosus, superficial transverse perineal and external anal sphincter muscles. Above this level there is a contribution from the longitudinal muscle of the anorectum and the medial fibres of the puborectalis muscle. Therefore, the support of the pelvic structures and, to some extent, of the urogenital hiatus between the levator ani muscles depends upon the integrity of the perineal body. To obstetricians, the term 'perineum' refers largely to this important fibromuscular perineal body between the vagina and anal canal.[4]

PERINEORRHAPHY

Traditionally, the pelvic floor is divided into anterior, middle and posterior compartments. However, injuries to the pelvic floor (especially during parturition) tend to involve more than one compartment and, not infrequently, all three. Perineal surgery is, therefore, more

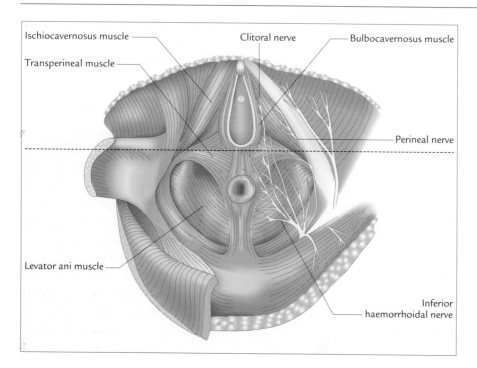

Figure 50.1. *Structures covering the pelvic outlet, as viewed from below. The broken line demarcates the anterior urogenital triangle from the posterior anal triangle. The bulbocavernosus muscle is now known as the bulbospongiosus muscle.*

frequently performed concurrent with (or after) other vaginal, vulval or anorectal surgery. As the vagina is, in effect, a cylinder, surgical correction may cause anatomical distortion in another dimension:

1. Augmentation of the perineal body and vaginal length could result in reduction of the cross-sectional area of the vaginal lumen and genital hiatus (e.g. after perineorrhaphy commonly performed with posterior colporrhaphy, complete perineal lacerations with the cruciate advancement flap and V-Y perineoplasties performed with anal sphincter repairs).
2. Relief of congenital and iatrogenic vaginal stenosis at the expense of vaginal and perineal length (e.g. after Fenton's operation and Z-plasty).

Technique

By horizontally closing a denuded diamond of tissue, the perineorrhaphy enlarges the perineal body[7–9] and lengthens the vagina (Fig. 50.2). Normally, no preoperative preparation other than prophylactic antibiotics is required.

The future calibre of the vaginal introitus is estimated by placing Allis clamps bilaterally on the labia minora and approximating them in the midline. The final hiatus should admit three fingerbreadths easily to avoid postoperative constriction. The superior and inferior apices of a diamond are noted along the vertical axis of the vagina and perineal body (Fig. 50.3a, b). After sharp excision of this diamond of perineal skin and vaginal mucosa, the bulbospongiosus and transverse perineal muscles are also dissected free of the overlying vagina and perineum (Fig 50.3c). These muscles and the fascia of the pubococcygeus are then approximated with 0 deep sutures (Fig. 50.3d, e). The vagina is closed with a 00 running locked stitch which is continued as the wide lateral 'crown' stitch of episiotomy repair. Continuous subcutaneous and subcuticular stitches complete the repair (Fig. 50.3f, g).

Postoperative course

The most common postoperative complication of perineal surgery (especially if combined with other posterior vaginal or anorectal surgery) is urinary retention.[10] Urethral catheterization is usually required for 24 hours. The use of stool softeners is advised for 6 weeks.

Obstetric dehiscence

Dehiscence of episiotomies and obstetric lacerations results in various combinations of perineal, anal sphincter and rectal wall defects. Type I defects retain a perineal body but have breaks in the lowermost fibres of the rectovaginal fascia, puborectalis, transverse perineal muscles and anterior anal sphincter. Type II defects display total absence of the perineal body, resulting from breakdown of third-degree lacerations (through the perineum and anal sphincter) or fourth-degree lacerations (through the perineum, anal sphincter and rectal mucosa)[11] (Fig. 39.4).

Timing of repair and perioperative care

Traditional repair after post-partum breakdown is delayed for 2–3 months to allow maximal revascularization and reinnervation of the affected tissues. However, investigators from Wilford Hall reported their results of early repair of 22 women with fourth-degree dehiscence within 10 days of delivery.[12,13] All wounds were debrided and cleansed according to the degree of necrosis and infection and re-repaired within 1–6 days. Mechanical bowel preparation and broad-spectrum antibiotic prophylaxis were used in all cases. The women consumed nothing orally for 72 hours, followed by a week of a low-residue diet. They were discharged on stool

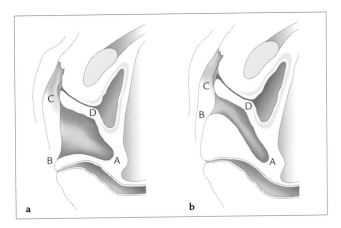

Figure 50.2. *(a) Points AB and CD in the posterior and anterior vaginal wall before perineorrhaphy. (b) Corresponding points AB and CD after perineorrhaphy, demonstrating lengthening of the vagina after reconstruction of the perineum.*

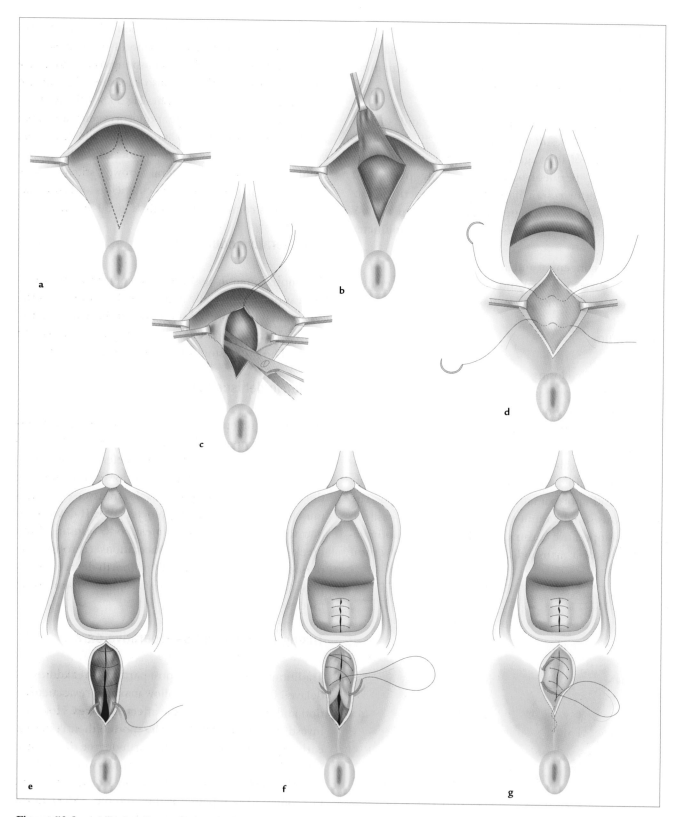

Figure 50.3. *(a) Broken line outlining the diamond area of (b) excision of vaginal and perineal skin. (c) The bulbospongiosus and transverse perineal muscles being dissected free from the overlying vaginal epithelium. (d, e) Plication of (d) perineal muscles and (e) puborectalis fascia. (f) Continuation of the running locked stitch of the vagina to the subcutaneous perineal stitch. (g) The subcuticular stitch.*

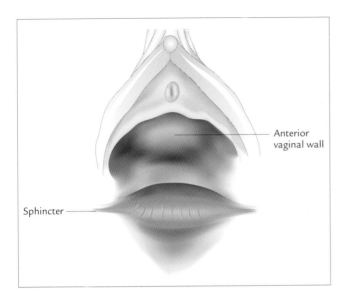

Anterior
vaginal wall

Sphincter

Figure 50.4. *Type II perineal defect. Note the absence of the perineum and the retracted anal sphincter.*

softeners for 6 weeks. Two women developed pinpoint rectovaginal fistulas in the hospital that were repaired easily with anal advancement flaps. By 9 months, all women were totally continent.

The same perioperative management applies to the delayed repairs described below.

Types of repairs

Three types of repairs are described for complete perineal laceration: these are the layered method, the Warren flap[14] and the Noble–Mengert–Fish[15,16] operation. The layered method essentially re-creates the original fourth-degree laceration, with sutures placed in the rectal mucosa. The Warren flap utilizes a segment of vaginal mucosa that is flipped over where it is continuous with the rectal wall and becomes part of the rectum and perineum. In the Noble–Mengert–Fish operation, the rectum is mobilized to the apex of the vagina so that it may be advanced just distal to the anal sphincter; there, it is sutured without tension to the sphincter and perineal skin. The two latter techniques avoid sutures in the rectal mucosa – an important factor in the pre-antibiotic era when they were first described. The disadvantage to these techniques is that the most distal part of rectum is increased in breadth at the very point where the anal sphincter is to be approximated or overlapped. Unless the anterior rectal wall is imbricated

at this point, it also becomes more difficult to approximate the transverse perineal muscles. A paradoxical relaxing incision[17] is no longer used because of the increased potential for anal incontinence.[7] The Noble–Mengert–Fish operation is particularly useful for complex fistulae with an anatomical success rate of 94% and a complete continence rate of 76%.[18]

Layered repair

The operative area is extensively infiltrated with a solution of 20 units of vasopressin in 100 ml normal saline. A curvilinear or cruciate incision is made at the junction of the rectal and anal mucosa, just past the skin dimples formed from the retracted anal sphincter ends (Fig. 50.5a). Extension of the incision to the ischiorectal fat aids in identification of the sphincter ends. The vaginal and rectal walls grasped with Allis clamps are sharply dissected superiorly, until the rectovaginal fascia is visualized, and laterally, until the scarred edges of the anal sphincter are identified. Care must be taken to avoid the posterolateral area where the inferior haemorrhoidal nerves and vessels join the anal sphincter. The junction of the transverse perineal muscles with the anal sphincter is often seen at this point (Fig. 50.5b). Scar tissue is excised from the free margin followed by closure of the defect in the rectal mucosa with a continuous 000 delayed absorbable suture. The suture line is imbricated with interrupted sutures incorporating the submucosa and muscularis of the rectum which, at the anus, includes the inner circular muscle of the sphincter. The external anal sphincter and adherent scar are overlapped or approximated. Puborectalis fascia and transverse perineal muscles are approximated in the midline with 00 delayed absorbable sutures (Fig. 50.5c). The rectovaginal fascia is then joined to these muscles to reconstitute the perineal body. Scarred vaginal mucosa is trimmed and the vagina closed with a running delayed absorbable suture. The remainder of the repair is as in standard episiotomy repair with subcutaneous plication and subcuticular stitches[19] (Fig. 50.5d).

The cruciate incision

A cruciate incision is particularly useful when there has been much destruction of tissue by infection or when there is a congenital lack of tissue, as follows previous surgery for congenital imperforate anus. Advancement and transposition of the V-shaped flaps allows

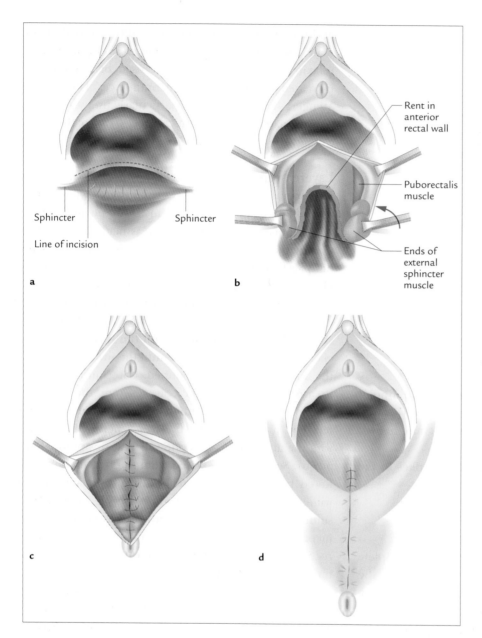

Figure 50.5. *(a) The initial incision for both the layered repair and the rectal advancement repair. (b) After extensive superior and lateral dissection, the junction of the transverse perineal muscle (curved arrow) and the external anal sphincter is seen. (c) Reconstruction of the original fourth-degree laceration. The rectal mucosa has been closed with a running locked stitch. This layer has been covered by imbricating interrupted stitches. The anal sphincter has been reapproximated. (d) Final result as in perineorrhaphy or episiotomy, but after plication of perineal muscles and re-attachment of rectovaginal fascia.*

tension-free reconstruction and augmentation of the perineum[20,21] (Fig. 50.6a, b).

The Warren flap

An inverted V-shaped flap of vaginal mucosa with the sides just lateral to the anal sphincter dimples is dissected off the rectum (Fig. 50.7a, b). Just shy of its junction with the free margin of the rectum, the flap is folded over this hinge-like junction to hang over the anus. This junction must not be injured or the blood supply to the pedicle will be compromised. The anal

sphincter and perineal muscles are plicated (Fig. 50.7c, d) and the vaginal mucosa closed in the customary manner. The vaginal graft is then sutured to the perineal skin (Fig. 50.7e). The tip of the graft retracts with healing.

The Noble–Mengert–Fish operation or rectal advancement

Rectal advancement is begun as in the layered repair. However, instead of closing the defect in the rectal mucosa, the dissection in the rectovaginal space is car-

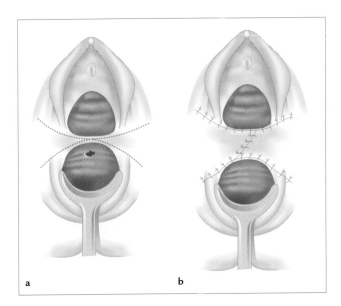

Figure 50.6. *(a) Initial cruciate incision for re-creation of perineum. (b) V-shaped flaps have been advanced and transposed.*

ried out superiorly and laterally enough so that the rectum may be advanced without tension and the free edge is sutured to the perineal skin (Fig. 50.8).

V-Y plasty

After isolated anal sphincter repair, the curvilinear perineal incision becomes distorted from overlapping the ends of the anal sphincter. If one chooses to close the skin, a V-Y plasty may be performed to achieve a better cosmetic result [22] (Fig. 50.9).

Relief of vaginal stenosis

The vaginal introitus may be congenitally narrowed, preventing initial coitus or may be narrowed from previous posterior colpoperineorrhaphy[23] or vulvar surgery.[24]

Relaxing perineoplasties

The simplest relaxing perineoplasty, sometimes called a Fenton's operation, is a vertical incision closed horizontally.[24,25] This widens a tight vaginal introitus and shortens the perineal body (Fig. 50.10a–c). This is the converse of the diamond incision closed vertically in the perineorrhaphy operation. If more than one incision is needed to relieve the stenosis, bilateral transverse incisions may be closed vertically[25] (Fig. 50.10d). An alternative is the Z-plasty (Fig. 50.11)[26] which may be

performed at the time of vulvectomy. A Z is drawn in ink at the 3 o'clock and 9 o'clock positions to produce a symmetrical scar. Each arm of the Z is 1 inch long and the angles of the Z are 60 degrees. Figure 50.11 shows the demarcation and transposition of the flaps required to produce the enlarged introitus.

Y-V flaps,[27] rhomboid flaps[28] or muscular flaps may be utilized if extensive tissue damage from radiation or previous surgery has occurred. The rare perineal hernia following exenteration or rectosigmoid resection may also require such flaps or artificial mesh.[29]

With all plastic repairs, wide dissection and closure of flaps without tension are essential. However, if the skin breaks down, subsequent granulation usually results in an acceptable cosmetic result.

PRIMARY ANAL SPHINCTER REPAIR

Definition

The terms 'primary' and 'secondary' anal sphincter repair can be confusing. Following obstetric anal sphincter rupture (ASR), a repair of the anal sphincter in the immediate post-partum period is usually performed as a primary procedure. When a repair of the anal sphincter is performed to treat faecal incontinence (usually months or years later), it is regarded as a secondary sphincter repair even though a direct primary repair may or may not have been attempted in the post-partum period. Indeed, there is now considerable evidence to suggest that occult or missed mechanical trauma to the anal sphincter during childbirth[1,30,31] is a major aetiological factor in the development of faecal incontinence.[32] In the UK, primary repair is conducted by obstetricians whereas secondary repairs are predominantly performed by colorectal surgeons.

Classification of perineal tears

There is considerable inconsistency in the literature regarding the classification of perineal tears, especially relating to third- and fourth-degree tears.[4] In an attempt to standardize and produce the most descriptive classification, Sultan[33] proposed the following:

- First degree: laceration of the vaginal epithelium or perineal skin only.

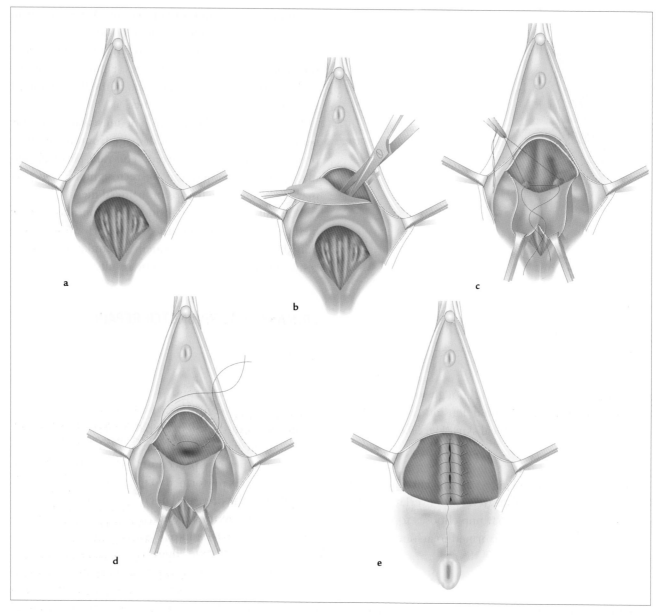

Figure 50.7. *(a) Initial incision for Warren flap. (b) The flap is dissected sharply from the underlying rectum taking care to preserve the free rectovaginal 'hinge'. (c) The anal sphincter ends are joined. (d) The puborectalis muscle may be plicated. (e) The perineal skin is sewn to either side of the flap. The extra tissue protruding will be absorbed with healing.*

- Second degree: involvement of the vaginal epithelium, perineal skin, perineal muscles and fascia but not the anal sphincter.
- Third degree: disruption of the vaginal epithelium, perineal skin, perineal body and anal sphincter muscles. This should be subdivided into:
  - 3a: partial tear of the external sphincter involving less than 50% thickness;
  - 3b: complete tear of the external sphincter;
  - 3c: internal sphincter torn as well.
- Fourth degree: a third-degree tear with disruption of the anal epithelium

Incidence of ASR and outcome of repair

The reported incidence of tears involving the anal sphincter varies between 0.5 and 2.5% in centres where mediolateral episiotomy is practised[3,34,35] and 11% in centres where midline episiotomy is practised.[36] Since 1988, 13 studies[3,34,35,38–47] have evaluated outcome

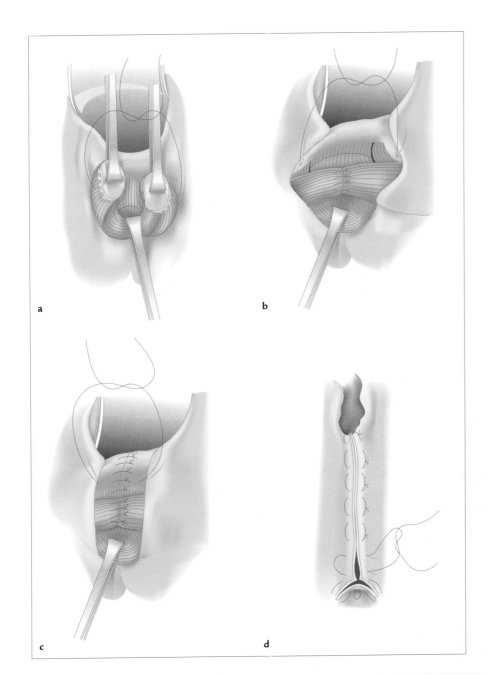

a

b

c

d

Figure 50.8. *(a) The Noble–Mengert–Fish operation begins as in layered closure, but the dissection is extended to the apex of the vagina and the rectum advanced. Each end of the anal sphincter is attached to the rectal wall before plication. (b) The puborectalis muscles are approximated in the midline. (c) The transverse perineal muscles are plicated. (d) The perineal skin is attached in the midline and to the rectal mucosa with horizontal mattress sutures.*

following ASR (Table 50.1). All but one of these studies[40] were performed in centres practising mainly mediolateral episiotomy. On average, about 37% of women continue to suffer from anal incontinence despite primary sphincter repair (Table 50.1). The morbidity would be much higher if other symptoms such as faecal urgency,[3] anal discomfort and dyspareunia[38] were evaluated. The embarrassing symptom of anal incontinence during sexual intercourse is encountered in 72% of symptomatic women.[38]

Anal resting and squeeze pressures are consistently lower in women who previously sustained ASR.[3,35,41,45,46] The anal canal is shorter after repair.[3,35] The development of incontinence does not appear to be directly related to a pelvic neuropathy, as demonstrated by EMG[42,45] and pudendal nerve motor latency conduction studies.[3,32,34] Tetzschner[45] reported that 3-month pudendal latency measurements are longer in women with a risk of incontinence. However, these measurements were still within the normal range and no relationship

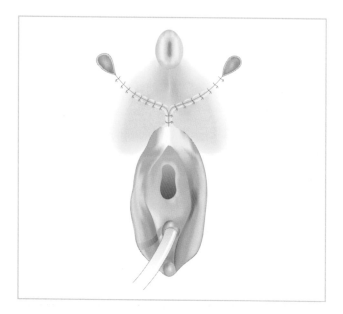

Figure 50.9. *V-Y plasty following anal sphincter repair. The patient is in the prone position.*

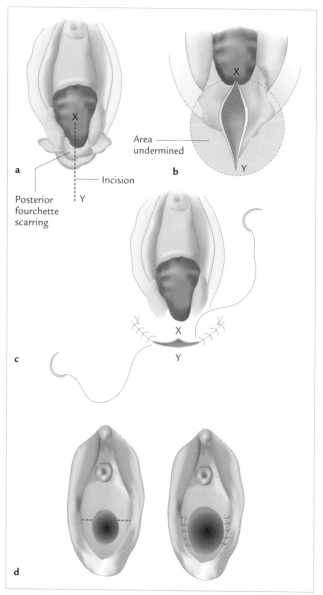

Figure 50.10. *(a) A vertical incision is (b) undermined and (c) closed horizontally (as shown also in the upper part of (d)) to enlarge the vaginal opening. (d) Two lateral horizontal incisions (lower part of illustration) may be closed vertically for further relaxation.*

was demonstrated between abnormal latency and incontinence. Although ASR and repair is invariably associated with some degree of denervation and atrophy, in our opinion none of the current neurophysiological tests available is sensitive or specific enough to quantify pudendal neuropathy. There is, however, strong evidence that poor outcome following primary[3,34,42] and secondary[32] repair is related to persistent mechanical disruption, as demonstrated by anal endosonography, rather than 'pudendal neuropathy'.

The possible reasons for the unsatisfactory outcome following primary sphincter repair are either operator inexperience or inappropriate technique of repair and subsequent management. Neither of these factors has been evaluated by a randomized trial; however, the lack of training and experience of clinicians performing perineal repair has been questioned[48,49] and could well contribute to adverse outcome.

Technique of primary repair

Approximation of the external anal sphincter by placing sutures in the outer fascial layer without traversing the muscle substance was described by Fulsher and Fearl in 1955;[50] however, proper evaluation of outcome with this technique is lacking. The most common type of repair performed by obstetricians is an end-to-end approximation of the anal sphincter by either inter-

rupted or 'figure-of-eight' sutures (Fig.50.12).[3,12] However, as shown in Table 50.1, up to 57% of women have some degree of persistent anal incontinence.

By contrast, when faecal incontinence is due to sphincter disruption, colorectal surgeons favour the 'overlap technique' of sphincter repair (secondary) as described by Parks and McPartlin.[51] Jorge and Wexner[52] reviewed the literature and reported on 21

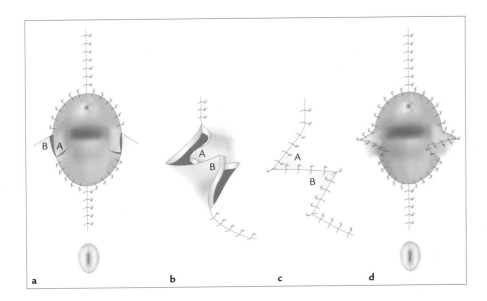

Figure 50.11. *(a) Z-plasty: the initial incisions are (a) made, (b) undermined and (c) transposed; (d) the final result*

studies using the overlap repair with good results ranging from 74 to 100%. Engel *et al.*[32] prospectively studied 55 patients with faecal incontinence undergoing overlap anterior anal sphincter repair and reported a good clinical outcome in 80%. A poor result was associated with an external sphincter defect demonstrated by anal endosonography. By contrast, when overlapping of the external sphincter was demonstrated by anal sonography, it correlated with a favourable outcome.

Despite scepticism from surgeons that overlapping friable torn muscle as a primary procedure is not possible, Sultan *et al.*[49] evaluated the feasibility of this technique in 27 women.

Principles and technique of repair

The principles and technique of repair of ASR are as follows:[49]

1. Repair should be conducted in the operating theatre where there is access to good lighting, appropriate equipment and aseptic conditions.
2. General or regional (spinal, epidural, caudal) anaesthesia is a prerequisite, particularly for overlap repair, as the inherent tone in the sphincter muscle can cause the torn muscle ends to retract within its sheath. Muscle relaxation is necessary to retrieve the ends and overlap without tension.
3. Repair is conducted in the lithotomy position under routine aseptic conditions. The first step is to evalu-

ate the full extent of the injury by a careful vaginal and rectal examination.

4. In the presence of a fourth-degree tear, the torn anal epithelium is repaired with interrupted vicryl 3/0 sutures with the knots tied in the anal lumen. A subcuticular repair of the anal epithelium using 3/0 polydioxanone sulphate (PDS) sutures via the transvaginal approach has also been used, with equal success.
5. The sphincter muscles are repaired with 3/0 PDS clear, monofilamentous sutures, which are less likely than a braided suture to precipitate infection. Non-absorbable monofilament sutures such as nylon or polypropylene (Prolene) are preferred by colorectal surgeons and can be equally effective;

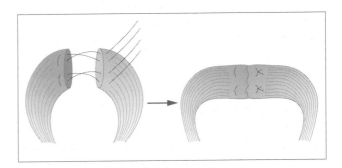

Figure 50.12. *Diagrammatic illustration demonstrating conventional end-to-end approximation of the disrupted anal sphincter with two figure-of-eight sutures.*

Table 50.1. *Incidence of anal incontinence (excluding faecal urgency) following anal sphincter rupture*

Authors*	Year	Country	n	Follow-up (months)	Anal incontinence (%)
Walsh et al.[39]	1996	UK	81	3	20
Crawford et al.[40]	1993	USA	35	12	23
Sorensen et al.[41]	1993	Denmark	38	3	24
Nielsen et al.[42]	1992	Denmark	24	12	29
Go and Dunselman[43]	1988	Netherlands	20	6	33
Uustal Fornell et al.[44]	1996	Sweden	51	6	40
Poen et al.[34]	1998	Netherlands	117	56	40
Sultan et al.[3]	1994	UK	34	2	41
Sorensen et al.[35]	1988	Denmark	25	78	42
Tetzschner et al.[45]	1996	Denmark	72	24–48	42
Haadem et al.[46]	1988	Sweden	62	3	44
Bek and Laurberg[47]	1992	Denmark	121	?	50
Gjessing H et al.[38]	1998	Norway	38	12–60	57

In all studies except those of Crawford et al.[40] (and in some patients in the study by Go and Dunselman[43]), mediolateral episiotomy was practised.

however, they can cause stitch abscesses and the sharp ends of the suture can cause discomfort, necessitating removal.

6. The internal anal sphincter should be identified and any tear should be repaired separately from the external sphincter. The internal anal sphincter lies between the external sphincter and the anal epithelium. It is paler than the striated external sphincter and the muscle fibres run in a circular fashion. The appearance of the internal sphincter can be described as being analogous to the white meat of chicken breast as opposed to the red meat appearance of the external sphincter. The ends of the torn muscle are grasped with Allis forceps and an end-to-end repair is performed with interrupted 3/0 PDS sutures (Fig. 50.13). A torn internal sphincter should be approximated with interrupted sutures, as overlapping can be technically difficult. We advocate primary surgical repair of the internal sphincter, as it has been shown to be beneficial in patients with established anal incontinence.[53]

7. The torn ends of the external anal sphincter are then identified and grasped with Allis tissue forceps. In order that an overlap may be achieved, the muscle may need to be mobilized by dissection with a pair of McIndoe scissors, separating it from the ischio-anal fat laterally. The external sphincter can now be pulled across to overlap in a 'double-breasted' fashion. The torn ends of the external sphincter are then overlapped, as shown in Figures 50.14–50.18, using PDS 3/0 sutures. A conventional end-to-end repair of the external sphincter using figure-of-eight sutures is shown in Figure 50.12.

8. Great care should be exercised in reconstructing the perineal muscles to provide support to the sphincter repair. The anal sphincter is more likely to be traumatized during a subsequent vaginal delivery in the presence of a short deficient perineum. Muscles of the perineal body are reconstructed with interrupted vicryl 2/0 sutures after closing the vaginal epithelium with a continuous vicryl 3/0 suture. Lastly, the perineal skin is approximated with a vicryl 3/0 subcuticular suture.

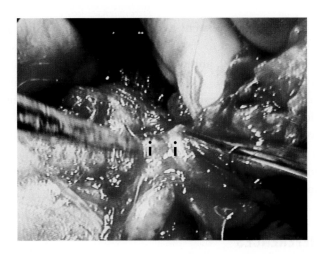

Figure 50.13. *End-to-end approximation of the torn ends of the internal anal sphincter (i). (Reproduced from ref. 49 with permission.)*

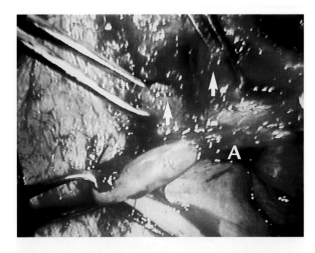

Figure 50.15. *The torn ends of the external anal sphincter (arrows) are being elevated with two pairs of Allis forceps (A, anal epithelium). (Reproduced from ref. 49 with permission.)*

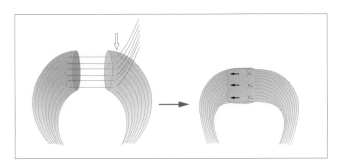

Figure 50.14. *The technique of overlap repair of the external anal sphincter. The first suture is inserted about 1.5 cm from the torn edge of the muscle (open arrow) and carried through to within 0.5 cm of the edge of the other arm of external sphincter. A second row of sutures (small arrows) is inserted to attach the loose end of the overlapped muscle.*

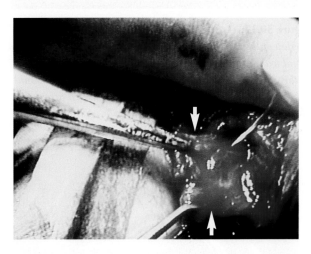

Figure 50.16. *The full width of the external sphincter (arrows) after mobilization. (Reproduced from ref. 49 with permission.)*

9. Intravenous antibiotics (cefuroxime 1.5 g and metronidazole 1 g) should be commenced intra-operatively and continued orally (cefuroxime 500 mg three times daily; metronidazole 400 mg three times daily) for 1 week. Although there are no randomized trials to substantiate benefit of this practice, the development of infection may jeopardize repair and lead to incontinence or fistula formation.

10. As passage of a large bolus of hard stool may disrupt the repair, a stool softener (lactulose 10 ml three times daily) and a bulking agent such as Fybogel (ispaghula husk, one sachet twice daily) is prescribed for at least 2 weeks postoperatively. Bowel confinement (medical colostomy) is still being practised by some clinicians, who are concerned that the passage of formed stool might disrupt a freshly repaired anal epithelium and sphincter muscle. However, a prospective, randomized, surgeon-blinded trial (n = 54) revealed that outcome of reconstructive anorectal surgery was not adversely affected by omission of bowel confinement.[54]

Tetzschner *et al.*[45] found that the frequency of anal incontinence increased from 17% at 3 months (n = 94) to 42% at 2–4 years *post partum* (n = 72). Five of the 17

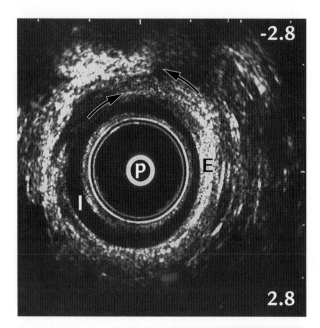

Figure 50.17. *Anal endosonographic image demonstrating overlap of the two ends of the external sphincter. P, probe in anal canal with arrow showing its outer limit. Immediately adjacent to this is the anal epithelium. I, internal sphincter; E, external sphincter. The overlap can be seen between the open arrows. (Reproduced from ref. 49 with permission.)*

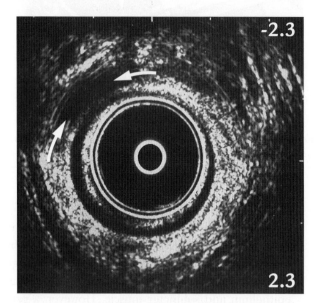

Figure 50.18. *Anal endosonographic image demonstrating an external sphincter defect (between arrows) in a woman complaining of faecal incontinence following an end-to-end repair. The arrows overlie the two retracted ends of the muscle. (Reproduced from ref. 49 with permission.)*

women who underwent a subsequent vaginal delivery were incontinent to flatus before delivery: two of these five experienced an increase in frequency of flatus incontinence; in the remaining three, symptoms remained unchanged. Only one (6%) of the 17 women developed anal incontinence (flatus only) *de novo*. No woman developed frank faecal incontinence following a subsequent vaginal delivery. This is important information for clinicians counselling women about the mode of delivery in a subsequent pregnancy.

REFERENCES

1. Sultan AH, Kamm MA, Hudson CN *et al.* Anal sphincter disruption during vaginal delivery. *N Engl J Med 1993;* 329: 1905–1911

2. Sultan AH, Johanson RB, Carter JE. Occult anal sphincter trauma following randomized forceps and vacuum delivery. *Int J Gynecol Obstet* 1998; 61: 113–119

3. Sultan AH, Kamm MA, Hudson CN, Bartram CI. Third degree obstetric anal sphincter tears: risk factors and outcome of primary repair. *Br Med J* 1994; 308: 887–891

4. Sultan AH, Kamm MA, Bartram CI, Hudson CN. Perineal damage at delivery. *Contemp Rev Obstet Gynaecol* 1994; 6: 18–24

5. Snooks SJ, Swash M, Mathers SE, Henry MM. Effect of vaginal delivery on the pelvic floor: a 5-year follow-up. *Br J Surg* 1990; 77: 1358–1360

6. Last RJ. *Anatomy, Regional and Applied.* 7th edn. London: Churchill Livingstone, 1984; 345–356

7. Wiskind AK, Thompson JD. Fecal incontinence and rectovaginal fistulas. In: Rock JA, Thompson JA (eds) *Te Linde's Operative Gynecology.* Philadelphia: Lippincott/ Raven, 1996; 1207–1236

8. Nichols DH. Posterior colporrhaphy and perineorrhaphy: separate and distinct operations. *Am J Obstet Gynecol* 1991; 164: 714–721

9. Nichols DH, Randall CL. Posterior colporrhaphy and perineorrhaphy. In: Nichols DH, Randall CL (eds) *Vaginal Surgery.* Baltimore: Williams and Wilkins: 1989; 269–293

10. Arnold MW, Stewart WR, Aguilar PS. Rectocele repair. Four years' experience. *Dis Colon Rectum* 1990; 33: 684–687

11. Rosenheim NB, Genadry RR, Woodruff JD. An anatomic classification of rectovaginal septal defects. *Am J Obstet Gynecol* 1980; 137: 439–442

12. Hauth JC, Gilstrap LC III, Ward SC, Hankins GD. Early repair of an external sphincter ani muscle and rectal mucosal dehiscence. *Obstet Gynecol* 1986; 67: 806–809

13. Hankins GDV, Hauth JC, Gilstrap LC III *et al.* Early repair of episiotomy dehiscence. *Obstet Gynecol* 1990; 75: 48–51

14. Warren JC. A new method of operation for the relief of rupture of the perineum through the sphincter and rectum. *Gynecol Soc* 1882; 7: 322–330

15. Noble GH. A new operation for complete laceration of the perineum designed for the purpose of eliminating danger of infection from the rectum. *Trans Am Gynecol Soc* 1902; 27: 357–363

16. Mengert WF, Fish SA. Anterior rectal wall advancement. Technic for repair of complete perineal laceration and rectovaginal fistula. *Obstet Gynecol* 1955; 3: 262–267

17. Miller NF, Brown W. The surgical treatment of complete perineal tears in the female. *Am J Obstet Gynecol* 1937; 34: 196–209

18. Veronikis DK, Nichols DH, Spino C. The Noble–Mengert–Fish operation revisited: a composite approach for persistent rectovaginal fistulas and complex perineal defects. *Am J Obstet Gynecol* 1998; 179: 1411–1417

19. Cunningham FG, MacDonald PC, Grant NF *et al.* *Williams Obstetrics*, 20th edn. Stamford: Appleton and Lange, 1997; 344–346

20. Corman H, Lowe R. Colon and rectal trauma. *Surg Clin North Am* 1978; 58: 519

21. Corman, ML. Anal incontinence following obstetrical injury. *Dis Colon Rectum* 1985; 28: 86–89

22. Cherry DA, Greenwald ML. Anal incontinence. In: Beck DE, Wexner SD (eds). *Fundamentals of Anorectal Surgery*. New York: McGraw-Hill, 1992; 104–130

23. Jeffcoate TNA. Posterior colpoperineorrhaphy. *Am J Obstet Gynecol* 1959; 77: 490–502

24. Copeland LJ. Reconstructive surgery in gynecologic oncology In: Gershenson DM, DeCherney AH, Curry SL (eds) *Operative Gynecology*. Philadelphia: Saunders, 1993; 607–627

25. Jimerson GK. Management of postoperative introital and vaginal stenosis. *Obstet Gynecol.* 1977; 50: 719–722

26. Scott JW, Gilpin CR, Vence CS, Vulvectomy, introital stenosis, and Z plasty. *Am J Obstet Gynecol* 1963; 85: 132–133

27. Braren V. Vaginal amplification using a posterolateral Y-V plasty. *Pediatr Articles* 1981; 126: 645–647

28. Helm CW, Hatch KD, Partridge EE. The rhomboid transposition flap for repair of the perineal defect after radical vulvar surgery. *Gynecol Oncol* 1993; 50: 164–167

29. So JB, Palmer MT, Shellito PC. Postoperative perineal hernia. *Dis Colon Rectum* 1997; 40: 954–957

30. Donnelly V, Fynes M, Campbell D *et al.* Obstetric events leading to anal sphincter damage. *Obstet Gynecol* 1998; 92: 955–961

31. Chaliha C, Kalia V, Sultan AH *et al.* Anal function: effect of pregnancy and delivery. *Neurourol Urodyn* 1998; 17: 417–418

32. Engel AF, Kamm MA, Sultan AH *et al.* Anterior anal sphincter repair in patients with obstetric trauma. *Br J Surg* 1994; 81: 1231–1234

33. Sultan AH. Obstetrical perineal injury and anal incontinence. *Clin Risk* 1999; 5: 193–196

34. Poen AC, Felt-Bersma RJF, Strijers RLM *et al.* Third-degree obstetric perineal tear: long-term clinical and functional results after primary repair. *Br J Surg* 1998; 85: 1433–1438

35. Sorensen SM, Bondesen H, Istre O, Vilmann P. Perineal rupture following vaginal delivery. *Acta Obstet Gynecol Scand* 1988; 67: 315–318

36. Hueston WJ. Factors associated with the use of episiotomy during vaginal delivery. *Obstet Gynecol* 1996; 87: 1001–1005

37. Sultan AH. Anal incontinence after childbirth. *Curr Opin Obstet Gynecol* 1997; 9: 320–324

38. Gjessing H, Backe B, Sahlin Y. Third degree obstetric tears; outcome after primary repair. *Acta Obstet Gynecol Scand* 1998; 77: 736–740

39. Walsh CJ, Mooney EF, Upton GJ, Motson RW. Incidence of third-degree perineal tears in labour and outcome after primary repair. *Br J Surg* 1996; 83: 218–221

40. Crawford LA, Quint EH, Pearl ML, DeLancey JOL. Incontinence following rupture of the anal sphincter during delivery. *Obstet Gynecol* 1993; 82: 527–531

41. Sorensen M, Tetzschner T, Rasmussen OO *et al.* Sphincter rupture in childbirth. *Br J Surg* 1993; 80: 392–394

42. Nielsen MB, Hauge C, Rasmussen OO *et al.* Anal endosonographic findings in the follow-up of primarily sutured sphincteric ruptures. *Br J Surg* 1992; 79: 104–106

43. Go PMNYH, Dunselman GAJ. Anatomic and functional results of surgical repair after total perineal rupture at delivery. *Surg Gynecol Obstet* 1988; 166: 121–124

44. Uustal Fornell EK, Berg G, Hallbook O *et al.* Clinical consequences of anal sphincter rupture during vaginal delivery. *J Am Coll Surg* 1996; 183: 553–558

45. Tetzschner T, Sorensen M, Lose G, Christiansen J. Anal and urinary incontinence in women with obstetric anal sphincter rupture. *Br J Obstet Gynaecol* 1996; 103: 1034–1040

46. Haadem K, Ohrlander S, Lingman G. Long-term ailments due to anal sphincter rupture caused by delivery – a hidden problem. *Eur J Obstet Gynecol Reprod Biol* 1988; 27: 27–32

47. Bek KM, Laurberg S. Risks of anal incontinence from subsequent vaginal delivery after a complete obstetric anal sphincter tear. *Br J Obstet Gynaecol* 1992; 99: 724–726

48. Sultan AH, Kamm MA, Hudson CN. Obstetric perineal tears: an audit of training. *J Obstet Gynaecol* 1995; 15: 19–23

49. Sultan AH, Monga AK, Kumar D, Stanton SL. Primary repair of obstetric anal sphincter rupture using the overlap technique. *Br J Obstet Gynaecol* 1999; 106: 318–323

50. Fulsher RW, Fearl CL. The third-degree laceration in modern obstetrics. *Am J Obstet Gynecol* 1955; 69: 786–793

51. Parks AG, McPartlin JF. Late repairs of injuries of the anal sphincter. *Proc R Soc Med* 1971; 64: 1187–1189

52. Jorge JMN, Wexner SD. Etiology and management of fecal incontinence. *Dis Colon Rectum* 1993; 36: 77–97

53. Meyenberger C, Bertschinger P, Zala GF, Buchmann P. Anal sphincter defects in fecal incontinence: correlation between endosonography and surgery. *Endoscopy* 1996; 28: 217–224

54. Nessim A, Wexner SD, Agachan F *et al.* Is bowel confinement necessary after anorectal reconstructive surgery? A prospective, randomized, surgeon-blinded trial. *Dis Colon Rectum* 1999; 42: 16–23

51

Faecal incontinence: postanal and direct sphincter repair

D. Kumar, M. Lamah

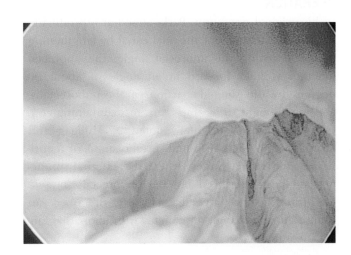

INTRODUCTION

Faecal incontinence is a complex and multifactorial problem. Surgical treatment can be expected to deal with only limited aspects of this complex problem. In order to achieve a successful outcome the patient must be carefully evaluated; in particular, a general neurological disorder should be excluded. It must also be ensured that an adequate trial of medical therapy has been carried out and that there are clear indications to perform surgical intervention. In patients with neuropathic faecal incontinence with no evidence of sphincter trauma, a postanal repair should probably be the initial operation. If, however, there is evidence of sphincter injury and this is confirmed on endoanal ultrasonography, a direct sphincter repair should be carried out.

Posterior plication of the external anal sphincter without attention to the puborectalis was first suggested by Nesselrod[1] in 1950. The importance of including the puborectalis in this procedure was later noted by Sir Alan Parks, who modified Nesselrod's original operation and introduced the operation of postanal repair. His original paper[2] should be obligatory reading for anyone contemplating this form of surgery. Parks used postanal repair in patients with rectal prolapse in order to avoid entering the pelvis in young women and to avoid the risk of developing an ivalon sponge sarcoma. It was also considered the operation of choice in patients with idiopathic or neurogenic incontinence.

ANATOMICOPHYSIOLOGICAL BASIS OF THE OPERATION

In his original operation, Parks aimed at reproducing the normal anatomy of the anal canal by lengthening it and restoring the anorectal angle: the anorectal junction is held forward at an angle of about 90 degrees by the sling-like action of the puborectalis, and was thought to be important in maintaining continence. This was originally noted by Milligan and Morgan, who demonstrated preservation of continence after fistula surgery where the external sphincter had been sacrificed but the puborectalis muscle was intact. Many investigators have described an obtuse anorectal angle in patients with idiopathic faecal incontinence.

Different theories have been postulated to explain the importance of the puborectalis and anorectal angle in maintaining faecal continence. Parks thought that this angle was vital to continence through the creation of a 'flap valve' mechanism,[3] in which increased intra-abdominal pressure compressed the anterior rectal wall against the pelvic floor. The essential part of this operation was, therefore, the reconstruction of the anorectal angle, with the restoration of a reliable flap valve mechanism which would not give way under stress. A subsidiary effect of the procedure was that shortening of the effective length of the puborectalis would allow those muscle fibres that were still innervated to function more efficiently. In addition, the repair includes ileococcygeus and pubococcygeus muscles, which are usually less degenerate than the lower muscles.

More recent work has cast doubts upon these concepts, suggesting that the anorectal angle has little, if any, role in the continence mechanism, for the following reasons:

- Some patients with idiopathic faecal incontinence do not have an obtuse anorectal angle.[4,5]
- Studies of pressure changes in the anal canal during the Valsalva manoeuvre suggest that continence is maintained by sphincteric action rather than a flap valve effect.[6]
- Proctographic techniques have demonstrated that, during periods of increased intra-abdominal pressure, the anterior rectal wall is not in contact with, and does not occlude, the upper anal canal.
- Anal pressures have been found to be at least $10\,cmH_2O$ higher than rectal pressures, which is the opposite gradient to that expected in the operation of a flap valve.

The importance of the anorectal angle in maintaining continence thus remains questionable and, as discussed below, has cast doubts on the anatomical rationale of postanal repair in restoring continence.

The operation is performed by approximating the pelvic floor and sphincter muscles behind the anorectal junction, displacing them anteriorly and increasing the angulation at this point. The repair is best performed by approaching the muscles from their inner surface so that sutures can be placed from the limb of one side of each muscle across to the equivalent part of the other side.

OPERATIVE TECHNIQUE

Preoperative preparation consists of a full bowel preparation and prophylactic antibiotics. The patient is placed in the lithotomy position and the area prepared. Some surgeons prefer to infiltrate the site with a mixture of saline solution and adrenaline (1:200 000); this helps to reduce capillary bleeding and aids the dissection between internal and external sphincters. A V- or U-shaped circumanal incision is made in the perineum at a distance approximately 6 cm behind the anus (if placed closer to the anal canal, the wound may be pulled towards the anal canal, increasing the risk of infection). The skin anterior to the incision is then raised until the anal verge is reached.

The inferior borders of the internal and external sphincters are then exposed and the relatively avascular plane between the two muscles is dissected. The external sphincter is usually red, whereas the internal sphincter is white; however, when the external sphincter is degenerate, the distinction between the two muscles may become blurred. The internal sphincter is separated from the lower part of the external sphincter for approximately half of its circumference. The dissection is continued upwards in the same plane, lifting the rectum upwards and medially, until the sling of the puborectalis muscle is reached at the anorectal junction. At this point, the condensation of Waldeyer's fascia and the levator fascia is encountered where it is attached to both the rectal wall and the puborectalis muscle.

The Waldeyer's fascia is incised near the muscle to enable the rectum to be separated from the pelvic floor, so providing access to the superior aspect of the pelvic floor muscles. The rectum is then held forwards by retractors, enabling access to the origin of the levator ani on both sides. The highest and most lateral points of the levators are then identified on each sides. Nonabsorbable polypropylene sutures are placed under the ileococcygeus muscle on one side, and then on the other side. About three layers are placed at this level and tied loosely, to form a lattice across the pelvis.

A second layer of sutures is then placed in the upper part of the pubococcygeus and again tied lightly to form a lattice. The most important layer is the one inserted into the puborectalis muscle. The latter is the strongest and thickest, and the sutures are again placed as near to the pubis as possible and tied so that the muscles are approximated. Finally, another layer of sutures is placed in the external sphincter below the puborectalis. A suction drain is placed in the supralevator space.

As a result of the repair, the anterior skin flap becomes drawn forward, and cannot be sutured to the posterior skin edge without undue tension. The wound is, therefore, best reconstituted in the shape of a V-Y plasty and partially closed, allowing the central defect to heal by secondary intention.

Postoperatively, it is essential that the patient does not strain during defecation as this might disrupt the repair. This is achieved by prescribing a combination of an osmotic and bulk-forming laxative for a period of approximately 2 weeks. In the longer term, it is essential that straining habits are not resumed as this will weaken the repair. A combination of bulk-forming agents and glycerine suppositories may be necessary in the intermediate-to-long term

RESULTS OF POSTANAL REPAIR

Following encouraging results in its early years, postanal repair was established as the standard operation for idiopathic faecal incontinence. In his original series, Parks reported excellent function in 83% of patients.[2]

Similarly, Braun et al.[7] have found an improvement in continence in 26 (84%) of 31 patients undergoing the procedure for idiopathic incontinence, although the mean follow-up was only 12 months, and a successful clinical outcome did not appear to be related to an improvement in sphincter pressures or to a reduction of the anorectal angle.

These results have not been reproduced, subsequent series reporting success rates varying from 13 to 88% in restoring continence to both solid and liquid stool. Furthermore, results are thought to deteriorate further with time, less than one-third of patients still having good function after 3 years. In a long-term follow-up study of 124 patients undergoing postanal repair for faecal incontinence, Yoshioka and Keighley[8] found that, even though incontinence was improved in 81% of patients at a median follow-up of 5 years, 60% of patients still claimed urgency, 76% still leaked faeces and 52% continued to wear pads after the operation, indicating a poor quality of continence after postanal repair. Maximum resting anal pressure and maximum squeeze pressure did not change significantly after the operation, either in patients whose symptoms improved or in those who had no improvement.

In a long-term follow-up of 36 patients who had undergone postanal repair for major faecal incontinence, Jameson *et al.*[9] found that, at a median of 25 months after the procedure, only 53% of patients had maintained some improvement in continence, compared with 83% at 6 months. There was a trend toward a more favourable outcome in patients with greater squeeze pressures preoperatively, but other tests were not found to have any of long-term predictive value.

In a retrospective study of 38 patients, Engel *et al.*[10] found that 50% of patients were satisfied after a median follow-up period of 43 months, although only 21% were fully continent. Similarly, in a retrospective study of 37 patients,[11] only 46% of patients were found to be continent after a median follow-up of 38 months. Setti Carraro *et al.*[12] followed patients for a median period of 6.2 years and found that, in one-third of patients, incontinence was relieved and in another third there was improved frequency of incontinent episodes; these authors maintain that the procedure still has an important place in the management of neurogenic faecal incontinence. They found that there was no correlation between preoperative clinical and physiological factors and clinical outcome, pudendal nerve terminal motor latency (PNTML) being the only preoperative physiological variable that correlated significantly with long-term outcome. They also found that the presence of an anterior defect did not relate to outcome.

More recently, Rieger *et al.*[13] have found improvement in symptoms in only 11 of 19 (58%) patients at a median follow-up period of 8 years, although this was still felt to be important as these patients had few alternatives other than complicated reconstructive procedures or a stoma. Furthermore, the outcome in this series was not influenced by the results of preoperative anal manometry, and although five sphincter defects were found by ultrasonography in six patients, such defects did not preclude improvement from postanal repair.

SIGNIFICANCE OF ANATOMICAL AND PHYSIOLOGIC PARAMETERS

Athanasiadis *et al.*[14] have studied the long-term results of postanal repair for idiopathic faecal incontinence

in 31 patients and, at median 4.2 years' follow-up, found no significant change in resting and maximum squeeze pressures, pelvic descent or anorectal angle postoperatively. Electromyographic (EMG) parameters did not change significantly after the operation, although the mean PNTML increased from 2.38 to 2.59 ms after surgery ($p > 0.05$). In an attempt to determine the reasons for failure to improve faecal incontinence after postanal repair, Snooks *et al.*[15] studied differences in electrophysiological and manometric parameters before and after surgery, but found no significant differences between resting and voluntary contraction anal canal pressures and single-fibre EMG fibre density values before and after postanal repair. However, a significant increase in PNTML after postanal repair suggested that, in patients with no improvement following the operation, a continuing neuropathic process may be taking place. This finding has been confirmed by an independent study by Laurberg *et al.*,[16] who found increased fibre density in the external anal sphincter and PNTML after surgery in patients who were symptomatically improved. They suggested that progression of neurogenic damage to the pelvic floor muscles after postanal repair may be caused by the operation, and that it may be responsible for the poor functional outcome noted in some patients.

Rainey *et al.*[17] also found that neither the anorectal angle nor anal canal length bore any relation to the results of surgery in 42 patients treated with postanal repair, although pudendal neuropathy, identified in 74% of subjects, slightly reduced the chance of success. Similarly, Womack *et al.*[18] found no significant change in the anorectal angle postoperatively, suggesting that postanal repair need not be restricted to patients with widening of the anorectal angle, as its beneficial effects did not appear to be related to reduction of this angle. In contrast to the foregoing evidence against a significant effect of the operation on anatomical and physiological parameters, Browning and Parks[19] found an increase in anal canal length and anal pressures in patients who had a successful clinical outcome following postanal repair.

In summary, the criticism of this operation is that it may restore anatomy rather than function, because an inconsistent relationship exists between clinical results and the effect of the procedure on the anorectal angle, squeeze pressure and length of anal canal postoperatively, and a success outcome does not necessarily depend on a resultant increase in anal pressures or change in anorectal angle.

The poor results obtained with postanal repair, together with the more recent realization that the commonest cause of anal incontinence in healthy women is unrecognized damage to the anal sphincter during childbirth,[20] has led to the development of direct sphincter repairs, alone or in combination with levatorplasty.

DIRECT ANTERIOR SPHINCTER REPAIR

Sphincter repair is the procedure of choice where there is a defined defect in the external anal sphincter ring. Anterior sphincter injuries usually follow obstetric trauma and are best managed by direct primary repair, when possible. Most sphincter repairs are done secondarily, however, because of unrecognized injury, contraindication to primary repair at the time of injury, or failed primary repair. Preoperative EMG mapping and endoanal ultrasonography assist in the identification of divided ends.

Historically, delayed repair of anal sphincter injury has involved excision of the scar, with direct apposition of the muscle ends.[21,22] Difficulty in identifying cut ends and poor suture-holding ability of muscle led to failures, and alternative methods were later suggested where scar tissue was not excised but the sphincter muscle ring was tightened by plication. The results were equally disappointing, but a technical advance came in the early 1970s, when Parks and McPartlin described the overlapping suture technique.[23] The procedure was later modified by Slade *et al.*[24] and has since been widely adopted. The principle of the procedure includes adequate mobilization of the external anal sphincter to avoid tension in the repair, preservation of the scar tissue to anchor the sutures and overlapping of the fibromuscular divided ends, creating a bulking effect, thus increasing the area of contact and reducing the chance of suture disruption. The other aims of the operation are to lengthen and tighten the anal canal (thereby increasing resting pressure) and restoration of the position of the transition zone (thus improving sensation and reducing incontinence).

Operative technique

Preoperatively, the patient undergoes a mechanical bowel preparation and receives prophylactic antibiotics. The procedure is carried out under general anaesthesia with the patient positioned in the lithotomy or prone jackknife position.

A curvilinear circumanal incision is made (Fig. 51.1). The intersphincteric space is entered, as in the operation of postanal repair, and scar tissue in the midline is divided. Dissection is carried out on the outer surface of the sphincter for 1.5–2 cm with countertraction applied by a tissue-holding forceps. Care is taken not to damage the nerve supply that enters the muscle between the 2 and 3 o'clock positions. Reconstruction consists of an overlapping repair with interrupted mattress sutures of a non-absorbable material (Fig. 51.2). Some surgeons prefer to use absorbable sutures. The skin is closed in a V-Y manner (Fig. 51.3) in order to increase the anovaginal distance, but the central portion is left open (Fig. 51.4). Postoperatively, laxatives are prescribed, as for postanal repair.

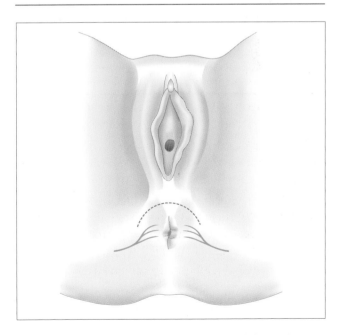

Figure 51.1. *The site of the circumanal incision. Care must be taken to avoid the branches of the pudendal nerve.*

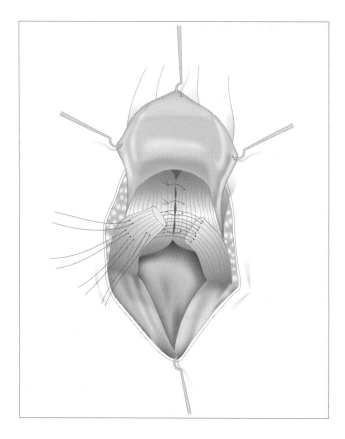

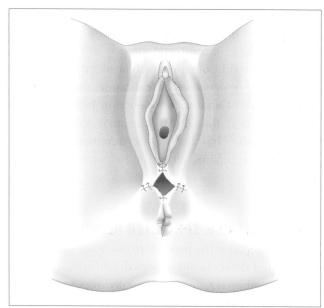

Figure 51.4. *The incision is closed partly to cover the Prolene suture knots. Part of the incision is left open to provide adequate drainage.*

Figure 51.2. *Mattress sutures are placed through the mobilized external sphincter muscle ends to achieve an overlap sphincter repair.*

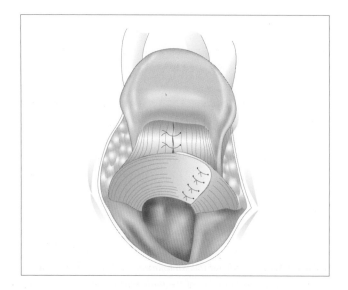

Figure 51.3. *The sutures are tied firmly but not tightly, overlapping the muscle ends.*

Results of direct sphincter repair

Many authors using this procedure have now published their results, and these have generally been encouraging, continence to solid and liquid stool being reported in approximately 70–80% of patients[25–29] (Table 51.1). Some studies have also shown good correlation between functional improvement of continence, objective physiological measures and ultrasonographic appearance.

Factors affecting the outcome include age, obesity, sepsis, the cause of sphincter damage and previous attempts at repair. Repeated sphincter repair can be performed after one or more failed attempts, especially if suture disruption is suspected.

Although sphincter repair has also been advocated in idiopathic or neurogenic incontinence, the results are generally poor. Patients with obstetric injury and prolonged PNTML should, therefore, be advised of the limited success of sphincter repair. In these patients, sphincter repair may, however, be combined with postanal repair (see below).

Table 51.1. *Functional results of overlapping sphincteroplasty*

Author and ref. no.	Results (%)		
	Continent of solids and liquids	Continent of solids only	Poor
Browning and Motson[25]	78	13	9
Fang[26]	89	7	1
Ctercteko et al.[27]	64	5	26
Fieshman et al.[28]	72	22	6
Wexner et al.[29]	76	19	5

The use of diverting colostomy at the time of primary repair is still controversial It is considered desirable in the presence of a large sphincter defect or in a previously failed repair, but successful results of sphincter repair have been reported without a defunctioning colostomy irrespective of the indication.

An alternative to postanal repair is an anterior approach, which has two theoretical advantages: an overlooked anterior sphincter injury can be repaired at the same time, and a coexisting rectocele is corrected by the levatorplasty.

A transverse incision is made midway between the vagina and anus. A careful, sharp dissection is then made between the posterior wall of the vagina and anterior wall of the rectum, allowing the anorectum to be pushed anteriorly. Both limbs of the puborectal and pubococcygeal muscles are then exposed on either side of the midline, and two layers of two or three sutures are used to approximate the levator ani muscles across the midline, giving a perineal body 2–3 cm high. The skin is closed with a perineoplasty, whereby the perineum is lengthened and elevated.

Good short-term results have been obtained by some groups,[30] and long-term follow-up by Osterberg et al.[31] has shown an excellent or good result in 74% of patients with an obstetric injury and in 45% of patients in the idiopathic group. The presence of a cloaca and a young age were associated with a favourable outcome in the obstetric and idiopathic groups, respectively. This study was retrospective, however, and anorectal physiological studies were not performed on these patients. In a study to determine the effectiveness of combined anterior sphincter repair and levatorplasty in the treatment of faecal incontinence, regardless of aetiology,

Miller et al.[32] found a satisfactory clinical result in 71% of patients who had developed problems as a result of trauma and in 62% of patients in the idiopathic group (compared with a 59% success rate using postanal repair on the same unit). This was associated with a significant increase in maximum voluntary contraction pressure in the traumatic group and in those patients who had a good result in the idiopathic group. Miller et al.[32] concluded that the type of approach (anterior or posterior) and the anorectal angle were irrelevant to the outcome of surgery for idiopathic faecal incontinence, and that success appeared to be related more to improved sphincter pressure and anal sensation.

COMBINED PLICATION (TOTAL PELVIC FLOOR REPAIR)

Since 1987, a combined procedure (postanal repair and anterior levatorplasty) pioneered by Keighley and termed total pelvic floor repair (TPFR), has been developed to reconstruct the entire pelvic floor. The rationale of the operation is to repair the anterior part of the levator ani in the rectovaginal septum and the posterior fibres of the puborectalis, as in postanal repair. Early experience was that this procedure successfully restored continence of both solids and liquids in 55% of 22 non-randomized patients,[33] a slight improvement on the results of postanal repair performed in the previous decade. However, in the only study so far looking at the long-term results of TPFR for neuropathic faecal incontinence,[34] the results were disappointing: only half of the patients benefited from long-term success, which is no better than the long-term outcome of postanal repair reported in other studies. Obesity and a history of straining or perineal descent were associated with a poor outcome.

In a prospective randomized trial comparing postanal repair, anterior levatorplasty and TPFR, it was found that the functional outcome after TPFR was significantly better than that after postanal repair or anterior levatorplasty alone; however, numbers were small and follow-up relatively short.[35,36]

If patients have impaired rectal evacuation demonstrated during preoperative videoproctography without a rectocele or rectal intussusception, TPFR is generally not recommended as this may further impair the evacuation of faeces. In addition, this procedure is inappropriate for patients with an isolated sphincter defect, which may be amenable to sphincter repair alone.

REFERENCES

1. Nesselrod JP. *Proctology in General Practice*. Philadelphia: Saunders

2. Parks AG. Anorectal incontinence. *J R Soc Med* 1975; 68: 681–690

3. Parks AG, Porter NH Hardcastle J. The syndrome of the descending perineum *Proc R Soc Med* 1966; 59: 477–482

4. Miller R, Bartolo DC, Locke-Edmunds JC, Mortensen NJ. A prospective study of conservative and operative treatment for faecal incontinence. *Br J Surg* 1988; 75: 101–105

5. Bannister JJ, Gibbons C, Read NW. Preservation of fecal continence during rises in intra-abdominal pressure: is there a role for the flap valve? *Gut* 1987; 28: 1242–1245

6. Bartolo DCC, Roe AM, Locke-Edmunds JC *et al.* Flapvalve theory of anorectal incontinence. *Br J Surg* 1986; 73: 1012–1014

7. Braun J, Tons C, Schippers E *et al.* Results of Parks postanal repair in idiopathic anal insufficiency. *Chirurg* 1991; 62: 206–210

8. Yoshioka K, Keighley MR. Critical assessment of the quality of continence after postanal repair for faecal incontinence. *Br J Surg* 1989; 76: 1054–1057

9. Jameson JS, Speakman CT, Darzi A *et al.* Audit of postanal repair in the treatment of fecal incontinence. *Dis Colon Rectum* 1994, 37: 369–372

10. Engel AF, van Baal SJ, Brummelkamp WH. Late results of postanal repair for idiopathic faecal incontinence. *Eur J Surg* 1994; 160: 637–640

11. Briel JW, Schouten WR. Disappointing results of postanal repair in the treatment of fecal incontinence. *Ned Tijdschr Geneeskd* 1995; 139: 23–26

12. Setti Carraro P, Kamm MA, Nicholis RJ. Long-term results of postanal repair for neurogenic faecal incontinence. *Br J Surg* 1994; 81: 140–144

13. Rieger NA, Sarre RG, Saccone GT *et al.* Hunter A, Toouli J. Postanal repair for faecal incontinence: long-term follow-up. *Aust N Z J Surg* 1997; 67: 566–570

14. Athanasiadis S, Sanchez M, Kuprian A. Long-term follow-up of Park's posterior repair. An electromyographic, manometric and radiologic study of 31 patients. *Langenbecks Arch Chir* 1995; 380: 22–30

15. Snooks SJ, Swash M, Henry M. Electrophysiologic and manometric assessment of failed postanal repair for anorectal incontinence. *Dis Colon Rectum* 1984; 27: 733–736

16. Laurberg S, Swash M, Henry M. Effect of postanal repair on progress of neurogenic damage to the pelvic floor. *Br J Surg* 1990; 77: 519–522

17. Rainey JB, Donaldson DR, Thomson JP. Postanal repair: which patients derive most benefit? *J R Coll Surg Edinb* 1990; 35: 101–105

18. Womack NR, Morrison JF, Williams NS. Prospective study of the effects of postanal repair in neurogenic faecal incontinence. *Br J Surg* 1988; 75: 48–52

19. Browning GG, Parks AG. Postanal repair for idiopathic faecal incontinence: correlation of clinical result and anal canal pressures. *Br J Surg* 1983; 70: 101–104

20. Kamm MA. Obstetric damage and faecal incontinence. *Lancet* 1994; 344: 730–733

21. Turrell R, Gordon JB, David K. Plastic repair for postoperative anal incontinence. *Am J Surg* 1948; 76: 89–91

22. Birnbaum W. A method of repair for a common type of traumatic incontinence of the anal sphincter. *Surg Gynecol Obstet* 1948; 87: 716–718

23. Parks AG, McPartlin JF. Late repair of injuries of the anal sphincter. *Proc R Soc Med* 1971; 64: 1187–1189

24. Slade MS, Goldberg SM, Schottler JL *et al.* Sphincteroplasty for acquired anal incontinence. *Dis Colon Rectum* 1977; 20: 33–35

25. Browning GG, Motson RW. Anal sphincter injury: management and results of Parks sphincter repair. *Ann Surg* 1984; 199: 351–357

26. Fang DT, Nivatvongs S, Vermeulen FD *et al.* Overlapping sphincteroplasty for acquired anal incontinence. *Dis Colon Rectum* 1984; 27: 720–722

27. Ctercteko GC, Fazio VW, Jagelman DG *et al.* Anal sphincter repair: a report of 60 cases and a review of the literature. *Aust N Z J Surg* 1988; 58: 703–710

28. Fieshman JW, Peters WR, Shemesh EL *et al.* Anal sphincter reconstruction: anterior overlapping muscle repair. *Dis Colon Rectum* 1991; 34: 739–743

29. Wexner SD, Marchetti F, Jagelman DG. The role of sphincteroplasty for fecal incontinence reevaluated: a prospective physiologic and functional review. *Dis Colon Rectum* 1991; 34: 22–30

30. Miller R, Orrom WJ, Cornes H *et al.* Anterior sphincter plication and levatorplasty in the treatment of faecal incontinence. *Br J Surg* 1989; 76: 1058–1060

31. Osterberg A, Graf W, Holmberg A *et al.* Long-term results of anterior levatorplasty for fecal incontinence: a retrospective study. *Dis Colon Rectum* 1996; 39: 671–675

32. Miller R, Orrom WJ, Cornes H *et al.* Anterior sphincter plication and levatorplasty in the treatment of faecal incontinence. *Br J Surg* 1989; 76: 1058–1060

33. Pinho M Ortiz J, Oya M *et al.* Total pelvic floor repair for the treatment of neuropathic fecal incontinence. *Am J Surg* 1992; 163: 340–343

34. Korsgen S, Deen KI, Keighley MRB. Long-term results of total pelvic floor repair for postobstetric fecal incontinence. *Dis Colon Rectum* 1997; 40: 835–839

35. Deen KI, Oya M Ortiz J, Keighley MRB. Randomized trial comparing three forms of pelvic floor repair for neuropathic faecal incontinence. *Br J Surg* 1993; 80: 794–798

36. Keighley MR, Oya M, Oritz J *et al.* What is the optimum pelvic floor repair for neuropathic fecal incontinence? *Dis Colon Rectum* 1991; 34: P6

52

Sacrospinous colpopexy for support of the vaginal apex

M. C. Slack

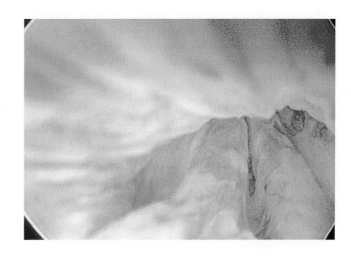

INTRODUCTION

A marked increase in the age of the population, coupled with a more active lifestyle and awareness of available therapy, have resulted in a greater specialist referral rate for the management of symptomatic urogenital prolapse. Most of these patients will prefer a permanent solution to conservative measures such as vaginal pessaries. They will also expect any surgical procedure to correct their symptoms while maintaining body image and coital function.

For some time, surgeons have been less than satisfied with the outcome of many of the procedures currently performed for the correction of marked uterovaginal prolapse. The recurrence of prolapse following surgical repair remains a significant problem and one that is generally poorly managed. The mainstay of therapy used by majority of gynaecologists is a vaginal repair incorporating an anterior and posterior colporrhaphy with dissection and closure of the enterocele. There is a remarkable paucity of recent literature supporting the continued use of these procedures for the management of post-hysterectomy or massive uterovaginal prolapse. The interest shown in new surgical procedures probably reflects less than satisfactory results in individual personal practice and the desire to improve outcome. This may have been prompted by a willingness on the part of patients to report less than satisfactory outcomes: although previous generations have accepted failure in stoical silence, it is unlikely that the modern patient will be as tolerant. Prolapse surgery will be expected to correct the anatomical problem, relieve symptoms and restore function. Previous surgeons have reported dissatisfaction with surgical results.

Te Linde,[1] writing in 1966, stated:

> It is probably true that every honest surgeon of extensive and long experience will have to admit that he is not entirely satisfied with his long-term results of all of his operations for prolapse and allied conditions.

Many recent publications have described improvements aimed at more effective vault support.[2,3] In this chapter I will discuss the most established of these: the transvaginal sacrospinous colpopexy.[4] It has received an enthusiastic reception but its true place in the management of prolapse has yet to be established.

HISTORY

The history of genital prolapse can be traced to records in Egyptian papyri in 1550BC.[5] A rich array of interventions and operations were prescribed for the treatment of this condition over the years. The best described, the vaginal hysterectomy, became an established procedure from 1861.[5]

The sacrospinous colpopexy, for the management of post-hysterectomy vault prolapse, evolved from Zweifel's first attempts in 1892 to secure the vault to the sacrotuberous ligament.[6] Its success was described by Richter[7] in 1968, following earlier unsuccessful attempts with the sacrotuberous ligament. Randall and Nichols[8] introduced the operation to the United States in 1971, since when it has become increasingly popular.

ANATOMICAL CONSIDERATIONS

Recent work on the pelvic floor anatomy has shown that the support of the pelvic viscera is dependent on two mechanisms.[9] The uterus and vagina are attached to the pelvic sidewall by the endopelvic fascia. This is divided into three regions which, although individually named, are one continuous unit. The level 1 (upper) fibres are the principal supporting structures for the upper vagina. Damage at this level will result in eversion of the vault or procidentia if the uterus is still *in situ*. In addition, the muscles of the levator ani fuse behind the anal canal and anterior to the coccyx to form the levator plate. This acts as a shelf against which the pelvic viscera are supported during rises in intra-abdominal pressure.

In cases of procidentia and post-hysterectomy vault eversion, any surgical procedure should seek to replace the damaged or absent upper supports while fixing the upper third of the vagina over the levator plate.

ANATOMY OF THE SACROSPINOUS LIGAMENT

Damage to nerves and vessels in this region is commonly cited as a possible complication of the sacrospinous colpopexy. A good understanding of the anatomy of the sacrospinous ligament will help minimize complications at the time of surgery. Reappraisal of the anatomy demonstrates how easy it is to avoid injury to these structures and how few structures are truly at risk of injury in a correctly performed procedure.

The sacrospinous ligament is thin and triangular. It attaches laterally to the spine of the ischium and medially by a broad base to the lateral margins of the sacrum and coccyx (Fig. 52.1). The sacrotuberous ligament, with which its fibres are intermingled, lies immediately behind it. The sacrospinous ligament may represent the degenerated dorsal lamina of the coccygeus, which lies in front of it. The sciatic notch is divided by the ligament into the greater and lesser sciatic foramina, of which it forms the inferior and superior borders, respectively.[10,11]

Most standard texts describe the pudendal nerve leaving the pelvis medial to the sciatic nerve and internal pudendal vessels, between piriformis and coccygeus and crossing the sacrospinous ligament close to its attachment to the ischial spine. The pudendal vessels usually lie on the spine itself[10,11] (Fig. 52.1). Verdeja *et al.*[12] dissected 24 human cadavers to assess the relationship of surrounding structures, and noted a direct relationship between the obstetric conjugate and the length of the ligament. In their dissections they noted that the pudendal complex and sciatic nerve were found 0.90–3.30 cm medial to the ischial spine, making injury during surgery a possibility. The inferior gluteal artery, which usually passes behind the pudendal artery, has been described as lying immediately posterior to the middle portion of the ligament.[13] This is not a common position and is therefore unlikely to pose a problem during surgery.

The histology of the sacrospinous ligament has been studied to determine whether nerves exist within the substance of the ligament itself.[14] Although nerve tissue is concentrated within the medial portion of the ligament, nerves are found in all segments. The size and myelination of these nerves suggest that they may carry pain sensation. It remains possible, therefore, that nerve pain may be an unavoidable complication of the procedure.

PATIENT SELECTION

Patients should be assessed in the normal fashion, including a good history, a detailed examination and preoperative urodynamic studies. The examination should aim to identify all the site-specific vaginal defects present.[15]

The operative correction of severe vault prolapse may result in the development of postoperative urinary incontinence – prospective studies have shown a 15–80% incidence after successful reduction of the prolapse.[16] It has been suggested that an accurate identification of the at-risk patient would determine which patients should have an anti-incontinence procedure performed at the time of surgery. Reduction of the prolapse during urodynamic studies may expose stress incontinence, which is otherwise masked by the descent and rotation of the anterior vaginal wall. Although, in my opinion, it is sensible to perform urodynamic studies in all patients who are to undergo pelvic floor surgery, it remains unclear how successfully these tests will identify these patients who will subsequently develop stress incontinence. In a prospective study, Veronikis *et al.*[17] demonstrated that reduction of the prolapse prior to urodynamic studies revealed a high incidence of low-pressure urethra and an even higher incidence of genuine stress incontinence (GSI). They concluded that these patients should be offered a suburethral sling at the time of surgery. This is in agreement with the study of Wall and Hewitt.[18] Bump and colleagues[16] used barrier testing to try to predict which patients should have a simultaneous suspending urethropexy at the time of prolapse surgery, concluding that this did not predict the functional status after surgery nor did it indicate which women required

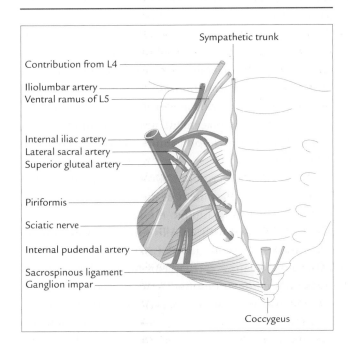

Figure 52.1. *Anatomy of the sacrospinous ligament and related structures.*

Labels:
Sympathetic trunk
Contribution from L4
Iliolumbar artery
Ventral ramus of L5
Internal iliac artery
Lateral sacral artery
Superior gluteal artery
Piriformis
Sciatic nerve
Internal pudendal artery
Sacrospinous ligament
Ganglion impar
Coccygeus

anti-incontinence procedures. There is a fear that barrier tests may overestimate the risk of potential GSI, resulting in the addition of unnecessary surgical procedures (see below).

The only specific preoperative requirement for a sacrospinous colpopexy is adequate vaginal length. The surgeon needs to ensure that there is sufficient vaginal depth to allow easy approximation of the vault to the ligament. Reduction in vaginal volume, such as occurs when there have been numerous previous attempts at repair, will be a contraindication to a sacrospinous colpopexy.

INDICATIONS

The principal indication for the sacrospinous colpopexy is symptomatic prolapse of the vaginal vault. It is done as part of the vaginal repair for patients with complex post-hysterectomy prolapse.[19] It has also been proposed as an adjunctive step during a hysterectomy for procidentia. More controversially, some surgeons use sacrospinous colpopexy at the time of a vaginal hysterectomy as a prophylactic step against subsequent vaginal vault eversion.[20] The procedure has also been used in young patients with marked degrees of prolapse when there was a desire to retain fertility.[21–23]

These various indications are discussed below in the Results section.

SURGICAL TECHNIQUE

All women have a standard preoperative preparation, which will include prophylactic antibiotics and prophylactic anticoagulation.

Surgery is performed with the patient in the lithotomy position. An examination under anaesthesia allows the surgeon to confirm that the vault can be comfortably attached to the sacrospinous ligament.

In patients with marked uterovaginal prolapse, the vaginal hysterectomy is performed first. If the anterior compartment has a defect it is addressed next. Most surgeons will perform a standard anterior repair with suburethral buttressing sutures.[4,19] A transvaginal paravaginal repair is advocated by some if there is evidence of a paravaginal defect.[24]

The sacrospinous colpopexy begins with a longitudinal incision in the posterior vaginal wall from introitus to vault. The epithelium is dissected laterally on both

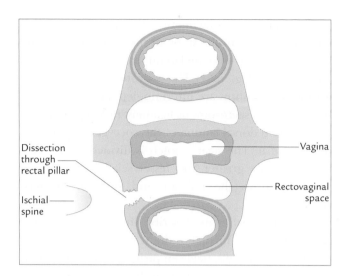

Figure 52.2. *Schematic representation of the rectovaginal space.*

sides. If an enterocele is identified, it is dissected free, opened and a high ligation performed with a purse-string suture. The right ischial spine is palpated and then a window is created between it and the rectovaginal space using a combination of blunt and sharp dissection (Fig. 52.2). The ischial spine is then palpated and the window developed along the ligament. Care must be taken to limit the blunt dissection to the area immediately in front of the ligament. It is important to split the fascia overlying the ligament to ensure that suture placement will be into the body of the ligament. Sutures are placed into the ligament two fingerbreadths medial to the spine, thus avoiding injury to the pudendal complex. In placing the suture, the surgeon must take care to avoid penetrating the full thickness of the ligament or risk injuring any structures behind the ligament. Meticulous placement will avoid injury to any major structures. A second suture can be placed at the same site.

The earliest descriptions involved exposure of the ligament before placement of the sutures under direct vision.[4,7,25] In this technique the ligament is visualized and then grasped with an Allis forceps before placing the suture. This is most easily achieved with a Deschamps ligature carrier. This method has required more dissection, prompting some surgeons to design specific instrumentation to facilitate suture placement.

Suture placement can be more easily achieved with the aid of the Miya hook ligature carrier[26] (Fig. 52.3). This is loaded with a suture, then passed through the window in the rectal pillar, allowing placement of the

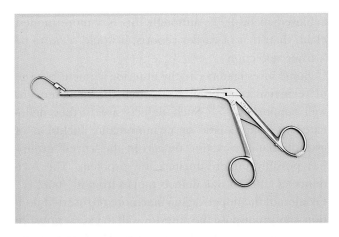

Figure 52.3. *Miya hook.*

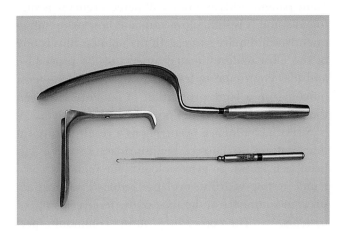

Figure 52.4. *Additional instruments used for a sacrospinous colpopexy: (a) Breisky–Navratill retractor; (b) notched speculum; (c) nerve hook.*

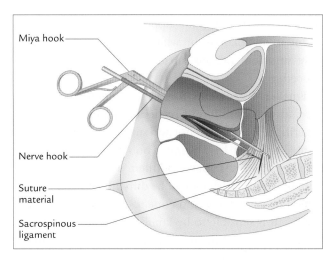

Figure 52.5. *Retrieval of suture material after successful placement with a Miya hook.*

Once this has been completed, the rectovaginal septum is reconstituted by a continuous locking suture through Denonvillier's fascia. The upper third of the vagina is closed with interrupted sutures. A second full-length absorbable suture is tied at the apex of the open epithelium and held. The sacrospinous sutures are then tied, taking the vault onto the ligament. It is important to gain a close approximation and not to allow a suture bridge between these two structures. Finally, the lower vagina is closed with the previously placed absorbable suture.

If the uterus is to be conserved, the posterior vaginal wall is opened to the level of the cervix. The dissection then proceeds as described above. Following placement, the sacrospinous sutures are attached to the posterior aspect of the cervix in the region of the uterosacral ligament attachments. This is achieved by loading the ligature onto a Mayo needle, which is then passed through the posterior aspect of the cervix. The suture is then passed through the vaginal epithelium at the level of insertion to the cervix. The other end of the suture is passed through the epithelium just lateral to the cervix. This step is repeated on the other side of the midline with the second suture. The operation then proceeds in a similar fashion to the above.[19]

The earlier descriptions advocated a unilateral approach, with most favouring the right-hand side. Morley and DeLancey concluded that there was no reason to perform a bilateral attachment.[4] Subsequently, a few authors have proposed that a bilateral sacrospinous fixation should be the procedure of choice, as it

tip of the hook two fingerbreadths medial to the spine and just inferior to the superior border of the ligament. The hook is pushed into the ligament with the right index finger. When the hook is closed, the tip describes an arc and takes a firm bite of the ligament. The handle of the hook is swept upwards, bringing the tip out of the ligament. The rectum is retracted medially by an 18 × 4 cm Breisky–Navratill vaginal retractor. Use of an 18 × 2 cm retractor will not provide effective retraction. A notched vaginal speculum is placed just below the tip of the hook and the suture is collected with a nerve hook (Fig. 52.4). This procedure is repeated, so that two sutures are placed through the ligament (Fig. 52.5). The sutures are then loaded onto a Mayo needle, passed through the vaginal epithelium at the level of the vault and held for later tying.

provides superior vaginal support. A recent description includes an analysis of what percentage of patients have sufficient vaginal capacity to undergo a bilateral procedure.[27-29]

Further instruments for the placement of the ligature, as well as different retrieval methods, have been described.[30-35] They do not add substantially to the technique designed by Miyazaki, but surgeons struggling with the above style may find them useful. In the obese patient, suture retrieval can be difficult and can be simplified by using an amnioscope to display the tip of the hook.[33] It is sensible to be familiar with more than one method, so that the procedure does not have to be abandoned in difficult cases.

Consensus does not exist over the choice of suture material. Initially, absorbable sutures were used,[4,7,36] whereas more recent papers advocate the use of a combination of absorbable and non-absorbable sutures.[29,37,38] This is one of the many issues that need more formal evaluation.

RESULTS

Sacrospinous colpopexy

A number of studies on the sacrospinous colpopexy have been reported[4,13,15,19,20,25,27,29,35-56] (Table 52.1.), involving more than 2000 procedures; these include cases of post-hysterectomy prolapse and procidentia and some in which the procedure was performed while preserving the uterus. Unfortunately, a lack of objective outcome measures and a variety of definitions of success make the data difficult to collate. Analysis in a similar format to that presented by Sze and Karram[57] has been utilized: they published a thorough description of the available literature with an analysis of the results. A good proportion (87%) were followed up for from 1 month to 11 years although, in a substantial group, the duration of follow-up was not specified. The cure rate, depending on the definition of cure, ranged from 8[46] to 97%.[25]

The first few papers published claimed outstanding results but classified success on a fairly superficial basis,[4,25] with the authors concentrating more on vault correction than on other sites of relaxation. However, most authors would agree that, if vault support is used as the sole parameter of evaluation, success is

achieved in 80–90%; although this is a more modest claim than that of earlier reports, it would seem to be a truer reflection.

Some investigators cite the anterior segment as a site of recurrent relaxation, even when the vault remains well supported.[19,29,46] Such defects are further delineated as symptomatic or asymptomatic. Inclusion of asymptomatic relaxation defects in the 'cured' groups has possibly underestimated the problem. The incidence of anterior wall defects ranges from 0[40] to 92%.[46] Fixation of the upper vagina in a more retroverted position may predispose the anterior wall to excess pressure and subsequent cystocele formation. The Burch colposuspension has a similar effect on the posterior wall.[58] Many patients with anterior wall defects remain asymptomatic and it is difficult to estimate how many subsequently will require surgery. In my opinion, this is one of the most underestimated aspects of the procedure and may contribute to less than satisfactory long-term outcomes in a large proportion of patients. However, the posterior wall does not pose the same problem.

Stress incontinence occurring as a result of surgical interventions to correct genitourinary prolapse has been well known to gynaecologists for years.[59] Urodynamic testing with the prolapse reduced will identify stress incontinence at the time of the test in 30–80% of patients.[17,60] The procedure most commonly performed on the anterior wall is an anterior repair with suburethral buttressing.[4,19] Some authors have suggested that this should be replaced by a suspending urethropexy[17] for the patients with urodynamic evidence of occult stress incontinence. In the largest single series of sacrospinous colpopexies, Paraiso *et al.*[50] described new-onset urinary incontinence in 12% of patients; however, 32/36 patients (89%), who had preexisting incontinence, were dry after the procedure. These were subjective results that were not backed up by urodynamic analysis. In the majority of papers, the described incidence of *de-novo* stress incontinence ranges from zero to 10% (Table 52.2.). It would seem that, despite predictions, the actual incidence of incontinence following sacrospinous colpopexy is very low.

Considering the low incidence of stress incontinence after sacrospinous colpopexy, it would seem that barrier testing may overestimate the incidence of incontinence. To include an anti-incontinence step as a routine procedure in all women with urodynamic evidence of stress incontinence is, therefore, unjustified. Bump *et al.*[16]

Table 52.1. *Long-term results after sacrospinous vault suspension*

Investigators and ref. no.	Year	Duration of follow-up*	No. available for follow-up	Repeated surgical repair/recurrent prolapse required (n)				No. cured†	Cure assessment‡
				Vault	Ant. wall	Post. wall	Not specified		
Richter and Albright[39]	1981	1–10 y	81	2/2	0/12	0/10		57 (70)	O
Nichols[25]	1982	2y	163	5/5				158 (97)	
Morley and DeLancey[4]	1988	1 m–11 y	92	3/3	2/11	0/0	0/3	75 (82)	S/O
Brown et al.[40]	1989	8–21 m	11	1/1	0/0	0/0		10 (91)	O
Kettel and Hebertson[13]	1989		31	2/6				25 (81)	S/O
Cruikshank and Cox[20]	1990	8 m–3.2 y	48	0/1	0/5	0/2		40 (83)	O
Monk et al.[41]	1991	1 m–8.6 y	61	1/1	0/6	0/2		52 (85)	O
Backer[42]	1992		51	0/0	0/3	0/0		48 (94)	O
Heinonen[43]	1992	6 m–5.6 y	22	0/0	0/1	0/2		19 (86)	O
Imparato et al.[38]	1992		155	0/4			0/11	140 (90)	O
Shull et al.[15]	1992	2–5 y	81	0/1	4/20	0/1	0/6	53 (65)	O
Kaminski et al.[44]	1993		23	2/2	0/1	0/0		20 (87)	O
Carey and Slack[19]	1994	2 m–1 y	63	1/1	0/16	0/0		46 (73)	O
Porges and Smilen[45]	1994		76						O
Holley et al.[46]	1995	15–79 m	36				0/33	3 (8)	O
Sauer and Klutke[47]	1995	4–26 m	24	3/5	1/3	0/1		15 (63)	O
Peters and Christenson[48]	1995	median = 48 m	30	0/0	0/0	4/6	0/1	23 (77)	S/O
Elkins et al.[49]	1995	3–6 m	14		0/2			12 (86)	O
Brieger et al.[36]	1995		100	0/5	0/0	0/2		92 (92)	O
Paraiso et al.[50]	1996	1–190 m	243	11/17	0/65	0/17		144 (59)	O
Benson et al.[29]	1996	1–5.5 y	42	5/5	1/12	1/1		24 (57)	O
Hoffman et al.[37]	1996	12–66 m	39	2/2	1/2	0/0		35 (90)	O
Pohl and Frattarelli[27]	1997	6–40 m	40	0/0	1/3			39 (98)	O
Chapin[51]	1997	1–11 y	112	5/5				107 (96)	O
Febbraro et al.[35]	1997	9–32 m	24	1/1	1/1		0/3	21 (88)	O
Schlesinger[52]	1997	2–18 m	17	0/2				15 (88)	O

cont.

Table 52.1. *Long-term results after sacrospinous vault suspension (cont.)*

Investigators and ref. no.	year	Duration of follow-up*	No. available for follow-up	Repeated surgical repair/recurrent prolapse required (n)				No. cured[†]	Cure assessment[‡]
				Vault	Ant. wall	Post. wall	Not specified		
Penalver et al.[53]	1998	18–78 m	160	?/10	?/10	?/4		136 (85)	O
Ozcan et al.[54]	1999	4–54 m	54	2/2	3/3	1/1	5/0	43 (79)	O
Meschia et al.[55]	1999	1–6.8 m	91	?/6	?/41	?/9	?/6	85 (93)	O
Vigano et al.[56]	2000	5–108 m	78	?/5	?/10	?/5		58 (74)	O

* m, months; y, years.
† Percentages in parentheses.
‡ Subjective (S) or objective (O) assessment.

showed that the inclusion of a retropubic suspending urethropexy increased the short-term complications without providing any additional protection from *de-novo* stress incontinence. More importantly, because the combination of sacrospinous colpopexy with retropubic suspension may predispose to failure of the prolapse procedure;[16,61] the approach to *de-novo* stress incontinence should be expectant. In some cases the condition will settle over a period of time without any further intervention; this probably reflects a gradual relaxation of the anterior wall supports, leaving only a small number of patients who will require a second procedure to deal with the incontinence.

A shortcoming of most studies is a failure to evaluate sexual function following surgery. Clinically, the patients retain normal vaginal depth with only a minimally reduced volume. Postoperative vaginal volume will depend in part on the preoperative characteristics. Pohl *et al.*[27] showed that, in a group who underwent bilateral fixation, the average vaginal depth was between 7.5 and 11 cm and the width 5 cm. Some authors have reported a low incidence of stenotic vagina after the procedure, but the majority of sexually active patients seem unaffected.[20,39–41,49] Given[62] did not find any alteration in function in the sexually active group.

Sacrospinous colpopexy with preservation of the uterus

There are two possible indications for the preservation of the uterus at the time of the procedure. Preservation of fertility is the primary indication but the technique

could also be used in elderly patients as a means of reducing surgical time and operative intervention and, by so doing, reducing morbidity.

Kovac and Cruikshank[21] presented a series of 19 women who underwent sacrospinous fixation with preservation of the uterus. This was performed as a bilateral procedure in 15 and as a unilateral procedure in the remainder. Most patients had good results and five attained normal pregnancies, all delivering vaginally. This procedure is much less likely to affect fertility than the Manchester repair, which can result in cervical stenosis or incompetence.

In one group, the uterus was preserved because of the frailty of the patients. The operating time was marginally reduced in the group with uterine preservation, but there was little difference in the blood loss or postoperative complications between the groups.[19]

Ongoing follow-up of this study group demonstrated continued success for both groups. With the inclusion of new patients a significantly shorter operating time with significantly less blood loss was demonstrated in the uterine preservation group.[63]

COMPLICATIONS

The most commonly reported complication is haemorrhage. It is difficult to isolate the loss directly attributable to the sacrospinous portion of the procedure, as most authors report blood loss for the whole operation which, naturally, includes loss incurred at the time of hysterectomy or repair. Of the 1901 cases reviewed, 64 required transfusion. This represents a very small proportion of the total cases but it must be remembered

Table 52.2. *Intra-operative and postoperative complications of sacrospinous colpopexy*

Investigators and ref. no.	Year	n	Cystotomy	Rectal injury	Haemorrhage	Nerve injury	GSI*	Buttock pain
Richter and Albright[39]	1981	81	1	0	0	1	1	
Nichols[25]	1982	163	0	1	0	2	0	
Miyazaki[26]	1987	74	0	0	0	0		
Morley and DeLancey[4]	1988	100	1	0	6	1	4	
Brown et al.[40]	1989	11	0	1	0	0	0	
Kettel and Hebertson[13]	1989	31			2			
Cruikshank and Cox[20]	1990	48	0	0	2		0	20
Monk et al.[41]	1991	69	2	2	1	1	3	1
Backer[42]	1992	51	0	0	0	0	2	5
Heinonen[43]	1992	25	0	0	7	0	0	
Imparato et al.[38]	1992	179	0	0	1	0	–	2
Kaminski et al.[44]	1993	24	0	0	8		0	
Carey and Slack[19]	1994	64	0	0	2	0	0	3
Porges and Smilen[45]	1994	76	0	0	0	0		
Holley et al.[46]	1995	36						
Sauer and Klutke[47]	1995	24	0	1	0	0		2
Peters and Christenson[48]	1995	30	0	0	0	0	1	1
Brieger et al.[36]	1995	104				?4		
Paraiso et al.[50]	1996	243	0	0	20	0	29	
Benson et al.[29]	1996	48	1	0	0	0	5	
Hoffman et al.[37]	1996	45	2	0	4	0	4	
Pohl and Frattarelli[27]	1997	40	0	0	5	0	0	
Chapin[51]	1997	134	0	0	1	0		
Febbraro et al.[35]	1997	24	0	3				
Schlesinger[52]	1997	17	0	0	0	0	0	
Penalver et al.[53]	1998	160	0	2	7	1	0	
Ozcan et al.[54]	1999	54	0	1	0	0	0	?
Meschina et al.[55]	1999	91	0	0	1	0	0	6
Vigano et al.[56]	2000	78	0	1	0	1	7	?

* GSI, genuine stress incontinence.

that severe intra-operative blood loss (more than 2 litres) was reported by three authors.[4,19,41] In one case, where laceration of the pudendal vessels occurred, the haemorrhage was controlled with a low-pressure hydrostatic balloon. In the same series a patient experienced blood loss of 650 ml which occurred as a result of laceration of sacral veins; this was controlled with Liga clips.[19] A multifire Liga clip applicator is particularly useful for controlling this type of bleeding.

Nerve injury is often cited as a complication of the procedure. Direct injury to major nerves is, however, very rare. Nichols describes injury to the sciatic nerve in two patients:[25] one required reoperation while the other resolved spontaneously; no details of the degree of injury are supplied. One case of pudendal nerve entrapment is described by Alevizon and Finon.[64] The pain resolved spontaneously following release of the sacrospinous sutures. Any evidence of direct injury to the sciatic or pudendal nerves would require immediate reoperation to remove the suture. Re-positioning could be achieved at the same time, thus ensuring a successful outcome.

Buttock pain is a much more commonly described complication, occuring in as many as 10–15% of patients.[19,21,42] Evaluation includes exclusion of motor nerve damage. The pain can be very severe but usually responds to non-steroidal anti-inflammatory drugs and is usually self-limiting, with very few cases persisting beyond 6 weeks. The pain could be due to haematoma formation at the site of suture insertion or could be secondary to trauma to nerve fibres in the substance of the ligament.[14] If the latter is the cause, pain may remain an unpredictable but inevitable complication in some patients.

One rare reported complication was evisceration through the vaginal incision.[65] Non-specific complications, such as injury to bladder and bowel, are also reported, although these are well-described complications of vaginal repair and are not unique to the sacrospinous colpopexy.[4,25,41]

FAILURES

Failure to maintain support of the vault could occur for a variety of reasons. A possible cause is poor approximation between the vault and the ligament. The presence of a suture bridge will prevent a tight attachment. Subsequent fibrosis between the vault and the ligament will not occur, leaving the suture material as the principal

supporting structure. For this reason the procedure is not suitable for a patient with a short vagina where stretch is needed to fix the vagina to the ligament.

Many authors have suggested using non-absorbable sutures to reduce the likelihood of failure; however, it is not obvious from the literature whether this is of any advantage. Other efforts to reduce failure rates have included performing a bilateral procedure; however, this cannot be done in all patients and does not appear to offer substantial increases in success rates.[27] A bilateral procedure does reproduce the anatomy more accurately and provides an increased surface area for attachment of the vault to the ligaments; however, it will take longer and is associated with increased blood loss.

If a unilateral procedure fails, it can be repeated on the contralateral side. Fibrosis and scarring make a repeat procedure on the same side virtually impossible.

ALTERNATIVE TRANSVAGINAL VAULT SUSPENSION PROCEDURES

Various transvaginal procedures have been described for the correction of procidentia and post-hysterectomy vaginal vault prolapse. Symmonds and Pratt obtained good success with endopelvic fascia vaginal vault fixation. They did, however, intentionally narrow and shorten the vagina in 12% of patients.[66]

Concern has been expressed that the marked retroversion of the upper vagina caused by the sacrospinous colpopexy may predispose to prolapse of the anterior vaginal segment.[46] With this in mind, investigators have proposed using the iliococcygeus fixation. In 1963, Inmon[67] described the use of iliococcygeus fascia to suspend the vaginal cuff in three patients who had inadequate uterosacral ligaments. Because the fascia is not as deep in the pelvis, it produces less retroversion and the problem of excessive stretching is eliminated.[24] It is hoped that the more neutral position, combined with bilateral attachments, will minimize the anterior wall defects. The iliococcygeus fascia suspension is easier to perform than the sacrospinous fixation as less dissection is required. Furthermore, the absence of major vessels or nerves traversing the iliococcygeus muscle should make it a safer procedure.

In a series of 110 patients undergoing this procedure, Meeks and colleagues[69] showed that the anterior wall remained susceptible to prolapse. Despite the theoretical advantages, two patients had bleeding in excess of 750 ml.

In a case-controlled study comparing the two techniques, equivalent outcomes were achieved for the correction of prolapse. Despite the theoretical advantages there were no differences in perioperative morbidity. The sacrospinous group had a quicker return to normal activity and a significantly higher patient satisfaction. Both had good symptomatic success with no statistical differences in outcome. Contrary to perceived wisdom, cystocele formation was no more prevalent following sacrospinous fixation.[68] Follow-up on the iliococcygeus fixation is too limited to draw any meaningful conclusions.

COMPARISON WITH ABDOMINAL PROCEDURES

Comparison with the intra-abdominal procedures is inevitable and appropriate. Vaginal hysterectomy is commonly believed to have a lower morbidity than the equivalent abdominal procedure. It is probably this belief that encourages us to view the vaginal procedures for the treatment of prolapse as carrying less potential for morbidity than the abdominal alternatives.

Many reasons are cited for choosing a vaginal rather than an abdominal approach. The theoretical advantages are shorter operating time, less postoperative pain and shorter hospital stay. The discomfort and side effects accompanying the abdominal incision are believed to account for most of these differences. More importantly, the vaginal approach allows a symptomatic cystocele or rectocele to be repaired with the same surgical approach.

Apart from the disadvantages mentioned above, complications of the abdominal procedure include infection and erosion of the synthetic graft material.

Very few studies have drawn any sort of comparison between the two approaches. The presence of an adnexal mass or a shortened vagina would favour an abdominal procedure; factors that would favour a vaginal approach include compromised health, obesity and multiple previous laparotomies. The literature would suggest that the two approaches have similar success rates.[4,25,70–72] What is less obvious is the difference in morbidity between the two procedures.

Two authors who compared the two procedures in a retrospective fashion concluded that the vaginal approach was preferable to the abdominal.[40,43] Numer-

ous others have stopped using the abdominal approach in favour of sacrospinous colpopexy.[4,25,47,53]

The only prospective evaluation is the study by Benson *et al.*[29] which is a truly prospective randomized trial of the abdominal versus the vaginal approach. Follow-up was performed by a non-surgeon co-author, thus eliminating some aspects of subjective evaluation. Interim analysis of the data to look for trends identified a disparity in outcome between the groups and so the study was stopped for ethical reasons. Surprisingly, there was no difference in complication rates between the groups and no difference in hospital stay. The operating time was less for the vaginal group. However, the effectiveness of surgical outcome was so much better for the abdominal group than for the vaginal group that the study was discontinued. Once again, the main reason for failure was recurrence involving the anterior vaginal wall. This represents a small number of women but highlights the need for large randomized trials.

CONCLUSIONS

Since its introduction, the sacrospinous colpopexy has received an enthusiastic reception from surgeons with a special interest in urogenital prolapse. This, in part, almost certainly reflects personal disappointment with the more traditional surgical methods employed to manage these conditions. Another reason is the excellent immediate postoperative result obtained after the newer procedure. At the completion of surgery these patients have reduction of the prolapse without any loss of vaginal volume. It is very pleasing to tie the vault sutures and watch the vault retract from view. Unfortunately, in common with so many new surgical procedures, sacrospinous colpopexy has gained widespread introduction before adequate long-term follow-up and validation.

The results confirm that sacrospinous colpopexy is easy to both learn and teach. Contrary to early warnings, it is a safe procedure with a low incidence of complications. In most series it achieves good success with reduction of the vault. Unfortunately, because of lack of standardization of follow-up, it is difficult to be confident that the operation satisfies all the principles of surgery. The aims of prolapse surgery are to relieve the symptoms, restore the anatomy and retain function. With careful follow-up it is apparent that the final position of the vault is anatomically exaggerated: it is more retroverted and the distance from the introitus to the apex of the vault is increased. The operation does re-create the upper vaginal supports but, by doing so, stretches the vagina and displaces the position of the apex. It has long been known that alteration of the vaginal axis is associated with the development of defects in other segments of the vagina. This was first described by Bonney[73] but has also been noted with other procedures that place pressure on only one segment of the vagina.[58] This could account for the high rate of cystocele after the procedure. For this reason it is probably wise to avoid the procedure at the time of vaginal hysterectomy for lesser degrees of prolapse. The incidence of post-hysterectomy vault prolapse in this group does not justify the inclusion of a procedure that may lead to a high incidence of cystocele formation which may require reoperation.

The development of support defects in other segments following successful vault correction also raises questions over the introduction of steps to prevent stress urinary incontinence. It would appear that, when the procedure is performed in conjunction with routine anterior colporrhaphy and suburethral buttressing, there is a very low incidence of *de-novo* stress incontinence. The introduction of procedures that pull the para-urethral tissues anteriorly appears to increase complication rates while simultaneously reducing the success of the prolapse repair.

It remains unclear whether the procedure is best performed as a bilateral or unilateral procedure, or which is the best suture material. These factors, together with studies aimed at assessing quality-of-life issues and subsequent sexual function, require exploration in properly designed prospective trials.

Other operations for the management of this condition also have good results. Operations such as the iliococcygeus fixation, which provides upper vaginal support without the marked posterior displacement, should be compared with the sacrospinous fixation. The abdominal operations using grafts or meshes may be shown to confer a longer-lasting cure, but it must be established that rates of complications such as stress incontinence are no higher. The abdominal operations currently use artificial mesh which may, with time, increase the complication rates.

I do not believe that the decision to proceed abdominally or vaginally should be a competitive one. Like so many other areas in medicine, the decision will take into account the medical history and condition of the patient. A thin, young patient may be ideally served by an abdominal approach; in contrast, patients who have had multiple laparotomies, or the medically infirm and obese, may be better suited to a vaginal approach.

In due course, those authors who produced the earliest series will be in a position to present long-term objective follow-up according to agreed guidelines. By so doing, they may help to resolve some of the current controversies.

REFERENCES

1. Te Linde RW. Prolapse of the uterus and allied conditions. *Am J Obstet Gynecol* 1982; 142: 901–904

2. Addison WA, Livengood CH, Sutton GP, Parker RT. Abdominal sacral colpopexy with Mersiline mesh in the retroperitoneal position in the management of post hysterectomy vaginal vault prolapse and enterocele. *Am J Obstet Gynecol* 1985; 153: 140–146

3. Maloney JC, Dunton CJ, Smith K. Repair of vaginal vault prolapse with abdominal sacropexy. *J Reprod Med* 1990; 35: 6–10

4. Morley GN, DeLancey JO. Sacrospinous ligament fixation for eversion of the vagina. *Am J Obstet Gynecol* 1988; 158: 872–879

5. Emge LA, Durfee RB. Pelvic organ prolapse: four thousand years of treatment. *Clin Obstet Gynecol* 1966; 9: 997–1032

6. Zweifel P. Vorlesungen uber Klinische Gynaecologie. Berlin: Hirschwald, 1892; 407–415

7. Richter K. Die Chirurgische anatomie der vaginaefixatio sacrospinous vaginalis. Ein Beitrag zur operativen Behandlung des Scheidenblindsach prolapses. *Geburtshilfe frauenheilkd* 1968; 78: 321–327

8. Randall CL, Nichols DH. Surgical treatment of vaginal eversion. *Obstet Gynecol* 1971; 38: 327–332

9. DeLancey JO. Anatomic aspects of vaginal erosion after hysterectomy. *Am J Obstet Gynecol* 1992; 166: 1717–1728

10. Tobias PV, Arnold M. Thorax and abdomen. *Man's Anatomy*. Johannesburg: Witwatersrand University Press, 1981; 347–366

11. Warwick R, Williams PL. *Gray's Anatomy*. Edinburgh; Longman, 1973; 444

12. Verdeja AM, Elkins TE, Odoi A *et al.* Transvaginal sacrospinous colpopexy: anatomic landmarks to be aware of to minimise complications. *Am J Obstet Gynecol* 1995; 173: 1468–1469

13. Kettel ML, Hebertson RM. An anatomic evaluation of the sacrospinous ligament colpopexy. *Surg Gynecol Obstet* 1989; 168: 318–322

14. Barksdale PA, Gasser RF, Gauthier CM *et al.* Intraligamentous nerves as a potential source of pain after sacrospinous ligament fixation of the vaginal apex. *Int Urogynecol J* 1997; 8: 121–125

15. Shull BT, Capen CV, Riggs MW, Kuch TJ. Preoperative and postoperative analysis of site-specific pelvic support defects in 81 women treated with sacrospinous ligament suspension and pelvic reconstruction. *Am J Obstet Gynecol* 1992; 166: 1764–1771

16. Bump RC, Hurt GW, Theofrastous JP *et al.* Randomised prospective comparison of needle colposuspension versus endopelvic fascia plication for potential stress incontinence prophylaxis in women undergoing vaginal reconstruction for stage III or IV pelvic organ prolapse. *Am J Obstet Gynecol* 1996; 175: 326–335

17. Veronikis DK, Nichols MD, Wakamatsu MM. The incidence of low-pressure urethra as a function of prolapse-reducing technique in patients with massive pelvic organ prolapse (maximum descent at all vaginal sites). *Am J Obstet Gynecol* 1997; 177: 1305–1314

18. Wall LL, Hewitt JK. Urodynamic characteristics of women with complete posthysterectomy vaginal vault prolapse. *Urology* 1994; 44: 336–341

19. Carey MP, Slack MC. Transvaginal sacrospinous colpopexy for vault and marked uterovaginal prolapse. *Br J Obstet Gynaecol* 1994; 101: 536–540

20. Cruikshank SH, Cox DW. Sacrospinous ligament fixation at the time of transvaginal hysterectomy. *Am J Obstet Gynecol* 1990; 162: 1611–1619

21. Kovac RS, Cruikshank SH. Successful pregnancies and vaginal deliveries after sacrospinous uterosacral fixation in five of nineteen patients. *Am J Obstet Gynecol* 1993; 168: 1778–1790

22. Richardson DA, Scott RJ, Ostergard DR. Surgical management of uterine prolapse in young women. *J Reprod Med* 1989; 34: 388–392

23. Nichols DH. Fertility retention in the patient with genital prolapse. *Am J Obstet Gynecol* 1991; 164: 1155–1158

24. Shull BL, Capen CV, Riggs MW, Kuehl TJ. Bilateral attachment of the vaginal cuff to iliococcygeus fascia: an effective method of cuff suspension. *Am J Obstet Gynecol* 1993; 168: 1669–1677

25. Nichols DH. Sacrospinous fixation for massive eversion of the vagina. *Am J Obstet Gynecol.* 1982; 142: 901–904

26. Miyazaki FS. Miya hook ligature carrier for sacrospinous ligament suspension. *Obstet Gynecol* 1987; 70: 286–288

27. Pohl JF, Frattarelli JL. Bilateral transvaginal sacrospinous colpopexy: preliminary experience. *Am J Obstet Gynecol* 1997; 177: 1356–1362

28. Nichols DH. Transvaginal sacrospinous colpopexy. *J Pelvic Surg* 1996; 2: 87–91

29. Benson TJ, Lucente V, McClellan E. Vaginal versus abdominal reconstructive surgery for the treatment of pelvic support defects: a prospective randomised study with long-term outcome evaluation. *Am J Obstet Gynecol* 1996; 175: 1418–1422

30. Mattox TF, Kelly T, Bhatia NN. Modification of the Miya hook in vaginal colpopexy. *J Reprod Med* 1995; 40: 681–683

31. Veronikis DK, Nichols DH. Ligature carrier specifically designed for transvaginal sacrospinous colpopexy. *Obstet Gynecol* 1997; 89: 478–481

32. Watson JD. Sacrospinous ligament colpopexy: new instrumentation applied to a standard gynaecologic procedure. *Obstet Gynecol* 1996; 88: 883–885

33. Hughes GW, Freeman RM. A modification of the technique of sacrospinous ligament fixation. *Br J Obstet Gynaecol* 1995; 102: 669–670

34. Lind LR, Choe J, Bhatia NN. An in-line suturing device to simplify sacrospinous vaginal vault suspension. *Obstet Gynecol* 1977; 89: 129–132

35. Febbraro W, Beucher G, Von Theobold P *et al.* Feasibility of bilateral sacrospinous ligament vaginal suspension with a stapler. Prospective study with the 34 first cases. *J Gynecol Obstet Biol Reprod (Paris)* 1997; 26: 815–821

36. Brieger GM, MacGibbon AL, Atkinson KH. Sacrospinous colpopexy. *Aust N Z J Obstet Gynaecol.* 1995; 35: 86–87

37. Hoffman MS, Harris MS, Bouis PJ. Sacrospinous colpopexy in the management of uterovaginal prolapse. *J Reprod Med* 1996; 41: 299–303

38. Imparato E, Aspesi G, Rovetta E, Presti M. Surgical management and prevention of vaginal vault prolapse. *Surg Gynecol Obstet* 1992; 175: 233–237

39. Richter K, Albright W. Long term results following fixation of the vagina on the sacrospinous ligament by the vaginal route. *Am J Obstet Gynecol* 1981; 141: 811–816

40. Brown WE, Hoffman MS, Bouis PJ *et al.* Management of vaginal vault prolapse; retrospective comparison of abdominal versus vaginal approach. *J Fla Med Assoc* 1989; 76: 249–252

41. Monk BJ, Ramp JF, Montz FJ, Febherz TB. Sacrospinous fixation for vaginal vault prolapse. Complications and results. *J Gynecol Surg* 1991; 7: 87–92

42. Backer MH. Success with sacrospinous suspension of the prolapsed vaginal vault. *Surg Gynecol Obstet* 1992; 175: 419–420

43. Heinonen PK. Transvaginal sacrospinous colpopexy for vaginal vault and complete genital prolapse in aged women. *Acta Obstet Gynecol Scand* 1992; 71: 377–381

44. Kaminski PF, Sorosky JI, Pees RC, Podczkski ES. Correction of massive vaginal prolapse in aged women. *J Am Geriatr Soc* 1993; 41: 42–44

45. Porges RF, Smilen SW. Long-term analysis of the surgical management of pelvic support defects. *Am J Obstet Gynecol* 1994; 171: 1518–1528

46. Holley RJ, Varner RE, Gleason BP *et al.* Recurrent pelvic support defects after sacrospinous ligament fixation for vaginal vault prolapse. *J Am Coll Surg* 1995; 180: 444–448

47. Sauer HA, Klutke CG. Transvaginal sacrospinous ligament fixation for treatment of vaginal prolapse. *J Urol* 1995; 154: 1008–1012

48. Peters WA, Christenson ML. Fixation of the vaginal apex to the coccygeal fascia during repair of vaginal vault eversion with enterocele. *Am J Obstet Gynecol* 1995; 172: 1894–1902

49. Elkins TE, Hopper JB, Goodfellow K *et al.* Initial report of anatomic and clinical comparison of the sacrospinous ligament fixation to the high McCall culdoplasty for vaginal cuff fixation at hysterectomy for uterine prolapse. *J Pelvic Surg* 1995; 1: 12–17

50. Paraiso MF, Ballard LA, Walters MD *et al.* Pelvic support defects and visceral and sexual function in women treated with sacrospinous ligament suspension and pelvic reconstruction. *Am J Obstet Gynecol* 1996; 175: 1423–1431

51. Chapin DS. Teaching sacrospinous colpopexy. *Am J Obstet Gynecol* 1997; 177: 1330–1336

52. Schlesinger RE. Vaginal sacrospinous ligament fixation with the Autosuture Endostitch device. *Am J Obstet Gynecol* 1997; 176: 1358–1362

53. Penalver M, Mekki Y, Laferty H *et al.* Should sacrospinous ligament fixation for the management of pelvic support defects be part of a residency program procedure? *Am J Obstet Gynecol* 1998; 178: 326–330

54. Ozcan U, Gungor T, Ekin M, Eken S. Sacrospinous fixation for the prolapsed vaginal vault. *Gynecol Obstet Invest* 1999; 47: 65–68

55. Meschia M, Bruschi F, Amicarelli F *et al.* The sacrospinous vaginal vault suspension: critical analysis of outcomes. *Int Urogynecol J* 1999; 10: 155–159

56. Vigano R, Ferrari A, Quellari P, Frigerio L. Sacrospinous ligament fixation: long term follow up. *Int Urogynecol J* 2000; 11: i–ii

57. Sze EH, Karram MM. Transvaginal repair of vault prolapse. *Am J Obstet Gynecol* 1997; 89: 466–475

58. Stanton SL, Williams JB, Ritchie D. The colposuspension operation for urinary incontinence. *Br J Obstet Gynaecol* 1976; 83: 890–895

59. Symmonds RE, Jordan LT. Iatrogenic stress incontinence of urine. *Am J Obstet Gynecol* 1961; 82: 1231–1237

60. Bergman A, Koonings PP, Ballard CA. Predicting postoperative urinary incontinence development in women undergoing operation for genitourinary prolapse. *Am J Obstet Gynecol* 1988; 158: 1171–1175

61. Sze EH, Miklos JR, Partoll L *et al.* Sacrospinous ligament fixation with transvaginal needle suspension for advanced pelvic organ prolapse and stress incontinence. *Obstet Gynecol* 1997; 89: 94–96

62. Given FT, Muhlendorf K, Browning GM. Vaginal length and sexual function after colpopexy for complete uterovaginal eversion. *Am J Obstet Gynecol* 1993; 169: 284–288

63. Maher CF, Carey MP, Slack MC *et al.* Uterine preservation or hysterectomy at prolapse surgery – a case control study (abstract). *Int Urogynecol J* 1999; 10: i–ix

64. Alevizon JS, Finon MA. Sacrospinous colpopexy: management of postoperative pudendal nerve entrapment. *Obstet Gynecol* 1996; 88: 713–715

65. Farrell SA, Scotti RJ, Ostergaard DR, Bart AE. Massive evisceration: a complication following sacrospinous vaginal vault fixation. *Obstet Gynecol* 1991; 78: 560–562

66. Symmonds RE, Pratt JH. Vaginal prolapse following hysterectomy. *Am J Obstet Gynecol* 1960; 79: 899–909

67. Inmon WB. Pelvic relaxation and repair including prolapse of vagina following hysterectomy. *Am J Obstet Gynecol* 1963; 56: 577–582

68. Maher CF, Murray CJ, Carey MP, Dwyer PL. Prespinous versus sacrospinous fixation for vault and marked uterovaginal prolapse – a case control study (abstract). *Int Urogynecol J* 1999; 10: i–ix

69. Meeks RG, Washburne JF, McGhee RP, Wiser WL. Repair of vaginal vault prolapse by suspension of the vagina to iliococcygeus (prespinous) fascia. *Am J Obstet Gynecol* 1994; 171: 1444–1454

70. Creighton SM, Stanton SL. The surgical management of vaginal vault prolapse. *Br J Obstet Gynaecol* 1991; 98: 1150–1154

71. Snyder TE, Krantz KE. Abdominal–retroperitoneal sacral colpopexy for the correction of vaginal prolapse. *Obstet Gynecol* 1991; 77: 944–949

72. Timmons CM, Addison WA, Addison SB, Cavenar MG. Abdominal sacral colpopexy in 163 women with posthysterectomy vaginal vault prolapse and enterocele. *J Reprod Med* 1992; 37: 323–327

73. Bonney V. The principles that should underlie all operations for prolapse. *J Obstet Gynaecol Br Commonw.* 1934; 41: 669–683

53

Abdominal sacral colpopexy

M. C. Timmons

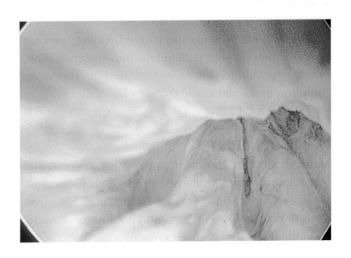

INTRODUCTION

Complete post-hysterectomy vaginal vault or uterovaginal prolapse are conditions with associated medical problems and impaired quality of life. In 1973, Birnbaum[1] estimated the incidence of post-hysterectomy vaginal vault prolapse to be 900 to 1400 per year. It is unlikely, however, that this number has remained constant. The incidence of total vault prolapse is likely to have risen with the increased life expectancy and active lifestyle of women today.

Mild to moderate degrees of prolapse can be treated with a variety of non-surgical means, including Kegel exercises (with or without biofeedback programmes), weighted vaginal devices, electrostimulation and pessaries. Complete prolapse with actual protrusion of the vaginal vault or uterus beyond the introitus of the vagina can only be treated effectively with pessaries or surgery. In a study of pessary use, Sulak[2] found that, of 58 women not desiring surgery over a 3-year study period, 22 discontinued pessary use with 10 choosing to have corrective surgery. In general, pessaries are more accepted by women who are elderly and sedentary, have medical conditions that make surgery high risk, or do not desire corrective surgery.

Because complete vaginal eversion and uterovaginal prolapse are always associated with prolapse of other pelvic organs and defects of support (i.e. cystoceles, rectoceles, enteroceles, and paravaginal defects), many different surgical techniques, both abdominal and vaginal, have been developed to treat this complex condition. Abdominal sacral colpopexy (ASC) is a well-accepted method to treat complete vaginal vault prolapse. The basic principle of this surgical technique is attachment of a synthetic material to the vaginal apex and the sacrum, thereby providing a suspensory hammock to prevent vaginal eversion and prolapse.

This chapter presents the pathophysiology of vault prolapse, preoperative patient selection and evaluation, surgical technique, intra-operative and postoperative complications, and expected results for ASC.

PATHOPHYSIOLOGY

Many factors are known to contribute to vaginal and uterovaginal vault prolapse. Previous hysterectomy, stretching and tearing of tissues during childbirth, medical conditions leading to repetitive increased intra-abdominal pressure (chronic coughing, obesity, chronic vomiting, etc.), abnormalities of support tissue such as collagen defects, and occupational or recreational activities leading to repetitive Valsalva manoeuvres are well-recognized predisposing factors to vaginal vault prolapse. Nevertheless, the exact pathophysiology of complete vault prolapse is not completely understood.

On the basis of a cadaveric study, DeLancey[3] elegantly described the support mechanisms of the different thirds of the vagina. He showed that the vaginal vault and cervix share support from vertically orientated fibres that have a broad origin from the pelvic sidewall and extend downwards to insert at the paracervical and paracolpial levels. Disruption of this superior support mechanism is necessary for vaginal vault and cervical prolapse. It is precisely this support mechanism that the suspensory hammock of ASC is meant to restore. The middle part of the vagina is supported by horizontal fibres; an increased degree of vaginal and cervical descent is the result of loss of support of these fibres. Finally, the lower third of the vagina was found to be fused to the adjacent pelvic structures, and loss of support at this level reflects displacement or attenuation of these organs. When this occurs, with formation of cystocele and rectocele, surgical procedures in addition to ASC may be necessary to correct these lower levels of loss of support. Complete vaginal eversion or uterovaginal prolapse represents disruption of the supports at all three levels.

Vaginal and uterine support are also affected by the pelvic floor musculature. Supporting muscles can be altered in position and function by displacement or attenuation from direct damage or denervation. Harris and Bent[4] discussed funnelling of the pelvic floor with resultant prolapse of the vaginal vault or uterus which can occur with changes in pelvic floor muscle support. These structural alterations are also associated with gynaecological surgical procedures for incontinence that alter the vaginal angle, such as retropubic suspension.

PATIENT SELECTION AND PREOPERATIVE EVALUATION

The woman with complete vaginal eversion presents with a consistent constellation of symptoms (Fig. 53.1). Complete vaginal vault eversion is easily recognized at pelvic examination (Fig. 53.2). If a patient presents with the symptoms suggestive of vaginal vault prolapse, and severe prolapse is not evident on the pelvic examination

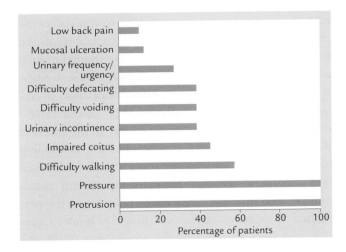

Figure 53.1 *Vaginal prolapse: percentage of patients presenting with various symptoms.*

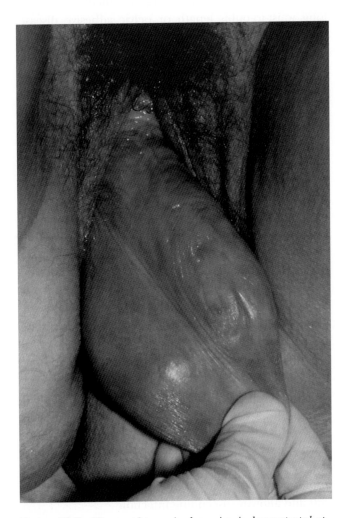

Figure 53.2. *The complete vaginal eversion is demonstrated at pelvic examination.*

in the dorsal lithotomy position, the patient should be examined in the standing position with Valsalva manoeuvre as needed. Because complete vaginal vault eversion or uterovaginal prolapse cannot, by definition, be an isolated prolapse, the examiner should note the associated defects of support (cystocele, rectocele, enterocele, paravaginal defects and perineal detachment) to add the necessary surgical procedures to correct all defects at the time of ASC. Preoperative imaging techniques such as contrast studies (delineating bladder, vagina and bowel) or defecography are rarely necessary. In some patients, however, there can be a question of residual support in either the anterior or posterior vaginal compartments, often because of previous corrective surgery for prolapse, which can be ascertained with imaging studies. Furthermore, some patients may have symptoms such as stool incontinence or bowel dysfunction that would require imaging studies for complete evaluation and accurate diagnosis.

Studies of bladder function, however, are indicated in the patient with vaginal eversion, whether or not urinary incontinence is a symptom. With complete prolapse, the patient may have obstructive uropathy, as demonstrated by Jay *et al.*,[5] with symptoms of voiding dysfunction (difficulty initiating the urinary stream; prolonged and intermittent voids) or overflow incontinence. An obstructive voiding pattern, however, may also be present because of previous anti-incontinence surgery and not because of severe prolapse. Stress incontinence with or without intrinsic sphincteric defect, may be masked by the obstructive uropathy from the prolapse, and the patient may not complain of any urinary incontinence. Reduction of the prolapse, however, without providing bladder-neck support with an anti-incontinence procedure, may result in postoperative urinary incontinence. Detrusor instability and urge incontinence are commonly present in elderly patients and should be diagnosed prior to ASC. For these reasons, optimal preoperative bladder evaluation prior to ASC would include urodynamic tests.

Standard preoperative laboratory tests for an abdominal operation should be performed according to the patient's health status and medical problems. Mechanical and antibiotic bowel preparation may be accomplished on the day before surgery; this is especially important in patients with known adhesive disease or those who previously have undergone multiple abdominal operations.

Vaginal eversion can be corrected by a number of surgical techniques, either abdominal or vaginal. Most defects of support can be corrected through either approach. A pelvic reconstructive surgeon should be at ease with techniques for both abdominal and vaginal corrective procedures. Patient selection criteria for ASC are shown in Table 53.1. These are guidelines and do not represent absolute indications or contraindications.

ASC TECHNIQUE

Because patients given epidural anaesthesia have experienced discomfort and sensation of respiratory compromise associated with extensive bowel packing high into the abdomen, general anaesthesia is recommended. After the patient is asleep, she is placed in the modified lithotomy position with Allen stirrups used to support the legs. This positioning is important because it allows an assistant to stand between the patient's legs and provide effective retraction in the operative field without compromising the surgeon's range of motion. The modified lithotomy position also permits the insertion of the vaginal stent. Finally, the operator can assess suspensory tension, elevate the vagina for retropubic or paravaginal procedures and perform procedures on the

posterior vaginal wall without having to reposition the patient. After preparation with antimicrobial solutions, the abdomen, perineum and vagina are draped in such a way as to give sterile access to all three fields. A drape is placed under the patient's buttocks because instruments and the operator's digits will be placed in and out of the vagina during the procedure. Sterile access to the perineum and vagina can be obtained by draping with a urology or laparoscopy sheet with an abdominal and a perineal opening. Standard laparotomy sheets may be used with a separate drape placed over the perineum. A triple-lumen Foley catheter is inserted sterilely and held aside for sterile access later to fill and flush the bladder during and after the ASC.

Although the standard reported incision for ASC has been vertical, transverse incisions can be used in many patients. The determinants for use of a transverse incision are patients without a large panniculus or with a long waist-to-pubis length or pelvic adhesive disease. After entry into the abdominal cavity, a self-retaining retractor is placed. A deep-bladed Balfour retractor can be rotated 180 degrees to provide retraction of the bowel packed out of the pelvis without having the retractor frame in the field of the retropubic space and deep pelvis – areas needing maximal exposure during ASC. Bowel packing above the level of the sacral promontory is essential for adequate exposure of the presacral space. At this point, adjunctive procedures such as abdominal hysterectomy or salpingo-oophorectomy can be performed. If hysterectomy is performed for complete uterovaginal prolapse, the cuff is closed in a standard fashion, but an additional imbricating closure layer is placed (Fig. 53.3) to prevent the theoretical risk of bacterial seeding of the synthetic material by vaginal flora introduced via the cuff. Although initially there was concern that hysterectomy at the time of ASC would increase postoperative morbidity, Fedorkow and Kalbfleisch[6] showed that this did not occur, by comparing febrile morbidity postoperatively and delayed infection, mesh erosion or need for mesh removal in a group of 86 women undergoing hysterectomy with ASC compared with those in 149 women undergoing ASC alone over a 5-year study period. Placing the stitches attaching the mesh to the vagina away from the cuff suture line is another way to prevent the mesh from pulling open the cuff and allowing ascending infection.

A vaginal stent is placed in the vagina and used to replace the everted vagina in the pelvis. Different types

Table 53.1. *Patient selection criteria for abdominal sacral colpopexy*

Indications

- Active lifestyle
- Factors predisposing to recurrent prolapse
  - Medical conditions:
    Pulmonary disease causing chronic coughing (COPD, chronic bronchitis, emphysema)
    Collagen disorders
    Hypo-oestrogenism
    Obesity
  - Repetitive occupational or recreational straining
- Desire to preserve or restore vaginal coital potential

Contraindications

- Sedentary, very elderly patients
- Dementia
- Sexually inactive patients of long standing who do not desire preservation of vaginal coital potential
- Medical conditions posing specific risk for abdominal surgery

COPD, chronic obstructive pulmonary disease.

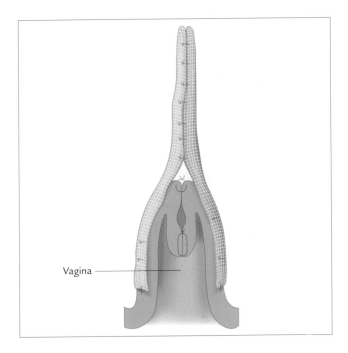

Vagina

Figure 53.3. *The cuff closure after hysterectomy. Note the closure of the cuff through the total thickness of the vaginal wall, followed by an imbricating closure that does not go through the complete vaginal wall proximal to the cuff closure layer. The flaps of the suspensory mesh are attached anteriorly and posteriorly peripheral to the cuff.*

of instruments can be used to do this. A simple Lucite stent can be fashioned in a tubular mould; the edges are rounded, permitting insertion of the lubricated stent without vaginal abrasion. The advantage of this instrument is that it has a smooth, firm surface that allows the vaginal apical stitches to be placed through the wall of the vagina and out again. When the stent has been placed, the peritoneum over the vaginal apex is opened and the bladder is sharply dissected off the anterior vagina. Because the vaginal apex in complete eversion is often thin and devascularized, minimal dissection is performed. The posterior vaginal peritoneum is not dissected away to allow mesh attachment; rather, the mesh is attached through the posterior peritoneum and vaginal wall. Sometimes, the vaginal apex is so thinned that it consists of little more than vaginal mucosa and peritoneum. In these instances, the vaginal apex can be opened with resection of attenuated tissue until the vaginal walls can be reapproximated, as one would a hysterectomy cuff, or the apical tissue can be imbricated with purse-string sutures of delayed absorb-

able suture without opening or resecting the vaginal apex. If the vaginal eversion is large, the vaginal apex may have redundant, thickened tissue; in this situation, upper colpectomy can be performed with a cuff-type closure to restore the vagina to a more normal size. Care must be taken to avoid removing an excess amount of tissue and leaving a foreshortened vagina with potential coital impairment.

Different synthetic materials have been used to suspend the vaginal apex to the sacral promontory. Mersilene mesh is strong, pliable and relatively inexpensive. The advantage of using any mesh is that it allows fibroblasts to grow into the mesh, form tissue and neovascularize. It will eventually be similar to native tissue.[7] The configuration of the mesh has varied over time. Because of concern about increased mesh erosion into the vagina[8] after instituting a double-thickness circumferential attachment,[9] the mesh was fashioned in an inverted-T configuration with an anterior and posterior flap of single thickness (Fig. 53.3). The width of the mesh and the length of the flaps can be tailored to each patient's prolapse. The flaps are attached to the anterior and posterior vagina with interrupted stitches of monofilament permanent suture. Although the stitches may penetrate through the full thickness of the vaginal wall with the surgeon's expectation of re-epithelialization from the vaginal mucosa, particular care is taken to minimize the amount of suture left exposed in the vagina because of the potential for mesh erosion with stitches if re-epithelialization does not occur. After the mesh is attached to the vagina, the stent is removed, and the mesh is held aside.

The rectosigmoid colon is then retracted to the left, and the posterior peritoneum is elevated over the sacral promontory and opened sharply with vertical extension of the incision (Fig. 53.4). Extreme care must be taken in dissecting the underlying adipose/areolar tissue away from the sacrum. This should be done with sharp, digital or cautery dissection gently to avoid tearing the presacral vessels with resultant haemorrhage.[10] Blunt dissection of this space with gauze is ill-advised. If presacral haemorrhage should occur, application of a thumb tack to the bleeding site can be effective.[11] When the sacrum is cleaned, four to six interrupted stitches are placed in a T configuration with the arms of the T on the sacral promontory. The stitches are placed securely in the periosteum, encircling rather than perforating presacral vessels. The ideal needle in terms of

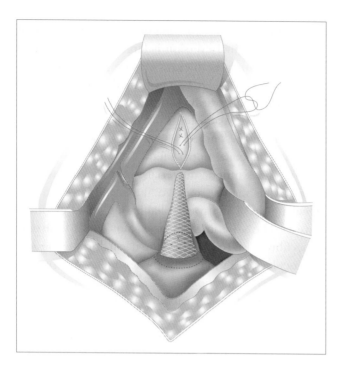

Figure 53.4. *The suspensory mesh has been attached anteriorly and posteriorly to the vagina; the rectosigmoid has been retracted to the left; the posterior peritoneum has been opened vertically, and the initial sacral stitches have been placed.*

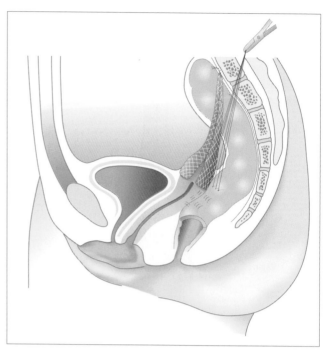

Figure 53.5. *A Halban cul-de-plasty has been placed with the stitches brought out through the mesh. When these stitches are tied, the top of the mesh will be attached to the sacrum.*

curvature and strength is the TT-20. These stitches are not tied at this time, unless there is bleeding associated with the stitch. The ends of these stitches are held aside.

Because all complete vaginal eversions are associated with enteroceles, and altering the vaginal axis anteriorly can predispose to enterocele formation, a cul-de-plasty is performed at the time. The type of cul-de-plasty performed should be based on the anatomy of the pelvis. In general, a broad pelvis and cul-de-sac might be better closed with a Halban anterior-to-posterior closure. A deep conical cul-de-sac can be ideally closed with a Moschowitz cul-de-plasty. The principles of this closure remain the same, despite the type of cul-de-plasty performed. Multiple, interrupted stitches of permanent, monofilament suture should be used. The stitches should be brought up through the mesh at the vaginal attachment (Fig. 53.5), apposing the cul-de-sac closure to the mesh to prevent enterocele formation between the vaginal mesh attachment and the cul-de-plasty.[12]

The final step in ASC is attaching the top of the mesh to the sacrum. The surgeon puts tension on the top of the mesh, bringing it to the sacrum, while assessing the axis and suspension of the vagina manually. To allow

the vagina to lie towards the hollow of the sacrum, there should be minimal or no tension on the vaginal apex. The tendency is to pull the mesh up too tightly to the sacrum, with resulting straightening of the anterior vaginal wall and severe urinary incontinence. If a retropubic or paravaginal suspension is to be performed after the ASC, there will not be enough mobility of the anterior vagina to allow effective suspension in these areas. When the mesh is approximated to the lowest sacral stitch and marked, the ends of the sacral stitches are pulled through the mesh in the order placed. After all the stitches are pulled through, they are tied. Pulling these stitches through the mesh can be facilitated with a small metal crochet hook (no. 7 or no. 8, depending on the suture used). Excess mesh is then trimmed. The posterior peritoneum is then closed with a running stitch of fine, delayed absorbable suture, and the rectosigmoid is replaced over the closure and any remaining exposed mesh. At this time, any additional procedures such as retropubic urethropexy or paravaginal defect repair can be performed. Because of the dissection of the bladder off the anterior vagina and the extensive nature of the cul-de-plasty with the potential for ureteral incorporation or kinking by cul-de-plastic stitches, a suprapubic teloscopy (transabdominal cystoscopy) is always performed with modifications as described by Timmons,[12] to ensure bladder integrity and ureteral patency at the end of the procedure. The abdominal incision is closed in a standard fashion. Finally, the posterior vaginal wall is assessed. If there is residual posterior vaginal relaxation or frank rectocele after the vaginal suspension, the surgeon performs a vaginal procedure to correct this problem.

COMPLICATIONS

Complications of ASC are listed in Table 53.2. The intra-operative complications are those that would be expected with any complex abdominal pelvic reconstructive surgery: these include haemorrhage and injury to the bowel, bladder and ureter. The risks of these complications are increased because of the technique of ASC, the areas of dissection and the frequent incidence of pelvic adhesive disease in women who have had multiple previous operations. The postoperative complication of ileus is related to the extensive bowel manipulation and packing out of the pelvis.

Two rare complications are specific to ASC. The first is mesh erosion into adjacent organs, specifically the vagina and bladder.[8] The actual incidence of mesh erosion into the vagina, the most common site, cannot be calculated but has been reported consistently. The principal symptom is blood-tinged vaginal discharge, with or without malodour. Systemic infection has not been reported, despite the potential for abdominopelvic infection from ascending vaginal flora. On examination, the mesh is often visible or a sinus tract is present. The recommended treatment of this complication is

Table 53.2. *Reported complications of abdominal sacral colpopexy*

Intraoperative
- Haemorrhage
- Bowel injury
- Bladder and ureteral injuries

Postoperative
- Ileus
- Urinary incontinence
- Mesh erosion into adjacent organs
- Sacral osteomyelitis

conservative transvaginal resection of the exposed mesh. This should be performed in the operating room to allow total patient relaxation and adequate retraction to perform the resection high at the vaginal apex. Half of the patients with eroded vaginal mesh will need only one procedure; others will require repeat transvaginal resections. There has been one instance of erosion into the bladder in a patient who presented with asymptomatic urinary infection. The diagnosis was made by cystoscopy, and the eroded mesh was resected at a combined abdominal and vaginal procedure. The mesh re-eroded, and the patient did not desire repeat surgery. She was continuing to have bladder infections at last contact, but she has since been lost to follow-up. Transabdominal resection of the mesh is not recommended unless there is systemic infection or inflammatory foreign body reaction. The greatest risk of haemorrhage occurs when the mesh is resected off the sacrum.

The second rare complication of ASC is osteomyelitis of the sacrum. The presenting symptom for this complication is severe back pain. Magnetic resonance imaging has revealed sacral erosions, and radiographically guided needle aspirates of these areas can be obtained to allow culture of the specific infecting organism. Intravenous antibiotic therapy for 6–8 weeks is recommended for full recovery.

CONCLUSIONS

ASC is an effective surgical technique for resuspending the prolapsed vaginal vault after hysterectomy or complete uterovaginal prolapse. The advantages and disadvantages of ASC over other pelvic reconstructive procedures for complete vaginal eversion are shown in Table 53.3. The durability of ASC for vault support has been documented in large studies with long follow-up by Snyder[13] and Timmons,[9] with good postoperative vaginal vault support in 93 and 99%, respectively. In addition, ASC does not compromise vaginal coital function or potential. In patients who have vaginal compromise from previous vaginal prolapse procedures, the suspension and elongation of the vagina may even restore vaginal function. Some of the disadvantages of ASC are directly related to the abdominal procedure and incision, with increased risk of postoperative ileus, slower recovery and need to perform additional surgical procedures vaginally to correct posterior vaginal

Table 53.3. *Advantages and disadvantages of abdominal sacral colpopexy*

Advantages

- Proven durability
- Non-reliance on patients' supporting tissues
- Preservation or restoration of vaginal coital function
- Access for additional abdominal procedures

Disadvantages

- Abdominal incision with associated slower recovery
- Insertion of synthetic material with potential for infection, foreign body reaction or erosion into adjacent organs
- Need for additional vaginal procedures to correct posterior vaginal relaxation

relaxation. A specific disadvantage of ASC, however, is the introduction of foreign material into the abdominal cavity. This material has the potential (albeit rare) to cause foreign body reaction, infection and erosion into adjacent organs; nevertheless, it undoubtedly contributes to the durability of the vaginal suspension. ASC, as with other abdominal and vaginal procedures for correction of vaginal vault prolapse, is very effective in resuspending the vagina. It must be noted, however, that the greatest challenge to surgeons treating complete vaginal eversion or uterovaginal prolapse is not the suspension of the vaginal apex but the restoration of the prolapsed bladder to normal position and function. ASC is rarely performed, therefore, without some form of bladder procedure to achieve the above goals.

Finally, each patient presents with different needs, medical conditions and pelvic pathology. The pelvic reconstructive surgeon must be able to perform different types of surgical procedures to treat complete vaginal eversion or uterovaginal prolapse and to tailor the approach and treatment to the individual patient. For vaginal eversion and resuspension of the vaginal apex, ASC is an effective surgical option.

REFERENCES

1. Birnbaum SJ. Rational therapy for the prolapsed vagina. *Am J Obstet Gynecol* 1973; 115: 411–419

2. Sulak PJ, Kuehl TJ, Shull BL. Vaginal pessaries and their use in pelvic relaxation. *J Reprod Med* 1993; 38: 919–923

3. DeLancey JOL. Anatomic aspects of vaginal eversion after hysterectomy. *Am J Obstet Gynecol* 1992; 166: 1717–1728

4. Harris TA, Bent AE. Genital prolapse with and without urinary incontinence. *J Reprod Med* 1990; 35: 792–798

5. Jay GD, Kinkead T, Hopkins T, Vollin M. Obstructive uropathy from uterine prolapse: a preventable problem in the elderly. *J Am Geriatr Soc* 1992; 40: 1156–1160

6. Fedorkow DM, Kalbfleisch RE. Total abdominal hysterectomy at abdominal sacrovaginopexy: a comparative study. *Am J Obstet Gynecol* 1993; 169: 641–643

7. Addison WA, Timmons MC, Wall LL *et al.* Failed abdominal sacral colpopexy: observations and recommendations. *Obstet Gynecol* 1989; 74: 480–482

8. Timmons MC, Addison WA. Mesh erosion after abdominal sacral colpopexy. *J Pelvic Surg* 1997; 3: 75–80

9. Timmons MC, Addison WA, Addison SB *et al.* Abdominal sacral colpopexy in 163 women with posthysterectomy vaginal vault prolapse and enterocele. *J Reprod Med* 1992; 37: 323–327

10. Sutton GP, Addison WA, Livengood CH *et al.* Life-threatening hemorrhage complicating sacral colpopexy. *Am J Obstet Gynecol* 1981; 140: 835–857

11. Patsner B, Orr JW. Intractable venous sacral hemorrhage: use of stainless steel thumbtacks to obtain hemostasis. *Am J Obstet Gynecol* 1990; 162: 452

12. Timmons MC. Transabdominal sacral colpopexy. *Op Tech Gynecol Surg* 1996; 1: 92–96

13. Snyder TE, Krantz KE. Abdominal–retroperitoneal sacral colpopexy for the correction of vaginal prolapse. *Obstet Gynecol* 1991; 77: 944–949

54

Hysterectomy

T. Miskry, A. Magos

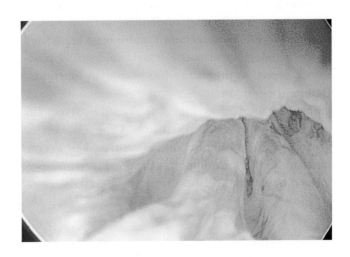

INTRODUCTION

Vaginal hysterectomy is one of the oldest major operations, with references dating from the time of Hippocrates in the 5th century BC and later described by Soranus of Ephesus in AD 120.[1,2] In comparison, the abdominal approach has been developed only in the last 150 years, with Burnham performing the first successful abdominal hysterectomy in 1853.[3] Although both procedures were initially associated with high morbidity and mortality, modifications in technique (not least, the use of sutures), as well as advances in antisepsis and anaesthesia and the introduction of antibiotics, have led to hysterectomy becoming both safe and the commonest major operation in the world after caesarean section. There are wide variations in hysterectomy rates, both nationally and internationally, which are not easily explained by differences in population or pathology characteristics.[4,5] The implication is that recourse to hysterectomy depends on physician preference, patient expectations and values and, perhaps, availability of alternatives. Recently, innovations such as development of intra-uterine hormone-delivery systems and the expanding role of minimally invasive surgical techniques such as endometrial ablation have been predicted to result in a reduction in hysterectomy rates.[6] In the USA the annual rate reached 592 000 in 1990[7] while 72 362 hysterectomies were performed in England alone in 1994.[8] Although there is some evidence that these rates have peaked, it has been estimated that, in the UK, 20% of women will undergo a hysterectomy by the age of 55,[9] while more than one-third of women in the USA have their uterus removed by the age of 60.[10] In contrast, hysterectomy rates are consistently low in the Scandinavian countries.[5]

Although satisfaction rates are high after surgery,[11,12] between one-quarter and one-half of patients sustain complications.[13] Hysterectomy has also been implicated in the aetiology of urinary,[14] bowel[15] and sexual problems,[16] as well as premature loss of ovarian function.[17] Despite these disadvantages and the continuing development of alternatives, for many women hysterectomy remains the end stage of treatment for a variety of gynaecological conditions and, as such, is likely to continue to be the most important major procedure performed by gynaecologists.

INDICATIONS FOR HYSTERECTOMY

There are universally accepted indications for hysterectomy, such as menorrhagia, uterine leiomyomata, prolapse and genital tract malignancy. Unfortunately, however, there is no universally accepted classification system for these indications, such that national and international epidemiological comparisons are fraught with inaccuracies. We would advocate wider use of the classification system suggested by Carlson *et al.*[18] (Table 54.1). Accepting this limitation on descriptive series, the majority of hysterectomies are performed for benign disease, with dysfunctional uterine bleeding and leiomyomata accounting for between 50 and 70% of cases (Fig. 54.1).[9] In 20% of hysterectomies for benign disease, no pathology is identified in the operative specimen.[19] This figure is increased where multiple

Table 54.1. *Classification system for the indications for hysterectomy*

- Uterine leiomyoma
- Dysfunctional uterine bleeding
- Genital prolapse
- Endometriosis and adenomyosis
- Chronic pelvic pain
- Pelvic inflammatory disease
- Endometrial hyperplasia
- Genital tract malignancy (including cervical intra-epithelial neoplasia)
- Obstetric indications

After ref. 18.

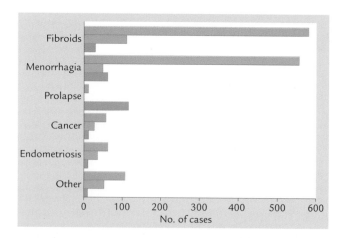

Figure 54.1. *Indications for hysterectomy (after ref. 9;)* ■, *abdominal hysterectomy;* ■, *abdominal hysterectomy with bilateral salpingo-oophorectomy;* ■, *vaginal hysterectomy.*

preoperative indications are listed, perhaps reflecting uncertainty of diagnosis.[20]

Particularly in cases with dysfunctional uterine bleeding or small leiomyomata, it is likely that improve-|ments in medical management (e.g. levonorgestrel intra-uterine system[21]) and wider use of minimal-access surgical techniques (e.g. endometrial ablation,[22,23] hysteroscopic myomectomy[24, 25]) will have the effect of reducing the number of women treated by hysterectomy. It is likely, none the less, that hysterectomy will remain a relatively common operation for women with pelvic pathology.

PRE-OPERATIVE GnRH ANALOGUES

The place of gonadotropin-releasing hormone (GnRH) analogues in patients with dysfunctional uterine bleeding or endometriosis prior to hysterectomy has not been established. However, there is evidence of a role in the pretreatment of the fibroid uterus. GnRH therapy results in a 40–60% reduction in uterine volume, the maximal effect occurring within 12 weeks of treatment.[26] Such reduction may allow borderline cases to be treated vaginally rather than abdominally. In one study, 50 patients with uteri greater than 14-week size were randomized to either no treatment or preoperative GnRH analogue. In the treated group, a significantly higher proportion of patients were able to undergo vaginal hysterectomy, which was associated with shorter postoperative hospital stay.[27]

Another benefit of GnRH pretreatment is that patients often become amenorrhoeic, which facilitates correction of pre-existing anaemia;[26,27] the need for intra-operative or postoperative transfusion is thus reduced.

ANTIBIOTIC PROPHYLAXIS

The introduction of antibiotics in the management of sepsis following gynaecological surgery was a major factor in reducing mortality rates associated with hysterectomy. Antibiotic prophylaxis is believed to reduce the number of contaminating organisms and to render tissue fluid less suitable as a culture medium, the effect being maximal if antibiotics are in the tissue before contamination occurs. The effectiveness of prophylaxis in reducing pelvic infection and febrile morbidity at vaginal hysterectomy has been consistently demonstrated with a variety of regimens,[28] whereas not all

reports have consistently demonstrated the benefit of prophylaxis prior to abdominal hysterectomy;[28,29] however, a meta-analysis of 25 randomized trials concluded that prophylaxis should be used routinely.[30] Although the UK does not have national guidelines, the American College of Obstetricians and Gynecologists recommends single-dose antibiotic prophylaxis with a penicillin or cephalosporin, depending on local efficacy, prior to both vaginal and abdominal hysterectomy.[31]

TYPES OF HYSTERECTOMY

After 150 years of concurrent practice of abdominal and vaginal hysterectomy, gynaecologists still cannot agree on appropriate criteria for route selection. In 1989, Reich first described laparoscopic hysterectomy[32] as an alternative to abdominal hysterectomy, but the route of surgery remains abdominal for the overwhelming majority of cases; typically, more than 70% of hysterectomies, both in the UK and elsewhere, are currently performed by this route (Figs 54.1, 54.2).[8,33]

ABDOMINAL HYSTERECTOMY

Following the introduction of laparoscopic hysterectomy and its subsequent modifications, together with the rekindling of interest in vaginal hysterectomy, an abdominal incision should be necessary only in a minority of patients. At present, this would include cases of genital tract malignancy, enormous uterine

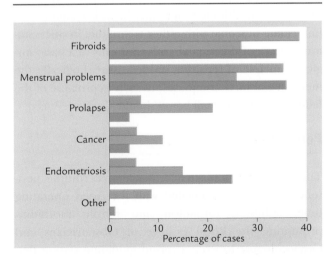

Figure 54.2. *Indications for laparoscopic (■)** hysterectomy compared with abdominal and vaginal hysterectomy in the UK (■)* and the USA (■) **.(*signifies ref. 9; ** signifies ref. 33.)*

enlargement or gross extra-uterine disease not amenable to the laparoscope. Many techniques for, and modifications to, total abdominal hysterectomy have been described and it is beyond the scope of this chapter to give a detailed review of all these alternatives. From a urological perspective, identification of the ureter in the pelvis is of particular importance. In addition, aggressive blunt dissection during bladder mobilization should be avoided in favour of sharp dissection, especially in cases of previous caesarean section, as this risks bladder damage.

Although this sequence of events is fairly standard, the further management of the vaginal vault and peritoneum is the subject of some controversy.

Management of the vaginal vault

Surgical textbooks fail to agree on whether closure or non-closure of the vaginal vault is associated with advantages. Proponents of vault closure argue that this policy reduces the risk of ascending infection, whereas those who favour leaving the vault open suggest that this allows drainage of the pelvis, preventing haematoma and reducing the risk of postoperative infectious morbidity. Unfortunately, this argument has not been resolved in the published literature: although Korn et al.[34] reported an increased risk of wound infection when the vault was left open, Colombo et al.[35] found no difference in rates of pelvic and wound infection rates or the incidence of vault haematomas and granulation tissue in 273 women randomized to open or closed vaginal vault at abdominal hysterectomy. Although there may be little difference in immediate outcome with either technique, in our opinion, closure of the vaginal vault conforms to a basic surgical principle of repairing divided tissue. Logically, the incidence of rarer complications such as prolapse of the fallopian tubes or small bowel should also be reduced.

Peritoneum

There is some published evidence that routine peritoneal closure is associated with increased operating time, adhesion formation and febrile morbidity, prompting the Royal College of Obstetricians and Gynaecologists to issue a recent guideline stating that '... non-closure [of peritoneum] appears to have few associated risks and may be recommended in many obstetric and gynaecological operations ....'[36] However,

during hysterectomy, a central principle behind peritoneal closure is to make vascular pedicles retroperitoneal so that postoperative bleeding is revealed. Occult blood loss may delay recognition of haemorrhage, resulting in significant morbidity. Korn et al.[34] also noted that the relative risk of wound infection was trebled if the parietal peritoneum (as well as the vault) was left open at hysterectomy.[34]

VAGINAL HYSTERECTOMY

Despite potential advantages of vaginal surgery, the majority of hysterectomies remain abdominal. One explanation for this is a list of contraindications to vaginal surgery, cited by proponents of abdominal and laparoscopic surgery. These have included a need for concurrent oophorectomy, presence of an enlarged uterus, previous pelvic surgery (including caesarean section), lack of prolapse, suspected endometriosis, adnexal pathology and malignancy.

However, there is evidence in the literature that many of these contraindications are no longer valid. For instance, vaginal oophorectomy is reported as being successful in more than 95% of patients.[37,38] Kovac graded the degree of ovarian descent at vaginal hysterectomy and reported that vaginal oophorectomy was possible in 99% of patients with ovaries of grade I or higher.[39] In simple cases, the fundamental principle involves division of the round ligament separate to the infundibulopelvic ligament, as this allows further mobilization and descent of the adnexa.[40] If this is insufficient to allow salpingo-oophorectomy, then, in the majority of cases, oophorectomy alone is achievable and acceptable. Even ovaries with no descent (grade 0 according to Kovac) can be removed vaginally, using minimal-access techniques such as transvaginal endoscopic oophorectomy.[41,42]

Simple debulking techniques such as bisection, coring, morcellation and myomectomy mean that even large uteri can be removed vaginally.[43–46] In our own series, successful vaginal hysterectomy was performed in uteri weighing 380–1100 g.[47] There is also good evidence in the literature that lack of prolapse[48] and previous pelvic surgery[49,50] do not contraindicate vaginal surgery. It has even been suggested that the vaginal approach facilitates dissection of the bladder from the cervix in patients who have undergone previous caesarean section[29]

LAPAROSCOPIC HYSTERECTOMY (AND ITS DERIVATIVES)

Although the majority of hysterectomies are suitable for vaginal surgery, there are clear indications for the laparoscopic approach in certain cases: these include the further evaluation and management of adnexal masses, pelvic adhesiolysis and ablation of symptomatic endometriosis, and in the treatment of certain cancers of the upper genital tract when combined with lymph-node sampling and other staging procedures. Since its inception, modifications of the original operation have proliferated, leading to a bewildering array of nomenclature. However, these derivatives can be grouped using a simple classification system (Table 54.2).[51] In addition, the operation can be staged to indicate the degree of surgery performed laparoscopically (Fig. 54.3).[52]

Table 54.2. *Simple classification of laparoscopic hysterectomy*
1. Laparovaginal hysterectomy
2. Laparoscopic subtotal hysterectomy
3. Laparoscopic total hysterectomy
4. Operative laparoscopy before vaginal hysterectomy
(5. Diagnostic laparoscopy before vaginal hysterectomy)*

* We have added category 5 to reflect the suggestion of Kovac *et al.*[106]
After ref. 51.

Operating time has been clearly demonstrated to increase with increasing stage of laparoscopic hysterectomy.[53] As well as being time consuming, management of the uterine artery laparoscopically is technically difficult and risks haemorrhage and injury to the ureter. It follows that, where indicated, laparoscopic surgery should be converted to a vaginal procedure as soon as possible; in practical terms, this means conversion to vaginal surgery once the uterovesical fold of peritoneum has been opened (stage 3 laparoscopic hysterectomy). Accepting this, there are two surgical approaches. In the first, an essentially Heaney vaginal hysterectomy with a laparoscopic component is performed (Fig. 54.4). The ovarian pedicles are divided laparoscopically, while the round ligaments are left intact. In this way, the uterine pedicles are supported, preventing avulsion secondary to traction during vaginal dissection. Alternatively, when the uterus is not grossly enlarged, a Doderlein–Kronig approach can be used (Fig. 54.5). In this technique, division of the round ligaments facilitates anteflexion of the uterus into the anterior colpotomy. The uterine vessels are then secured prior to division of the uterosacral and cardinal ligaments, the latter structures providing support and reducing the risk of vascular avulsion.

Electrosurgical desiccation, sutures and staples have all been described to secure vascular pedicles. Although stapling devices allow these steps to be performed

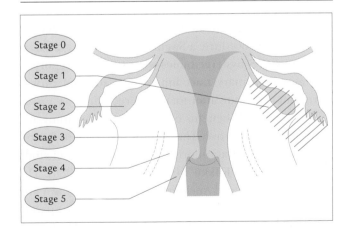

Figure 54.3. *Staging of laparoscopic hysterectomy : stage 0: diagnostic laparoscopy; stage 1: adhesiolysis and other preparative procedures; stage 2: ovarian pedicle; stage 3: uterovesical fold; stage 4: uterine pedicle; stage 5: vault pedicle.*

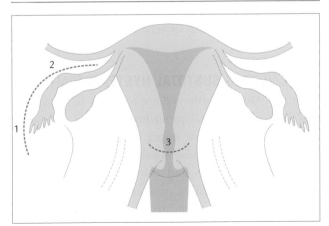

Figure 54.4. *Stage III laparoscopic hysterectomy with a Heaney-type vaginal component: (1) ovarian pedicle is divided; (2) broad ligament divided lateral to ovary but round ligament left intact; (3) uterovesical fold is opened, prior to Heaney vaginal hysterectomy.*

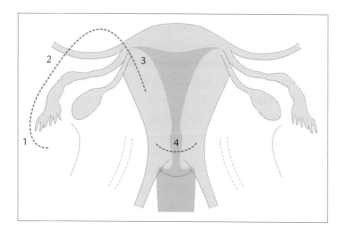

Figure 54.5. *Stage III laparoscopic hysterectomy with a Doderlein-type vaginal component: (1) ovarian pedicle is divided; (2) broad ligament divided lateral to ovary followed by round ligament; (3) peritoneal dissection continued anteriorly towards bladder; (4) uterovesical fold is opened, prior to Doderlein vaginal hysterectomy.*

rapidly, they require 12 mm cannulae with higher port placement. In addition, they are expensive and increase the risk of damage to the ureter. Electrosurgery, although involving an initial capital outlay, is versatile and effective and does not require expensive disposable instruments. In situations where vital structures such as bowel or ureter are close to the vascular pedicle, laparoscopic suturing may be the safest option.

Paradoxically, the development of laparoscopic hysterectomy has led to a re-evaluation of the role of vaginal hysterectomy. In the same way, difficulty in managing the uterine artery laparoscopically has rekindled interest in subtotal hysterectomy.

TOTAL VERSUS SUBTOTAL HYSTERECTOMY

Prior to 1940, the universal approach to hysterectomy had been the subtotal procedure with the associated reduced risk of ureteric injury, haemorrhage and – in particular – postoperative sepsis.[3] Following the introduction of antibiotics and consequent fall in febrile morbidity and mortality, total hysterectomy became established, partly as a means of preventing the occurrence of cervical stump carcinoma at a time when detection of pre-invasive lesions was not possible.[54] Indeed, in surgical textbooks of the time, subtotal hysterectomy was rarely mentioned and the operation itself was often regarded as evidence of a lack of surgical skill![55] Although there remain some well-established

indications for subtotal hysterectomy (e.g. caesarean hysterectomy, severe endometriosis with cul-de-sac obliteration), the rationale of removing the cervix at hysterectomy is now being questioned.

Although removal of the cervix is undoubtably indicated in the treatment of conditions such as malignancy and uterine prolapse, it is evident that, in the majority of patients undergoing hysterectomy, there is no cervical disease. Following the recognition that pre-invasive lesions of the cervix can be identified from cervical cytology and treated at colposcopy, routine removal of the cervix to prevent stump carcinoma has become a less persuasive argument for total hysterectomy. In a Danish study of over 1000 women undergoing subtotal hysterectomy, the incidence of subsequent cervical stump carcinoma was only 0.3%,[56] and simultaneous treatment of the transformation zone may reduce this risk further.[57] Although carcinoma arising in the cervical stump may complicate treatment because of distorted anatomy, this does not appear to affect prognosis. Several case series have been published that consistently report that, stage for stage, treatment results for cervical stump cancer do not differ from those for women with an intact uterus.[58–60]

Rather than subtotal hysterectomy being an incomplete procedure, retention of the cervix may confer benefits. The ureter, bladder and (to a lesser extent) the rectum are all anatomically related to the cervix and may be injured during dissection. In addition, the nerve supply to pelvic organs via the pelvic plexus is at risk during total hysterectomy which, in theory, could lead to symptoms.[61] As one indication of the relative safety of the subtotal procedure, a Swedish study (where 21% of a series of 678 hysterectomies were subtotal) reported no cases of urinary tract injury after subtotal procedures but a 1% rate after total hysterectomy.[62]

The long-term benefits of subtotal hysterectomy are more difficult to prove. The most quoted data in favour of cervical conservation originate from a series of studies published by Kilkku in Finland in the 1980s. He reported a reduced incidence of subjective urinary symptoms in women undergoing subtotal compared with those undergoing total hysterectomy.[63] He found statistically significant differences in the sensation of incomplete bladder emptying postoperatively (10.3 vs 22.1%), urinary incontinence at one year (22.6 vs 28.8%) and a trend towards reduced urinary frequency in the subtotal hysterectomy group. These results must be interpreted with some caution, however, as although the study was prospective it was non-randomized and the patient groups may have been dissimilar.

Objective measurement of bladder function by urodynamic studies has failed to demonstrate a benefit from subtotal hysterectomy. Kujansuu and colleagues[64] assessed urethral closure function pre- and postoperatively in a small non-randomized study and were unable to find any differences between subtotal and total hysterectomy. In a randomized comparison of 22 patients, Lalos and Bjerle[65] found no difference in either urodynamic evaluation or subjective symptoms between subtotal and total hysterectomy.

Increased media interest in the subtotal procedure was aroused by Kilkku's series of papers when he reported that total hysterectomy resulted in a reduced frequency of orgasm and was associated with less improvement in dyspareunia.[16,66] However, there is no consistent evidence that hysterectomy *per se* has any significant effects on libido or sexual enjoyment.[54,55,67] Furthermore, two more recent studies of sexual function after subtotal hysterectomy have also failed to demonstrate any benefit. Helstrom *et al.*[68] compared sexual experience pre- and postoperatively in 104 women undergoing the subtotal procedure and reported improvement in 50%, with deterioration in 21%. Nathorst-Boos *et al.*[62] compared total with subtotal hysterectomy and found no difference in sexual satisfaction between the two groups. As with urinary symptoms, the available evidence in favour of cervical conservation is inconclusive.

There is no doubt regarding some advantages to the subtotal approach: complications such as vault haematomas are reduced,[62] while fallopian tube[69] and small bowel[70] prolapse become impossible; in addition, granulation tissue of the vault, which is said to complicate 21% of hysterectomies and invariably causes symptoms, is also avoided.[71] Conversely, retaining the cervical stump can give rise to clinical symptoms secondary to endometriosis, chronic cervicitis or prolapse. In one series, 11/12 women required cervicectomy after subtotal hysterectomy.[72] Finally, there remains a small but significant risk of subsequent cervical malignancy and the patient is committed to continued cervical surveillance.

OOPHORECTOMY AT HYSTERECTOMY

As with the cervix, the ovaries are usually disease free at hysterectomy but have malignant potential. Unlike the situation with cervical cancer, however, satisfactory screening strategies for premalignant lesions are, as yet, unavailable. In addition, as 75% of patients present with extra-ovarian disease (which has a 5–year survival rate of only 15%),[73] there is a case for elective oophorectomy at hysterectomy. It has been suggested that at least 10% of ovarian cancers could be prevented by such a strategy;[73] there is also evidence that hysterectomy alone reduces the risk of subsequent ovarian malignancy.[74-76] An explanation for this may be that clinical inspection at hysterectomy screens out abnormal or suspicious ovaries and these are removed at the time. An additional factor may be surgical impairment of ovarian blood flow and subsequent function.

Apart from the hazard of subsequent malignancy, conservation of the ovaries at hysterectomy may result in morbidity. Pelvic pain and dyspareunia secondary to the residual ovary syndrome results in further surgery in 1–2% of patients after hysterectomy.[29] In certain patient groups this figure may be higher: for example, Namnoum *et al.*[77] found that women who had ovarian conservation at the time of hysterectomy for endometriosis had a relative risk of reoperation of 8.1 compared with those who underwent oophorectomy. However, in a survey of the attitudes of gynaecologists to oophorectomy at hysterectomy, 85% would recommend elective oophorectomy in post-menopausal women, whereas only 20% would do the same in premenopausal women over the age of 45 years.[73] This is because oophorectomy itself has disadvantages. Loss of ovarian function, whether through surgical or natural menopause, is associated with short-term problems such as vasomotor symptoms and, more importantly, in the long term has detrimental effects on bone density, the cardiovascular system and urogenital tract. In addition, reduction in circulating androgens may be responsible for psychological symptoms and loss of libido.[78] Although these effects can be countered by hormone-replacement therapy, some women are reluctant to commit to drug treatment and compliance may be poor. Oestrogen replacement may also be associated with short-term side effects as well as an increased risk of thromboembolism[79] and, possibly, breast cancer.[80]

Overall, it seems likely that, in postmenopausal and immediately perimenopausal women, the evidence is in favour of elective oophorectomy. In premenopausal women an individual decision should be made with the patient; in the majority of cases, ovarian conservation may be preferable. Elective oophorectomy is indicated, however, in premenopausal patients in certain high-risk groups, such as women with a strong family history of ovarian malignancy or a history of prolonged ovulation induction.

COMPLICATIONS OF HYSTERECTOMY

Little more than 100 years ago the mortality rate following hysterectomy was as high as 70%.[1] Major advances in surgical and anaesthetic technique, together with the introduction of antisepsis and antibiotics, have meant that the overall mortality rate is now as low as 10–20/10 000 patients.[33] This rate is, however, age related. Wingo *et al.*[81] reported that the mortality rate ranged from 3–7/10 000 below the age of 55 years to 173/10 000 for age 75 years and above. In addition, mortality is higher in certain subsets of women, even when corrected for age: for example, in women undergoing pregnancy-related hysterectomy the mortality rate is 29.2/10 000 and, where the indication is cancer, the mortality rate is 37.8/10 000.[81]

Morbidity is more difficult to analyse, as different definitions and classification systems of complications are reported in the literature. Dicker *et al.*[13] stated that a complication should have the following characteristics: it should be as objective as possible, should be uniformly documented in hospital records and should be clinically reasonable and acceptable. Using these criteria, the Collaborative Review of Sterilization (CREST) study defined six categorial complications (Table 54.3).[13] The Health Technology Assessment Information Service in the recent ECRI report used these categories to compare contemporary data for vaginal, abdominal and laparoscopic hysterectomy.[33] In addition, they contrasted this with the historical data from the CREST study (Fig. 54.6). It is clear from these fig-

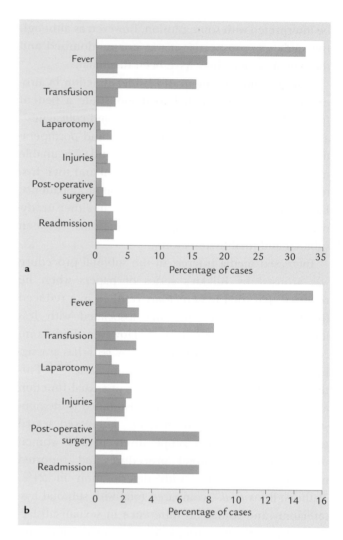

a

b

Figure 54.6. *Complications of (a) abdominal (■* and ■**) laparoscopic (■***) hysterectomy and (b) vaginal (■* and ■**) and laproscopic hysterectomy (■***). * Signifies ref. 13; ** signifies ref. 33 (Laproscopy in Hysterectomy (LH) reports 1992–1995); *** signifies ref. 33 (LH reports 1990–1995).*

ures that fever and need for transfusion are the commonest complications associated with hysterectomy.

The frequency of blood transfusion has also decreased since the CREST report, although this may reflect a higher threshold for treatment following increased concern over the transmission of viral infections and reduced blood stocks. In contrast, the incidence of unintended major surgical procedures to manage intra-operative injury to bowel or bladder or to control haemorrhage is relatively unchanged. This rate is also relatively independent of route, occurring in approximately 2% of hysterectomies.[33]

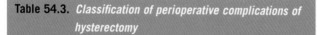

Table 54.3. *Classification of perioperative complications of hysterectomy*

- Febrile morbidity
- Haemorrhage requiring transfusion
- Unintended major surgical procedure
- Life-threatening event
- Death
- Rehospitalization

After ref. 13.

Table 54.4. *Complications of hysterectomy*

Genital tract complications

- Vault prolapse
- Incisional hernia at vaginal apex
- Vaginal vault rupture
- Eversion of vagina
- Prolapse of fallopian tube
- Foreign body granuloma
- Residual ovarian syndrome
- Ectopic pregnancy
- Adnexal abscess
- Consort glans laceration

Urinary tract complications

- Ureteric fistula
- Salpingovesical fistula
- Hydronephrosis
- Chronic renal failure
- Wissler–Fanconi syndrome
- Incisional bladder hernia

Gastrointestinal complications

- Necrotizing colitis
- Constipation
- Irritable bowel syndrome
- Bowel obstruction
- Colovaginal fistula
- Sigmoidovesical fistula
- Perforation of duodenal ulcer

Other complications

- Sexual difficulties
- Recurrent pneumoperitoneum
- Femoral neuropathy
- Premature ovarian failure
- Ischaemic heart disease
- Osteoporosis

As well as the categorial complications described by Dicke,[13] numerous complications – both immediate and delayed – have been documented in the literature (Table 54.4). As this is a textbook of urology and urogynaecology, we concentrate here on the potential urological complications of hysterectomy.

Urological complications

Immediate complications

Urinary tract injuries are the commonest cause of litigation following hysterectomy,[82] and are increasingly seen as indefensible.[83] Ureteric injuries, either ligation or transection, are reported to occur in 0.5–3% of cases, most frequently involving the lowest 3 cm close to the cervix. If unrecognized, damage may be associated with considerable morbidity and potential loss of kidney function, or fistula formation. Although most series report that ureteric injuries are more common with abdominal than with vaginal hysterectomy, this may be secondary to case selection.[84] None the less, it has been postulated that inherent advantages in the technique of vaginal hysterectomy may protect the ureter from damage.[85] In a systematic review of laparoscopic hysterectomy, Meikle *et al.*[86] reported a significantly higher rate of ureteric injury during laparoscopic than with abdominal hysterectomy. This risk may be related to difficulty in securing the uterine arteries laparoscopically, especially when linear stapling devices are used.[87]

Mobilization of the bladder is an integral part of hysterectomy by whatever route and, not surprisingly, bladder injury has been reported in 0.3–0.8% of cases.[88] As with ureteric transection, unrecognized bladder perforation will lead to the formation of a vesicovaginal fistula.

Lesser immediate complications include acute postoperative urinary retention, affecting 15% of patients after vaginal and 4.8% after abdominal hysterectomy in the CREST study.[13] However, 44.5% of the vaginal hysterectomy patients in this study underwent concurrent colporrhaphy. In theory, reduced pain and increased early mobilization associated with simple vaginal hysterectomy should reduce the incidence of acute retention. Urinary tract infection (UTI) occurred in 7% of abdominal and 3.4% of vaginal hysterectomy patients in the CREST report, where fewer than 50% of patients received antibiotics.[13] The incidence of UTI is related to the use of prophylactic antibiotics and duration of catheterization.[28] Avoidance of an indwelling catheter is possible following laparoscopic and vaginal hysterectomy,[89] and may result in a reduction in risk of UTI.

Late complications

The uterus has a close anatomical relationship with the bladder and the pelvic plexus. Disruption of this anatomical relationship and/or damage to the autonomic innervation of the pelvis, as a consequence of gynaecological surgery, may potentially give rise to urinary outflow tract dysfunction. The pelvic plexus is particularly at risk during total hysterectomy – when injury may occur during division of the cardinal ligaments, dissection of the bladder from the uterus and cervix, paravaginal dissection and removal of the cervix.[67]

Conversely, urinary symptoms may resolve if hysterectomy removes pathology such as fibroids or endometriosis.

In contrast to radical hysterectomy, which is associated with almost universal neural damage to the bladder, hysterectomy for benign conditions is associated with inconsistent damage to the pelvic plexus and thus a spectrum of symptoms postoperatively. In a retrospective survey of 946 women, 40.9% of those who had undergone hysterectomy reported urinary symptoms, compared with 40.8% of women who had undergone laparoscopic sterilization only.[90] In a similar study, Griffith-Jones et al.[91] found no difference in symptoms in women undergoing hysterectomy compared with those having dilatation and curettage. However, retrospective questionnaires have also reported both an increased[92] and a decreased[93,94] incidence of urinary symptoms following hysterectomy. Unfortunately, the value of these surveys is questionable, as bladder dysfunction prior to surgery may differ in the groups assessed.

Objective evaluation of function both pre- and postoperatively has been reported by various authors, although in most studies the patient numbers have been small. Parys et al.[95] performed urodynamic and nerve conduction studies in 42 patients, before and after hysterectomy, and correlated the results with subjective symptoms. After hysterectomy, the incidence of urinary symptoms increased from 58 to 75%, while 30% of patients developed new urodynamic abnormalities, of whom 72% had evidence of pelvic neuropathy as detected by sacral reflex latencies. In contrast, Langer et al.[96] reported no significant differences in symptoms or urodynamic findings in 16 patients before and after hysterectomy. Other studies have also failed to demonstrate measurable changes in objective endpoints.[64,65] Some have questioned the relevance of objective assessments. Prior et al.[97] examined 26 patients and found a postoperative increase in vesical sensitivity which was not always associated with symptoms; Vervest et al.[98] reported decreased cystometric capacity and reduced bladder compliance but concluded that this was of no clinical importance.

Most published evidence on the effect of hysterectomy on urinary function relies either on retrospective data or prospective studies with small numbers. In addition, there is a high prevalence of urinary symptoms in women undergoing hysterectomy. As a result,

at present it is not possible to conclude if hysterectomy has an overall effect – either positive or negative. However, it seems likely that postoperative symptoms will depend greatly on the patient's preoperative urological status.

Comparison of abdominal, vaginal and laparoscopic hysterectomy

Accepting the fact that abdominal, vaginal and laparoscopic hysterectomies tend to be performed on different populations of patients, most observational and comparative studies have come to broadly similar conclusions. Laparascopic hysterectomy generally takes longer than either of the two other approaches, usually by a factor of 1 hour, but is associated with faster recovery and less discomfort than abdominal hysterectomy.[99,100] However, there is no such advantage of laparoscopic over vaginal hysterectomy.[53,89]

With respect to complications, the most quoted data regarding abdominal and vaginal hysterectomy derive from the 1982 CREST study surveying hysterectomy practice in the USA.[13] Complication rates of 42.8 and 24.5% were reported for abdominal and vaginal hysterectomy, respectively. At first sight, these figures compare unfavourably with recent data for laparoscopic hysterectomy, such as the overall rate of 15.6% reported by Garry and Phillips.[101] The CREST study, however, took place between 1978 and 1981, involving surgeons of all grades (including trainees), with a high proportion of women who were obese (42.6%) and who underwent additional surgical procedures (74.1%). Only 47.3% of patients received prophylactic antibiotics, and febrile morbidity represented the most frequent complication of both abdominal and vaginal hysterectomy. In contrast, many of the early publications about laparoscopic hysterectomy summarized outcome of individual and expert laparoscopic surgeons.

Extreme care has, therefore, to be taken if any comparison between the different types of hysterectomies is to be fair and valid. A careful and detailed analysis of all published data to date was presented in 1995 by the Health Technology Assessment Service of ECRI in the USA, involving over 6000 hysterectomies performed in the late 1980s and early 1990s.[33] The analysis showed that the complication rates for abdominal and vaginal hysterectomies are considerably less than in the CREST study of the 1980s: in particular, febrile morbidity and transfusion have become much less common, especially following vaginal surgery. As a result, whereas the complication rate of laparoscopic hysterectomy remains superior to that of abdominal hysterectomy, there is little (if any) difference between laparoscopic and vaginal hysterectomy. The ECRI report also confirmed that laparoscopic and vaginal hysterectomy are associated with shorter inpatient hospital stay than abdominal hysterectomy. Cost analysis of the three procedures demonstrated that vaginal hysterectomy is the cheapest, and laparoscopic hysterectomy the most expensive, because of the longer operating time and use of expensive disposable instruments.

These findings have been replicated by other, more recent (albeit smaller) studies. Although both laparoscopic and vaginal hysterectomy have been shown to be potentially outpatient procedures,[89] vaginal hysterectomy is consistently reported in the literature as the most cost-effective procedure.[102,103] From this evidence it appears that the vaginal route should be considered superior to both abdominal and laparoscopic hysterectomy.

DECISION ABOUT THE ROUTE OF HYSTERECTOMY

Many factors determine the route of hysterectomy. In some cases there is no doubt about the route of hysterectomy (e.g. laparotomy for enormous uterine fibroids); however, in many cases, any of the three routes – abdominal, vaginal or laparoscopic – could be suitable. Then it is a matter of personal judgement and preference based on history, indications, clinical findings and – above all – experience. The importance of the latter was well demonstrated by Kovac and colleagues,[104] addressing the issue of why relatively few hysterectomies are performed vaginally. Limitations in training and experience appear to lead to a lack of confidence in the ability to perform vaginal surgery, with a resultant preference for abdominal hysterectomy for many gynaecologists. Surgeons with a preference for the vaginal route, for instance, are more likely to assess uterine mobility and size as part of their preoperative assessment,[104] knowing (as they do) the importance of these two variables in terms of successful vaginal surgery. In contrast, gynaecologists with a preference for abdominal surgery make less effort to discriminate between cases suitable for either route. Where appro-

priate preoperative assessment is used, the vaginal route is successful in over 99% of cases and the present ratio of abdominal to vaginal hysterectomy of 3 : 1 could be reversed.[105] In uncertain cases, laparoscopy immediately before hysterectomy can provide useful information about the optimum route of surgery, which can be logically based on the state of the pelvis and extent of pathology (Tables 54.5, 54.6).[106] In most cases the experienced vaginal surgeon can dispense with laparoscopy and, in the absence of extra-uterine disease or malignancy, can decide whether to proceed vaginally on two cardinal criteria – namely, uterine mobility (which is not synonymous with prolapse) and vaginal access. As already discussed, nulliparity, uterine enlargement (within reason), absence of prolapse, history of pelvic surgery, or the need for oophorectomy should not be perceived as contraindications to the vaginal route.

It should not, therefore, be surprising that Kovac in the USA[105] and Querleu in France[107] clearly showed that many patients currently managed by abdominal or laparoscopic hysterectomy are suitable for vaginal surgery. They report rates of vaginal hysterectomy for

Table 54.5. *Laparoscopic scoring for determining operative approach to hysterectomy*

Parameter	Points
Uterine size	
Grade I: 8 weeks or less	1
Grade II: 8–12 weeks	3
Grade III: 12–16 weeks	5
Mobility of adnexa*	
Good: > 5 cm	1
Moderate: 2–5 cm	3
Poor: < 2 cm	5
Adnexal adhesions	
None	1
Moderate	3
Severe	5
Status of cul-de-sac	
Accessible	0
Obliterated	5
Endometriosis†	
Stage I	1
Stage II	2
Stage III	3
Stage IV	4

* As judged by stretched length of infundibulopelvic ligament.
†American Fertility Society classification.
After ref. 106.

Table 54.6. *Route of hysterectomy according to laparoscopy score*

Parameter	Weighted score
Uterine size	1, 3 or 5
Mobility of adnexa	1 or 5
Adnexal adhesions	1, 3 or 5
Status of cul-de-sac	0 or 5
Endometriosis	1, 2, 3 or 4
Total*	< 11 VH
	11–19 LAVH
	> 19 LH

* VH, vaginal hysterectomy; LAVH, laparoscopic-assisted vaginal hysterectomy; LH, laparoscopic hysterectomy. After ref. 106.

benign indications of 88% (97% if women undergoing intra-operative diagnostic laparoscopy are included) and 77%, respectively. Similarly, the conclusion of the comprehensive ECRI report was unequivocal:

> Specific guidelines should be largely to replace abdominal hysterectomy not with laparoscopic hysterectomy but with vaginal hysterectomy. Based on available evidence, laparoscopic hysterectomy has an established place, but only in a minority of patients, with laparoscopy confined to diagnostic uses in most of these cases.[33]

To achieve these rates, a gynaecologist has, in particular, to master vaginal surgery when there is no uterine prolapse, in cases of uterine enlargement with leiomyomata, and also has to have the ability to carry out oophorectomy vaginally.[108]

CONCLUSIONS

Hysterectomy is (and is likely to remain) a common gynaecological procedure. It is the most effective management for several chronic conditions; it is relatively safe, and long-term patient satisfaction is high. Arguably, the major change in hysterectomy practice as we head into the next millennium will be in surgical approach, with an increasing proportion of cases managed laparoscopically and (in particular), vaginally.

REFERENCES

1. Sutton C. Hysterectomy: a historical perspective. In: Wood C, Maher PJ (eds) Hysterectomy. *Bailliere's Clin Obstet Gynaecol* 1997; 11: 1–22

2. Leonardo RA. *History of Gynecology* New York: Foben Press, 1944

3. Benrubi GI. History of hysterectomy. *J Fla Med Assoc* 1988; 75: 533–542

4. McPherson K. International differences in medical care practices. *Health Care Finance Rev Annu Suppl* 1989; 9–20

5. McPherson K, Wennberg JE, Hovind OB, Clifford P. Small-area variation in the use of common surgical procedures: an international comparison of New England, England and Norway. *N Engl J Med* 1982; 307: 1310–1314

6. Lilford RJ. Hysterectomy: will it pay the bills in 2007? *Br Med J* 1997; 314: 160–161

7. Wilcox LS, Koonin LM, Pokras R *et al*. Hysterectomy in the United States, 1988–1990. *Obstet Gynecol* 1994; 83: 549–555

8. Hospital Episode Statistics. *Finished Consultant Episodes by Diagnosis Operation and Speciality. Financial year 1993–1994*, Volume 1. UK: Government Statistics Service.

9. Vessey MP, Villard-MacKintosh L, McPherson K *et al*. The epidemiology of hysterectomy: findings in a large cohort study. *Br J Obstet Gynaecol* 1992; 99: 402–407

10. National Center for Health Statistics, Pokras R, Hufnagel VG. Hysterectomies in the United States,1965–84. *Vital Health stat* [13] 1987; 92

11. Schofield MJ, Bennett A, Redman S, Walters WAW, Sanson-Fisher RW. Self-reported long-term outcomes of hysterectomy. *Br J Obstet Gynaecol* 1991; 98: 1129–1136

12. Carlson KJ, Miller BA, Fowler FJ. The Maine Women's health study: 1. Outcomes of hysterectomy. *Obstet Gynecol* 1994; 83: 556–565

13. Dicker RC, Greenspan JR, Strauss LT *et al*. Complications of abdominal and vaginal hysterectomy among women of reproductive age in the United States. The Collaborative Review of Sterilization. *Am J Obstet Gynecol* 1982; 144: 841–848

14. Parys BT, Haylen BT, Hutton JL, Parsons KF. Urodynamic evaluation of lower urinary tract function in relation to total hysterectomy. *Aust N Z J Obstet Gynaecol* 1990; 30: 161–165

15. Taylor T, Smith AN, Fulton PM. Effect of hysterectomy on bowel function. *Br Med J* 1989; 299: 300–301

16. Kilkku P, Gronroos M, Hirvonen T, Rauramo L. Supravaginal uterine amputation vs. hysterectomy. Effects on libido and orgasm. *Acta Obstet Gynecol Scand* 1983; 62: 147–152

17. Siddle N, Sarrel P, Whitehead M. The effect of hysterectomy on the age at ovarian failure: identification of a subgroup of women with premature loss of ovarian function and literature review. *Fertil Steril* 1987; 47: 94–100

18. Carlson KJ, Nichols DH, Schiff I. Indications for hysterectomy. *N Engl J Med* 1993; 328: 856–860

19. Lee NC, Dicker RC, Rubin MB, Ory HW. Confirmation of the preoperative diagnoses for hysterectomy. *Am J Obstet Gynecol* 1984; 150: 283–287

20. Reiter RC, Gambone JC, Lench JB. Appropriateness of hysterectomies performed for multiple preoperative indications. *Obstet Gynecol* 1992; 80: 902–905

21. Andersson D, Rybo G. Levonorgestrel-releasing intrauterine system in the treatment of menorrhagia. *Br J Obstet Gynaecol* 1990; 97: 690–694

22. O'Connor H, Magos AL. Endometrial resection for menorrhagia: evaluation of the results at 5 years. *N Engl J Med* 1996; 335: 151–156

23. Phillips G, Chien PFW, Garry R. Risk of hysterectomy after 1000 consecutive endometrial ablations. *Br J Obstet Gynaecol* 1998; 105: 897–903

24. Derman SG, Rehnstrom J, Neuwirth RS. The long term effectiveness of hysteroscopic treatment of menorrhagia and leiomyomas. *Obstet Gynecol* 1991; 77: 591–594

25. Donnez J, Clerck X, Gillerot S *et al.* Neodymium: YAG laser hysteroscopy in large submucous fibroids. *Fertil Steril* 1990; 54: 999–1003

26. Stovall TG, Ling FW, Henry LC, Woodruff MR. A randomised trial evaluating leuprolide acetate before hysterectomy as treatment for leiomyomas. *Am J Obstet Gynecol* 1991; 164: 1420–1425

27. Candiani GB, Vercellini P, Fedele L *et al.* Use of goserelin depot, a gonadotropin-releasing hormone agonist, for the treatment of menorrhagia and severe anemia in women with leiomyomata uteri. *Acta Obstet Gynecol Scand* 1990; 69: 413–415

28. Houang ET. Antibiotic prophylaxis in hysterectomy and induced abortion: a review of the evidence. *Drugs* 1991; 41: 19–37

29. Thompson JD, Warshaw J. Hysterectomy. In: Rock JA, Thompson JK (eds) *Te Linde's Operative Gynecology*, 8th edn. Philadelphia: Lippincott-Raven, 1997: 771–854

30. Mittendorf R, Aronson MP, Berry RE *et al.* Avoiding serious infections associated with abdominal hysterectomy: a meta-analysis of antibiotic prophylaxis. *Am J Obstet Gynecol* 1993; 169: 1119–1124

31. ACOG educational bulletin. Antibiotics and gynecologic infections. *Int J Gynecol Obstet* 1997; 58: 333–340

32. Reich H, DeCaprio J, McGlynn F. Laparoscopic hysterectomy. *J Gynecol Surg* 1989; 5: 213–216

33. Report by the Health Technology Assessment Service of ECRI. *Laparoscopy in Hysterectomy for Benign Conditions.* Pennsylvania: ECRI, 1995

34. Korn AP, Grullon K, Hessol N *et al.* Does vaginal cuff closure decrease the infectious morbidity associated with abdominal hysterectomy? *J Am Coll Surg* 1997; 185: 404–407

35. Colombo M, Maggioni A, Zanini A *et al.* A randomised trial of open versus closed vaginal vault in the prevention of postoperative morbidity after abdominal hysterectomy. *Am J Obstet Gynecol* 1995; 173: 1807–1811

36. Royal College of Obstetricians and Gynaecologists. *Peritoneal Closure.* Guideline No 15: London: RCOG, 1998

37. Davies A, O'Connor H, Magos AL. A prospective study to evaluate oophorectomy at the time of vaginal hysterectomy. *Br J Obstet Gynaecol* 1996; 103: 915–920

38. Sheth SS. The place of oophorectomy at vaginal hysterectomy. *Br J Obstet Gynaecol* 1991; 98: 662–666

39. Kovac SR, Cruikshank SH. Guidelines to determine the route of oophorectomy with hysterectomy. *Am J Obstet Gynecology* 1996; 175: 1483–1488

40. Sheth SS, Malpani A. Technique of vaginal oophorectomy during vaginal hysterectomy. *J Gynecol Surg* 1994; 10: 197–202

41. Magos AL, Bournas N, Sinha R *et al.* Transvaginal endoscopic oophorectomy. *Am J Obstet Gynecol* 1995; 172: 123–124

42. Hefni MA, Davies AE. Vaginal endoscopic oophorectomy: a simple minimal access surgery technique. *Br J Obstet Gynaecol* 1997; 104: 621–622

43. Kovac RS. Intramyometrial coring as an adjunct to vaginal hysterectomy. *Obstet Gynecol* 1986; 67: 131–136

44. Brill HM, Golden M. Vaginal hysterectomy, the treatment of choice for benign enlargement of the uterus. *Am J Obstet Gynecol* 1941; 62: 528–538

45. Grody MHT. Vaginal hysterectomy: the large uterus. *J Gynecol Surg* 1989; 5: 301–312

46. Mazdisnian F, Kurzel RB, Coe S *et al.* Vaginal hysterectomy by uterine morcellation: an efficient, non-morbid procedure. *Obstet Gynecol* 1995; 86: 60–64

47. Magos A, Bournas N, Sinha R *et al.* Vaginal hysterectomy for the large uterus. *Br J Obstet Gynaecol* 1996; 103: 246–251

48. Sheth SS. Vaginal hysterectomy. *Prog Obstet Gynecol* 1993; 10: 317–340

49. Coulam CB, Pratt JH. Vaginal hysterectomy: is previous pelvic operation a contraindication? *Am J Obstet Gynecol* 1973; 116: 252–260

50. Ingram JM, Withers RW, Wright HL. Vaginal hysterectomy after previous pelvic surgery. *Am J Obstet Gynecol* 1957; 74: 1181–1186

51. Wood C, Maher PJ. Laparoscopic hysterectomy. In: Wood C, Maher PJ (eds). Hysterectomy. *Baillière's Clin Obstet Gynaecol* 1997; 11: 111–136

52. Johns DA. Laparoscopic assisted vaginal hysterectomy. In: Sutton CJG, Diamond MP (eds) *Gynaecological Endoscopy.* London: Baillière Tindall 1993: 179–186

53. Richardson RE, Bournas N, Magos AL. Is laparoscopic hysterectomy a waste of time? *Lancet* 1995; 345: 36–41

54. Munro MG. Supracervical hysterectomy: A time for reappraisal. *Obstet Gynecol* 1997; 89: 133–139

55. Drife J. Conserving the cervix at hysterectomy. *Br J Obstet Gynaecol* 1994; 101: 563–564

56. Storm HH, Clemmenson IH, Manders T, Brinton LA. Supravaginal uterine amputation in Denmark 1978–1988 and risk of cancer. *Gynecol Oncol* 1992; 45: 198–201

57. Kilkku P, Gronroos M, Rauramo L. Supravaginal uterine amputation with preoperative electrocoagulation of endocervical mucosa: description of the method. *Acta Obstet Gynecol Scand* 1985; 64: 175–177

58. Miller BE, Copeland LJ, Hamberger AD *et al.* Carcinoma of the cervical stump. *Gynecol Oncol* 1984; 18: 100

59. Peterson LK, Mamsen A, Jakobsen A. Carcinoma of the cervical stump. *Gynecol Oncol* 1992; 46: 199

60. Porpora MG, Nobili F, Pietrangeli D *et al.* Cervical stump carcinoma therapy. *Eur J Gynaecol Oncol* 1991; 12: 45–50

61. Mundy AR. An anatomical explanation for bladder dysfunction following rectal and uterine surgery. *Br J Urol* 1982; 54: 501–504

62. Nathorst-Boos J, Fuchs T, von Schoultz B. Consumer's attitude to hysterectomy: the experience of 678 women. *Acta Obstet Gynecol Scand* 1992; 71: 230–234

63. Kilkku P. Supravaginal uterine amputation versus hysterectomy with reference to bladder symptoms and incontinence. *Acta Obstet Gynecol Scand* 1985; 64: 375–379

64. Kujansuu E, Teisala K, Punnonen R. Urethral closure function after total and subtotal hysterectomy measured by urethrocystometry. *Gynecol Obstet Invest* 1989; 27: 105–6

65. Lalos O, Bjerle P. Bladder wall mechanics and micturition before and after subtotal and total hysterectomy. *Eur J Obstet Gynecol Reprod Biol* 1986; 21: 143–150

66. Kilkku P. Supravaginal uterine amputation vs hysterectomy: effects on coital frequency and dyspareunia. *Acta Obstet Gynecol Scand* 1983; 62: 141–145

67. Thakar R, Manyonda I, Stanton SL, *et al.* Bladder, bowel and sexual function after hysterectomy for benign conditions. *Br J Obstet Gynaecol* 1997; 104: 983–987

68. Helstrom L, Lundberg PO, Sorbom D, Backstrom T. Sexuality after hysterectomy: a factor analysis of women's sexual lives before and after subtotal hysterectomy. *Obstet Gynecol* 993; 81: 357–362

69. Muntz HG, Falkenberry S, Fuller AF Jr. Fallopian tube prolapse after hysterectomy. A report of two cases. *J Reprod Med* 1988; 33: 467–469

70. Astill AN. Small bowel prolapse through the vaginal vault. *Aust N Z J Obstet Gynaecol* 1982; 22: 59–60

71. Manyonda IT, Welsh CR, McWhinney NA, Ross CD. The influence of suture materials on vaginal vault granulations after abdominal hysterectomy. *Br J Obstet Gynaecol* 1990; 97: 608–612

72. van Coeverden de Groot HA, Zabow P. The cervical stump. *S Afr Med J* 1993; 64: 745–746

73. Jacobs I, Oram D. Prevention of ovarian cancer: a survey of the practice of prophylactic oophorectomy by fellows and members of the Royal College of Obstetricians and Gynaecologists. *Br J Obstet Gynaecol* 1989; 96: 510–515

74. Hankinson S, Hunter D, Colditz G *et al.* Tubal ligation, hysterectomy, and risk of ovarian cancer: a prospective study. *J Am Med Assoc* 1993; 270; 2813

75. Parazzini F, Negri E, Vecchia C et al. Hysterectomy, oophorectomy, and subsequent ovarian cancer risk. *Obstet Gynecol* 1993; 81: 363–366

76. Loft A, Lidegaard O, Tabor A. Incidence of ovarian cancer after hysterectomy: a nationwide controlled follow up. *Br J Obstet Gynaecol* 1997; 104: 1296–1301

77. Namnoum AB, Hickman TN, Goodman SB, Gehlbach DL. Incidence of symptom recurrence after hysterectomy for endometriosis. *Fertil Steril* 1995; 64: 898–902

78. Sands R, Studd J. Exogenous androgens in postmenopausal women. *Am J Med* 1995; 98: 76–79

79. Perez Gutthann S, Garcia Rodriguez LA, Castellsague J, Duque Oliart A. Hormone replacement therapy and risk of venous thromboembolism: population based case–control study. *Br Med J* 1997; 314: 796–800

80. Speroff L. Postmenopausal hormone therapy and breast cancer. *Obstet Gynaecol* 1996; 87S: 44–54

81. Wingo PA, Huezo CM, Rubin GL *et al.* The mortality risk associated with hysterectomy. *Am J Obstet Gynecol* 1985; 144: 803–808

82. Whitelaw JM. Hysterectomy: a medical-legal perspective, 1975 to 1985. *Am J Obstet Gynecol* 1990; 162: 1451–1458

83. Brudenell M. Medico-legal aspects of ureteric damage during abdominal hysterectomy. *Br J Obstet Gynaecol* 1996; 103: 1180–1183

84. Thompson JD. Operative injuries to the ureter: prevention, recognition and management. In: Rock JA, Thompson JK (eds) *Te Linde's Operative Gynecology*, 8th edn. Philadelphia: Lippincott-Raven 1997: 1135–1173

85. Cruikshank SH, Kovac SR. Role of the uterosacral–cardinal ligament complex in protecting the ureter during vaginal hysterectomy. *Int J Gynaecol Obstet* 1993; 40: 141–144

86. Meikle SF, Nugent EW, Orleans M. Complications and recovery from laparoscopy-assisted vaginal hysterectomy compared with abdominal and vaginal hysterectomy. *Obstet Gynecol* 1997; 89: 304–311

87. Woodland MB. Ureter injury during laparoscopy-assisted vaginal hysterectomy with the endoscopic linear stapler. *Am J Obstet Gynecol* 1994; 167: 756–757

88. Bachman GA. Hysterectomy: a critical review. *J Reprod Med* 1990; 35; 839–862

89. Summitt RL Jr, Stovall TG, Lipscomb GH, Ling FW. Randomized comparison of laparoscopy-assisted vaginal hysterectomy with standard vaginal hysterectomy in an outpatient setting. *Obstet Gynecol* 1992; 80: 895–901

90. Iosif CS, Bekassy, Z, Rydhstrom H. Prevalence of urinary incontinence in middle-aged women. *Int J Gynaecol Obstet* 1988; 26: 255–259

91. Griffith-Jones MD, Jarvis GJ, McNamara HM. Adverse urinary symptoms after total abdominal hysterectomy: fact or fiction *Br J Urol* 1991; 67: 295–297

92. Milsom I, Ekelund P, Monlander U *et al.* The influence of age, parity, oral contraception, hysterectomy and menopause on the prevalence of urinary incontinence in women. *J Urol* 1993; 149: 1459–1462

93. Jequier AM. Urinary symptoms and total hysterectomy. *Br J Urol* 1976; 48: 437–441

94. Virtanen HS, Makinen JI, Tenho T *et al.* Effects of abdominal hysterectomy on urinary and sexual symptoms. *Br J Urol* 1993; 72: 868–872

95. Parys BT, Haylen B, Hutton JL, Parsons KF. The effect of simple hysterectomy on vesicourethral function. *Br J Urol* 1989; 64: 594–599

96. Langer R, Neuman M, Ron-el R *et al.* The effect of total abdominal hysterectomy on bladder function in asymptomatic women. *Obstet Gynecol* 1989; 74: 205–207

97. Prior A, Stanley K, Smith AR, Read NW. Effect of hysterectomy on anorectal and urethrovesical physiology. *Gut* 1992; 33: 264–267

98. Vervest HA, van Venrooij GE, Barents JW *et al.* Nonradical hysterectomy and the function of the lower urinary tract: urodynamic quantification of changes in storage function. *Acta Obstet Gynecol Scand* 1989; 68: 221–229

99. Nezhat F, Nezhat C, Gordon S, Wilkins S. Laparoscopic versus abdominal hysterectomy. *J Reprod Med* 1992; 37: 247–250

100. Howard FM, Sanchez R. A comparison of laparoscopically assisted vaginal hysterectomy and abdominal hysterectomy. *J Gynecol Surg* 1993; 9: 83–90

101. Garry R, Phillips G. How safe is the laparoscopic approach to hysterectomy? *Gynaecol Endosc* 1995; 4: 77–79

102. Dorsey JH, Holtz RN, Griffiths RI *et al.* Costs and charges associated with three alternative techniques of hysterectomy. *N Engl J Med* 1996; 335: 476–482

103. Ransom, SB, McNeeley SG, White C, Diamond MP. A cost analysis of endometrial ablation, abdominal hysterectomy, vaginal hysterectomy, and laparoscopic-assisted vaginal hysterectomy in the treatment of primary menorrhagia. *J Am Assoc Gynecol Laparosc* 1996; 4: 29–32

104. Kovac SR, Christie SJ, Bindbeutel GA. Abdominal versus vaginal hysterectomy: a statistical model for determining physician decision making and patient outcome. *Med Decis Making* 1991; 11; 19–28

105. Kovac SR. Guidelines to determine the route of hysterectomy. *Obstet Gynecol* 1995; 85: 18–22

106. Kovac SR, Cruikshank SH, Retto HF. Laparoscopy-assisted vaginal hysterectomy. *J Gynecol Surg* 1990; 6: 185–193

107. Querleu D, Cosson M, Parmentier D, Debodinance P. The impact of laparoscopic surgery on vaginal hysterectomy. *Gynecol Endosc* 1993; 2: 89–91

108. Davies A, Vizza E, Bournas N *et al.* How to increase the proportion of hysterectomies performed vaginally. *Am J Obstet Gynecol* 1998; 179: 1008–1012

55

Surgical fistulae

P. Hilton

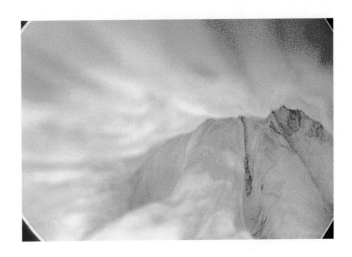

AETIOLOGY AND EPIDEMIOLOGY

Urogenital fistulae may occur congenitally, but are most often acquired from obstetric, surgical, radiation, malignant and miscellaneous causes. The same factors may be responsible for intestinogenital fistulae, although inflammatory bowel disease is an additional important aetiological factor here. In most developing countries, over 90% of fistulae are of obstetric aetiology,[1–4] whereas in the UK and USA over 70% follow pelvic surgery.[5–6] (see Table 55.1). Obstetric fistulae are

Table 55.1. *Aetiology of urogenital fistulae in two series, from north-east England and from south-east Nigeria**

Aetiology	NE England (n = 140)		SE Nigeria (n = 2389)[†]	
	%	n	%	n
Obstetric: obstructed labour	2			1918
caesarean section		3		165
ruptured uterus		5		119
forceps/ventouse		5		
breech extraction		1		
placental abruption		1		
Total obstetric	12.1	17	92.2	2202
Surgical: abdominal hysterectomy		59		33
radical hysterectomy		11		
urethral diverticulectomy		10		
colporrhaphy		1		35
vaginal hysterectomy		4		25
TAH + colporrhaphy		1		
TAH + colposuspension		1		
LAVH		3		
cystoplasty + colposuspension		2		
colposuspension		1		
sling		1		
needle suspension		1		
cervical stumpectomy		1		
subtrigonal phenol injection		1		
transurethral resection (tb)		1		
lithoclast		1		
unknown surgery in childhood		1		
suture to vaginal laceration				12
Total surgical	71.4	100	4.4	105
Radiation	12.6	18	0.0	0
Malignancy	0.0	0	1.8	42
Miscellaneous: catheter associated		2		
foreign body		2		
trauma		1		11
infection				7
coital injury				22
Total miscellaneous	3.6	5	1.7	40
Total	100.0		100.0	

LAVH, laparoscopically assisted vaginal hysterectomy; TAH, total abdominal hysterectomy.
[†] No. of patients for whom notes were available, out of a total of 2484 patients.
* from ref. 4.

covered in chapter 56; although the present chapter deals primarily with surgical fistulae, other aetiologies are mentioned briefly for the sake of completeness.

Surgical fistulae

Genital fistulae may occur following a wide range of surgical procedures within the pelvis (Fig. 55.1 a–f). It is often supposed that this complication results from direct injury to the lower urinary tract at the time of operation. Certainly, on occasions, this may be the case: careless, hurried or rough surgical technique makes injury to the lower urinary tract much more likely. However, of 140 urogenital fistulae referred to me over the last 10 years, 100 have been associated with pelvic surgery 79 of which followed hysterectomy; of these 100

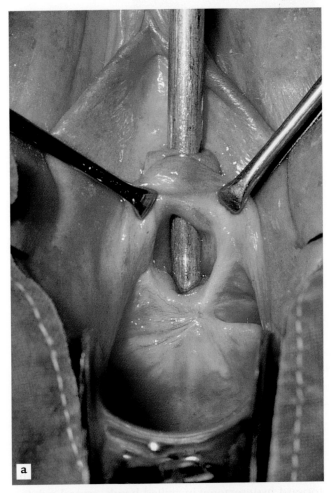

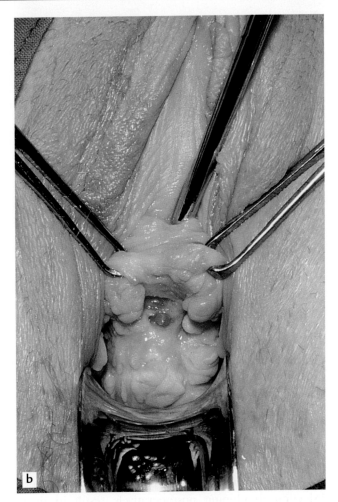

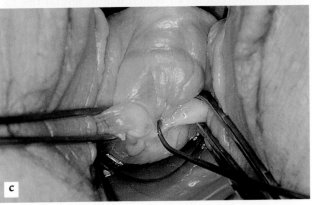

Figure 55.1. *Postoperative urogenital fistulae following various procedures: (a) anterior colporrhaphy; (b) urethral diverticulectomy; (c) simple abdominal hysterectomy.*

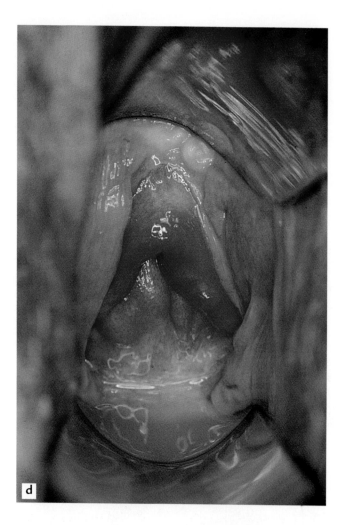

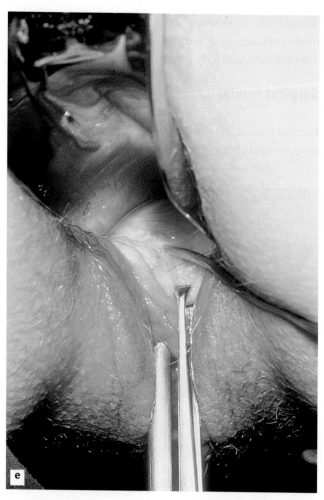

Figure 55.1. *Postoperative urogenital fistulae following various procedures: (cont.) (d) radical hysterectomy; (e) colposuspension (the fistula in this case was fixed retropubically in the midline at the bladder neck, and the photograph shows the patient prone, in the reverse lithotomy position); (f, facing page) subtrigonal phenol injection.*

only four (4%) presented with leakage of urine on the first day postoperatively. In other cases it is presumed that tissue devascularization during dissection, inadvertent suture placement, pelvic haematoma formation or infection developing postoperatively result in tissue necrosis, with leakage developing most usually 5–14 days later. Overdistension of the bladder postoperatively may be an additional factor in many of these cases. It has recently been shown that there is a high incidence of abnormalities of lower urinary tract function in patients with fistulae;[7] whether these abnormalities antedate the surgery, or develop with or as a consequence of the fistula, is unclear. It is likely that patients with a habit of infrequent voiding, or those with inefficient detrusor contractility, may be at increased risk of postoperative urinary retention; if this

is not recognized at an early stage and managed appropriately, the risk of fistula formation may be increased.

Although it is important to remember that the majority of surgical fistulae follow apparently straightforward hysterectomy in skilled hands, several risk factors that make direct injury more likely may be identified (see Table 55.2). Obviously, anatomical distortion within the pelvis by ovarian tumour or fibroid will increase the difficulty, and abnormal adhesions between bladder and uterus or cervix following previous surgery or associated with previous sepsis, endometriosis or malignancy may make fistula formation more likely. Preoperative or early radiotherapy may decrease vascularity, and make the tissues in general less forgiving of poor technique.

Issues of training and surgical technique are, of

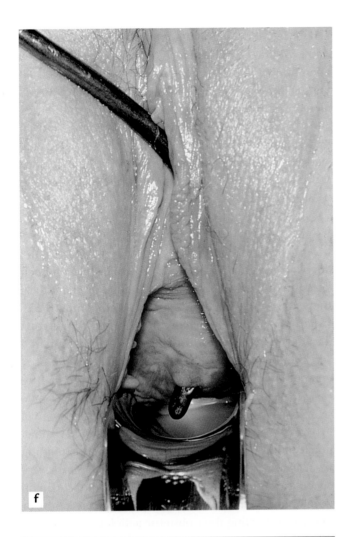

f

course, also important. The ability to locate and, if necessary, dissect out the ureter must be part of our routine gynaecological training, as should the first-aid management of lower urinary tract injury when it arises. The use of gauze swabs to separate the bladder from the cervix at caesarean section or hysterectomy should be discouraged: sharp dissection with knife or scissors does less harm, especially where the tissues are abnormally adherent.

Radiation

The obliterative endarteritis associated with ionizing radiation in therapeutic dosage proceeds over many years and may be aetiological in fistula formation long after the primary malignancy has been treated. Of the 18 radiation fistulae in my series, the fistula has developed at intervals between 1 and 30 years following radiotherapy. The associated devascularization in the adjacent tissues means that ordinary surgical repair has a high likelihood of failure, and modified surgical techniques are required.

Malignancy

Excluding the effects of treatment, malignant disease itself may result in genital tract fistula. Carcinoma of cervix, vagina and rectum are the most common malig-

Table 55.2. *Risk factors for postoperative fistulae*

Risk factor	Pathology	Specific example
Anatomical distortion		Fibroids Ovarian mass
Abnormal tissue adhesion	Inflammation	Infection Endometriosis
	Previous surgery	Caesarean section Cone biopsy Colporrhaphy
	Malignancy	
Impaired vascularity	Ionizing radiation Metabolic abnormality Radical surgery	Preoperative radiotherapy Diabetes mellitus
Compromised healing		Anaemia Nutritional deficiency
Abnormality of bladder function		Voiding dysfunction

nancies to present in this way. It is relatively unusual for urothelial tumours to present with fistula formation, other than following surgery or radiotherapy. The development of a fistula may be a distressing part of the terminal phase of malignant disease; it is, nevertheless, one deserving not simply compassion, but full consideration of the therapeutic or palliative possibilities.

Inflammatory bowel disease

Inflammatory bowel disease is the most significant cause of intestinogenital fistulae in the UK, although these rarely present directly to the gynaecologist. Diverticular disease can produce colovaginal fistulae and, rarely, colouterine fistulae with surprisingly few symptoms attributable to the intestinal pathology. The possibility should not be overlooked if an elderly woman complains of feculent discharge or becomes incontinent without concomitant urinary problems. Crohn's disease appears to be increasing in frequency in the western world, and a total fistula rate approaching 40% has been reported; the genital tract may be involved in up to 7% of women. Ulcerative colitis has a small incidence of low rectovaginal fistulae. In my own series of cases of rectovaginal fistulae, 65% are of obstetric aetiology, 21% relate to inflammatory bowel disease, 7% follow radiotherapy and 7% are of uncertain cause.

Miscellaneous

Other miscellaneous causes of fistulae in the genital tract include infection (lymphogranuloma venereum, schistosomiasis, tuberculosis, actinomycosis, measles, noma vaginae), trauma (penetrating trauma, coital injury, neglected pessary or other foreign bodies) and catheter-related injuries.

PREVALENCE

The prevalence of genital fistulae obviously varies from country to country and continent to continent as the main causative factors vary. Recent data from the Regional Health Authority Information Units in England and Wales suggest an average of 10 fistula repairs per health region per year over the last few years, and a national figure of approximately 152 repair procedures per year.[8]

The rate of fistula formation following hysterectomy in the UK has been calculated as approximately 1/1300 operations (0.08%).[9] Following laparoscopic-assisted vaginal hysterectomy the incidence of fistula development may approach 1%.[10–12] Figures of between 1% and 4% fistulae have been reported following radical hysterectomy,[13,14] with a similar incidence following radiation for gynaecological malignancies.[15] The incidence of fistula formation following pelvic exenteration may be as high as 10%.[16]

CLASSIFICATION

Many different fistula classifications have been described in the literature on the basis of anatomical site; these are often subclassified into simple cases (where the tissues are healthy and access good) or complicated (where there is tissue loss, scarring, impaired access, involvement of the ureteric orifices or the presence of coexistent rectovaginal fistula). Urogenital fistulae may be classified into urethral, bladder neck, subsymphysial (a complex form involving circumferential loss of the urethra with fixity to bone), mid-vaginal, juxtacervical or vault fistulae, massive fistulae extending from bladder neck to vault, and vesicouterine or vesicocervical fistulae. Whereas over 60% of fistulae in developing countries are mid-vaginal, juxtacervical or massive (reflecting their obstetric aetiology), such cases are relatively rare in fistula practice in the western world; by contrast, 50% of the fistulae managed in the UK are situated in the vaginal vault (reflecting their surgical aetiology).[5]

PRESENTATION

Fistulae between the urinary tract and the genital tract in women are characteristically said to present with continuous urinary incontinence, with limited sensation of bladder fullness and with infrequent voiding. Where there is extensive tissue loss, as in obstetric or radiation fistulae, this typical history is usually present, the clinical findings gross, and the diagnosis rarely in doubt. With post-surgical fistulae, however, the history may be atypical and the orifice small, elusive or occasionally completely invisible. Under these circumstances the diagnosis can be much more difficult, and a high index of clinical suspicion must be maintained.

Occasionally, a patient with an obvious fistula may

deny incontinence, and this is presumed to reflect the ability of the levator ani muscles to occlude the vagina below the level of the fistula. Some patients with vesico-cervical or vesicouterine fistula following caesarean section may maintain continence at the level of the uterine isthmus, and complain of cyclical haematuria at the time of menstruation, or menouria.[17,18] In other cases patients may complain of little more than a watery vaginal discharge, or intermittent leakage that seems to be posturally related. Leakage may appear to occur specifically on standing or on lying supine, prone, or in left or right lateral positions, presumably reflecting the degree of bladder distension and the position of the fistula within the bladder; such a pattern is most unlikely to be found with ureteric fistulae.

Although, in the case of direct surgical injury, leakage may occur from day 1, in most surgical and obstetric fistulae symptoms develop between 5 and 14 days after the causative injury; the time of presentation, however, may be quite variable. This will depend to some extent on the severity of symptoms but, as far as obstetric fistulae in developing countries are concerned, is determined more by access to health care. In a recent review of cases from Nigeria the average time for presentation was more than 5 years, and in some cases more than 35 years, after the causative pregnancy.[4]

Urethrovaginal fistulae distal to the sphincter mechanism will often be asymptomatic and require no specific treatment. Some may lead to obstruction, and are more likely to present with post-micturition dribbling than other types of incontinence; they can, therefore, be very difficult to recognize. More proximally situated urethral fistulae are perhaps most likely to present with stress incontinence, since bladder-neck competence is frequently impaired.

With intestinal fistulae the history may be much more misleading. A small communication with the large bowel may cause only an offensive discharge. Even fistulae of obstetric origin may be rendered relatively asymptomatic by the cicatrization of the vagina that occurs following sloughing. A small, high, posterior horseshoe-shaped fistula may become apparent only during division of constricting bands for the repair of a vesicovaginal fistula. Most typically, however, patients will complain of incontinence of liquid stool, and flatus; whereas they may often be unsure as to whether stool is from the vagina or

anus, the sensation of flatus from the vagina is rarely misinterpreted.

INVESTIGATIONS

If there is suspicion of a fistula, but its presence is not easily confirmed by clinical examination with a Sims' speculum, further investigation will be necessary to confirm or fully exclude the possibility. Even where the diagnosis is clinically obvious, additional investigation may be appropriate for full evaluation prior to deciding treatment. The main principles of investigation therefore are:

- to confirm that the discharge is urinary,
- to establish that the leakage is extra-urethral rather than urethral,
- to establish the site of leakage.

Biochemistry and microbiology

Excessive vaginal discharge, or the drainage of serum from a pelvic haematoma postoperatively, may simulate a urinary fistula. If the fluid is in sufficient quantity to be collected, biochemical analysis of its urea content in comparison with that of urine and serum will confirm its origin.

Urinary infection is surprisingly uncommon in patients with fistulae, although (especially where there have been previous attempts at surgery) urine culture should be undertaken and appropriate antibiotic therapy instituted.

Dye studies

Although other imaging techniques undoubtedly have a role (see below), carefully conducted dye studies remain the investigation of first choice. Phenazopyridine may be used orally, or indigo carmine intravenously, to stain the urine and hence to confirm the presence of a fistula. The identification of the site of a fistula is best carried out by the instillation of coloured dye (methylene blue or indigo carmine) into the bladder via catheter with the patient in the lithotomy position. The traditional 'three swab test' has its limitations and is not recommended: the examination is best carried out with direct inspection; multiple fistulae may be located in this way. If leakage of clear fluid continues after dye instillation, a ureteric fistula is likely; this is most easily confirmed by a 'two dye test', using phenazopyridine to stain the renal urine and methylene blue to stain the bladder contents.[19]

Dye tests are less useful for intestinal fistulae, although a carmine marker taken orally may confirm their presence. Rectal distension with air via a sigmoidoscope may be of more value; if the patient is kept in a slightly head-down position and the vagina is filled with saline, the bubbling of any air leaked through a low fistula may be detected.

Imaging

Excretion urography

Although intravenous urography is a particularly insensitive investigation in the diagnosis of vesicovaginal fistula, knowledge of upper urinary tract status may have a significant influence on treatment measures applied, and should therefore be looked on as an essential investigation for any suspected or confirmed urinary fistula. Compromise to ureteric function is a particularly common finding when a fistula occurs in relation to malignant disease or its treatment (by radiation or surgery).

Dilatation of the ureter is characteristic in ureteric fistula, and its finding in association with a known vesicovaginal fistula should raise suspicion of a complex ureterovesicovaginal lesion (see Fig. 55.2). Although it is essential for the diagnosis of ureteric fistula, intravenous urography is not completely sensitive; the presence of a periureteric flare is, however, highly suggestive of extravasation at this site.

Retrograde pyelography

Retrograde pyelography is a more reliable way of identifying the exact site of a ureterovaginal fistula, and may be undertaken simultaneously with either retrograde or percutaneous catheterization for therapeutic stenting of the ureter.

Cystography

Cystography is not particularly helpful in the basic diagnosis of vesicovaginal fistulae, and a dye test carried out under direct vision is likely to be more sensitive. It may, however, occasionally be useful in achieving a diagnosis in complex or vesicouterine fistulae.

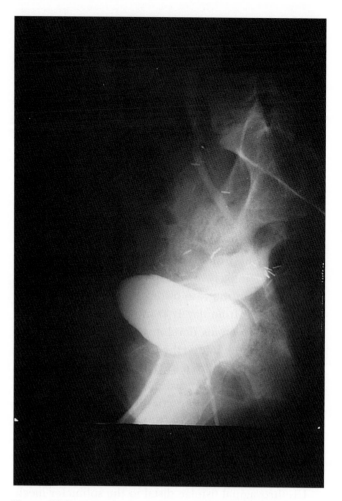

Figure 55.2. *Intravenous urogram (with simultaneous cystogram) demonstrating a complex surgical fistula occurring after radical hysterectomy. After further investigation (including cystourethroscopy, sigmoidoscopy, barium enema, and retrograde cannulation of the vaginal vault to perform fistulography,) the lesion was defined as a ureterocolovesicovaginal fistula.*

Fistulography

Fistulography is a special example of the radiographic technique commonly referred to as sinography. For small fistulae a ureteric catheter is suitable, although if the hole is large enough a small Foley catheter may be used to deliver the radiopaque dye; this is of particular value for fistulae for which there is an intervening abscess cavity. If a catheter will pass through a small vaginal aperture into an adjacent loop of bowel, its nature may become apparent from the radiological appearance of the lumen and haustrations, although further imaging studies are usually required to demonstrate the underlying pathology.

Ultrasonography, computerized tomography and magnetic resonance imaging (MRI)

Ultrasonography, computed tomography and MRI may occasionally be appropriate for the complete assessment of complex fistulae. Endo-anal ultrasonography and MRI are particularly useful in the investigation of anorectal and perineal fistulae.

Examination under anaesthesia

Careful examination, if necessary under anaesthesia, may be required to determine the presence of a fistula; it is deemed by several authorities to be an essential preliminary to definitive surgical treatment.[5,20–23] It is important at the time of examination to assess both the available access for repair vaginally and the mobility of the tissues. The decision between the vaginal and abdominal approaches to surgery is thus made; when the vaginal route is chosen, it may be appropriate to select between the more conventional supine lithotomy with a head-down tilt, and the prone (reverse lithotomy) with head-up tilt. This may be particularly useful in allowing the operator to look down on to bladder-neck and subsymphysial fistulae, and is also of advantage in some massive fistulae in encouraging the reduction of the prolapsed bladder mucosa.[24]

ENDOSCOPY

Cystoscopy

Although some authorities suggest that endoscopy has little role in the evaluation of fistulae, it is my practice to perform cystourethroscopy in all but the largest defects. In some obstetric and radiation fistulae, the size of the defect and the extent of tissue loss and scarring may make it difficult to distend the bladder: nevertheless, much useful information is obtained. The exact level and position of the fistula should be determined; its relationship to the ureteric orifices and bladder neck is particularly important. With urethral and bladder-neck fistulae the failure to pass a cystoscope or sound may indicate that there has been circumferential loss of the proximal urethra, a circumstance that is of considerable importance in determining the appropriate surgical technique and the likelihood of subsequent urethral incompetence.[2,7]

The condition of the tissues must be carefully assessed. Persistence of slough means that surgery should be deferred; this is particularly important in obstetric and post-radiation cases. Biopsy from the edge of a fistula should be taken in radiation fistulae if persistent of recurrent malignancy is suspected. Malignant change has been reported in a long-standing benign fistula therefore, where there is any doubt at all about the nature of the tissues, biopsy should be undertaken.[25] In areas of endemicity, evidence of schistosomiasis, tuberculosis and lymphogranuloma may become apparent in biopsy material; again, it is important that specific antimicrobial treatment is instituted prior to definitive surgery.

Sigmoidoscopy and proctoscopy

Sigmoidoscopic and proctoscopic examinations are important for the diagnosis of inflammatory bowel disease, which may not have been suspected before the occurrence of a fistula. Biopsies of the fistula edge or any unhealthy looking area should always be obtained.

PREOPERATIVE MANAGEMENT

Before epithelialization is complete, an abnormal communication between viscera will tend to close spontaneously, provided that the natural outflow is unobstructed. Bypassing the sphincter mechanisms, for example by urinary catheterization or defunctioning colostomy, may encourage closure. The early management is critical and depends on the aetiology and site of the lesion. If surgical trauma is recognized within the first 24 hours postoperatively, immediate repair may be appropriate, provided that extravasation of urine into the tissues has not been great. Most surgical fistulae are, however, recognized between 5 and 14 days postoperatively, and these should be treated with continuous bladder drainage. It is worth persisting with this line of management in vesicovaginal or urethrovaginal fistulae for 6–8 weeks, since spontaneous closure in both surgical and obstetric cases may occur within this period.[26,27]

It is important to appreciate that some fistulae may be associated with few or minor symptoms and, even if persistent, these do not require surgical treatment. Small distal urethrovaginal fistulae, uterovesical fistulae with menouria, and some low rectovaginal fistulae may fall into this category.

Palliation and skin care

During the waiting period from diagnosis to repair, incontinence pads should be provided in generous quantities so that the patient can continue to function socially to some extent. Patients with fistulae usually leak very much greater quantities of urine than those with urethral incontinence from whatever cause, and this must be recognized in terms of provision of supplies.

The vulval skin may be at considerable risk from ammoniacal dermatitis, and liberal use of silicone barrier cream should be encouraged. Steroid therapy has been advocated in the past as a means of reducing tissue oedema and fibrosis, although these benefits are refuted and there may be a risk of compromise to subsequent healing. Local oestrogen has been recommended by some; however, although empirically one might expect benefit in postmenopausal women or in those patients with obstetric fistulae and prolonged amenorrhoea, the evidence for this is lacking.

Antimicrobial therapy

Opinions differ on the desirability of prophylactic antibiotic cover for surgery: some avoid their use other than in the treatment of specific infection; others advocate broad-spectrum treatment in all cases. My current practice is to use single-dose prophylaxis in urinary fistulae, and 5 days' cover for intestinal fistulae, in each case using metronidazole and cefuroxime.

Bowel preparation

Although surgeons vary in the extent to which they prepare the bowel prior to rectovaginal fistula repair, I prefer to carry out formal preparation in all cases of intestinogenital fistula, whatever the level of the lesion. A low-residue diet should be advised for a week prior to admission, followed by a fluid-only diet for 48 hours preoperatively. Polyethylene glycol 3350 (Kleneprep; four sachets in 4 litres of water over a 4-hour period) or, alternatively, sodium picosulphate (Picolax; 10 mg repeated after 6 hours) is given orally on the day before operation. Bowel washout should be performed on the evening before surgery; if the bowel content is not completely clear, this should be repeated on the morning of surgery.

Counselling

Patients with surgical fistulae are usually previously healthy individuals who entered hospital for what was expected to be a routine procedure, and who ultimately have symptoms infinitely worse than their initial complaint; they are invariably devastated by their situation. It is vital that they understand the nature of the problem, why it has arisen, and the plan for management at all stages. Confident but realistic counselling by the surgeon is essential, and the involvement of nursing staff or counsellors with experience of patients with fistulae is also highly desirable. The support given by previously treated sufferers can also be of immense value in maintaining patient morale, especially where a delay prior to definitive treatment is required.

GENERAL PRINCIPLES OF SURGICAL TREATMENT

Timing of repair

The timing of surgical repair is perhaps the single most contentious aspect of fistula management. Although curtailing the waiting period is of both social and psychological benefit to what are always very distressed patients, one must not trade these issues for compromise to surgical success. The benefit of delay is to allow slough to separate and inflammatory change to resolve. In both obstetric and radiation fistulae there is considerable sloughing of tissues, and it is imperative that this should have settled before repair is undertaken. In radiation fistulae it may be necessary to wait 12 months or more. In obstetric cases most authorities suggest that a minimum of 3 months should be allowed to elapse, although others have advocated surgery as soon as slough is separated.

With surgical fistulae the same principles should apply and, although the extent of sloughing is limited, extravasation of urine into the pelvic tissues inevitably sets up some inflammatory response. Although early repair is advocated by several authors, again most would agree that 10–12 weeks postoperatively is the earliest appropriate time for repair.

Pressure from patients to undertake repair at the earliest opportunity is always understandably great, but is never more so than in the case of previous surgical failure. Such pressure must, however, be resisted, and

8 weeks is the minimum time that should be allowed between attempts at closure.

Route of repair

Many urologists advocate an abdominal approach for all fistula repairs, claiming the possibility of earlier intervention and higher success rates in justification; others suggest that all fistulae can be successfully closed by the vaginal route. Surgeons involved in fistula management must be capable of both approaches, and should have the versatility to modify their techniques to select that which is most appropriate to the individual case. Where access is good and the vaginal tissues are sufficiently mobile, the vaginal route is usually most appropriate (see Fig. 55.3a, b). If access is poor and the fistula cannot be brought down, the abdominal approach should be used. Overall, more surgical than obstetric fistulae are likely to require an abdominal repair, although in my series of cases from the UK, and those reviewed from Nigeria, two-thirds of patients were satisfactorily treated by the vaginal route, regardless of aetiology.

Instruments

All operators have their own favoured instruments, although those described by Chassar Moir,[20] and Lawson[24] are eminently suitable for repair by any route. The following are particularly useful:

- Series of fine scalpel blades on the No. 7 handle, especially the curved No. 12 bistoury blade;

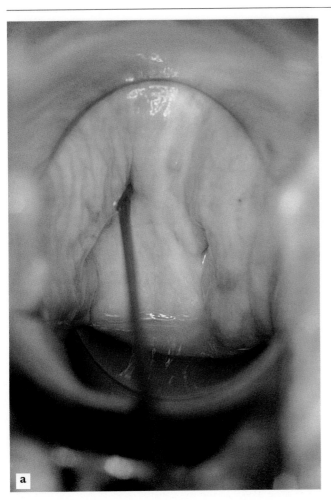
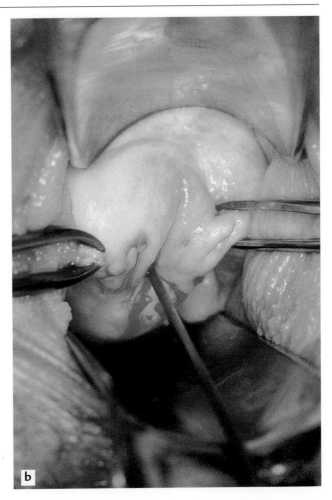

Figure 55.3. *Simple post-hysterectomy vault vesicovaginal fistula, and steps in vaginal repair procedure by dissection and closure in layers: (a) fistula visible in vaginal vault; (b) tissue forceps applied illustrating tissue mobility, and ease of access for repair per vaginam. (Reproduced from ref. 8 with permission.)*

- Chassar Moir 30-degree angled-on-flat and 90-degree curved-on-flat scissors;
- cleft-palate forceps;
- Judd–Allis, Stiles and Duval tissue forceps;
- Millin's retractor for use in transvesical procedures, and Currie's retractors for vaginal repairs;
- Skin hooks to put the tissues on tension during dissection;
- A Turner-Warwick double-curved needle-holder is particularly useful in areas of awkward access, and has the advantage of allowing needle placement without the operator's hand or the instrument obstructing the view.

Dissection

Great care must be taken over the initial dissection of the fistula, and one should probably take as long over this as over the repair itself. The fistula should be circumcised in the most convenient orientation, depending on size and access. All things being equal, a longitudinal incision should be made around urethral or mid-vaginal fistulae; conversely, vault fistulae are better handled by a transverse elliptical incision (see Fig. 55.3c). The tissue planes are often obliterated by scarring, and dissection close to a fistula should therefore be undertaken with a scalpel or scissors (see Fig. 55.3d). Sharp dissection is easier with countertraction applied by skin hooks, tissue forceps or retraction sutures. Blunt dissection with small pledgets may be

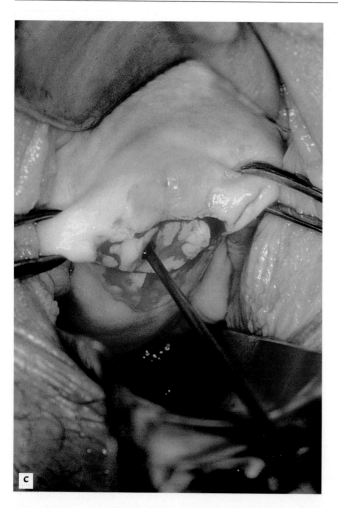

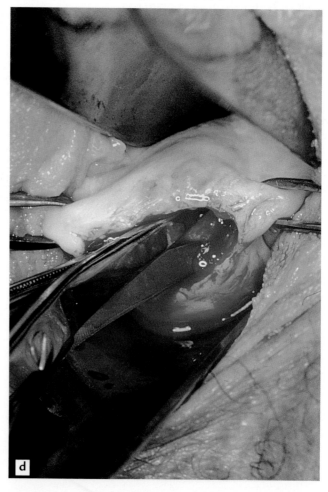

Figure 55.3. *Simple post-hysterectomy vault vesicovaginal fistula, and steps in vaginal repair procedure by dissection and closure in layers: (cont.) (c) fistula circumcised using no. 12 scalpel; (d) sharp dissection around fistula edge; (e) fistula fully mobilized; (f) vaginal scar edge trimmed. (Reproduced from ref. 8 with permission.)*

helpful once the planes are established, and provided one is away from the fistula edge. Wide mobilization should be performed, so that tension on the repair is minimized (see Fig. 55.3e). Bleeding is rarely troublesome with vaginal procedures, except occasionally with proximal urethrovaginal fistulae. Diathermy is best avoided – pressure or under-running sutures are preferred.

Suture materials

Although a range of suture materials have been advocated over the years, and a range of opinion still exists, my view is that absorbable sutures should be used throughout all urinary fistula repair procedures.

- Polyglactin (Vicryl) 2/0 suture on a 25 mm heavy tapercut needle is preferred for both the bladder and vagina;

- polydioxanone (PDS) 4/0 on a 13 mm round-bodied needle is used for the ureter;
- 3/0 sutures on a 30 mm round-bodied needle are used for bowel surgery – PDS for the small bowel, and either PDS or braided polyamide (Nurolon) for large bowel reanastomosis.

SPECIFIC REPAIR TECHNIQUES

Vaginal procedures

The two main types of closure technique applied to the repair of urinary fistulae are the classic saucerization technique described by Sims[27] and the much more commonly used dissection and repair in layers.

Dissection and repair in layers

Sutures must be placed with meticulous accuracy in the bladder wall, care being taken not to penetrate the mucosa, which should be inverted as far as possible.

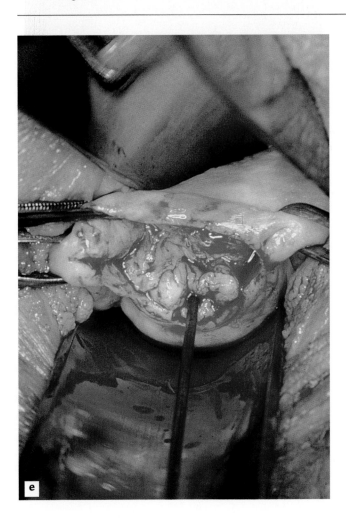

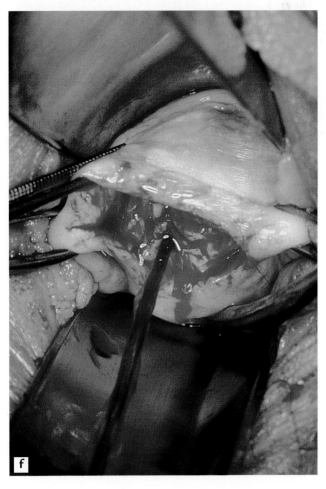

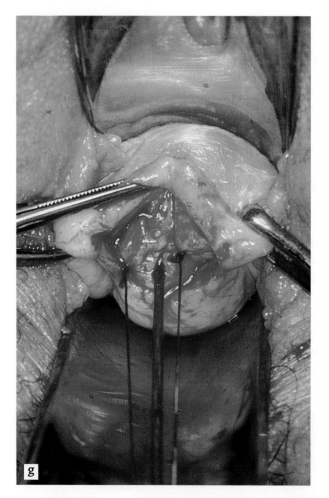
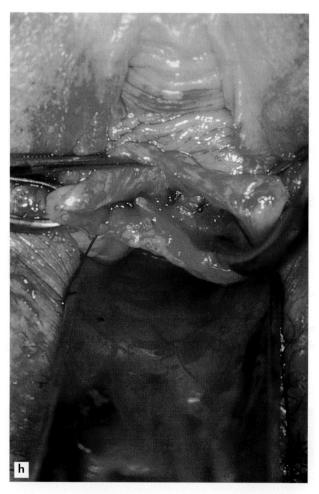

Figure 55.3. *Simple post-hysterectomy vault vesicovaginal fistula, and steps in vaginal repair procedure by dissection and closure in layers: (cont.) (g) first two sutures of first layer of repair in place lateral to the angles of the repair; (h) second layer completed, sutures catching back of vaginal flaps to close off dead space; (i, facing page) testing the repair with methylene blue dye instillation; (j, facing page) final layer of mattress sutures in the vaginal wall. (Reproduced from ref. 8 with permission.)*

The repair should be started at either end, working towards the midline, so that the least accessible aspects are sutured first (see Fig. 55.3g). Interrupted sutures are preferred and should be placed approximately 3 mm apart, taking as large a bite of tissue as feasible. Stitches that are too close together, or the use of continuous or purse-string sutures, tend to impair blood supply and interfere with healing. Knots must be secured with three hitches, so that they can be cut short, leaving the minimum amount of material within the body of the repair.

With dissection and repair in layers, the first layer of sutures in the bladder should invert the edges; the second adds bulk to the repair by taking a wide bite of bladder wall, but also closes off dead space by catching the back of the vaginal flaps (Fig. 55.3h). After the repair has been tested (see Fig. 55.3i and below), a third layer of interrupted mattress sutures is used to evert and close the vaginal wall, consolidating the repair by picking up the underlying bladder wall (see Fig. 55.3j).

Saucerization

The saucerization technique involves converting the track into a shallow crater, which is closed without dissection of bladder from vagina using a single row of interrupted sutures. The method is applicable only to small fistulae and, perhaps, residual fistulae after closure of a larger defect; in other situations the technique does not allow secure closure without tension.

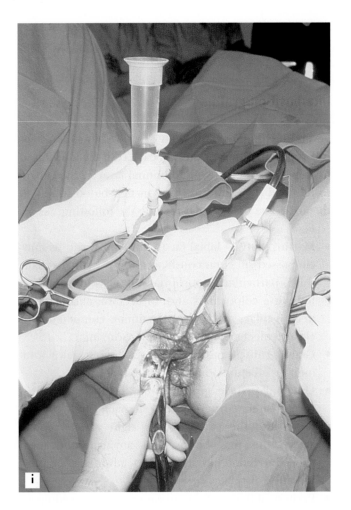

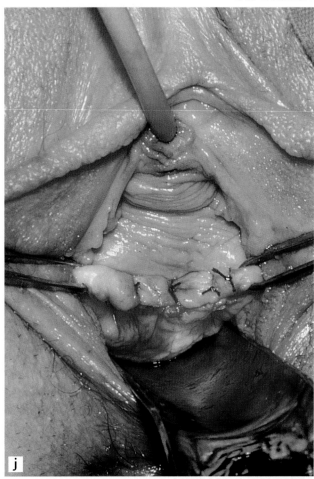

Vaginal repair procedures in specific circumstances

The conventional dissection and repair in layers, as described above, is entirely appropriate for the majority of mid-vaginal fistulae, although modifications may be necessary in specific circumstances. In juxtacervical fistulae in the anterior fornix, vaginal repair may be feasible if the cervix can be drawn down to provide access. Dissection should include mobilization of the bladder from the cervix. The repair must be undertaken transversely to reconstruct the underlying trigone and prevent distortion of the ureteric orifices.

Vault fistulae, particularly those following hysterectomy, can also usually be managed vaginally. The vault is incised transversely and mobilization of the fistula is often aided by deliberate opening of the pouch of Douglas.[29] The peritoneal opening does not need separate closure, but is incorporated into the vaginal closure.

With subsymphysial fistulae involving the bladder neck and proximal urethra as a consequence of obstructed labour, tissue loss may be extensive and fixity to underlying bone a common problem. The lateral aspects of the fistula require careful mobilization to overcome disproportion between the defect in the bladder and the urethral stump. A racquet-shaped extension of the incision facilitates exposure of the proximal urethra. Although transverse repair is often necessary, longitudinal closure gives better prospects for urethral competence.

Where there is substantial urethral loss, reconstruction may be undertaken using the method described by Chassar Moir[20] or by Hamlin and Nicholson.[30] A strip of anterior vaginal wall is constructed into a tube over a catheter. Plication behind the bladder neck is probably important if continence is to be achieved. The interposition of a labial fat or muscle graft not only fills up the potential dead space but also provides additional bladder-neck support and improves continence by reducing scarring between bladder neck and vagina.

With very large fistulae extending from bladder neck to vault, the extensive dissection required may produce considerable bleeding. The main surgical difficulty is to avoid the ureters. They are usually situated close to the superolateral angles of the fistula and, if they can be identified, they should be catheterized. Straight ureteric catheters passed transurethrally, or double-pigtail catheters, may both be useful in directing the intramural portion of the ureters internally; nevertheless, great care must be taken during dissection.

Radiation fistulae present particular problems in that the area of devitalized tissue is usually considerably larger than the fistula itself. Mobilization is often impossible and if repair in layers is attempted, the flaps are likely to slough; closure by colpocleisis is therefore required. Some have advocated total closure of the vagina, although it is preferable to avoid dissection entirely in the devitalized tissue, and to perform a lower partial colpocleisis converting the upper vagina into a diverticulum of the bladder. It is usually necessary to fill the dead space below this with an interposition graft (see below).

Abdominal procedures

Transvesical repair

Repair by the abdominal route is indicated when high fistulae are fixed in the vault and are therefore inaccessible *per vaginam*. Transvesical repair has the advantage of being entirely extraperitoneal. It is often helpful to elevate the fistula site by a vaginal pack, and the ureters should be catheterized under direct vision. The technique of closure is similar to that of the transvaginal flap-splitting repair except that, for haemostasis, the bladder mucosa is closed with a continuous suture.

Transperitoneal repair

It is often said that there is little place for a simple transperitoneal repair, although a combined transperitoneal and transvesical procedure is favoured by urologists and is particularly useful for vesicouterine fistulae following caesarean section. A midline split is made in the vault of the bladder; this is extended downwards in a racquet shape around the fistula. The fistulous track is excised and the vaginal or cervical defect closed in a single layer. The bladder is then closed in two layers.

Interposition grafting

Several techniques have been described to support fistula repair in different sites. In each case the interposed tissue serves to create an additional layer in the repair, to fill dead space and to bring in new blood supply to the area. The tissues used include the following:

* Martius graft[31] – labial fat and bulbocavernosus muscle passed subcutaneously to cover a vaginal repair; this is particularly appropriate to provide additional bulk in a colpocleisis and, in urethral and bladder-neck fistulae, may help to maintain competence of closure mechanisms by reducing scarring;
* Gracilis muscle passed either via the obturator foramen or subcutaneously[30] is used as above;
* Omental pedicle grafts[32,33] may be dissected from the greater curve of the stomach and rotated down into the pelvis on the right gastro-epiploic artery; this may be used at any transperitoneal procedure, but has its greatest advantage in post-radiation fistulae;
* Peritoneal flap graft[21] is an easier way of providing an additional layer at transperitoneal repair procedures, by taking a flap of peritoneum from any available surface, most usually the paravesical area.

Testing the repair

The closure must be watertight and so should be tested at the end of vaginal repairs by the instillation of dye into the bladder under minimal pressure; a previously unsuspected second fistula is occasionally identified this way. Testing after abdominal procedures is impractical.

POSTOPERATIVE MANAGEMENT

Fluid balance

Nursing care of patients who have undergone urogenital fistula repair is critical, and obsessional postoperative management may do much to secure success. As a corollary, however, poor nursing may easily undermine what has been achieved by the surgeon. Strict fluid balance must be kept and a daily fluid intake of at least 3 litres, and output of 100 ml/h, should be maintained until the urine is clear of blood. Haematuria is more persistent following abdominal than vaginal procedures, and intravenous fluid is therefore likely to be required for longer in this situation.

Bladder drainage

Continuous bladder drainage in the postoperative period is crucial to success, and nursing staff should check catheters hourly throughout each day to confirm free drainage, and check output. Bladder irrigation and suction drainage are not recommended. Views differ as to the ideal type of catheter: the calibre must be sufficient to prevent blockage, although whether the suprapubic or urethral route is used is, to a large extent, a matter of individual preference. My usual practice is to use a 'belt and braces' approach of both urethral and suprapubic drainage initially, so that, if one route becomes blocked, free drainage is still maintained. The urethral catheter is removed first, and the suprapubic retained and used to assess residual volume until the patient is voiding normally.[34]

The duration of free drainage depends on the fistula type: following repair of surgical fistulae, 12 days is adequate; with obstetric fistulae, up to 21 days' drainage may be appropriate and, following repair of radiation fistulae, 21–42 days is required. If there is any doubt about the integrity of the repair it is wise to carry out dye testing prior to catheter removal. Where a persistent leak is identified, free drainage should be maintained for 6 weeks.

Mobility and thromboprophylaxis

The greatest problem in ensuring free catheter drainage lies in preventing kinking or drag on the catheter. Restricting patient mobility in the postoperative period helps with this, and some advocate continuous bedrest during the period of catheter drainage. If this approach is chosen, patients should be looked on as being at moderate-to-high risk for thromboembolism, and appropiate prophylaxis must be employed.[35]

Antibiotics

Antibiotic cover is advised for all intestinovaginal fistula repairs. If prophylactic antibiotics are not used at urogenital fistula repair, catheter urine specimens should be collected for culture and sensitivity tests every 48 hours; only symptomatic infection need be treated in the catheterized patient.

Bowel management

If patients are restricted to bed following urogenital fistula repair, a laxative should be administered to prevent excessive straining at stool. Following abdominal repair of intestinovaginal fistulae, patients should either have a nasogastric tube inserted or remain 'nil by mouth' until they are passing flatus; the majority prefer the latter approach. Once oral intake is allowed, or following vaginal repair of rectovaginal fistulae, a low-residue diet should be administered until at least the fifth postoperative day. Some authorities advocate total parenteral nutrition throughout the first week postoperatively for all cases of intestinovaginal fistulae. Enemas and suppositories should be avoided, although a mild aperient such as docusate sodium is advised to ease initial bowel movements.

Subsequent management

On removal of catheters most patients will feel the desire to void frequently, as the bladder capacity will be functionally reduced, having been relatively empty for so long. In any case, it is important that patients do not become overdistended: hourly voiding should be encouraged and fluid intake limited. It may also be necessary to wake them once or twice through the night for the same reason. After discharge from hospital, patients should be advised to increase gradually the period between voiding, aiming to be back to a normal pattern by 4 weeks postoperatively.

Tampons, pessaries, douching, and penetrative sex should be avoided until 3 months postoperatively.

PROGNOSIS

Results

It is difficult to compare the results of treatment in different series, as the lesions involved and the techniques of repair vary so greatly. Cure rates should be considered in terms of closure at first operation, and vary from 60 to 98%.[4–6,30,36–42] Of the 140 patients in my series managed in the UK, six (4.3%) healed without operation, four declined surgery; one (with coexistent detrusor instability) was asymptomatic on medical treatment; three (2.1%) underwent primary urinary diversion; two patients with radiotherapy fistulae died without being operated upon (one from recurrent disease and one from cachexia without recurrence). Of the remaining 124 who have undergone repair surgery, 118 (95%) were cured by the first operation; of the 59 patients with fistulae following simple hysterectomy, all have been cured at their first operation.

A law of diminishing returns is evident in fistula surgery, as in many other forms of surgery. Although repeat operations are certainly justified, the success rate decreases progressively with increasing numbers of previous unsuccessful procedures. Surgical series are rarely large enough for this to be evident: in a series of 2484 largely obstetric fistulae, the success rate fell from 81.2% for first procedures to 65.0% for those requiring two or more procedures.[4] It cannot be overemphasized that the best prospect for cure is at the first operation, and there is no place for the well-intentioned occasional fistula surgeon, whether gynaecologist or urologist.[8]

Post-fistula stress incontinence

Stress incontinence has long been recognized as a complication of vesicovaginal fistulae.[24] It is most likely to occur in patients with obstetric fistulae when the injury involves the sphincter mechanism, particularly if there is tissue loss,[43] although it has also been reported in a large proportion of surgical fistulae involving the urethra or bladder neck.[7] It affects at least 10% of all patients with fistulae.

REFERENCES

1. Zacharin R. *Obstetric Fistula*. Vienna: Springer-Verlag, 1988

2. Waaldijk K. The surgical management of bladder fistula in 775 women in Northern Nigeria. MD thesis, University of Utrecht, Nijmegen, 1989

3. Danso K, Martey J, Wall L, Elkins T. The epidemiology of genitourinary fistulae in Kumasi, Ghana, 1977–1992. *Int Urogynecol J Pelvic Floor Dysfunct* 1996; 7: 117–120

4. Hilton P, Ward A. Epidemiological and surgical aspects of urogenital fistulae: a review of 25 years experience in Nigeria. *Int Urogynecol J Pelvic Floor Dysfunct* 1998; 9: 189–194.

5. Hilton P. Fistulae. In: Shaw R, Souter W, Stanton S (eds) *Gynaecology*, 2nd edn. London: Churchill Livingstone, 1997; 779–801

6. Lee R, Symmonds R, Williams T. Current status of genitourinary fistula. *Obstet Gynecol* 1988; 71: 313–319

7. Hilton P. Urodynamic findings in patients with urogenital fistulae. *Br J Urol* 1998; 81: 539–542

8. Hilton P. Post-operative urogenital fistulae are best managed by gynaecologists in specialist centres. *Br J Urol* 1997; 80, (Suppl 1): 35–42

9. Lawson J. Personal communication, 1990

10. Price JH, Nassief SA. Laparoscopic-assisted vaginal hysterectomy: initial experience. *Ulster Med J* 1996; 65: 149–151

11. Malik E, Schmidt M, Schneidel P. Complications following 106 laparoscopic hysterectomies. *Zentralbl Gynakol* 1997; 119: 611–615

12. Chapron CM, Dubuisson JB, Ansquer Y. Is total laparoscopic hysterectomy a safe surgical procedure? *Hum Reprod* 1996; 11: 2422–2424

13. Averette H, Nguyen H, Donato D *et al.* Radical hysterectomy for invasive cervical cancer. A 25–year prospective experience with the Miami technique. *Cancer* 1993; 71(Suppl 4): 1422–1437

14. Emmert C, Köhler U. Management of genital fistulas in patients with cervical cancer. *Arch Gynecol Obstet* 1996; 259: 19–24

15. White A, Buchsbaum H, Blythe J, Lifshitz S. Use of the bulbocavernosus muscle (Martius procedure) for repair of radiation-induced rectovaginal fistulas. *Obstet Gynecol* 1982; 60: 114–118

16. Bladou F, Houvenaeghel G, Delpero J, Guerinel G. Incidence and management of major urinary complications after pelvic exenteration for gynecological malignancies. *J Surg Oncol* 1995; 58: 91–96

17. Youssef A. 'Menouria' following lower segment caesarean section: a syndrome. *Am J Obstet Gynecol* 1957; 73: 759–767

18. Falk F, Tancer M. Management of vesical fistulas after cae-sarean section. *Am J Obstet Gynecol* 1956; 71: 97–106

19. Raghavaiah N. Double-dye test to diagnose various types of vaginal fistulas. *J Urol* 1974; 112: 811–812

20. Chassar Moir J. *The Vesico-vaginal Fistula*, 2nd edn. London: Baillière, 1967

21. Jonas U, Petri E. Genitourinary fistulae. In: Stanton S (ed) *Clinical Gynecologic Urology*. St Louis: Mosby, 1984; 238–255

22. Lawson J. The management of genito-urinary fistulae. *Clin Obstet Gynecol* 1978; 6: 209–236

23. Lawson J, Hudson C. The management of vesico-vaginal and urethral fistulae. In: Stanton S, Tanagho E (eds) *Surgery for Female Urinary Incontinence*. Berlin: Springer-Verlag, 1987; 193–209

24. Lawson J. Injuries to the urinary tract. In: Lawson J, Stewart D (eds) *Obstetrics and Gynaecology in the Tropics and Developing Countries*. London: Edward Arnold, 1967: 481–522

25. Hudson C. Malignant change in an obstetric vesico-vaginal fistula. *Proc R Soc Med* 1968; 61: 121–124

26. Waaldijk K. Immediate indwelling catheterization at post-partum urine leakage – personal experience of 1200 patients. *Trop Doct* 1993; 27: 227–228

27. Davits R, Miranda S. Conservative treatment of vesico-vaginal fistulas by bladder drainage alone. *Br J Urol* 1991; 68: 155–156

28. Sims J. On the treatment of vesico-vaginal fistula. *Am J Med Sci* 1852; 23: 59–82

29. Lawson J. Vesical fistulae into the vaginal vault. *Br J Urol* 1972; 44: 623–631

30. Hamlin R, Nicholson E. Reconstruction of urethra totally destroyed in labour. *Br Med J* 1969; 2: 147–150

31. Martius H. Die operative Wiederherstellung der vollkommen fehlenden Harnrohie und des Schiessmuskels derselben. *Zentralbl Gynakol* 1928; 52: 480

32. Turner-Warwick R. The use of the omental pedicle graft in urinary tract reconstruction. *J Urol* 1976; 116: 341–347

33. Kiricuta I, Goldstein A. The repair of extensive vesico-vaginal fistulas with pedicled omentum: a review of 27 cases. *J Urol* 1972; 108: 724–727

34. Hilton P. Bladder drainage. In: Stanton S, Monga A (eds) *Clinical Urogynaecology*, 2nd edn. London: Churchill Livingstone, 1999; 541–550

35. Thromboembolic Risk Factors (THRIFT) Consensus Group. Risk of and prophylaxis for venous thromboembolism in hospital patients. *Br Med J* 1992; 305: 567–574

36. Turner-Warwick RT, Wynne EJ, Handley-Ashken M. The use of the omental pedicle graft in the repair and reconstruction of the urinary tract. *Br J Surg* 1967; 54: 849–853

37. Chassar Moir J. Vesico-vaginal fistulae as seen in Britain. *J Obstet Gynaecol Br Commonw* 1973; 80: 598–602

38. Hudson C, Hendrickse J. An operation for restoration of urinary continence following total loss of the urethra. *Br J Obstet Gynaecol* 1975; 82: 501–504

39. Kelly J. Vesico-vaginal fistulae. *Br J Urol* 1979; 51: 208–210

40. Goodwin WE, Scardino PT. Vesicovaginal and ureterovaginal fistulas: a summary of 25 years of experience. *J Urol* 1980; 123: 370–374

41. Elkins T, Drescheer C, Martey J, Fort D. Vesicovaginal fistula revisited. *Obstet Gynecol* 1988; 72: 307–312

42. O'Conor VJ J. Review of experience with vesicovaginal fistula repair. *J Urol* 1980; 123: 367–369

43. Waaldijk K. *Step-by-step Surgery for Vesico-vaginal Fistulas*. Edinburgh: Campion, 1994

56

Obstetric fistulae

P. Hilton

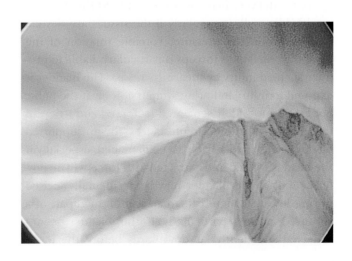

AETIOLOGY AND EPIDEMIOLOGY

As emphasized in chapter 55, in the UK and USA over 70% of fistulae follow pelvic surgery,[1,2] whereas in most developing countries over 90% are of obstetric aetiology[3-6] (see Table 55.1).

The underlying factors responsible for the development of obstetric fistulae may be considered in physical, biosocial, cultural, and geographical or political terms. The basic physical factors responsible for obstetric fistula development include obstructed labour, accidental injury at the time of caesarean section, forceps delivery, craniotomy or symphysiotomy, traditional surgical practices including circumcision and gishiri, and complications of criminal abortion.

The overwhelming proportion of cases are complications of neglected obstructed labour. During normal labour the bladder is displaced upwards and the anterior vaginal wall, bladder base and urethra are compressed between the fetal head and the posterior surface of the pubis. No harm results if this occurs for a short time; however, in prolonged obstructed labour, the intervening tissues are devitalized by ischaemia. Usually, the anterior vaginal wall and underlying bladder neck are affected, although sometimes the area of necrosis is higher, in which case the anterior lip of the cervix and underlying trigone are involved. Compression of the soft tissues posteriorly between the sacral promontory and the presenting part may occur at the same time, with necrosis at the posterior vaginal wall and underlying rectum. The devitalized area separates as a slough, usually between days 3 and 10 of the puerperium, with resulting incontinence (see Fig. 56. 1).

Accidental injury to the vaginal wall during a difficult operative delivery may involve damage to the underlying bladder wall, particularly if the tissues are devitalized by prolonged pressure. Forcible rotation of the head with Kielland's forceps is particularly liable to produce such an injury by shearing stresses. The bladder is exposed to injury following symphysiotomy if the pubic bones are too widely separated by forced abduction of the thighs. In these circumstances the unsupported bladder neck is very likely to be damaged, especially if the head is rotated and extracted with forceps. The posterior wall of the bladder may be accidentally incised during lower segment caesarean section or repair of a ruptured uterus, particularly if the bladder is not reflected sufficiently far downwards before the lower

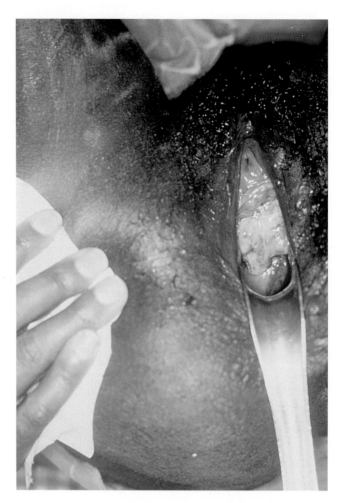

Figure 56.1. *Puerperal patient following prolonged obstructed labour. An area of devitalized tissue is seen on the anterior vaginal wall, about to slough, with resultant fistula formation. (Reproduced from ref. 2 with permission.)*

segment is opened. During the reflection itself the bladder may be torn, especially if a previous operation has made it densely adherent to the lower segment. If the bladder injury goes undetected at the time, urinary leakage through the abdominal wound soon develops. This is usually followed by incontinence vaginally when the urine finds its way through the uterine incision. The abdominal leakage then dries up as the bladder drains through the resulting vesicocervical fistula. Alternatively, sutures may be passed through the posterior bladder wall during repair of the uterine incision. The appearance of urinary incontinence in these cases is delayed until sloughing of the intervening bladder tissue caught up in the suture.

The perineum and posterior vaginal wall are, of

course, at risk from even the most straightforward delivery, although primiparity, forceps delivery, birth weight over 4 kg and occipitoposterior position have been found to be significant risk factors associated with third-degree tears.[7] Even when identified and repaired, such tears increase the risk of rectovaginal fistula.

Traditional surgical practices play a significant role in the aetiology of obstetric fistulae in several parts of Africa. Among the Hausa, Fulani and Kanuri tribes of Northern Nigeria, the practice of gishiri is commonly employed to treat a wide variety of conditions including obstructed labour, infertility, dyspareunia, amenorrhoea, goitre, backache and dysuria. The traditional cut made with a razor blade or knife through the vaginal introitus is sometimes superficial, but may result in fistula formation (see Fig. 56.2). Since these cuts are usually made by linear incision into healthy tissues, repair is often much easier than those resulting from pressure necrosis.

Circumcision has been practised in various forms in much of North Africa, and is still practised widely in Sudan and other Moslem cultures. The most extreme form – pharaonic circumcision – involves removal of the labia minora, most of the labia majora, the mons veneris and, often, the clitoris (see Fig. 56.3), the introitus being reduced to pinhole size. The effect in labour is to produce significant delay in the second stage. This will often necessitate wide episiotomy, often with an anterior incision to allow delivery, and contributes to the development of both vesicovaginal fistulae, and rectovaginal fistulae or third-degree tears.

Tahzib reported on the epidemiological determinants of vesicovaginal fistulae in Northern Nigeria.[8,9] In over 80% of cases, obstructed labour was the major aetiological factor; one-third had undergone gishiri, and in 15% this was felt to be the main aetiological factor.

In considering obstetric fistulae, however, it is perhaps as relevant (if not more so) to consider not simply the direct physical injury to the lower urinary tract but also the social, cultural and geographical influences. Obstructed labour is most often due to a contracted pelvis; this usually results from stunting of growth by malnutrition and untreated infections in childhood and adolescence. Where women retain a subservient role in society, and standards of education are limited, early marriage and the absence of family planning services result in an early start to childbearing; where first pregnancies occur soon after the menarche, before

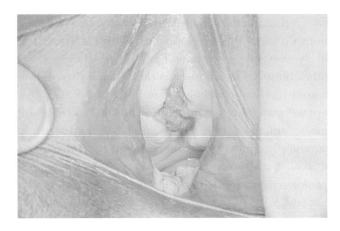

Figure 56.2. *Vesicovaginal fistula resulting from gishiri cut in a young Hausa girl. (Reproduced from ref. 2 with permission.)*

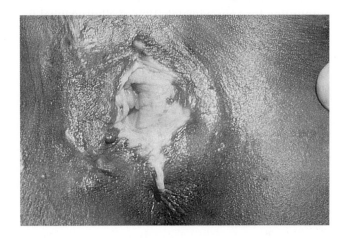

Figure 56.3. *Pharaonic circumcision. (Reproduced from ref. 2 with permission.)*

growth of the pelvis is complete, this also contributes to obstruction in labour.

The influence of these factors is illustrated in the epidemiological studies alluded to earlier. Tahzib[8] reported that, in over 50% of the cases of vesicovaginal fistulae seen in northern Nigeria, the mothers were aged under 20 years; over 50% were in their first pregnancy, and only 1 in 500 had received any formal education.[8] Murphy,[10] from the same area, reported that 88% of patients had married at 15 years of age or less and 33% had delivered their first child before the age of 15 years. In different developing societies, however, these factors do seem to have variable influence: for example, in south-east Nigeria[4] and the north-west frontier of Pakistan,[11] patients with a fistula seem to be somewhat older and of higher party; they also appear to have a higher literacy rate and to be more likely to remain in a married relationship after the development of their fistula. It is likely that the development of fistulae here reflects other biosocial variations. It is clear that in these populations, even where skilled maternity care is available, uptake may be poor: mistrust of hospital is commonplace, antenatal care poorly attended, and delivery commonly conducted at home by elderly relatives or unskilled traditional birth attendants. Where labour is prolonged, transfer to hospital may be used only as a last resort.

PREVALENCE

In western practice, obstetric fistulae are uncommon, accounting for approximately 10% of all urogenital fistulae (see Table 55.1). Third-degree tears have been reported to follow 0.6% of vaginal deliveries, and in 6% of these (1 in 3000 deliveries overall) a rectovaginal fistula may result.[7]

In developing countries, many women with fistulae are unknown to medical services, being separated from their husbands and ostracized from society. Although the true prevalence of fistulae in developing countries is unknown, particularly high prevalence rates have been reported from Sudan,[12] Ethiopia,[13] Chad,[14] Ghana[3] and Nigeria.[8] An incidence of 1–2/1000 deliveries has been estimated, with a worldwide annual incidence of 50 000–100 000 and a prevalence of untreated fistulae of 500 000–2 000 000.[15] The incidence of fistulae clearly relates to the level of maternity care provision, those areas with high maternal mortality tending also to have high fistula rates. Danso and colleagues[3] have suggested that a more realistic estimate of the incidence of fistulae in any community might be that it approaches the maternal mortality rate. This might indicate an annual incidence worldwide of up to 500 000. Harrison[16,17] reported an overall maternal and perinatal mortality rate of 10/1000 and 90/1000, respectively, and 34/10000 and 125/1000 in primipara under 16 years of age in northern Nigeria.

CLASSIFICATION

The classification of fistulae types and sites is discussed in Chapter 55. Over 70% of obstetric fistulae are located in the mid-vaginal or juxtacervical areas, or are massive (extending from bladder neck to vaginal vault – see Fig. 56.4)[4] (Table 56.1).

PRESENTATION

Although surgical fistulae may often present less typically, most obstetric fistulae resulting from ischaemic

Table 56.1. *Fistula site in two groups of patients: the first are largely those with surgical fistulae from north-east England;* the second largely patients with obstetric fistulae from south-east Nigeria[†]*

Fistula site	NE England (n = 140)*		SE Nigeria (n = 2484)[†]	
	n	%	n	%
Urethral	18	12.9	70	2.8
Subsymphyseal			75	3.0
Bladder neck	13	9.3	132	5.3
Mid-vaginal	11	7.9	579	23.3
Large	4	2.9	432	17.4
Juxtacervical	2	1.4	773	31.1
Vault	75	53.6	5	0.2
Uterus/cervix	6	4.3	77	3.1
Multiple			89	3.6
Ureteric	11	7.9		
Unspecified			252	10.2
Total	140	100.0	2484	100.0

* Hilton P, unpublished data.
[†] From ref. 4.

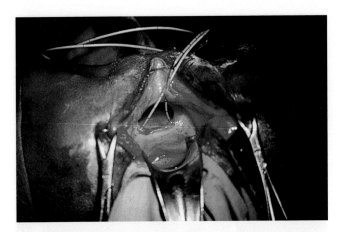

Figure 56.4. *Massive complex obstetric fistula: both ureteric orifices are visible within the upper edge of the fistula; there is a concurrent rectovaginal fistula, the patient having already undergone defunctioning colostomy.*

necrosis will have the characteristic presentation with continuous urinary incontinence, limited sensation of bladder fullness and infrequent voiding. Some patients with vesicocervical or vesicouterine fistula following caesarean section may maintain continence at the level of the uterine isthmus, and complain of cyclical haematuria at the time of menstruation (menouria).[18,19]

Although symptoms usually develop 5–14 days after the causative injury, the time of presentation may be quite variable. This will depend to some extent on the severity of symptoms, but as far as obstetric fistulae in developing countries are concerned, is determined more by access to healthcare. In a recent review of cases from Nigeria, the average time for presentation was more than 5 years – in some cases, more than 35 years – after the causative pregnancy.[4] Many patients with obstetric fistulae are amenorrhoeic at the time of presentation.[4,20] It is not clearly established whether the amenorrhoea reflects the gross tissue loss within the pelvis, or a hypothalamic influence as a result of the physical and emotional effects of a traumatic labour, stillbirth and fistula development. Since the live-birth rate is so low, clearly lactation is unlikely to be a significant factor. In the epidemiological studies of Hilton and Ward,[4] 44% of patients were amenorrhoeic at the time of referral. The average time to presentation in those who had resumed menstruation was over 4 years, compared with 2 years in those who remained amenorrhoeic. This might be taken to imply that the natural history of the hypothalamic

suppressive effect of developing a fistula tends towards spontaneous resolution after 2 years, even if the fistula remains untreated. Alternatively, however, these findings may simply reflect the fact that the more dramatically affected patients (who are more likely to develop amenorrhoea) are also more likely to present earlier for treatment than less-traumatized women, who may have resumed menstruation at any stage.

INVESTIGATIONS

The investigation and treatment of most obstetric vesicovaginal fistulae will follow principles similar to those described for surgical fistulae in chapter 55; only those areas where the two fistula types differ in their implications for management are included in this chapter.

If a patient with a vesicouterine fistula has no history of incontinence but complains of cyclical haematuria, contrast studies carried out through the uterus (i.e. hysterosalpinography) may be more rewarding than cystography; a lateral or oblique view may be necessary to detect the anterior leak (see Fig. 56.5).

PREOPERATIVE MANAGEMENT

The role of catheterization in the immediate management of surgical fistulae has already been emphasized. Obstetric fistulae developing after obstructed labour should also be treated by continuous bladder drainage, combined with antibiotics to limit tissue damage from infection. Indeed, if a patient is known to have been in

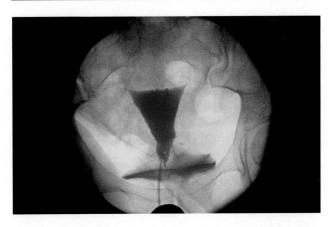

Figure 56.5. *Hysterosalpingogram in a patient presenting with menouria and urinary incontinence following caesarean section; cystography failed to demonstrate the uterovesical fistula.*

obstructed labour for any significant length of time, or is recognized to have areas of slough on the vaginal walls in the puerperium, prophylactic catheterization should be undertaken to reduce the likelihood of fistula development. This should be maintained for 6–8 weeks, since spontaneous closure in both surgical and obstetric cases may occur within this period.[21,22] If sloughing of the rectal wall has also occurred, faecal discharge will adversely affect spontaneous healing and temporary defunctioning colostomy should be performed.

The principles of pallation and skin care are outlined in chapter 55.

Nutrition

Because of social ostracism and the effects of prolonged sepsis, patients with obstetric fistulae may also suffer from malnutrition and anaemia. To maximize the prospects for postoperative healing it is essential, therefore, that the general health of the patient should be optimized. The admission of patients with fistulae to preoperative hostel facilities is encouraged by several of the larger fistula units in developing countries.[6] Where nursing staff is limited, family members may also be admitted to such facilities to help with the provision of supplies and cooking etc.

Physiotherapy

Obstetric fistulae are commonly associated with lower-limb weakness, foot drop and limb contracture (see Fig. 56.6). In a group of 479 patients studied prospectively, 27% had signs of peroneal nerve weakness at presentation; a further 38%, although having no current signs, gave a history of relevant symptoms.[23] Early involvement of the physiotherapist in preoperative management and rehabilitation of such patients is essential.

GENERAL PRINCIPLES OF SURGICAL TREATMENT

Timing of repair

In timing the surgical repair of obstetric fistulae, most authorities suggest that a minimum of 3 months should be allowed to elapse, although others have advocated surgery as soon as slough is separated.[22]

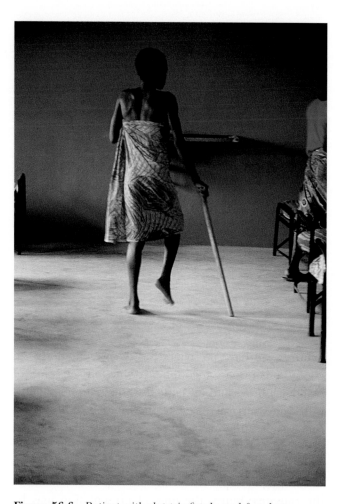

Figure 56.6. *Patient with obstetric fistula and foot drop.*

Route of repair

There is clearly always benefit in avoiding the abdominal approach to surgery, and this advantage is undoubtedly greater in developing countries. Although many urologists advocate an abdominal approach for all fistula repairs, those experienced in developing countries suggest that most obstetric fistulae can (and should) be managed by the vaginal route.[24] In my series of cases from the UK, and those reviewed from Nigeria,[4] two-thirds of patients were satisfactorily treated by the vaginal route, regardless of aetiology (see Table 56.2).

Interposition grafting

The use of interposition grafting to support fistula repair is discussed in chapter 55. This type of grafting serves to create an additional layer in the repair, to fill

Table 56.2. *Route of primary repair (i.e. first repair at referral centre) of urogenital fistulae in two series, from north-east England* and from south-east Nigeria[†]*

Route of repair (primary procedure)	Percentage			
	NE England (n = 140)*		SE Nigeria (n = 2484)[†]	
Abdominal	30.8		17.0	
transperitoneal		15.0		
transvesical		8.3		13.4
ureteric reimplantation/stenting		5.8		3.0
ureterosigmoid transplantation		0.0		0.6
primary ileal conduit		1.7		0.0
Vaginal lithotomy	67.5		80.0	
layer dissection		41.7		
layer dissection + Maritus graft		18.3		
colpocleisis		7.5		
Vaginal reverse lithotomy	1.7		3.0	
Total	100.0		100.0	

* Hilton P, unpublished, data.
[†] from ref. 4.

dead space, and to bring in new blood supply to the area. In the case of obstetric fistulae, especially those involving the bladder neck or urethra, interposition grafting may have the additional benefit of reducing scarring in the area and therefore limiting the incidence of post-fistula stress incontinence. The procedures most commonly advocated in this context are the Martius (labial fat and bulbocavernosus muscle) graft,[25] and the gracilis muscle graft.[26]

PROGNOSIS

Results

As reported in chapter 55, cure rates at first operation recorded in the literature vary between 60 and 98%, averaging approximately 80% regardless of aetiology or technique used. The success rate has been shown to fall from 81.2% for first procedures to 65.0% where multiple repair procedures are required.[4]

Post-fistula stress incontinence

Stress incontinence has long been recognized as a complication of vesicovaginal fistulae.[27] It is most likely to occur in patients with obstetric fistula when the injury involves the sphincter mechanism, particularly if there is tissue loss.[5] It affects at least 10% of all patients with fistulae.

The extent of scarring in the area means that conventional approaches to bladder-neck elevation may be technically difficult, and of limited success. The use of a labial muscle–fat graft in the initial repair may reduce the likelihood of this complication,[24] and a number of other techniques have been attempted.[24,28] The implantation of an artificial urinary sphincter, or neourethral reconstruction, might be appropriate from a theoretical point of view;[29] however, the former would be prohibitively expensive, and both cause excessive morbidity, for use in the developing countries. Periurethral injection holds promise as a minimally invasive technique that may be particularly appropriate in the situation of urethral insufficiency with a relatively fixed immobile urethra; initial success with this technique in patients with stress incontinence following fistula has been reported.[30]

Subsequent pregnancy

Although many patients with obstetric vesicovaginal fistula will experience amenorrhoea for 2 years or more after the causative pregnancy,[4] nevertheless, where tissue loss is not great, hypothalamic function often returns to normal immediately after successful repair and fertility may be relatively normal. Most authorities emphasize the need for caesarean section in any subsequent pregnancy.[31] Kelly,[32] however, reported on 33 women who became pregnant within 1 year of fistula repair, 12 of whom delivered vaginally without damage to the repair. The criteria he used for attempting vaginal delivery were: that the fistula arose from a non-recurrent cause (i.e. malpresentation as opposed to pelvic contraction), that an interposition graft had been utilized in the repair, and that the labour is conducted under skilled supervision in hospital.

The management of delivery in women who have had a previous third-degree tear has not been prospectively studied, although it has been suggested that there may be benefit in assessing the sphincter prior to delivery by endo-anal ultrasonography: where minor defects are present, potentially traumatic vaginal delivery should be avoided; where more major defects are identified, caesarean section might be offered.[7]

PREVENTION

It is estimated by the World Health Organization (WHO) that there are approximately 500 000 maternal deaths/year worldwide, and it is clear that the prevalence of obstetric fistulae and maternal mortality rates are closely related. Indeed, one might look on the patient with vesicovaginal fistula as being a 'near-miss' maternal death. In recognition of this fact, the WHO established, through their 'Safe Motherhood Initiative', a technical working group to investigate the problems of prevention and management of obstetric fistulae. The recommendations from that working group included the extension of antenatal and intrapartum care; the transfer of women in prolonged labour for delivery by skilled personnel; the identification of regions where fistulae are still prevalent, so that resources could be mobilized to deal with fistulae more effectively; and the creation of specialized centres for management, training and research.[11]

Certainly, obstetric fistulae would disappear if early intervention in obstructed labour were available and acceptable throughout the world. It has been pointed out, however, that in Nigeria alone this would require the establishment of some 75 000 obstetric units.[33] Clearly, the achievement of the aims and recommendations of the WHO is critically dependent on major

social change in areas of endemicity. Without improvement in the status of women, an extension of primary education, deferment of marriage and childbearing, the abolition of female genital mutilation, improved nutritional status and contraceptive services, and skilled attendants in childbirth throughout the world, the problem of obstetric fistulae will remain with us for many years to come.

REFERENCES

1. Lee R, Symmonds R, Williams T. Current status of genitourinary fistula. *Obstet Gynecol* 1988; 71: 313–319

2. Hilton P. Fistulae. In: Shaw R, Souter W, Stanton S (eds) *Gynaecology*, 2nd edn. London: Churchill Livingstone, 1997; 779–801

3. Danso K, Martey J, Wall L, Elkins T. The epidemiology of genitourinary fistulae in Kumasi, Ghana, 1977–1992. *Int Urogynecol J Pelvic Floor Dysfunct* 1996; 7: 117–120

4. Hilton P, Ward A. Epidemiological and surgical aspects of urogenital fistulae: a review of 25 years experience in south-east Nigeria. *Int Urogynecol J Pelvic Floor Dysfunct* 1998; 9: 189–194

5. Waaldijk K. The surgical management of bladder fistula in 775 women in Northern Nigeria. MD thesis, University of Utrecht, Nijmegen, 1989

6. Zacharin R. *Obstetric Fistula*. Vienna: Springer-Verlag, 1988

7. Sultan AH, Kamm MA, Hudson CN, Bartram CI. Third degree obstetric and sphincter tears: risk factors and outcome of primary repair. *Br Med J* 1994; 308: 887–891

8. Tahzib F. Epidemiological determinants of vesicovaginal fistulas. *Br J Obstet Gynaecol* 1983; 90: 387–391

9. Tahzib F. Vesicovaginal fistula in Nigerian children. *Lancet* 1985; 2: 1291–1293

10. Murphy M. Social consequences of vesico-vaginal fistula in Northern Nigeria. *J Biosoc Sci* 1981; 13: 139–150

11. World Health Organization. *The Prevention and Treatment of Obstetric Fistulae: Report of a Technical Working Group*. Geneva: WHO, 1989

12. Abbo A. New trends in the operative management of urinary fistulae. *Sudan Med J* 1975; 13: 126–132

13. Hamlin R, Nicholson E. Experiences in the treatment of 600 vaginal fistulas and in the management of 80 labours which have followed the repair of these injuries. *Ethiop Med J* 1966; 4: 189–192

14. Barnaud P, Veillard J, Richard J et al. Les fistulas vesicovaginales Africaines. *Med Trop Mars* 1980; 40: 389–401

15. Waaldijk K, Armiya'u Y. The obstetric fistula: a major

public health problem still unsolved. *Int Urogynecol J* 1993; 4: 126–128

16. Harrison KA. *Childbearing in Zaria. Public Health Lecture, 1978;* Zaria: Amadu Bello University, 1978

17. Harrison KA. Approaches to reducing maternal and perinatal mortality in Africa. In: Philpott RH (ed) *Maternity Services in the Developing World. What the Community Needs.* Proceedings of the 7th RCOG Study Group. London: RCOG, 1979; 52–69

18. Falk F, Tancer M. Management of vesical fistulas after caesarean section. *Am J Obstet Gynecol* 1956; 71: 97–106

19. Youssef A. 'Menouria' following lower segment caesarean section: a syndrome. *Am J Obstet Gynecol* 1957; 73: 759–767

20. Evoh NJ, Akinla O. Reproductive performance after the repair of obstetric vesico-vaginal fistulae. *Ann Clin Res* 1978; 10: 303–306

21. Davits R, Miranda S. Conservative treatment of vesicovaginal fistulas by bladder drainage alone. *Br J Urol* 1991; 68: 155–156

22. Waaldijk K. The immediate surgical management of fresh obstetric fistulas with catheter and/or early closure. *Int J Gynaecol Obstet* 1994; 45: 11–16

23. Waaldijk K, Elkins T. The obstetric fistula and peroneal nerve injury: an analysis of 947 consecutive patients. *Int Urogynecol J* 1994; 5: 12–14

24. Waaldijk K. *Step-by-step Surgery for Vesico-vaginal Fistulas.* Edinburgh: Campion, 1994

25. Martius H. Die operative Wiederherstellung der vollkommen fehlenden Harnrohre und des Schiessmuskels derselben. *Zentralbl Gynakol* 1928; 52: 480

26. Hamlin R, Nicholson E. Reconstruction of urethra totally destroyed in labour. *Br Med J* 1969; 2: 147–150

27. Lawson J. Injuries to the urinary tract. In: Lawson J, Stewart D (eds) *Obstetrics and Gynaecology in the Tropics and Developing Countries.* London: Edward Arnold, 1967; 481–522

28. Hudson C, Hendrickse J, Ward A. An operation for restoration of urinary continence following total loss of the urethra. *Br J Obstet Gynaecol* 1975; 82: 501–504

29. Hilton P. Surgery for genuine stress incontinence: which operation and for which patient? In: Drife J, Hilton P, Stanton S (eds) *Micturition.* Proceedings of the 21st RCOG Study Group. London: Springer-Verlag, 1990; 225–246

30. Hilton P, Ward A, Molloy M, Umana O. Periurethral injection of autologous fat for the treatment of post-fistula repair stress incontinence: a preliminary report. *Int Urogynecol J Pelvic Floor Dysfunct* 1998; 9: 118–121

31. Lawson J. The management of genito-urinary fistulae. *Clin Obstet Gynecol* 1978; 6: 209–236

32. Kelly J. Vesicovaginal fistulae. *Br J Urol* 1979; 51: 208–210

33. Waaldijk K. Personal communication, 1988

57

Urethral diverticulum and fistula

G. E. Leach, K. C. Kobashi

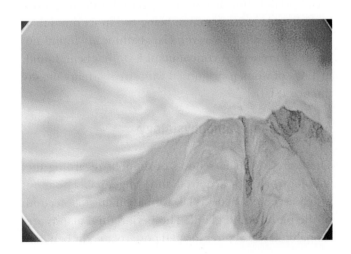

Urethral Diverticulum

INTRODUCTION

Female urethral diverticulum (UD) has been a historically underdiagnosed condition. Novak[1] stated, 'This is a relatively rare condition and no gynecologist will see more than a few in a lifetime'. However, with higher clinical suspicion and improved diagnostic techniques, the frequency of diagnosis has increased.

History

The existence of UD has been known since at least the early 19th century, when Hey reported the first case in 1805.[2] In 1938, Hunner[3] reported three cases associated with calculi and commented on the rarity of the condition. In 1956, Davis and Cian[4] reported 50 cases, more than had been reported previously in the entire history of the Johns Hopkins Hospital. They also developed a double-balloon catheter to be used in conjunction with positive-pressure profilometry to facilitate diagnosis of UD.

Incidence and patient profile

The incidence of female UD is reported in the urological literature as 0.6–6%[5,6] and in the gynaecological literature as 5%.[7] However, these numbers are probably an underestimate and, with increasing clinical suspicion, the true incidence may prove to be higher.[8]

Patients typically present in the third to sixth decades of life, with a mean age of 45 years.[9] Rarely, UD has been diagnosed in neonates and children.[10,11] A racial predilection has been suggested, with diagnosis in African-American women being two to six times that in white women;[12] however, Ganabathi *et al.*[9] found no racial differences. A concomitant UD[13] has been found in 1.4% of women diagnosed with stress urinary incontinence (SUI).

Aetiology and pathophysiology

There are two main schools of thought regarding the aetiology of UD – acquired and congenital. The most widely accepted theory is UD formation due to infection of the periurethral gland. The periurethral glands are tuboalveolar structures located posterolaterally beneath the periurethral fascia. They are found in the proximal two-thirds of the urethra and drain into the distal third of the urethra.[14] Infection leads to obstruction of the glands, local abscess formation and eventual rupture into the urethral lumen, as first described by Routh[15] in 1890.

Trauma secondary to childbirth or forceps delivery[16] remains a problem in developing countries, possibly contributing to UD formation.[17] However, with current obstetric technology, traumatic delivery is no longer a prevalent factor in developed nations. In fact, 15–20% of patients diagnosed with UD are nulliparous, thereby completely refuting this aetiologic theory.[11]

A congenital aetiology is doubtful, although there has been some evidence supporting this theory.[10] Faulty union of primordial folds, genesis from cell rests or Gartner's duct remnants, and müllerian remnants causing vaginal cysts have all been suggested as possible aetiologies.[17] The discovery of mesonephric adenoma and adenocarcinoma has implicated Gartner's duct remnants. Paneth cell metaplasia lining a UD also supports a congenital basis.[18] Blind-ending ureters resulting from an aborted ureteral duplication may rarely lead to an anterior UD.[19] Other suggested aetiologies of UD include high-pressure voiding against outlet obstruction, urethral calculi, instrumentation, and complications of previous anterior vaginal surgery.[17]

Associated complications

Complications associated with UD include incontinence, infection, stones and malignancy. Urinary incontinence is common in patients with UD. In fact, Ganabathi *et al.*[9] reported a 65% incidence of SUI among patients with UD (57% with SUI as the presenting complaint). These patients may also suffer from urge incontinence or 'paradoxical incontinence', in which urine stored in the UD is lost during stress.[5]

About 25–33% of patients present with recurrent urinary tract infections, including some who suffer from systemic infections. The most common infecting organisms of UD are *Escherichia coli*, chlamydia and gonococcus; however, multiple organisms have been cultured.[17,20] Up to 13% of patients present with calculi in the UD, and this can be confirmed by plain radiograph.[21,22] Stones form secondary to stasis, infection and chronic inflammation in the UD.[6] Urethrovaginal fistula secondary to rupture of a UD is also a potential complication.[23,24]

Approximately 100 cases of neoplasm within a UD have been reported in the world literature.[25–28] There have also been reports of 16 cases of nephrogenic adenoma, a benign metaplastic condition.[29–34] Malignancy must be considered whenever a UD is diagnosed, particularly when accompanied by haematuria, induration or firmness of a UD on physical examination, non-calcified filling defects within the UD on radiography, or a visible lesion on cystoscopic examination. Despite the fact that squamous epithelium lines most of the urethra, adenocarcinoma is by far the most common histopathological condition demonstrated within UD.[30] More than 80% of the diverticular cancers seen are either adenocarcinoma (61%) or transitional cell carcinoma (27%), which is the second most common malignancy seen in UD.[35] Squamous cell carcinoma is rare, comprising only 12% of UD malignancies.[35] Treatment of diverticular carcinoma includes wide local excision for localized disease.[27] Adjuvant radiation therapy or chemotherapy may also be indicated for extensive malignancy or for non-surgical candidates.[36,37] Survival is a function of stage[37] and grade[36] of the disease.

PRESENTATION

Clinical symptoms

Patients found to have UD present with a variety of symptoms ranging from irritative voiding complaints to pelvic pain and dyspareunia (Table 57.1).[5] The classic triad of UD is known as the '3 Ds' – dysuria, dyspareunia and dribbling. However, many patients are asymptomatic.

Physical examination

Patients with UD most commonly have anterior vaginal wall tenderness, with or without a concomitant palpable suburethral mass.[38] Pressure on the mass may demonstrate expressable purulence or blood from the UD (Fig. 57.1), and firmness of the area may indicate a diverticular stone or neoplasm. Rarely, some patients are without any pertinent physical findings and work-up is based only on clinical suspicion established by the patient's history. Importantly, the clinician must also examine patients for urethral hypermobility with or without SUI, which can be addressed at the time of repair of the UD if deemed necessary.

Table 57.1. *Presenting symptoms in 627 women with urethral diverticula from published reports*

Symptom	n (%)
Frequency	351 (56)
Dysuria	345 (55)
Recurrent infection	251 (40)
Tender mass	219 (35)
Stress incontinence	201 (32)
Post-void dribbling	160 (26)
Urge incontinence	157 (25)
Haematuria	107 (17)
Dyspareunia	376 (16)
Pus *per urethram*	75 (12)
Retention	25 (4)
Asymptomatic	38 (6)

From ref. 5.

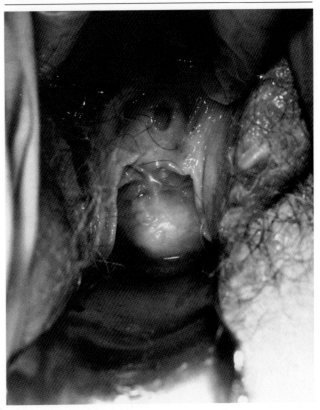

Figure 57.1. *Urethral diverticulum presenting as an anterior vaginal mass. (Reproduced from ref. 9 with permission.)*

Differential diagnosis

The differential diagnosis of urethral and meatal/perimeatal masses (Figs 57.2, 57.3) is illustrated in Tables 57.2 and 57.3, respectively. Note that Table 57.3 includes conditions that occur in locations distal to the majority of UD; however, they should be considered in the differential diagnosis.[39]

Classification system

Leach and coworkers[43] created a system for classification of female UD known as the L/N/S/C3 system. This acronym represents Location, Number, Size, Configuration, Communication, and Continence. This system facilitates preoperative assessment of UD and standardizes the classification, thereby simplifying

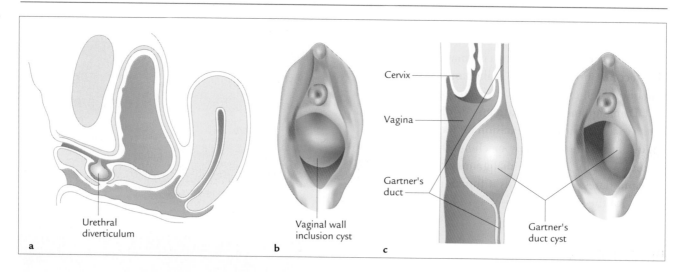

Figure 57.2. *Differential diagnosis of urethral and anterior vaginal wall masses: (a) urethral diverticulum; (b) vaginal wall inclusion cyst; (c) Gartner's duct cyst.*

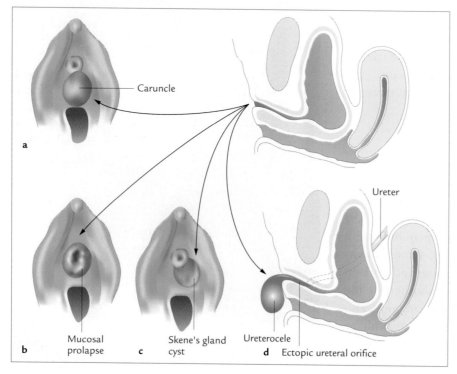

Figure 57.3. *Differential diagnosis of meatal and perimeatal lesions: (a) caruncle; (b) mucosal prolapse; (c) Skene's gland (or duct) cyst; (d) ureterocele.*

Table 57.2. *Differential diagnosis of urethral and anterior vaginal wall lesions*

Lesion	Location	Symptoms/physical exam	Cystoscopy/radiography	Comments
Urethral diverticulum	Anterior vaginal wall, midline	UTI, dysuria, dyspareunia, post-void dribbling, cystic mass	Orifice of diverticulum visible on urethral floor; VCUG opacifies lesion	May be multilocular
Vaginal wall cyst	Anterior vaginal wall, midline or eccentric	Cystic mass; may be loculated	None or extrinsic compression	–
Gartner's duct cyst	Anterolateral vaginal wall	Cystic mass	None or extrinsic compression; IVP may indicate ectopic ureteral drainage	Rule out ectopic ureter prior to excision
Müllerian remnant cyst	Midline	Cystic mass	None or extrinsic compression	–
Ectopic ureterocele[40]	Anywhere in bladder, urethra, vagina (upper third), uterus, Fallopian tubes	Cystic mass	May be seen on IVP, US, or cystoscopy	–
Leiomyoma, hamartoma	Vaginal wall	Solid mass	None or extrinsic compression	Rule out malignancy
Malignant urethral or vaginal neoplasms	Urethral or vaginal wall or haematuria	Solid mass; may have pain cystoscopy may show	None or extrinsic compression; ± adjuvant therapy erythema, obvious lesion or tumour growing from the diverticulum into the urethral lumen	Wide local excision

UTI, urinary tract infection; VCUG, voiding cystourethrogram; IVP, intravenous pyelography; US, ultrasonography.
Adapted from ref. 39.

Table 57.3. *Differential diagnosis of meatal and perimeatal lesions*

Lesion	Location	Presentation	Comments
Caruncle	Inferior to meatus	Asymptomatic or dysuria/pain with atrophic or ischaemic mucosal changes	Post-menopausal age group
Skene's gland cyst or abscess[41]	Inferior and lateral to meatus	Painful, orifice of duct visible at urethral meatus	–
Mucosal prolapse	Circumferential mucosal prolapse with central meatus	Pain and dysuria, atrophic or ischaemic mucosal changes	Young girls or post-menopausal women
Prolapsed ureterocele[42]	Submeatal, prolapsed through meatus	Glistening mucosa, may be fluid filled, may be ischaemic, may be asymptomatic	IVP to evaluate upper tract status

IVP, intravenous pyelography.
Adapted from ref. 39.

Table 57.4. *L/N/S/C3 Classification system[43] applied to 63 patients with urethral diverticula*

Location (L)	Number (N)	Size (S)	Configuration (C1)	Communication (C2)	Continence (C3)
Proximal, beneath bladder neck (9)	Single	0.2 × 0.2 cm to 6.0 × 4.5 cm	Multiloculated (22)	Proximal urethral (16)	Complete (26)
Proximal urethra (7)	Multiple		Single (41)	Midurethra (35)	SUI only (30)
Mid-urethra (36)			Saddle-shaped (14)*	Distal urethra (12)	Urge incontinence only (3)
Distal urethra (11)					SUI and urge incontinence (4)

* These patients are also included in the 'simple' or 'multiloculated' groups.
SUI, Stress urinary incontinence.
Adapted from ref. 43.

comparison between series. Table 57.4 illustrates the classification of 63 patients.

DIAGNOSIS

Endoscopic examination

A blunt-tip female urethroscope with a 0 or 30-degree lens is used. The anterior vaginal wall is compressed with a finger in the vagina, and the urethral lumen is inspected for any expression of pus from the floor or roof of the urethra (Fig. 57.4). In 50% of patients there will be multiple diverticula and more than half of the UDs will communicate with the middle third of the urethra.[7]

Urodynamic evaluation

Urodynamic studies are not always required in the evaluation of all patients with UD. The indications include patients with symptoms of SUI or bladder dysfunction.[44,45] These symptoms may include urinary leakage with increased intra-abdominal pressure, urge incontinence, or spontaneous loss of urine, which may represent intrinsic sphincter deficiency, paradoxical incontinence (i.e. loss of urine that has 'pooled' in the UD), or detrusor instability. Identification of these problems is critical in proper surgical planning. If a patient has a work-up indicative of SUI, appropriate correctional surgery can be performed at the time of diverticulectomy. The urodynamic findings in 55 women studied by Leach and Ganabathi[44] are noted in Table 57.5.

Table 57.5. *Urodynamic findings in 55 women with urethral diverticula*

Urodynamic finding	n (%)
Normal	22 (40)
SUI alone	18 (32.7)
SUI + DI	8 (14.5)
DI alone	5 (9)
Sensory urgecy	1 (2)
Myogenic decompensation	1 (2)

DI, detrusor instability; SUI, stress urinary incontinence.
From ref. 44, with modifications.

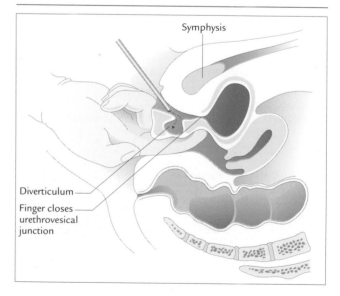

Figure 57.4. *The technique of endoscopic examination of the urethra while 'milking' the anterior vaginal wall and urethral roof.*

Radiological studies

Voiding cystourethrogram

The voiding cystourethrogram (VCUG) is the study of choice for the diagnosis of UD, with an accuracy of 95% (Fig. 57.5). The VCUG is performed under fluoroscopic visualization with the patient standing. Assessment of the bladder neck and proximal urethra as well as bladder-neck competency is imperative to document incontinence that may be treated at the time of diverticulectomy. Filling defects within a UD may represent tumour or stones[5] (Fig. 57.6). An air–fluid level in the UD may indicate a UD that is much larger than it appears radiographically. In 50% of patients there will be multiple UD. Correct identification is critical to ensure complete excision of all components of the UD.

Ultrasonography

We use ultrasonography in the evaluation of the upper tracts or, occasionally, in conjunction with VCUG to confirm the number and size of diverticula, especially in those not completely filled during urethrography[22,47,48] (Fig. 57.7). Vargas-Serrano *et al.*[48] advocate transrectal ultrasonography (TRUS) as the most sensitive tool in the diagnosis of female UD. Keefe *et al.*[47] support transperineal or transvaginal sonography, stating 100% sensitivity in their small series and stressing the non-invasive nature of the technique. Multiple approaches to ultrasonography have been employed, including transvaginal,[49,50] translabial,[51] suprapubic,[47] perineal[47] and TRUS.[48] Intra-operative endoluminal ultrasonography has been described for localization of the UD;[52,53] however, this is very difficult to perform.

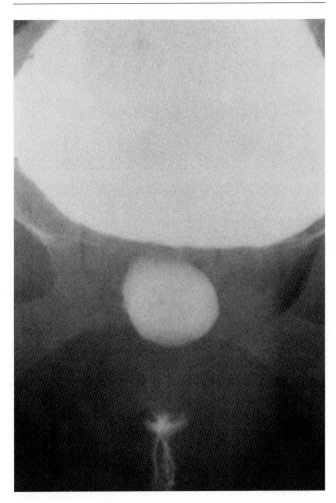

Figure 57.5. *A voiding cystourethrogram demonstrating a multiloculated diverticulum. (Reproduced from ref. 43 with permission.)*

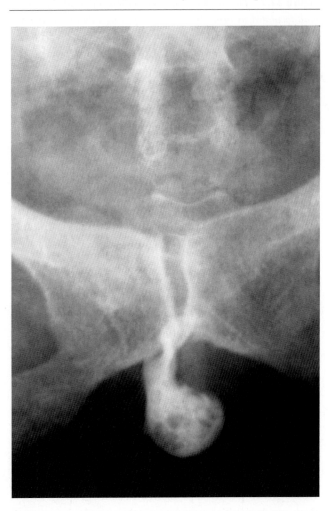

Figure 57.6. *A post-void film demonstrating filling defects within a urethral diverticulum suggestive of stones or tumour. (Reproduced from ref. 46 with permission.)*

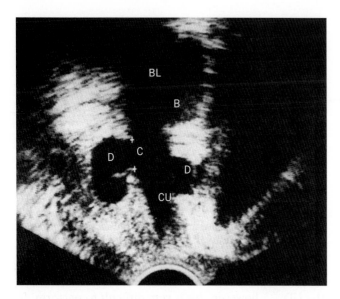

Figure 57.7. *Transvaginal ultrasonography demonstrating a multiloculated urethral diverticulum opening into the proximal urethra. BL, bladder; B, Foley catheter balloon; C, diverticular communication; D, diverticulum; CU, intraurethral Foley catheter. (Reproduced from ref. 9 with permission.)*

Intravenous pyelography

Intravenous pyelography (IVP) can be useful to evaluate the upper tracts and rule out an ectopic ureterocele.[54–56] Ectopic ureterocele may be considered when there is an abnormal protrusion into the urethra or from the meatus. It is important to obtain a low pelvic view in order to visualize the urethra completely (Fig. 57.8).

Magnetic resonance imaging

Magnetic resonance imaging (MRI) has recently been found to be a useful diagnostic tool with a high sensitivity for identifying fluid-filled cavities.[29,57–60] Kim *et al.*[61] reported 100% sensitivity of MRI in the detection of UD. The signal intensity of fluid is high on T2-weighted images and isointense on T1-weighted images (Fig. 57.9). MRI is being advocated as helpful in defining the extent of a UD and differentiating it from other urethral or vaginal masses, such as malignancy, paraurethral cysts and Gartner's duct cysts.

Retrograde positive-pressure urethrography

Retrograde positive-pressure urethrography is reported by Robertson[7] to have a 90% accuracy. However, we never use this technique and, in urological practice today, it is employed only as a last resort, when high-

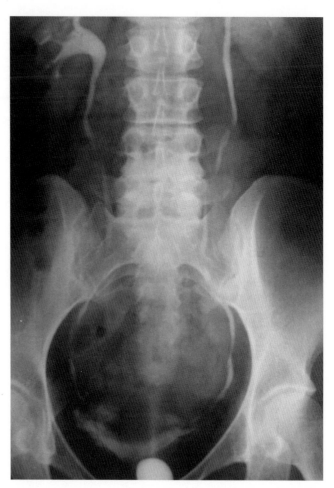

Figure 57.8. *Intravenous pyelogram demonstrates the urethral diverticulum and the upper tracts.*

quality VCUG is not available. It is a painful procedure for patients, often necessitating anaesthesia; it is also technically difficult to obtain an adequate study, requiring a special catheter known as the Davis or Tratner catheter[7,62] (Fig. 57.10). This catheter has a double balloon: one balloon is placed in the bladder; the distal (wedge-shaped) balloon slides to occlude the external meatus during injection of contrast via ports located between the balloons (Fig. 57.10).

THERAPY

History

Numerous techniques for identification and repair of UD have been described. Intradiverticular placement of a sound,[3,63] a Foley catheter,[64] a Fogarty catheter,[65]

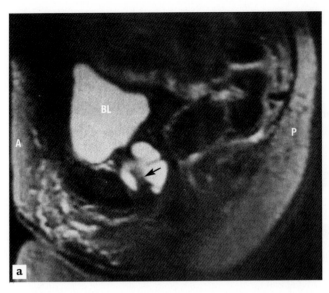
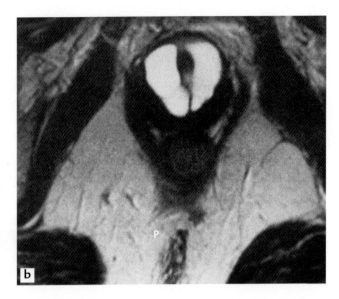

Figure 57.9. *T2-weighted magnetic resonance imaging illustrates a multiloculated diverticulum (arrow) posterolateral to the urethra: (a) sagittal view; (b) axial view. (BL, bladder; A, anterior; P, posterior.) (Reproduced from ref. 59 with permission.)*

gauze,[66] or silicone or blood products[67] has been used to faciliate identification of the defect. Repair has been performed endoscopically and transvaginally by incision of the urethral floor with layered reconstruction,[33] marsupialization,[68,69] packing of the UD with various materials to obliterate the cavity,[70,71] and transvaginal flap creation with layered closure.[44,64,72,73]

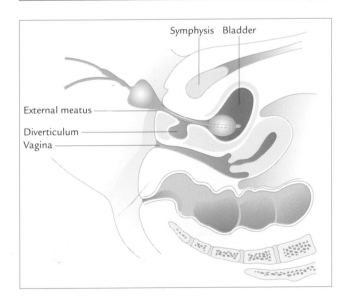

Figure 57.10. *Placement of Tratner/Davis double-balloon catheter for positive-pressure retrograde urethrography.*

Observation

Surgical resection and reconstruction is frequently necessary in the treatment of UD. However, observation is an option in the asymptomatic or very small UD. Marshall,[74] reported that UD in young girls may regress spontaneously; therefore, in this rare situation, observation may be a reasonable option.

Endoscopic therapy

Endoscopic treatment should be utilized only for distal UD to avoid injury to the proximally located continence mechanism. Transurethral saucerization with incision of the urethral floor[75,76] or of the anterior urethra overlying the UD,[77] with a Collins' knife through a paediatric resectoscope can be performed with minimal risk of complication. The major risk is incontinence and can be avoided by limiting this technique to distal UD.[5] This risk also applies to transvaginal marsupialization (Fig. 57.11), an outpatient procedure often referred to as the Spence procedure.[7] One blade of the scissors is placed in the vagina, the other in the urethra to marsupialize the cavity.

Excision with vaginal flap technique

We prefer the transvaginal flap technique for all midurethral or proximal UDs. This technique allows

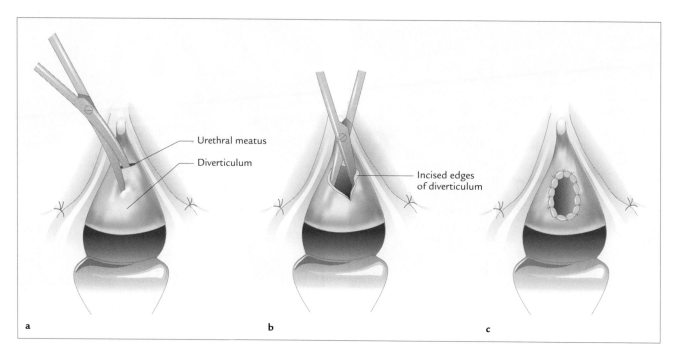

Figure 57.11. *The Spence technique for marsupialization of a urethral diverticulum (UD): (a) one blade of the scissors is inserted into the UD and the other into the vagina; (b) the full thickness of the diverticular septum is incised; (c) a running locking absorbable suture ensures haemostasis.*

complete resection of the UD with a three-layer closure and no overlapping suture lines. Simultaneous needle bladder-neck suspension (BNS) can easily be performed when deemed necessary (in cases of SUI or bladder-neck/proximal-urethral hypermobility).

Preoperative preparation

Preoperatively, the risks of diverticulectomy – including bleeding, infection, recurrence, urethrovaginal fistula formation and incontinence – are explained to the patient in detail. Patients may benefit from a short course of oral antibiotics, and all receive perioperative intravenous antibiotics. Vaginal douching and lower abdominal scrubbing are performed the night before and on the morning of surgery.

Surgical technique

The patient is placed in the lithotomy position, and a suprapubic tube (SPT) is placed with a modified Lowsley tractor. A 14F urethral Foley catheter is passed and a weighted vaginal speculum and a Scott ring retractor facilitate exposure. The anterior vaginal wall (Fig. 57.12) is infiltrated with saline to facilitate dissection in the proper plane. A U-shaped incision is made with the apex located distal to the UD (Fig. 57.13).

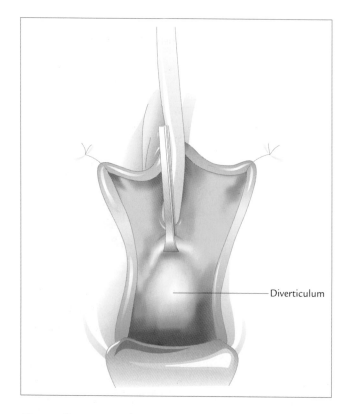

Figure 57.12. *Anterior vaginal wall and urethral diverticulum. (Reproduced from ref. 44 with permission.)*

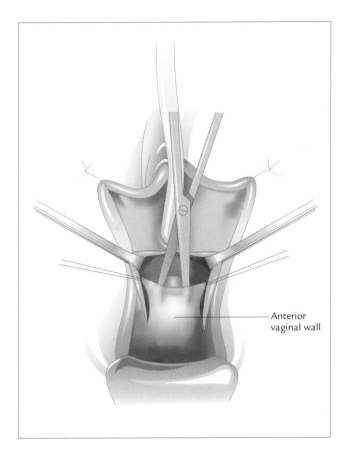

Figure 57.13. *An inverted U-incision is made in the anterior vaginal wall, and the vaginal wall is dissected off the underlying periurethral fascia.*

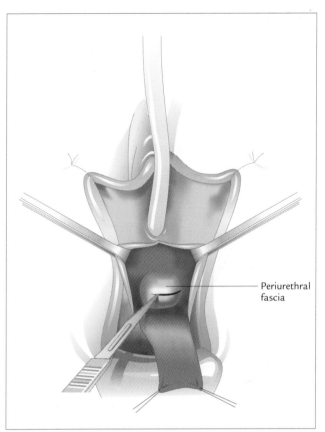

Figure 57.14. *The periurethral fascia is incised transversely.*

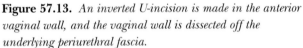

If concomitant BNS is performed, the vaginal dissection is extended laterally beneath the vaginal wall to the pubic bone on each side. The suspension sutures should be placed prior to manipulation or decompression of the UD, to avoid postoperative infection. The endopelvic fascia is perforated with the bladder completely emptied and the retropubic space is developed. Helical 1/0 Prolene sutures are placed in the vaginal wall and directed with a Pereyra needle into the suprapubic incision. Cystoscopy is performed to ensure that no suture has passed into the bladder or urethra. *Care must be taken to avoid entry into the UD during suture placement. If the UD is large and/or proximally located, it may be difficult to avoid; in this situation, the BNS should be postponed.* The use of bone anchors for the BNS has been described;[72] however, we do not advocate this when diverticulectomy is being performed, in view of the risk of infection. Additionally, Swierzewski and McGuire[78] have recommended a pubovaginal sling concomitant with diverticulectomy, but we avoid the use of a sling procedure because of concerns of urethral erosion of the sling and breakdown of the reconstruction site.

The diverticulectomy is continued with creation of a vaginal flap with sharp dissection directly on the shiny white layer of the vaginal wall. *Dissection in the wrong plane can result in significant bleeding or inadvertent entry into the periurethral fascia or the UD, thereby rendering the remainder of the dissection very difficult.* Mobilization of the vaginal flap towards the bladder neck, followed by a transverse incision in the periurethral fascia (Fig. 57.14) exposes the UD, which lies directly beneath this layer. The periurethral fascia is then sharply dissected off the UD (Fig. 57.15), which is then exposed circumferentially until the diverticular neck is encountered (Fig. 57.16). *Difficulty in identification of the urethral communication site can result in incomplete resection of the UD and subsequent recurrence. Identification can be facilitated by insertion of a paediatric sound into the UD.*

731

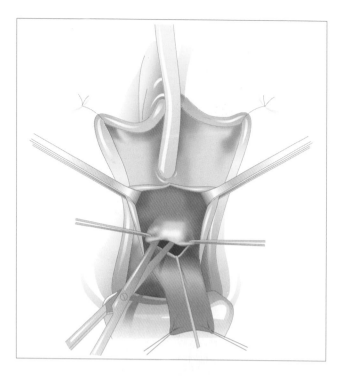

Figure 57.15. *The periurethral tissue is dissected from the diverticulum.*

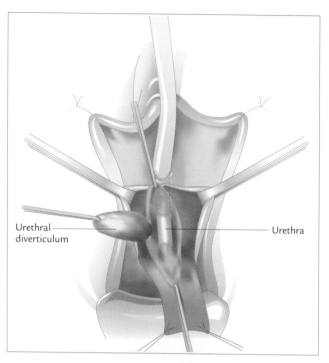

Figure 57.17. *The diverticulum is amputated at its communication site, thereby exposing the urethral Foley catheter and leaving a urethral defect.*

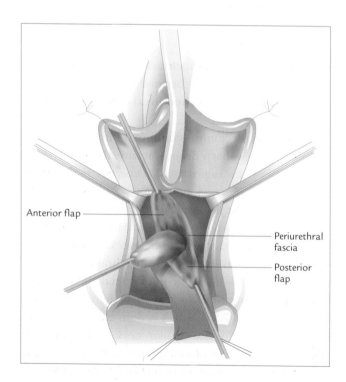

Figure 57.16. *The diverticulum is isolated and carefully dissected until the communication is identified.*

Complete excision of both the UD and its neck creates a significant urethral defect (Fig. 57.17). *Incomplete resection of the diverticulum can lead to recurrence. However, where the UD is large, extensive dissection beneath the trigone can endanger the ureters and bladder base, sometimes necessitating leaving the most proximal portion of the UD behind. In these cases, cautery to the inner epithelial surface will obliterate the cavity.* The urethral defect is closed vertically over a 14F catheter without tension using a full-thickness 4/0 Vicryl stitch, incorporating both urethral mucosa and the urethral wall (Fig. 57.18). *In cases in which there is not enough tissue for closure of a second layer, or when the vaginal tissue is tenuous or fibrotic (such as secondary to previous surgery or radiation), a well-vascularized 8–12 cm Martius fat-pad graft may be placed between the vagina and urethra.* The periurethral fascia is closed transversely with running 3/0 Vicryl (Fig. 57.19). Dead space should be obliterated beneath this layer. If a Martius flap is employed, it is placed at this point, between the urethra and vagina. The third and final layer is the vaginal wall, which is closed with 2/0 absorbable suture. *The three layers of closure include the urethral wall vertically, the periurethral fascia transversely, and the vaginal U-incision. There are no overlapping suture lines (Fig. 57.20).* Antibiotic-soaked vaginal packing is

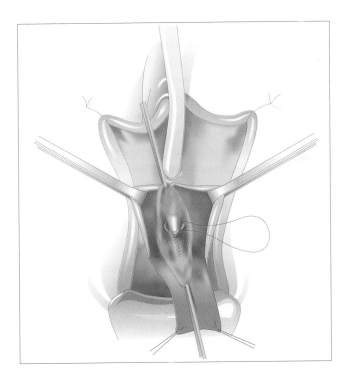

Figure 57.18. *The urethra is reapproximated longitudinally with 4/0 absorbable suture.*

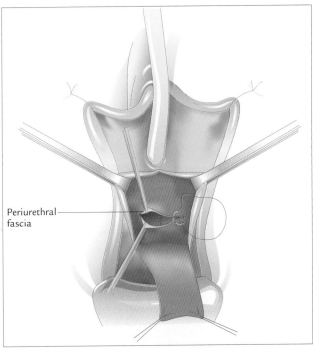

Periurethral fascia

Figure 57.19. *The periurethral tissue is closed transversely with 3/0 absorbable suture.*

inserted, and the SPT and Foley catheter are placed to gravity drainage.

Postoperative management

The vaginal packing is removed on postoperative day 1. All patients receive 24 hours of intravenous antibiotics followed by oral antibiotics until the catheters are removed. Anticholinergics are given to relieve bladder spasms but are discontinued 24 hours prior to the VCUG, which is performed 7–10 days postoperatively. At the time of this first VCUG, approximately 50% of patients have some extravasation from the urethral reconstruction site.[5] When extravasation is evident, the SPT is left in place, and the urethral catheter is not reinserted. A follow-up VCUG is obtained in a week's time. When there is no extravasation, the SPT is clamped and a post-void residual (PVR) is checked. If it is 100 ml or less, the SPT is removed; if the PVR exceeds 100 ml, the SPT is left in place until this volume decreases.

RESULTS AND COMPLICATIONS

Potential complications following a urethral diverticulectomy include incontinence, UD recurrence, ure-

throvaginal fistula, irritative symptoms, urethral stricture, and general postoperative complications (Table 57.6).[79]

Ganabathi *et al.*[9] evaluated 63 women who had been treated for UD between 1982 and 1992: 56 were treated operatively and seven were observed. The specific treatment modalities employed are shown in Table 57.7. Patients were followed-up for a mean of 70 months, with a range of 10–124 months. Table 57.8 reports the complications encountered. The two recurrences of the UD occurred distal to the initial repair site.

Overall continence status, shown in Table 57.9, indicates that the majority of patients were totally continent. A greater percentage of the patients who underwent diverticulectomy alone were reported as continent, than were those who underwent diverticulectomy with concomitant BNS (Table 57.10). It was reported that incontinence was more frequently secondary to SUI than to detrusor instability, despite the presumed increase in bladder-neck support.

Incontinence may be secondary to persistent SUI that was present preoperatively. This situation can be avoided by a comprehensive preoperative evaluation so that it can be addressed at the time of diverticulectomy.[9,80,81] Incontinence can also be a result of

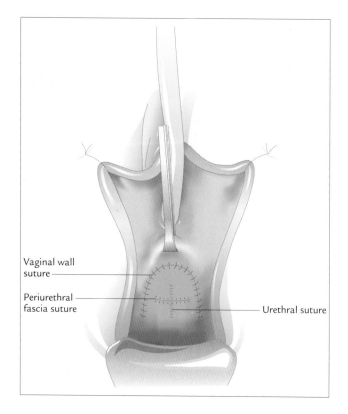

Vaginal wall
suture

Periurethral
fascia suture

Urethral suture

Figure 57.20. *The vaginal wall flap is closed, resulting in a three-layer closure with no overlapping suture lines.*

urethrovaginal fistula, recurrent diverticulum with paradoxical loss of urine with stress, infection, persistent detrusor instability or new-onset SUI. The first two conditions may require surgical intervention. New-onset SUI may be a result of the urethral dissection, which may compromise urethral support, or secondary to dissection beneath the proximal urethra and bladder neck, which is often necessary when removing a large UD. Detrusor instability can be treated successfully in many cases with anticholinergic therapy or the addition of a tricyclic antidepressant such as imipramine; this not

Table 57.6. *Complications of urethral diverticulectomy*

Complication	Possible causes
Incontinence	Failure to identify SUI preoperatively New onset SUI DI Recurrent diverticulum leading to 'paradoxical incontinence' Urethrovaginal fistula
Recurrent diverticulum	Failure to identify multiple diverticula preoperatively Incomplete excision Faulty closure
Urethrovaginal fistula	Closure under tension Tenuous, unhealthy tissue Failure to close in layers Overlapping suture lines
Irritative symptoms	Urinary tract infection Bladder dysfunction (DI) Outlet obstruction
Urethral stricture	Extensive urethral wall excision Closure under tension

SUI, stress urinary incontinence; DI, detrusor instability.

Table 57.7. *Treatment modalities for 63 patients*

Operative treatment	56 (88.9%)
Diverticulectomy alone	29 (51.8%)
Diverticulectomy +BNS	27 (48.2%)
Martius fat-pad graft	7 (11.1%)
No operative treatment	7* (11.1%)

*In three cases surgery was refused; there were four cases of small asymptomatic diverticula not requiring surgery.
BNS, bladder-neck suspension.
(Reproduced, with modifications, from ref. 9 with permission.)

Table 57.8. *Complications*

Recurrence (distal repair site)	2
Suprapubic tenderness*	1
Early UTI (none recurrent)	6
Urethrovaginal fistula†	1
Wound infection/urethral stricture	0

UTI, urinary tract infection.
* Patient had concomitant bladder-neck suspension.
† Required subsequent surgical repair

Table 57.9. *Overall continence of 56 patients with mean follow-up of 70 months*

Incontinence	n (%)
Nil or moderate (dry or 0 pads/day)	45 (80.4)
Moderate (1–2 minipads/day)	10 (17.9)
Severe (several pads/day)	1 (1.8)

Table 57.10. *Continence status of 56 patients with mean follow-up of 70 months*

	Diverticulectomy alone (n=29)	Diverticulectomy and BNS (n=27)
Continent	25 (86.2%)	20 (74%)
Incontinent	4 (13.8%)	7 (26%)
DI	1 (3.4%)	1 (3.7%)
SUI	3 (10.3%)	6 (22.2%)

DI, detrusor instability; SUI, stress urinary incontinence; BNS, bladder-neck support. (Reproduced, with modifications, from ref. 9 with permission.)

only increases bladder-outlet tone but also decreases detrusor contractility.

Recurrent UD is often a result of failure to identify multiple UD preoperatively, secondary to lack of either suspicion or proper high-quality studies.[9,82] Incomplete excision of the diverticular neck, as well as faulty closure of the urethral defect, are also possible causes. This problem can be managed with interposition of a Martius fat-pad graft between the vagina and urethra.[9] For small, distal recurrences, endoscopic saucerization or Spence marsupialization may suffice;[5] however, caution must be exercised not to injur the proximally located continence mechanism. Urethrovaginal fistula (UVF) formation, another potential complication, is managed in much the same manner and may be prevented by intra-operative Martius flap if tissues appear tenuous or under tension. UVF is discussed in more detail in the next section.

Finally, urethral stricture may result from extensive excision of the urethral wall at the time of diverticulectomy and can be prevented by a tension-free urethral closure over a 14F catheter. If this is not possible, reconstruction using vaginal wall can be contemplated, again with consideration of a Martius labial fat-pad graft.

Urethrovaginal Fistula

INTRODUCTION

UVF is a rare condition. Fistulae range from small communications between the urethra and the vagina to total loss of the urethra and bladder neck.[5,82–84] A distal fistula may present with vaginal voiding or a splayed urinary stream. Midurethral or proximal fistulae can present with varying degrees of continence, depending upon fistula location and bladder-neck competence.[85,86] Urethral fistulae are most commonly caused by complications of previous surgery, such as anterior colporrhaphy or urethral diverticulectomy (see previous section). Other causes include radiation therapy and birth trauma, although this is rare with modern obstetric techniques. Obstructed labour remains the most common cause of urethral injury in developing countries.[16]

DIAGNOSIS

The differential diagnosis of UVF includes SUI, intrinsic sphincter deficiency (ISD), or vaginal voiding due to other conditions.

A careful history and physical examination can help to differentiate between the above conditions. A history may reveal previous vaginal or pelvic surgery or symptoms of stress versus urge incontinence. Physical examination is important to assess urethral loss, location and size of the fistula, urethral and bladder-neck mobility, and quality of vaginal tissue, including scarring and atrophy.

Studies which may aid in the diagnosis include cystourethroscopy, IVP to evaluate the upper tracts, renal ultrasonography, VCUG and urodynamic studies. Cystoscopy is performed with a 20F female urethroscope with a 0-degree lens. It is essential to examine the urethra, bladder neck, trigone, and quality of the tissue. A concomitant vesicovaginal fistula must be excluded. If identification of the UVF is difficult, simultaneous vaginal examination with a speculum may identify fluid spraying into the vagina through the communication.

Upper tract evaluation is essential when the trigone is involved and may be accomplished with IVP or renal ultrasonography. A standing fluoroscopic VCUG is often helpful in identification of the urethral defect and in excluding a vesicovaginal fistula. The VCUG also aids in assessment of urethral hypermobility and/or leakage of urine across the bladder neck during stress. Finally, urodynamic studies may be of benefit in evaluation of bladder function and sphincter integrity when the UVF is in the distal third of the vagina.

TREATMENT

The goal of treatment of urethral fistulae is to create a competent neourethra of adequate length to permit unobstructed passage of urine and urinary continence.[83] Additionally, urethrovaginal repair must be tension free. Distal fistulae may be managed with an extended meatotomy.[5] The postoperative incontinence rate may be as high as 50% if SUI is not considered at the time of fistula repair.[5] Some authors have suggested concomitant sling at the time of fistula repair.[83] We are concerned about the risks of erosion of the sling at the time of mid- or proximal UVF repair; we therefore avoid performing a sling simultaneously with UVF repair.

Operative technique

Preoperative preparation is similar to that for urethral diverticulectomy (see previous section). Oestrogens are administered preoperatively, if indicated, to treat atrophic vaginitis. Urine culture is performed to ensure that the urine is sterile preoperatively. If necessary, a short course of oral antibiotics is given. All patients receive perioperative intravenous ampicillin and gentamycin, unless contraindicated. Additionally, all patients perform a vaginal betadine douche the night before and the morning of surgery.

Essentially all types of urethral and bladder-neck defects can be approached from the transvaginal approach, often in conjunction with a Martius fat-pad graft.[85,87] This includes simple fistula repair and vaginal flap total urethral reconstruction.

Our preferred technique for transvaginal fistula closure and vaginal flap urethral reconstruction requires placement of the patient in the lithotomy position (Fig. 57.21). A 20–24F SPT is placed over a modified Lowsley tractor and a 14F urethral catheter is inserted. Self-catheterization of the neourethra must be avoided; hence, the necessity of the SPT. The SPT also serves as a 'safety valve' if the urethral catheter becomes obstructed. The vaginal wall is infiltrated with saline to develop the proper plane, and an inverted U-incision is made. The apex of the incision is located just proximal to the fistula for fistulectomy and at the meatus for total urethral reconstruction. Dissection in the avascular plane exposes the shiny white surface of the interior vaginal wall. Excessive bleeding and bladder perforation are risks if dissection is too deep.

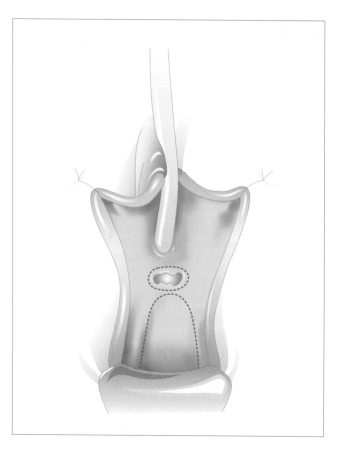

Figure 57.21. *An inverted U-incision is made in the vaginal wall with the apex just proximal to the fistula.*

When concomitant BNS is necessary, lateral dissection and perforation of the endopelvic fascia is performed. The suspension sutures in the anterior vaginal wall and periurethral tissue are placed but not tied. We do not recommend simultaneous sling procedures, owing to the risk of erosion through the reconstructed urethra.

The fistula is circumscribed but not excised (Fig. 57.22). Scarred tissue margins are freed to allow a tension-free closure of the tract. A portion of the vaginal wall just distal to the fistula is then mobilized to create a flap. The fistula is closed with running locking absorbable suture (Fig. 57.23). For total reconstruction of the urethra, two vaginal wall incisions are made parallel to and on either side of the urethra to create medially based flaps (Fig. 57.24). The flaps are tubularized around a 14F urethral catheter and approximated at the midline with 4/0 absorbable sutures (Fig. 57.25).

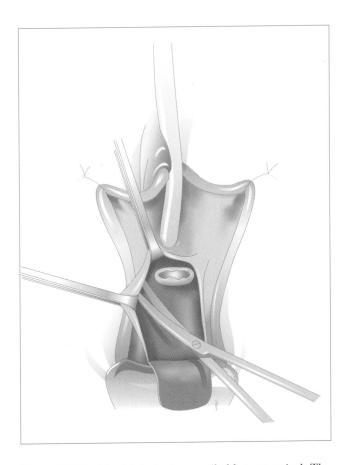

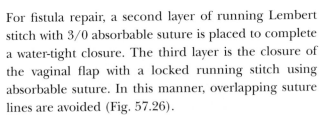

Figure 57.22. *The fistula is circumscribed but not excised. The avascular plane beneath the lateral vaginal wall is developed.*

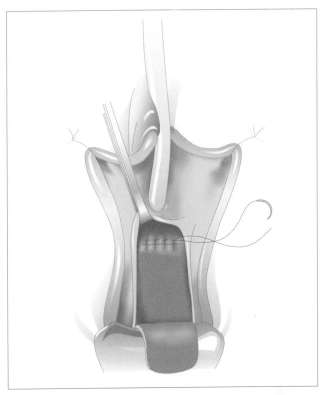

Figure 57.23. *The fistula is closed with absorbable suture.*

For fistula repair, a second layer of running Lembert stitch with 3/0 absorbable suture is placed to complete a water-tight closure. The third layer is the closure of the vaginal flap with a locked running stitch using absorbable suture. In this manner, overlapping suture lines are avoided (Fig. 57.26).

If the tissues are tenuous or inadequate, a Martius fat-pad graft may be interposed between the urethra and the vagina. The labium majus is incised to expose the underlying fat pad. The flap is mobilized, preserving the pudendal vessels, located posteriorly (Fig. 57.27). The fat pad is passed through a subcutaneous tunnel from the labia to the vagina and secured over the fistula repair site with absorbable sutures (Fig. 57.28). A ¼-inch Penrose drain is placed deep into the labial wound, and the labial incision is closed in layers. The vaginal flap (described above) is closed over the Martius flap (Fig. 57.29).

When a Martius fat-pad graft is not feasible a meatal-based vaginal flap can be rotated distally (Fig. 57.30)[83] or a neourethra can be created from a cutaneous portion of the gracilis muscle or a perineal artery-based myocutaneous flap.[83] Finally, in selected cases, one may resort to closure of the bladder neck with creation of a catheterizable stoma or placement of a suprapubic catheter.[88]

The urethral Foley catheter and SPT are placed to gravity drainage, and an antibiotic-soaked vaginal pack is placed. Patients receive perioperative intravenous antibiotics, which are converted to oral medication on postoperative day 1. Anticholinergics are administered to prevent bladder spasm. These must be discontinued at least 24 hours prior to the VCUG, which is performed between postoperative days 7 and 10. If extravasation is noted, the SPT is left to gravity and the urethral catheter is not replaced. The VCUG is repeated after 1–2 weeks and the SPT is removed when there is no extravasation and PVRs are minimal (<100 ml).

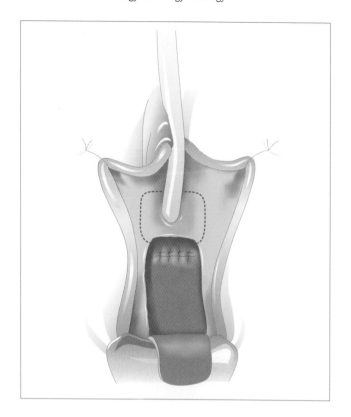

Figure 57.24. *Two longitudinal incisions are made to create medially based flaps.*

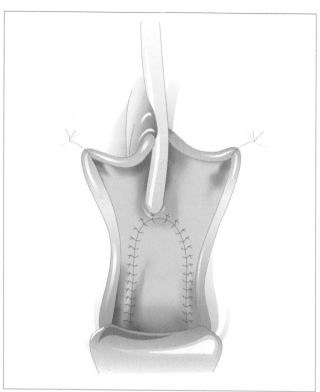

Figure 57.26. *The vaginal flap is closed with a running, locking absorbable suture.*

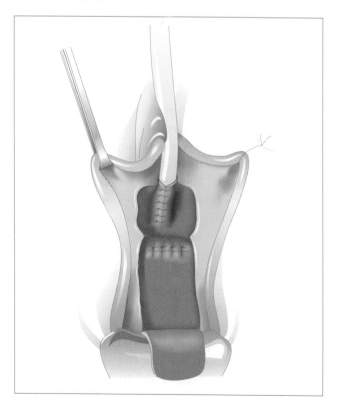

Figure 57.25. *The flaps are rolled over a 14F urethral catheter.*

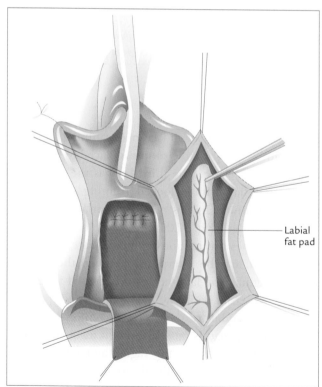

Labial fat pad

Figure 57.27. *The labium majus is incised, and the Martius fat-pad graft is mobilized with care to preserve the posteriorly located pudendal vessels.*

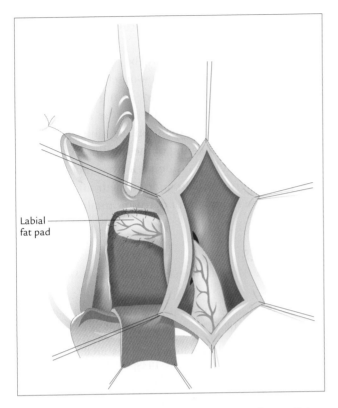

Figure 57.28. *The labial fat pad is passed through a medial tunnel and secured over the fistula repair site.*

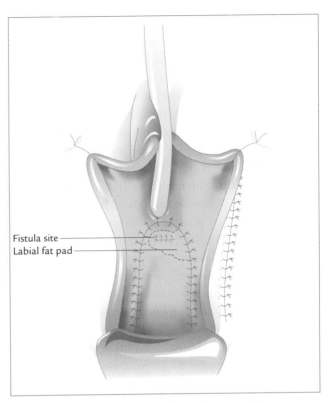

Figure 57.29. *The vaginal wall flap is advanced over the fat-pad graft, resulting in closure with no overlapping suture lines.*

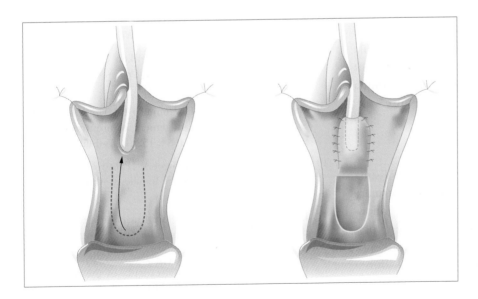

Figure 57.30. *A meatus-based vaginal flap is rotated distally.*

RESULTS

Few series in the literature report the results of UVF repair. Most series include ten or fewer patients, and continence rates range from 30 to 80%, including patients who underwent a single operation or multiple repairs.

Blaivas[83] reported on his experience with 24 women with bladder-neck and urethral defects. The patients ranged from 36 to 80 years of age and were followed-up for 9 months to 7 years: 23 patients underwent a concomitant anti-incontinence procedure, including pubovaginal sling in 20, needle suspension in three and Kelly plication in one. A pedicle graft was performed in all patients, with 18 unilateral Martius fat-pad grafts, one bilateral Martius fat-pad graft and one gracilis flap. Nineteen (79%) patients were continent after one operation. Goodwin and Scardino[89] similarly reported a 70% success rate following one operation in 24 patients treated for vesicovaginal or UVF. Their success rate was 92% following a second operation. Keetel *et al.*[90] reviewed their results in 24 patients with UVF and reported an overall success rate of 87.5%. Lee[86] claimed a 92% correction rate of UVF in 50 patients after one surgery and 100% success rate with two operations. Each of the series favoured the vaginal approach over the abdominal approach: the vaginal approach generally involves a lower blood loss, shorter hospital stay and shorter operating time.[89,90]

In Blaivas' series, two patients developed necrosis of the vaginal flaps requiring subsequent surgery. One patient was found, after her urethral reconstruction, to have a previously undiagnosed vesicovaginal fistula. She was reportedly continent following vesicovaginal fistula repair. Finally, two of the three patients who underwent bladder-neck needle suspension developed ISD, which was corrected with a pubovaginal sling procedure.

COMPLICATIONS

Postoperative complications following urethral fistula repair may include urinary retention, and urinary incontinence. High PVRs are not uncommon following urethral reconstruction, especially when performed with a simultaneous anti-incontinence procedure. Urinary retention usually resolves within a few weeks and can be managed by keeping the SPT in place until the PVRs reduce to 100 ml or less. If retention persists, the patient may be instructed on how to perform clean intermittent catheterization, which

should not be initiated until the urethra has healed completely.

Urinary incontinence may be secondary to undetected preoperative SUI, new-onset SUI if extensive dissection has been performed, or urge incontinence due to detrusor instability. SUI may be managed with concomitant needle suspension or sling procedure following adequate healing of the urethra. Periurethral collagen may also be considered if hypermobility is not a major concern. Anticholinergic medications may be helpful in the treatment of detrusor instability.

REFERENCES

1. Novak R. Editorial comment. *Obstet Gynecol Surv* 1953; 8: 423

2. Hey W. *Practical Observations in Surgery*, Philadelphia: J. Humphries, 1805

3. Hunner GL. Calculus formation in a urethral diverticulum in women. *Urol Cut Rev* 1938; 42: 336

4. Davis HJ, Cian LG. Positive pressure urethrography: a new diagnostic method. *J Urol* 1956: 75: 753–757

5. Leach GE, Trockman BA. In: Walsh PC, Retik AB, Vaughan ED, Wein AJ (eds) *Campbell's Urology*, 7th edn. Philadelphia: Saunders, 1997; 1141–1151

6. Wittich AC. Excision of urethral diverticulum calculi in a pregnant patient on an outpatient basis. *J Am Osteopath Assoc* 1997; 97: 461–462

7. Robertson JR. Urethral diverticula. In: Ostergard DR (ed) *Gynecologic Urology and Urodynamics: Theory and Practice*, 2nd edn. Baltimore: Williams and Wilkins, 1985; 329–338

8. Levinson ED, Spackman TJ, Henken EM. Diagnosis of urethral diverticula in females. *Urol Radiol* 1979–80; 1: 165–167

9. Ganabathi K, Leach GE, Zimmern PE, Dmochowski RR. Experience with the management of urethral diverticulum in 63 women. *J Urol* 1994; 152: 1445–1452

10. Hesserdorfer E, Kuhn R, Sigel A. [Pathogenetic synopsis of diverticular disease of the female urethra] (abstract). *Urologe* 1988; 27: 343–347

11. Lee RA. Diverticulum of the urethra: clinical presentation, diagnosis, and management. *Clin Obstet Gynecol* 1984; 27: 490–498

12. Davis BL, Robinson DG. Diverticula of the female urethra: assay of 120 cases. *J Urol* 1970; 104: 850–853

13. Aldridge CW, Beaton JH, Nanzig RP. A review of office urethroscopy and cystometry. *Am J Obstet Gynecol* 1978; 131: 432–437

14. Huffman AB. The detailed anatomy of the paraurethral ducts in the adult human female. *Am J Obstet Gynecol* 1948; 55: 86

15. Routh A. Urethral diverticula. *Br J Urol* 1890; 1: 361

16. McNally A. Diverticula of the female urethra. *Am J Surg* 1935; 28: 177

17. Raz S, Little NA, Juma S. Female urology. In: Walsh, PC, Retick AB, Stamey TA, Vaughan ED (eds) *Campbell's Urology*, 6th edn. Philadelphia: Saunders, 1992; 2782–2788

18. Niemic TR, Mercer LJ, Stephens JK *et al.* Unusual urethral diverticulum lined with colonic epithelium with paneth cell metaplasia. *Am J Obstet Gynecol* 1989; 260: 186–188

19. Silk MR, Lebowitz JM. Anterior urethral diverticulum. *J Urol* 1969; 101: 66–67

20. Peters WH, Vaughan ED. Urethral diverticulum in the female. *Obstet Gynecol* 1976; 47: 549–552

21. Aragona F, Mangano M, Artibani W, Passerini GG. Stone formation in a female urethral diverticulum. Review of the literature. *Int Urol Nephrol* 1989; 21: 621–625

22. Pavlica P, Viglietta F, Losinno F *et al.* [Diverticula of the female urethra. A radiological and ultrasound study] (abstract). *Radiol Med* 1988; 75: 521–527

23. Ginsberg S, Geneandry R. Suburethral diverticulum: classification and therapeutic considerations. *Obstet Gynecol* 1983; 61: 685–688

24. Nielsen VM, Nielsen KK, Vedel P. Spontaneous rupture of a diverticulum of the female urethra presenting with a fistula to the vagina. *Acta Obstet Gynecol Scand* 1987; 66: 87–88

25. Evans KJ, McCarthy MP, Sands JP. Adenocarcinoma of a female urethral diverticulum case report and review of the literature. *J Urol* 1981; 126: 124–126

26. Okubo Y, Fukui I, Sakano Y *et al.* [Mesonephric adenocarcinoma arising in the female urethral diverticulum (abstract)]. *Nippon Hinyokika Gakkai Zasshi* 1996; 87: 1138–1141

27. Seballos RM, Rich RR. Clear cell adenocarcinoma arising from a urethral diverticulum. *J Urol* 1995; 153: 1914–1915

28. Srinivas V, Dow D. Transitional cell carcinoma in a urethral diverticulum with a calculus. *J Urol* 1983; 129: 372–373

29. Klutke CG, Akdmna EI, Brown JJ. Nephrogenic adenoma arising from a urethral diverticulum: magnetic resonance features. *Urology* 1995; 45: 323–325

30. Materne R, Dardenne AN, Opsomer RJ *et al.* [Apropos of a case of nephrogenic adenoma in a urethral diverticulum in a woman] (abstract). *Acta Urol Belg* 1995; 63: 13–18

31. Medeiros LJ, Young RH. Nephrogenic adenoma arising in urethral diverticula. A report of five cases. *Arch Pathol Lab Med* 1989; 113: 125–128

32. Paik SS, Lee JD. Nephrogenic adenoma arising in an urethral diverticulum. *Br J Urol* 1997; 80: 150

33. Parks J. Section of the urethral wall for correction of urethrovaginal fistula and urethral diverticula. *Am J Obstet Gynecol* 1965; 93: 683–692

34. Summit RL, Murrmann SG, Flax SD. Nephrogenic adenoma in a urethral diverticulum: a case report. *J Reprod Med* 1994; 39: 473–476

35. Poore RE, McCullough DL. Urethral carcinoma. In: Gillenwater JY, Grayhack JT, Howards SS, Duckett JW (eds) *Adult and Pediatric Urology*, 3rd edn. Salem, MA: Mosby, 1996; 1846–1847

36. Gonzalez MO, Harrison ML, Boileau MA. Carcinoma in diverticulum of female urethra. *Urology* 1985; 26: 328–332

37. Jimenez de Leon J, Luz Picazo M, Mora MM *et al.* [Intradiverticular adenocarcinoma of the urethra in women] (abstract). *Arch Exp Urol* 1989; 42: L931–935

38. Jensen LM, Aabech J, Lundvall F, Iversen HG. Female urethral diverticulum. Clinical aspects and a presentation of 15 cases. *Acta Obstet Gynecol Scand* 1996; 75: 748–752

39. Dmochowski RR, Ganabathi K, Zimmern PE, Leach GE. Benign female periurethral masses. *J Urol* 1994; 152: 1943–1951

40. Curry NS. Ectopic ureteral orifice masquedaring as a urethral diverticulum. *Am J Roentgenol* 1983; 141: 1325–1326

41. Dias P, Hillard P, Rauh J. Skene's gland abscess with suburethral diverticulum in an adolescent. *J Adolesc Health Care* 1987; 8: 372–375

42. Konami T, Wakabayashi Y, Takeuchi J, Tomoyoshi T. Female wide urethra masquerading as a urethral diverticulum in association with ectopic ureterocele. *Hinyokika Kiyo* 1988; 34: 1437–1441

43. Leach GE, Sirls LT, Ganabathi K *et al.* LNSC3: a proposed classification system for female urethral diverticula. *Neurourol Urodyn* 1993; 12: 523–531

44. Leach GE, Ganabathi K. Urethral diverticulectomy. *Atlas Urol Clin North Am* 1994; 2: 73–85

45. Leach GE, Bavenden TG. Female urethral diverticula. *Urology* 1987; 30: 407–415

46. Reid RE, Gill B, Laor E *et al.* Role of urodynamics in management of urethral diverticulum in females. *Urology* 1986; 28: 342–346

47. Keefe B, Warshauer DM, Tucker MS, Mittelstaedt CA. Diverticula of the female urethra: diagnosis by endovaginal and transperineal sonography. *Am J Roentgenol* 1991; 156: 1195–1197

48. Vargas-Serrano B, Cortina-Moreno B, Rodriguez-Romero R, Ferreiro-Arguees I. Transrectal ultrasonography in the

diagnosis of urethral diverticula in women. *J Clin Ultrasound*, 1997; 25: 21–28

49. Iula G, Stefano ML, Castaldi L, del Vecchio E. Post-irradiation female urethral diverticula: diagnosis by voiding endovaginal sonography. *J Clin Ultrasound* 1995; 23: 63–65

50. Mouritsen L, Bernstein I. Vaginal ultrasonography: a diagnostic tool for urethral diverticulum. *Acta Obstet Gynecol Scand* 1996; 75: 188–190

51. Martensson O, Duchek M. Translabial ultrasonography with pulsed colour Doppler in the diagnosis of female urethral diverticulum. *Scand J Urol Nephrol* 1994; 28: 101–104

52. Chancellor MB, Liu JB, Rivas DA *et al.* Intraoperative endo-luminal ultrasound evaluation of urethral diverticula. *J Urol* 1995; 153: 72–75

53. Lopez Rasines G, Rico Guttierez M, Abascal Abascal F, Calbia de Diego A. Female urethral diverticula: value of transrectal ultrasound. *J Clin Ultrasound* 1996; 24: 90–92

54. Blacklock ARE, Shaw RE, Geddes JR. Late presentation of ectopic ureter. *Br J Urol* 1982; 54: 106–110

55. Boyd SD, Raz S. Ectopic ureter presenting in midline urethral diverticulum. *Urology* 1993; 41: 571–574

56. Goldfarb S, Mieza M, Leiter E. Postvoid film of intravenous pyelogram in diagnosis of urethral diverticulum. *Urology* 1981; 17: 390–392

57. Debaere C, Rigauts H, Steyaert L *et al.* MR imaging of a diverticulum in a female urethra. *J Belge Radiol* 1995; 78: 345–346

58. Hricak H, Secaf E, Buckley DW *et al.* Female urethra: MR imaging. *Radiology* 1991; 178: 527

59. Neitlich JD, Foster HE, Glickman MG, Smith RC. Detection of urethral diverticula in women: comparison of a high resolution fast spin echo technique with double balloon urethrography. *J Urol* 1998; 159: 408–410

60. Siegelman ES, Banner MP, Ramchandani P, Schneall MD. Multicoil MR imaging of symptomatic female urethral and periurethral disease. *Radiographics* 1997; 17: 349–365

61. Kim B, Hricak H, Tanagho EA. Diagnosis of urethral diverticula in women: value of MR imaging. *Am J Roentgenol* 1993; 161: 809

62. Greenberg M, Stone D, Cochran ST *et al.* Female urethral diverticula: double-balloon catheter study. *Am J Roentgenol* 1981; 136: 259–264

63. Young HH. Treatment of urethral diverticulum. *South Am J* 1938; 31: 1043–1047

64. Moore TD. Diverticulum of the female urethra. An improved technique of surgical excision. *J Urol* 1952; 68: 611–616

65. Wear JB. Urethral diverticulectomy in females. *Urol Times* 1976; 4: 2–3

66. Hyams JA, Hyams MN. New operative procedures for treatment of diverticulum of female urethra. *Urol Cutan Rev* 1939; 43: 573

67. Feldstein MS. Cryoprecipititate coagulum as an adjunct to surgery for diverticula of the female urethra. *J Urol* 1981; 126: 698–699

68. Downs RA. Urethral diverticula in females: alternative surgical treatment. *Urology* 1987: 2: 201–203

69. Spence HM, Duckett JW. Diverticulum of the female urethra: clinical aspects and presentation of a simple operative technique for cure. *J Urol* 1970; 14: 432–437

70. Ellik M. Diverticulum of the female urethra: a new method of ablation. *J Urol* 1957; 77: 234

71. Mizrahi S, Bitterman W. Transvaginal, periurethral injection of polytetrafluoroethylene (polytef) in the treatment of urethral diverticula. *Br J Urol* 1988; 62: 280

72. Fall M. Vaginal wall bipedicled flap and other tehniques in complicated urethral diverticulum and urethrovaginal fistula. *J Am Coll Surg* 1995; 180: 150–156

73. Leach GE, Schmidbauer CP, Hadley HR *et al.* Surgical treatment of female urethral diverticulum. *Semin Urol* 1986; 4: 33–42

74. Marshall S. Urethral diverticula in young girls. *Urology* 1981; 17: 243–245

75. Lapides J. Transurethral treatment of urethral diverticula in women. *J Urol* 1979: 121: 736–738

76. Vergunst H, Blom JH, De Spiegeleer AH, Miranda SI. Management of female urethral diverticula by transurethral incision. *Br J Urol* 1996; 77: 745–746

77. Spencer WF, Streem SB. Diverticula of the female urethra roof managed endoscopically. *J Urol* 1987; 138: 157–158

78. Swierzewski SJ, McGuire EJ. Pubovaginal sling for treatment of female stress urinary incontinence complicated by urethral diverticulum. *J Urol* 1993; 149: 1012–1014

79. Coddington CC, Knab DR. Urethral diverticulum: a review. *Obstet Gynecol Surv* 1983; 38: 357–364

80. Bass JS, Leach GE. Surgical treatment of concomitant urethral diverticulum and stress urinary incontincence. *Urol Clin North Am* 1991; 18: 365–373

81. Ganabathi K, Sirls L, Zimmern PE, Leach GE: Operative management of female urethral diverticulum. In: McGuire E (ed) *Advances in Urology.* Chicago: Mosby, 1994; 199–228

82. Blaivas JG. Vaginal flap urethral reconstruction: an alternative to the bladder flap neourethra. *J Urol* 1989; 141: 542–545

83. Blaivas JG. Treatment of female incontinence secondary to urethral damage or loss. *Urol Clin North Am* 1991; 18: 355–363

84. Robertson JR. Urinary fistulas. In: Ostergard DR (ed) *Gynecologic Urology and Urodynamics: Theory and Practice*, 2nd edn. Baltimore: Williams and Wilkins, 1985; 323–328

85. Leach GE. Urethrovaginal fistula repair with Martius labial fat pad graft. *Urol Clin North Am* 1991; 18: 409–413

86. Lee RA. Current status of genitourinary fistula. *Obstet Gynecol* 1988; 72: 313–319

87. Chassagne S, Haav F, Zimmern. [The Martius flap in vaginal surgery: technic and indications] (abstract). *Prog Urol* 1997; 7: 120–125

88. Zimmern PE, Hadley HR, Leach GE *et al.* Transvaginal closure of the bladder neck and placement of a suprapubic catheter for destroyed urethra after long-term indwelling catheter. *J Urol* 1985; 134: 554

89. Goodwin WE, Scardino PT. Vesicovaginal and urethrovaginal fistulas: a summary of 25 years of experience. *Trans Am Assoc GU Surg* 1979; 71: 123–129

90. Keetel WC, Schring FG, deProsse CA, Scott JR. Surgical management of urethrovaginal and vesicovaginal fistulas. *Am J Obstet Gynecol* 1978; 131: 425–431

58

Electrical implants in the treatment of voiding dysfunction

Ph. E. V. Van Kerrebroeck

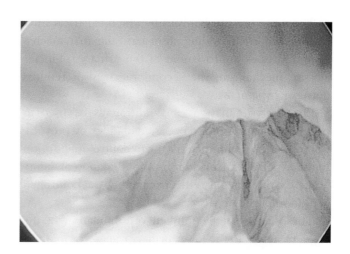

INTRODUCTION

A multitude of neurological disorders can affect the bladder and, although the incidence of lower urinary tract dysfunction differs among the various neurological entities, an important percentage of patients develop voiding dysfunction.[1] Incontinence and poor evacuation of urine, with residual urine and recurrent urinary tract infections, can cause important morbidity and affect patients' quality of life. In patients with spinal cord injury, the lack of ability to control the storage and evacuation function of the bladder is one of the most prominent aspects of their disability.

Although many bladder problems have a proven neurological basis, a vast group of patients suffer from lower urinary tract dysfunction without an evident neurological cause. These patients present with different forms of so-called 'idiopathic' dysfunctional voiding. Therapeutic modalities include pharmacological treatment, eventually in combination with clean intermittent catheterization. Lifelong continuation of this therapy, however, is a major issue, primarily because of side effects. Furthermore, in most patients, especially in females, urge incontinence remains a problem even with maximal pharmacological treatment. The failure of pharmacological manipulation has led to the development of surgical approaches such as augmentation cystoplasty, sphincteric incisions and artificial sphincter implantation. However, a considerable number of patients with neurogenic bladder dysfunction continue to have significant urological problems even though maximal classical therapy is applied. Therefore, the use of electrical stimulation to control storage and evacuation of urine has become an important tool in the urological treatment of refractory voiding dysfunction.

There are two mechanisms by which electrical stimulation can treat voiding disorders: the first mechanism addresses improvement of the urinary sphincter closure mechanism; the second mechanism reduces detrusor hyperactivity.

Electrical stimulation can additionally be used to permit evacuation of a paraplegic bladder by provocation of detrusor contractions, or to control micturition in the hyperreflexic bladder by a combination of dampening of spontaneous reflex excitability and controlled activation of the detrusor.

These aims can be fulfilled by stimulation of the efferent nerves to the lower urinary tract or by modulation of reflex activity as a consequence of stimulation of afferent nerves. Different modalities to apply electrical current to the lower urinary tract are available. Surface electrodes can be used as non-implantable devices.[2] Plugs inserted in the anal canal or the vagina are applied to treat incontinence.[3–5] Intravesical electrostimulation is performed in children with meningomyelocele.[6–8] Implantable prostheses are available to induce bladder contraction in order to evacuate urine in paraplegic patients or to control detrusor contraction in hyperreflexic bladders.[9–11] Another type of prosthesis permits the modulation of symptomatic voiding dysfunction such as urge incontinence, urgency–frequency and retention.[12,13]

ELECTRICAL STIMULATION IN SPINAL CORD INJURY

The development of systems for electrical stimulation of the bladder in spinal cord injury coincided with a better knowledge of the pathophysiology of neurogenic bladder dysfunction. In patients with complete spinal cord injury and bladder hyperreflexia the complete micturition cycle must be controlled. This means that, supplementary to electrostimulation for evacuation, an increase in bladder capacity and compliance must be realized. Two approaches for stimulation of the bladder in patients with spinal cord injury are available: intradural and extradural.

In 1969, Brindley[14] from London initially used animal models in an attempt to develop a system for intradural sacral anterior root stimulation. The first successful sacral anterior root stimulator for a patient with traumatic paraplegia was implanted in 1978.[15] The clinical results have been greatly improved since the introduction in 1986 of complete intradural sacral posterior root rhizotomies to control the reservoir function of the bladder in combination with implantation of the sacral posterior root stimulator.[16]

Technique

Owing to the anatomical features of the sacral roots, the anterior (motor) aspect and the posterior (sensory) aspect of the sacral roots can be separated. Therefore, the actual technique of intradural sacral anterior root stimulation consists of the combination of complete posterior rhizotomy with implantation of electrodes on the remaining anterior roots.[17] After a development period of 14 years in the Neurological Prostheses Unit in London, an anterior root stimulator device has been commercially available in Europe since 1986 (Finetech Ltd, Welwyn Garden City, England/Neuro-Control Inc., Brussels, Belgium). The Finetech–Brindley bladder controller consists of an implanted system of electrodes for sacral anterior root stimulation which contains no implanted power supply but is driven by an external radio transmitter (Fig. 58.1).

The implanted device (Fig. 58.2) consists of three parts. The anterior sacral roots are placed intradurally into the electrodes (termed 'books') at about the level of the intervertebral disc L5–S1. The radio-receiver block, which contains three radio receivers, is implanted subcutaneously in a pouch in the lower thoracic or abdominal wall. Three silicone-coated cables form the connection between the electrode book and the radio-receiver block. In combination with the implanted device, a sleeve is delivered to pass the cables through the dura mater and to prevent leakage of cerebrospinal fluid.

The external equipment (Fig. 58.3) consists of a transmitter block with three coils connected through an isolated cable with the control box that contains the electronics and the rechargeable batteries. The control box generates electrical impulses that are transmitted to the transmitter block, which transforms the impulses into high-frequency signals. The implanted radio-receiver transforms these high-frequency signals back into electrical impulses that are transmitted to the motor spinal nerve roots.

The control box permits the installation of three different stimulation programmes that are individually tailored by the physician for each patient. Normally, the first programme serves for micturition (Fig. 58.4), the second is designated for defecation and the third can be used for erection in men and lubrication of the vagina in women. After the stimulation programme has been installed, the patient can initiate the device for voluntary micturition, defecation or erection/lubrication.

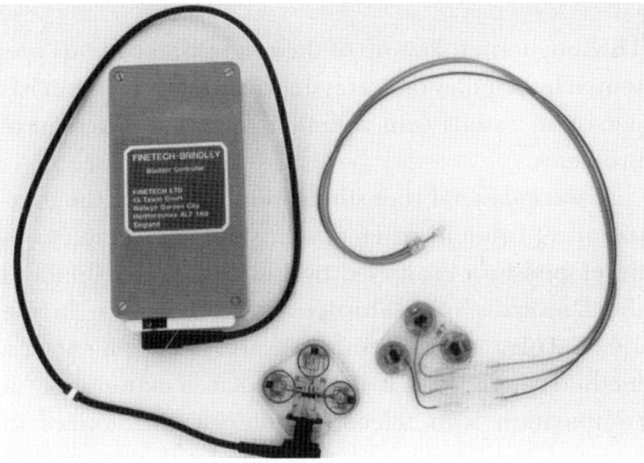

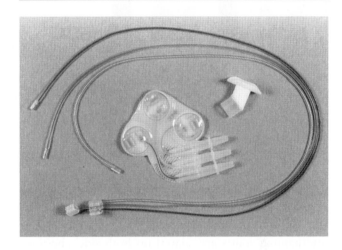

Figure 58.2. *The internal equipment with the electrode mounts connected to the connection cables. In the middle are the radio-receiver block and the sleeve to pass the connection cables through the dura.*

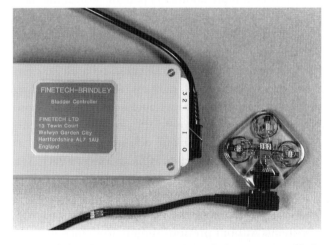

Figure 58.1. *The internal equipment (implant) along with the electrode mounts, the cables and the radio-receiver block are shown on the right. The external stimulation unit together with the control box and the transmitter block are on the left.*

Figure 58.3. *The external equipment with the transmitter block to the right and the control box to the left.*

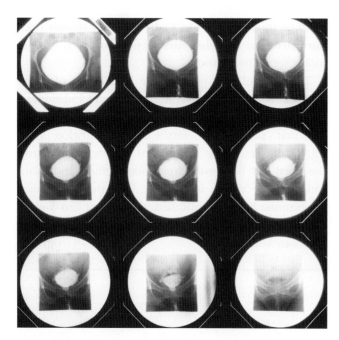

Figure 58.4. *Videocystography during micturition following stimulation of the sacral roots. Urine is evacuated in spurts of about 100 ml per stimulation period until evacuation is complete.*

A laminectomy from the third or the fourth lumbar vertebra to the second sacral vertebra is necessary (Fig. 58.5) in order to implant the material intradurally. The interlaminar joints are spared on both sides, because they are essential for the stability of the spine.

Results

With this technique about 700 patients worldwide have undergone this procedure.[18] In a personal series of 52 patients, and also in a review of 184 patients from different centres, more than 80% of the patients were able to achieve adequate intravesical pressure and efficient voiding.[19] In nearly all patients with a functioning implant, the incidence of infection is decreased. In those patients who have had posterior rhizotomies, the occurrence of reflex uninhibited detrusor contractions is abolished because the reflex arc is no longer intact. As a result, patients have an increased functional capacity without involuntary detrusor contractions (Fig. 58.6). Therefore, continence can be achieved in the majority of patients without previous surgery to reduce the urethral closure function. Most patients will become appliance free, which enhances dignity and self-image.[20,21]

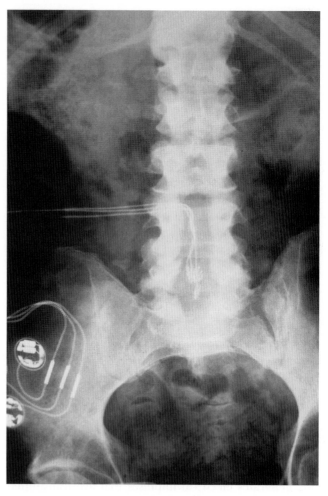

Figure 58.5. *Plain radiograph of the abdomen, showing the electrodes in the spinal canal and the cables connected with the receiver block on the right lower abdomen.*

The long-term follow-up of the original 50 patients presented by Brindley indicates that bladder stimulation has persistent results with a limited number of technical problems.[22]

A second sacral root stimulation device for the evacuation of urine in patients with spinal cord injury was developed by a group led by Tanagho and Schmidt at the University of California at San Francisco in the 1980s. This research resulted in the development of a method whereby electrodes were placed extradurally in combination with selective posterior rhizotomies of sacral roots S3 and/or S4. Compared with the Brindley technique, the extradural approach has the primary advantage of minimized risk of leakage of cerebrospinal fluid. However, precise separation of the anterior and posterior aspects of the sacral nerve roots is more

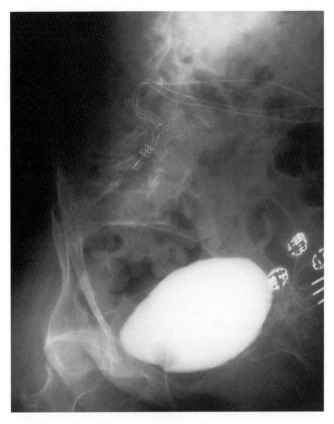

Figure 58.6. *Control cystography 6 weeks after complete posterior rhizotomies and implantation of intradural electrodes and a subcutaneous receiver.*

difficult in the extradural segment of S3 and nearly impossible at the S4 level. In a group of 22 patients there was a complete success in 8 patients (36%) resulting in normal reservoir function, continence and evacuation of urine with sacral root stimulation therapy.[11] Voiding with this type of stimulation is claimed to be synchronous with a low associated voiding pressure. This extradural stimulation system is not commercially available. Further experimental and clinical work continues.

ELECTRICAL STIMULATION FOR CHRONIC LOWER URINARY TRACT DYSFUNCTION

Chronic types of lower urinary tract dysfunction, including urge incontinence, urgency–frequency and retention, present a challenge. Most patients are initially treated with conservative therapies including bladder retraining, pelvic floor exercises and biofeedback. In the majority of patients, this standard regimen is supplemented with pharmacological therapy (anticholin-

ergics, tricyclic antidepressants, antibiotics). However, approximately 40% of patients either do not achieve an acceptable level of therapeutic benefit or remain completely refractory to treatment. Alternative surgical procedures such as bladder transection, transvesical phenol injection of the pelvic plexus, augmentation cystoplasty and even urinary diversion, are often advocated for chronic conditions. These surgical procedures have variable efficacy and they have associated morbidity and risk.

During the last decade, use of electrical stimulation for the treatment of lower urinary tract dysfunction has gained interest. External electrical stimulation of the pelvic floor using electrical probes placed in the vagina or the anus has been associated with favourable results for the indication of incontinence. Long-term efficacy, however, has not been established and is believed to be influenced by lack of standardization and patient compliance.

Since the 1960s, transcutaneous stimulation of the sacral nerves, which are accessed through the third or fourth sacral foramen, has been tried as a method to control functional lower urinary tract disorders.[23] Sacral nerve stimulation therapy offers a reversible mode of treatment for patients presenting with voiding dysfunction and secondary chronic pelvic pain in patients refractory to conservative treatment.

The goal of sacral nerve stimulation therapy is to relieve dysfunctional voiding symptoms by rebalancing micturition control. Long-term therapy with the InterStim system (Medtronic, Inc., Minneapolis, Minnesota, USA) is accomplished with a surgically implanted lead electrode at the level of the sacral foramen (S3 or S4).

In the 1980s a feasibility trial was performed to optimize surgical techniques and to focus on patient selection criteria. Since that time, valuable experience has been gathered in the evaluation, surgery and follow-up of patients presenting with voiding dysfunction and secondary pelvic pain who have been treated with sacral foramen electrode implants.[24]

Mode of action

The mode of action of this so-called 'sacral neuromodulation' is still unclear, but it has been hypothesized that the electrical current modulates reflex pathways involved in the filling and evacuation phase of the micturition cycle.[25] Stimulation of myelinated Aδ-fibres of the S3 and S4 sacral nerves decreases the spastic behaviour of the pelvic floor and enhances the tone of the urethral sphincter. In many patients, the primary voiding dysfunction appears to begin with unstable urethral activity, which overfacilitates the voiding reflexes, leading to detrusor instability and associated urgency, frequency and incontinence.[26] For patients presenting with urinary retention, it is believed that unstable urethral activity may actually inhibit the voiding reflex, leading to an underfacilitated or acontractile detrusor. Sacral nerve stimulation therapy is believed to modulate pelvic floor spasticity and therefore stabilizes overactive or underactive detrusor function.[27] The threshold for the somatic component of the spinal nerve that innervates the pelvic floor is lower than that for the autonomic component to the bladder; simultaneous bladder contraction and high-pressure storage problems are therefore avoided during sacral nerve stimulation therapy.

Ideal candidates for sacral neuromodulation are patients presenting with refractory voiding disorders (urge incontinence, urinary urgency–frequency and retention), who have neurologically intact sacral nerves, and who are amenable to long-term therapy. Patients in whom numerous other forms of therapy have failed should not be excluded from neuromodulation as they often show an excellent response to this technique.

Procedure: test stimulation

Although sacral neuromodulation is planned as a long-term treatment, the therapy incorporates a unique temporary test stimulation procedure that allows patients and physicians to assess sacral nerve stimulation over a trial period.[28] Results of the trial are used by the physician to assess viability of surgical implantation. The test stimulation is conducted as an outpatient procedure and comprises two steps – acute testing and the home evaluation phase. The purpose of the acute testing procedure is to locate and identify the sacral nerves and verify neural integrity. Home evaluation affords the patient an opportunity to feel the stimulation and enables the physician to assess the effects of therapy on dysfunctional voiding behaviour.

During an outpatient acute testing procedure, under local anaesthesia, a targeted sacral nerve (preferably

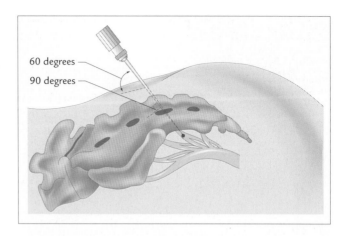

Figure 58.7. *Left S3 is accessible through the sacral foramen using an insulated 22-gauge needle.*

S3) is accessed with a 22-gauge foramen needle (Fig. 58.7). Focused electrical stimulation is applied to the sacral nerve by delivery of current to the uninsulated (proximal and distal) portions of the needle.

Typical motor responses to stimulation of each nerve level are seen at both the local (perineum) and distant (foot and toe) sites (Table 58.1). S3 stimulation produces a contraction of the levator muscles (bellows-like contraction) as well as detrusor and urethral sphincter contraction. Signs of S3 stimulation in the lower extremities include plantar flexion of the great toe. Subjectively, patients report a pulling sensation in the rectum during S3 stimulation, with variable tingling or vibrating sensations being perceived in the scrotum and the tip of the penis by men or in the labia and vagina in women. S4 stimulation results in a contraction of the levator ani muscle (bellows-like contraction) with no activity being noted in the foot or leg. The sacral nerve at either site with the best clinical (subjective) or urodynamic response is selected and the intensity of the current can be readily adapted to the sensation of stimulation.

Once the appropriate motor and sensory responses have been obtained, a test stimulation lead is implanted adjacent to the targeted sacral nerve through the cannula of the foramen needle. The needle is then removed. The lead remains in the vicinity of the targeted sacral nerve and passes posteriorly through the sacral foramen, subcutaneous tissue and the skin. Upon reconfirmation of the acute motor and sensory responses to stimulation, the lead is connected to an

Table 58.1. *Typical motor and sensory responses to sacral nerve stimulation*

Nerve innervation	Response		Sensation
	Pelvic floor	Foot/calf/leg	
S2 Primary somatic contributor of pudendal nerve for external sphincter, leg, foot	'Clamp'* of anal sphincter	Leg/hip rotation, plantar flexation of entire foot, contraction of calf	Contraction of base of penis, vagina
S3 Virtually all pelvic autonomic functions and striated muscle (levator ani)	'Bellows'* of perineum	Plantar flexion of great toe, occasionally other toes	Pulling in rectum, extending forwards to scrotum or labia
S4 Pelvic autonomic and somatic No leg or foot	'Bellows'**	No lower extremity motor stimulation	Pulling in rectum only

* Clamp: contraction of anal spincter and, in males, retraction of base of penis. Move buttocks aside and look for anterior/posterior shortening of the perianal structures

** Bellows: lifting and dropping of pelvic floor. Look for deepening and flattening of buttock groove. With a levator ani contraction, the levator muscles lift and drop, producing a deepening and relaxation of the buttock groove. A strong bellows response is preferred over a strong toe response.

external test stimulation device and the patient will conduct the home evaluation for a period of 3–7 days. Changes in dysfunctional voiding behaviour can be quantified in patient voiding diaries or by urodynamic examination.

Patients with a favourable clinical outcome (and, preferably, urodynamic result) during the test stimulation procedure are considered candidates for long-term therapy.

Procedure for long-term therapy

The surgically implanted InterStim device consists of a quadripolar lead, neurostimulator, and an extension that connects the lead to the neurostimulator.

Surgical implantation is performed under general anaesthesia. After a midline incision over the sacrum, the fascia overlying the sacral foramina is opened, permitting access to the targeted sacral foramen. The targeted sacral nerve is given acute stimulation with an insulated foramen needle to confirm the motor responses observed during test stimulation. The lead is positioned within the foraminal canal to allow adjacent placement to the sacral nerve. The lead is sutured to the periostial tissue overlying the posterior aspect of the sacrum with non-absorbable sutures. The proximal end of the lead is then passed subcutaneously to a flank incision. A subcutaneous pocket is created in the upper buttock region, away from bony structures, for implan-

tation of the neurostimulator and extension. For patients with minimal adipose tissue, implantation of the neurostimulator in the lower abdominal region should be considered.

Relatively low amplitudes (1.5–5.5 V, 210 μs pulse width, 10–15 pulses/s, cycling mode) are sufficient for stimulation of the somatic nerve fibres and to minimize the potential for nerve damage due to overstimulation. Within these recommended stimulation parameters, dyssynergia of the bladder and striated urethral musculature is not induced – even when voiding is initiated during active stimulation.

Results

Previous reports indicate an overall success rate of 60–75% on initial trial stimulation.[24] Recent improvements to the design of the test stimulation lead appear to have resolved previous problems with lead migration and subsequent loss of stimulation sensation. Of the patients who qualified for surgical implantation after a successful test, up to 83% have derived major clinical benefit from the definitive procedure.[25,29] This effect appears to be durable, as shown by the latest results. However, about 20% of patients who respond well on trial stimulation fail to reproduce the same result after long-term stimulation. On the basis of clinical parameters, it appears that patients with detrusor overactivity and urethral instability have the best clinical outcome.[30]

Recently, the results of an international, multicentre, randomized clinical trial of the InterStim system have been presented.[31] In a group of 155 patients with refractory urge incontinence, 98 (63%) responded to test stimulation. Compared with a concurrent control group who did not receive stimulation therapy, patients treated with sacral nerve stimulation therapy demonstrated clinically and statistically significant reductions in urge incontinent symptoms at 6 months. Moreover, 47% of the patients with implants were completely dry and an additional 29% reduced incontinence symptoms by more than 50%. Of these patients, 38 were followed for a year after implantation with a successful outcome in 30 (79%).

Acute and chronic efficacy profiles for the indications of urgency–frequency and retention have borne similar results in the multicentre trial.[32] At 6 months after implantation, statistically significant reductions were documented in the patients with urgency–frequency who received implants compared with control group patients with respect to number of voids/day, the volume/void and the degree of urgency ranking (all $p < 0.0001$). Clinical success was achieved in 88% of the treated patients at 6 months, with a concomitant reduction in secondary pelvic/bladder discomfort. For the patients with retention, 69% of the patients who received implants had eliminated use of catheterization by 6 months, with significant reductions in the incidence of urinary tract infection by 12 months after implantation.

These compelling results were obtained in populations which were highly refractory to pharmacological therapy, non-surgical interventions, and even surgery. Improvement in quality of life and significantly favourable perceptions of health status over time on the basis of the Short Form 36 Health Outcome Survey were additionally demonstrated for each of the groups of implanted patients evaluated in the multicentre trial.

Safety of the InterStim system was established in over 2300 months of device experience from 157 patients.[32] No reports of nerve injury or adverse change in voiding function were noted in the multicentre study. Post-implantation events reported in the trial that had an incidence of 5% or higher included pain at the lead implant site (21.0%), pain at the neurostimulator site (17%), lead migration (9%), infection/skin irritation (7.0%), technical problem (7.0%), increased electrical stimulation sensation (6%), and adverse change in bowel function (5%). The majority of events resolved either spontaneously or with treatment.

Adverse events that necessitated surgical reintervention occurred in approximately one-third of the patients with implants. Surgical reintervention, however, did not appear to preclude a patient from having a good clinical outcome. The safety profile of the InterStim system is comparable to that of other implantable urological neuroprostheses such as the urinary sphincter with respect to the potential for surgical reintervention and infection. The advent of new technical advances in the therapy, including implantation of the neurostimulator in the upper buttock region and availability of a patient hand-held programmer, may reduce the potential for adverse events in future patients.

Conclusions

Sacral neuromodulation seems to be an effective treatment modality in patients with various forms of lower urinary tract dysfunction. This technology is a valuable addition to our treatment options when conservative measures fail.

REFERENCES

1. Wein AT, Raezer DM, Benson GS. Management of neurogenic bladder dysfunction in the adult. *Urology* 1976; 8: 432–443

2. Bradley WE, Timm GW, Chou SN. A decade of experience with electronic stimulation of the micturition reflex. *Urol Int* 1971; 26: 283–303

3. Godec C, Cass AS, Ayala GF. Electrical stimulation for incontinence: technique, selection and results. *Urology* 1976; 7: 388–397

4. Merrill DC. The treatment of detrusor incontinence by electrical stimulation. *J Urol* 1979; 122: 515–517

5. Fall M. Does electrical stimulation control incontinence? *J Urol* 1984; 131: 664–667

6. Katona F. Stages of vegetative afferentiation in reorganization of bladder control during intravesical electrotherapy. *Urol Int* 1975; 30: 192–199

7. Seiferth J, Heising I, Larkamp H: Experiences and critical comments on the temporary intravesical electrostimulation of neurogenic bladder in spina bifida children. *Urol Int* 1978; 33: 279–284

8. Madersbacher H, Pauer W, Reiner E. Rehabilitation of micturition by transurethral electrostimulation of the

bladder in patients with incomplete spinal cord lesions. *Paraplegia* 1982; 20: 191–195

9. Caldwell KPS. Urinary incontinence following spinal injury treated by electronic implant. *Lancet* 1985; 1: 846

10. Brindley GS, Polkey CE, Rushton DN, Cardozo L. Sacral anterior root stimulators for bladder control in paraplegia. The first 50 cases. *J Neurol Neurosurg Psychiatry* 1986; 49: 1104–1114

11. Tanagho EA, Schmidt RA, Orvis BR. Neural stimulation for control of voiding dysfunction: a preliminary report in 22 patients with serious neuropathic voiding disorders. *J Urol* 1989; 142: 340–345

12. Markland C, Merrill D, Chou S, Bradley W. Sacral nerve root stimulation: a clinical test of detrusor innervation. *J Urol* 1972; 107: 772–776

13. Schmidt RA. Advances in genitourinary neurostimulation. *Neurosurgery* 1986; 18: 10–41

14. Brindley GS. Experiments directed towards a prosthesis which controls the bladder and the external sphincter from a single site of stimulation. *Proc Biol Eng Soc 46th Meeting, Liverpool 1972*

15. Brindley GS, Polkey CE, Rushton DN. Sacral anterior root stimulation for bladder control in paraplegia. *Paraplegia* 1982; 20: 365–381

16. Sauerwein D. Die operative Behandlung der spastischen Blasenlahmung bei Querschnittlahmung. *Urologe[A]* 1990; 29: 196–203

17. Van Kerrebroeck PhEV, Koldewijn EL, Wijkstra H, Debruyne FMJ. Intradural sacral rhizotomies and implantation of an anterior sacral root stimulator in the treatment of neurogenic bladder dysfunction after spinal cord injury. *World J Urol* 1991; 9: 126–132

18. Van Kerrebroeck PhEV, Debruyne FMJ. World-wide experience with the Finetech–Brindley bladder stimulator. *Neurourol Urodyn* 1993; 12: 497–503

19. Van Kerrebroeck PhEV, Koldewijn EL, Rosier P *et al.* Results of the treatment of neurogenic bladder dysfunction in spinal cord injury by sacral posterior root rhizotomy and anterior sacral root stimulation. *J Urol* 1996; 155: 1378–1381

20. Van Kerrebroeck PhEV, van der Aa HE, Bosch JLHR *et al.* Sacral rhizotomies and electrical bladder stimulation in spinal cord injury. Part II: clinical and urodynamic analysis. *Eur Urol,* 1997; 31: 263–271

21. Wielink G, Essink-Bot ML, Van Kerrebroeck PhEV *et al.* Sacral rhizotomies and electrical bladder stimulation in spinal cord injury. Part II: cost-effectiveness and quality of life analysis. *Eur Urol* 1997; 31: 441–446

22. Brindley GS, Rushton DN. Long-term follow-up of patients with sacral anterior root stimulator implants. *Paraplegia* 1990; 28: 469–475

23. Habib TIN. Experiences and recent contributions in sacral nerve stimulation for both human and animal. *Br J Urol* 1967; 39: 73–83

24. Schmidt RA. Applications of neurostimulation in urology. *Neurourol Urodyn* 1988; 7: 585

25. Thon WF, Baskin LS, Jonas U *et al.* Neuromodulation of voiding dysfunction and pelvic pain. *World J Urol* 1991; 9: 38

26. Park JM, Bloon DA, McGuire EJ. The guarding reflex revisited. *Br J Urol* 1997; 80: 940–945

27. Schmidt RA, Doggweiler R. Neurostimulation and neuromodulation: a guide to selecting the right urologic patient. *Eur Urol* 1998; 34 (Suppl 1): 23

28. Schmidt RA, Senn E, Tanagho EA. Functional evaluation of sacral nerve root integrity. Report of a technique. *Urology* 1990; 35: 388–392

29. Bosch JLHR, Groen J. Sacral (S3) segmental nerve stimulation as a treatment for urge incontinence in patients with detrusor instability: results of chronic electrical stimulation using an implantable neural prosthesis. *J Urol* 1995; 154: 504–507

30. Koldewijn EL, Rosier PFWM, Meuleman EJH *et al.* Predictors of success with neuromodulation in lower urinary tract dysfunction: results of trial stimulation in 100 patients. *J Urol* 1994; 152: 2071–2075

31. Janknegt RA, Van Kerrebroeck PhEV, Lycklama à Nijeholt A *et al.* Sacral nerve modulation for urge incontinence: a multinational, multicenter randomized study. *J Urol* 1997; 157: 1237

32. Medtronic, Inc., Minneapolis, Minnesota, USA: data on file

59

Complex reconstructive urological surgery

C. R. Chapple, P. J. R. Shah, S. C. Radley, D. Png

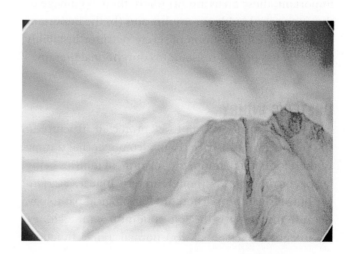

INTRODUCTION

Complex reconstructive surgery may be more appropriately considered as surgical restoration of lower urinary tract function. Preoperative evaluation relies upon accurate functional assessment and hence knowledge and understanding of the principles and practice of urodynamic investigation. An appreciation of lower urinary tract anatomy and pelvic surgery, with some understanding of both gynaecological and urological pathology, is essential. The basic surgical principles are those underlying any form of successful surgical reconstruction – namely, an understanding of anatomy and function, with attention to excision of ischaemic tissue, obliteration of dead space, interposition of vascularized tissue, avoidance of infection and haematoma, and tension-free anastomosis.

The term 'reconstructive surgery' inspires images of difficult and esoteric surgical practice best confined to specialist centres. Although there is no doubt that subspecialization increases the success of such surgery, the basic underlying principles are fundamental to the practice of all surgery, namely:

- a detailed knowledge of normal anatomy and a clear definition of abnormal radiology;
- comprehensive and appropriate assessment of upper and lower urinary tract function;
- good surgical technique, with good access and exposure and a full appreciation of available surgical techniques.

In this brief exposition on the subject, it is our intention to consider areas in urogynaecological practice where functional and anatomical reconstruction is important; these areas are (a) where there is damage to the ureter, the bladder or urethra and (b) the important area of surgical resolution of severe detrusor instability (DI) that has proved resistant to conventional therapy.

URETERIC INJURY

The ureter is an elastic and well-protected structure in the retroperitoneal space. Injury from external trauma is, therefore, uncommon, the majority of injuries being iatrogenic in origin. Although ureteric injuries account for only a small proportion of all urological pathology, because the ureter is the sole conduit from the kidney, its integrity is essential for normal renal function.

Ureteric injuries, therefore, demand careful appraisal and timely intervention.

True incidence of injury

A number of iatrogenic ureteric injuries may never become clinically apparent; the true incidence of ureteric injury is, therefore, difficult to estimate. The incidence of clinical ureteric injury in routine gynaecological surgery has been reported to vary from 0.2 to 1.5% in retrospective studies.[1-5] This rises to 2.5% for prospective studies where postoperative urograms are done and up to 30–35% when radical pelvic surgery is involved.[6-10]

In a major study by Goodno *et al.*,[2] the incidence of ureteric injuries involving 4665 surgical operations was noted to be 0.4% – a figure that has not changed significantly over the years.[11] In most series, gynaecological surgery accounts for about two-thirds of iatrogenic ureteric injuries. Most are related to abdominal, radical or vaginal hysterectomy, ovarian tumour surgery and incontinence surgery. Non-gynaecological causes of iatrogenic injuries include colorectal surgery (15%), ureteroscopic surgery (2–17%), vascular surgery (6%), laminectomy/spinal fusion (1%); bladder-neck suspension procedures (3%), appendicectomy (1%) and caesarean section (1%).[12] Rare causes of ureteric injury following procedures such as open herniorrhaphy, computed tomography (CT)-guided chemical sympathectomy, termination of pregnancy and Kirschner wire application for hip dislocation in a child have also been reported.[13-16]

In recent years, with the development and proliferation of new laparoscopic techniques, there has been a significant increase in associated injuries, especially in gynaecology, where laparoscopy now accounts for 25% of all gynaecological injuries to the ureter.[17] This rise parallels the rise of ureteric injuries associated with a similar expansion in endoscopic approaches to complex ureteric problems in urological practice. In a recent review by Selzman and Spirnak[18] of 165 ureteric injuries, urological surgery accounted for 42% of the total compared with 34% for gynaecological surgery and 24% for general surgery. Most injuries to the ureter in this series followed endoscopic urological surgery (79%) compared with gynaecological surgery and general surgery where the majority occurred during open procedures.

Risk factors for iatrogenic ureteric injuries

Previous surgery, bulky or invasive tumours, ureteric duplication, ectopic ureters, endometriosis, retroperitoneal fibrosis and inflammatory conditions such as chronic pelvic infection all predispose to iatrogenic ureteric injury. Situations when life is threatened owing to haemorrhage or during emergency caesarean section, when speed becomes critical, can also predispose to iatrogenic ureteric injury.

Types of iatrogenic injury

1. *Avulsion.* This occurs when forceful retraction is used, especially when tissues are soft as a result of infection or necrosis.
2. *Transection.* This is caused by the scissors or scalpel, especially when the ureters are enveloped within a tumour or fibrous tissue. Common sites of such injuries during gynaecologic surgery include:
   - the pelvic brim, where the vascular pedicle to the ovary is in close proximity to the ureter;
   - the broad ligament, where the ureter is crossed by the uterine artery;
   - the ureteric canal in the cardinal ligament, 1 cm lateral to the supravaginal cervix and 1 cm above the lateral vaginal fornix.

   In surgery of the rectum and sigmoid colon, the left ureter is more commonly involved in iatrogenic ureteric injuries. Invasive tumour, dense fibrosis and inflammatory conditions all contribute to ureteric trauma even in the hands of experienced surgeons. Retrocaecal appendicitis has been known to result in similar iatrogenic ureteric injuries on the right.

   During vascular surgery, ureteric injury can occur with aorto-iliac and aortofemoral bypass. Predisposing factors include retroperitoneal fibrosis, radiation exposure, long-term ureteric stents, graft infections or graft dilatations.
3. *Ligation.* This occurs when the ureters are mistaken for bleeding vessels. It can also occur during vaginal hysterectomy when the uterine arteries are being ligated and in procidentia when the ureters prolapse with the uterus.
4. *Crushing.* This may occur when clamps are used blindly to control haemorrhage and is seen at similar sites to transection injury, especially during radical

hysterectomy for cancer. Necrosis and ultimately stricture or fistula formation can result.

5. *Devascularization.* This occurs when extensive or overenthusiastic dissection of the ureter is performed. In 80% of individuals the ureter is supplied by a single artery along its entire length, with anastomotic feeding vessels at each end and in the middle. Devascularization results in ischaemic necrosis, which ultimately leads to fistula or stricture.
6. *Perforation.* This is commonly caused by ureteroscopy and associated endoscopic manipulation for ureteric stones. Oedematous tissue surrounding the stone, or tissue traumatized by lithotripsy, are predisposing factors. Needle injury during open surgery may result in perforation but is rarely a cause of problems in healthy tissues.
7. *Fulguration.* This can occur during transurethral resection of bladder cancers taken too close to the ureteric orifices. Laparoscopic diathermy or laser treatment of endometriotic lesions are increasingly important causes of thermal injury to the urinary tract that have seen an increase in parallel with the rise of laparoscopic surgery in gynaecology.
8. *Fistula formation.* This can follow transection, ischaemic necrosis or perforation if the distal end of the ureter is not in continuity or is obstructed. Urine will then discharge from the vagina, operative wound or drain site, or into the peritoneal cavity or retroperitoneal space.
9. *Stricture formation.* This can follow any of the above injuries and ultimately lead to obstruction of the ureters, hydronephrosis and renal damage.

Non-iatrogenic ureteric injury

Non-iatrogenic ureteric injuries are uncommon, but are found in 2.3–17% of cases of penetrating abdominal trauma, most commonly gunshot or stab wounds.[19] Associated injuries to the colon, duodenum, pancreas and great vessels make such injuries potentially life threatening.

Blunt or avulsion injuries are very rare, most commonly occurring in patients who have fallen from a height or have been thrown from a car. Severe compression injuries, such as those related to the steering wheel and seat belts, can also cause ureteric injuries, which may even present with a soft, non-tender abdomen. Most blunt trauma involves the pelviureteric junction and often presents late with a ureteric fistula or urinoma as a result of an avulsion injury.[20,21]

Radiation injury to the ureters is rare but can occur in radiotherapy for cervical, bladder, rectal and other pelvic tumours. Most post-irradiation ureteric strictures, however, are due to recurrent tumour. Presentation may be from 3 months up to 10 years, usually with a long thread-like stenotic lesion or a localized constriction 4–6 cm from the bladder. These are thought to be due to the endarteritis obliterans resulting from radiotherapy. Subsequent surgery on such poor tissues also predisposes to a higher complication rate involving the ureters.[22]

Presentation

Approximately 15–25% of iatrogenic ureteric injuries during open surgery are discovered intra-operatively. The majority present postoperatively, delays in diagnosis being the rule rather than the exception. Delays can vary from 2 days to 12 years.[23–27] Early signs of ureteric injuries are subtle and usually missed, the injury being discovered several days or weeks later when a complication occurs. In urological surgery, however, where injury is most commonly associated with ureteroscopic procedures for stone disease, 77% are diagnosed intra-operatively. Of such ureteric injuries, 91% occur in the lower third, 7% in the middle third and 2% in the upper third of the ureter.

Fever is a common feature after any surgery but, if persistent, may be a sign of urinary sepsis which occurs in 10% of those with ureteric obstruction. Flank pain occurs in 36–90% of cases of hydronephrosis.[25,27,28] Fistulae of the vagina and skin tend to present 7–10 days after surgery, with urinary leakage.[23–25,27,28] Those involving the peritoneum may leak urine from the wound or drains. An abdominal or pelvic mass, urinoma or pelvic abscess may also result. Malaise and gastrointestinal upset or ileus are often accompanying features. These do not settle spontaneously and an abdomen distended as a consequence of ileus and supposed 'ascites' should raise the suspicion of urinary leakage. Ureteric injuries must first be suspected if they are to be detected.

Penetrating injuries involving the ureter usually present with the associated injuries and in most cases are identified intra-operatively during exploration of the wound. Gross haematuria is present in approximately one-third of the patients, whereas in about one-third no blood is detected on urinalysis.[20,21,29,30]

Diagnosis

Ureteric injuries recognized intra-operatively and repaired immediately carry a better prognosis of cure than those which become manifest postoperatively as a result of complications.[18,23,25,31] In a recent review by Selzman et al.,[18] of 165 ureteral injuries, the number of procedures required to repair urological injuries was 1.2 for those diagnosed intra-operatively compared with 1.6 for those diagnosed postoperatively. A total of 77% of urological injuries were diagnosed intra-operatively compared with 16% in gynaecological surgery and 56% in general surgery. This difference is due mainly to the different procedures that cause such injuries in these specialities, in addition to the greater familiarity of working with ureters for most urologists.

A high index of suspicion is required for the diagnosis of iatrogenic ureteric injury in the immediate postoperative period, especially in non-urological operations. Fever, flank pain and ileus are highly suspicious but non-specific features. Excessive wound drainage or leakage *per vaginam* should be collected, analysed and its electrolytes compared with in those in the patient's urine to establish the likely origin of this fluid.

An intravenous urogram (IVU) or retrograde study is mandatory whenever ureteric injury is suspected. This will usually demonstrate the site of injury as well as associated pathology such as hydronephrosis and ureteric fistula. Cystoscopy and bilateral retrograde pyelograms should be performed in all cases. Antegrade nephrostogram may be useful. Higher concentrations of contrast in these studies allow demonstration of leakage and establish the diagnosis in most cases.

Following penetrating trauma, the ureters should be explored if injury is suspected. IVUs using high doses of contrast have not been helpful: in a series of 12 patients with penetrating injuries of the ureter, only 25% were diagnosed on IVU.[19] Features of extravasation of contrast, ureteric obstruction, deviation, dilatation or non-visualization are diagnostic. In 75% of such cases, IVU demonstrated only kidney presence and function.[19–21] Conversely, direct exploration of the ureter and the use of indigo carmine dye intra-operatively provided the diagnosis in 83% of cases.[19] CT scans are of limited value in demonstrating ureteric injuries *per se* but may be helpful when extravasation is seen or when urinomas have developed. The primary role of CT remains in the assessment of other associated abdominal and pelvic injuries. The absence of haematuria in one-third of ureteric injuries and a negative IVU in about three-quarters of penetrating ureteric injuries implies that, in such cases, even in the presence of negative preoperative diagnostic radiology, the suspicion of ureteric injury warrants exploration.[20,21,29]

Following blunt trauma, delays in diagnosis are relatively common, owing to the lack of early characteristic features and the association of other severe life-threatening injuries warranting more immediate attention.

Prevention

Iatrogenic injuries are best managed by preventative rather than corrective measures. Avoidance of ureteric injuries begins with a thorough knowledge of the course of the ureters, the nature and site of potential ureteric injuries and adequate preoperative evaluation. This may include an IVU or contrast-enhanced CT scans if major pelvic or retroperitoneal surgery is planned. Congenital anomalies, ectopic ureters and ureteric duplications may be diagnosed on IVU; more importantly, where radical surgery is indicated and ureters are involved or displaced by the pathology, their course can be mapped and the necessary precautions taken. Preoperative, or more commonly intra-operative, placement of ureteric catheters may facilitate their identification during difficult anatomical dissection. Such manoeuvres should not induce complacency, since injuries are known to occur despite the presence of a ureteric catheter.[32]

A preoperative IVU allows for comparative studies should a postoperative IVU become necessary. However, preoperative IVUs have not been shown to be of value prior to routine hysterectomy and cannot substitute for good surgical technique and identification of anatomical landmarks.[33,34] Palpation of the ureter should not be relied on.

Identification of the length of ureter within the operative field should significantly reduce the risk of damage. The ureters are recognized by the glistening appearance of their sheaths, peristalsis on stimulation and characteristic feel on palpation. Dissection of the ureters may be necessary, especially when in close proximity to resection margins. Sharp dissection along the line of the ureter, incorporating a generous cuff of peri-ureteric adventitia, should reduce the risk of an ischaemic injury.

The close relationship of the uterine artery to the last 3 cm of the ureter makes the latter vulnerable to injury when mass ligatures and blind clamping of an injured artery occurs. Proper identification and isolation of the uterine artery before ligation and digital compression of the internal iliac artery to control haemorrhage can avoid the need for blind clamping. Most unexpected haemorrhage can be controlled by suitable compression of the bleeding point until the ureter is identified.

If ureteric injury is suspected during open surgery, indigo carmine dye may be useful in identifying the presence and site of the lesion. Contrast solution with intra-operative imaging is more useful during ureteroscopic procedures. Most ureteroscopic injuries occur during stone extraction and fragmentation. The experience of the urologist has also been shown to be an important risk factor.[35] Other important principles in the prevention of ureteroscopic injuries include careful patient selection, availability of good endoscopic instrumentation and the use of intra-operative fluoroscopy. Large and high stones may be better managed by open surgery.

Management of ureteric injury

The management of a ureteric injury depends on its extent and location, its aetiology, associated injuries and the time of its discovery (Fig. 59.1).

Timing of surgery

Ureteric injuries discovered intra-operatively and repaired immediately have an excellent prognosis, probably due to the absence of sequelae following urine leak and complications such as infection.[18,36] If the injury is incurred during a ureteroscopic procedure, an internal stent placed retrogradely across the defect may be all that is required. Small perforations usually heal within 1–2 weeks, whereas larger defects and thermal injuries require up to 6 weeks of internal stenting. If immediate stenting is impossible, initial percutaneous

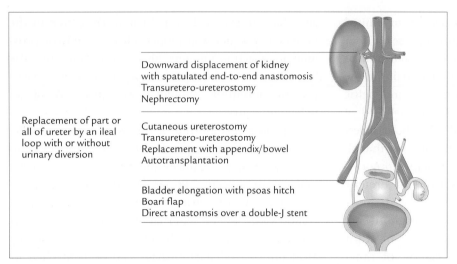

Replacement of part or all of ureter by an ileal loop with or without urinary diversion

Downward displacement of kidney with spatulated end-to-end anastomosis
Transuretero-ureterostomy
Nephrectomy

Cutaneous ureterostomy
Transuretero-ureterostomy
Replacement with appendix/bowel
Autotransplantation

Bladder elongation with psoas hitch
Boari flap
Direct anastomsis over a double-J stent

Figure 59.1. *Options for ureteric repair according to the level of injury.*

nephrostomy and subsequent antegrade placement of the ureteric stent are indicated.[17]

Injuries diagnosed postoperatively may initially be managed conservatively using nephrostomy drainage and/or subsequent ureteric stenting, if the ureteric defect is short (<2.5 cm) and a stent can be passed across the defect, either retrogradely or antegradely.[26] About one-half of all ureteric injuries can be treated by such endoscopic stenting, whereas the remainder will require an open procedure for definitive repair. In a series of 165 iatrogenic ureteric injuries, 49% were treated with 6 weeks' internal stenting, 89% showing no evidence of obstruction on follow-up lasting 1–20 years (mean of 8.5 years).[18] In a further series of 50 ureteric injuries it was found that endoscopic treatment performed for defects of less than 2 cm required less operating time and had fewer complications and shorter hospital stays than those undergoing open surgery.[37] No recurrences were noted over a 2-year follow-up period. However, in 14 of the 30 patients selected for endoscopic treatment, ureteric catheterization failed, and open repair was subsequently required. (All were ureteric injuries diagnosed after 3 weeks.) The authors concluded that endoscopic management of ureteric injuries should be carried out only in those with defects less than 2 cm in length diagnosed within 3 weeks of injury. In a further series of 27 patients, it was reported that percutaneous nephrostomy alone or in conjunction with ureteric stenting was successful in treating 11 (65%) of the 17 ureteric injuries considered suitable for endoscopic stenting.[24] As reported by Cormio *et al.*,[37] only 1/20 retrograde ureteric catheterizations

attempted was successful in those with delayed diagnoses. All ureteric fistulae required ureteric stenting for healing, and percutaneous nephrostomy was successful only in those with demonstrable ureteric obstruction. These cases presumably represent ligation or crush injuries requiring time for dissolution of sutures and tissue healing. Ureteric obstruction persisting after 8 weeks of percutaneous drainage will require open exploration and repair.[24] In a series of 20 patients with ureteric injuries who had percutaneous nephrostomy with or without a stent as a primary procedure, 80% had spontaneous recovery of the injured ureter without further intervention. Morbidity and reoperation rates were reduced compared with 24 ureteric injuries treated by immediate open ureteric repair.[38]

For those that require open surgical correction, immediate repair is increasingly shown to have results similar to (if not better than) those obtained with the traditional approach of waiting for 6 weeks to 3 months before definitive repair. A number of series support early surgical intervention within 3 weeks.[23,25,26,30,31,39,40] Selzman and Spirnak[18] also found that the rate of complications was five times higher in the group treated by delayed rather than immediate repair for urologically injured ureters.

Open surgical management

Ureteral transection is best repaired by immediate spatulated ureteroureterostomy. This should be carried out with a tension-free anastomosis, using interrupted absorbable sutures. Sutures should not be too close together (in an attempt to achieve a watertight anastomosis), as ischaemia and subsequent stricture formation may result. A double-J stent is often used as a splint and is removed after 2–6 weeks. Ligation injuries are simply de-ligated, but crush injuries may be of greater extent, owing to ischaemia, and must be handled carefully.[28] If doubt exists as to the viability of the ureter, partial excision and spatulated reanastomosis may be required.

For injuries at or below the pelvic brim, an antireflux ureteroneocystostomy is the treatment of choice, for which various methods have been described. In the event of a gap between the end of the ureter and the bladder, extra length can be obtained with a psoas hitch.[41] Alternatively, a Boari flap may be employed to achieve a tension-free anastomosis[42,43] (Fig. 59.2). A graft length-to-width ratio of 3:2 is necessary, using a vascular pedicle based on the superior vesical artery. As

the tubularized flap has no functional activity, the tube should be open-mouthed for adequate drainage.[44] The theoretical advantage of the psoas hitch is the better preservation of the blood supply, which may be more precarious in the Boari flap. Other practical advantages include the relative ease of closure of the incision in thick-walled bladders. The incision is relatively smaller to produce an equivalent length of tube, thereby facilitating a non-refluxing reimplantation, and the subsequent ureteric positioning facilitates ureteroscopy.

For ureteric defects above the pelvic brim, an additional length of ureter of a few centimetres can be obtained by mobilization of the kidney, allowing spatulated ureteroureterostomy. Other options to foreshorten the ureteric course include calycoureterostomy, transureterostomy and autotransplantation.[45–47] If all else fails, nephrectomy is a final resort which, although previously an acceptable form of management

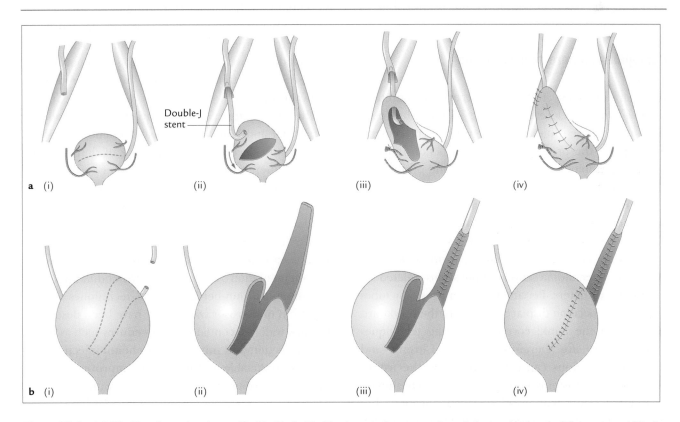

Figure 59.2. *(a) Bladder elongation (psoas hitch): (i) the bladder is opened transversely and the proximal end of the ureter mobilized; (ii) following spatulation, a double-J stent is inserted and the bladder brought up to be anastomosed; (iii) the ureter is anastomosed to the bladder over a stent; (iv) the bladder is closed longitudinally and sutured to the psoas muscle to eliminate any chance of tension at the anastomosis. (b) Construction of a Boari flap: (i,ii) a posteriorly based full-thickness flap of bladder is raised on the distal side of the injury; (iii) the flap is 'tubed' over a stent and anastomosed to the ureter; (iv) the defect is closed. Absorbable sutures (e.g. 3/0 vicryl) are used throughout.*

for such injuries, is now less acceptable, given the other options available.

Alternatives for substantial ureteric defects involve the use of substitutes. These may be biological or non-biological.

A number of non-biological substitutes have been reported; however, their use is overshadowed by the ileal ureter, which has proved the most reliable ureteric replacement to date.[48,49] The main drawbacks to the use of bowel (as in other bowel replacement surgery) relates to the production of mucus (which can cause obstruction), inadequate peristalsis, anastomotic stricture and reabsorption of excretory waste products. Consequently, contraindications to ileoureteric substitution include uncorrected bladder outlet obstruction and impaired renal function. Recurrent urinary tract infection and subsequent renal impairment are potential complications.[44] The appendix is an alternative biological substitute but is of limited length.[50] The fallopian tube has been employed but is limited by its relatively small calibre.

Postoperative care and follow-up

Postoperative care following surgery for ureteric injuries requires close monitoring of renal function, with appropriate fluid and electrolyte replacement, especially in the presence of postobstruction diuresis. Adequate antibiotic cover, wound care and prophylaxis for deep vein thrombosis follow standard surgical practice. Meticulous care of catheters and drains is critical, given the dependence of renal function and uneventful postoperative recovery on these devices.

Common complications include urinary leakage, infection, haematoma and complications related to drains and catheters. Percutaneous nephrostomy tubes may kink or become displaced, owing to their awkward locations in the flank; correct anchoring techniques and after-care are therefore essential. Chronic and recurrent infections can also result from the use of long-term nephrostomy drainage. Alternatively, the use of internal stents may avoid such complications but often causes irritative symptoms; in the long term, such stents may become encrusted if they are not changed every 6–8 weeks. Vesicoureteric reflux may occur following reimplantation and may present with recurrent infection and dilatation of the pelvicalyceal system.

Monitoring of wound drainage and contrast radiography immediately after placement of stents or drains is essential. Tube nephrostograms are useful for diagnostic purposes. A repeat IVU following stent removal and long-term follow-up (including IVU at 3 months and possibly subsequently) are recommended.

SURGERY FOR DETRUSOR OVERACTIVITY

Detrusor overactivity can result in considerable morbidity in patients with idiopathic DI and also those with neurogenic bladder dysfunction (NBD). In patients with DI, marked bladder overactivity leads to disabling frequency and incontinence, whereas, in NBD, renal impairment is a consequence of poor bladder compliance, ureteric reflux and/or ureteric obstruction caused by the thick-walled bladder, a consequence of hyperreflexic contractions against detrusor sphincter dyssynergia. In both conditions, the cornerstone of pharmacotherapy remains anticholinergic agents. This is combined with bladder retraining in DI. In the context of NBD, the clinical picture is complicated by an admixture of other functional problems associated with the bladder overactivity, including uncoordinated detrusor contraction and varying degrees of bladder outflow obstruction.

The aim of surgical therapy directed at the detrusor in both DI and NBD is to increase functional bladder capacity and decrease the amplitude of detrusor contractions, thereby preventing incontinence and protecting the upper tracts in patients with NBD.

In recent years, the mainstay of therapy for bladder overactivity has been augmentation cystoplasty, most usually using the 'clam' technique.[51] Two further options have been explored recently – namely, bladder autoaugmentation[52] and sacral neuromodulation.[53]

Although a number of surgical techniques for the treatment of detrusor overactivity have been described, it is now widely accepted that procedures such as detrusor transection and transtrigonal phenol injection produce unpredictable and temporary improvement, with potentially serious side effects. Their routine use can, therefore, no longer be supported.

Augmentation cystoplasty

Until the middle of the 20th century, patients with refractory incontinence were treated by either an indwelling catheter or urinary diversion, mainly in the form of an ileal conduit. Anticholinergic drugs were used with variable success, with oxybutynin being launched in the early 1980s. Surgically, two main strategies were adopted: the first was to disrupt the nerve supply to the bladder; the second was to increase its capacity. Partial sacral parasympathectomy,[54] bladder denervation,[55] cystolysis,[56] bladder transection (which was modified from cystolysis by Yeates) and transvesical infiltration of the pelvic plexuses with phenol, as described by Ewing *et al.*,[57] were all designed to disrupt the nerve supply. Bladder distension, developed by Smith and Higson,[58] was thought to cause ischaemic changes in the nerves or their endings. 'Clam' ileocystoplasty was described by Bramble[59] and was later popularized by Mundy and Stephenson.[60] The procedure works by producing an increase in bladder capacity and the interposed bowel segment 'absorbs' any residual detrusor activity. Many reports over the past decade have supported the results of the clam procedure,[60–62] and the procedure has become well accepted as that most effective for the treatment of intractable DI and hyperreflexia.

Ileocystoplasty and 'double-clam' ileocystoplasty may be effectively used for the treatment of patients with hyperreflexic and poorly compliant neuropathic bladders and DI. Although 'clam' ileocystoplasty has been used in patients with interstitial cystitis and for small-capacity bladders, the results are less certain.

Prior to augmentation ileocystoplasty, medical management should have been tried, with anticholinergic medication being the most effective method of management. Bladder distension[63] does not produce long-term benefits, and transtrigonal phenol has been shown to be ineffective for long-term relief of symptoms.[64]

The principle underlying augmentation cystoplasty is that, by bivalving a functionally overactive bladder and introducing a segment of detubularized intestine, a low-pressure bladder with an increased functional capacity will result.

The three intestinal segments commonly used are ileum, right colon and sigmoid colon. The sigmoid is usually used in patients where a short small-bowel mesentery impedes the use of ileum. Ileum is preferred, as it produces lower reservoir pressures and better compliance.[65]

The original technique described for clam cystoplasty is still widely used but modifications to this include opening the bladder in the sagittal plane, which appears to be equally effective, or opening the bladder as a 'star'.[66] This particular modification can be particularly useful in patients with NBD where the bladder is small and thick-walled. A double-dam is also effective. An alternative surgical technique popularized by McGuire is his modification of the hemi-Kock procedure. This utilizes a transverse 'smile' incision (looking posteriorly) which is fashioned 3 cm above the ureteral orifices, creating an anteriorly based detrusor flap.[67] Most workers find coronal or sagittal bivalving of the bladder to be effective and acceptable, provided that adequate opening of the bladder is performed right down to the ureteral orifices, in order both to open the bladder adequately and to prevent 'diverticulation' of the cystoplasty segment.

A number of studies attest to the efficacy of augmentation cystoplasty in children, adolescents and adults with DI and NBD.[68–73] Mundy and Stephenson[68] reported a series of 40 cases of whom 90% were cured at a mean follow-up of 1 year. Mean functional bladder capacity was increased from 280 to 440 ml, reduced compliance was improved in 70% of patients and DI abolished in 50%, the remainder having low-pressure detrusor overactivity. In a series of 26 adolescents undergoing enterocystoplasty, of whom 19 had a 'clam' cystoplasty, results were satisfactory in all three male but poor in five of the 16 female patients. In three patients, difficulty was experienced with clean intermittent self-catheterization (CISC).[69] In a series of 39 children with spina bifida, bladder capacity at safe storage pressures of less than 29 cm of saline was achieved in all patients, with a reduction in upper tract distension in 91.7% of kidneys.[70] A satisfactory result was achieved in all but one patient. Singh and Thomas in 1995 reviewed 67 patients who underwent augmentation cystoplasty:[71] of these, 47 had an ileal segment and 20 a sigmoid segment. These data are presented in combination with those from a further 11 patients who had an ileocaecal cystoplasty: 52 patients had an artificial sphincter, nine had a colposuspension and one had both. Acceptable continence was achieved in 93.6% of patients. Hasan *et al.*,[73] in 1995, reported on 48 patients who underwent augmentation cystoplasty for DI (n = 35) or NBD (n = 13): the mean follow-up was 38 months, with 83% achieving a good outcome, 15% a moderate outcome and 2% an unsatisfactory result. Flood *et al.*,[72] in 1995, reported 122 augmentation cystoplasties. It must, however, be borne in mind that the 'McGuire' technique used differed from the standard clam procedure reported for all the other series described above and this was a very mixed group of patients: 67% had an ileal augmentation, 30% a detubularized caecocystoplasty and 3% a sigmoid augmentation. In 19 patients this procedure was related to undiversion and 17% had interstitial cystitis, 7% radiation cystitis, 13% miscellaneous conditions; the remainder had either NBD or DI. The mean follow-up was 37 months. Bladder capacity was increased from a preoperative mean of 108 ml to 438 ml; of 106 patients in whom surgery was successful, 75% had an excellent result, 20% were improved and 5% had major, persistent problems.

The above results support augmentation cystoplasty as being an effective form of therapy with a low operative morbidity and satisfactory long-term results, although most of the reported series have a follow-up of less than 5 years. It must be remembered that this is major surgery and, despite adequate preoperative counselling, many patients take some months to adapt to their new bladder and to learn to void effectively by abdominal straining. It is important to monitor postoperative residual urine volumes. CISC is almost invariably the rule in those with NBD and is variably necessary after cystoplasty for DI. The reported incidence of CISC varies from 15% up to 85% of cases.[68] It is evident that a number of factors contribute to the need for CISC: these include the level of residual deemed acceptable by the supervising urologist and the concomitant use of procedures directed at the bladder outflow – either urethral dilatation (rebalancing) or treatments for stress incontinence. A particular debate centres around the treatment of coexisting stress incontinence at the time of clam cystoplasty; contemporary opinion remains divided on this matter, as measures designed to treat stress incontinence will generally increase the need for CISC. However, in women a colposuspension at the time of cystoplasty is an appropriate approach where necessary.

Other problems encountered with augmentation cystoplasty include persistent mucus production, recurrent or persistent urinary tract infections and metabolic disorders (which are usually mild and subclinical). Provided that patients are counselled preoperatively, mucus is rarely a problem. Persistent urinary infection can be troublesome, particularly in female patients, and has been reported in up to 30% of cases, often requiring long-term antibiotic therapy. Long-term bowel dysfunction occurs in up to one-third of patients and is thought to be related to the interruption of the normal enterohepatic circulation.[71,73,74] Bladder perforations have been reported in up to 10% of patients.[66] At present, lifelong follow-up of these patients is recommended, not only because of the above complications but also in view of the suggestion that augmentation cystoplasty predisposes to the subsequent development of malignancy.[75] However, there remains no convincing evidence to support an association with tumour in the absence of other predisposing factors, such as previous tuberculosis or chronic urinary stasis such as that associated with paraplegia.

Augmentation cystoplasty is an effective management option in contemporary practice in patients with intractable DI or NBD resistant to conventional therapy. In addition, cystoplasty can be used as part of an undiversion procedure. A proportion of patients are not significantly improved by this procedure: one series found a 'good-to-moderate' outcome in only 58% of patients with DI.[73] It must be borne in mind that up to 30% of patients experience increased frequency and looseness of bowel motions and a tendency to incontinent episodes, with a significant number of patients requiring long-term ISC. With these observations in mind, alternative therapies have been explored, bladder autoaugmentation in particular.[52]

Technique (Fig. 59.3)

The patient is admitted to hospital one day before the operation for bowel preparation with one or two sachets of sodium picosulphate and is restricted to fluids only. The patient should be prehydrated with intravenous fluids prior to surgery.

A Pfannenstiel incision or lower midline incision may be used. The bladder is mobilized extraperitoneally with approximately 2–3 cm of peritoneum being separated from the dome. The side of the bladder is measured from the pelvic floor to the dome on each side. This length forms the basis for preparation of an appropriate length of small bowel. The bladder is then bisected in the coronal plane. The anterior segment is usually smaller than the posterior one. This is taken down to 1 cm from the bladder neck and 1–2 cm anterior to the ureteric orifices. A segment of ileum is isolated 60 cm or more proximal to the ileocaecal valve. Bowel continuity is re-established using a one- or two-layered anastomosis depending on the surgeon's pref-

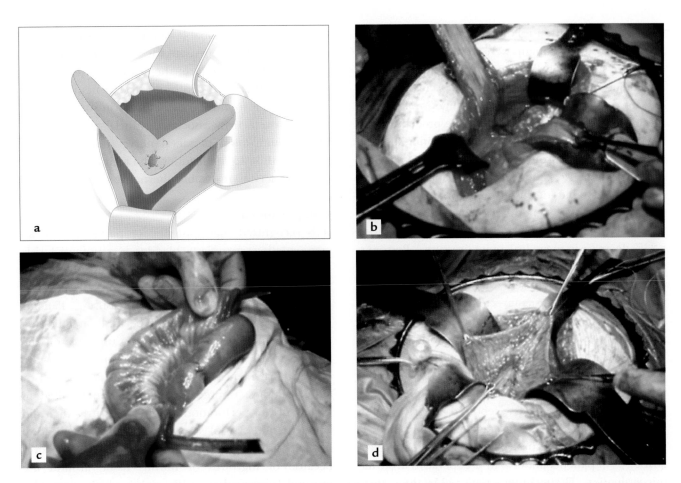

Figure 59.3. *The technique of clam ileocystoplasty. (a) Schematic of the 'clam'. The bladder is bivalved to within 1 cm of the bladder neck, anterior to the ureters. (b) The bladder has been divided 'à la clam' down its corners; (c) a section of small bowel isolated from its mesentery is being prepared for the clam; (d) the bowel sutured on to the back wall of the bladder.*

erence. A short ileal mesentery may make it impossible to bring the bowel segment down (although this is unusual). In this situation sigmoid colon should be used. The isolated bowel segment is then detubularized using diathermy over plastic suction tubing. The bowel is sutured to the opened bladder using a single extramucosal layer of 3/0 polyglycolic acid. For high-pressure neuropathic bladders a 'double-clam' is recommended. Urethral and suprapubic catheters are left in the bladder. The latter is brought out through the anterior bladder wall. A wound drain is left in the pelvis. Postoperatively, the bladder may be irrigated for 24 hours. The urethral catheter is removed on day 3 or 4. The suprapubic catheter is clamped on postoperative day 10. Cystography is not usually necessary.

Bladder autoaugmentation

Cartwright and Snow in 1989 reported a technique which they named bladder autoaugmentation.[76] This procedure involves the excision of the detrusor muscle over the entire dome of the bladder, leaving the underlying bladder urothelium intact. A large epithelial 'bulge' is created, which functions by augmenting the storage capacity of the bladder; this is referred to as autoaugmentation.

Following initial studies in six dogs, this technique was extended to seven patients aged 4–17 years, all of whom had poorly compliant bladders as shown by pressure–flow urodynamic studies. Following excision of the dome detrusor muscle, the lateral margins of the detrusor were fixed bilaterally to the psoas muscles. The follow-up of patients was short. A subsequent report by these workers after studying a total of 19 patients concluded that, with a follow-up of between 3 months and 4 years, 80% of patients were continent and another 10% were significantly improved. A significant increase in bladder capacity of more than 50 ml occurred in only 40% of patients, with a minimal change in 35%; 25% actually had a decrease in capacity. The procedure was, however, accompanied by improved continence and reduced rates of hydronephrosis.[80]

In 12 paediatric patients with low-capacity bladders and demonstrable detrusor overactivity (aged 4–14 years, 10 with NBD), 6 months following autoaugmentation the mean increase in bladder capacity was 40%, with a 33% decrease in mean leak-point pressure.[77] Postoperative complications were minor. A modification of the previous technique was used, whereby a vesicomyotomy was used rather than vesicomyectomy, with no fixation of the bladder laterally to the psoas muscles. A subsequent preliminary report on five adult patients, with the follow-up ranging from 12 to 82 weeks, claimed an increase in bladder capacity varying from 40% up to 310%; this was measured at an intravesical pressure of 40 cmH$_2$O.

Stohrer and colleagues[78] reported a series of 29 patients aged 14–64 years (average age of 35 years). It was thought that 24 of these patients were likely to have NBD.[78,79] All patients underwent preoperative urodynamic evaluation. The technique reported by these authors is based on the original one described by Cartwright and Snow,[76] with an extraperitoneal approach, filling the bladder to 200–250 ml. A section of the detrusor around the urachus, 7–8 cm in diameter, is dissected completely and removed, leaving the mucosa intact. The detrusor is not fixed to the psoas muscle and all bands of detrusor overlying the urethelium are removed.

Follow-up data to 7 years show that whereas 50% of patients can void without significant residual, up to one-half require ISC. The authors found an improved compliance and increased capacity of 130–600 ml.

An alternative surgical approach that has been explored in case reports is laparoscopically assisted autoaugmentation, but no comment on this is possible in the absence of adequate numbers of patients and no significant follow-up.[80]

At present, although autoaugmentation has a number of attractive features, it is clear that the resultant increase in bladder capacity and reduction in detrusor overactivity are far less pronounced than those following augmentation cystoplasty. The number of cases reported in the literature is small, with relatively short follow-up. It is questionable whether the associated benefits adequately compensate for the limited long-term efficacy of the procedure; the search for less-invasive techniques therefore continues. Sacral neuromodulation has been found to have efficacy in some cases of detrusor overactivity associated with DI and NBD, acting via stimulation of sacral nerve roots and sacral neural outflow to the bladder. The technique offers an organ-preserving reversible alternative to cystoplasty.

Complications

It is recognized that spontaneous perforation of an augmentation cystoplasty bladder is a potential risk, occurring in up to 10% of cases. This may be due to high intravesical pressure,[81] and can usually be managed successfully by conservative measures.[82] Patients may be at even greater risk of perforation following autoaugmentation because of the thinness of the mucosa in the bulging 'diverticulum' produced by the operation. Evidence in support of this is provided by animal studies, where autoaugmentation resulted in higher risk of perforation at lower pressures than did augmentation cystoplasty.[83] To date, this complication has yet to be reported in clinical series, possibly because of ingrowth of fibrous tissue around the mucosal diverticulum with time, which may also account for the limited increase in capacity seen following the procedure. This phenomenon, if progressive, may limit the durability of this operation.

URINARY DIVERSION

Investigation

The majority of patients that present with the need for urinary augmentation and diversion are either those who have neurological dysfunction as a primary cause of their urinary abnormality or in whom previous surgical procedures have failed. Some of these patients will have undergone a number of operations that have failed to resolve incontinence or obstruction. The necessity to proceed to more major surgery will be guided by the need to provide continence (Table 59.1). Videourodynamic studies provide the most comprehensive information about bladder and urethral function and will also demonstrate the presence or absence of vesicoureteric reflux. If videourodynamics

Table 59.1. *Indications for urinary diversion*

Temporary

- Drainage of retention of urine
- Drainage of an obstructed upper urinary tract caused by ureteric obstruction (ligated ureter, cancer, retroperitoneal fibrosis, stone)

Permanent, where reconstructive surgery is not possible or not desired

- After cystectomy for bladder cancer or after pelvic exenteration
- For intractable incontinence
- After failed continent diversion and augmentation or substitution cystoplasty

are not available, simple cystometry with the added information from a separately performed cystometrogram (CMG) should be obtained. Each patient considered for bladder reconstruction should undergo a pressure study of the bladder. Information about the upper urinary tract must also be obtained. Although an ultrasound scan of the kidneys will provide useful information, intravenous urography should be performed to demonstrate the presence of normally functioning kidneys and the anatomy of ureteric drainage.

Urinary diversion in association with the repair of urogenital fistulae

Indications for bladder substitution

1. *Bladder and pelvic cancers.* In gynaecological practice the principal indications for bladder excision or substitution follow radical surgery for cervical cancer (81% of a series of 86 patients had cervical cancer).[84] Radical pelvic exenteration was possible in 55% of this series, with 12% undergoing palliative diversion. Other indications quoted for urinary diversion were urinary fistulae (19%), ureteric or urethral obstruction (7%), ureteric injury (1%) and overflow incontinence (2%). Female patients who require cystectomy for treatment of bladder cancer usually undergo ileal conduit urinary diversion. However, recent experience has demonstrated that orthotopic neobladders after cystectomy for transitional cell carcinoma of the bladder are successful in producing continence during both day and night.[85,86]

2. *Interstitial cystitis.* This rare and distressing condition affects women in middle age. The symptoms of urinary frequency, nocturia and pain cause severe debilitation. Medical therapy may palliate the symptoms but do not usually cure. Surgical therapy includes augmentation (controversial), bladder excision and substitution or cystectomy and urinary diversion.[87]

Surface urinary diversion has certain attractions, as the procedure is simpler to perform and the long-term complications are well recognized. For the obese, surgically difficult, or immobile patient, or for the patient in whom multiple procedures have failed or who cannot tolerate ISC, diversion is an attractive option. Undiversion may be used at a future time but is rarely necessary in this difficult patient group.

Most patients can be cured of their incontinence using one of the several procedures that have been described in the preceding chapters. However, there will always be a few patients who remain incontinent. Urinary diversion may be contemplated in these patients if they are sufficiently motivated to become continent again.

The simplest diversion is a catheter, preferably the long-term all-silicon suprapubic catheter. However, for patients who wish to avoid long-term catheterization or those who wish to have greater control of 'bladder-emptying', reconstructive diversion should be considered after appropriate counselling.

Ureterosigmoidostomy

The first record of a urinary diversion to the intestine was in 1852 when Simon[88] diverted the urine into the rectum in a patient with ectopia vesicae. Coffey described a technique for diversion of the ureters into the colon in 1911.[89] This form of urinary diversion, ureterosigmoidostomy, was the most popular method of urinary diversion until 1950. The surgical technique up to 1950 left a freely refluxing ureteric anastomosis which gave rise to the problems of infection, stenosis, obstruction and acid–base balance disorders. The tunnelled reimplantation of the ureters described by Leadbetter in 1950[90] allowed ureterosigmoidostomy to continue in clinical practice, although this technique rapidly became replaced by the ileal conduit urinary diversion, described in 1950 by Bricker.[91]

Ureterosigmoidostomy lost favour in many centres over the years in the western world and remained popular in others.[92] A recent resurgence in interest has taken place since the description of the Mainz 2 pouch (see Fig. 59.4). In countries where surface incontinent stoma are unpopular and where stoma care facilities are not readily available and long-term follow-up of patients is difficult, ureterosigmoidostomy still has a place. There are still patients who prefer this method of urinary diversion, which avoids a collecting device or the need for regular catheterization of a continent stoma. Those patients who wish to undergo ureterosigmoidostomy require good anal sphincter tone, which must be assessed before surgery. One effective way of assessing rectal continence is with the Weetabix test in which Weetabix in water (or porridge) is inserted into the rectum. Provided that patient selection is correct, surgical technique is meticulous and follow-up carefully supervised, the long-term results should be excellent. Stockle *et al.*[93] claimed that, of 46 children with bladder extrophy treated by ureterosigmoidostomy, '39 were alive with a functioning ureterosigmoidostomy after 14.7 years', with a continence rate of 92%. Of the 46 patients treated, 45 had normal renal function. Connor *et al.*[94] did not experience the same good results with ureterosigmoidostomy. Their review of 40 patients showed renal deterioration in 92% with unilateral nephrectomy necessary in 40%. More recently, Bissada *et al.*[92] have shown that short- to medium-term results with ureterosigmoidostomy are the same as those for an ileal conduit.[95]

Follow-up should take place every 3 months for a year and then yearly subsequently. A protocol for follow-up should be followed. The electrolytes should be measured and the urinary tract followed by a plain abdominal radiograph and renal ultrasound scan. A radionuclide scintigram at 3 months after surgery is valuable to demonstrate unobstructed renal function.

Apart from the general complications associated with abdominal surgery, few additional complications may be expected. Urinary fistulae, bowel obstruction, pyelonephritis and ureteric obstruction may occur in the early postoperative period, with an approximate overall rate of complications of 13%.

Regular long-term follow-up is necessary, as previously mentioned. Electrolyte disturbance is likely to be due to hyperchloraemic acidosis and is corrected by the use of sodium bicarbonate in a dose of 1–6 g daily. The acid–base balance should be checked regularly in order to assess the need for, and the appropriate dose of, bicarbonate. The majority of patients may be expected to need a bicarbonate supplement.

The incidence of neoplasia in association with ureterosigmoidoscopy is significantly higher than that in the general population, with a 8.5–10.5-fold increased risk.[96] Annual colonoscopic inspection of the sigmoid colon and ureteric anastomotic site is therefore necessary in all patients with ureterosigmoidostomies after 5 years have elapsed since the primary procedure.[93] The incidence of tumours at the anastomotic site is small; early diagnosis and treatment will avoid the development of bowel neoplasia and enable early treatment of any abnormality.

Mainz 2 pouch (Fig. 59.4)

The Mainz 2 pouch involves a detubularization of the sigmoid colon to enable low-pressure storage in a sigmo-rectum of larger capacity, and has become popular when ureterosigmoidostomy is contemplated.

Double-barrelled wet colostomy

For patients that undergo pelvic exenteration, a double-barrelled colostomy may be created to which the ureters are anastomosed. A single collection appliance is then necessary and may be an advantage for those patients who wish to avoid multiple stomata.[97]

Surface diversion (Fig. 59.5)

Patient preparation

The simple principles for preparation for diversion should apply, whether the patient is to undergo bladder augmentation or substitution, continent or incontinent.

Stomal siting

It is worth considering the important aspects of preparation of the patient for an incontinent stoma. The patient should be counselled prior to surgery. This is when an experienced stomatherapist is most valuable: the stomatherapist, together with the surgeon, will choose the stomal site according to the mobility, obesity, deformity and manual dexterity of the patient. The conduit should be brought out through the rectus muscle just at or below the level of the umbilicus. However, in the patient with a spinal deformity it may be

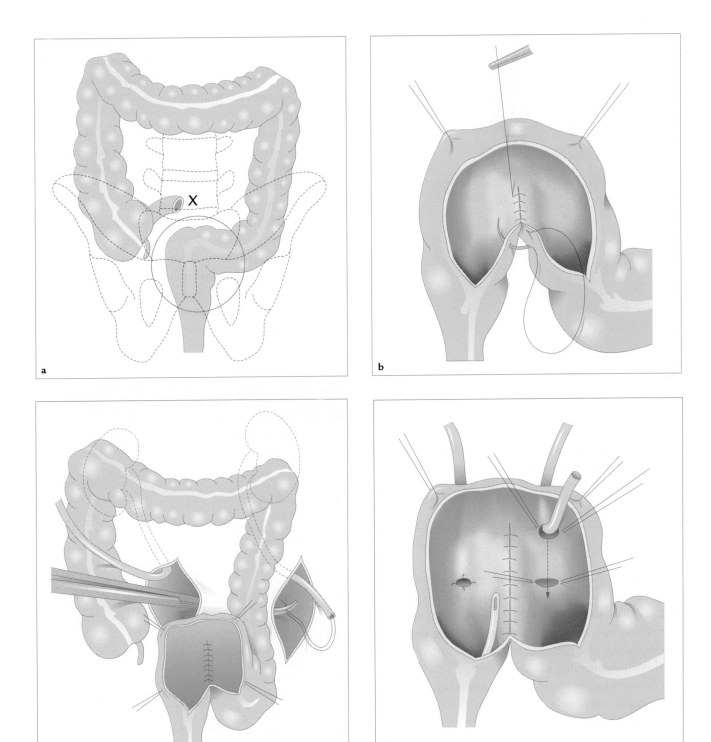

Figure 59.4. *Modified ureterosigmoidostomy (Mainz II pouch): (a) the area of the rectosigmoid junction is outlined. The X marks the later point of pouch fixation to the promontory; (b) a pouch plate is created by side-to-side anastomosis of the posterior wall by means of two running sutures; (c) the left ureter is pulled through to the right side retroperitoneally; (d) the ureters are implanted via a submucosal tunnel 3.5–4 cm in length using the Goodwin–Hohenfellner technique. (Continued overleaf.)*

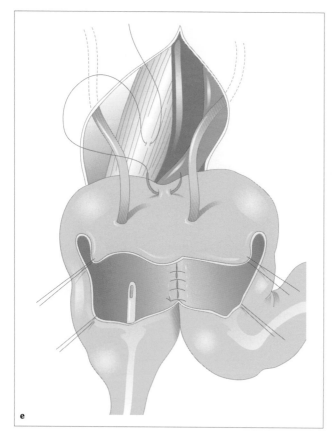

e

Figure 59.4. *Modified ureterosigmoidostomy (Mainz II pouch) (cont.): (e) pouch fixation to the anterior longitudinal cord in the area of the promontory without the risk of compromising the blood supply. Alternatively, the pouch may be fixed to the psoas muscle.*

necessary to site the stoma in the upper abdomen on any area of flat skin that will support a stoma appliance and which is accessible to the patient. A flat skin surface is very important, so that skin dimpling or irregularities do not give rise to later problems with adhesion of the urine-collecting devices.

The commonest bowel–urinary diversion procedure is the ileal conduit urinary diversion. The ileal conduit does not need to be very long, the length being determined by the size of the patient and level of abdominal wall thickness; however, 15–20 cm of ileum is usually adequate. Recently, interest has been shown in the minimally invasive creation of an ileal conduit, which has been achieved using a laparoscopic technique.[98]

Ileal conduit urinary diversion has provided effective urinary tract drainage for many patients in the 35 years since it was first introduced. Although it is a

major procedure, it is also relatively straightforward. Complications arising from the procedure are similar to those seen after surgery to the abdomen (Table 59.2).[99–111] Careful long-term follow-up is recommended for patients undergoing ileal conduit urinary diversion.

If urinary diversion is performed and the native bladder is left behind (as is the case in patients with neuropathic bladders), the bladder should not be ignored. There is a reported risk of bladder infection and the formation of pyocystitis in 20% of patients.[112] A surgically created vesicovaginal fistula for recurrent cystitis and pyocystitis helps the defunctioned bladder to drain if the urethra is competent. Later cystectomy may be necessary for the patient who becomes intermittently ill because of pyocystitis and may be performed through a Pfanenstiel incision with an extraperitoneal approach.

Table 59.2. *Late complications of urinary tract reconstruction and diversion[99–101]*
Bladder augmentation
• Urinary tract infection[99]
• Stones – upper urinary tract[102] and bladder
• Excess mucus
• Voiding dysfunction
• (Tumours)
• Hour-glass deformity
• Bladder rupture[103]
Conduits[104]
• Adhesive obstruction
• Urinary tract infection
• Stomal prolapse and stenosis[105]
• Mid-ileal stenosis[106]
• Metabolic acidosis
• Urinary tract stone disease
• Skin dermatitis
Continent diversion
• Stomal stenosis
• Prolapse of the continent nipple
• Ureteric obstruction and/or reflux
• Pouch stone formation
• Urinary leakage from pouch
• Metabolic complications – metabolic acidosis, renal tubular dysfunction and bone demineralization[107–111]
• Excess mucus production
• Urinary infection
• Pouch rupture

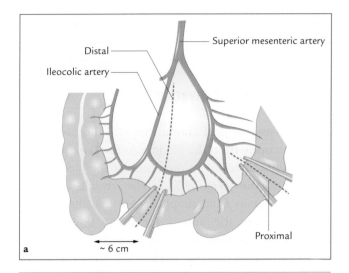

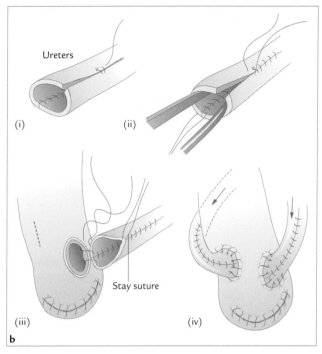

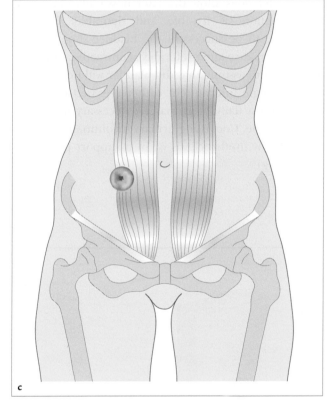

Figure 59.5. *(a) Isolation of the ileal conduit. Note the distal mesenteric incision in an avascular plane between the ileocolic and superior mesenteric arterial supplies, facilitating mobility of the distal end of the ileal segment; (b) Bricker procedure for uretero-ileal anastomosis. The spatulated ureter is anastomosed end-to-side to the proximal end of the ileal conduit using interrupted fine absorbable suture. The more frequent technique in the UK is the Wallace 66 in which the ureters are anastomused together side to side and then to the end of the ileum; (c) the ideal stoma site is to the right of the midline just medial to the border of the rectus and between the umbilicus and the anterior superior iliac spine.*

CONTINENT VESICOSTOMY

Continent vesicostomy (Fig. 59.6) is more suitable for long-term access to the bladder by means of intermittent catheterization using the Mitrofanoff principle, employing attachment of the appendix or other structure to the bladder for access by catheterization.[113] When appendix is not available, a continent tube can be made from the bladder (bladder tube Mitrofanoff) or from a segment of ileum, tailored either longitudinally or by means of the transverse tubularized technique.[114,115] This is very appropriate for the patient with an acontractile bladder who cannot (or does not wish to) perform urethral catheterization. Such a diversion is suitable for patients with disability that makes them unable to gain access to the urethra.

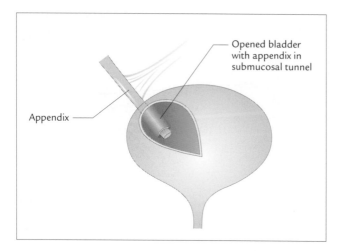

Figure 59.6. *Continent vesicostomy: the Mitrofanoff procedure. The appendix is separated from the caecum and is attached to the skin in the right iliac fossa or to the umbilicus, with or without bladder augmentation.*

NEPHROSTOMY AND PYELOSTOMY

Nephrostomy has an important place in relieving upper urinary tract obstruction for the temporary relief of ureteric obstruction after surgical obstruction, or where pelvic malignancy has led to renal failure due to ureteric obstruction.[116]

Pyelostomy is appropriate for the grossly dilated upper urinary tract only when urinary tract surgery is proposed in the future. Pyelostomy is preferred to ureterostomy, particularly if the pelvis is extrarenal and large. Pyelostomy affects neither the ureter nor its blood supply and does not preclude any further ureteric procedures, whereas ill-performed ureterostomy can make later reconstructive procedures very difficult. However, with the advent of percutaneous drainage of the upper urinary tract and the longevity of percutaneous stenting, open pyelostomy is very rarely necessary.

Ureterostomy

Cutaneous ureteric diversion is used for the treatment of ureteric obstruction when the ureters are dilated and may be adequately brought to the skin surface. There is very little place for ureterostomies, which have a tendency to stenose at skin level. However, in the rare case of dilated ureter(s) in a patient with inoperable malig-

nancy in the pelvis, where stents cannot be placed, ureterostomy(ies) may provide a solution for the remaining life and avoid the need for nephrostomies.

Bladder-to-surface diversion

An alternative to ileal conduit urinary diversion is to divert the urine from the bladder to the skin by means of a conduit attached to the dome of the bladder – a bladder chimney (Fig. 59.7).[117] The advantages of this procedure, apart from simplicity, are that the bladder is retained and the ureters remain in their normal position and are thus protected from the problems of reflux or obstruction (or both). The preservation of the bladder does allow the later possibility of urinary reconstruction, if feasible and desirable. For the procedure to be successful the bladder should be of good compliance and preferably acontractile. Although it is logical to assume that the bladder will not drain, it does. A single intermittent catheter passed down the conduit on a daily basis may be necessary if there is residual urine. Coexisting urinary incontinence may be corrected by urethrocleisis or by a support procedure (i.e. a sling).

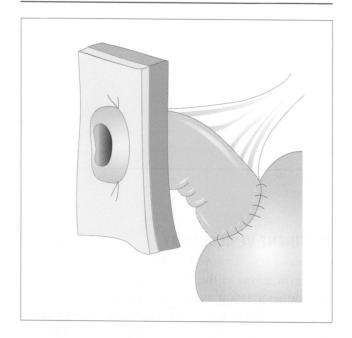

Figure 59.7. *Bladder chimney.*

Orthotopic neobladders

Reconstruction of the urinary tract after removal of the bladder for cancer or interstitial cystitis has become increasingly popular in women. Once the bladder has been removed and the urethra preserved to provide continence, the bladder may be reconstructed using the Kock principle with small bowel segments or by using detubularized large bowel (Fig. 59.8). Ileocaecocystoplasty is generally used for this purpose.[85,118–122] After cystectomy for transitional cell carcinoma, if the urethra is preserved for orthotopic reconstruction, in appropriately selected cases the risk of tumour in the remaining urethra is unlikely.[123]

Continent diversion

Provision of a continent catheterizable reservoir for the storage of urine is an attractive option for patients who are intractably incontinent and who wish to avoid surface urinary diversion. Many procedures are available for continent diversion (Table 59.3), all of which involve modification of the principle described by Kock (Fig. 59.9). The remaining bladder may be used as a base for bowel reconstruction (substitution cystoplasty), or a neobladder may be created from bowel segments independent from the bladder. The patient is able to catheterize the bowel pouch through a connection to the abdominal wall. This connection may be made via a continent port made from tailored bowel, or via the appendix which, in turn, is tunnelled into the pouch (Mitrofanoff principle) (Table 59.4). Continent diver-

Table 59.4. *Structures used to fashion the catheterization point*

Appendix*
Fallopian tube
Ureter
Labial tube reconstruction
Tailored ileum
Terminal ileum
Transverse tubularized ileum

sion involves more intricate and time-consuming surgery than surface diversion, although it is reported to be associated with a similar risk of complications.[124–126]

Bladder-neck and urethral closure

The patient with intractable urinary incontinence that is not resolved by suspension, injectables, urethrocleisis or artificial urinary sphincter – or where these options are neither applicable nor possible – should be offered urethral closure. The majority of patients that require urethral closure have neurological dysfunction as the primary cause of urethral incompetence, or have developed urethral damage as a consequence of an indwelling urethral catheter. Urethral closure via a vaginal approach carries a minimum surgical morbidity but has a lower success rate,[127–129] although it can be performed as a day-stay procedure. If the repair fails it can be repeated through the vaginal approach. Abdominal bladder-neck closure, although more effective,[130] can be difficult in the very obese bedridden patient with a catheter-related urethral injury. Bladder-neck closure is usually combined with the insertion of a suprapubic catheter for long-term bladder drainage. The Mitrofanoff principle, with or without augmentation, may be adopted in association with bladder-neck closure.

PREGNANCY AFTER AUGMENTATION AND DIVERSION

There are a number of reports of successful pregnancy after diversionary surgery. There is no need to counsel against pregnancy in young women who have undergone urinary tract reconstruction. Urinary tract infection should be kept under control. Bladder emptying should be ensured and the upper urinary tracts surveyed by ultrasonography. Successful vaginal delivery

Table 59.3. *Types of continent neobladder reconstruction*

Chosen bowel segment	Neobladder
Stomach	Gastric neobladder
Ileum	Kock pouch and its various modifications (Camey, Hautmann, Studer, Stanford, Le Duc
Right colon	Caecal reservoir or detubularized ileocaecocystoplasty
Sigmoid colon	Sigma–rectum pouch – Mainz 2 Modified rectal bladder – Ghoneim

Variations on theme: Mainz pouch, Indiana pouch, Ileocolonic 'Le Bag'

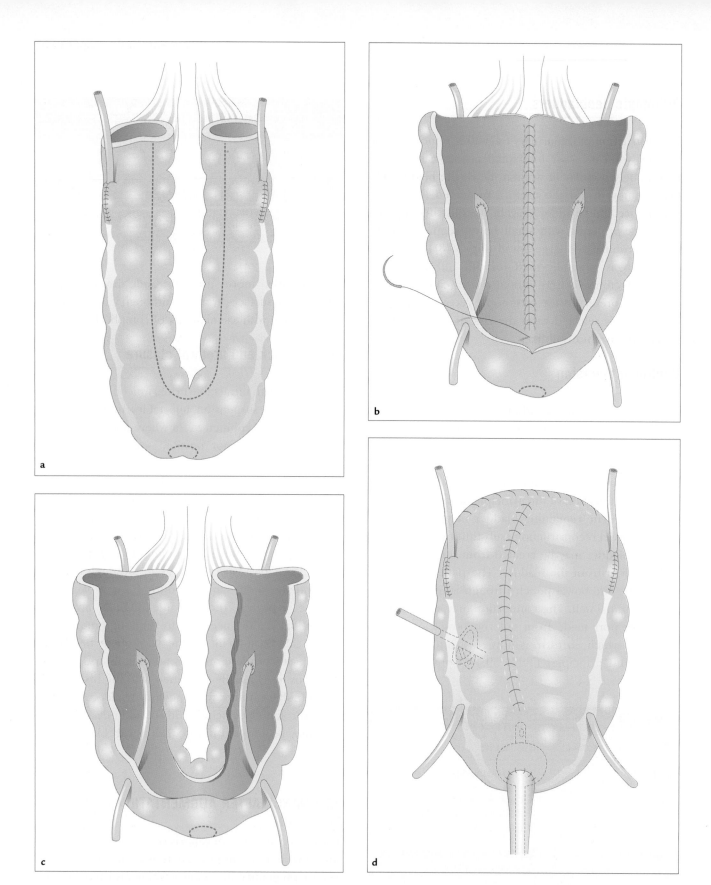

Figure 59.8. *Orthotopic neobladder. (a) The colon segment is placed in a U-shaped configuration. The most dependent part is marked for anastomosis to the urethra. The urethral reimplantation is anterior along the lateral tenia. The dashed line indicates the incision to detubularize the segment. (b) The reservoir is constructed by approximating the posterior edges and anterior edges separately. The ureters have been reimplanted posteriorly and intubated with feeding tubes exiting the reservoir anteriorly. (c) The neobladder viewed from within to demonstrate the reimplanted ureters intubated by infant feeding tubes. (d) The completed neobladder with antirefluxing ureteral anastomosis intubated with infant feeding tubes exiting interiorly; both a urethral catheter and a Malecot catheter drain the neobladder.*

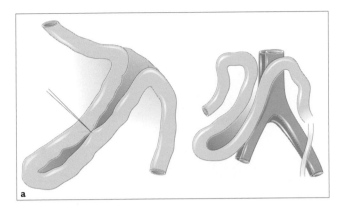

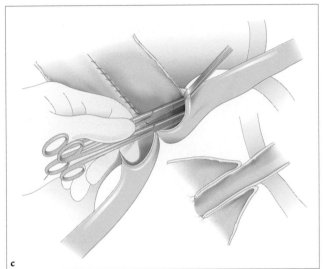

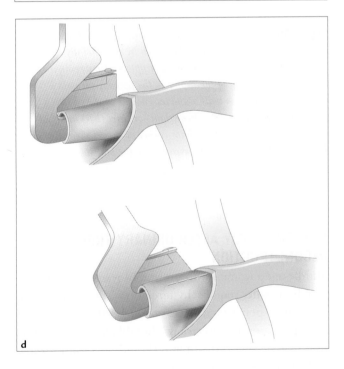

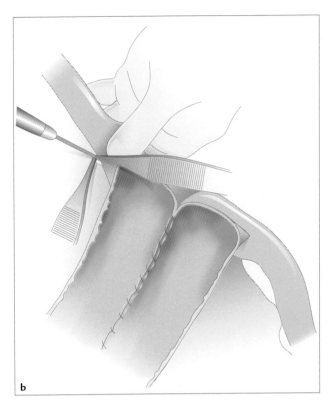

Figure 59.9. *Continent diversion. (a) The reservoir segment is isolated in the right lower quadrant in a U-shape and the serosal walls of the 22 cm segments are approximated with running 3/0 polyglycolic acid (PGA) sutures approximately 1 cm away from the mesenteric attachment to the bowel. The bowel is opened adjacent to this suture line to allow watertight closure of the back wall. (b) The windows of Deaver are made by dividing the mesentery of the ileum proximal and distal to the pouch for 7–8 cm. After two or three vascular arcades are spared, another small mesenteric opening is made to accommodate the PGA mesh that will act as the anchoring collar at the base of the nipple. (c) The nipple valves are intussuscepted into the reservoir lumen with Allis clamps. A third Allis clamp on the cut edge of the ileum provides countertraction. (d) Two rows of staples are placed in the anterior 180 degrees of the nipple lying in the lumen of the reservoir, taking care to use the entire length of the stapler for nipple construction. (Continued overleaf.)*

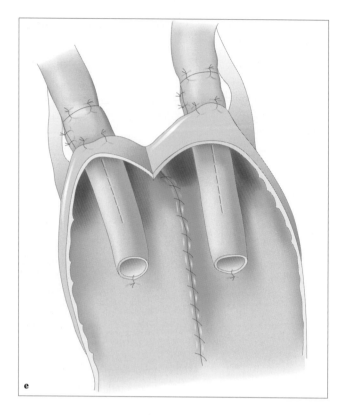

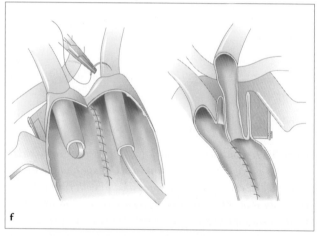

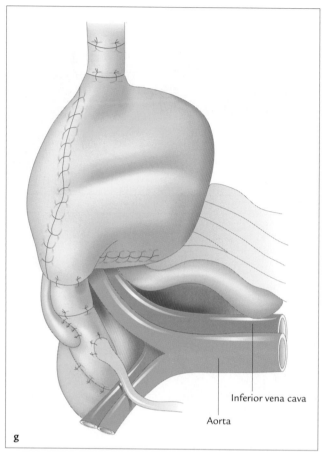

Figure 59.9. *Continent diversion (cont.): (e) The finished nipples are further secured to the pouch by superficially cauterizing the mucosa of opposing nipple and reservoir surfaces and suturing the tip of the nipple to the pouch wall with 2/0 chromic. (f) The back wall of the reservoir is attached to the nipple incorporating either two (right) or three (left) layers of bowel wall. (g) The right inferior corner of the reservoir is invaginated medial to its mesentery into the pouch.*

has taken place after urinary reconstruction and diversion. If necessary, caesarean section should be performed as an elective procedure. The mesentery of the bowel reconstruction must be carefully avoided, as its division may give rise to necrosis of the bowel segment. The obstetrician should enlist the assistance of the urologist responsible for initial care.[131]

HYSTERECTOMY AFTER URINARY TRACT RECONSTRUCTION

Middle-aged women with uterine fibroids or menstrual problems who require hysterectomy should have the procedure performed in association with any bladder surgery. Later hysterectomy after bladder reconstruction may be very difficult and should be a joint urological/gynaecological procedure.

QUALITY OF LIFE AFTER URINARY DIVERSION AND RECONSTRUCTION

There is increasing evidence from validated questionnaire surveys[132-134] that quality of life is substantially improved following urinary diversion, whether this is by a continent or an incontinent stoma.[135] Bladder substitution has appeared to improve quality of life more effectively than surface urinary diversion, although the differences were not found to be substantial.[133] Problems with the skin around the stoma are prevalent in incontinent stoma, affecting 37% of patients.[136]

REFERENCES

1. Daly JW, Higgins KA. Injury to the ureter during gynaecological surgical procedures. *Surg Gynecol Obstet* 1988; 167: 19–22

2. Goodno JA, Powers TW, Harris VD. Ureteral injury in gynecology surgery. A ten year review in a community hospital. *Am J Obstet Gynecol* 1995; 172: 1817–1820

3. Amirikia H, Evans TN. Ten year review of hysterectomies: trends, indications, risks. *Am J Obstet Gynecol.* 1979; 134: 431–434

4. Newell QU. Injury to the ureters during pelvic operations. *Ann Surg* 1939; 109: 981–986

5. Benson RC, Hinman F. Urinary tract injuries in obstetrics and gynaecology. *Am J Obstet Gynecol* 1956; 70: 467–485

6. St Martin EC, Trichel BE, Campbell JH, Locke CH. Ureteral injuries in gynaecologic surgery. *J Urol* 1953; 70: 51–57

7. Solomons E, Levin EJ, Bauman J, Baron J. A pyelographic study of ureteric injuries sustained during hysterectomy for benign conditions. *Surg Gynecol Obstet* 1960; 111: 41–48

8. Gangai MP, Agee RE, Spence CR. Surgical injury to ureter. *Urology* 1976; 8: 22–27

9. Mattsson T. Frequency and management of urological and some other complications following radical surgery for carcinoma of the cervix uteri, stages I and II. *Acta Obstet Gynecol Scandinavia* 1975; 54: 271–280

10. Underwood PB, Wilson WC, Kreutner A *et al.* Radical hysterectomy: a critical review of twenty-two years' experience. *Am J Obstet Gynecol* 1979; 134: 889–898

11. Thompson JD. Operative injuries to the ureter: prevention, recognition and management. In: Gershenson DM, Decherney AH, Curry SL (eds) *Te Linde's Operative Gynecology.* 7th edn. Philadelphia: Lippincott, 1992; 749–783

12. Lezin MA, Stoller ML. Surgical ureteral injuries. *Urology* 1991; 38: 497–506

13. Spence HM, Boone T. Surgical injuries to the ureter. *J Am Med Assoc* 1961; 176: 1070

14. Trigaux JP, Decoene B, Van Beers B. Focal necrosis of the ureter following CT-guided chemical sympathectomy. *Cardiovasc Intervent Radiol* 1992; 15: 180–182

15. Meyer NL, Lipscomb GH, Ling FW. Ureteral injury during elective pregnancy termination. A case report. *J Reprod Med* 1994; 39: 743–746

16. Altin MA, Gundogdu ZH. Ureteral injury due to Kirschner wire in a five year-old girl. A case report. *Turk J Pediatr* 1994; 36: 77–79

17. Assimos DG, Patterson LC, Taylor CL. Changing incidence and etiology of iatrogenic ureteral injuries. *J Urol* 1994; 152: 2240–2246

18. Selzman AA, Spirnak JP. Iatrogenic ureteral injuries: a 20 year experience in treating 165 injuries. *J Urol* 1996; 155: 878–881

19. Brandes SB, Chelsky MJ, Buckman RF, Hanno PM. Ureteral injuries from penetrating trauma. *J Trauma* 1994; 36: 766–769

20. Presti JC, Carroll PR, McAninch JW. Ureteral and renal pelvic injuries from external trauma: diagnosis and treatment. *J Trauma* 1989; 29: 370–374

21. Campbell EW, Filderman PS, Jacobs SC. Ureteral injury due to blunt and penetrating trauma. *Urology* 1992; 40: 216–220

22. Brady LW. Ureteral injury as a consequence of radiation treatment. In: Bergman H (ed) *The Ureter.* New York: Springer-Verlag, 1981; 421–426

23. Witters S, Cornelissen M, Vereecken R. Iatrogenic ureteral injury: aggressive or conservative treatment. *Am J Obstet Gynecol* 1986; 155: 582–584

24. Dowling RA, Corriere JN, Sandler CM. Iatrogenic ureteral injury. *J Urol* 1986; 135: 912–915

25. Hoch WH, Kursh ED, Persky L. Early, aggressive management of intraoperative ureteral injuries. *J Urol* 1975; 114: 530–532

26. Badenoch DF, Tiptaft RC, Fowler CG, Blandy JP. Early repair of accidental injury to the ureter or bladder following gynaecological surgery. *Br J Urol* 1987; 59: 516–518

27. Higgins CC. Ureteral injuries. *J Am Med Assoc* 1967; 199: 82–88

28. Zinman LM, Libertino JA, Roth RA. Management of operative ureteral injury. *Urology* 1978; 12: 290–303

29. Walker JA. Injuries of the ureter due to external violence. *J Urol* 1969; 102: 410

30. Bright TC, Peters PC. Ureteral injuries due to external violence: 10 years experience with 59 cases. *J Trauma* 1977; 17: 616–620

31. Flynn JT, Tiptaft RC, Woodhouse CRJ *et al.* The early and aggressive repair of iatrogenic ureteric injuries. *Br J Urol* 1979; 51: 454–457

32. Guerriero WG. Ureteral injury. *Urol Clin North Am* 1989; 16: 237–248

33. Larson DM, Malone JM, Copeland LJ *et al.* Ureteral assessment after radical hysterectomy. *Obstet Gynecol* 1987; 69: 612–616

34. Piscitelli JT, Simel DL, Addison WA. Who should have intravenous pyelograms before hysterectomy for benign disease? *Obstet Gynecol* 1987; 69: 541–545

35. Weinberg JJ, Ansong K, Smith AD. Complications of ureteroscopy in relation to experience: report of survey and author experience. *J Urol* 1987; 137: 384–385

36. Fry DE, Milholen L, Harbrecht PJ. Iatrogenic ureteral injury. *Arch Surg* 1983; 118: 454–457

37. Cormio L, Battaglia M, Traficante A, Selvaggi FP. Endourological treatment of ureteric injuries. *Br J Urol* 1993; 72: 165–168

38. Lask D, Abarbanel J, Luttwak Z *et al.* Changing trends in the management of iatrogenic ureteral injuries. *J Urol* 1995; 154: 1693–1695

39. Belande G. Early treatment of ureteral injuries found after gynaecological surgery. *J Urol* 1977; 118: 25–27

40. Blandy JP, Badenoch DF, Fowler CG *et al.* Early repair of iatrogenic injury to the ureter or bladder after gynaecological surgery. *J Urol* 1991; 146: 761–765

41. Turner-Warwick RT, Worth PHL. The psoas bladder hitch procedure for the replacement of the lower third of the ureter. *Br J Urol* 1969; 41: 701

42. Spies JW, Johnson CE, Wilson CS. Reconstruction of the ureter by means of bladder flaps. *Proc Soc Exp Biol Med* 1933; 30: 425

43. Ockerblad NF. Reimplantation of the ureter into the bladder by a flap method. *J Urol* 1947; 57: 845

44. Benson MC, Ring KS, Olsson CA. Ureteral reconstruction and bypass: experience with ileal interposition, Boari flap–psoas hitch and autotransplantation. *J Urol* 1990; 143: 20–23

45. Hodges CV, Barry JM, Fuchs EF *et al.* Transureteroureterostomy: 25 year experience with 100 patients. *J Urol* 1980; 123: 834–838

46. Hendren WH, Hensle TW. Transureteroureterostomy: experience with 75 cases. *J Urol* 1980; 123: 826–833

47. Bodie B, Novick AC, Rose M, Straffon RA. Long-term results with renal autotransplantation for ureteral replacement. *J Urol* 1986; 136: 1187–1189

48. Thorne ID, Resnic MI. The use of bowel in urologic surgery: a historical perspective. *Urol Clin North Am* 1986; 13: 179–191

49. Boxer RJ, Fritzsche P, Skinner DG *et al.* Replacement of the ureter by small intestine: clinical application and results of the ileal ureter in 89 patients. *J Urol* 1979; 121: 728–731

50. Mesrobian HG, Azizkhan RG. Pyeloureterostomy with appendiceal interposition. *J Urol* 1989; 142: 1288–1289

51. Bramble FJ. The treatment of adult enuresis and urge incontinence by enterocystoplasty. *Br J Urol* 1992; 54: 693–696

52. Cartwright PC, Snow BW. Bladder autoaugmentation: early clinical experience. *J Urol* 1989; 142: 505–507

53. Schmidt RA. Advances in genitourinary neurostimulation. *Neurosurgery* 1986; 18: 1041–1044

54. Marshall CJ. Persistent adult bed-wetting treated by sacral neurectomy. *Br Med J* 1954; 1: 308–311

55. Ingleman Sundberg A. Partial denervation of the bladder. A new operation for the treatment of urge incontinence and similar conditions in women. *Acta Obstet Gynecol Scand* 1959; 38: 487–502

56. Worth PHL, Turner-Warwick RT. The treatment of interstitial cystitis by cystolysis with observations on cystoplasty. *Br J Urol* 1973; 45: 65–71

57. Ewing R, Bultitude MI, Shuttleworth KE. Subtrigonal phenol injection for incontinence in female patients with multiple sclerosis. *Lancet* 1983; 11: 1304–1306

58. Smith JC, Higson RH. Cystodistension. In: Smith JC, Higson RH, Stanton SL, Tanagho EA (eds) *Surgery of Female Incontinence*. Berlin: Springer Verlag, 1980; 99–109

59. Bramble FJ. The treatment of adult enuresis and urge incontinence by enterocystoplasty. *Br J Urol* 1982; 54: 693–696

60. Mundy AR, Stephenson TP. 'Clam' ileocystoplasty for the treatment of refractory urge incontinence. *Br J Urol* 1985; 57: 641–646

61. Lewis DK, Morgan JR, Weston PT, Stephenson TP. The 'clam': indications and complications. *Br J Urol* 1990; 65: 488–491

62. George VK, Russell GL, Shutt A *et al.* Clam ileocystoplasty. *Br J Urol* 1987; 60: 523–525

63. Pengelly A. Effect of prolonged bladder distension on detrusor function. *Urol Clin North Am* 1979; 6: 279–281

64. Rosenbaum TP, Shah PJR, Worth PHL. Trans-trigonal phenol failed the test of time. *Br J Urol* 1990; 66: 164–169

65. Rodomski SB, Herschorn S, Stone AR. Urodynamic comparison of ileum vs augmentation cystoplasty for neurogenic bladder dysfunction. *Neurourol Urodynam*, 1995 14: 231–237

66. Keating MA, Ludlow JK, Rich MA. Enterocystoplasty: the star modification. *J Urol* 1996; 155: 1723–1725

67. Weinberg AC, Boyd SD, Lieskovsky G *et al*. The hemi-Kock ileocystoplasty: a low pressure anti-refluxing system. *J Urol* 1988; 140: 1380–1384

68. Mundy AR, Stephenson TP. 'Clam' ileocystoplasty for the treatment of refractory urge incontinence. *Br J Urol* 1985; 57: 641–646

69. Woodhouse CRJ. Reconstruction of the lower urinary tract for neurogenic bladder: lessons from the adolescent age group. *Br J Urol* 1992; 69: 589–593

70. Krishna A, Gough DC, Fishwick J, Bruce J. Ileocystoplasty in children: assessing safety and success. *Eur Urol* 1995; 27: 62–66

71. Singh G, Thomas DG. Enteroplasty in neuropathic bladder. *Neurourol Urodyn* 1995; 14: 5–10

72. Flood HD, Malhotra SJ, O'Connell HF *et al*. Long-term results and complications using augmentation cystoplasty in reconstructive urology. *Neurourol Urodyn* 1995; 14: 297–309

73. Hasan ST, Marshall C, Robson WA, Neal DE. Clinical outcome and quality of life following enterocystoplasty for idiopathic detrusor instability and neurogenic bladder dysfunction. *Br J Urol* 1995; 76: 551–557

74. Barrington JW, Fern-Davies H, Adams RJ *et al*. Bile acid dysfunction after clam enterocystoplasty. *Br J Urol* 1995; 76: 169–171

75. Barrington JW, Fulford S, Griffiths D. Pro-mutagenic methylation damage and repair in bladder and bowel DNA following clam enterocystoplasty. *J Urol* 1997; 157: 254

76. Cartwright PC, Snow BW. Bladder autoaugmentation. *Urol Clin North Am* 1992; 23: 323–331

77. Stothers L, Johnson H, Arnold W *et al*. Bladder autoaugmentation by vesicomyotomy in the pediatric neurogenic bladder. *Urology* 1994; 44: 110–113

78. Stohrer M, Kramer A, Goepel M *et al*. Bladder auto-augmentation – an alternative for enterocystoplasty: preliminary results. *Neurourol Urodyn* 1995; 14: 11–23

79. Kramer G, Stohrer M. Neurourology. *Curr Opin Urol* 1996; 6: 176–183

80. McDougall EM, Clayman RV, Figenshaw RS, Pearle MS. Laparoscopic retropubic auto-augmentation of the bladder. *J Urol* 1995; 153: 123–126

81. Anderson PAM, Rickwood AMK. Detrusor hyper-reflexia as factor in spontaneous perforation of augmentation cystoplasty for neuropathic bladder. *Br J Urol* 1991; 67: 210–212

82. Slaton JW, Kropp KA. Conservative management of suspected bladder rupture after augmentation enterocystoplasty. *J Urol* 1994; 152: 713–715

83. Rivas DA, Chancellor MB, Huang B *et al*. Comparison of bladder rupture pressure after intestinal bladder augmentation (ileocystoplasty) and myomyotomy (autoaugmentation). *Urology* 1996; 48: 40–46

84. Segreti EM, Morris M, Levenback C *et al*. Transverse colon urinary diversion in gynecologic oncology. *Gynecol Oncol* 1996; 63: 66–70

85. Stein JP, Stenzl A, Grossfield GD *et al*. The use of orthotopic neobladders in women undergoing cystectomy for pelvic malignancy. *World J Urol* 1996; 14: 9–14

86. Stenzl A, Colleselli K, Poisel S *et al*. The use of neobladders in women undergoing cystectomy for transitional cell cancer. *World J Urol* 1996; 14: 15–21

87. Thompson AC, Christmas TJ. Interstitial cystitis – an update. *Br J Urol* 1996; 78: 813–820

88. Simon J. Ectopic vesical operation for diverting the orifices of the ureters into the rectum: temporary success: subsequent death: autopsy (abstr) *Lancet* 1852; 2: 568

89. Coffey RC. Physiological implantation of the severed ureter or common bile duct into the intestine. *J Am Med Assoc* 1911; 56: 397

90. Leadbetter WF. Considerations of the problems incident to the performance of uretero-enterostomy – a report of a technique. *Trans Am Assoc Genitourin Surg* 1950; 42: 39

91. Bricker EM. Bladder substitution after pelvic evisceration. *Gynecol Obstet* 1950; 30: 1511

92. Bissada NK, Morcos RR, Morgan WM, Hanash KA. Ureterosigmoidostomy: is it a viable procedure in the age of continent urinary diversion and bladder substitution? *J Urol* 1995; 153: 1439–1440

93. Stockle M, Becht E, Voges G *et al*. Ureterosigmoidostomy: an outdated approach to bladder extrophy? *J Urol* 1990; 143: 770

94. Connor JP, Hensle TW, Lattimer JK, Burbige K. Long-term follow up of 207 patients with bladder exstrophy: an evolution in treatment. *J Urol* 1989; 142: 793–795

95. Bazeed M, Nabeeh A, el-Kenaway M, Ashmallan A. Urovaginal fistulae: 20 years experience. *Eur Urol* 1995; 27: 34–38

96. Kalbe T, Tricker AR, Freidl P. Ureterosigmoidostomy: long-term results, risk of carcinoma and aetiological factors for carcinogenesis. *J Urol* 1990; 145: 1110

97. Takada H, Yoshioka K, Boku T *et al.* Double-barrelled wet colostomy. A simple method of urinary diversion for patients undergoing pelvic exenteration. *Dis Colon Rectum* 1995; 38: 1235–1236

98. Vara-Thorbeck C, Sanchez de Badajoz E. Laparoscopic ileal conduit. *Surg Endosc* 1994; 8: 114–115

99. Ackerlund S, Campanello M, Kaijser B, Jonsson O. Bacteriuria in patients with a continent ileal reservoir for urinary diversion does not regularly require antibiotic treatment. *Br J Urol* 1994; 74: 177–181

100. Okada Y, Shichiri Y, Terai A *et al.* Management of late complications of continent urinary diversion using the Kock pouch and the Indiana pouch procedures. *Int J Urol* 1996; 77: 334–339

101. Nurse DE, McInerney PD, Thomas PJ, Mundy AR. Stones in enterocystoplasties. *Br J Urol* 1996; 77: 684–687

102. Cohen TD, Streem SB, Lammert G. Long-term incidence and risks for recurrent stones following contemporary management of upper urinary tract calculi in patients with a urinary diversion. *J Urol* 1996; 155: 69–70

103. Chancellor MB, Rivas DA, Bourgeois IM. Laplace's law and the risks and prevention of bladder rupture after enterocystoplasty and bladder autoaugmentation. *Neurourol Urodyn* 1996; 15: 223–233

104. Cheung MT. Complications of abdominal stoma: an analysis of 322 stomas. *Aust N Z J Surg* 1995; 65: 808–811

105. Khoury AE, Van Savage JG, McLorie GA, Churchill BM. Minimising stomal stenosis in appendicovesicostomy using the modified umbilical stoma. *J Urol* 1996; 155: 2050–2051

106. Shandera KC, Thompson IM, Wong RW, Cossi AF. Delayed development of mid-ileal conduit stenosis: the importance of life-long urologic follow-up. *South Med J* 1998; 88: 1118–1120

107. Kristjansson A, Grubb A, Mansson W. Renal tubular dysfunction after urinary diversion. *Scand J Urol Nephrol* 1995; 29: 407–412

108. Pannek J, Haupt G, Schulze H, Senge T. Influence of continent ileal urinary diversion on vitamin B12 absorption. *J Urol* 1996; 155: 1206–1208

109. Davidsson T, Lindergard B, Mansson W. Long-term metabolic and nutritional effects of urinary diversion. *Urology* 1995; 46; 804–809

110. Davidsson T, Lindergard B, Obrant K, Mansson W. Long-term metabolic effects of urinary diversion on skeletal bone; histomorphometric and mineralogic analysis. *Urology* 1995; 46: 804–809

111. Campanello A, Herlitz H, Lindstedt G *et al.* Bone mineral and related biochemical variables in patients with Koch ileal reservoir or Bricker conduit for urinary diversion. *J Urol* 1996; 155: 1209–1213

112. Granados EA, Salvador J, Vicente J, Villavicencio H. Follow-up of the remaining bladder after supravesical urinary diversion. *Eur Urol* 1996; 29: 308–311

113. Woodhouse CRJ. The Mitrofanoff Principle for continent urinary diversion. *World J Urol* 1996; 14: 99–104

114. Monti PR, Lara RC, Dutra MA, de Carvalho JR. New techniques for construction of efferent conduits based on the Mitrofanoff principle. *Urology* 1997; 49: 112–115

115. Gerharz EW, Tassadaq T, Pickard RS *et al.* Transverse retubularised ileum: early clinical experience with a new second line Mitrofanoff tube. *J Urol* 1998; 159: 525–528

116. Hyppolite JC, Daniels ID, Friedman EA. Obstructive uropathy in gynaecological malignancy. Detrimental effect of intraureteral stent placement and value of percutaneous nephrostomy. *ASAIO Trans* 1995; 41: 318–323

117. Rivas DA, Karasick S, Chancellor MB. Cutaneous ileocystostomy (a bladder chimney) for the treatment of severe neurogenic vesical dysfunction. *Paraplegia* 1995; 33: 530–535

118. Smith AY, Borden T. Excisional plication of the ileocaecal valve: a useful adjunct for the construction of continent urinary diversions. *J Urol* 1996; 156: 1118–1119

119. Davidsson T, Hedlund H, Mansson W. Detubularised right colonic reservoir with intussuscepted ileal nipple valve or stapled ileal ('Lundiana') outlet. Clinical and urodynamic results in a prospective randomised study. *World J Urol* 1996; 14: 78–84

120. Elmajian DA, Stein JP, Skinner DG. Orthotopic urinary diversion: the Koch ileal neobladder. *World J Urol* 1996; 14: 40–46

121. Boyd SD, Skinner E, Liesokovsky G, Skinner DG. Continent and orthotopic urinary diversion following radical cystectomy. Should these reconstructive procedures now be considered standard of care? *Surg Oncol Clin North Am* 1995; 4: 277–286

122. Barre PH, Herve JM, Botto H, Camey M. Update on the Camey II procedure. *World J Urol* 1996; 14: 27–28

123. Stenzl A, Draxl H, Posch B *et al.* The risk of urethral tumours in female bladder cancer: can the urethra be used for orthotopic reconstruction of the lower urinary tract? *J Urol* 1995; 153: 950–955

124. Carr LK, Webster GD. Koch versus right colon continent urinary diversion: comparison of outcome and reoperation rate. *Urology* 1996; 48: 711–714

125. Lampel A, Fisch M, Stein R *et al.* Continent diversion with the Mainz pouch. *World J Urol* 1996; 14: 85–91

126. Rowland RG. Present experience with the Indiana pouch. *World J Urol* 1996; 14: 92–98

127. Andrews HO, Shah PJR. Surgical management of urethral damage in neurologically impaired female patients with chronic indwelling catheters. *Br J Urol* 1998; 82: 820–824

128. Eckford SB, Kohler-Ockmore J, Feneley RC. Long-term follow-up of transvaginal urethral closure and suprapubic cystostomy for urinary incontinence in women with multiple sclerosis. *Br J Urol* 1994; 74: 319–321

129. Levy JB, Jacobs JA, Wein AJ. Combined abdominal and vaginal approach for bladder neck closure and permanent suprapubic tube: urinary diversion in the neurologically impaired woman. *J Urol* 1994; 152: 2081–2082

130. Hensle TW, Kirsch AJ, Kennedy WA, Reiley EA. Bladder neck closure in association with continent urinary diversion. *J Urol* 1995; 154: 883–885

131. Voges GE, Orestano L, Schumacher S, Hohenfellner R. Continent urinary diversion and pregnancy. *Geburtshilfe Frauenheilkd* 1995; 55: 711–715

132. Moreno JG, Chancellor MB, Karasick S *et al.* Improved quality of life and sexuality with continent urinary diversion in quadriplegic women with umbilical stoma. *Arch Phys Med Rehabil* 1995; 76: 758–762

133. Bjerre BD, Johansen C, Steven K. Health related quality of life after urinary diversion: continent diversion with the Kock pouch compared with the ileal conduit. *Scand J Urol Nephrol* 1994; 157: 113–118

134. Schurmans JR, Weerman PC, Bosch JL *et al.* Quality of life assessment in heterotopic and orthotopic neobladder construction: a comparison. *Acta Urol Belg* 1995; 63: 55–58

135. Castagnola C, Marechal JM, Hanauer MT *et al.* Quality of life and skin diversions. Results of a questionnaire completed by 73 patients. *Prog Urol* 1996; 6: 207–216

136. Momose H, Hirao Y, Tanaka N *et al.* Complications and quality of life in patients with ileal conduit. *Hinyokika Kiyo* 1995; 41: 927–935

60

Gynaecological developmental anomalies

K. Edmonds

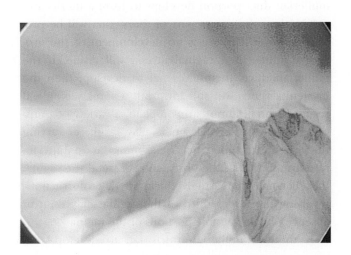

INTRODUCTION

The relationship between the development of the urological tract and the gynaecological organs is well described. This needs to be understood clearly prior to understanding the aetiology of these linked abnormalities. A summary of the embryology is included here to remind the reader of this important area of study, but greater detail can be found in chapters 9 and 10. It is imperative that clinicians, particularly when dealing with teenagers, have a clear and exact understanding of the abnormalities with which they are dealing. Failure to achieve this means that the clinician will ill-advise a patient or her parents; such misinformation may lead to very great difficulties in coping with the psychological side effects that are associated with these problems.

The embryology of the female genital tract

The müllerian ducts fuse at their lower parts and extend caudally to reach the urogenital sinus by week 9 of gestation. The lower end of this duct is solid and forms the müllerian tubercle; this does not open into the urogenital sinus but makes contact with the sinovaginal bulbs, which are solid protuberances of the sinus. As the hind part of the fetus unfolds, so the sinus and the müllerian tubercle become increasingly distanced from the müllerian ducts. A solid epithelial plate develops, which will subsequently become the vagina. This solid piece of tissue then develops lacunae and these gradually fuse to canalize the vagina. It is believed that most of the upper vagina develops from the müllerian structures and the lower part arises from the urogenital sinus. Canalization of the vagina is usually complete by around 20 weeks of gestation. If the müllerian duct portion develops to form a uterus and cervix, then the upper part of the vagina will be present; however, if there is no development of the urogenital sinus, then vaginal atresia will ensue. If the müllerian ducts themselves fail to develop, then the urogenital sinus will still form but a short vagina will result. If canalization is incomplete, a variety of transverse septae or sagittal septae may result, of varying thickness. Such septae may be as minor as an imperforate hymen but, as the obstructions ascend the vagina, they become increasingly thick, so that obstructions involving the upper third of the vagina may result in absence of considerable portions of the vagina.

If the two müllerian ducts fail to develop and, therefore, there is incomplete fusion, the uterus itself will develop as two halves with two cervices and two vaginas; this condition is known as uterus didelphus.

The external genitalia develop from the genital ridge, the genital tubercle giving rise to the clitoris, the genital folds to the labia minora and the genital swellings to the labia majora. More detailed embryology can be found in chapters 9 and 10. The intimate relationship between the development of the urological tract and the gynaecological system means that there are occasions when defects in the development of one system are closely associated with defects in the other.

ABNORMAL DEVELOPMENT OF THE VAGINA

When defects of vaginal development occur they do so in one of three ways. The classification that is used is as follows:

1. Congenital absence of the vagina (the Mayer–Rokitanksy–Kuster–Hauser syndrome) (Figs 60.1, 60.2);
2. Disorders of lateral fusion (Figs 60.3, 60.4);
3. Disorders of vertical fusion (Fig. 60.5).

Vaginal abnormalities, particularly those with congenital absence of the vagina, have been very rarely reported in siblings.[1] There is only one report of monozygotic twins with one child affected.[2] It is extremely unlikely that simple inheritance is the

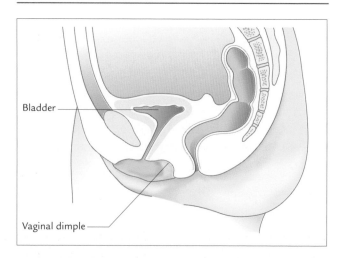

Figure 60.1. *Congenital absence of the uterus and vagina.*

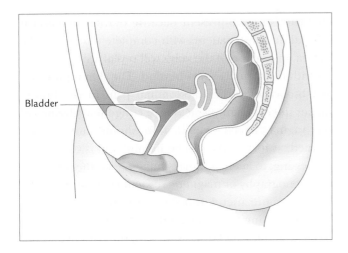

Figure 60.2. *Congenital absence of the vagina, with rudimentary uterus or functional uterus.*

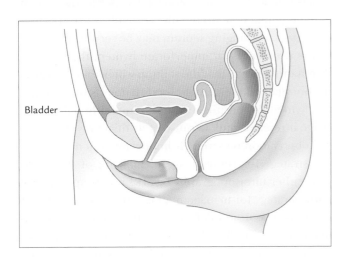

Figure 60.3. *Uterus didelphys with complete vaginal septum.*

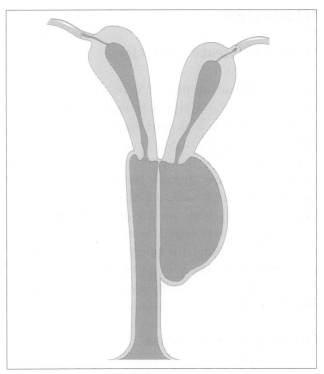

Figure 60.4. *Uterus didelphys with obstructed hemivagina.*

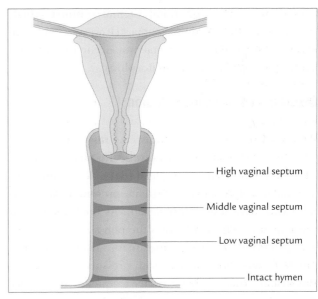

High vaginal septum

Middle vaginal septum

Low vaginal septum

Intact hymen

Figure 60.5. *Disorders of vertical fusion.*

genetic aetiology. An autosomal dominant trait that was suggested by Shokeir[3] is no longer deemed plausible. Proband studies by Carson *et al.*[4] suggest a polygenic multifactorial inheritance, which suggests a recurrence risk in first-degree relatives of between 1 and 5%. Although it is possible that müllerian duct defects could be the result of teratogens, no definite association has been demonstrated.

Epidemiology

The incidence of vaginal malformation is variously reported at between 1 in 4000 and 1 in 10 000 female births.[5] However, as there is no national register in any country for this congenital abnormality, its true incidence remains speculative. When considered as a cause of primary amenorrhoea, however, vaginal malformation is the second commonest cause (second only to gonadal dysgenesis).

PRESENTATION

Congenital absence of the vagina

Vaginal atresia usually presents at puberty with primary amenorrhoea; the symptom complex depends on whether there is an associated functional uterus. If the uterus is non-functional or absent, there are no associated symptoms other than primary amenorrhoea. However, a functional uterus may be present and haematometra may develop, which causes cyclical abdominal pain. Rarely, uterine distention may occur, but this is extremely unusual as menstrual blood retrogradely passes through the fallopian tubes and into the peritoneal cavity, where is it absorbed. Occasionally, haematosalpinges may form, which may cause pelvic masses.

Disorders of vertical fusion

Vertical fusion disorders may involve the uterus as well as the vagina and, in some circumstances, may lead to complete duplication of the genital tract. In this condition there is a longitudinal vaginal septum, which usually presents as dyspareunia. However, complete cannulation of the vagina may not occur in one half, leading to a unilateral haematocolpos.

Disorders of transverse fusion

Patients with disorders of transverse fusion have transverse vaginal septae which prevent the escape of menstrual blood and, therefore, lead to the development of a haematocolpos. These patients present post-pubertally with cyclical abdominal pain. As the haematocolpos expands, a mass occupies the pelvis and eventually will extend to an abdominal mass arising from the pelvis. Patients may present with pressure symptoms of the urinary tract; either urinary frequency or urinary retention may occur as a result of obstruction of the urethra. Transverse fusion defects may occur at three levels: in the largest reported series, 46% of defects were high, 35% mid and 19% low septae.[6]

INVESTIGATION

All the patients described above present with primary amenorrhoea. In all circumstances secondary sexual characteristics are present because ovarian function is normal. In those patients with complete absence of the vagina, inspection of the vulva will reveal a small vaginal pit with no normal vagina beyond. The skin is pink and an absence of cyclical abdominal pain in the history makes the clinician suspicious of congenital absence of the vagina. Rectal examination should not be performed, as it is unlikely to be helpful and is considered distressing to teenage girls. Imaging of the pelvis by ultrasonography or magnetic resonance imaging (MRI) is much more useful and describes the anatomy with accuracy, giving the clinician the information necessary to have an informed discussion with the patient and her parents. Laparoscopy is unnecessary in these patients and does not give any useful information with regard to management.

Disorders of vertical fusion lead to pelvic masses that may be palpable abdominally; certainly, on inspection of the vulva, a bulging septum may be seen. If the cause of the problem is an imperforate hymen, then its very thin nature means that the septum will be blue, because of the retained menstrual blood that is visible through the hymen. When it is a true septum, although it may bulge it remains pink because of its thickness. This clinical observation is extremely important, as it determines the strategy for surgery. Again, imaging of the pelvis with either ultrasonography or MRI is extremely useful and a strategy for management can then be described.

Transverse fusion defects are often more difficult to diagnose or certainly there is a longer delay in diagnosis. In these circumstances one hemivagina is occluded and, because the patient reports that she has a menstrual cycle which is painful, delay in diagnosis may occur. However, once the clinician is alerted to this possibility, an ultrasound scan of the pelvis will reveal the obstruction; clinical examination of the vagina (which should be performed only under general anaesthesia, unless the patient is sexually active) will reveal a bulging vaginal septum.

Associated abnormalities

In 40% of patients with vaginal abnormalities there will be associated urinary tract abnormalities.[7] Curiously Thompson and Lynn[8] reported that 40% of patients with congenital absence of a kidney will be found to have associated genital abnormalities. The renal abnormalities are severe in some 15% of patients with the Rokitansky syndrome, and these major defects include absence of a kidney or a pelvic kidney.

Patients with disorders of lateral fusion commonly have unilateral renal agenesis which is usually ipsilateral to the vaginal abnormality. Rarely, partial vaginal agenesis with a urinary vaginal fistula may occur; these patients usually present with cyclical recurrent haematuria. It is theorized that this results from failure of canalization of the vagina and partial persistence of the urogenital sinus.[9]

An associated problem relating to the urinary tract is occurrence of urethral coitus in patients with vaginal agenesis. In this condition, penile penetration gradually leads to dilatation of the urethra, such that fully penetrative sex may occur in some patients. Of interest is the observation that this does not usually result in any degree of urinary incontinence. However, following corrective surgery for the absent vagina, the urethra remains patulous; long-term follow up of these women is lacking.

The presence of urinary tract abnormalities in association with this condition of maldevelopment of the vagina emphasizes the need for thorough evaluation of the urological tract in these women. Conversely, congenital aberrations of the urinary tract should prompt the urologist to image the internal genitalia to assess whether there are significant abnormalities present that would benefit from future management.

TREATMENT OF VAGINAL ATRESIA

Patients with absence of the vagina require extremely careful management in centres with appropriate expertise. Psychologically, these patients cope extremely poorly with the news that they have no fertility and are unable to embark on intercourse without reconstructive help. The initial information is usually received with a considerable degree of shock by both the patient and her parents. This is followed by a period of marked depression and despair, when they question their femininity and look upon themselves as quite abnormal females. Some even question their gender. They cannot understand how they would ever be able to enter into a heterosexual relationship, or that any male would be interested in them because of their congenital abnormality. Counselling of both parents and the patient is extremely important in their manage-

ment and certainly needs to occur before any surgical or non-surgical process is embarked upon. If patients are well managed, then their subsequent sex life will be excellent, comparable to that of women in a normal population.

The approach to management of the congenital abnormality may be either non-surgical or surgical.

The non-surgical management of these patients, when the vagina is between 0.5 and 1 cm in length, involves the use of graduated dilators (Frank's procedure).[10] A small vaginal dilator is pressed firmly against the vaginal dimple for about 20 minutes, three times a day.; pressure is exerted, but pain should not be induced. Some 85% of patients will have success over about an 8-week period, to the extent that sexual intercourse by this stage is usually quite satisfactory.

In those patients with a vagina less than 1 cm long, or in whom Frank's procedure fails, a formal vaginoplasty will be required. Here three techniques may be employed. The McIndoe–Reed procedure involves the use of a split-thickness skin graft over a solid mould which is placed in a surgically created neovagina created between the urethra and rectum. This space is created digitally following a transverse incision in the vaginal dimple. This exploration of the neovaginal space must be performed with immense care, as damage to the bladder or rectum can easily occur. The space must reach the peritoneum of the pouch of Douglas if an adequate length of vagina is to be created. A partial-thickness skin graft is taken from a donor site and the mould is covered with the skin graft, which is then fashioned over the mould and sutured with the skin surface next to the mould. The mould with its graft is then placed into the neovagina, and sutured into place. Reported outcomes by McIndoe,[11] and by Cali and Pratt[12] suggest that 80% of patients achieve good sexual function. Subsequent reconstructive surgery was necessary in about 10% of patients, and a further 10% had other complications, such as urinary neovaginal fistula.

The problem with the skin graft technique is that, although it gives a functional vagina in the majority of cases, the patient is left with a graft site that is visible. Psychologically, this is something most patients deplore: it is an open, visual reminder of their congenital abnormality. Alternative materials have, therefore, been suggested: these have included the use of amnion[13] and Intercede (Johnson & Johnson Medical Inc.). These techniques have resulted in an equally successful functional sexual vagina in 85% of patients.

In the Williams vulvovaginoplasty,[14] the labia are used to create a skin pouch to allow intercourse to occur at the level of the vulva. In those patients with severe abnormalities of the vulva this may be the only approach that can be adopted; however, for those women with simple congenital absence of the vagina, this procedure should not be performed.

Occasionally, patients with an absent vagina have a coexistent functional uterus, and this actually creates considerable problems. It is often the wish of the patients (and their parents) that the uterus should be salvaged at all costs in an attempt to keep their fertility. In these circumstances the surgery can be extremely complicated, involving the initial creation of a neo-vagina and then a subsequent uterovaginal anastomosis in an attempt to create a fistula between the uterus and the vagina, and subsequently the discharge of menstrual flow through this fistula. If this attempt at surgery fails, the uterus should be removed.

Some 25% of women who have a surgical approach to their problem will have some degree of dyspareunia,[15] and this most commonly involves scarring of the upper margin of the vagina which involves the peritoneum and, during sexual intercourse, causes some degree of discomfort. It is difficult to know how best to avoid this, as all series and all techniques seem to incur a small degree of problem. Attempts to use a full-thickness skin graft have been less successful, even though the complication rates of dyspareunia may be less. Again, the donor site is a massive defect, which the patient has to come to terms with.

In disorders of transverse fusion, the surgical procedure is to remove the obstruction, and this procedure varies in its complexity. If the obstruction is caused by an imperforate hymen, then incision of this and drainage of the haematocolpos is simple. In patients with lower-third absence of the vagina there is a reasonably straightforward surgical solution, with surgical excision and a reanastomosis of the vagina. These patients should use vaginal dilators postoperatively; if this technique is used over 2–4 weeks, excellent healing will occur and a functional vagina will result, without any further complications. Patients with middle- and upper-third vaginal obstructions need much more complex surgery, primarily because there is much greater absence of vagina, which requires reconstruction.

Excision must be performed with enormous care if damage to the bladder is to be avoided. Again, excision and anastomosis of the vagina will have a functional result, with drainage of the obstruction. The incidence of fistula formation between the bladder and the vagina remains undocumented, but these fistulae do occur and can require complex closure techniques if vaginal function is to be maintained. The difficulty is that closure of the fistula may result in some reduction in vaginal length and also in increased scarring involving the peritoneum, which, in itself, leads to dyspareunia.

Finally, patients with vertical fusion defects require excision of the vaginal septum. The vaginal septum must be excised in its entirety if a successful result is to ensue; failure to do this will result in the reaccumulation of the haematocolpos. Sepsis may also occur, resulting in formation of pelvic abscess and subsequent septicaemia.

ABNORMAL DEVELOPMENT OF THE UTERUS

The uterus develops as a result of fusion of the two müllerian ducts at their lower part; failure of this fusion may result in two uterine horns, two cervices and two vaginas. This complete failure of fusion is less common than partial failure of fusion, which can result in single vaginas, single or double cervices and complete or partial duplication of the uterus (Fig. 60.6). The uterine body itself unifies by reabsorption of the midline fusion, and failure of this process may lead to septate uteri.

Presentation

Uterus didelphus (complete uterine duplication) is usually diagnosed when a patient presents with two cervices and a longitudinal vaginal septum. When the vagina is single and the uterus has an anomaly, the abnormality can only usually be diagnosed by some form of imaging. This may be by hysterosalpingography, ultrasonography[16] or MRI.[17] The indication for this investigation would be either dysmenorrhoea or some form of reproductive failure. Occasionally, a single uterine horn may not develop a passage of drainage; an obstructive uterine abnormality may, therefore, result. This is known as a rudimentary uterine horn, and usually presents with dysmenorrhoea in adolescence. These rudimentary horns must be removed surgically in order to alleviate the symptoms.

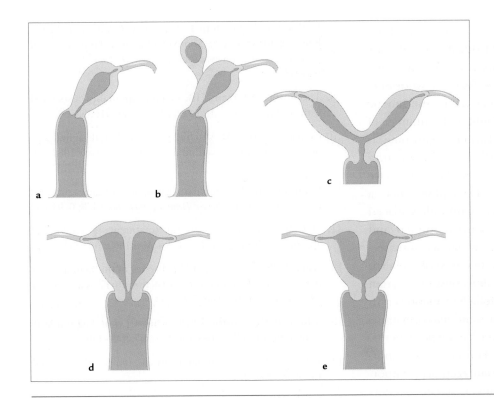

Figure 60.6. *A variety of uterine anomalies: (a) unicornuate uterus; (b) unicornuate uterus with rudimentary horn; (c) bicornuate uterus; (d) complete septate uterus; (e) partial or incomplete septate uterus.*

Associated anomalies

Uterine abnormalities are associated with the same incidence of renal abnormalities as congenital vaginal abnormalities. Again, a patient with a uterine abnormality should be screened for renal problems. The presence of a single kidney is an important medical finding and, therefore, must be determined in all these cases. In cases of unicornuate uterus the renal anomaly will usually arise on the contralateral side to the unicornuate uterus,[18] consistent with the developmental absence of the ipsilateral uterine horn.

Treatment

Uterine abnormalities do not, in general, need any treatment at all, and only if they are symptomatic should surgical intervention be considered. As mentioned above, rudimentary horns should be removed if they are causing dysmenorrhoea. Patients with recurrent pregnancy loss should be fully investigated for all causes of this problem before any uterine surgery is considered, although the association between uterine abnormalities and recurrent miscarriage is established.[19]

However, evidence from randomized controlled trials of surgery in the treatment of this condition is completely lacking. In patients with a uterine septum, surgical removal is best performed hysteroscopically; this may be done either with a resectoscope[20] or using the laser under hysteroscopic direct vision.[21] Simultaneous laparoscopy should be performed in order to prevent uterine perforation, but the surgical results from this are usually very good. In patients with duplication of the uterine body, excluding uterus didelphus, excision hysteroscopically can be very difficult, and I do not recommend this approach. Treatment should be by metroplasty, using either a Strassman's operation or Tomkins' procedure. These two operations are used to unify the uterine body following excision of the septum or removal of the medial portions of the uterus, and subsequent surgical reunion. Again, results of this procedure are usually good, but patients must be warned that subsequent development of intra-uterine synechiae is possible and this can also result in Asherman's syndrome.[22] If this does occur, fertility may be lost. It is this risk that makes the surgical approach to the union in these uteri something that must be carefully justified in each individual case.

OVARIAN DYSGENESIS

Ovarian dysgenesis, which results from absence of a sex chromosome, occurs in individuals with a chromosomal complement of 45XO, known as Turner's syndrome. The short arm of the X chromosome carries the genetic information influencing adult height and a number of skeletal system developments. Turner's syndrome is characterized by skeletal abnormalities and premature atresia of the ovarian follicles. At birth, these girls have characteristic physical findings of lymphoedema, a webbed neck, a wide carrying angle and widely spaced nipples. During development, stature is stunted and primary amenorrhoea and failure of characteristic secondary sexual development are features of puberty. Their gonads are streaks of tissue that consist of ovarian stroma and there are no ovarian follicles whatsoever. In a recent study,[23] renal abnormalities and malformations were found in 53% of pure 45XO karyotype patients, but only 7% of mosaic patients. However, the importance of the association with ovarian agenesis is important and, again, prompts clinicians to screen patients with Turner's syndrome for renal abnormalities.

REFERENCES

1. Jones HW, Mermut S. Familial occurrence of congenital absence of the vagina. *Am J Obstet Gynecol* 1972; 114: 1100–1101

2. Lischke JH, Curtis CH, Lamb EJ. Discordance of vaginal agenesis in monozygotic twins. *Obstet Gynecol* 1973; 41: 920–924

3. Shokeir MH. Aplasia of the Müllerian system: evidence for probable sex-limited autosomal dominant inheritance. *Birth Defects Orig Artic Ser* 1978; 14: 147–165

4. Carson SA, Simpson JL, Malinak LR *et al.* Heritable aspects of uterine anomalies. II. Genetic analysis of Müllerian aplasia. *Fertil Steril* 1983; 40: 86–90

5. Evans TN, Poland ML, Boving RL. Vaginal malformations. *Am J Obstet Gynecol* 1981; 141: 910–920

6. Rock JA, Zacur HA, Dlugi AM *et al.* Pregnancy success following surgical correction of imperforate hymen and complete transverse vaginal septum. *Obstet Gynecol* 1982; 59: 448–451

7. D'Alberton A, Reschini E, Ferrari N, Candiani P. Prevalence of urinary tract abnormalities in a large series of patients with uterovaginal atresia. *J Urol* 1981; 126: 623–624

8. Thompson DP, Lynn HB. Genital anomalies associated with solitary kidney. *Mayo Clin Proc* 1966; 41: 538–548

9. Genest D, Farber M, Mitchell GW *et al.* Partial vaginal agenesis with a urinary–vaginal fistula. *Obstet Gynecol* 1981; 58: 130–134

10. Edmonds DK. Congenital malformations of the vagina and their management. *Semin Reprod Endocrinol* 1988; 6: 91–96

11. McIndoe AH. Discussion on treatment of congenital absence of the vagina. *Proc R Soc Med* 1959; 52: 952–957

12. Cali RW, Pratt JH. Congenital absence of the vagina. Long term results of vaginal reconstruction in 175 cases. *Am J Obstet Gynecol* 1968; 100: 752–763

13. Ashworth MF, Morton KE, Dewhurst J *et al.* Vaginoplasty using amnion. *Obstet Gynecol* 1986; 67: 443–446

14. Williams AE. Uterovaginal agenesis. *Ann R Coll Surg Engl* 1976; 58: 266–272

15. Smith MR. Vaginal aplasia: therapeutic options. *Am J Obstet Gynecol* 1983; 146: 488–494

16. Jurkovic D, Gruboeck K, Tailor A, Nicolaides KH. Ultrasound screening for congenial uterine anomalies. *Br J Obstet Gynaecol* 1997; 104: 1320–1321

17. Doyle MB. Magnetic resonance imaging in Müllerian fusion defects. *J Reprod Med* 1992; 37: 33–38

18. Rock JA, Murphy AA. Anatomic abnormalities. *Clin Obstet Gynecol* 1986; 29: 886–911

19. Daya S. Evaluation and management of recurrent spontaneous abortion. *Curr Opin Obstet Gynecol* 1996; 8: 188–192

20. Vercellini P, Vendola N, Colombo A *et al.* Hysteroscopic metroplasty with resectoscope or microscissors for the correction of septate uterus. *Surg Gynecol Obstet* 1993; 176: 439–442

21. Donnez J, Nisolle M. Endoscopic laser treatment of uterine malformations. *Hum Reprod* 1997; 12: 1381–1387

22. Elchalal U, Schenker JG. Hysteroscopic resection of uterus septus versus abdominal metroplasty. *J Am Coll Surg* 1994; 178: 637–644

23. Flynn MT, Ekstrom L, De-Arce M *et al.* Prevalence of renal malformation in Turner syndrome. *Pediatr Nephrol* 1996; 10: 498–500

61

Paediatric urogynaecology

A. J. Kirsch, H. M. Snyder

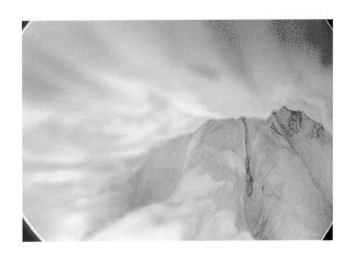

INTRODUCTION

The wide spectrum of anomalies of female embryogenesis result in problems related to the development of the urinary and genital tracts. Many of the clinical disorders seen in girls and young women that appear to involve the genitalia alone may be the harbinger of related urinary tract disorders. Abnormalities presenting in infancy may be easy to recognize secondary to an abnormal antenatal ultrasonographic or physical examination in the newborn period. Many urogenital malformations, however, are elusive and may become evident only when a clinical problem arises.

The most common urogynaecological disorders prompting childhood evaluation focus on problems of urinary continence and introital abnormalities. Interlabial masses, often included in the differential diagnosis of urinary incontinence, as well as difficulties with appropriate gender identification in genetic and phenotypic females, are discussed in this chapter. As congenital abnormalities result from abnormal embryogenesis, it is appropriate to begin with a brief overview of normal female embryology (also see chapter 9).

FEMALE EMBRYOLOGY

Congenital abnormalities commonly involve both the urinary and genital tracts. An understanding of normal embryogenesis is a prerequisite for understanding congenital abnormalities. A detailed discussion of the embryology of the lower urinary tract is provided by Marshall[1] and by Stephens *et al.*[2]

The divergence of normal sexual differential into male and female phenotypes begins in week 9 of gestation. If no Y chromosome is present, the ovaries develop whereas the testis and Sertoli cells do not. As a result, the wolffian system regresses (absence of androgen production) and the müllerian ducts form the fallopian tubes, uterus and proximal part of the vagina (absence of müllerian inhibiting factor). The embryological origins and adult counterparts of the female genital tract are shown in Figure 61.1 and described in the Table 61.1.

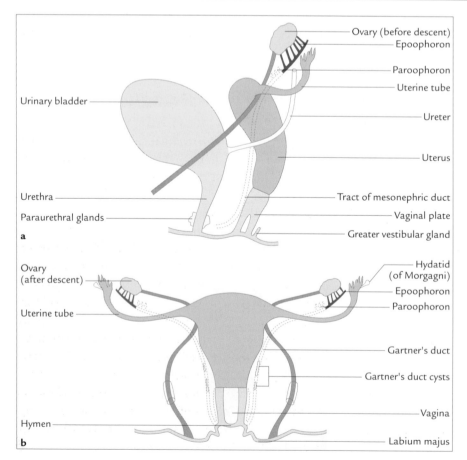

Figure 61.1. *Embryology and development of the female genital tracts: (a) a 12-week fetus; (b) a newborn female (urogenital sinus; ▪ mesonephric duct; paramesonephric duct).*

Table 61.1. *Female embryology*

Weeks of gestation	Embryonic structure/event	Adult counterpart
7–8	Genital ridge transformed	Ovary
9–10	Müllerian ducts fuse distally	Fallopian tubes, uterus, cervix, proximal vagina
12–20	Sinovaginal bulbs elongate, form vaginal plate; canalization of plate at urogenital sinus	Distal vagina
	Genital tubercle elongates	Clitoris, hymen
	Urethral folds do not fuse	Labia minora
	Labial swellings enlarge	Labia majora
	urogenital groove remains	Introitus
	Mesonephric ducts	Ureters
	Vestigial structures: Mesonephric duct Proximal end	Appendix vesiculosa, paroöphoron and epoöphoron
	Distal end	Gartner's duct/cysts

URINARY INCONTINENCE IN GIRLS

Aetiology

Urinary incontinence in females may have functional or neurogenic causes, or may be secondary to congenital abnormalities of the lower urinary tract. The most common cause of severe urinary incontinence in children is related to a neurological deficit. The leading causes of neurogenic incontinence include myelomeningocele (spina bifida), sacral agenesis and vertebral or spinal cord lesions. In these conditions, changes within the spinal cord may occur over time and make careful evaluation and close follow-up essential.

In all children presenting with urinary incontinence urinalysis should be performed to assess the presence of infection, haematuria, proteinuria, glucosuria or renal concentrating defect (early morning specific gravity < 1.022). Chronic night-time wetting, polyuria or nocturia may indicate renal failure or diabetes and requires thorough medical evaluation.

Incontinence can be broadly divided between that requiring surgical intervention and that requiring medical or behavioural therapies. In general, incontinence related to primary nocturnal enuresis or infrequent voiding tends to resolve with time and does not require surgery. The following sections address the clinical presentation, evaluation and treatment of lower urinary tract abnormalities associated with urinary incontinence in girls.

FUNCTIONAL CAUSES OF URINARY INCONTINENCE

Functional causes of urinary incontinence include primary nocturnal enuresis, dysfunctional voiding and pseudo-incontinence (e.g. vaginal voiding).

Nocturnal enuresis

Primary nocturnal enuresis is defined as persistent night-time wetting past the age of 5 years. Nocturnal enuresis occurs in approximately 20% of 5-year-old children and is more common in boys than girls.[3] Daytime wetting, urinary urgency and frequency are more common in girls. Diagnosis and treatment of nocturnal enuresis is multifactorial, relying on both the pathophysiology and psychological analysis of the patient. Treatment using desmopressin, bedwetting alarm or combination therapy is often successful. Daytime symptoms such as enuresis, urgency and frequency may be treated with anticholinergic medications.

Dysfunctional voiding

Children with dysfunctional voiding have difficulty relaxing their pelvic floor musculature, which comprises the external urethral sphincter and which is traversed by the rectum. As a result, day- and night-time wetting, urinary frequency or infrequency, urgency, urinary tract infections, and constipation or encopresis are common.

It is helpful if patients and their families keep an elimination diary to ascertain the child's specific toileting habits. For example, many parents are not aware that their child has constipation unless specifically queried as to the frequency and calibre of the stool. Simple treatment of constipation with stool softeners (e.g. mineral oil, Kondremul) or laxatives (e.g. Milk of Magnesia or Dulcolax) permit better overall toileting behaviour. Voiding dysfunction may be treated by behaviour modification or pharmacological agents and does not require surgical intervention. A list of common pharmacotherapeutic agents for neurovesical dysfunction is provided in Table 61.2.

Vaginal voiding

Vaginal voiding is often confused with true urinary incontinence. Micturition into the vagina results in leakage when the child stands upright, allowing efflux of urine from the vaginal vault. Simple manoeuvres to direct the urinary stream more accurately by separating the legs further during voiding, and waiting a few minutes after micturition to allow efflux into the toilet, usually solve the problem.

CONGENITAL ABNORMALITIES CAUSING INCONTINENCE

Congenital anomalies may cause incontinence by interfering with the function of the sphincter mechanisms or the storage function of the bladder, or by anatomically bypassing normal sphincter mechanisms (Table 61.3).

Imaging studies are essential to define the anatomical abnormalities causing the incontinence. The first studies obtained are usually renal and bladder ultrasonography and the voiding cystourethrogram (VCUG). The plain abdominal scout film of the VCUG assesses bony abnormalities and the presence or absence of faecal impaction. An intravenous pyelogram is useful to identify ectopic ureters, duplication anomalies and ureteroceles, as well as providing useful information regarding renal function. Urodynamic studies are often useful in detecting sphincteric, storage and urinary flow abnormalities, and are essential in all patients with neurogenic incontinence.

The goals of treatment for congenital abnormalities of the female urogenital tract are restoration of physical appearance and function, preservation of renal function and achievement of manageable urine storage and continence.

Abnormal storage

Bladder exstrophy

Bladder exstrophy (Fig. 61.2) has an incidence of 1/30 000 live births and is less common in females than in males. Debate continues about the development of the bladder wall and matrix proteins. Why some children

Table 61.2. *Pharmacotherapy for neurovesical dysfunction*		
Drug	Action	Dose/frequency
Bethanechol	Cholinergic	0.6 mg/kg/day 3–4 times daily
Dicyclomine	Anticholinergic	5–10 mg 3–4 times daily
Oxybutynin	Anticholinergic	0.2 mg/kg 2–4 times daily
Propantheline	Anticholinergic	1.5 mg/kg/day 3–4 times daily

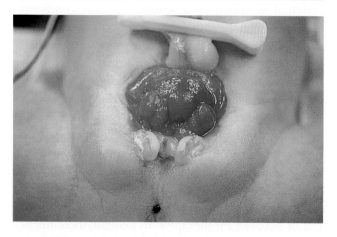

Figure 61.2. *A newborn girl with bladder exstrophy. Note separation of the labia and clitoris, and the normal vagina.*

Table 61.3. *Mechanisms of incontinence in congenital genitourinary anomalies**

Abnormal storage	Abnormal sphincter	Bypass sphincter
Bladder exstrophy	Epispadias	Ectopic ureters
Cloacal exstrophy	Urogenital sinus	Vesicovaginal fistulae
Bladder agenesis	Ectopic ureteroceles	
Bladder duplication	Neurogenic[†]	
Neurogenic[†]		

*Multiple mechanisms for incontinence often coexist in a given patient.
[†]Abnormalities of storage or sphincteric function may be seen with neurogenic bladders (e.g. spina bifida) and may be related to detrusor hypo- or hyperactivity, or from secondary changes within the detrusor muscle, resulting in stiff (non-compliant) or floppy (very compliant) bladders.

develop normal bladder capacities while others go on to develop small and poorly compliant bladders is incompletely understood. Treatment involves bladder closure within the first days of life. Bladder enhancement or diversion are surgical options later on. Bladder-neck reconstruction may be performed at the time of bladder closure or later on. Continence rates range from 43 to 87%.

Cloacal exstrophy

Cloacal exstrophy (Fig. 61.3) has an incidence of 1:200 000 and is much less common in females. Cloacal exstrophy is much more complex than bladder exstrophy and requires extensive evaluation for associated abnormalities of the nervous system, upper urinary tract and gastrointestinal tract.

The treatment of storage abnormalities of the bladder usually involves bladder augmentation with intestinal segments. Clean intermittent catheterization (CIC) may also be required to maintain urinary continence.

Myelomeningocele

In the paediatric population, myelomeningocele (Fig. 61.4) is a common cause of neurogenic bladder leading to problems with urinary storage, sphincteric function and elimination. In the United States, the prevalence is approximately 1/1000 births. CIC in conjunction with anticholinergic medication has brought about a dramatic improvement in the management of patients with myelomeningocele. The use of CIC has been shown to promote continence, preserve renal function and

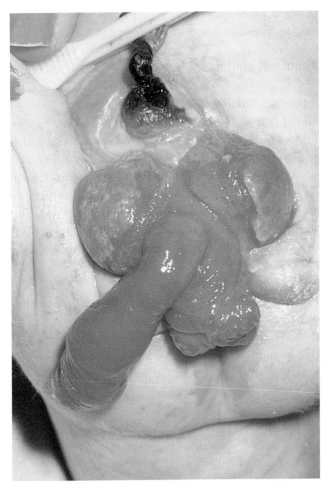

Figure 61.3. *Newborn with cloacal exstrophy illustrating separation of bladder halves, herniation of the hindgut and prolapse of the ileocaecal segment.*

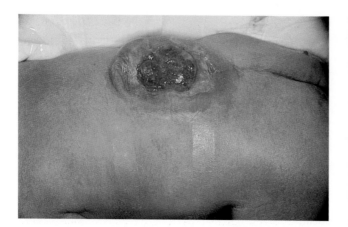

Figure 61.4. *A newborn with characteristic appearance of myelomeningocele protruding from the lower back*

decrease the incidence of symptomatic pyelonephritis.[4] McGuire and co-workers[5] determined that a leak-point pressure (LPP) greater than 40 cmH$_2$O was predictive of renal deterioration over time. CIC serves to keep bladder pressure low, avoiding high LPP.

Abnormal sphincter

Anatomical abnormalities may impede normal development of the bladder neck. Incompetence of the bladder neck may result in primary urinary incontinence and is seen in conditions such as female epispadias, urogenital sinus, bilateral ureteral ectopia and ectopic ureteroceles. Conservative measures to improve sphincteric function are limited and a surgical approach is needed. The surgical options focus on creation of an increase in bladder outlet resistance or of a new sphincter mechanism.

Female epispadias

Female epispadias (Fig. 61.5) may result in a variable presentation, depending on the severity of the urethral defect. In complete epispadias, incontinence results secondary to (a) a foreshortened and widened urethra, (b) a partially absent external urethral sphincter, and (c) a poorly developed bladder neck. Treatment is directed at reconstruction of these deficient structures and ureteral reimplantation proximal to the reconstructed bladder neck region.[6,7] Persistent incontinence may be treated with collagen injection at the bladder neck.

Urogenital sinus anomalies

The persistence of a urogenital sinus may result in the urethra emptying into the vaginal vault. This may not

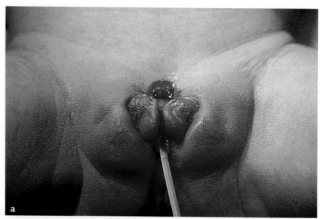

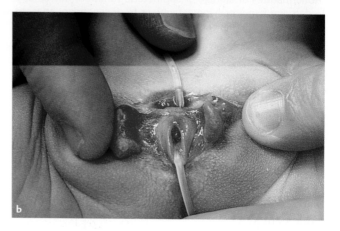

Figure 61.5. *Appearance of a newborn girl with epispadias (a); note the open bladder neck with a catheter introduced superior to a normal catheterized vagina, and separation of the labia and clitoris (b).*

be readily apparent unless the urethra is not seen during attempts at catheterization. Infants may present with a dilated vagina, possibly resulting in an abdominal mass, if the posterior lip of the hymen causes partial obstruction at the orifice of the urogenital sinus (Fig. 61.6). Retained urine in the vagina (urocolpos) and uterine canal may increase to enormous volumes. Drainage of urine with vaginal catheterization followed by a vaginogram showing contrast within the cervical canal and uterus, and possibly into the peritoneal cavity, is diagnostic. Treatment involves endoscopic division of the posterior hymenal lip. Further reconstructive surgery will usually be required.

Duplicated ectopic ureters

An ectopic upper pole ureter may join the lower end of the remnant mesonephric duct system comprising Gartner's ducts. These ureters are associated with non-function of the associated renal moiety and may result in cystic dilatation of Gartner's duct with eventual rupture of the cyst and drainage into the vaginal opening. Drainage of fluid or pus into the vagina prompts further investigation. A renal and pelvic ultrasound scan may show a dilated or abnormal upper pole renal moiety, and a cystic structure may be seen in the pelvis or vaginal area. Computed tomography scanning or magnetic resonance imaging are helpful in further delineating the anatomy, while retrograde fluoroscopic studies are diagnostic if the often elusive ectopic orifice can be identified (Fig. 61.7).

The appropriate treatment of ectopic ureters depends on whether the ureter is ectopic or bilateral and whether it drains into the genital or urinary tracts. Ectopic ureters to the genital tracts may be treated by simple upper pole nephrectomy; ectopia to the urinary tract usually involves ureterectomy in addition to heminephrectomy in order to prevent postoperative urinary reflux and infection (Fig. 61.8).

Bypass of sphincter mechanism

In instances where the bladder neck and sphincter mechanism have developed normally, urinary incontinence may develop as a result of ureteral ectopia distal to the continence mechanism. The most common cause of this abnormality is ectopic ureters. Incontinence may

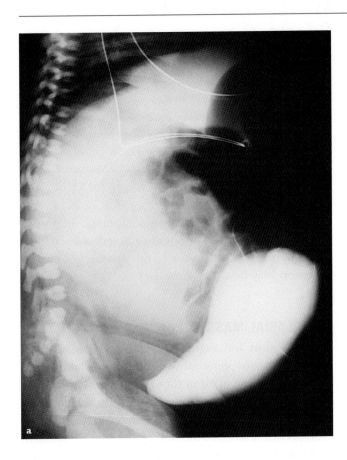

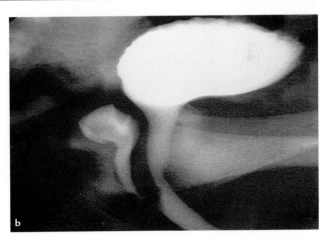

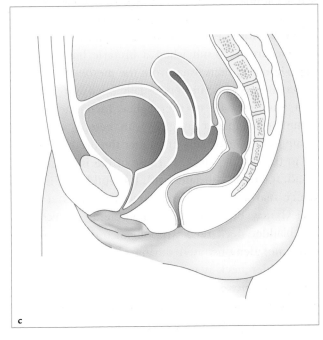

Figure 61.6. *(a) This contrast vaginogram in a newborn girl with an abdominal mass shows retained fluid and an obstructed vagina (urocolpos) secondary to a urogenital sinus abnormality. (b) A flush genitogram in another patient reveals a urogenital sinus with contrast seen within the bladder and vagina. (c) Line drawing showing the relationship between the urethra, narrow distal vagina and urogenital sinus.*

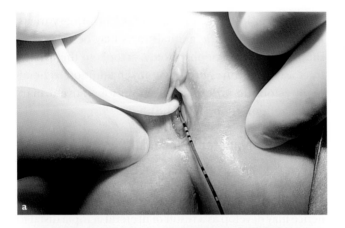

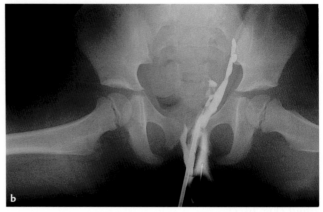

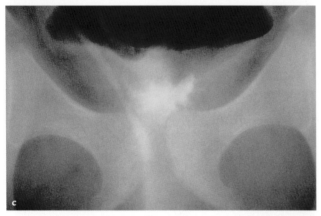

Figure 61.7. *A young girl with continuously damp underpants was found to have ureteral ectopia to her vagina: (a) photo of the vagina showing a ureteral stent placed within the ectopic ureter and a Foley catheter within the urethra; (b) retrograde pyelogram shows contrast within the ectopic ureter. (c) An intravenous urogram in another patient reveals an ectopic ureter of an upper pole moiety terminating beyond the bladder neck and into the vaginal introitus.*

not be purely secondary to a bypass mechanism, as abnormal urethral development may contribute to poor urinary control.

Bilateral single ectopic ureters

Ectopic ureters result when a ureteric bud develops more cranially than usual from the mesonephric duct. In females, ectopic ureters usually open into the urethra, the vestibule or the vagina. Incontinence is a common complaint in girls with ectopic ureter(s). Bilateral ectopic ureters may enter the urethra just distal to the bladder neck. Because of the inadequacy of urethral length associated with this condition, incontinence may result. In single ectopic ureters, a cyclic VCUG may demonstrate vesicoureteral reflux when the bladder neck relaxes upon micturition; reflux is often not demonstrated during bladder filling when the bladder neck is in a contracted state. Treatment involves ureteral reimplantation and bladder-neck reconstruction for bilateral single ectopic ureters and upper pole partial nephrectomy and lower pole reim-

plantation for duplicated ectopic ureters. In unsuccessful cases, use of a continent catheterizable channel (e.g. appendicovesicostomy) or continent urinary diversion may be considered.

INTERLABIAL MASSES

Masses within the vagina presenting in infants and young girls are generally referred to as interlabial masses. Although many of these lesions arise within the introitus, those arising in the urethra or bladder must be recognized to afford proper management. Many patients with masses within the vaginal area complain of leakage of fluid (e.g. urine, pus, transudate). A thorough physical examination of the introitus is part of the complete evaluation of urinary incontinence.

Skene's glands (para-urethral glands)

The tubular Skene's glands (Fig. 61.9) arise from the urethral epithelium and are the counterparts to the

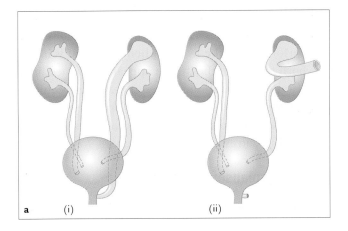

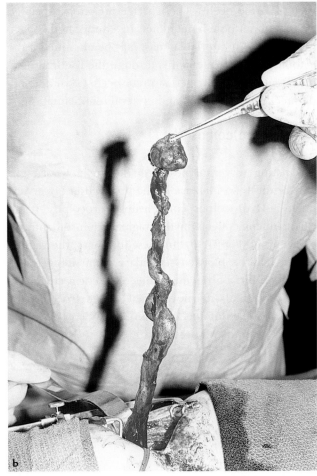

Figure 61.8. *(a) illustration of nephroureterectomy (i) preoperatively and (ii) postoperatively; (b) nephroureterectomy specimen from the patient in Figure 61.7.*

male prostate gland. In females, these glands may end up in the urethral meatus and hymen. Cysts (tense, yellow, thin-walled) partially arising within the urethral meatus but mostly external to it may resemble a bulging

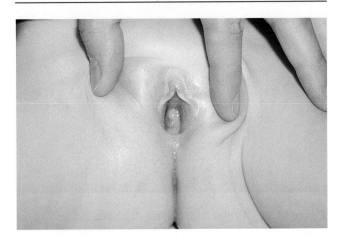

Figure 61.9. *Illustration of the Skene's glands in a newborn girl.*

hymen associated with hydrometrocolpos, or a prolapsing ureterocele (fleshy, compressible, protruding through the urethra).

Bartholin's glands

The major vestibular glands of Bartholin arise from the urogenital sinus and come to open into the vestibule on either side of the hymen. The main glands lie against the ischiopubic ramus deep to the bulbospongiosus muscle and cavernous tissue. Blockage of the main ducts of Bartholin's glands may lead to cystic dilatation at any age, but rarely become infected prior to puberty.[1]

Prolapsed ureterocele

A ureterocele is a dilated distal ureter within the detrusor muscle which may extend beyond the bladder neck (ectopic ureterocele). These ureters are often associated with an upper pole renal moiety of a duplicated collecting system.[8] An interlabial mass may be identified if the ectopic ureterocele extends through the urethral meatus. Treatment is directed at ureterocele excision, bladder-neck reconstruction and ureteral reimplantation.

Hydro(metro)colpos

Circulating maternal oestrogen in the newborn girl may result in an increase in the production of cervical mucus. Hydrocolpos and hydrometrocolpos result when mucus collects in the vaginal vault and uterus, respectively (Fig 61.10). In these instances, the vaginal orifice may be blocked secondary to an imperforate hymen, within a urogenital sinus, anatretic rectocloacal canal, or vaginal/uterine atresia. Hydrometrocolpos, by virtue of its abdominal extension, may compress the urethra, rectum and ureters.

Treatment of hydro(metro)colpos secondary to a normally located imperforate hymen may involve simple perforation of the hymen when the infant is in the newborn nursery. If the hymen appears thickened, incision under general anaesthesia may be required. Higher obstruction involves a more formal approach to treat the associated urogenital abnormalities (e.g. urogenital sinus, atresia, rectocloacal canal).

Urethral prolapse

Eversion of the distal urethral mucosa through the urethral meatus results in a circumferential interlabial lesion (Fig. 61.11). The lesion may be painful or may bleed or weep serosanguinous fluid, prompting medical attention; however, they do not lead to urinary incontinence. On examination, urethral prolapse

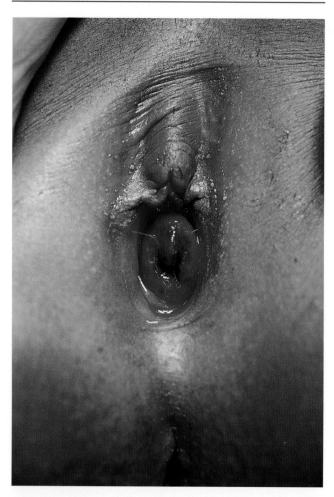

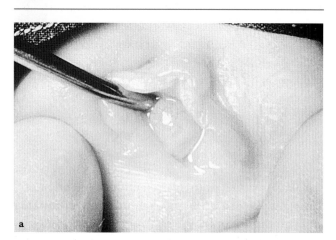

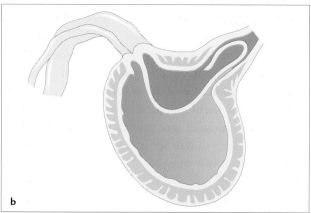

Figure 61.10. *A newborn girl with urinary obstruction: (a) external appearance of the prolapsing ectopic ureterocele (b) illustration depicting the ectopic ureterocele with extension into the urethra.*

Figure 61.11. *An 8-year-old African–American girl with urethral prolapse presented with 'vaginal' pain and blood spotting.*

appears oedematous or necrotic with the urethral meatus seen within its centre. This lesion should be distinguished from neoplasms of the vagina or bladder (see below). A prolapsed urethra associated with mild oedema without necrosis or significant pain may reasonably be treated conservatively with sitz-baths and oestrogen cream over a 2–3-week period. More significant lesions should be excised.[9]

Rhabdomyosarcoma of the vagina

Rhabdomyosarcoma of the vagina and bladder (Fig. 61.12) may present as a grape-like interlabial lesion associated with vaginal bleeding.[10] Because of the propensity of these lesions to spread, a complete endoscopic and radiographic evaluation is indicated to confirm the diagnosis and rule out local extension and distant lesions. Primary chemotherapy has resulted in better bladder salvage and can cure metastatic disease.[11] Surgical excision, with or without radiation therapy, is reserved for post-chemotherapy biopsy-proven residual masses.

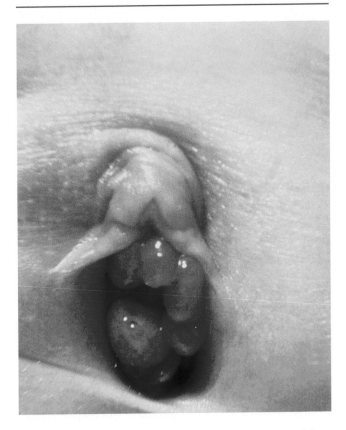

Figure 61.12. *A 5-year-old girl with rhabdomyosarcoma of the vagina (sarcoma botryoides) presented with blood spotting and dysuria.*

DISORDERS OF THE FEMALE GENITALIA

Intersex disorders

A complete description of the array of intersex disorders is beyond the scope of this chapter. However, urologists and gynaecologists must be familar with the more common intersex disorders whereby gender assignment and rearing is along female lines. These conditions include girls of normal appearance who are genetically male (male pseudohermaphrodites) and genetic females appearing as males (female pseudohermaphrodites).

Female pseudohermaphroditism

Female pseudohermaphrodites are genetic females (XX karyotype) but may appear as males without testes (Fig. 61.13). The most common cause of female pseudohermaphroditism is congenital adrenal hyperplasia (21-hydroxylase deficiency in >90%). In this disorder, the absence of 21-hydroxylase results in the overproduction of androgens and results in a wide spectrum of genital abnormalities, ranging from mild masculinization of the clitoris (clitoromegaly) to complete masculinization. The labioscrotal folds are rugated and hyperpigmented, giving the physical appearance of severe hypospadias with cryptorchidism. In all cases, however, the internal female anatomy is normal. After the diagnosis is established, surgical treatment involves feminizing genitoplasty (reduction clitoroplasty, vaginoplasty and labioplasty).

Male pseudohermaphroditism

Male pseudohermaphrodites are genetic males (XY karyotype) but may appear as normal females. Testicular feminization is the most common cause of male pseudohermaphroditism and results from the lack of androgen receptors at the cell surface of all tissues. The diagnosis should be suspected in all girls with inguinal hernias – the hernia sacs may be found to contain testes. The diagnosis should always be suspected in adolescent girls with normal development and primary amenorrhoea. Development and sexual identity is female. Treatment involves bilateral orchidectomy. Testes left in place will produce testosterone, which is converted to oestradiol, allowing spontaneous breast development. Testes should be removed because of the risk of gonadoblastoma. Oestrogen must be replaced at puberty in girls who have undergone prepubertal

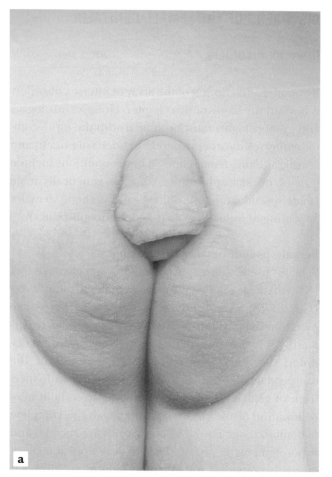

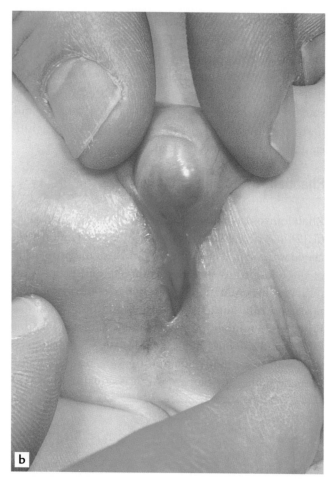

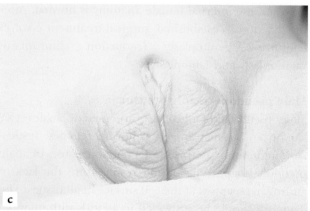

Figure 61.13 *This newborn with ambiguous genitalia, elevated 17-hydro-oxyprogesterone and XX chromosomes was diagnosed with congenital adrenal hyperplasia (21-hydroxylase deficiency): (a) preoperative appearance showing phallic structure and non-palpable gonads; (b) prominent scrotal folds and clitoromegaly; (c) appearance 6 months after reduction clitoroplasty and scrotoplasty.*

orchidectomy, which is the standard treatment when the diagnosis is made.

Vaginal agenesis and the Mayer–Rokitansky syndrome

Agenesis of the vagina in genetic females (Fig. 61.14) may be accompanied by various other defects in the genitourinary tract. Most patients present in adolescence with amenorrhoea or pain, but this condition may also present in young girls with urinary tract infection or hydrocolpos. Genital defects range from vaginal agenesis alone to agenesis of the uterus and fallopian tubes. These genital defects are associated with (ipsilateral) renal agenesis.[12] Some patients present after having urethral intercourse and stress urinary

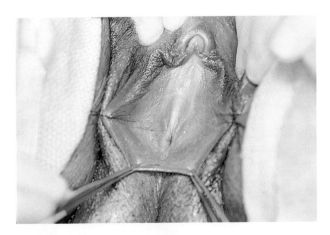

Figure 61.14. *Vaginal agenesis in a 16-year-old with Mayer–Rokitansky syndrome. The sexually active patient engaged in urethral coitus.*

incontinence. Treatment of the Mayer–Rokitansky syndrome includes vaginoplasty or neovaginal reconstruction with bowel.

URINARY TRACT RECONSTRUCTION

Lower urinary tract reconstruction

Since 1950, bowel segments have been used to replace entirely a diseased or dysfunctional bladder. The current success in reconstruction of the lower urinary tract reflects our improved understanding of the physiological principles involved in bladder and urethral function.[13-18] Spontaneous voiding can occasionally be achieved with a quite abnormal lower urinary tract. This, of course, is provided that the pressure gradient between the bladder and distal urethra is low. It follows, then, that even in cases where the bladder is replaced in part (intestinal cystoplasty) or entirely (neobladder), patients may still be able to empty their bladders satisfactorily. Many patients require bladder-neck reconstruction[19] to achieve continence and most will require CIC.[20]

Continent reconstruction of the lower urinary tract is often desired in the face of congenital or acquired anomalies of both the outlet and the bladder. Much of the principles and background of continent reconstruction is derived from experience with undiversion. The early work of Hendren, Mitrofanoff and others has

led to surgical approaches that produce both better reservoir function and a continent outlet.[21]

Continent urinary diversion encompasses three interrelated but independently functioning components. These include a channel by which urine is conducted to the skin, a reservoir or pouch, and a mechanism by which continence is achieved.[22] A host of tissues are available to the reconstructive surgeon (Table 61.4).

The flap valve principle for continence dictates that a portion of the continence channel be fixed on the inner wall of the reservoir. This is the same principle by which ureteral tunnelling in the bladder muscle prevents reflux during voiding. In general, a 5: 1 length-to-diameter ratio of the continence structure is required. This is the case whether the structure is ureter, ileum or appendix.

The Mitrofanoff principle of continent reconstruction describes a supple catheterizable structure (ureter, appendix, etc.) implanted into the inner wall of the reservoir to create a flap valve continence mechanism.[23] The most popular form of flap valve construction for urinary continence is the use of appendix implanted into the bladder or reservoir (appendicovesicostomy). The small stoma may be concealed within the umbilicus (Fig. 61.15). Assurance of complete bladder emptying is essential, as this type of continence channel is very

Table 61.4. *Tissues available for lower urinary tract reconstruction**

External conduit	Urinary reservoir	Continence mechanism
Appendix	Bladder	Anal sphincter
Fallopian tube	Caecum	Artificial urinary sphincter
Ileum	Colon	Benchekroun (hydraulic valve)
Ileal tube	Ileum	Ileocaecal valve
Skin tube	Rectum	Koch (nipple valve)
Stomach	Stomach	Mitrofanoff (flap valve)
Urethra		Urethral sphincter
Ureter		

In general, three components are required for continent diversion: these are (1) conduit from the reservoir to the skin, (2) a pouch or reservoir, and (3) a mechanism by which continence is attained.

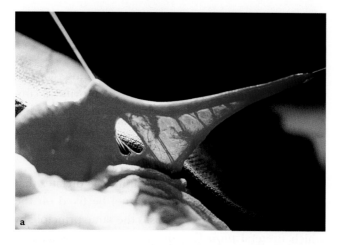

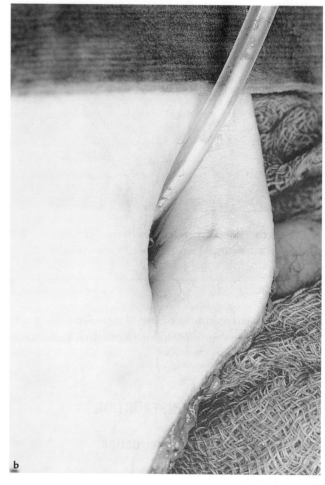

Figure 61.15. *In the Mitrofanoff procedure, the appendix is mobilized with its blood supply as illustrated in (a) and reimplanted into the bladder in a tunnelled non-refluxing fashion. The proximal appendix may be brought out to the umbilicus for clean intermittent catheterization (b).*

effective in its ability to withstand very high intraluminal pressure. In the non-compliant patient, pouch rupture or upper tract injury may result from failure to empty the reservoir regularly.

Urinary tract reconstruction and pregnancy

Future pregnancy must be kept in mind when reconstructing the genitourinary tract. Pregnancy may be complicated and requires care by both the obstetrician and urologist. Renal obstruction and incontinence may result as the uterus enlarges. Neobladder reconstruction has a good outcome, but chronic bacteriuria is frequent and occasionally requires an indwelling catheter in the third trimester.[24] Similarly, when suprapubic catheterizable continent stomas have been constructed, indwelling catheterization through the stoma during the third trimester may be needed to avoid serious urinary tract infections.[25]

Successful pregnancies and deliveries have been reported after both continent and loop urinary diversions.[26–28] The mode of delivery should be guided by obstetric indications,[27] although vaginal delivery has been successful in the majority of cases. Alternatively, if the bladder neck has been reconstructed it is usually advisable for delivery to be by caesarean section to avoid damage to the bladder-neck reconstruction. The urologist should be available to the obstetric team for consultation if caesarean section is deemed necessary, especially if a bladder augmentation with bowel has been carried out, in order to avoid injury to the vascular pedicle to the bowel segment.

REFERENCES

1. Marshall FF. Embryology of the lower genitourinary tract. *Urol Clin North Am* 1978; 5: 3–15.

2. Stephens FD, Smith ED, Hutson JM. *Congenital Abnormalities of the Urinary and Genital Tracts.* Oxford: Isis Medical Media, 1996

3. Miller FJW. Children who wet the bed. In: Kolvin I, MacKeith RC, Meadow SR (eds) *Bladder Control and Enuresis.* London: Heinemann Medical Books, 1973; 47–52

4. Scott JE, Deegan S. Management of neuropathic urinary incontinence in children by intermittent catheterization. *Arch Dis Child* 1982; 57: 253–258

5. McGuire EJ, Woodside JR, Borden TA *et al.* Prognostic value of urodynamic testing in myelodysplastic patients. *J Urol* 1981; 126: 205–209

6. Geahart JP, Peppas DS, Jeffs RD. Complete genitourinary reconstruction in female epispadias. *J Urol* 1993; 149: 1110–1113

7. Mollard P, Basset T, Mure PY. Female epispadias. *J Urol* 1997; 158: 1543–1546

8. Mandell J, Colodny AH, Lebowitz R *et al.* Ureteroceles in infants and children. *J Urol* 1980; 123: 921–926

9. Jerkins GR, Verheeck K, Noe HN. Treatment of girls with urethral prolapse. *J Urol* 1984; 132: 732–733

10. Hays DM. Pelvic rhabdomyosarcomas in childhood: diagnosis and concepts of management reviewed. *Cancer* 1980; 45: 1810–1814

11. Hays DM, Raney RB, Crist W *et al.* Improved survival and bladder preservation among patients with bladder– prostate rhabdomyosarcoma primary tumors in Intergroup Rhabdomyosarcoma Study III. *Proc Am Soc Clin Oncol* 1991; 10: 318 (abstr 1119)

12. Tarry WF, Duckett JW, Stephens FD. The Mayer–Rokitansky syndrome: pathogenesis, classification and management. *J Urol* 1986, 136: 648–657

13. Kass EJ, Koff SA. Bladder augmentation in the pediatric neuropathic bladder. *J Urol* 1983; 129: 552–555

14. Koch NG, Norlen L, Phillipson BM *et al.* The continent ileal reservoir (Koch pouch) for urinary diversion. *World J Urol* 1985; 3: 146–151

15. Koff SA. Guidelines to determine the size and shape of intestinal segments used for reconstruction. *J Urol* 1988; 140: 1150–1151

16. Hinman F Jr. Selection of intestinal segments for bladder substitution: physical and physiological characteristics. *J Urol* 1988; 139: 519–523

17. McDougal WS. Metabolic complications of urinary intestinal diversion. *J Urol* 1992; 147: 1199–1208

18. Hall MC, Koch MO, McDougal WS. Metabolic consequences of urinary diversion through intestinal segment. *Urol Clin North Am* 1991; 18: 725–735

19. Kropp KA, Angwafo FF. Urethral lengthening and reimplantation for neurogenic incontinence in children. *J Urol* 1986; 135: 553–536

20. Lapides J, Dionko AC, Silber SJ *et al.* Clean intermittent catheterization in the treatment of urinary tract disease. *J Urol* 1972; 107: 458–461

21. Hendren WH. Urinary tract refunctionalization after long-term diversion. *Ann Surg* 1990; 212: 478–495

22. Kirsch AJ, Snyder, HM. Trends in continent reconstruction of the lower urinary tract. *Contemp Urol* 1997; 9: 61–69

23. Duckett JW, Snyder HM. Use of the Mitrofanoff principle in urinary reconstruction. *World J Urol* 1985; 3: 191–193

24. Creagh TA, McInerney PD, Thomas PJ, Mundy AR. Pregnancy after lower urinary tract reconstruction in women. *J Urol* 1995, 154: 1323–1324

25. Hatch TR, Steinberg RW, Davis LE. Successful term delivery by Cesarean section in a patient with a continent ileocecal urinary reservoir. *J Urol* 1991: 146: 1111–1112

26. Greenberg M, Vaughan ED Jr, Pitts WR Jr. Normal pregnancy and delivery after ileal conduit urinary diversion. *J Urol* 1981; 125: 172–173

27. Barrett RJ, Peters WA. Pregnancy following urinary diversion. *Obstet Gynecol* 1983; 62: 582–586

28. Akerlund S, Bokstrom H, Jonson O *et al.* Pregnancy and delivery in patients with urinary diversion through the continent ileal reservoir. *Surg Gynecol Obstet* 1991; 173: 350–352

62

Complications of surgery for genuine stress incontinence

C. Chaliha, S. L. Stanton

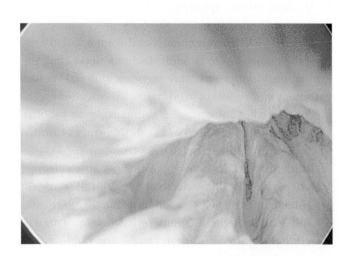

INTRODUCTION

Over 150 operations have been described for the cure of stress incontinence in women. The variety of procedures indicates that none is entirely satisfactory. The choice sometimes depends more on the training and skill of the surgeon than on the urodynamic characteristics of each patient.

The evaluation of any surgery should be based on the patient's clinical symptoms and signs, urodynamic studies and an analysis of short- and long-term success as well as immediate and delayed complications. The cure rate should be weighed against the risk of complications.

Operations for genuine stress incontinence

The criteria for surgical treatment of genuine stress incontinence (GSI) are an objective demonstration of urethral sphincter incompetence and failure of conservative treatment. Ideally, the woman should have completed her family. Relative contraindications include untreated detrusor instability (DI) and voiding disorder. As some operations predispose to prolapse, pre-existing prolapse must be evaluated.

The common operations to treat stress incontinence are as follows:

1. Open or laparoscopic Burch colposuspension;
2. Endoscopic bladder-neck suspension operations (Pereyra, Stamey and Raz procedures);
3. Sling procedures;
4. Periurethral or transurethral bulking injections;
5. Marshall–Marchetti–Krantz operation;
6. Anterior colporrhaphy;
7. Artificial urinary sphincter.

There is no single operation for all women and, therefore, the choice has to be individualized, depending on the clinical symptoms and signs, additional pelvic pathology and results of urodynamic investigations.

The complications may be summarized as follows: (1) immediate (0–24 hours); (2) short-term; (24 hours to 6 weeks); (3) long-term (6 weeks onwards).

To identify studies assessing outcome, an electronic search of the Medline database (1966–1997) of all English language articles was undertaken, together with a hand search of the citations revealed by this initial search. Randomized controlled trials, non-randomized trials, prospective and retrospective cohort studies and case–control studies were included.

IMMEDIATE COMPLICATIONS

Haemorrhage

Significant bleeding may occur from perivesical venous plexus trauma during anterior colporrhaphy and dissection of the retropubic space during colposuspension. A retropubic haematoma may result and serve as a nidus for infection and abscess formation. The mean blood loss following anterior colporrhaphy was 200 ml (standard deviation [SD] 135 ml) and following Burch colposuspension was 260 ml (SD 195 ml).[1] Alcalay et al.[2] surveyed 109 women who had undergone a Burch colposuspension. Although there was no difference in blood loss between primary and secondary surgery, blood loss of more than 1 litre was associated with a synchronous hysterectomy and more failures to cure stress incontinence. Blood loss with laparoscopic colposuspension is said to be minimal; however, the operation has a cure rate less than that of an open colposuspension.[3,4] The average blood loss with the Marshall–Marchetti–Krantz operation is 142 ml (range 20–500 ml), with the Stamey procedure is 53 ml (range 10–157 ml)[5] and with the Teflon (polytetrafluoroethylene) sling is 153 ml.[6] The frequency of significant haemorrhage following the different operations[1,2,5,7–15] is summarized in Table 62.1.

Urinary tract injuries

Bladder and ureteric injury can occur during dissection of the retropubic space or insertion of sutures. The bladder is most frequently damaged during endoscopic bladder-neck suspension, sling operations and laparoscopic colposuspension. Cystoscopy should always be performed during endoscopic bladder-neck suspension and, if in doubt, at time of sling and laparoscopic surgery. Mainprize and Drutz[11] found that 19 (0.7%) women who sustained lacerations to the bladder in a survey of 2712 women undergoing the Marshall–Marchetti–Krantz procedure; in addition, 13 women (0.5%) experienced urethral obstruction and 2 (0.1%) ureterovesical obstruction. Injury to the bladder and ureter have been reported in up to 6% at

Table 62.1. *Immediate complications of operations for genuine stress incontinence*

Complication	Operation	Number in study	Number of patients*	Reference
Haemorrhage	Anterior colporrhaphy	56	2 (3.6)	Van Geelen et al.[1]
	Burch colposuspension	180	1 (0.6)	Stanton and Cardozo[7]
	Burch colposuspension	109	8 (7.3)	Alcalay et al.[2]
	Sling	281	6 (2.1)	Morgan et al.[8]
	Needle suspension procedures	44	3 (6.8)	Peattie and Stanton[9]
	Needle suspension procedures	20	2 (10)	Varner[10]
	Marshall–Marchetti–Krantz	2712	7 (0.3)	Mainprize and Drutz[11]
	Marshall–Marchetti–Krantz	54	2 (3.7)	Spencer et al.[5]
	Marshall–Marchetti–Krantz	490	10 (2)	Riggs[12]
	Marshall–Marchetti–Krantz	21	2 (10)	Green et al.[13]
Urinary tract injury	Burch colposuspension	34	1 (2.9)	Van Geelen et al.[1]
	Burch colposuspension	180	2 (1.1)	Stanton and Cardozo[7]
	Burch colposuspension	38	2 (5.3)	Pow-Sang et al.[14]
	Sling	48	3 (6.3)	Summitt et al.[15]
	Needle suspension procedures	44	1 (2)	Peattie and Stanton[9]
	Needle suspension procedures	29	1 (3.4)	Green et al.[13]
	Marshall–Marchetti–Krantz	2712	34 (1.3)	Mainprize and Drutz[11]

* Percentages in parentheses.

open colposuspension,[1,7,14] but none was reported by Alcalay *et al.*[2] Laparoscopic surgery carries a greater risk of urinary tract injury, which can occur in up to 10% of women.[16–18] The incidence of urinary tract injuries during endoscopic bladder-neck suspension is 1–7%.[13,19,20] Urethral injury or unrecognized entry into a urethral diverticulum during anterior colporrhaphy may result in urethrovaginal fistula.

Trauma to the bladder and urethra can also occur at insertion of an artificial urinary sphincter. The rate of injury to the urinary tract following the different operations is summarized in Table 62.1.

Suprapubic catheterization has its risks: the catheter may kink, become obstructed, break or dislodge.[21,22] Perforation of the bowel may occur during suprapubic and transurethral insertion.[23–25] In one case, perfora-

tion of the caecum during endoscopic bladder-neck suspension was detected some 4 years later during abdominal surgery for stress urinary incontinence.[26]

Urinary tract infection

Voiding difficulties after surgery for GSI may require prolonged catheterization, which may lead to urinary tract infection. This is associated more with transurethral than with suprapubic catheterization. The rate of infection increases with the duration of catheterization by 6–7.5% per day.[27] In a randomized trial of suprapubic compared with transurethral drainage after colposuspension or vaginal repair, Anderson *et al.*[28] found that bacteriuria on postoperative day 5 was less common with suprapubic catheterization (21 vs 46%).

SHORT-TERM COMPLICATIONS

Wound infection

Following vaginal continence surgery, wound infection is more common when a hysterectomy is performed at the same time. Permanent sutures and synthetic grafts increase the likelihood of infection. The frequency of wound infection and abscess formation is summarized in Table 62.2.[7,11,29–41] Wound infection leads to short-term morbidity and delayed hospital discharge and may necessitate removal of inorganic slings. Pubovaginal slings with synthetic material increase the risk of infection and erosion rates by 21%.[42] Mundy[43] reported that 16% of patients required the removal of a Dacron rectus sheath buffer after a Stamey procedure. Jarvis[44] noted that 1.5% of women undergoing the same procedure had erosion of the suture, which sometimes had to be removed. Infection following periurethral Teflon, leading to granuloma and abscess formation has been reported.[33] Infection of the artificial urinary sphincter has been reported in up to 9.5% of cases and may lead to pump or cuff erosion, requiring subsequent removal of the sphincter.[45,46]

Osteitis pubis

Osteitis pubis is self-limiting non-infectious inflammation of the symphysis pubis, which can occur in up to 5% of patients who have undergone a Marshall–Marchetti–Krantz procedure. It may lead to osteomyelitis of the pubic bone. Its pathogenesis may be trauma to the periosteum, low-grade infection, trophic changes in the bone similar to causalgia, and venous thrombosis.[11] It has also been found after endoscopic bladder-neck suspension.[13]

Urogenital fistulae

Urogenital fistulae are rare complications and usually present within 10 days of surgery. They may occur following direct injury to the urinary tract, or infection or erosion of sling or suture material; the frequency of this complication is summarized in Table 62.2.

Nerve injuries

Endoscopic bladder-neck suspension may lead to injury to the common peroneal, sciatic, obturator, femoral, saphenous and ilio-inguinal nerves.[47] The ilio-inguinal nerve is particularly susceptible to damage as it emerges from the superficial inguinal ring, owing to insertion of the Stamey needle lateral to the pubic tubercle. The incidence of this complication is summarized in Table 62.2.

The femoral nerve can be directly injured during operation and is also susceptible to indirect injury due to retractor blades and to abduction and flexion of the thigh in the modified lithotomy position often used for operations for stress incontinence. This leads to weakness of the quadriceps, which is noticeable during walking, and decreased sensation over the anterior thigh and medial calf.

Voiding dysfunction

Most operations for stress incontinence are obstructive and may result in voiding difficulty. The true incidence is difficult to ascertain because definitions and treatment vary from mild disturbance to that requiring intermittent self-catheterization. Extreme elevation of the bladder neck – such as occurs with over-enthusiastic colposuspension or undue tension being applied to a sling – is the most likely cause of postoperative voiding difficulty.[48,49] In women with abnormal voiding patterns and who void by straining, an increased incidence of voiding disorder is seen after bladder-neck surgery.[50,51] The incidence of voiding dysfunction is summarized in Table 62.2. Delayed voiding is the most common complication after sling operations, especially when using synthetic materials,[40,52] and up to 8% of patients may require long-term self-catheterization.[53] Korda *et al.*[54] reported voiding disorders in 37% of patients, and 28% had to return to theatre for a sling release to allow voiding to take place.

Voiding difficulties after periurethral injections are uncommon, but temporary voiding disorder may occur in up to 2% of women.[55,56]

Suprapubic catheters are associated with a more rapid return to normal voiding than is achieved after transurethral catheterization.[57] Where voiding disorder is prolonged, self-catheterization is the simplest remedy, which may be helped by the addition of an α-adrenergic blocking agent.

Table 62.2. *Short-term complications of operations for genuine stress incontinence*

Complication	Operation	Number in study	Number of patients*	Reference
Wound infection	Anterior colporrhaphy	294	38 (12.9)	Peters and Thornton[29]
	Burch colposuspension	180	1 (0.6)	Stanton and Cardozo[7]
	Fascial sling	170	8 (4.7)	Beck et al.[30]
	Marlex sling	69	4 (5.8)	Bryans[31]
	Needle suspension procedures	98	7 (7.1)	Muznai et al.[32]
	Periurethral injections	27	1 (3.7)	Lotenfoe et al.[33]
	Marshall–Marchetti–Krantz	102	10 (9.8)	Peters and Thornton[29]
Osteitis pubis	Needle suspension procedures	29	1 (3.4)	Green et al.[13]
	Marshall–Marchetti–Krantz	2712	68 (2.5)	Mainprize and Drutz[11]
Urogenital fistulae	Anterior colporrhaphy	519	2 (0.4)	Beck et al.[34]
	Sling	105	1 (0.9)	Kersey[35]
	Needle suspension procedures	60	1 (1.7)	Guam et al.[36]
	Marshall–Marchetti–Krantz	2712	7 (0.3)	Mainprize and Drutz[11]
Nerve injuries	Needle suspension procedures	402	7 (1.7)	Miyazaki and Shook[37]
Voiding difficulty	Anterior repair	519	3 (0.6)	Beck et al.[34]
	Burch colposuspension	50	8 (16)	Galloway et al.[38]
	Burch colposuspension	80	20 (25)	Lose et al.[39]
	Sling	88	2 (2.3)	Chin and Stanton[40]
	Needle suspension procedures	93	14 (15)	Karram et al.[41]
	Marshall–Marchetti–Krantz	2712	98 (3.6)	Mainprize and Drutz[11]

* Percentages in parentheses.

LONG-TERM COMPLICATIONS

Detrusor instability

There is a 40–45% risk of preoperative DI persisting following continence surgery.[58] This has a deleterious effect on cure of stress incontinence and, ideally, drug treatment and bladder retraining should be carried out beforehand.

DI arising for the first time following continence surgery is a troublesome complication. In men, urethral obstruction secondary to prostatic hypertrophy induces DI. In women, decreased flow rates and increased pressure transmission ratios have been seen in women who develop postoperative DI.[49] This has been disputed by Cardozo et al.,[59] who found that flow rates were decreased in women who had both stable and unstable bladders and that maximum voiding pressure was increased in stable bladders but unaltered in unstable bladders. They suggested that instability arising for the first time was due to nerve damage following dissection of the bladder. Vierhout and Mulder[60] reviewed six studies involving 396 women without preoperative DI who had undergone

Table 62.3. *Long-term complications of operations for genuine stress incontinence*

Complication	Operation	Number in study	Number of patients*	Reference
De-novo detrusor instability	Anterior colporrhaphy	436	28 (6.4)	Beck et al.[34]
	Burch colposuspension	92	17 (18.4)	Cardozo et al.[59]
	Burch colposuspension	109	16 (14.7)	Alcalay et al.[2]
	Sling	80	22 (27.5)	Chin and Stanton[40]
	Sling	82	5 (6.1)	McGuire et al.[65]
	Needle suspension procedures	10	1 (10)	Hilton[66]
	Needle suspension procedures	206	11 (5.3)	Raz et al.[67]
Genital prolapse, vault prolapse	Burch colposuspension	50	4 (8)	Galloway et al.[38]
	Needle suspension procedures	206	2 (1)	Raz et al.[67]
Cystocele	Needle suspension procedures	206	4 (2)	Raz et al.[67]
Rectocele	Burch colposuspension	109	28 (25.7)	Alcalay et al.[2]
	Burch colposuspension	131	29 (22.1)	Wiskind et al.[68]
Enterocele	Burch colposuspension	109	5 (4.6)	Alcalay et al.[2]
	Burch colposuspension	131	14 (10.7)	Wiskind et al.[68]
	Needle suspension procedures	206	7 (3)	Raz et al.[67]
Pain	Burch colposuspension	50	6 (12)	Galloway et al.[38]
	Burch colposuspension	102	27 (26)	Wheelahan[69]
	Needle suspension procedures	17	1 (5.9)	Griffith-Jones and Abrams[70]
	Needle suspension procedures	206	7 (3.4)	Raz et al.[67]
Dyspareunia	Burch colposuspension	34	1 (0.3)	Van Geelen et al.[1]
	Burch colposuspension	50	2 (4)	Galloway et al.[38]
	Needle suspension procedures	206	3 (1.5)	Ra et al.[67]
	Needle suspension procedures	142	1 (0.7)	Kursh et al.[71]
	Marshall–Marchetti–Krantz	2712	10 (0.4)	Mainprize and Drutz[11]

* Percentages in parentheses.

Burch colposuspension: they found that instability occurred in 5–27% of women postoperatively, and concluded that the differences in prevalence rates were due to differences in cystometric and surgical techniques. The incidence of DI following laparoscopic Burch colposuspension is 10–12%,[61,62] and transient instability has been reported after periurethral injections.[63,64] The incidence of DI following other surgery for incontinence is summarized in Table 62.3.[1,2,11,34,38,40,59,65–71]

Genital prolapse

Burch[72] originally noted that enterocele occurred in 8% and cystocele in 3% of women following colposuspension. In a systematic review, Jarvis[73] found that prolapse occurred in 14% of women after colposuspension. In an uncontrolled case series the proportion was as high as 22%.[68] The incidence of this complication is summarized in Table 62.3.

Alcalay *et al.*[2] found that 33 of 109 women (30%) developed prolapse between 10 and 20 years after their Burch colposuspension. The development of prolapse is thought to be due to the elevation of the anterior vaginal wall, which exposes the vault and posterior vaginal wall to the direct force of intra-abdominal pressure. Colposuspension may also weaken the supports of these structures.

Dyspareunia and chronic suprapubic pain

The incidence of chronic pain and dyspareunia after surgery for stress incontinence is difficult to determine, as these symptoms may not always be reported. The incidence of these complications is summarized in Table 62.3.

Pain caused by sutures occurs in approximately 10% of women after endoscopic bladder-neck suspension and may be due to entrapment of the ilio-inguinal nerve within the stitch or inflammation around it.[70] About 5% of women require one or both stitches to be removed because of persistent pain or sinus formation. Chronic pain may occur in 12% of women after colposuspension and may be relieved by cutting the stitch on the affected side. In both operations there is a risk of recurrence of incontinence.

Dyspareunia has been reported in 0.4% of women after the Marshall–Marchetti–Krantz procedure and in up to 4% after colposuspension (Table 62.3).

Effect on quality of life

In a prospective study Black and colleagues[74,75] found that 7% of women reported deterioration in their general health 1 year after continence surgery; 25% of women reported worse mental health, which may be a reflection of disappointment on not achieving a cure, as only 28% of women in this group achieved continence. Postoperative recovery was longer than anticipated, with 24% of women still on sick or unpaid leave when they had previously been employed. Although this information is limited, as it assesses a heterogeneous group of women who have undergone different procedures by many different surgeons, it provides a valuable reminder that surgery for stress incontinence may have detrimental economic, psychological and social consequences.

CONCLUSIONS

Improved quality of life and success rate must significantly outweigh the risk of complications. Analysis of the true incidence of complications is difficult, as reporting and definitions of complications is not uniform and patient follow-up is too short for true assessment. The validity of outcome data is questionable as there have been few large randomized controlled trials.

In this present climate of increased litigation, counselling a woman prior to surgery must include information about the possible complications of the procedures as well as the success rates. Any new or experimental procedures must be disclosed to the patient. For any new procedure, the subjective and objective outcomes need to be measured over a follow-up period of at least 2 years. This rigorous assessment of each surgical procedure will allow both surgeon and patient to make an informed decision on consent.

REFERENCES

1. Van Geelen JM, Theeuwes AGM, Eskes TKAB, Martin CB. The clinical and urodynamic effects of anterior vaginal repair and Burch colposuspension. *Am J Obstet Gynecol* 1988; 159: 137–144

2. Alcalay M, Monga A, Stanton SL. Burch colposuspension: a 10–20 year follow up. *Br J Obstet Gynaecol* 1995; 102: 740–745

3. Burton G. A three year prospective randomised urodynamic study comparing open and laparoscopic colposuspension. *Neurourol Urodyn* 1997; 5: 353–354

4. Tsung-Hsien Su, Kuo-Gon Wang, Chin-Yan Hsu *et al.* Prospective comparison of laparoscopic and traditional colposuspension in the treatment of genuine stress incontinence. *Acta Obstet Gynecol Scand* 1997; 76: 576–582

5. Spencer JR, O'Connor J, Schaeffer AJ. A comparison of endoscopic suspension of the vesical neck with suprapubic vesico-urethropexy for the treatment of stress urinary incontinence. *J Urol* 1987; 137: 411–415

6. Horbach NS, Blanco JS, Ostergard DR *et al.* A suburethral sling procedure with polytetrafluoroethylene for the treatment of genuine stress incontinence in patients with low urethral closure pressure. *Obstet Gynecol* 1988; 71: 648–652

7. Stanton SL, Cardozo LD. Results of the colposuspension operation for incontinence and prolapse. *Br J Obstet Gynaecol* 1979; 86: 693–697

8. Morgan JE, Farrow GA, Stuart FE. The Marlex sling operation for the treatment of recurrent stress urinary incontinence: a sixteen year review. *Am J Obstet Gynecol* 1985; 151: 224–226

9. Peattie AB, Stanton SL. The Stamey operation for the correction of genuine stress incontinence in the elderly woman. *Br J Obstet Gynaecol* 1989; 96: 983–986

10. Varner RE. Retropubic long needle suspension procedures for stress urinary incontinence. *Am J Obstet Gynecol* 1990; 163: 551–557

11. Mainprize TC, Drutz HP. The Marshall–Marchetti–Krantz procedure. a clinical review. *Obstet Gynecol Surv* 1988; 43: 724–729

12. Riggs JA. Retropubic cystourethropexy: a review of two operative procedures with long-term follow-up. *Obstet Gynecol* 1986; 68: 98–105

13. Green DF, McGuire EJ, Lytton B. A comparison of endoscopic suspension of the vesical neck versus anterior urethropexy for the treatment of stress urinary incontinence. *J Urol* 1986; 136: 1205–1207.

14. Pow-Sang JM, Lockart JL, Suarez A *et al.* Female urinary incontinence, preoperative selection, surgical complications and results. *J Urol* 1986; 136: 831–833

15. Summitt RL, Bent AE, Ostergard DR, Harris TA. Suburethral sling procedure for genuine stress incontinence and low urethral closure pressure: a continued experience. *Int Urogynecol J* 1992; 3: 18–21

16. Liu CY, Paek W. Laparoscopic retropubic colposuspension (Burch procedure). *J Am Assoc Gynecol Laparosc* 1993; 1: 31–35

17. Vancaillie TG, Schuessler W. Laparoscopic bladder neck suspension. *J Laparoendosc Surg* 1991; 1: 169–173

18. McDougall EM, Klutke CG, Cornell T. Comparison of transvaginal versus laparoscopic bladder neck suspension for stress urinary incontinence. *Urology* 1995; 45: 641–646

19. Pereyra AJ, Lebherz TB, Growdon WA, Powers JA. Pubourethral supports in perspective: modified Pereyra procedure for urinary incontinence. *Obstet Gynecol* 1982; 59: 643–648

20. Backer MH Jr, Probst RE. The Pereyra procedure. favorable experience with 200 operations. *Am J Obstet Gynecol* 1976; 125: 346–351

21. Broberg C. Catheter drainage after gynecologic surgery; a comparison of methods. *Am J Obstet Gynecol* 1984; 149: 18–21

22. Drutz HP, Khosid HI. Complications with Bonanno suprapubic catheters. *Am J Obstet Gynecol* 1984; 149: 685–686

23. Noller KI, Pratt JH, Symmonds HE. Bowel perforation with suprapubic cystostomy; report of two cases. *Obstet Gynecol* 1976; 48: 675–695

24. Loughlin KR, Whitmore WF, Gittes RF, Richie JP. Review of an eight-year experience with modifications of endoscopic suspension of the bladder neck for female stress urinary incontinence. *J Urol* 1990; 143: 44–45

25. Cundiff G, Bent AE. Suprapubic catheterisation complicated by bowel injury. *Int Urogynecol J* 1995; 6: 110–113

26. Tamussino K, Zivkovic F, Lang PFJ, Ralph G. Unrecognised perforation of the cecum at needle suspension of the bladder neck: a case report. *Int Urogynecol J* 1995; 6: 355–356

27. Foucher JE, Marshall V. Nosocomial catheter associated urinary tract infections. *Infect Surg* 1983; 2: 43–45

28. Anderson JT, Heisterberg S, Hebjorn S *et al.* Suprapubic versus transurethral bladder drainage after colposuspension/vaginal repair. *Acta Obstet Gynecol Scand* 1985; 64: 139–143

29. Peters WA, Thornton WN. Selection of the primary operative procedure for stress urinary incontinence. *Am J Obstet Gynecol* 1980; 137: 923–930

30. Beck RP, McCormick S, Nordstrom L. The fascia lata sling procedure for treating recurrent genuine stress incontinence of urine. *Obstet Gynecol* 1988; 72: 699–703

31. Bryans FE. Marlex gauze hammock sling operation with Cooper's ligament attachment in the management of recurrent urinary stress incontinence. *Am J Obstet Gynecol* 1974; 133: 292–294

32. Muznai D, Carrill E, Dubin C, Silverman I. Retropubic vaginopexy for the correction of urinary stress incontinence. *Obstet Gynecol* 1992; 59: 113–118

33. Lotenfoe R, O'Kelly JK, Helal M, Lockart JL. Periurethral polytetrafluoroethylene paste injection in incontinent female subjects: surgical indications and improved surgical technique. *J Urol* 1993; 149: 279–282

34. Beck RP, McCormick S, Nordstrom L. A twenty five year experience with 519 anterior colporrhaphy procedures. *Obstet Gynecol* 1991; 78: 1011–1018

35. Kersey J. The gauze hammock sling operation in the treatment of stress incontinence. *Br J Obstet Gynaecol* 1983; 90: 945–949

36. Guam L, Ricciotti NA, Fair WR. Endoscopic bladder neck

suspension for stress urinary incontinence. *J Urol* 1984; 132: 1119–1121

37. Miyazaki F, Shook G. llioinguinal nerve entrapment during needle suspension for stress incontinence. *Obstet Gynecol* 1992; 80: 246–248

38. Galloway NTM, Davies N, Stephenson TP. The complications of colposuspension. *Br J Urol* 1987; 60: 122–124

39. Lose G, Jorgensen L, Mortensen SO *et al.* Voiding difficulties after colposuspension. *Obstet Gynecol* 1987; 69: 33–37

40. Chin YK, Stanton SL. A follow-up of silastic slings for genuine stress incontinence. *Br J Obstet Gynaecol* 1995; 102: 143–147

41. Karram MM, Angel O, Koonings P *et al.* The modified Peyrera procedure: a clinical and urodynamic review. *Br J Obstet Gynaecol* 1992; 99: 655–658

42. Bent AE, Ostergard DR, Zwick-Zaffulo M. Tissue reaction to expanded polytetrafluoroethylene suburethral sling for urinary incontinence. clinical and histological study. *Am J Obstet Gynecol* 1993; 169: 1198–1204

43. Mundy AR. A trial comparing Stamey bladder neck suspension procedure with colposuspension for the treatment of stress incontinence: *Br J Urol* 1983; 55: 687–690

44. Jarvis GJ. Re: Erosion of buttress following bladder suspension [letter, comment]. *Br J Urol* 1992; 70: 695

45. Appell RA. Techniques and results in the implantation of the artificial urinary sphincter in women with type III stress urinary incontinence by vaginal approach. *Neurourol Urodyn* 1988; 7: 613–619

46. Light JK. Abdominal approach for the implantation of the AS800 artificial urinary sphincter in females. *Neurourol Urodyn* 1988; 7: 603–611

47. Karram MM, Angel O, Koonings P *et al.* The modified Peyrera procedure. a clinical and urodynamic review. *Br J Obstet Gynaecol* 1992; 99: 655–658

48. Hertogs K, Stanton SL. Mechanism of urinary incontinence after colposuspension: barrier studies. *Br J Obstet Gynaecol* 1985; 92: 1184–1188

49. Bump RC, Fantl JA, Hurt WG. Dynamic urethral pressure profilometry pressure transmission ratio determinations after continence surgery: understanding the mechanisms of success, failure and complications. *Obstet Gynecol* 1988; 72: 870–877

50. Rud T, Ulmsten U, Anderssen KE. Initiation of voiding in healthy women and those with stress incontinence. *Acta Obstet Gynecol Scand* 1978; 57: 457–462

51. Bhatia NN, Bergman A. Urodynamic predictability of voiding following incontinence surgery. *Obstet Gynecol* 1984; 63: 85–91

52. Young SB, Rosenblatt PL, Pingeton DM *et al.* The Mersilene mesh suburethral sling: a clinical and urodynamic evaluation. *Am J Obstet Gynecol* 1995; 173: 1719–1726

53. Spence-Jones C, DeMarco E, Lemieux M-C, Drutz HP. Modified urethral sling for the treatment of genuine stress incontinence and latent incontinence. *Int Urogynecol J* 1994; 5: 69–75

54. Korda A, Peat B, Hunter P. Experience with silastic slings for female urinary incontinence. *Aust N Z J Obstet Gynaecol* 1989; 29: 150–154

55. Deane AM, English P, Hehir M *et al.* Teflon injection in stress incontinence. *J Urol* 1985; 57: 78–80

56. Stanton SL, Monga AK. Incontinence in elderly women: is periurethral collagen an advance? *Br J Obstet Gynaecol* 1997; 104: 154–157

57. Bergman A, Matthews L, Ballard CA, Roy S. Suprapubic versus transurethral bladder drainage after surgery for stress urinary incontinence. *Obstet Gynecol* 1987; 69: 546–549

58. Langer R, Ron-El R, Newman M *et al.* Detrusor instability following colposuspension for urinary stress incontinence. *Br J Obstet Gynaecol* 1988; 95: 607–610

59. Cardozo LC, Stanton SL, Williams JE. Detrusor instability following surgery for genuine stress incontinence. *Br J Urol* 1979; 51: 204–207

60. Vierhout ME, Mulder APF. De novo detrusor instability after Burch colposuspension. *Acta Obstet Gynecol Scand* 1992; 71: 414–416

61. Radomski SB, Herschorn S. Laparoscopic Burch bladder neck suspension: early results. *J Urol* 1996; 155: 515–518

62. Polascik T, Moore R, Rosenberg M, Kavoussi L. Comparison of laparoscopic and open retropubic urethropexy for treatment of stress urinary incontinence. *Urology* 1995; 45: 647–652

63. Politano VA. Periurethral polytetrafluoroethylene injection for urinary incontinence. *J Urol* 1982; 127: 439–442

64. Stricker P, Haylen B. Injectable collagen for type III female stress incontinence: the first 50 Australian patients. *Med J Aust* 1993; 151: 89–91

65. McGuire EJ, Bennett CJ, Konnak JA *et al.* Experience with pubovaginal slings for urinary incontinence at the University of Michigan. *J Urol* 1987; 138: 525–526

66. Hilton P. A clinical and urodynamic study comparing the Stamey bladder neck suspension and suburethral sling procedures in the treatment of genuine stress incontinence. *Br J Obstet Gynaecol* 1989; 96: 213–220

67. Raz S, Sussman EM, Eriksen DB *et al.* The Raz bladder neck suspension: results in 206 patients. *J Urol* 1992; 148: 845–850

68. Wiskind AK, Creighton SM, Stanton SL. The incidence of genital prolapse after Burch colposuspension. *Am J Obstet Gynecol* 1992; 167: 399–405

69. Wheelahan JB. Long-term results of colposuspension. *Br J Urol* 1990; 65: 329–332

70. Griffith-Jones MD, Abrams PH. The Stamey endoscopic bladder neck suspension in the elderly. *Br J Urol* 1990; 65: 170–172

71. Kursh ED, Angell AH, Resnick MI. Evolution of endoscopic urethropexy: seven year experience with various techniques. *Urology* 1991; 37: 428–431

72. Burch JC. Cooper's ligament urethrovesical suspension for stress incontinence. nine years' experience. Results, complications, technique. *Am J Obstet Gynecol* 1968; 100: 764–772.

73. Jarvis GJ. Surgery for genuine stress incontinence. *Br J Obstet Gynaecol* 1994; 101: 371–374

74. Black NA, Griffiths JM, Pope C *et al.* Impact of surgery for stress incontinence on morbidity: cohort study. *Br Med J* 1997; 15: 1493–1498

75. Black NA, Bowling A, Griffiths JM, Abel PD. Impact of surgery for stress incontinence on the social lives of women. *Br J Obstet Gynaecol* 1998; 105: 605–612

63

Effects of pelvic surgery on the lower urinary tract

M. E. Vierhout

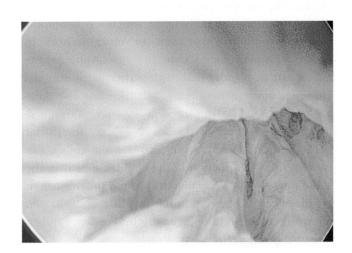

INTRODUCTION

The lower urinary tract (urethra, bladder and lower ureter) is positioned deep in the female pelvis, in close proximity to the uterus and vagina as well as to the rectum. Pelvic surgery involving either the uterus and adnexa or the colorectal system has a profound influence on the lower urinary tract, not only through this anatomical proximity but also through a functional interrelationship.[1–5] Embryologically, there is also a common origin between the female reproductive system and the urinary tract.

A number of mechanisms are responsible for the effects of surgery of the female pelvis on the lower urinary tract. By removal of the uterus, the bladder will have a new anatomical position. When a large fibroid or ovarian cyst is removed, the anatomical changes will be even more pronounced. Sometimes a relatively abnormal position will become more physiological after removal of these, sometimes major, deformations of the normal anatomy.

In (radical) hysterectomy the proximity is so close that accidental perforation of the bladder is a well-known complication. In cases that are not well recognized and treated, a vesicovaginal fistula can occur, as can direct damage to the bladder wall with its neurogenic structures. However, it is more common for the neurological damage to the lower urinary tract to be caused by trauma to the common autonomic and somatic innervation of the bladder, uterus and rectum. The lower urinary tract is innervated by autonomic parasympathetic (S2–4), autonomic sympathetic (T10–L2) and somatic (S2–4) nerves. In particular, dissection low in the pelvis, below the level of the cardinal ligaments, will cause neurological damage.[6] Depending on the precise nature of the trauma – parasympathetic, sympathetic or somatic – symptoms will be hypotonic, hypertonic or more sensory in nature. This neurological damage is responsible for the major part of bladder dysfunction after pelvic surgery. However, not only neurological damage but also damage to the blood or lymph vessels (or both) is responsible for dysfunction of the lower urinary tract after pelvic surgery. Furthermore, major haematomas can cause serious dysfunction of the bladder, mostly in the acute phase when a haematoma around the urethra or bladder neck will be responsible for the inabilty to void after surgery. In addition, para-urethral oedema and an awkward position for micturition, in combination with the effects of certain drugs and pain, will be responsible for this phenomenon which is, however, usually temporary. Nevertheless, if it leads to overdistension of the bladder it can cause serious damage, such as a poorly functioning detrusor giving rise, in turn, to chronic retention.

Urinary tract infections are common after pelvic surgery. They can easily occur, and not only after catheterization; however, if they are recognized at an early stage and dealt with appropriately, they should not lead to any long-term damage. However, failure to recognize or to treat urinary tract infection can lead to chronic infection with subsequent long-term damage. Repeated catheterization can lead to urethral damage with strictures and stenosis.

In daily practice, the effect of pelvic surgery on the lower urinary tract is sometimes difficult to interpret because of the effects of other treatment modalities: for example, radiotherapy has a severely damaging effect on the lower urinary tract and can cause irritation, haematuria and bladder fibrosis.[1]

In this chapter the major gynaecological and colorectal operations and their effects on the lower urinary tract are discussed, omitting any mention of surgical procedures that are specifically aimed at correcting an abnormally functioning bladder or urethra (such as the Burch colposuspension).

RADICAL HYSTERECTOMY

Radical or Wertheim's hysterectomy is currently the primary treatment for cervical carcinoma stages IB and IIA. It includes (in addition to removal of the uterus), pelvic lymphadenectomy, removal of the upper part of the vagina and removal of the parametrium and higher paracolpium. The 5-year survival rate is over 85%. In relation to the effects on the lower urinary tract, it must be borne in mind that often these patients also receive radiotherapy, which has also a negative effect.

Radical hysterectomy has a well-known and accepted adverse effect on the lower urinary tract, generally described as occurring in over 50% of patients but in some series to 80%.[6–20] In early series, more attention was given to the formation and prevention of fistulae between the urinary tract and the vagina. In the current series, the incidence of fistulae has decreased to less than 1%,[11] in sharp contrast to the incidence of 13% that was quoted in earlier series.[1] The reason for this lower incidence of fistulae is probably multifactorial and may include a less-radical procedure, greater emphasis on atramautic surgery (especially with respect to the ureter and its blood supply), greater care in the prevention of infection by the use of prophylactic antibiotics and, more recently, the technique of transposition of the omentum, which improves the blood supply to the pelvis.

Currently, neurological damage is considered to be the main cause of the high incidence of lower urinary tract dysfunction. Anatomically, the area where the damage occurs is in the deeper cardinal–uterosacral complex (sacro-uterine web), where there are branches of parasympathetic and sympathetic as well as somatic nerves. Various studies have shown that protection of this area by a lesser degree of dissection gives rise to fewer adverse effects on the lower urinary tract; however, this is disputed by other authors.[17] Apart from neurological damage, fibrosis, haematoma and lymphoedema of the area can be held responsible for lower urinary tract dysfunction. Although it is possible that loss of urethral support could cause stress incontinence after radical hysterectomy, in an elegant study by Westby this was not confirmed.[19]

The symptoms of lower urinary tract dysfunction after radical hysterectomy are diverse. In general, a concept of parasympathetic denervation with sympathetic dominance is accepted. Loss of the sensation of micturition, poor stream and a feeling of incomplete emptying, stress incontinence and urge symptoms are prominent; these can be mild or extremely bothersome. In urodynamic studies generally a decreased compliance is seen with a poor flow rate, residual, loss of sensation with an increased bladder capacity and decreased urethral closure pressure.[1]

To prevent these lower urinary tract symptoms it will be necessary to perform less-radical surgery, with long-term initial bladder drainage after surgery to prevent overdistension and with atraumatic and sparing surgical techniques, especially in relation to the urinary tract, and prevention of urinary tract and other types of pelvic infection.

The symptoms may be considered as those that occur (a) in the early phase (first month), (b) in the intermediate phase (up to 1 year) and (c) in the later phase (more than 1 year). The long-term symptoms, in particular, are considered to be of neurological origin. It has been shown that after a year there is little or no improvement in symptoms and urodynamic parameters.[21]

Treatment of lower urinary tract symptoms after radical hysterectomy is symptomatic and dependent on the most prominent symptom. In particular, regular (scheduled) voiding is advised in patients with lack of bladder sensation. Sometimes intermittent catheterization and long-term antibiotic therapy are advised. Where there are irritative symptoms, anticholinergics have a place but can increase an already existent residual. Colposuspension is not usually indicated in the treatment of stress incontinence.

SIMPLE (NON-RADICAL) HYSTERECTOMY

Simple hysterectomy is often mentioned as a cause of dysfunction of the lower urinary tract;[22,23] however, this accusation is not supported by data from the literature. The first to mention this detrimental effect of hysterectomy was Hanley in 1969.[24] Since his publication, numerous studies and opinions have appeared in the literature.[25–45] However, most of these have failed to demonstrate any clinically significant effect of simple hysterectomy on the lower urinary tract. This apparent discrepancy between clinical experience and scientific evidence could be caused by a number of factors:

1. The majority of women in whom hysterectomy is performed are in the perimenopausal age group in which lower urinary tract symptoms have a high prevalence. It is not surprising, therefore, that, when a post-hysterectomy group is studied, a high prevalence will be found.

2. The individual patient will often relate the onset of the symptoms to the moment of hysterectomy; however, this does not necessarily have to be a causational relationship – patients will often date the onset of their symptoms in relation to a life event such as hysterectomy.

3. Less-prominent symptoms already present, such as mild stress incontinence, can become more dominant when major symptoms such as menorrhagia have been abolished by the hysterectomy, thus giving a seemingly causal relationship.

4. When hysterectomy is performed because of prolapse in combination with an anterior repair with latent stress incontinence, developing stress incontinence

will be blamed on the hysterectomy whereas, in fact, the anterior repair is the culprit.

5. Certainly, hysterectomy is known to have a short-term effect on lower urinary tract function but these symptoms, which are due to irritation, haematoma and oedema, generally will not persist.

6. In contrast to radical hysterectomy, there is far less reason to suspect lower urinary tract damage during simple hysterectomy because no dissection of the innervation of the bladder and urethra is involved. Also no change to the vascular and lymphatic drainage can usually be expected.

Because of the aforementioned arguments, it is clear that only studies in which women are studied prospectively are valid. Those studies in which urodynamics is performed before and after hysterectomy are of particular value. An overview of these studies is given in Table 63.1: in only one of the eight studies was there a detrimental effect;[37] the other studies showed no major clinical effects on bladder and/or urethral function. Objective findings of bladder dysfunction after simple hysterectomy are therefore scarce .

A number of studies have assessed the effects of hysterectomy, using a surgical control group: in one such study the control group underwent dilatation and curettage;[40] in another, the control group consisted of women undergoing sterilization,[34] and the last and most recent was an elegant and randomized study comparing groups undergoing hysterectomy or endometrial ablation.[45] In all these studies there was no difference in the prevalence of urinary symptoms between the hysterectomy and the control group.

Much attention has been devoted in the literature to the problem of subtotal (supracervical, supravaginal) hysterectomy as opposed to total hysterectomy (including the cervix). Kilkku[30] concluded that total hysterectomy had more adverse effects than subtotal hysterectomy; however, his study has been criticized on methodological grounds, and three other studies[28,34,36] have failed to find such a difference. The results of the first randomized study comparing total and subtotal hysterectomy were published recently.[46] Subtotal hysterectomy showed no benefits over total hysterectomy with respect to bladder or bowel function one year after the operation. No clear differences between abdominal and vaginal hysterectomy in relation to lower urinary tract dysfunction have been documented; although four studies[8,33,41,44] specifically looked at this question, none found any difference between the two methods.

COLORECTAL SURGERY

Lower urinary tract dysfunction after colorectal surgery is well known.[47–53] In particular, abdominoperineal resection (anteroposterior) is associated with a high incidence of bladder dysfunction. The exact prevalence is not known because of the difficulty in comparing reports describing different types of operations and studies, with different lengths of follow-up. The overall

Table 63.1. *Overview of clinically relevant changes in prospective studies with urodynamic data before and after hysterectomy*

Study (ref. no)	Flow	Cystometry	UPP	Duration (weeks)	No. of patients
Hansen[29]	Improved (Ns)	Improved (compl)	–	68	35
Vervest[38,39]	Unchanged (F_{max})	Unchanged (cap, compl)	Unchanged (MUCP, FUL)	12–26	22
Coughlan[33]	–	Improved (DI)	–	52	25
Parys[37]	–	Deteriorated (DI, SI)	Deteriorated (Ns)	12–24	44
Kujansuu[36]	–	–	Unchanged (MUCP, FUL, TR)	12	31
Langer[35]	Unchanged (F_{max})	Unchanged (cap, compl)	Unchanged (MUCP, FUL, TR)	>52	16
Lalos[28]	Unchanged (F_{max}, resid)	Unchanged (compl, cap)	–	26	35
Prior[41]	–	Unchanged (compl)	–	26	26

Ns, not specified; F_{max}, maximum flow rate; cap, cystometric capacity; MUCP, maximum urethral closure pressure; FUL, functional urethral length; DI, detrusor instability; SI, stress incontinence; TR, transmission ratio; UPP, urethral pressure profile; compl, compliance; resid, residual.

prevalence varies between 10 and 60%,[5] the higher rate being generally attributed to autonomic nerve damage in the pelvic plexus, analogous to the damage brought about by radical hysterectomy. More recently, low anterior resection with the use of stapling instruments has gained popularity. In general, this is less damaging to the pelvic nerves than are the abdominal perineal resection techniques. However, one study still found an prevalence of 25% after low anterior resection.[48] Neverthless, in another study[51] a far lower was found. In general, the reason for resection (either tumour or infection) appears to have little effect on subsequent lower urinary tract dysfunction.

In general, these symptoms are similar to those noted after radical hysterectomy, atony, residual and stress incontinence being the most marked. Treatment is analogous to treatment of the symptoms that occur after radical hysterectomy. Scheduled micturition with, if necessary, self-catheterization and prevention of infection are the mainstays of treatment.

RADICAL VULVECTOMY

Radical vulvectomy remains the primary treatment for squamous cell vulvar carcinoma, stages I and II. The operation has an 80–85% 5-year survival rate.[54,55]

Currently, there is a shift towards less-radical surgical techniques, especially with a separate groin incision. Vulva tumours are often situated near the meatus urethrae; wide excision, therefore, often involves the distal part of the urethra. However, interruption of the blood and nerve supply to the urethra, as well as interference with the support mechanism and removal of part of the the pelvic floor, are held responsible for prolapse and urinary incontinence after radical vulvectomy. The most frequently seen complication, however, is misdirection or spraying of the urinary stream, which occurs in 17–65% of patients,[4] is difficult to correct and can be bothersome. Urinary incontinence has been noted after radical vulvectomy in 40% of cases,[56] and pelvic relaxation with cystocele and rectocele in 17%.[55] However, it is also possible that an already existing mild prolapse will become more visible because of the widely gaping vulvar opening. The development of stress incontinence has been closely related to involvement of the distal urethra in the dissection. In these patients there was a decrease in the functional ure-

thral length and in the distal transmission ratios, without a change in the maximum urethral closure pressure.[58] In this study, patients developed genuine stress incontinence only when the distal urethra was removed, indicating that the distal urethra has an important role in the continence mechanism.

PROLAPSE SURGERY

Prolapse surgery, which is not specifically directed towards correction of a malfunctioning lower urinary tract, can adversely affect it.[58–62] Well-known sequelae are urinary retention and urinary incontinence. Urinary retention is often a temporary effect of anterior repair caused by oedema, pain and mild obstruction. It will generally be alleviated by time and by permanent (either suprapubic or transurethral) or intermittent bladder drainage.

Urinary incontinence can be unmasked when there is occult stress incontinence due to kinking of the urethra in a major cystocele. In these patients the normal continence mechanism is destroyed by pelvic relaxation, and continence is dependent on the prolapse. When testing these patients preoperatively with a pessary, or on reduction of the prolapse, a decrease in the closure pressure of the urethra with subsequent stress incontinence is seen. An additional procedure to rectify this occult stress incontinence is often suggested.

REFERENCES

1. Koonings PP. The effects of gynecologic cancer and its treatment on the lower urinary tract. In: Walters MD, Karram MM (eds) *Clinical Urogynecology*. St Louis: Mosby, 1993; 373–387

2. Petri E. Bladder dysfunction after intra-abdominal or vaginal surgery. In: Ostergard DR, Bent AE (eds) *Urogynecology and Urodynamics. Theory and Practice.* Baltimore: Williams and Wilkins, 1996; 609–615

3. Zimmern PE. Bladder dysfunction after radiation and radical pelvic surgery. In: Raz S (ed) *Female Urology.* Philadelphia: Saunders, 1996; 214–218

4. Barnick C. Urinary tract involment by benign and malignant gynecological disease. In: Cardozo L (ed) *Urogynecology.* New York: Churchill Livingstone, 1997; 529–550

5. Aronson MP, Sant GR. Urinary incontinence after pelvic surgery. In: O'Donnell PD (ed) *Urinary Incontinence.* St Louis: Mosby, 1997; 325–331

6. Mundy AR. An anatomical explanation for bladder dysfunction following rectal and uterine surgery. *Br J Urol* 1982; 54: 501–504

7. Fraser AC. The late effects of Wertheim's hysterectomy on the lower urinary tract. *J Obstet Gynaecol Br Commonw* 1966; 73: 1002–1007

8. Vervest HAM, Barents JW, Haspels AA, Debruyne FMJ. Radical hysterectomy and the function of the lower urinary tract: urodynamic quantification in storage and evacuation function. *Acta Obstet Gynecol Scand* 1989; 68: 331–339

9. Fishman IJ, Swabsigh R, Kaplan AL. Lower urinary tract dysfunction after radical hysterectomy for carcinoma of the cervix. *Urology* 1986; 28: 462–468

10. Halaska M, Voigt R, Bauer J et al. Urogynecologic follow up after abdominal radical hysterectomy for cervical cancer. *Zentralbl Gynakol* 1988; 110: 1117–1123

11. Forney JP. The effect of radical hysterectomy on bladder physiology. *Am J Obstet Gynecol* 1980; 138: 374–382

12. Low JA, Mauger GM, Carmichael JA. The effect of Wertheim hysterectomy upon bladder and urethral function. *Am J Obstet Gynecol* 1981; 139: 826–834

13. Carenza L, Nobili F, Giacobini S. Voiding disorders after radical hysterectomy. *Gynecol Oncol* 1982; 13: 213–219

14. Sasaki H, Yoshida T, Noda K et al. Urethral pressure profiles following radical hysterectomy. *Obstet Gynecol* 1982; 59: 101–104

15. Debus-Thiede G, Maassen V, Dimpf T et al. Bladder function disturbances following Wertheim hysterectomy – an analysis of urodynamic parameters in considering operative radicality. *Geburtshilfe Frauenheilkd* 1993; 53; 525–531

16. Farquaharson DI, Shingleton HM, Soong SJ et al. The adverse effects of cervical cancer treatment on bladder function. *Gynecol Oncol* 1987; 27: 15–23

17. Scotti RJ, Bergman A, Bhatia N, Ostergard DR. Urodynamic changes in urethrovesical function after radical hysterectomy. *Obstet Gynecol* 1986; 68: 111–119

18. Vierhout ME, Schreuder HWB, Veen HF. The relation between colorectal and lower urinary tract dysfunction following radical hysterectomy for carcinoma of the cervix. *Int Urogynecol J* 1994; 5: 82–85

19. Westby M, Asmussen M. Anatomical and functional changes in the lower urinary tract after radical hysterectomy with lymph node dissection as studied by dynamic urethrocystography and simultaneous urethrocystometry. *Gynecol Oncol* 1985; 21: 261–276

20. Gerdin E, Cnattingius S, Johnson P. Complications after radiotherapy and radical hysterectomy in early stage cervical carcinoma. *Acta Obstet Gynecol Scand* 1995; 74: 554–561

21. Dwyer PL, O'Callaghan D. Urinary dysfunction following radical hysterectomy: is there spontaneous improvement with time? *Neurourol Urodyn* 1993; 12: 429 (abstr 72)

22. Griffith-Jones MD, Tufnell D. Urinary symptoms after total abdominal hysterectomy – a review. *Int Urogynecol J* 1994: 5: 61–63

23. Thakar R, Manyonda I, Stanton SL et al. Bladder bowel and sexual function after hysterectomy for benign conditions. *Br J Obstet Gynecol* 1997; 104: 983–987

24. Hanley HG. The late urological complications of total hysterectomy. *Br J Urol* 1969; 41: 682–684

25. Farghaly SA, Hindmarsh JR, Worth PHL. Post hysterectomy urethral dysfunction: evaluation and management. *Br J Urol* 1986; 58: 299–302

26. Jequier AM. Urinary symptoms and total hysterectomy. *Br J Urol* 1976; 48: 437–441

27. Wake CR. The immediate effect of abdominal hysterectomy on intravesical pressure and detrusor activity. *Br J Obstet Gynecol* 1980; 87: 901–902

28. Lalos O, Bjerle P. Bladder wall mechanics and micturition before and after subtotal and total hysterectomy. *Eur J Obstet Gynecol Reprod Biol* 1986; 21: 143–150

29. Hansen BM, Bonnesen T, Jorgenesen E et al. Changes in symptoms and colpo-cystourethrography in 35 patients before and after total abdominal hysterectomy: a prospective study. *Urol Int* 1985; 40: 224–226

30. Kilkku P. Supravaginal uterine amputation versus hysterectomy with reference to subjective bladder symptoms and incontinence. *Acta Obstet Gynecol Scand* 1985; 64: 375–379

31. Vervest HAM, Kiewiet de Jonge M, Vervest TMJS et al. Micturition symptoms and urinary incontinence after non-radical hysterectomy. *Acta Obstet Gynecol Scand* 1988; 67: 141–146

32. Parys BT, Haylen BT, Hutton JL, Parsons KF. The effects of simple hysterectomy on vesicourethral function. *Br J Urol* 1989; 64: 594–599

33. Coughlan BM, Smith JM, Moriarty CT. Does simple hysterectomy affect lower urinary tract function – a urodynamic investigation. *Ir J Med Sci* 1989; 20: 215–218

34. Iosif CS, Bekassy Z, Rydhstrom H. Prevalence of urinary incontinence in middle aged women. *Int J Gynaecol Obstet* 1988; 26: 255–259

35. Langer R, Neuman M, Ron-El R et al. The effect of total abdominal hysterectomy on bladder function in asymptomatic women. *Obstet Gynecol* 1989; 74: 205–207

36. Kujansuu E, Teisala K, Punnonen R. Urethral closure function after total and subtotal hysterectomy measured by urethrocystometry. *Gynecol Obstet Invest* 1989; 27: 105–106

37. Parys BT, Haylen BT, Hutton JL, Parsons KF. Urodynamic evaluation of lower urinary tract function in relation to total hysterectomy. *Aust N Z J Obstet Gynaecol* 1990; 30: 161–165

38. Vervest HAM, van Venrooy GEPM, Barents JW *et al.* Non radical hysterectomy and the function of the lower urinary tract. Part 1: Urodynamic quantification of changes in storage function. *Acta Obstet Gynecol Scand* 1989; 68: 221–230

39. Vervest HAM, van Venrooy GEPM, Barents JW *et al.* Non radical hysterectomy and the function of the lower urinary tract. Part 2: Urodynamic quantification of changes in evacuation function. *Acta Obstet Gynecol Scand* 1989; 68: 231–238

40. Griffith-Jones MD, Jarvis GJ, McNamara M. Adverse urinary symptoms after total abdominal hysterectomy – fact or fiction? *Br J Urol* 1991; 67: 295–297

41. Prior A, Stanley K, Smith ARB, Read NW. Effect of hysterectomy on anorectal and urethrovesical physiology. *Gut* 1992; 33: 264–267

42. Narushima M, Otani T, Itoh I *et al.* Clinical effects of transbdominal simple hysterectomy on micturition function. *Hinyokika Kiyo* 1993; 39: 797–800

43. Virtanen H, Makinen J, Tenho T *et al.* Effects of abdominal hysterectomy on urinary and sexual symptoms. *Br J Urol* 1993; 72: 868–872

44. Voigt R, Scheffel F, Michels W *et al.* The influence of hysterectomy on urodynamic parameters. *Proceedings of the International Continence Society,* Sydney 1995; 244–245

45. Bhattacharya S, Mollison J, Pinion S *et al.* A comparison of bladder function two years following hysterectomy or endometrial ablation. *Br J Obstet Gynaecol* 1996; 103: 898–903

46. Thakar R, Manyonda I, Stanton S *et al.* A randomised study of total and subtotal hysterectomy: effect on bladder and bowel function. *Int Urogynecol J* 2000; 11 (Suppl 1): S21

47. Petrelli NJ, Nagel S, Rodriguez-Bigas M *et al.* Morbidity and mortality following abdominoperineal resection for rectal adenocarcinoma. *J Urol* 1983; 59: 400–404

48. Kirkegaard P, Hjortrup A, Sanders S. Bladder dysfunction after low anterior resection for mid-rectal cancer. *Am J Surg* 1981; 1141: 266–268

49. Neal DE, Parker AJ, Johnston D. The long term effects of proctectomy on bladder function in patients with inflammatory bowel disease. *Br J Surg* 1982; 69: 349–352

50. Chang PL, Fan HA. Urodynamic studies before and/or after abdominoperineal resection of the rectum for carcinoma. *J Urol* 1983; 130: 948–951

51. Kinn A, Ohman U. Bladder and sexual function after surgery for rectal cancer. *Dis Colon Rectum* 1986; 29: 43–48

52. Varma JS. Autonomic influences on colorectal motility and pelvic surgery. *World J Surg* 1992; 16: 811–819

53. Cunsolo A, Bragaglia RB, Manara G *et al.* Urogenital dysfunction after abdominoperineal resection for carcinoma of the rectum. *Dis Colon Rectum* 1990; 33: 918–922

54. Calame RJ. Pelvic relaxation as a complication of the radical vulvectomy. *Obstet Gynecol* 1980; 55: 716–719

55. Burke TW, Stringer CA, Gershenson DM *et al.* Radical wide excision and selective inguinal node dissection for squamous cell carcinoma of the vulva. *Gynecol Oncol* 1990; 38: 328–332

56. Boutselis JG, Ullery JC, Teteris NJ. Epidermoid carcinoma of the vulva. *Obstet Gynecol* 1963; 22: 713–724

57. Reid GC, DeLancey JOL, Hopkins MP *et al.* Urinary incontinence following radical vulvectomy. *Obstet Gynecol* 1990; 75: 852–858

58. Richardson DA, Bent AE, Ostergard DA. The effect of uterovaginal prolapse on urethrovesical pressure dynamics. *Am J Obstet Gynecol* 1983; 146: 901–910

59. Bump RC, Fantl JA, Hurt WG. The mechanism of urinary incontinence in women with severe uterovaginal prolapse: results of barrier studies. *Obstet Gynecol* 1988; 72: 291–295

60. Bergman A, Koonings PP, Ballard CA. Predicting post operative urinary incontinence development in women undergoing operation for genitourinary prolapse. *Am J Obstet Gynecol* 1988; 158: 1171–1178

61. Borstad E. The risk of urinary stress incontinence after anterior repair. *Int Urogynecol J* 1992; 3: 163–167

62. Fianu S, Kjaeldegaard A, Larsson B. Preoperative screening for latent stress incontinence in women with cystocele. *Neurourol Urodyn* 1985; 4: 3–7

64

Urological complications of gynaecological surgery

K. R. Loughlin

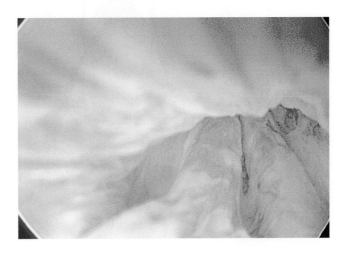

INTRODUCTION

The management of urological injuries during gynaecological surgery represents a challenging problem to the surgeon. In this chapter, the methods of operative repair that are necessary to manage these injuries are reviewed. First, the female pelvic anatomy is described; the techniques necessary to manage these iatrogenic injuries (whether they are recognized intraoperatively or postoperatively) are then discussed.

FEMALE PELVIC ANATOMY AND ITS RELATIONSHIP TO THE URINARY TRACT

Ureteral injuries are less likely to occur if the operating surgeon has a thorough knowledge of the female pelvic anatomy and its relationship to the urinary tract. To that end, some of the female pelvic anatomy as it relates to ureteral injuries is reviewed briefly here.

The ureters cross over the pelvic brim and enter the pelvis in close proximity to the ovarian vessels. This is one of the three most common sites of urological injury during gynaecological surgery.[1] The ureter then courses medially into the lower and medial portions of the broad ligament. At this juncture, the ureter is crossed by the uterine artery and this is the second area of the ureter that is commonly injured during gynaecological operations.[2] The ureter then continues its medial course and enters the bladder in the deep pelvis. The ureterovesical junction is the third common site of ureteral injury during female pelvic surgery. An outline of female pelvic anatomy and its relationship to the urinary tract appears in Figure 64.1.

URETERAL INJURIES – INTRAOPERATIVE RECOGNITION AND REPAIR

Ureteral injuries occur in 0.5–2.5% of routine pelvic operations and in as many as 30% of radical pelvic procedures performed for malignancy.[3] However, less than one-third of these injuries are identified intraoperatively.[4] Ideally, the ureters should be identified and isolated prior to any extensive pelvic dissection. A useful manoeuvre is to identify the ureters as they cross the iliac vessels and then place Vascu-ties (vesiloop)

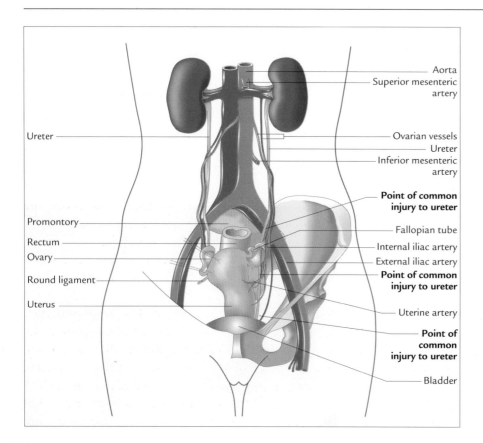

Figure 64.1. *An overview of the course of the ureters in the pelvis. The three most common sites of injury are at the pelvic brim near the ovarian vessels, at the point where the uterine artery crosses the ureter and at the ureterovesical junction.*

around each ureter for later reference as the operation proceeds. Most ureteral injuries occur when there is extensive bleeding, or when the anatomy is distorted from previous surgery or radiation treatment. If the surgeon encounters extensive bleeding or there is a question of ureteral injury, the gynaecologist or urological consultant should identify the ureter from above and trace out its course to the bladder.

THE ROLE OF THE UROLOGICAL CONSULTANT

When the urologist is called to the operating room for consultation on a possible urological injury, he should do several things before scrubbing up. First, he should read the chart for any relevant history that may affect the patient's urological status. Second, he should ask if any preoperative radiological studies, such as an intravenous pyelogram (IVP), are available for review. It is my practice to take a 'urology bag' with me when called for an intra-operative consultation. This bag contains ureteral stents, infant feeding tubes, Malecot catheters and three-way uretheral catheters, which are often unfamiliar to non-urological nurses.

After the urologist scrubs up, he should assess the situation. If exposure is poor, he should not be shy about repositioning retractors or extending the surgical incision, if necessary. In addition, if haemostasis is inadequate, the urologist should make sure he achieves a relatively dry surgical field before proceeding. The urologist should then identify the ureter and trace it out above and below the area of concern. The urologist should be aware that, if a ureter has been injured, the contralateral ureter or bladder may also have been injured; depending on the circumstances, these structures should also be examined intra-operatively. Indigo carmine or methylene blue may be given intravenously to aid in checking the integrity of the ureters and these dyes may be instilled via a uretheral catheter to help identify or confirm bladder injuries.

INTRA-OPERATIVE REPAIR – BLADDER INJURIES

Most bladder injuries are relatively straightforward to repair. They usually occur during a hysterectomy and usually involve the anterior bladder wall. Most bladder injuries are satisfactorily repaired with two layers of absorbable suture. Occasionally, the bladder wall will need to be debrided before closure. If a Foley catheter

is not in place, one should be inserted and either indigo carmine or methylene blue can be injected to verify the adequacy of the closure. The urologist should remember the caveat of associated ureteral injuries. If there is uncertainty about a ureteral injury at the time of a bladder injury, 5F or 8F infant feeding tubes can be inserted into the ureteral orifices prior to closure of the bladder. This often makes identification of the ureters easier.

Bladder injuries associated with caesarean section are often more difficult to manage. These bladder injuries are often more posterior and often are near the vaginal wall. Such injuries are hard to close because the exposure is difficult and these injuries carry an increased risk of postoperative vesicovaginal fistula formation. It is often prudent, when faced with a posterior bladder wall repair, to interpose omentum between the bladder repair and vaginal wall to decrease the likelihood of postoperative fistula formation. All bladder injuries should be drained with an indwelling bladder catheter and either a closed or an open drainage system from the space of Retzius. The customary postoperative regimen is to remove the drain from the space of Retzius on postoperative day 2 or 3 and to perform a cystogram about a week postoperatively to confirm satisfactory bladder repair before discontinuing the urethral catheter.

INTRA-OPERATIVE REPAIR – LOWER URETER

Injuries to the distal 4 cm of the ureter can be handled in one of three ways, outlined below.

Ureteroureterostomy

If the ureteral injury is within 3–4 cm above the ureterovesical junction it can often be repaired by a primary ureteral anastomosis. It is important to resect a small portion of both the proximal and distal ureteral segments to ensure that viable tissue is being anastomosed. It is preferable to spatulate either end of the ureter that is being repaired and to use interrupted, absorbable sutures (Fig. 64.2). Whether to stent the anastomosis is best left to the discretion of the surgeon, but all anastomoses should be drained. Non-transecting injuries of the ureter, such as ureteral tears or inadvertent ureteral clamping, are also best left to the judgement of the individual surgeon; however, in most cases,

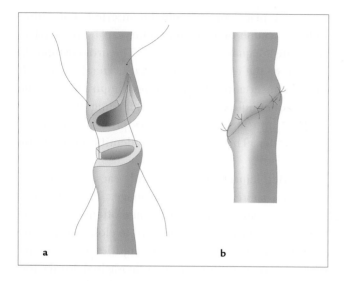

Figure 64.2. *A primary ureteroureterostomy is best performed after each ureteral segment has been resected back to viable tissue and with each end spatulated.*

such injuries are best excised and a ureteral anastomosis performed to complete the repair.

Ureteral implant

When the ureteral injury is quite low – in the distal 2 cm – primary ureteral repair is usually difficult. In these situations, a ureteral reimplant is usually preferable. I prefer to utilize the Leadbetter–Politano technique of ureteral reimplantation (Fig. 64.3), but any method of reimplantation with which the surgeon feels comfortable is acceptable. A non-refluxing reimplantation is preferable in women who are in the age group where sexual activity is likely. Whether to stent the reimplanted ureter is, again, best left to the individual surgeon's judgement; however, all ureteral reimplants should be drained.

Psoas hitch

If the primary ureteroureterostomy or ureteral implant cannot be performed with a tension-free anastomosis, then a psoas hitch is a very good solution for lower ureteral injuries.[5–7] The techniques used for performing the psoas hitch have been described previously; below, I describe the technique that I have used over the years.[8,9]

Bladder mobilization is important in order to pro-

vide a tension-free ureteral reimplantation. It is usually necessary to mobilize the bladder bilaterally, not just on the side of the ureteral injury. The cystostomy should be made on the anterior wall of the bladder, away from the dome. This enables the surgeon's fingers to be placed in the bladder dome, thus aiding mobilization of the bladder as well as placement of the anchoring stitches in the psoas muscle (Fig. 64.4). My own preference is to use non-absorbable stitches to anchor the bladder to the psoas muscle. During this manoeuvre, care should be taken to avoid injury to the genitofemoral nerve or inadvertent incorporation of the nerve within the sutures. In most cases I use the Leadbetter–Politano technique for ureteral reimplantation and, in these cases, I find it preferable to leave an indwelling ureteral stent (Fig. 64.5). The cystostomy is closed in the usual manner. A urethral catheter is left in place and a suprapubic tube is usually not necessary. An external drain is left near the reimplantation site.

INTRA-OPERATIVE REPAIR – MIDURETER

Midureteral injuries that are not extensive can be repaired with a ureteroureterostomy, as described above. However, when a primary repair is not possible, other operative techniques are useful.

Transureteroureterostomy

The technique of transureteroureterostomy was first described in 1934 by Higgins to manage persistent unilateral ureteral reflux.[10] Since that time it has been used to treat unilateral ureteral injuries.[6,9,10] However, the concern has been that, if a complication occurs following a transureteroureterostomy, then both ureters are jeopardized.[11,12] A history of stone disease is a contraindication to this procedure.

The technique of transureteroureterostomy is straightforward. Both the donor and recipient ureters should be mobilized to prepare for a tension-free anastomosis. Under no circumstances should the recipient ureter be angulated in order to reach the donor ureter. My own preference is to spatulate the donor ureter and then to place stay sutures in the recipient ureter and perform the ureteroureterostomy between the stay sutures (Fig. 64.6a). I prefer to use 4/0 chromic sutures for the anastomosis: I perform a running suture line, with the knots on the outside on the posterior wall, and

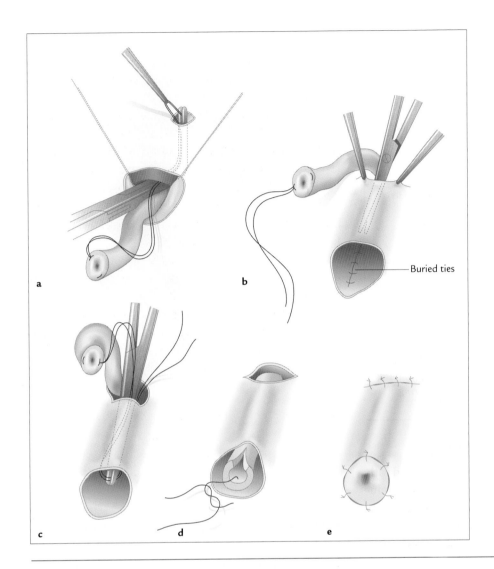

Figure 64.3. *The Leadbetter–Politano ureteral reimplantation technique.*

use interrupted sutures on the anterior wall (Fig. 64.6b). Because stenting a transureteroureterostomy is usually an awkward procedure, in most cases the anastomosis is left unstented; however, an external drain is always used.

Boari flap

The Boari flap is an attractive solution for repair of extensive midureteral injuries. Boari first described his operative technique for ureteral replacement in a canine model in 1894.[13] Subsequently, the Boari flap has been incorporated into clinical practice and is particularly adaptable to the management of injuries to the midureter.[14–17] As with preparation for a psoas hitch, the bladder must be thoroughly mobilized.

Before the flap is created, the bladder should be distended with saline and the flap carefully planned with a sterile marker. The most critical manoeuvre is to make sure that the base of the flap is wide enough to prevent distal ischaemia in the flap: the flap should have its blood supply based on the superior vesicle artery; usually, the base of the flap should be at least 4 cm wide, depending on the length of the flap required (Fig. 64.7a).

After the flap is created, it is tubularized with running absorbable sutures. The distal ureter is then anastomosed to the flap (Fig. 64.7b) in the standard fashion. These anastomoses are preferably stented and all are drained. A urethral catheter is left indwelling to drain the bladder and a suprapubic tube is used at the surgeon's discretion.

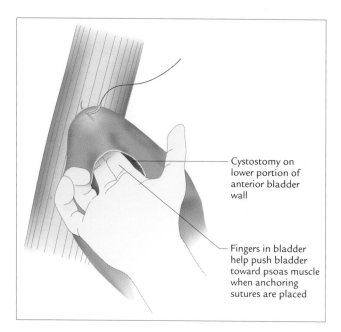

Cystostomy on lower portion of anterior bladder wall

Fingers in bladder help push bladder toward psoas muscle when anchoring sutures are placed

Figure 64.4. *The cystostomy should be made on the interior portion of the anterior bladder wall to permit the surgeon's finger to aid in bladder mobilization and guide in the anchoring stitches to the psoas muscle.*

INTRAOPERATIVE REPAIR – UPPER URETER

Injuries to the upper ureter that cannot be repaired with a straightforward ureteroureterostomy can be problematic. In most cases, a Boari flap will not reach an upper ureteral injury; therefore, the choices usually include autotransplantation, ileal ureter or nephrectomy.

Autotransplantation

Autotransplantation of the kidney is a formidable procedure and should not be undertaken if other options exist.[16,18,19] It is usually considered when the contralateral kidney is absent or poorly functioning. The kidney is harvested with maximal vessel length and the vascular anastomoses to the iliac vessels are performed in the standard fashion. The upper ureter or renal pelvis can then be anastomosed directly to the bladder.

Ileal ureter

The use of ileal interposition for extensive upper ureteral injuries has also been reported.[6,16,20] As with autotransplantation, ileal interposition should be considered only when simpler alternatives are not practical. It is preferable to create an ileal ureter in patients

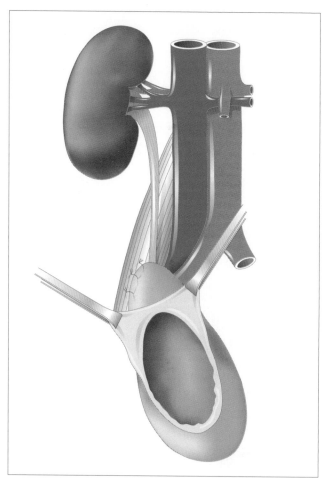

Figure 64.5. *Completed psoas hitch and ureteral implant.*

who have had thorough preoperative bowel preparation; in emergency situations, however, an ileal segment can be isolated without such preparation. The techniques used for creation of an ileal ureter are similar to those used in an ileal conduit. The proximal and distal ureteral segments should be fully mobilized and the ureteral–ileal anastomoses are performed with absorbable sutures (Fig. 64.8). No stents are utilized and an external drain is necessary.

Nephrectomy

When a normal contralateral kidney is present, a simple nephrectomy should be considered as an expeditious solution to extensive upper ureteral injury.[6,21] A nephrectomy is often attractive because it obviates the postoperative complications, such as urinary leak or infection, that can be seen with other techniques used to manage upper ureteral injuries.

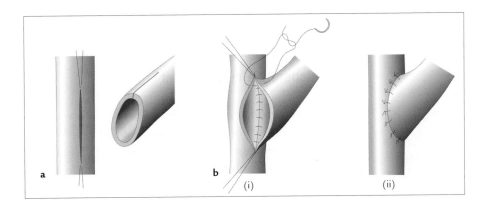

Figure 64.6. *(a) Stay sutures mark the area of planned ureterotomy; (b) The transuretero-ureterostomy anastomosis: anastomosis of the posterior (i) and anterior (ii) walls of the ureter.*

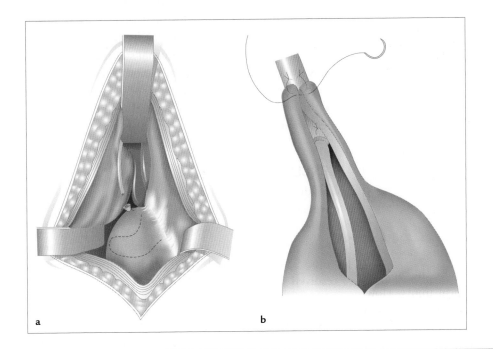

Figure 64.7. *(a) The Boari flap is planned out on the distended bladder wall; (b) the proximal ureter is anastomosed to the tubularized Boari flap.*

POSTOPERATIVE PROCEDURES

Postoperative recognition of bladder injuries

Postoperative symptoms associated with delayed recognition of bladder injuries include fever, abdominal pain, abdominal distension, infection, decreased urine output and rising serum creatinine. The management of these cases should be individualized, since the patient's overall condition is an important consideration. In general, however, extraperitoneal injuries can be managed with a trial of catheter drainage, whereas intraperitoneal injuries merit surgical exploration and repair. The most direct way to diagnose the presence and location of a bladder injury is a cystogram.

Postoperative recognition of ureteral injuries

Postoperative symptoms of ureteral injuries may include flank pain, fever, sepsis, decreased urine output, abdominal mass, elevated creatinine or urinary fistula. However, ureteral injuries can also be asymptomatic. If a ureteral injury is suspected, an IVP is the diagnostic study of choice,[21,22] although an abdominal ultrasound or computed tomography scan may also be helpful.

Once a diagnosis of ureteral injury is suspected or confirmed, a retrograde pyelogram can give more information regarding the precise location of the injury. There is genuine debate as to whether stent placement should be attempted at the time of a retrograde pyelogram. Dowling and associates[21] found that,

831

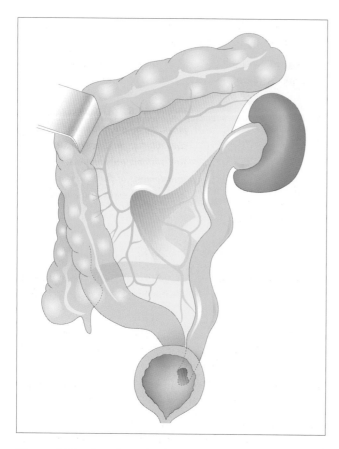

Figure 64.8. *Completed ileal ureter.*

in 19 of 20 patients, a retrograde stent could not be placed beyond the site of the urological injury. However, others feel that, if a stent can be negotiated through the area of injury, in some cases this will promote satisfactory ureteral healing and avoid the need for open surgery.[23]

When ureteral stent placement is not possible, nephrostomy tube placement is an option.[21,24] Nephrostomy tube placement has two potential benefits. First, if the patient is septic or in other ways not ideally suitable for surgical re-exploration, the nephrostomy tube can temporize until the patient's condition improves to the point where surgery is a more realistic alternative. Second, some cases of ureteral obstruction secondary to suture entrapment have been reported to resolve successfully with nephrostomy tube drainage alone.[25] Again, which cases can be adequately managed with nephrostomy tube drainage can best be judged by the individual surgeon.

If conservative measures are unsuccessful, and surgical re-exploration is required, the options available are identical to those mentioned previously for the management of injuries recognized intra-operatively.

Postoperative management

The urological consultant should always dictate a separate operative note. He should meet the family members and explain his role in the surgery. He should make postoperative visits to the patient and he should be the only physician to order urological radiographic studies or the removal of tubes. In general, suprapubic tubes are removed on postoperative day 2 or 3, or when the urine is clear. Urethral catheters are removed after a cystogram shows no leak – this is usually on about postoperative day 7. Internal stents and nephrostomy tubes are ordinarily removed later, about 2–3 weeks postoperatively and after either an IVP or a nephrostogram has confirmed good healing of the surgical repair.

CONCLUSIONS

Bladder and ureteral injuries during gynaecological surgery present a difficult challenge to both the gynaecologist and urologist. If the guidelines reviewed above – together with good judgement and good technique – are employed, most of these injuries can be resolved successfully.

REFERENCES

1. Tarkington MA, Detjer SW, Bresette JF. Early surgical management of extensive gynecologic ureteral injuries. *Surg Gynecol Obstet* 1991; 173: 17–21

2. Gangi MP, Agee RE, Spence CR. Surgical injury to ureter. *Urology* 1976; 8: 22–27

3. Neuman M, Eidelman A, Langer R *et al.* Iatrogenic injuries to the ureter during gynecologic and obstetric operations. *Surg Gynecol Obstet* 1991; 173: 268–272

4. Turner-Warwick R, Worth PHL. The psoas bladder hitch procedure for the replacement of the lower third of the ureter. *Br J Urol* 1969; 41: 701–709

5. Gross M, Peng B, Waterhouse K. Use of the mobilized bladder to replace the pelvic ureter. *J Urol* 1969; 101: 40

6. Zinman LM, Libertino JA, Ruth RA. Management of operative ureteral injury. *Urology* 1978; 12: 290–303

7. Ehrlich RM, Melman A, Skinner DG. The use of vesico-psoas hitch in urologic surgery. *J Urol* 1978; 119: 322–325

8. Matthews R, Marshall FF. Versatility of the adult psoas hitch ureteral reimplantation. *J Urol* 1997; 158: 2078–2082

9. Hodges CV, Moore RJ, Lehman TH, Benham AM. Clinical experiences with transuretero-ureterostomy. *J Urol* 1963; 90: 552–562

10. Smith IB, Smith JC. Transuretero-ureterostomy: British experience. *Br J Urol* 1975; 47: 519–523

11. Ehrlich RM, Skinner DG. Complications of transuretero-ureterostomy. *J Urol* 1975; 113: 467–473

12. Sandoz IL, Paull DP, MacFarlane CA. Complications with transuretero-ureterostomy. *J Urol* 1977; 117: 39–42

13. Boari A. Chirurgia dell uretere, con pretazience de Dott: I. Albarran, 1, 900 contribute sperementale alla plastica delle uretere. *Atti Accad Med Ferrara* 1894; 14: 444

14. Konigsberg H, Blunt KJ, Muecke EC. Use of Boari flap in lower ureteral injuries. *Urology* 1975; 5: 751–755

15. Colimbu M, Block N, Morales P. Ureterovesical flap operation for middle and upper ureteral repair. *Invest Urol* 1973; 10: 313–317

16. Benson MC, Ring KS, Olsson CA. Ureteral reconstruction and bypass: experience with ileal interposition, the Boari flap–psoas hitch and renal autotransplantation. *J Urol* 1990; 143: 20–23

17. Bright TC III, Peters PC. Ureteral injuries secondary to operative procedures. *Urology* 1977; 9: 22–26

18. Hardy JD. High ureteral injuries: management by autotransplantation of the kidney. *J Am Med Assoc* 1963; 184: 97–101

19. Novick AC, Stewart BH. Experience with extracorporeal renal operations and autotransplantation in the management of complicated urologic disorders. *Surg Gynecol Obstet* 1981; 153: 10–18

20. McCullough DL, McLaughlin AP, Gittes RF, Kerr WS. Replacement of the damaged or neoplastic ureter by ileum. *J Urol* 1977; 118: 375–378

21. Dowling RA, Corriere JN, Sandler CM. Iatrogenic ureteral injury. *J Urol* 1986; 135: 912–915

22. Mann WJ. Intentional and unintentional ureteral surgical treatment in gynecologic procedures. *Surg Gynecol Obstet* 1991; 172: 453–456

23. Mitty HA, Train JS, Dan SJ. Antegrade ureteral stenting in the management of fistulas, strictures and calculi. *Radiology* 1983; 149: 433–438

24. Persky L, Hampel N, Kedia K. Percutaneous nephrostomy and ureteral injury. *J Urol* 1981; 125: 298–300

25. Harshman MW, Pollack HM, Banner MP, Wein AJ. Conservative management of ureteral obstruction secondary to suture entrapment. *J Urol* 1982; 127: 121–123

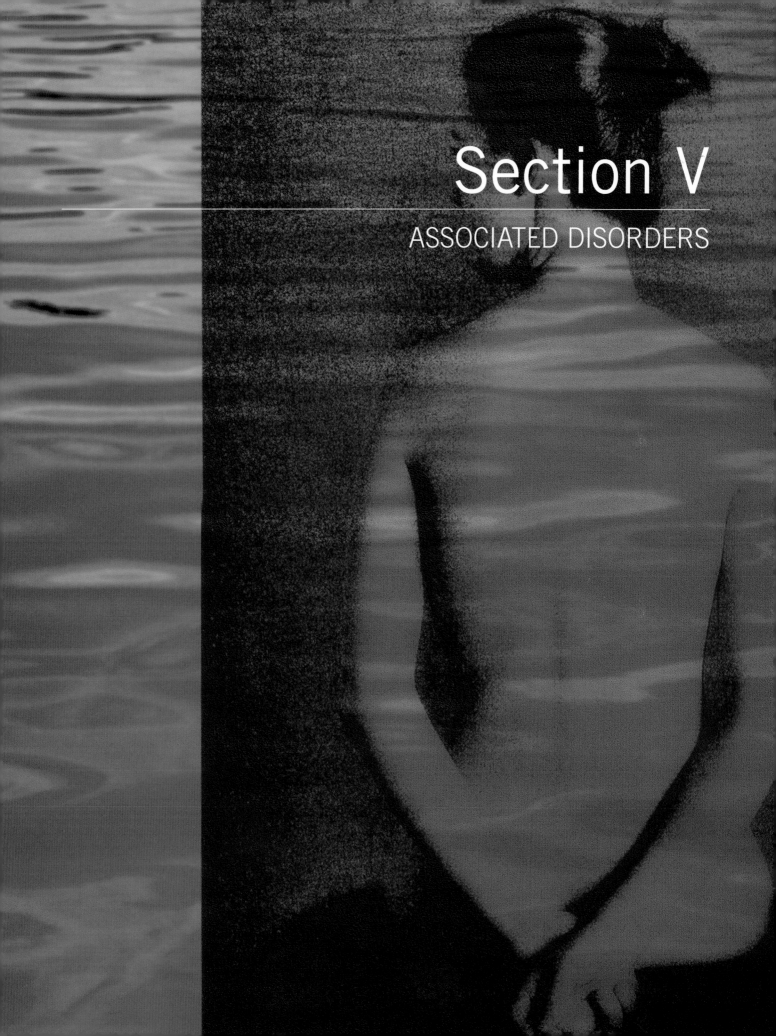

Section V

ASSOCIATED DISORDERS

65

Neurological disorders

S. Y. Jung, M. B. Chancellor

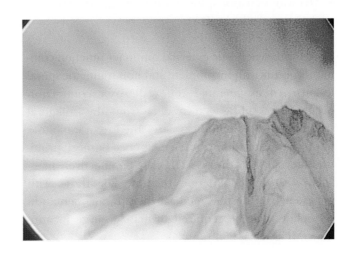

INTRODUCTION

The lower urinary tract can be divided into two functional areas: the bladder or detrusor, and the outlet – comprised of the bladder neck, internal sphincter and external sphincters. Under normal physiological circumstances these two areas accomplish the functions of urinary storage and emptying under neurological control. Neurological lesions produce either a loss of function – characterized as 'underactivity', areflexia or denervation – or release of reflex function, manifested as 'overactivity' or hyperreflexia. The functional effect of neurological lesions is generally determined by the anatomical level: cerebral (suprapontine), spinal (suprasacral) or peripheral (infrasacral).

In so far as voiding dysfunction is predictable on the basis of the level of neuron injury, injuries above the pons result in detrusor hyperreflexia (DH) with sphincter coordination; spinal lesions result in an upper motor neuron lesion and DH with or without sphincter coordination. Injuries involving either the sacral cord or the cauda equina result in a lower motor neuron lesion and detrusor areflexia (DA) with or without sphincter denervation. However, many patients, particularly those with multiple or incomplete injuries, have a mixed pattern which cannot be predicted by the neurological lesion.[1-3]

BLADDER FUNCTIONAL PATTERN AFTER NEUROLOGICAL DAMAGE

We believe that there are three general urodynamic patterns seen after neurological damage:

- detrusor hyperreflexia (DH)
- DH with detrusor sphincter dyssynergia (DSD)
- detrusor areflexia (DA).

DH with synergistic external sphincter function commonly occurs with incomplete and non-traumatic spinal lesions. An exaggerated reflex detrusor contraction occurs after suprasacral trauma from the collateral sprouting of new neural pathways, the loss of inhibitory impulse transmission or the emergence of more primitive alternative pathways.[4] DH may be effectively managed with anticholinergic therapy. For those with persistent DH despite medical therapy, augmentation cystoplasty may be required to manage urge incontinence (Figs 65.1, 65.2).

DH with DSD is frequently noted in those with complete thoracic- and cervical-level spinal cord injury (SCI). Approximately 10–20% of SCI patients with DSD also have coexistent dyssynergia of the internal sphincteric mechanism[5] (Fig. 65.3).

DH associated with DSD is best managed by decreasing detrusor activity medically or surgically to allow low-pressure urinary storage. This requires an intermittent catheterization programme to ensure complete low-pressure urinary drainage. An alternative management strategy is to establish low-pressure urinary drainage with surgical ablation of the external urinary sphincter, permitting unimpeded reflex detrusor activity to empty the bladder. Management with indwelling catheterization is to be avoided because upper tract deterioration may still occur, and chronic catheterization is associated with urolithiasis, chronic infection, tissue erosion and bladder cancer.

DA, or possibly only significantly impaired detrusor contractility, is frequently associated with sacral and lumbar injury. DA is characterized urodynamically by the absence of detrusor contraction, allowing low-pressure urinary storage. Management includes the use of an intermittent catheterization programme (Fig. 65.4).

DA may also occur in patients with upper motor neuron lesions, who would otherwise be expected to have DH, presumably because of a clinical or subclinical sacral lesion such as coexistent traumatic injury or syrinx.[6] Lower motor neuron injury may, however, result in 'adrenergic' overgrowth in the bladder, contributing to increased bladder tone and decreased bladder compliance.[7] Because upper tract damage varies directly with increasing time at or above the critical $40\,cmH_2O$ pressure,[8] diminished compliance requires the use of anticholinergic agents or surgical bladder augmentation to establish urinary storage under acceptable pressure.

Patients with lesions between the sacral spinal cord and the pons, in which the coordination reflex occurs, may have DH and contraction of the striated urethral sphincter during involuntary detrusor contraction.[9,10] This is DSD and can cause vesicoureteral reflux because of elevation in intravesical pressure. The diagnosis of DSD is crucial because there is a 50% or greater chance of developing urological complications within 5 years of DSD beginning.[11-13] Treatment must be directed at bladder sphincter dysfunction. Typical causes are SCI and multiple sclerosis (MS).[14-16]

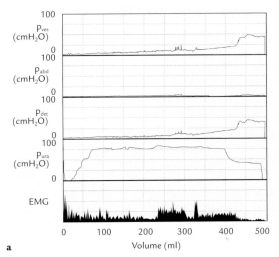

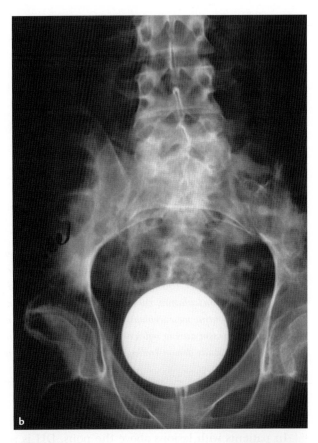

Figure 65.1. *(a) Normal urodynamic study in a 51-year-old woman after a cerebrovascular accident. Her only urological symptom is nocturia, one episode per night. The patient had normal sensation of filling and fullness at a volume of approximately 430 ml. At capacity she initiated a voluntary detrusor contraction with relaxation of her external sphincter. p_{ves}, intravesical pressure; p_{abd}, intra-abdominal pressure; p_{det}, subtracted detrusor pressure ($p_{det} = p_{ves} - p_{abd}$); p_{ura}, urethral sphincter pressure; EMG, electromyography of the external sphincter. (b) Cystogram reveals a smooth round bladder to capacity.*

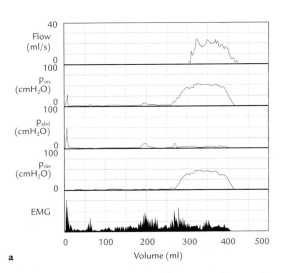

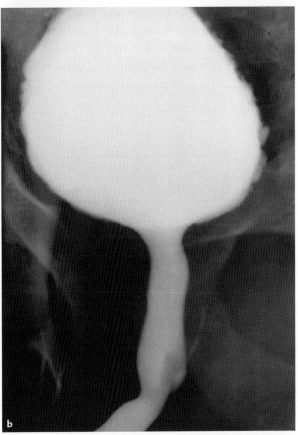

Figure 65.2. *(a) Detrusor hyperreflexia in a 52-year-old woman after a cerebrovascular accident with complaints of urgency, frequency, urge incontinence and nocturia, five episodes per night. An involuntary detrusor contraction occurred after 265 ml had been infused. The maximum voiding pressure was 48 cmH$_2$O and there was no evidence of bladder outlet obstruction with maximum flow rate of over 20 ml/sec. Abbreviations as Figure 65.1. (b) Voiding cystourethrogram phase of the videourodynamic study demonstrating a mildly trabeculated bladder with open bladder neck during the involuntary detrusor contraction.*

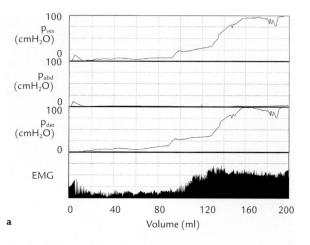
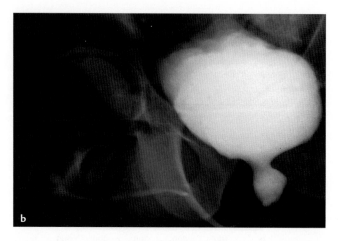

Figure 65.3. *(a) Detrusor hyperreflexia with detrusor sphincter dyssynergia in a 25-year-old man with a C6-level spinal cord injury (SCI) resulting from a gunshot wound. Electrical activity of the external sphincter increases dramatically with the onset of uninhibited detrusor contraction after 100 ml has been infused. Continued filling results in continued contraction of both the detrusor and external sphincter musculature, culminating in severe elevation of intravesical pressure to 100 cmH$_2$O. Disruption of the coordinating influence of the pontine mesencephalic reticular formation by suprasacral SCI can result in dyssynergic contraction of the external sphincteric mechanism during reflex detrusor contraction. Abbreviations as Figure 65.1. (b) Voiding cystourethrogram phase of the videourodynamic study demonstrating an open bladder neck and prostatic urethra but significant narrowing of the membranous urethra.*

In patients with lesions above the pons, DH is not associated with DSD because the lesion is above the level where detrusor contraction is coordinated with reflex urethral relaxation. Typical causes are cerebrovascular disease, Parkinson's disease and some cases of MS.[17,18] In patients with lumbosacral or peripheral nerve lesions, such as myelodysplasia, cauda equina injury and diabetes mellitus, DA with high or low bladder compliance may develop.[1,19,20] In cases of low compliance, increased resistance provided by the striated sphincter usually causes the bladder's response, which puts the upper urinary tract at risk. Again, this is a case of combined bladder and sphincter dysfunction.

These examples demonstrate a practical approach to the evaluation of neurological patients. It is important to keep in mind the concept of bladder and sphincter function and how they relate to urine storage (continence and storage pressures), emptying and effects on the upper urinary tract. This approach, as opposed to other complex neurourological classification systems, allows for accurate diagnosis and, more importantly, institution of appropriate treatment.

In this chapter, we will discuss motor neuron diseases that affect lower urinary tract function in detail.

Figure 65.4. *Detrusor areflexia in woman with a T12-level spinal cord injury with urinary retention. The patient was unable to generate any voluntary or involuntary detrusor contraction. She was able to 'void' a small amount with a Valsalva manoeuvre at 400 ml and 450 ml. Abbreviations as Figure 65.1.*

CONDITIONS OF THE BRAIN AFFECTING THE URINARY TRACT

Cerebrovascular accident

The annual incidence of cerebrovascular accidents has been estimated at 6–12 per 1000 individuals aged 65–74 years and at 40 per 1000 in those aged over 85 years.[21] The effects of cerebrovascular accident on the function of the lower urinary tract are variable, depending on the location of the neural injury, its size and aetiology.[22] Because the function of the neural arcs above the pontine level is to inhibit micturition, injury in this area decreases inhibitory control over detrusor function.[23] Although the most frequent long-term urological dysfunction of cerebrovascular accident is DH, a significant number of newly affected patients develop urinary retention for periods of several weeks. We have named this phase of acontractile detrusor 'cerebral shock', much like the classic acontractile bladder 'spinal shock' phase that immediately follows an SCI.[24]

As recovery ensues, patients may experience urinary urgency, with the incidence of incontinence reported to be as high as 51% within a year of injury. Urinary incontinence may also result from limitations in cognitive function and mobility resulting from neural injury.[25]

Although external sphincter function is preserved, urinary incontinence results from uninhibited detrusor contractions.[26] DH results from damage to the cerebral inhibitory centres. Patients with lesions above the level of the pons characteristically demonstrate synergetic activity of the external sphincter with detrusor activity.[22] Patients with suprapontine lesions may, however, *purposely* increase sphincteric activity during an uninhibited detrusor contraction to avoid urge incontinence. This guarding reflex or pseudodyssynergia may be confused with true dyssynergia by those not familiar with the interpretation of urodynamic studies.[27]

In the absence of other urinary disease, such as outflow obstruction, as long as external sphincter activity remains coordinated with detrusor contraction, intravesical pressure should remain physiological and therefore preserve the function of the urinary tracts.

Parkinson's disease

Parkinson's disease is one of the most frequent neurological entities causing voiding dysfunction, classically resulting in detrusor overactivity, sphincter bradykinesia and impairment of relaxation of the striated external sphincter muscle. In the United States this entity has a prevalence of 100–150 per 100 000, affecting men and women equally, chiefly in the sixth and seventh decades.[28]

Pathologically, degeneration of the pigmented neurons in the substantia nigra and locus caeruleus in the brain stem occurs. Clinical features of tremor, bradykinesia and muscular rigidity are probably due to focal dopamine deficiency in these areas, as well as the caudate nucleus, putamen and globus pallidus.[29]

Up to 75% of patients with Parkinson's disease experience some degree of voiding dysfunction.[30,31] Irritative symptoms of urinary frequency, urgency and urge incontinence are reported by 57% of patients with Parkinson's disease and voiding disturbance; 23% experience obstructive symptoms including hesitancy, incomplete emptying or urinary retention; 20% have mixed symptoms.[29]

Urodynamic evaluation has revealed DH in up to 90% of patients, with sporadic electrical activity of the external sphincter during uninhibited detrusor contractions in 61%.[18] A less frequent urodynamic finding in the patient with Parkinson's disease is impaired detrusor contractility.[32] Stress urinary incontinence was reported in 50% of women with Parkinson's disease in one study.[33]

Proper management will serve to protect the upper urinary tracts. Treatment of the patient with L-dopa can significantly improve symptoms; however, anticholinergic therapy can be added to suppress uninhibited detrusor contractions.

Brain neoplasms

Patients with intracranial neoplasms often maintain control over urinary tract function. As is the case with cerebrovascular accidents, alterations in lower urinary tract function will tend to relate directly to the area of the brain affected, rather than the type of neoplasm.

Because neural arcs above the pontine level, including the superior aspects of the frontal lobe[34] and frontoparietal areas,[35] are associated with the inhibition of detrusor activity, compression by tumour, or neural degeneration would induce DH with synergetic sphincter function.[22,36]

Dementia

Dementia occurs as a result of deterioration and atrophy of both grey and white matter in the brain, particularly of the frontal lobes. Although associated with syndromes such as head injury, hydrocephalus, encephalitis, syphilis and Alzheimer's, Pick's and Creutzfeldt–Jakob diseases, the aetiology of neuronal degeneration associated with dementia is poorly understood.[29]

The chief urinary symptom is that of incontinence, with a prevalence approaching 90% of patients in some series.[37] It has not, however, been established whether detrusor dysfunction or, more likely, a defect in cognitive function, is responsible for the lack of social continence in patients with dementia.

In one report, 71% of elderly patients with cognitive impairment showed DH; however, 65% of those with no impairment demonstrated hyperreflexia by the same criteria. Therefore, it is unlikely that the incontinence associated with dementia is due merely to detrusor overactivity.[38]

Shy–Drager syndrome (multiple system atrophy)

Shy and Drager described a neurological syndrome characterized by autonomic dysfunction consisting of orthostatic hypotension, anhydrosis, erectile dysfunction, extrapyramidal symptoms and poor urinary and faecal control.[39] The mean age of onset is 55 years, with a male predominance of 2 or 3:1.[40] This disease results in the symmetrical degeneration of neurons and associated fibres of motor and extrapyramidal systems, including the cerebellum and brain stem.[41] Disease progression results in death 7–20 years after the onset of neurological symptoms.[40]

Blaivas has reported that urinary symptoms of incontinence are caused by DH and some element of paralysis of the external sphincter, while an open bladder neck was noted during cystography, indicative of peripheral sympathetic dysfunction.[44] The combination of detrusor dysfunction and sphincter denervation contraindicates the surgical management of symptoms; currently recommended treatment is therefore that of a combination of intermittent catheterization and medical therapy, including anticholinergics and desmopressin.[39,42]

CONDITIONS OF THE SPINAL CORD AFFECTING THE URINARY TRACT

In general, the degree of dysfunction is related to the process of the condition or disease itself, the area of the spinal cord affected and the severity of neurological impairment. While the neurological process itself can result in urinary tract pathology, pre-existing conditions, such as pelvic floor prolapse or hysterectomy, must also be considered as contributing to altered radiographic and urodynamic parameters.[34,43,44]

Neurological injury, which can involve parasympathetic, sympathetic and somatic nerve fibres, can result in a complex array of signs and symptoms. The urodynamic investigation of those with neurological impairment can provide objective information regarding the nature and extent of the effect on lower urinary tract function. For this reason, urodynamic testing should be an integral part in the evaluation of all patients with complete and incomplete spinal cord dysfunction.

Spinal cord injury

SCI occurs at a rate of approximately 32 new injuries per million population in the United States, with a prevalence of approximately 906 per million.[45] With 85% of injuries occurring at or above the T12 level, nearly 55% of patients develop quadriplegia, while 45% become paraplegic. Neurologically incomplete injuries (53.8%) are slightly more frequent than are complete injuries (46.2%).[46] Patients with any type of SCI commonly develop lower urinary tract dysfunction, which often results in structural alterations, urolithiasis and infection.

Neurogenic lower urinary tract dysfunction resulting from SCI is an excellent model for the understanding of neurourological dysfunction. The principles of urological evaluation and management of traumatic SCI patients are applicable to those with other spinal cord pathology.[5] Lower urinary tract dysfunction, however, varies depending on the stage of recovery from SCI, which is best described in three phases: spinal shock, recovery and stable phases.

The *spinal shock phase* occurs immediately after spinal cord trauma, and is characterized by flaccid paralysis, absence of reflex activity below the level of the lesion, and DA. Although this may last for several weeks or even months, reflex detrusor activity usually appears within 2–12 weeks. Thomas and O'Flynn[47] confirmed that the most peripheral somatic reflexes of the sacral cord segments may never disappear or, if they do, return within minutes or hours of the injury. Urinary retention during this period is practically universal, and is best managed with an intermittent catheterization programme.

The return of reflex detrusor activity marks the beginning of the *recovery phase*, with the level of the neurological lesion frequently correlating with expected lower tract function. After a cervical- or thoracic-level injury, DH is anticipated, and is frequently associated with detrusor external sphincter dyssynergia. Lower urinary tract function after lumbar-level injuries is more difficult to predict, while those with sacral-level injuries commonly develop DA, although this may occasionally occur in patients with cervical or thoracic lesions.

The *stable phase* after SCI is typified by the absence of any further neurological recovery and an unchanging urodynamic pattern. Despite the progression to neurological stability after SCI, however, periodic urodynamic and radiographic assessment is required to safeguard the upper urinary tracts.

The relationship of lower urinary tract dysfunction to level of injury has been evaluated in an analysis of 489 consecutive SCI patients.[48] The bladder and sphincter behaviour of 284 patients with traumatic SCI is shown in Table 65.1 for cervical, thoracic, lumbar and sacral levels of injury. Of 104 patients with cervical SCI, 15% had DA. The remaining 88 patients (85%) had involuntary detrusor contractions, and 57 of 88 (65%) had DSD. All of the 87 thoracic SCI patients had DH, and 78 of 87 (90%) had DSD. Lumbar SCI resulted in the most mixed urodynamic patterns. Forty per cent

had DA, and 60% had DH (half with DSD and half without). Sacral SCI was the only group that had patients with normal urodynamic studies (12%); 64% of the patients had DA.

Autonomic dysreflexia

Autonomic dysreflexia (AD) represents an exaggerated response by the sympathetic nervous system to afferent visceral stimulation. The stimulus is usually noxious in nature, frquently emanating from bowel or bladder distention, although indwelling urinary catheters have been implicated. This response occurs chiefly in those with an SCI at the T7 level or higher, and the resultant cardiovascular response can be life-threatening.

The symptoms commonly associated with AD include a pounding headache associated with diaphoresis and flushing above the level of the injury, and paroxysmal, severe hypertension accompanied by reflex bradycardia. The labile hypertension associated with the AD response can result in intracranial haemorrhage and death.[49]

Multiple sclerosis

MS is a disease of focal inflammatory and demyelinating lesions of the nervous system, affecting those 20–50 years of age in the temperate climates. Prevalence in the United States varies from 6 to 122 per 100 000.[50] In approximately 60% of patients, the disease is initially manifested by exacerbations and remissions. The clinical courses of MS have been described as acute, progressive, chronic and benign.[51]

Table 65.1. *Urodynamic findings (%) in 284 patients with spinal cord injury, stratified to the level of the injury*

Level of injury	Detrusor hyperreflexia		Detrusor areflexia	Normal
	Without DSD	With DSD		
Cervical (n = 104)	30	55	15	0
Thoracic (n = 87)	10	90	0	0
Lumbar (n = 61)	30	30	40	0
Sacral (n = 32)	12	12	64	12

DSD, detrusor sphincter dyssynergia.
Data are modified from ref. 48.

Impairment of neurological function results from demyelinating plaques of the white matter of the brain and spinal cord, especially the posterior and lateral columns of the cervical cord, which serve as pathways for neurological control over vesical and urethral function.[52] Such plaque formation is probably the result of an autoimmune process.[53]

Symptoms of voiding dysfunction are experienced by 90% of patients with MS.[54] These include not only frequency, urgency and urge incontinence, but also urinary hesitancy, intermittency and poor urinary stream.

Urodynamically, the most frequent pattern seen is DH, which may occur in 50–99% of patients[54–56] (Table 65.2). Detrusor external sphincter dyssynergia is also documented in up to 50% of patients with DH.[16,57,58] DA, associated with lower cord and cauda equina plaques, is seen in 20–30% of patients; these patients usually strain to void.[59] This can be accounted for by degenerative plaque formation in the sacral cord, impairing motor impulse outflow to the detrusor. Although these patients may be managed effectively with an intermittent catheterization programme, periodic urodynamic re-evaluation is essential to ensure protection of the upper urinary tract.[60] This is because the neurourological status of the patient with MS may change over time.

Management of lower urinary tract dysfunction is based on the avoidance of indwelling catheters and minimizing intravesical storage pressure while assuring low-pressure urinary drainage.[60] Urinary storage pressure can be minimized with the use of anticholinergic medications, or augmentation cystoplasty if medical therapy is ineffective.[61] In men, external sphincterotomy is effective in assuring low-pressure drainage if an external collection device can be maintained.[60] In place of sphincterotomy or in patients who have had poor outcome after sphincterotomy, Urolume urethral stents can be used.[62] Unfortunately, sphincterotomy is not an option for women, and many women with neuropathic bladder dysfunction are treated in the community with indwelling urethral or suprapubic catheters.

Intervertebral disc disease

Herniation of intervertebral discs into the spinal canal as a result of degenerative disease or trauma may result in lower urinary tract dysfunction, with or without somatomotor symptoms. The resulting hyperexcitability of the sensory and motor fibres may result in the irritative urinary symptoms of frequency and urgency caused by DH.[63]

A more acute compression of the sacral nerve roots, however, impairs nerve conduction. Decreased autonomic outflow significantly decreases detrusor contractility and may result in DA, while interference with somatic outflow to the pudendal nerve can compromise function of the external sphincter mechanism, causing intrinsic sphincteric deficiency.[64]

Relief of nervous or cord compression may improve

Table 65.2. *Urodynamic patterns in patients with multiple sclerosis*					
Series	Sample size	Normal	DA	DH without DSD	DH and DSD
Blaivas et al.[55]	45 studies in 41 patients	2 (4)	18 (40)	14 (31)	11 (24)
McGuire and Savastano[54]	46 patients	0	13 (28) mean PVR 600 ml	12 (26) mean PVR 30 ml	21 (46) mean PVR 90 ml
Goldstein et al.[16]	94 studies in 84 patients	5 (5)	18 (19)	47 (50)	24 (26)
Awad et al.[56]	57 patients	7 (12)	12 (21)	21 (37)	17 (30)
Weinstein et al.[57]	89 patients	11 (12)	15 (17)	47 (53)	16 (18)
Sirls et al.[58]	113 patients	7 (6)	17 (15)	79 (70)	15/54 tested (28)

Percentages shown in parentheses. DA, detrusor areflexia; DH, detrusor hyperreflexia; DSD, detrusor sphincter dysnergia; PVR, post-void residual urine volume.

voiding function; however, recovery is generally slow, and may take years.[63–65] We have carefully reviewed our experience with urological dysfunction after lower-back disc disease.[3] We found that 41% of patients with very incomplete (American Spinal Injury Association Category E) injury impairment demonstrated neurogenic lower urinary tract dysfunction. Neural injury, which can involve parasympathetic, sympathetic and somatic nerve fibres, can result in a complex array of signs and symptoms.

The urodynamic investigation of those with neurological impairment can, however provide objective information about the nature and extent of the effect on lower urinary tract function (Fig. 65.5). Urodynamic testing should be an integral part of the evaluation of all patients with incomplete lumbosacral spinal injuries.

Ankylosing spondylitis

Ankylosing spondylitis, which affects predominantly men, is an inflammatory disease of the spine that results in fusion of the joints, and ligamentous calcification. Aberrations of neurological function generally result from spinal cord compression caused by atlantoaxial subluxation or trauma to the rigid spine.[66]

Neurogenic lower urinary tract dysfunction caused by ankylosing spondylitis will usually result in impaired detrusor contractility. More severe cases may result in DA, which can progress to upper tract deterioration as bladder compliance decreases. External sphincter activity may also be compromised as neuropathy progresses. Surgery to effect neural decompression has met with varying success.[67]

Guillain–Barré syndrome

The Guillain–Barré syndrome is an inflammatory demyelinating polyneuropathy which mainly affects the peripheral nervous system;[68] however, a predilection for the nerve roots may exist.[69] In severe cases, progression continues to affect central nervous, respiratory and autonomic function, which results in urinary retention.[70] Although recovery is a hallmark of Guillain–Barré syndrome, only 15% of patients suffer no residual neurological deficit, and mortality caused by secondary complications has been reported in up to 18% of patients.[71] Detrusor and sphincter motor and sensory

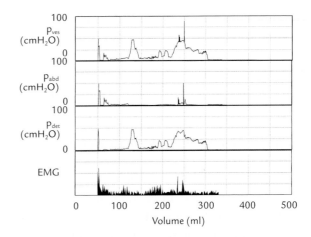

Figure 65.5. *A 44-year-old woman suffered a work-related back injury with magnetic resonance imaging documentation of a left-sided L3–4 level disc herniation. Since the back injury the patient complains of new-onset burning on urination, suprapubic pressure and urinary frequency. The urine analysis was normal. Post-void residual urine was less than 30 ml. Videourodynamic evaluations demonstrated several involuntary detrusor contractions between 100 ml and 300 ml. Electrical activity of the external sphincter did not increase during uninhibited detrusor contractions. The correct diagnosis is detrusor hyperreflexia. The patient was treated with oral oxybutynin and referred for neurosurgical evaluation. Abbreviations as Figure 65.1.*

deficits are encountered in the course of Guillain–Barré syndrome,[72] resulting in urinary retention, which is usually reversible.[44]

More recently, urodynamic evaluation has revealed DH in some patients with Guillain–Barré syndrome, accounted for by either central nervous system involvement, or the timing of the urodynamic study, perhaps during neural regeneration.[73]

Tabes dorsalis

Tabes dorsalis (locomotor ataxia) is a form of neurosyphilis in which demyelinating atrophy of the dorsal columns of the spinal cord and sensory nerve trunks is caused by infection of the central nervous system with *Treponema pallidum*.[74] Progression of the sacral root and dorsal column degeneration results in increasing residual urine and, ultimately, the development of urinary retention.[75]

More recently, urodynamic evaluation of patients with tabes dorsalis has revealed that detrusor hypertonicity may occur. It is postulated that involvement of the conus medullaris or cauda equina predisposes to a poorly compliant areflexic bladder, while suprasacral lesions are responsible for the DH in these cases.[76] These patients can be managed effectively with treatment of the primary infection with antibiotics and an intermittent catheterization programme.[77]

Acquired immune deficiency syndrome

Patients with acquired immune deficiency syndrome (AIDS) may be expected to have an increased incidence of voiding dysfunction. AIDS is associated with neurologic dysfunction in up to 40% of patients.[78,79]

Neurological symptoms may also be caused by non-viral opportunistic infection of the nervous system. Specifically, toxoplasmosis is reported frequently in AIDS patients, with a frequency of 14% in those with neurological disease.[79] Neoplasms may also account for neural disturbances, with primary central nervous system lymphoma, systemic lymphoma with central nervous system involvement, and Kaposi's sarcoma reported.[80–82]

In one series, 11 of 677 patients with AIDS reported significant voiding symptoms in a 1-year period, with urinary retention in 55% of patients.[83] Urodynamic evaluation revealed DA in 36%, DH in 27%, and bladder outlet obstruction in 18% of patients. The remaining 19% of patients had normal urodynamic parameters. Interestingly, the onset of urological disturbance represented a poor prognostic indicator, as 44% of patients died within 24 months.[84]

Tropical spastic paraparesis

Tropical spastic paraparesis is a condition of progressive paraparesis and back pain, with urinary hesitancy, urgency and incontinence in up to 60% of patients, associated with, and probably induced by, infection with the retrovirus human T-cell lymphotrophic virus type 1.[85] This clinical entity is caused by meningomyelitis with demyelinization and axonal loss, which can involve the corticospinal tracts.[86]

The urodynamic evaluation of patients with tropical spastic paraparesis has revealed both DA and DH.[87] The effect on lower urinary tract function may predispose to upper tract deterioration; therefore all patients should undergo urodynamic evaluation and appropriate urological therapy should be instituted.[77]

Transverse myelitis

Transverse myelitis is a rare inflammatory condition of the spinal cord which may affect children or adults.[88,89] The entire thickness of the cord is involved, including both the grey and white matter.[90]

The neurological deficit may be sudden in onset or progressive over several days to weeks. Affected individuals may suffer from residual neurological deficit, although complete recovery may occur within 3–18 months.[89,91] Lower urinary tract dysfunction may present as either urinary retention or incontinence.

Lyme disease

Lyme disease is caused by the spirochaete *Borrelia burghdor feri*, which has demonstrated the ability to invade numerous body tissues, including the nervous system. Neurological symptoms may be caused by encephalopathy, polyneuropathy and leukoencephalitis. Although initially associated with urinary retention, the urological symptoms of urinary urgency, urge incontinence and nocturia may occur at any time during the disease process.[93]

Urodynamic evaluation may reveal either DA or DH, although sphincter dyssynergia has not been documented.[94] Although the disease may respond to a 2-week course of antimicrobial therapy,[95] those with relapsing and remitting symptoms may require long-term administration of antimicrobials.[96]

Herpes zoster

Herpes zoster is a reactivation of the varicella virus, which proliferates in the dorsal root ganglion.[97] Sensory disturbances such as pain and paresthesia are common, although paralytic complications are rare.[98]

As the virus travels via the autonomic nerves of the bladder, irritative voiding symptoms of dysuria and frequency may develop. The sacral micturition reflex arc may be compromised as the virus affects afferent neurons.[99] Progression of viral involvement proximally to involve the anterior horns of the spinal cord can result in somatic and visceral motor neuropathy, and urinary retention may ensue.[100]

We see two or three patients each year, generally otherwise health young women, who develop lower urinary tract symptoms such as urgency or retention that turn out to be the initial clinical manifestation of a herpes infection. The course of the viral infection is usually self-limiting, with spontaneous recovery usually occurring within several months.[101]

Poliomyelitis

Poliomyelitis results in destruction of the grey matter of the anterior horn cells and selective destruction of large-diameter fast-conducting motor neurons.[102] Therefore, polio is essentially a pure motor neuropathy, and sensory function is usually normal.[103] Urinary retention may occur in up to 40% of patients, depending on disease severity. Although DA is noted urodynamically, bladder sensation and anal sphincter function remain intact.[43]

Over the past few years there has been a resurgence of interest in poliomyelitis. Some patients with moderate motor dysfunction and who have had adequate motor function for 30 years are developing late motor decompensation, including urinary incontinence and retention.

Tethered cord syndrome and short filum terminale

In the course of normal fetal development, the spinal cord initially reaches the inferior aspect of the sacrum. Growth of the vertebrae exceeds that of the spinal cord, therefore the conus medullaris must migrate cephalad.[104] At 2 years of age, the conus approximates the second lumbar vertebra and the T12 level by adulthood.[105] The tethered cord syndrome results from the impediment of the cephalad migration of the conus, and may be caused by a short filum terminale, intraspinal lipoma or fibrous adhesions resulting from the surgical repair of spinal dysraphism.[106] The syndrome is classically associated with children, especially during adolescence, but the process may occur in adulthood.[107,108]

DA has been reported in 60% of patients, although recovery of lower tract function approached 60% with surgical release of the cord.[107] Detrusor overactivity can also occur;[109] another study documented 22% of patients with DH, all with improvement following surgery.[110] Early and aggressive surgical correction therefore is indicated.[111]

CONDITIONS OF THE PERIPHERAL NERVOUS SYSTEM AFFECTING THE URINARY TRACT

We have recently focused our research on assessing the correlation between anatomical lesion, neurological examination and urological dysfunction[1-3] (Table 65.3). The most dorsolateral fibres in the spinothalamic tracts are located close to the autonomic system tracts; therefore, initial perianal pin sensation may be predictive of the potential for recovery of bladder function. In our study, all SCI patients with an absent or significantly diminished perianal pin sensation and bulbocavernosus reflex demonstrated lower urinary tract dysfunction; however, intact pin prick and bulbocavernosus reflex were not sensitive in predicting an absence of lower urinary tract dysfunction. Our most significant finding is that 41% of patients with very incomplete SCI impairment had neurogenic lower urinary tract dysfunction.

Table 65.3. *Neurological conditions that can cause urinary tract dysfunction*

Conditions affecting the brain

- Cerebrovascular accident
- Parkinson's disease
- Brain neoplasms
- Dementia
- Shy–Drager syndrome (multiple system atrophy)

Conditions affecting the spinal cord

- Spinal cord injury
- Multiple sclerosis
- Invertebral disc disease
- Ankylosing spondylitis
- Guillain–Barré syndrome
- Tabes dorsalis
- Acquired immune deficiency syndrome
- Tropical spastic paraparesis
- Transverse myelitis
- Lyme disease
- Herpes zoster
- Poliomyelitis
- Tethered cord syndrome and short filum terminale

Conditions affecting the peripheral nervous system

- Pelvic plexus injury
- Abdominoperineal resection
- Hysterectomy
- Diabetic neuropathy

Pelvic plexus injury

The pelvic plexus contains both parasympathetic and sympathetic fibres in a branching array, parasagittally adjacent to the rectum. Disruption of pelvic plexus function may occur with any major pelvic surgical procedure or traumatic pelvic fracture. Such traumatic injury to the hypogastric, pelvic and pudendal nerves results in damage to sympathetic, parasympathetic and somatic nerve fibres and, consequently, lower urinary tract dysfunction (Figure 65.6).

Decreased parasympathetic innervation generally results in decreased detrusor contractility and potentially DA, while impaired sympathetic transmission results in incomplete bladder-neck closure, internal sphincter dysfunction and stress incontinence. Up to 80% of patients with voiding disturbances after significant pelvic procedures will resume normal voiding within 6 months.[112]

Abdominoperineal resection

Abdominoperineal resection (APR) of the rectum has been associated with significant lower urinary tract dysfunction for over 50 years.[113] Postoperative urinary retention or incomplete bladder emptying may affect

up to 90% of patients.[114] Coursing in proximity to the rectum and its investing fascia, the pelvic plexus is susceptible to direct neural disruption and traction injury during rectal resection.[115]

One study revealed evidence of sympathetic denervation in 100%, parasympathetic denervation in 38% and pudendal denervation in 54% of patients postoperatively. Although the voiding dysfunction is usually transitory,[116] sphincteric insufficiency may be permanent. Internal sphincteric insufficiency, demonstrable by an open bladder neck on cystography, may respond to α-adrenergic therapy.[117]

If the APR has denervated the external sphincter, transurethral incision of the urethra in women or prostatectomy in men should be avoided because it may cause stress urinary incontinence. The most logical and safest urological treatment of post-APR retention is clean intermittent self-catheterization.

Hysterectomy

The effect on lower urinary tract function of radical hysterectomy and bilateral pelvic lymphadenectomy is similar to that of APR of the rectum. Because of the position of the pelvic nerves far posterior, with the pelvic plexus below the cardinal ligament,

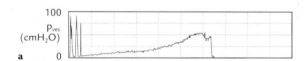

Figure 65.6. *A 49-year-old woman with recurrent left pyelonephritis and urinary incontinence after a radical hysterectomy 2 years previously. She reports having to strain to urinate and her residual urine volume is 185 ml. (a) Urodynamic evaluation reveals continual increase in intravesical pressure (p_{ves}) during slow-fill cystometry despite the absence of discrete detrusor contraction; p_{ves} exceeds the safe level of 40 cmH$_2$O at 255 ml, risking damage to the upper urinary tract. (b) The bladder is trabeculated on the voiding cystogram. The patient attempts voiding by Valsalva manoevre. She is able to partially empty her bladder but high-grade left vesicoureteral reflux develops. The diagnosis is detrusor areflexia with decreased detrusor compliance. She was started on oxybutynin and clean intermittent self-catheterization every 6 hours. We recommended a repeat of the urodynamic study after 3 months. If she continues to develop pyelonephritis and her detrusor compliance does not improve we will recommend an intestinal bladder augmentation procedure.*

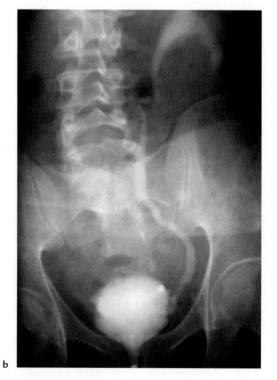

parasympathetic disturbance should be less frequently encountered after radical hysterectomy than after APR.

Management includes anticholinergic therapy to decrease intravesical storage pressure, with drainage provided by an intermittent catheterization programme. Although intravenous urography may demonstrate upper tract dilatation and a contracted bladder, effectively lowering intravesical pressure can stabilize or reverse upper tract changes.[118]

Diabetic neuFropathy

Diabetes mellitus is a common medical condition, affecting 1–2% of the population;[119] it is by far the most common disorder resulting in sensory neurogenic lower urinary tract dysfunction.[120] Voiding symptoms generally develop at least 10 years after the onset of the disease, as a result of peripheral and autonomic neuropathies.[44,121] Metabolic abnormalities of Schwann cell function result in segmental demyelinization and subsequent axonal degeneration, impairing nerve conduction.[122,123]

Chronic hyperglycaemia is associated with the loss of myelinated and unmyelinated fibres, Wallerian degeneration and blunted nerve fibre reproduction.[124] The proposed mechanisms include: (1) increased accumulation of polyols (sorbitol) from glucose through the aldolase reductase pathway, ultimately resulting in decreased activity of $Na^+-K^+-ATPase$ and (2) the formation of advanced glycosylation end-products from glucose.

Deficits in bladder sensation occur initially, with insidious onset, usually associated with other sensory impairment. Classically, patients experience decreased urinary frequency, urinary hesitancy and slowing of the urine stream. These symptoms may progress to include a sensation of incomplete emptying or even urinary dribbling from overflow incontinence.[125]

When questioned, up to 50% of unselected diabetes mellitus patients have subjective evidence of diabetic cystopathy. The urodynamic evaluation, however, suggests alterations in lower urinary tract function in 27–85% of these patients.[125,126] Although diabetics will frequently report urinary urgency and frequency, increased residual urine is the hallmark of the later stages of diabetic sensory neurogenic bladder dysfunction.

Urodynamic studies frequently reveal impaired bladder sensation, increased cystometric bladder capacity, decreased detrusor contractility, an impaired urine flow and an elevated post-void residual urine volume.[44] Upper tract changes depend upon the duration and severity of the process, as well as the effect on intravesical pressure. The effect of diabetes-induced lower urinary tract dysfunction on the upper urinary tract is difficult to determine because of the other effects of diabetes on renal function.

Urodynamic evaluation of 182 diabetic male and female patients referred for voiding symptoms demonstrated that 55% manifested DH, while only 33% had either impaired contractility or DA.[127] It must be remembered that diabetics with voiding symptoms are generally older, and are subject to infection, outlet obstruction and uninhibited detrusor contraction, as are others in their age group.

Similar to other neurourologic diseases, preservation of renal function is of greatest priority. A timed voiding schedule is effective in those with impaired contractility, while intermittent catheterization is reserved for those who experience greater difficulty with emptying. Anticholinergic therapy may be effective for those with DH or impaired bladder compliance.[120]

REFERENCES

1. Weiss DJ, Fried GW, Chancellor MB *et al*. Spinal cord injury and bladder recovery. *Arch Phy Med Rehab* 1996; 77: 1133–1135

2. Shenot PJ, Rivas DA, Watanabe T *et al*. Early predictors of bladder recovery and urodynamics after spinal cord injury. *Neurourol Urodyn*, 1998; 17: 25–29

3. Watanabe T, Vaccaro AR, Kumon H *et al*. High incidence of occult neurogenic bladder dysfunction in neurologically intact patients with thoracolumbar spinal injuries. *J Urol* 1998; 159; 965–968

4. de Groat WC, Kawatani M. Neural control of the urinary bladder: possible relationship between peptidergic inhibitory mechanisms and detrusor instability. *Neurourol Urodyn* 1985; 4: 285–300

5. Chancellor MB, Rivas DA, Ackman D. Multicenter trials of Urolume™ endourethral Wallstent® prosthesis for the urinary sphincter in spinal cord injured men. *J Urol* 1994; 152: 924–930

6. Tosi L, Righetti C, Terrini G, Zanette G. Atypical syndromes caudal to the injury site in patients following spinal cord injury. A clinical, neurophysiological and MRI study. *Paraplegia* 1993; 31: 751–756

7. Sundin T, Dahlstrom A. The sympathetic innervation of the urinary bladder and urethra in the normal state and after parasympathetic denervation at the spinal root level. An experimental study in cats. *Scand J Urol Nephrol* 1973; 7: 131–149

8. Staskin D, Nehra A, Siroky M. Hydroureteronephrosis after spinal cord injury: effects of lower urinary tract dysfunction on upper tract anatomy. *Urol Clin North Am* 1991; 18: 309–316

9. Blaivas JG. The neurophysiology of micturition: a clinical study of 550 patients. *J Urol* 1982; 127: 958–963

10. McGuire EJ, Brady S. Detrusor-sphincter dyssynergia. *J Urol* 1979; 121: 774–779

11 Blaivas JG, Barbalias GA. Detrusor-external sphincter dyssynergia in men with multiple sclerosis: an ominous urologic condition. *J Urol* 1984; 131: 91–94

12. Borges P, Hackler RH. The urologic status of the Vietnam war paraplegic: a 15-year prospective follow-up. *J Urol* 1982; 127: 710–711

13. Lloyd K. New trends in urologic management of spinal cord injured patients. *Central Nervous System Trauma* 1986; 3: 3–11

14. Anderson RU. Urodynamic patterns after acute spinal cord injury: association with bladder trabeculation in male patients. *J Urol* 1983; 129: 777–779

15. Ruutu M. Cystometrographic patterns in predicting bladder function after spinal cord injury. *Paraplegia* 1985; 23: 243–252

16. Goldstein I, Siroky MB, Sax DS, Krane RJ. Neurourologic abnormalities in multiple sclerosis. *J Urol* 1982; 128: 541–545

17. Ruch TC. The urinary bladder. In: Ruch TC, Patton HD *Physiology and Biophysics: Circulation, Respiration, and Fluid Balance*, 20th edn. Philadelphia: W.B. Saunders, 1974; 525–546

18. Berger Y, Blaivas JG, DeLaRocha ER, Salinas J. Urodynamic findings on Parkinson's disease. *J Urol* 1987; 138: 836–838

19. Blaivas JG. Techniques of evaluation. In: Yalla SV, McGuire EJ, Elbadasi A, Blaivas JG (eds) *Neurourology and Urodynamics: Principles and Practice*. New York: Macmillan, 1988; 155–198

20. McGuire EJ, Woodside JR, Borden TA *et al.* The prognostic significance of urodynamic testing in myelodysplastic patients. *J Urol* 1981; 125: 205–209

21. Khan Z, Starer P, Yang WC, Bhola A. Analysis of voiding disorders in patients with cerebrovascular accidents. *Urology* 1990; 35: 265–270

22. Tsuchida S, Noto H, Yamaguchi O, Itoh M. Urodynamic studies on hemiplegic patients after cerebrovascular accident. *Urology* 1983; 21: 315–318

23. Redding MJ, Winter SW, Hochrein SA. Urinary incontinence after unilateral hemispheric stroke: a neurologic epidemiologic perspective. *J Neurorehabil* 1987; 1: 25–31

24. Blaivas JG, Chancellor MB. Cerebrovascular accidents and other intracranial lesions. *Practical Neurourology – Genitourinary Complications in Neurologic Disease*. Boston: Butterworth–Heinemann, 1995; 119–125

25. Borrie MJ, Campbell AJ, Caradoc-Davies TH, Spears GFS. Urinary incontinence after stroke: a prospective study. *Age Ageing* 1986; 15: 177–181

26. Brocklehurst JC, Andrews K, Richards B *et al.* Incidence and correlates of incontinence in stroke patients. *J Am Geriatric Soc* 1985; 33: 540–542

27. Siroky MB, Krane RJ. Neurologic aspects of detrusor-sphincter dyssynergia, with reference to the guarding reflex. *J Urol* 1982; 127: 953–957

28. Yahr MD. Parkinson's disease – overview of its current status. *Mt Sinai J Med* 1977; 44: 183–191

29. Staskin DR. Intracranial lesions that affect lower urinary tact function. In: Krane RJ, Siroky MB (eds) *Clinical Neuro-Urology*, 2nd edn. Boston: Little Brown, 1991; 345–351

30. Antel JP, Arnason BW. Demyelinating diseases. In: Wilson JD, Braunwald EB, Isselbacher KJ (eds) *Harrison's Principles of Internal Medicine*. New York: McGraw-Hill, 1991; 2038–2065

31. Pavlakis AJ, Siroky MB, Goldstein I, Krane RJ. Neurourologic findings in Parkinson's disease. *J Urol* 1983; 129: 80–83

32. Blaivas JG, Chancellor MB. Parkinson's disease. *Practical Neurourology – Genitourinary Complications in Neurologic Disease.* Boston: Butterworth–Heinemann, 1995; 139–147

33. Kahn Z, Starr P, Bhola A. Urinary incontinence in female Parkinson's disease patients. *Urology* 1989; 33: 486–489

34. Hald T, Bradley WE. *The Urinary Bladder: Neurology and Dynamics.* Baltimore: Williams & Wilkins, 1982; 48–50: 157–159

35. Kahn Z, Hertanu J, Yang WC *et al.* Predictive correlation of urodynamic dysfunction and brain injury after cerebrovascular accident. *J Urol* 1981; 126: 86–88

36. Yalla SV, Fam BA. Spinal cord injury. In: Krane RJ, Siroky MB (eds) *Clinical Neuro-Urology* 2nd edn Boston: Little, Brown, 1991; 319–322

37. Skelly J, Flint AJ. Urinary incontinence associated with dementia. *J Am Geriatric Soc* 1995; 43: 286–294

38. Resnick NM, Yalla SV, Laurino E. The pathophysiology of urinary incontinence among institutionalized elderly persons. *New Engl J Med* 1989; 320: 1421–1422

39. Wulfsohn MA, Rubenstein A. The management of Shy–Drager syndrome with propantheline and intermittent self-catheterization: a case report. *J Urol* 1981; 126: 122–123

40. Abyad A. Shy–Drager syndrome: recognition and management. *J Am Board Fam Pract* 1995; 8: 325–330

41. Lockhart JL, Webster GD, Sheremata W *et al.* Neurogenic bladder dysfunction in the Shy–Drager syndrome. *J Urol* 1981; 126: 119–121

42. Beck RO, Betts CD, Fowler CJ. Genitourinary dysfunction in multiple system atrophy: clinical features and treatment in 62 cases. *J Urol* 1994; 151: 1336–1341

43. Bors E, Comarr AE. *Neurologic Urology.* Baltimore: University Park Press, 1971

44. Blaivas JG. Neurologic dysfunctions. In: Yalla SV, McGuire EJ, El-Badawi A, Blaivas JG (eds) *Neurourology and Urodynamics: Principles and Practice.* New York: Macmillan, 1988; 343–357

45. De Vivo MJ, Rutt RD, Black KJ *et al.* Trends in spinal cord injury demographics and treatment outcomes between 1973 and 1986. *Arch Phys Med Rehabil* 1982;7 3: 424–430

46. Watanabe T, Rivas DA, Chancellor MB. Urodynamics of spinal cord injury. *Urol Clin North Am* 1996; 23: 459–473

47. Thomas DG, O'Flynn KJ. Spinal cord injury. In: Mundy AR, Stephenson TP, Wein AJ (eds) *Urodynamics: Principles, Practice, Application.* London: Churchill Livingstone, 1994; 345–358

48. Kaplan SA, Chancellor MB, Blaivas JG. Bladder and sphincter behavior in patients with spinal cord lesions. *J Urol* 1991; 146: 113–117

49. Rivas DA, Chancellor MB, Huang B, Salzman SK. Autonomic dysreflexia in a rat model of spinal cord injury and the effect of pharmacologic agents. *Neurourol Urodyn* 1995; 14: 141–152

50. Poser CM. The epidemiology of multiple sclerosis: a general overview. *Ann Neurol* 1994; 36: S180–S193

51. McFarlin DE, McFarland HF. Multiple sclerosis. *New Engl J Med* 1982; 307: 1183–1188

52. Nathan PW, Smith NC. The centrifugal pathway for micturition with the spinal cord. *J Neurol Neurosurg Psychiatry* 1958; 21: 177–186

53. Lublin FD. Relapsing experimental allergic encephalitis: an autoimmune model of multiple sclerosis. *Semin Immunopathol* 1985; 8: 197–208

54. McGuire EJ, Savastano JA. Urodynamic findings and long-term outcome management of patients with multiple sclerosis-induced lower urinary tract dysfunction. *J Urol* 1984; 132: 713–715

55. Blaivas JG, Bhimani G, Labib KB. Vesicourethral dysfunction in multiple sclerosis. *J Urol* 1979; 122: 342–347

56. Awad SA, Gajewski JB, Sogbein SK *et al.* Relationship between neurological and urological status in patients with multiple sclerosis. *J Urol* 1984; 132: 499–502

57. Weinstein MS, Cardenas DD, O'Shaughnessy EJ, Catanzaro ML. Carbon dioxide cystometry and postural changes in patients with multiple sclerosis. *Arch Phys Med Rehabil* 1988; 69: 923–927

58. Sirls LT, Zimmern PE, Leach GE. Role of limited evaluation and aggressive medical management in multiple sclerosis: a review of 113 patients. *J Urol* 1994; 151: 946–950

59. Gonor SE, Carroll DJ, Metcalfe JB. Vesical dysfunction in multiple sclerosis. *Urology* 1985; 25: 429–431

60. Chancellor MB, Blaivas JG. Multiple sclerosis. *Practical Neurourology – Genitourinary Complications in Neurologic Disease.* Boston: Butterworth–Heinemann, 1995; 127–137

61. Fowler CJ, van Kerrebroeck PEV, Nordenbo A, van Poppel H. Treatment of lower urinary tract dysfunction in patients with multiple sclerosis. *J Neurol Neurosurg Psychiatry* 1992; 55: 986–989

62. Juma S, Niku SD, Brodak PP, Joseph AC. Urolume urethral wallstent in the treatment of detrusor sphincter dyssynergia. *Paraplegia* 1994; 32: 616–621

63. Jones DL, Moore T. The types of neuropathic bladder dysfunction associated with prolapsed lumbar intervertebral discs. *Br J Urol* 1973; 45: 39–43

64. Malloch JD. Acute retention due to intervertebral disc prolapse. *Br J Urol* 1965; 37: 578–585

65. Hellstrom P, Kortelainen P, Kontturi M. Late urodynamic findings after surgery for cauda equina syndrome caused a prolapsed lumbar intervertebral disk. *J Urol* 1986; 135: 308–312

66. Russell ML, Gordon DA, Ogryzlo MA, McPhedran RS. The cauda equina syndrome of ankylosing spondylitis. *Ann Int Med* 1973; 78: 551–554

67. Tyrrell PNM, Davies AM, Evans N. Neurological disturbances in ankylosing spondylitis. *Ann Rheumatic Dis* 1994; 53: 714–717

68. Asbury AK, Arnason BG, Adams RD. The inflammatory lesion in idiopathic polyneuritis: its role in pathogenesis. *Medicine* 1969; 48: 173–215

69. Haymaker W, Kernohan JW. The Landry–Guillan–Barré syndrome: clinicopathologic report of fifty fatal cases and a critique of the literature. *Medicine* 1949; 28: 59–65

70. Ropper AH. The Guillain–Barré syndrome. *New Engl J Med* 1992; 326: 1130–1136

71. Ng KKP, Howard RS, Fish DR *et al.* Management and outcome of severe Guillain–Barré syndrome. *Q J Med* 1995; 88: 243–250

72. Kogan BA, Solomon MH, Diokno AC. Urinary retention secondary to Landry–Guillain–Barré syndrome. *J Urol* 1981; 126: 643–644

73. Wheeler JS, Siroky MB, Pavlakis A, Krane RJ. The urodynamic aspects of the Guillain–Barré syndrome. *J Urol* 1984; 131: 917–919

74. Wheeler JS Jr, Culkin DJ, O'Hara RJ, Canning JR. Bladder dysfunction and neurosyphilis. *J Urol* 1986; 136: 903–905

75. Harper JM, Politano VA, Schwarcz . The FTA–ABS test in the diagnosis of the neurogenic bladder. *J Urol* 1967; 97: 862–863

76. Hattori T, Yasuda K, Kita K, Hirayama K. Disorders of micturition in tabes dorsalis. *Br J Urol* 1990; 65: 497–499

77. Chancellor MB, Blaivas JG. Infectious neurologic diseases. *Practical Neurourology – Genitourinary Complications in Neurologic Disease.* Boston: Butterworth–Heinemann, 1995; 179–185

78. Lange DJ, Britton CB, Younger DS, Hays AP. The neuromuscular manifestations of human immunodeficiency infections. *Arch Neurol* 1988; 45: 1084–1088

79. Levy RM, Bredesen DE, Rosenblum ML. Neurological manifestations of acquired immunodeficiency syndrome: experiences at UCSF and review of the literature. *J Neurosurg* 1985; 62: 475–495

80. Snider WD, Simpson DM, Aronyk KE. Primary lymphoma of the nervous system associated with acquired immunodeficiency syndrome (letter). *New Engl J Med* 1983; 308: 45

81. Levy RM, Pons VG, Rosenblum ML. Intracerebral-mass lesions in the acquired immunodeficiency syndrome (AIDS) (letter). *New Engl J Med* 1983; 309: 1454

82. Levy RM, Pons VG, Rosenblum ML. Central nervous system mass lesions in the acquired immunodeficiency syndrome (AIDS). *J Neurosurg* 1984; 61: 9–16

83. Khan Z, Singh VK, Yang WE. Neurogenic bladder in AIDS. *Urology* 1992; 40: 289–291

84. Hermieu JF, Delmas V, Boccon-Gibod L. Micturition disturbances and human immunodeficiency virus infection. *J Urol* 1996; 156: 157–159

85. Cruickshank JK, Rudge P, Dalgleish AG. Tropical spastic paraparesis and human T-cell lymphotrophic virus type 1 in the United Kingdom. *Brain* 1989; 112: 1057–1090

86. Montgomery RD, Cruickshank JK , Robertson WB. Clinical and pathological observations on Jamaican neuropathy. A report of 206 cases. *Brain* 1964; 87: 425–440

87. Eardley I, Fowler CJ, Nagendran K *et al.* The neurourology of tropical spastic paraparesis. *Br J Urol* 1991; 68: 598–603

88. Dunne K, Hopkins IJ, Shield LK. Acute transverse myelopathy in childhood. *Dev Med Child Neurol* 1986; 28: 198–204

89. Lipton HL, Teasdall RD. Acute transverse myelopathy in adults. *Arch Neurol* 1973; 28: 252–257

90. Adams RD, Victor M. *Principles of Neurology,* 3rd edn. New York: McGraw–Hill, 1985; 673–702

91. Ropper AH, Poskanzer DC. The prognosis of acute and subacute transverse myelopathy based on early signs and symptoms. *Ann Neurol* 1978; 4: 51–59

92. Logigian EL, Kaplan RF, Steere AC. Chronic neurologic manifestations of Lyme disease. *New Engl J Med* 1990; 323: 1438–1444

93. Chancellor MB, Dato VM, Yang J. Lyme disease presenting as urinary retention. *J Urol* 1990; 143: 1223–1224

94. Chancellor MB, McGinnis D, Shenot PJ *et al.* Urinary dysfunction in Lyme disease. *J Urol* 1993; 149: 26–30

95. Steere AC, Green J, Schoen RT *et al.* Successful penicillin therapy of Lyme arthritis. *New Engl J Med* 1985; 312: 869–874

96. Rahn DW, Malawista SE. Lyme disease: recommendations for diagnosis and treatment. *Ann Int Med* 1991; 114: 472–481

97. Weller TH. Varicella and herpes zoster: a perspective and overview. *J Infect Dis* 1992; 166(Suppl 1): S1–6

98. Thomas JE, Howard FM. Segmental zoster paresis – a disease profile. *Neurology* 1972; 22: 459–466

99. Izumi AK, Dewards J Jr. Herpes zoster and neurogenic bladder dysfunction. *J Am Med Assoc* 1973; 224: 1748–1749

100. Straus SE, Ostrove JM, Inchauspe G. Varicella zoster virus infections. Biology, natural history, treatment, and prevention. *Ann Int Med* 1988; 109: 438–439

101. Rosenfeld T, Price MA. Paralysis in herpes zoster *Aust N Z J Med* 1985; 15: 712–716

102. Hodes R. Selective destruction of large motor-neurons by poliomyelitis virus: I. Conduction velocity of motor nerve fibers of chronic poliomyelitis. *J Neurophysiol* 1949; 12: 257

103. So YT, Olney RK. AAEM case report #23: acute paralytic poliomyelitis. *Muscle Nerve* 1991; 14: 1159–1164

104. Pang D, Wilberger JE Jr. Tethered cord syndrome in adults. *J Neurosurg* 1982; 57: 32–47

105. Barson AJ. The vertebral level of termination of the spinal cord during normal and abnormal development. *J Anat* 1969; 106: 489–497

106. Al-Mefty O, Kandzari S, Fox JL. Neurogenic bladder and the tethered spinal cord syndrome. *J Urol* 1979; 179: 112–115

107. Kondo A, Kato K, Kanai S, Sakakibara T. Bladder dysfunction secondary to tethered cord syndrome in adults: is it curable? *J Urol* 1986; 135: 313–316

108. Adamson AS, Gelister J, Hayward R, Snell ME. Tethered cord syndrome: an unusual case of adult bladder dysfunction. *Br J Urol* 1993; 71: 417–421

109. Kondo A, Kato K, Sakakibar T *et al.* Tethered cord syndrome: cause for urge incontinence and pain in lower extremities. *Urology* 1992; 40: 143–146

110. Hellstrom WJG, Edwards MSB, Kogan BA. Urological aspects of the tethered cord syndrome. *J Urol* 1986; 135: 317–320

111. Fukui J, Kaizaki T. Urodynamic evaluation of tethered cord syndrome including tight filum terminale. *Urology* 1980; 16: 539–552

112. Blaivas JG, Chancellor MB. Cauda equina and pelvic plexus injury. *Practical Neurourology – Genitourinary Complications in Neurologic Disease.* Boston: Butterworth–Heinemann, 1995; 155–163

113. Marshal VF, Pollack RS, Miller C. Observations on urinary dysfunction after excision of the rectum. *J Urol* 1946; 55: 409–421

114. Fowler JW, Bremner DN, Moffat LEF. The incidence and consequences of damage to the parasympathetic nerve supply to the bladder after abdominoperineal resection of the rectum for carcinoma. *Br J Urol* 1978; 50: 95–98

115. Mundy AR. An anatomical explanation for bladder dysfunction following rectal and uterine surgery. *Br J Urol* 1982; 54: 501–504

116. Blaivas JG, Barbalias GA. Characteristics of neural injury after abdominoperineal resection. *J Urol* 1983; 129: 84–87

117. McGuire EJ. Urodynamic evaluation after abdominal–perineal resection and lumbar intervertebral disc herniation. *Urology* 1975; 6: 63–70

118. Tempkin A, Sullivan G, Paldi J, Perkash I. Radioisotope renography in spinal cord injury. *J Urol* 1985; 133: 228–230

119. Foster DW. Diabetes mellitus. In: Wilson JD, Braunwald EB, Isselbacher kJ *et al.* (eds) *Harrison's Principles of Internal Medicine.* New York: McGraw–Hill, 1991; 1739–1753

120. Chancellor MB, Blaivas JG. Diabetic neurogenic bladder. *Practical Neurourology – Genitourinary Complications in Neurologic Disease.* Boston: Butterworth–Heinemann, 1995; 149–154

121. Frimodt-Moller C, Hald T. A new method for quantitative evaluation of bladder sensibility. *Scand J Urol Nephrol* 1972; 15: 134–135

122. Faerman I. Autonomic nervous system and diabetes: histological and histochemical study of the autonomic nerve fibers of the urinary bladder in diabetic patients. *Diabetes* 1973; 22: 225–237

123. Thomas PK, Lascelles RG. The pathology of diabetic neuropathy. *Q J Med* 1978; 35: 449–457

124. Clark CMJ, Lee DA. Prevention and treatment of the complications of diabetes mellitus. *N Engl J Med* 1995; 332: 1210–1217

125. Appel RA, Whiteside HV. Diabetes and other peripheral neuropathies affecting lower urinary tract function. In: Krane RJ, Siroky MB (eds) *Clinical Neurourology* 2nd edn. Boston: Little, Brown, 1991; 365–373

126. Ueda T, Yoshimura N, Yoshida O. Diabetic cystopathy: relationship to autonomic neuropathy detected by sympathetic skin responses. *J Urol* 1997; 157: 580–584

127. Kaplan SA, Te AE, Blaivas JG. Urodynamic findings in patients with diabetic cystopathy. *J Urol* 1995; 153: 342–343

66

Non-neurogenic voiding difficulties and retention

A. K. Monga

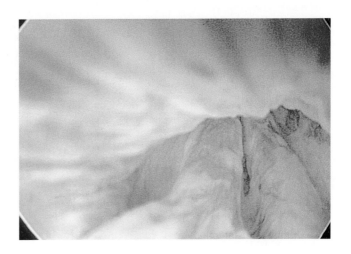

INTRODUCTION

Normal voiding occurs when a bladder contraction is initiated and the bladder neck and the urethra are synchronously relaxed. Depending on the relationship between the force of detrusor contraction and the residual urethral resistance, the intravesical pressure may rise to a variable extent. When the falling urethral pressure and increasing intravesical pressure equate, urine flow will commence. The act of micturition is governed by a number of contributory factors: control from higher centres, the sacral reflex arc, the innervation of the bladder muscle and sphincter mechanisms, the outflow resistance and the speed of contraction of the detrusor muscle fibres. Abnormalities of any component of this interactive mechanism may result in voiding dysfunction.

Voiding difficulties and retention represent a gradation of failure of bladder emptying. In the woman, these disorders are poorly documented mainly because they are frequently misdiagnosed until symptoms such as recurrent urinary tract infections or incontinence prevail. Since the conditions rarely progress to upper tract dilatation and renal failure, they are not associated with mortality, but it's morbidity is significant. The disorders are a spectrum, ranging from an asymptomatic condition diagnosed by ultrasonography or urodynamic studies to acute or chronic retention.

DEFINITIONS AND CLASSIFICATION

The absence of clear definitions presents further difficulty in attempting to classify and clarify these disorders. The standardization of terminology of lower urinary tract dysfunction, published by the International Continence Society,[1] does not provide a classification. Table 66.1 summarizes a working classification.

Acute retention

Acute retention is the sudden onset of painful or painless inability to void over 12 hours, requiring catheterization with removal of a volume equal to or greater than normal bladder capacity. Acute retention is usually painful but may be painless in the presence of a neurological lesion or following an epidural anaesthetic. It seems reasonable

Table 66.1. *Classification of voiding difficulty and retention*

Condition	Symptom	Urodynamic data
Asymptomatic voiding difficulty	Frequency UTI	Reduced flow Elevated, normal or reduced voiding pressure With or without residual urine
Symptomatic voiding difficulty	Poor stream Incomplete emptying Straining Frequency UTI	Peak flow < 15 ml/s Elevated voiding pressure With or without residual urine
Acute retention	Painful or painless	Residual urine
Chronic retention	Reduced sensation Poor stream Incomplete emptying Straining Frequency Nocturia Incontinence UTI	Flow < 15 ml/s Low or elevated voiding pressure Residual urine With or without upper tract dilatation
Acute or chronic retention	Painful or painless Frequency Incontinence	Residual urine With or without low voiding pressure

UTI, urinary tract infection.

to set a time limit and to state the requirement for catheterization to confirm the diagnosis. The volume should be at least equal to normal bladder capacity to avoid the misdiagnosis of acute retention.

Chronic retention

Chronic retention describes the insidious and painless failure of bladder emptying where catheterization yields a volume equal to at least 50% of normal bladder capacity. Shah *et al.* suggested that normal bladders do not retain residual urine;[2] however, it seems reasonable to suggest 50% of normal capacity as a working definition. Chronic retention may cause urinary incontinence and occur without obvious cause.

There are usually two phases through which women pass before developing acute or chronic urinary retention. The first is asymptomatic voiding difficulty where the woman is unaware of impaired bladder emptying. The urinary stream is reduced, and the peak flow rate is less than 15 ml/s. The maximum voiding pressure is usually normal, although it may be raised in the presence of urethral obstruction, and there is no residual urine. The second stage is that of bladder decompensation when symptoms of voiding difficulty appear such as hesitancy, poor stream, straining to void and incomplete emptying, with or without urinary tract infection. The peak flow is less than 15 ml/s, the voiding pressure is reduced and there is residual urine.

There is a paucity of data on the incidence or prevalence of voiding disorders in the absence of neuropathy. Of 600 women with symptoms of bladder dysfunction attending a urodynamic clinic, 2% had asymptomatic and 14% had symptomatic voiding difficulty. The symptomatic group tended to be older and were more likely to have had previous pelvic surgery.[3] Dwyer and Desmedt[4] examined the clinical and urodynamic findings of 1193 consecutive women referred for investigation of symptoms of lower urinary tract dysfunction: 165 women had voiding difficulties, one-third of whom were asymptomatic.

AETIOLOGY AND PATHOPHYSIOLOGY

In the female, voiding can occur via one of three mechanisms: contraction of the detrusor muscle, a rise in abdominal pressure, and relaxation of the urethral sphincter and pelvic floor musculature. Therefore,

voiding disorders result when these mechanisms fail, that is when the detrusor muscle is unable to maintain an effective contraction, the urethra fails to relax and lower urethral resistance, or if there is a failure in the synchronization of these two actions, resulting in detrusor sphincter dyssynergia. The latter occurs in suprasacral neurological lesions; neurogenic voiding dysfunction is discussed in chapter 65. Table 66.2 lists the causes of voiding difficulty.

Pharmacological causes

Obstetric epidural anaesthesia is the most frequent pharmacological cause of voiding dysfunction. If retention is overlooked, overdistension injury may result in long-term voiding difficulty.[5] Drugs that interfere with the release and action of acetylcholine at cholinergic synapses or neuromuscular junctions result in voiding difficulty, especially when mild impairment is already present. Anticholinergic agents used to treat urgency and frequency are frequent causes, for example tolterodine, oxybutynin, probanthine and imipramine. It is therefore vital to exclude urinary residual before prescribing this class of agent. In women with a combination of poor voiding and detrusor instability these drugs may be used in conjunction with intermittent selfcatheterization. Ganglion-blocking drugs have a similar effect to anticholinergics, and α-adrenergic agents increase urethral resistance.

Inflammatory causes

Any painful vulvovaginal lesion may result in disturbance of normal micturition. The most frequent causes of inflammation are infective, chemical or allergic (local or systemic allergens). Voiding difficulties may result from painful stimuli produced by urine coming into contact with the inflamed mucosa of either the urethra or vagina. This may be aggravated by urethral oedema. Primary anogenital herpetic infection may produce urinary retention by both the effect of local inflammatory lesions and lumbosacral meningomyelitis affecting the central nervous system.[6,7]

Obstructive causes

Urethral stenosis is rare in the female. Distal urethral stenosis usually results from urogenital atrophy in the

Table 66.2. *Non-neurogenic causes of voiding difficulty and retention*

Pharmacological
- Anticholinergic agents
- α-Adrenergic agents
- Epidural and spinal anaesthesia
- Ganglion-blocking agents
- Tricyclic antidepressants

Acute inflammation
- Acute urethritis (infective and chemical)
- Acute cystitis
- Acute vulvovaginitis (e.g. herpes)
- Acute anogenital infection
- Acute allergy

Obstruction
- Distal urethral stenosis
- Post-surgical urethral oedema
- Chronic urethral fibrosis
- Foreign body, calculus
- Post-stress incontinence surgery (e.g. sling)
- Allergic response to collagen injection
- Prolapse causing urethral distortion:
    Cystocele
    Vault prolapse
    Uterovaginal prolapse
    Rectocele
- Impacted pelvic mass:
    Haematocolpos
    Retroverted gravid uterus
    Uterine fibroid
    Ovarian cyst
    Faecal impaction
- Ectopic ureterocele

Endocrine
- Hypothyroidism
- Diabetic neuropathy

Overdistension
- Most common post-surgically or after epidural anaesthesia

Post-surgical
- Stress-incontinence surgery
- Pelvic surgery (especially radical)
- Anorectal surgery
- Other surgery (e.g. orthopaedic procedures)

Others
- Psychogenic
- Urethral sphincter hypertrophy
- Detrusor myopathy
- Iatrogenic

post-menopausal woman but can result from chronic fibrosis following chronic inflammation, urethral instrumentation (e.g. urethrotomy) and scarring following surgery (e.g. anterior colporrhaphy). This condition is detected during urethral catheterization or cystourethroscopy. Acute urethral oedema may occur after bladder-neck surgery or, rarely, secondary to premenstrual fluid retention. Foreign bodies and calculi are rare causes of obstruction in women. Bladder-neck surgery (e.g. sling procedures) may cause compression, and obstruction due a late allergy reaction to collagen injections has been reported (unpublished data).

Extrinsic causes of obstruction include impaction of a retroverted gravid uterus, particularly in association with a posterior uterine wall fibroid.[8] Pelvic masses, for example uterine fibroids and ovarian cysts, and faecal impaction can also cause urethral compression. Haematocolpos associated with cryptomenorrhoea may present with retention due to urethral obstruction.

Urethral distortion due to genital prolapse occurs more frequently than previously believed. Chaikin *et al.*[9] investigated 84 women with genital prolapse: 2% of women with grades 1 and 2, and 33% of women with grades 3 and 4 prolapse had evidence of urethral obstruction.

Finally ectopic ureterocele is a cause of urethral obstruction in children.

Endocrine causes

Hypothyroidism and diabetes mellitus can cause peripheral neuropathy, resulting in urinary retention as a consequence of bladder atony.

Overdistension

Bladder overdistension as a result of mismanagement of acute or chronic retention develops insidiously and is more frequent in women than in men. It often results after failure to detect retention after pelvic surgery (e.g. hysterectomy) or epidural anaesthesia. Overdistension may occur without obvious cause and is frequently observed in elderly women with large acontractile bladders.

Overdistension beyond normal bladder capacity leads to ischaemic damage to the detrusor muscle. The prime affected site is the basal urothelium.[10] Continued ischaemia leads to a proliferative vascular response, laying down of new collagen and irreversible damage.

Urethral sphincter hypertrophy

Fowler and Kirby have described a group of women who present with voiding difficulties due to a primary defect within the striated urethral sphincter.[11] The muscle is hypertrophied and fails to relax, and characteristic electromyographic patterns are observed with complex repetitive discharges and decelerating bursts. There appears to be an association with polycystic ovarian syndrome.

Detrusor myopathy

Primary changes in the detrusor muscle have been reported as a cause of retention. Lipid inclusion bodies are observed within the muscle cells.[12]

Psychogenic causes

Psychogenic causes of urinary retention are well documented.[13,14] Criteria for this diagnosis are an absence of neurological and or other significant organic disease, correlation of psychological disturbance with onset of symptoms, and a response to psychotherapy or psychopharmacological agents. This diagnosis should be made only after careful evaluation and exclusion of other causes, because of the social stigma attached to such disturbance. Psychiatric diagnoses include hysteria and depression.

PRESENTATION

Symptoms

Impaired voiding may be asymptomatic in a few patients but the majority present with infrequent voiding, poor flow, intermittent stream, incomplete emptying, straining to void and/or hesitancy. Others may present with overflow incontinence and frequency or urinary tract infection due to stasis. Hilton and Laor[15] compared presenting symptoms with urodynamic evidence of voiding difficulty and found that the symptom of poor or intermittent stream correlated best with diagnosis. Acute retention may present with pain.

History taking should be directed towards determination of a primary cause. Neuropathy should be enquired about and a detailed drug, medical and surgical history, including genital and urinary tract infection, should be obtained. Continence surgery is well recognized as a causative factor.

Signs

A careful general abdominal and pelvic examination should be performed to exclude the causes listed in Table 66.2. A neurological examination should be performed and the lumbar region examined for stigmata of an underlying spinal disorder. Abdominal and pelvic examination should be performed after bladder emptying and masses noted (e.g. ovarian cyst, fibroids etc.). The bladder may be palpable and will characteristically be dull to percussion.

Any urethral or vulvovaginal inflammation is noted and the urethra is palpated for tenderness and scarring. Infected urethral diverticulum or vaginal cysts are excluded and any genital prolapse demonstrated. Finally the patient's general demeanour should be carefully monitored to detect any signs of psychiatric disorder.

INVESTIGATIONS

Urinary tract infection should be excluded as it may predispose to voiding difficulty. The simplest investigations are uroflowmetry and ultrasonography for residual, but cystometry and other investigations may required to make a more accurate diagnosis.

Frequency volume chart

An accurate record of fluid intake and output is important and can usually be maintained by the patient. Infrequent voiding should be discouraged as it may lead to long-term voiding difficulty. When catheterization is performed for acute retention the residual volume should be recorded. This will confirm the diagnosis and give a guide to the severity of bladder overdistension, and may be useful in assessing prognosis.

Uroflowmetry

Uroflowmetry is the most important initial screening procedure and is simple and non-invasive. The measurement should be made in privacy and the patient should attend with a comfortably full bladder. At maximum capacity the flow rate may be lower than the norm for an individual. Measurements may need to be repeated as a single measurement may be unreliable. Flow rates consistently below 15 ml/s for a volume of greater than 150 ml indicate impaired voiding and this may be a precusor of retention. A normal flow pattern is shown in Figure 66.1. Obstructed voiding may occur in the presence of normal uroflowmetry because the detrusor may compensate by increasing the voiding pressure. Subtracted cystometry is required to detect this.

Cystometry

The filling phase of cystometry may indicate a lower or upper motor neuron lesion. The voiding phase will confirm any disorder of bladder emptying. The following changes may be observed in cases of voiding difficulty and retention (changes found in association with neuropathy are discussed elsewhere):

- difficulty catheterizing in presence of obstruction;
- residual urine greater than 50 ml;
- delayed first sensation (early first sensation in upper motor neuron lesions);
- increased bladder capacity;
- pressure rise during filling and compliance usually normal;
- maximum voiding pressure will be raised in the presence of obstruction prior to decompensation (it

will be low or non-existent when detrusor failure occurs);
- isometric pressure is usually reduced or non-existent, demonstrating poor detrusor reserve.

The residual urine volume is a good indicator of bladder efficiency after a patient voids normally in privacy. While absence of residual urine does not exclude voiding dysfunction, the presence of residual urine greater than 50 ml is not normal. The interpretation and management will depend on the clinical situation and other urodynamic data. An isolated residual urine is not usually clinically significant.

Pressure measurement during uroflowmetry allows detection of a poorly contractile bladder and will also demonstrate voiding by straining. Figure 66.2 shows a normal void with normal voiding pressure, flow rate and isometric detrusor pressure. Figure 66.3 shows a prolonged void with a poor maximum voiding pressure. Figure 66.4 shows complete absence of any detrusor voiding pressure, with voiding accomplished by straining.

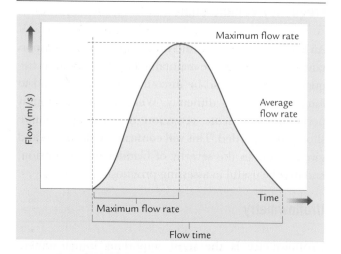

Figure 66.1. *Uroflowmetry: a normal flow pattern.*

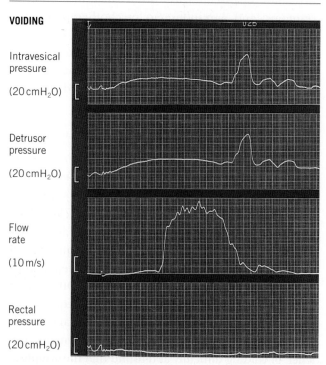

Figure 66.2. *Normal voiding with normal voiding pressure, flow rate and isometric detrusor pressure.*

VOIDING

Intravesical
pressure
(20 cmH₂O)

Detrusor
pressure
(20 cmH₂O)

Flow
rate
(10 m/s)

Rectal
pressure
(20 cmH₂O)

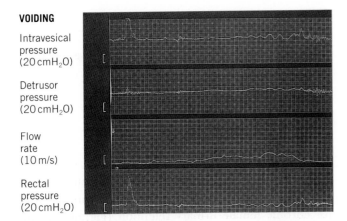

Figure 66.3. *Prolonged void with poor maximum voiding pressure.*

VOIDING

Intravesical
pressure
(20 cmH₂O)

Detrusor
pressure
(20 cmH₂O)

Flow
rate
(10 m/s)

Rectal
pressure
(20 cmH₂O)

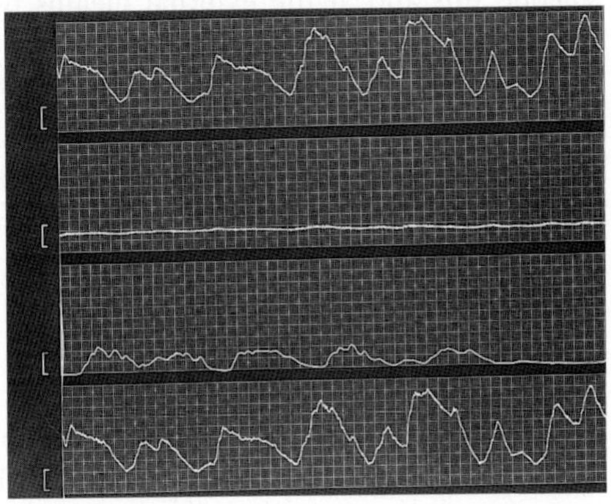

Figure 66.4. *Complete absence of any detrusor voiding pressure; voiding is accomplished by straining.*

Radiology

A plain abdominal radiograph will disclose a full bladder, and lumbosacral film will demonstrate congenital conditions such as spina bifida occulta or acquired conditions such as intervertebral disc prolapse. Video-cystourethrography can provide additional information at the time of cystometry. Trabeculation diverticula and ureteric reflux can be detected and distal urethral stenosis identified.

Ultrasonography

Abdominal ultrasonography allows non-invasive measurement of urinary residual and also assessment of the upper urinary tract.

Cystourethroscopy

Difficulty in instrumentation of the urethra will suggest stenosis. Cystoscopy will allow visualization of intravesical pathology such as trabeculation, sacculation and diverticula.

Electromyography

Single or concentric needle electromyography can be used to demonstrate the characteristic decelerating bursts and complex repetitive discharges due to ephaptic transmission seen in Fowler's syndrome associated with urethral sphincter hypertrophy and retention.

Electromyography will also allow diagnosis of multiple system atrophy with signs suggestive of denervation injury, including prolonged, high amplitude polyphasic action potentials.

TREATMENT

Prophylaxis

Prevention or early recognition of retention may avoid long-term voiding difficulty. Difficulty in resumption of spontaneous voiding occurs in over 45% of patients after radical pelvic surgery for gynaecological malignancy,[16,17] in 60% of women undergoing continence surgery (e.g. colposuspension or sling procedures), and also after epidural anaesthesia. This indicates a pre-emptive need to drain the bladder after these procedures.

If a catheter is intended to be placed for a short period then a urethral catheter will suffice, for example after epidural anaesthesia. Where longer term problems may ensue (e.g. after continence surgery) a suprapubic catheter allows better assessment of voiding and residual volumes and is associated with a lower rate of urinary tract infection. In women with evidence of voiding difficulty prior to continence surgery (e.g. low flow rate and low maximum voiding pressure [less than 15 cmH₂O]) it is reasonable to counsel appropriately and teach intermittent self-catheterization. The case for routine urethral catheterization for 24 hours after all pelvic surgery remains unresolved. Dobbs *et al.*[18] observed a high rate of catheterization after hysterectomy and suggested that catheterization be used pre-emptively.

Intermittent self-catheterization

Intermittent self-catheterization as a non-sterile procedure was first described by Lapides in 1972.[19] Originally used in neurogenic conditions, it is now the principal treatment for chronic urinary retention. It allows women to lead independent lives with efficient bladder emptying and low rates of urinary tract infection. Although patients are often initially hesitant at the idea of such a technique, if properly counselled by trained professional staff, most will easily master the technique and appreciate the consequent improvement in quality of life.

There are two forms of intermittent self-catheterization: sterile and clean. The former is usually reserved for patients with neuropathic bladders in a hospital environment to prevent cross infection.

Clean intermittent self-catheterization (CISC)

This technique is usually performed by the patient but can be performed by a carer or relative. The technique is designed for everyday use. The patient has to be reasonably dextrous and is taught using a clean technique and mirror: the patient lies down initially, and inserts a fine-bore catheter. When proficient with the mirror, she is taught to insert the catheter by feel in the sitting or standing position. Disposable catheters are available but reusable ones do not pose a significant risk of infection. A salt coating allows easier insertion with less urethral friction. The frequency of catheterization varies, with the aim being to avoid incontinence and filling beyond normal bladder capacity. The procedure has good long-term results.[20]

Pharmacotherapy

Cholinergic agents (e.g. bethanechol chloride) distigmine bromide (an anticholinesterase) and prostaglandins have been advocated but there is no real evidence that they are of any clinical benefit. Alpha-adrenergic blocking agents (e.g. phenoxybenzamine) have no proven benefit in women. Diazepam used as an anxiolytic may help with postoperative voiding problems.[21]

In women with combined urge incontinence and retention, anticholinergic agents such as tolterodine may be used effectively in conjunction with CISC.

Surgery

If voiding difficulty is due to urethral stenosis, urethral dilatation using Hegar dilators or the Otis urethrotome are appropriate options.

Alternatives

Turbine valve

Monga *et al.*[22] described a new replaceable intraurethral sphincter prosthesis with a self-contained urinary pump for chronic female urinary retention (Fig. 66.5). The prosthesis consists of a valve and pump mounted inside a tube-shaped, catheter-like, soft polycarbonate casing. It is secured at the bladder neck by soft expandable silicone fins and at the external meatus by a flexible flange. Activation is achieved by turning on a small battery-operated remote-control unit placed over the lower abdomen: the valve opens and the pump actively draws urine from the bladder and the patient 'voids'. At the end of urination the valve closes, restoring continence. Early results have been encouraging and larger trial have confirmed this.[23]

Neuromodulation

This two-stage procedure involves stimulation of the S3 nerve root through the S3 foramen. The first stage is that of percutaneous nerve evaluation using a temporary stimulation wire. If this has a beneficial effect then a permanent stimulator is implanted. Early results are encouraging, especially in patients with Fowler's

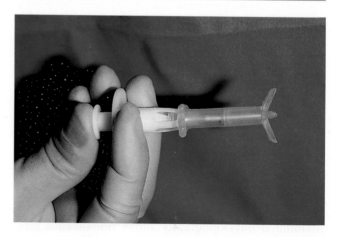

Figure 66.5. *Self-contained urinary pump for chronic female urinary retention.*

syndrome (unpublished findings) but the mechanism of action is not understood.

CONCLUSIONS

Voiding difficulties in women are poorly understood. Prompt treatment of acute retention and pre-emptive management to avoid overdistension are essential. CISC remains the most effective therapy for chronic retention although newer modalities are being investigated. The role of pharmacological agents and surgery in women is limited.

REFERENCES

1. Abrams P, Blaivas G, Stanton SL *et al.* Standardisation of terminology of lower urinary tract function. *Scand J Urol Nephrol Suppl* 1988; 114: 5–19

2. Shah PJR, Whiteside CG, Milroy EJG, Turner-Warwick R. Radiological assessment of the male bladder—a clinical and urodynamic assessment. *Br J Urol* 1980; 53: 567–570

3. Stanton SL, Ozsoy C, Hilton P. Voiding difficulties in the female: prevalence, clinical and urodynamic review. *Obstet Gynecol* 1983; 61: 144–147

4. Dwyer PL, Desmedt E. Impaired bladder emptying in women. *Aust N Z J Ostet Gynaecol* 1994; 34: 73–78

5. Jackson SR, Barry C, Davies G *et al.* Length of labour and epidural anaesthesia: long term effects on urinary symptoms. *Int Urogynecol J* 1995; 6: 244

6. Oates J, Greenhouse PR. Retention of urine in ano-genital herpetic infection. *Lancet* 1978; 1: 691–692

7. Hemrika DJ, Schutte MF, Bleker OP. Elsberg syndrome: a neurologic basis for acute urinary retention in patients with genital herpes. *Obstet Gynecol* 1986; 68: 37S–39S

8. Monga AK, Woodhouse C, Stanton SL. A case of simultaneous urethral and ureteric obstruction. *Br J Urol* 1995; 77: 606–607

9. Chaikin DC, Romanzi L, Rosenthal J *et al.* The effects of genital prolapse on micturition. *Neurourol Urodyn* 1998; 17: 426–427

10. Tong YC, Monson FC, Erika B, Levin RM. Effects of acute in vitro overdistension of the rabbit urinary bladder on DNA synthesis. *J Urol* 1992; 148: 1347–1350

11. Fowler CJ, Kirby RS. Abnormal electromyographic activity (decelerating burst and complex repetitive discharges) in the striated urethral sphincter in 5 women with urinary retention. *Br J Urol* 1985; 57: 67–70

12. Martin JE, Sobeh M, Swash C *et al.* Detrusor myopathy: a cause of detrusor weakness with retention. *Br J Urol* 1993; 71: 235–236

13. Barrett DM. Evaluation of psychogenic urinary retention. *J Urol* 1978; 120: 191–192

14. Krane R, Siroky M. Psychogenic voiding dysfunction. *Clinical Neuro-urology* Boston: Little, Brown & Co., 1978

15. Hilton P, Laor D. Voiding symptoms in the female: the correlation with urodynamic voiding characteristics. *Neurourol Urodyn* 1989; 8: 308–310

16. Fraser AC. The late effects of Wertheims hysterectomy on the urinary tract. *Br J Obstet Gynaecol* 1966; 73: 1002–1007

17. Smith PH, Turnbull GA, Currie DW, Peel KR. The urological complications of Wertheims hysterectomy. *Br J Urol* 1969; 41: 685–688

18. Dobbs SP, Jackson SR, Wilson AM *et al.* A prospective randomised trial comparing continuous bladder drainage with catheterization at abdominal hysterectomy. *Br J Urol* 1997; 80: 554–556

19. Lapides J, Diokno C, Silber SJ, Lowe BS. Clean intermittent self catheterization in the treatment of lower urinary tract disease. *J Urol* 1972; 107: 458–461

20. Wyndaele J, Maes D. Clean intermittent self-catheterization: a 12-year follow up. *J Urol* 1990; 143: 906–908

21. Stanton SL, Cardozo L, Kerr-Wilson R. Treatment of delayed onset of spontaneous voiding after surgery for incontinence. *Urology* 1979; 13: 494–496

22. Monga AK, Madjar S, Stanton SL *et al.* A new intraurethral pump for urinary retention. *Neurourol Urodyn* 1996; 4: 363–364

23. Madjar S, Sabo E, Halachmi S *et al.* Predictors of treatment success of the remote controlled intraurethral insert in women with voiding dysfunction. *Neurourol Urodyn* 1998; 4: 348–349

CONCLUSIONS

Voiding difficulties in women are poorly understood. Prompt assessment of acute retention and prompt management to avoid decompensation are essential. CISC remains the most effective therapy for chronic retention although newer modalities are being investigated. The role of pharmacological agents and surgery in women is limited.

REFERENCES

67

Cystitis and urethritis

K. Boos

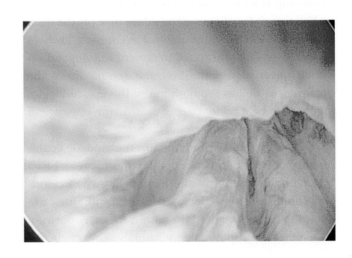

Cystitis

INTRODUCTION

Cystitis is a term used to describe inflammation of the urinary bladder. The inflammatory response arises in a variety of clinical situations and may have an infectious or non-infectious aetiology. Infectious cystitis may be classified as acute, chronic or recurrent infection. It broadly describes the inflammatory response to microbiological invasion of the bladder, encompassing not only the clinical symptoms of urinary frequency, urgency and dysuria but also the cystoscopic and histological appearance of the bladder wall.

Infection is characterized by large numbers of organisms and leucocytes in the urine, with varying significance and severity. The natural history of the disease depends on the type of urinary pathogen, its virulence and resistance to antimicrobial agents, as well as certain host factors and special circumstances. The pathogenesis is often unclear and the clinical course may be complicated or uncomplicated. A variety of specific factors interact between the host and invading organism and will determine the progress of the disease.

Diagnosis is based on the clinical manifestations, microscopic examinations, non-culture techniques and the results of urine culture. It may require the use of certain criteria to make an accurate diagnosis. The interpretation of results is often difficult and may be improved by the application of certain diagnostic criteria and the use of tests of antimicrobial susceptibility. In certain circumstances it may be necessary to carry out tests to localize the infection to the bladder, as opposed to the upper urinary tract, and to investigate the presence of underlying risk factors and secondary complications.

The principles of management are to verify the diagnosis and select the antimicrobial agent most likely to be effective. The efficacy of treatment will depend on the characteristics of the host and the nature of the organism, as well as the duration of therapy. Strategies may have to be modified depending on the presence of a complicated or recurrent infection.

Aside from these considerations, the ultimate goal is primary prevention. The scope for this is limited to a better understanding of the natural history of cystitis and eliminating or reducing the risk factors that are known to be important in the pathogenesis. Population screening of asymptomatic individuals as a strategy for secondary prevention is probably not cost-effective, and screening of at-risk individuals is also controversial. However, the appropriate use of low-dose prophylactic antimicrobial therapy is highly successful.

PREVALENCE

Cystitis in healthy women is a common problem throughout the world. In the USA, the National Center for Health Statistics recorded six million visits a year to general practitioners to manage urinary tract infections (UTIs).[1] Bacterial cystitis is the most frequent bacterial infection occurring in women. It has been estimated that women have at least a 50% chance of developing at least one UTI during their lifetime.[2] Studies have also shown that the prevalence of bacteriuria in schoolgirls is 1–2% – about ten times higher than in boys.[3]

PATHOGENESIS AND NATURAL HISTORY

In recent years our knowledge of the pathogenesis and natural history of cystitis has been enhanced and improved by methods of bacterial diagnosis. A number of epidemiological studies and prospective randomized clinical trials have determined the outcome of infection. Enteric bacteria that ascend into the bladder and establish bacteriuria, often at levels less than 10^5 bacteria per ml, are thought to cause cystitis, and studies support the hypothesis of a faecal–perineal–urethral route of infection. *Escherichia coli* is the main causative agent in all groups. In particular, strains of *E. coli* residing in the rectal flora serve as a reservoir for cystitis.[4]

Normally the urinary tract is sterile above the level of the distal urethra, but organisms do gain access to the bladder. The prevalence of colonization with, and the pathways to acquisition of, uropathogenic *E. coli* in the pathogenesis of cystitis is incompletely defined.[5] Organisms that gain access to the bladder and cause infection tend to do so from neighbouring sites. These sites include the bowel, perineum, vaginal vestibule, urethra and paraurethral tissues.

The most frequent route of infection is the ascending route after entry via the urethral meatus into the bladder. This may be spontaneous along the short female urethra or facilitated by sexual intercourse or catheterization. Transfer of organisms to the urinary tract may also be by way of lymphatics or the organisms may be blood-borne (but this is quite rare).

Kallenius *et al.*[6] proposed an explanation which has evolved as a model for the pathogenesis for infection of the lower urinary tract. Meatal colonization occurs, mediated by fimbriae and specific receptor proteins in the epithelial cells in the region of the external meatus of the urethra. The periurethral area is heavily colonized with bacteria and these ascend the urethra to enter the bladder and adhere to the urothelium.[6,7] Yamamoto *et al.*,[5] using precise genetic techniques to accurately characterize *E. coli* strains, also provided good evidence to support the faecal–perineal–urethral hypothesis, indicating that microorganisms residing in the rectal flora serve as a reservoir for cystitis. These observations have been confirmed in girls where colonization of the vaginal mucosa preceded the occurrence of bacteriuria.[8] In addition to simple carriage, colonization in susceptible women occurs in larger numbers and persists for longer periods.[9]

Other factors must be involved, since it is well known that several bacterial virulence factors occur more frequently among urinary *E. coli* isolates than among faecal isolates.[10] It has been suggested that specific local factors make individuals prone to recurrent cystitis. Possibly due to some permissive factor, pathogenic organisms colonize the vaginal vestibule and periurethral region of some women.[11] Another partial explanation was proposed by Lapides, who suggested that ischaemia of the bladder wall might reduce the resistance to invasion and infection. This may occur when there is increased intravesical pressure and/or overdistension of the bladder.[12]

Exactly how bacteria enter the bladder is uncertain, but it is suggested that bacteria may reflux into the bladder after voiding, or may ascend against the urinary stream during micturition because of turbulent flow, or milk back into the bladder after completion of voiding.[13,14]

A complicated relationship exists in the pathogenesis of cystitis in women as these factors *per se* do not necessarily stimulate infection within the bladder. It has been demonstrated that virulent organisms require some host susceptibility. Schlager *et al.* have found that, by itself, expression of virulence factors by *E. coli* that colonize the periurethra of healthy girls is not enough to predict subsequent cystitis.[15] There appears to be a multifactorial interplay between host factors determining susceptibility and the characteristic ability of the urinary pathogens to invade and colonize the bladder, which combine to allow the establishment and multi-

plication of microorganisms. Bacterial virulence factors, host defence mechanisms and various predisposing factors affect the course and severity of disease.[16]

HOST DEFENCE

The bacteriuria associated with urinary frequency and dysuria may clear spontaneously without antimicrobial therapy. In one study, 40% of women with bacteriuria became free of infection spontaneously within 12 months.[17] In another study, 80% of women with uncomplicated infections who received a placebo attained sterile urine spontaneously. However, almost half of these women subsequently experienced a reinfection within a year.[18]

The bladder possesses a number of mechanisms whereby it resists microbial invasion. One of the most important protective factors is the hydrokinetic or 'washout' effect. Diuresis and voiding tend to dilute the bacterial load and wash away pathogenic organisms. The initiation and persistence of infection in the bladder will depend on the size and rate of growth of the microbiological colony, the residual volume of urine, rate of urine flow and frequency of voiding.

Microbiological factors

The cellular mechanism by which uroepithelial cells of the bladder resist ascending infection is not completely understood. It has been shown, however, that activation of uroepithelial cell defence and suppression of bacterial growth depend on direct contact between the cells and bacteria. This ligand–receptor interaction is independent of the common pili expressed on *E. coli*.[19]

Unfortunately, urine is generally a good culture medium for bacteria, influenced by its pH, osmolality and biochemical content. The osmolality of the bladder urine is constantly fluctuating. A more hostile environment for growth of bacteria includes extremes of pH (<5.5; >7.5), high osmolality and the presence of certain diet-derived weak organic acids. However, bacterial growth is poor in concentrated urine. Urea is the principal antibacterial electrolyte in urine and its effect is modulated by its concentration and the pH.[20]

Another compound, betaine, is present in bladder urine and is osmoprotective. Culham *et al.* have provided evidence that uropathogenic *E. coli* take up betaine, utilizing its osmoprotective effect, thereby facilitating their growth and colonization of the urinary tract.[21]

Bladder epithelium

The intact bladder mucosa has a bactericidal action on organisms present in small residual volumes of urine.[22] However, in general terms, healthy bladder epithelial cells are not phagocytic. If damage occurs and the epithelium is regenerating, the rapidly dividing cells can engulf cells and debris, but it is unlikely that these cells are phagocytic to invading organisms in any great capacity.[23] A role for nitric oxide (NO) in bladder wall inflammation and host defence has been suggested. NO produced locally in the bladder has cytotoxic effects that may be directed against microorganisms. Lundberg *et al.* found that NO levels, measured directly in the bladder, were 30–50 times higher in all varieties of cystitis compared with controls. They concluded that NO might contribute as a host defence mechanism in the bladder during infection and may be a marker of bladder mucosal inflammation.[24]

Natural killer cells also become activated in the inflamed urothelium, with increased cytolytic activity enhancing the immunological defence mechanisms of the bladder.[25] The bladder also produces a surface secretion of mucus to inhibit bacterial adhesions to the mucosal cells, providing an antibacterial barrier to infection.[26]

Hormonal effects

Local oestrogen may contribute to the host defence mechanisms since oestrogen deprivation has an unfavourable effect, increasing susceptibility to cystitis. This may be linked to decreased production of bladder mucus.[27]

It is interesting to note the effect of the menstrual cycle on the normal resident flora of the vagina: the mean concentration of anaerobes is relatively constrained throughout, whereas the mean concentration of aerobes decreases 100 fold in the last week of the cycle.[28]

Humoral factors

Secretory IgA is synthesized by plasma cells in the lamina propria adjacent to the mucous membranes of the bladder and provides some degree of humoral immunity and bactericidal effect. Burdon[29] found that a significant proportion of this secretory IgA originates in the urethra and may have an inhibitory effect on ascending bacteria.

Immunoglobulins

A marked and rapid antibody response is elicited in women with pyelonephritis whereas there is, at most, only a moderate response in cystitis or asymptomatic bacteriuria. However, local production of secretory IgA has been shown to prevent microbial invasion by interfering with bacterial adherence.[30] Secretory IgA and IgG antibodies to bacterial pili are also excreted into bladder urine and can prevent adhesion of *E. coli* to the bladder urothelium.[31] These urinary antibodies may be detected in the absence of circulating IgA antibodies. It has also been shown that production of IgA may be deficient in some women and predispose them to recurrent infections.[32]

Tamm–Horsfall protein

Tamm–Horsfall is a mucoprotein shed from renal tubular cells and excreted in bladder urine. Using electrophoresis Jerkins[33] demonstrated that it could easily be detected in concentrated urine. This uromucoid protein can trap or bind type I fimbriated *E. coli* in bladder urine, providing a natural defence mechanism.[34,35] Levels of antibodies (IgG) to this protein are significantly higher in patients with acute pyelonephritis and those with vesicoureteric reflux (VUR) than in healthy patients. Less is known about the response in acute cystitis without upper tract infection.[36,37]

Major histocompatibility complex and red blood cell antigens

Hopkins *et al.*[38] performed a comparative study of major histocompatibility complex and red blood cell antigen phenotypes to determine if host characteristics were significant risk factors in the development of recurrent infection. They found that the overall risk for women to develop recurrent UTIs did not appear to be associated with any single HLA, ABO or Lewis phenotype.[38]

ROLE OF THE ORGANISM

Microbes are pathogenic by virtue of their ability to survive and multiply in bladder urine and adhere to the mucosal surfaces. Some unique qualities also make them particularly virulent to the lower urinary tract. Each virulence factor has a role in the causation of UTI and the presence of additional virulence factors acts in an additive or synergistic fashion, enhancing the impact of the uropathogens.[39]

Adherence

The ability of microorganisms to adhere to uroepithelial cells of the bladder wall is an important initial step in the pathogenesis and progression of cystitis. In studies of introital colonization in women with recurrent UTIs, vaginal and periurethral cells showed greater ability to bind bacteria and allow adherence than did cells from healthy subjects.[40] This has also been investigated by Kozody *et al.*,[41] who found evidence of increased receptivity of uroepithelial cells for bacteria and increased frequency of vaginal colonization and subsequent infection in women with recurrent UTIs.

Bacterial adhesins bind their ligands with a high degree of specificity and this interaction triggers transmembrane events that cause cell activation, followed by an acute inflammatory response.[42] Adherence of the organism stimulates the inflammatory response by activation of cytokines. These are hormone-like chemical messengers that mediate the immune response. Cytokines stimulate the production of intercellular adhesion molecule, which, by leucocyte adhesion, causes migration of these cells to the site of infection.[43] The attached microbes can then avoid 'washout' and the attached state enhances their ability to trap nutrients and allows more efficient multiplication.

Antigenic structure and fimbriae

A variety of host-specific factors such as glycosphingolipids on the surface of cells in the bladder also determine the virulence of pathogenic organisms and the natural history of cystitis. Enterobacteriaceae have an antigenic structure which tends to induce an antibody immune response. This antigenic structure partly contributes to the invasiveness and virulence of these bacteria.

The outer membrane of the cell wall contains complex polysaccharide polymers termed O antigens. The bacteria also contain cell wall lipopolysaccharide or endotoxin. Both endotoxin and O antigens initiate the inflammatory response in the host by inducing macrophages to produce increased amounts of cytokines.[44] Capsular or K antigens on the surface of the bacteria help it to inhibit phagocytosis and resist IgA and IgG in the urothelium.

Pili and fimbriae on uropathogenic bacteria are structures that project from their outer membrane and contain, on their distal tip, an adhesion protein. This is responsible for the binding of the bacterium to the surface of epithelial cells lining the bladder. P-fimbriae and specific receptors for their protein in the epithelial cells of the bladder mediate adherence of bacteria to urothelium.[45] Type I fimbriae confer the ability for bacteria to adhere to mucus while P-fimbriae adhere to glycolipids on uroepithelial cells. Type I piliated strains of *E. coli* are more abundant and more often recovered in women with acute cystitis.

Bullitt and Makowski[46] have used electromicroscopy to distinguish morphologically different states of pili rods and to show that, despite similar architecture, they have specific differences designed to optimize their virulence. Blanco *et al.*[47] examined the relationship between the presence of bacterial virulence factors and the severity of UTIs. They found that *E. coli* strains causing pyelonephritis showed virulence factors more frequently than those causing cystitis or asymptomatic bacteriuria. Nevertheless, many cases of serious cystitis may be caused by a limited number of P-fimbriated *E. coli* strains that usually produce alpha-haemolysin.[47]

The characteristics and virulence-associated factors of *E. coli* in acute community-acquired cystitis in adult women have been studied and compared with strains isolated from stools of healthy women. The prevalence of virulence-associated factors for UTIs was significantly higher in cystitis isolates. The presence of P-fimbriae, type IC fimbriae and haemolysin production all contribute to the establishment of cystitis in adults.[48] Funfstruck *et al.*[49] suggested that other properties such as serum resistance, iron sequestration, hydroxamate production and the presence of K-antigen are found in strains that persist in the host without initiating clinical symptoms.

Another factor involved in the virulence of uropathogens is the ability of some organisms to break down bladder mucin and invade the endothelium beneath. This may also make the host susceptible to recurrent infections.[50]

IRON BUILDING AND HAEMOLYSIN

Microorganisms take up iron from their surroundings for survival. There is convincing evidence that the ability to acquire iron from the host is a critical determinant of the host–parasite relationship and is linked to virulence.[51] Haemolysins are produced by some strains of *E. coli* which are isolated more frequently from women with acute cystitis. These are cytolytic proteins but their function *in vivo* remains unclear. It seems that they break down erythrocytes, release haemoglobin and enhance the availability of iron. This may provide the organism with more iron, which then increases its virulence.[52] In women with cystitis the inflammatory response is associated with haemolysin production. Connell *et al.*[53] analysed the inflammatory response in patients with UTI and found no significant increase in the severity of inflammation caused by haemolytic-positive compared with haemolytic-negative *E. coli*. In contrast, the potential of uropathogenic *E. coli* to cause severe inflammation was better described by the presence or absence of P-fimbriae than by haemolysin.[53]

Microorganisms can also produce aerobactin, an iron-chelating compound (siderophore) which competes for excess iron. The ability to synthesize aerobactin is associated with increased virulence.[54]

Hull *et al.*[55] demonstrated that bacteria from patients with symptomatic UTI are more likely to be haemolytic than isolates from patients with asymptomatic bacteriuria ($p = 0.05$) or faecal isolates from healthy volunteers.

CLASSIFICATION

In 1975 Stamey proposed a clinical classification of UTIs into five groups:[56]

- First infection;
- Unresolved infections;
- Bacterial persistence;
- Reinfections;
- Recurrent UTI.

Acute cystitis in the adult should be considered uncomplicated if the woman is young, non-pregnant or

elderly, if there has been no recent instrumentation, catheterization or antimicrobial treatment and if there are no known functional or anatomical abnormalities of the urogenital tract.[57] In these cases cystitis is mostly caused by Gram-negative aerobic organisms originating from the gut.

In uncomplicated infection enterobacteriaceae are the most frequent organisms implicated, with *E. coli* accounting for 80–90% of infections; *Klebsiella pneumoniae* and *Proteus mirabilis* are the other species of this family of bacilli that produce UTIs in women.[49] *Staphylococcus saprophyticus* accounts for 10–15% of uncomplicated infections, and is more common in young women. *Streptococcus faecalis* may account for up to 5% of infections. These urinary pathogens are also linked to complicated UTIs and nosocomial infections, along with *Pseudomonas aeruginosa*, *Enterobacter* and *Candida*.[58] Enterobactericeae, enterococci and *Candida* species are often the cause of complicated cystitis.[59]

Overall, *E. coli* dominates as the causative organism in all patient groups, with *S. saprophyticus* as the second most common, accounting for 10–30% of infections in young adult women. Lactobacilli, alpha streptococci and coryne bacteria are common contaminants and, if found, should be considered as such.[60] The common uropathogens are listed in Table 67.1.

P. mirabilis is also a cause of complicated UTI and is a frequent cause of cystitis in catheterized patients and in those with structural abnormalities of the urinary tract. Tolson *et al.*[61] showed that factors such as the production of haemolysin and urease and non-agglutinating fimbriae-mediated adherence to uroepithelial cells contribute to its virulence.

Table 67.1. *Common uropathogens*

Gram-negative bacilli

- *Escherichia coli*
- *Klebsiella*
- *Proteus*
- *Pseudomonas*

Gram-positive cocci

- *Streptococcus faecalis*
- *Staphylococcus aureus*
- *Staphylococcus saprophyticus*
- *Staphylococcus epidermidis*

In neonates, complicated infections tend to occur with congenital anomalies of the urinary tract such as urethral valves, or in those with neurologic disease, resulting in urinary stasis.[62]

TERMINOLOGY

The renal system filters the blood, and the product – urine – is excreted free of microorganisms. The urinary stream may become contaminated by small numbers of bacteria hence the term 'bacteriuria', which means bacteria in the urine, regardless of source. Bacteriuria may or may not be associated with symptoms or pyuria. From a clean, freshly voided specimen of urine, one may expect less than 10 000 colony-forming units (cfu) per ml. 'Significant bacteriuria' describes the situation where organisms derived from infected tissues are multiplying in the urine.

Kass[63] proposed a useful cut-off point of 100 000 cfu per ml to define significant bacteriuria and to differentiate it from contamination. In his original work, Kass also reported that a single culture of 100 000 cfu per ml had a 20% chance of representing contamination.[64] This was based on the fact that most urinary infections are caused by enteric Gram-negative bacteria which grow well in urine. There is much debate regarding the significance of bacterial colonization of urine versus infection. Low bacterial counts of certain organisms should be considered significant, such as those which grow slowly in urine. These include coagulase-negative staphylococci and the tubercle bacilli. Low counts may also be the result of concurrent use of antimicrobial agents, and the pH and constituents of the urine that may suppress growth. Also, one may detect the early phase of an infection when growth is slow.[65,66] A concentration of 100 cfu per ml can cause an acute UTI in a healthy woman.[62]

Twenty to forty per cent of women with symptomatic UTIs present with bacterial counts of less than 100 000 cfu per ml of urine.[67,68] A statistically significant association has been found between low-count bacteriuria (>100 to 10 000 cfu per ml) and acute cystitis symptoms in young women.[69] Dilution of the urine or failure of the bacteria to grow well in the subject's urine could not explain these low counts. These findings suggest that the infection was not established in the bladder urine and that the so-called 'low-count' bacteriuria might be the early phase of a UTI.[69] Also, many women with dysuria and frequency have bacterial counts below 100 000 cfu per ml, but improve with treatment.[70] Stamm *et al.*[71] have proposed that, in symptomatic women, an appropriate threshold value for defining significant bacteriuria is in excess of 100 cfu per ml of a known pathogen. This criterion gives an acceptable sensitivity of 0.95 and a specificity of 0.85.[71]

This debate can only be resolved by making a judgement based on the interpretation of the results of laboratory tests as well as the presence of symptoms and clinical findings.

Urine collection

Urine samples constitute the largest single category of specimens examined in most medical microbiology laboratories. Despite this, there is no standard method of collection, transport or processing of specimens or of reporting results. There is also considerable variation between laboratories in the interpretation of quantitative culture results. In this section the best practice is presented.

Specimens should be obtained early in the morning whenever possible because the bacterial counts will be highest at this time. Contamination of the specimen may occur if the urine flushes onto the vulva and vagina. This can be minimized by instructing the woman to separate the labia and wash and dry the periurethral region. She should void with the labia spread and collect a mid-stream specimen. This method can provide reliable specimens but occasionally it may be necessary to perform urethral catheterization. Culture of the first 10 ml of voided urine is thought to represent urethral flora. Delivery to the laboratory should be prompt because delays of more than 2 hours may result in a rise in bacterial count in contaminated specimens to greater than 100 000 cfu per ml.[72] Otherwise refrigeration is necessary to ensure that the sample truly reflects the status of organisms in the bladder.

Suprapubic bladder puncture performed aseptically may yield urine with a low bacterial count and this should also be considered 'significant', because it cannot be accounted for by contamination.[73]

Collection in children

In making a diagnosis of cystitis in infants or children, the method of urine collection is paramount. Clean-catch specimens of urine are difficult to obtain from this group. Urethral catheterization is currently used but suprapubic needle aspiration has proved particularly useful because it bypasses organisms that contaminate the urethra, and is now accepted as the 'gold standard'.

Another method is collection from disposable diapers to detect chemical abnormalities and microscopic examination. Cohen *et al.* described a simple technique to obtain valid diaper samples of urine which was as accurate as suprapubic aspiration in the detection of UTI.[74] Another method is to cut out samples of urine-soaked diapers and mix with 20 ml of sterile saline. Culture of the supernatant provides accurate and reliable estimates of bacterial concentrations in the usual range for infected urine.[75]

URINALYSIS

In addition to irritative urinary symptoms of frequency, urgency and dysuria, urinalysis may provide additional supportive evidence of cystitis to allow a pre-emptive diagnosis of infection. In practice this allows empirical therapy to be started in uncomplicated cases. Some of the elements of information provided by urinalysis are more valuable than others. For instance, cloudy urine indicates white cells or crystals and can be due to the presence of bacteria but this is unreliable. The pH and specific gravity of urine are not helpful in diagnosing infections except in the case of *P. mirabilis* (pH 8).

Proteinuria

Dipstick tests for proteinuria have a poor predictive value in detecting renal disease because of their low specificity. Up to 6% of school children have proteinuria and the rate rises with age.[76] Proteinuria is generally a reflection of renal disease and is not normally judged to be a sign of bladder infection.

Pyuria

Pyuria implies the presence of polymorphonuclear (PMN) leucocytes or pus cells in the urine. Pyuria and the presence of urinary antibodies are indications of the host's response to inflammation but are not sensitive or specific enough as a screening test for acute cystitis. However, they may be helpful in the interpretation of the clinical significance of urine culture results, and the presence of leucocytes in the urine is of increasing

diagnostic value.[62,77] Infection is the most frequent cause of pyuria but there are also non-infections causes associated with a 'sterile pyuria'. These leucocytes appear secondary to an inflammatory response occurring in the urinary tract. Detection of pyuria is a helpful pointer to the presence of infection, with 96.6% of patients with symptomatic bacteriuria having 10 or more white cells per mm^3 compared with 1.6% of subjects who are asymptomatic and abacteriuric.[70] A midstream urine sample with greater than 10 pus cells per high-power field (hpf) has an 87% chance of being infected, compared with 10% in specimens with less than two pus cells per hpf.[78] In the absence of pyuria, one should question the diagnosis of infective cystitis.

A dipstick test for pyuria, termed the leucocyte esterase test, is used to screen urine. Bailey and Blake[79] compared this test with a chamber count method using a cut-off of 10 or more white cells per mm^3 and reported a high degree of sensitivity and specificity. The predictive value of this test is less good in women because of the possibility of contamination of the sample by leucocytes from the vagina.[80]

Haematuria

The presence of red blood cells in the urine frequently occurs when there is an infection in the mucosa of the bladder wall. It tends to occur in association with bacteriuria and pyuria. Dipstick urinalysis for the presence of haematuria is often used as a guide to the management of adults with suspected cystitis. Jou and Powers performed a study to determine whether patient-management decisions made on the basis of dipstick urinalysis are altered when results of urine microscopy become available.[81] In 94% of patients, subsequent findings on urine microscopy did not prompt a change in management. They concluded that primary use of dipstick urinalysis, with microscopy in selected cases, would likely result in considerable cost and time saving without compromising patient care.

Crystals

The formation of distinctive crystals in the urine may be associated with dysuria, frequency and flank or back pain, but crystalluria is not sensitive or specific for acute cystitis.[82] The presence of casts indicates renal disease.

Nitrite test

This is a chemical method to detect bacteriuria. Bacteria reduce nitrate in the urine to nitrite which can be tested for using a dipstick test strip. The test has a high sensitivity and specificity if performed on an early morning specimen and is useful for population screening.[83]

Urine microscopy

This involves examination of centrifuged urinary sediment for bacteria, or a Gram stain of unspun urine. The criterion for positive sediment is the presence of more than 20 bacteria while that of a Gram-stained specimen is one or more organisms per immersion field. These tests are shown to be reliable and correlate well with quantitative culture. However, to detect bacteria in this way, bacterial counts must be in excess of 30 000 per ml.[84,85]

Dipslide

Many different rapid automated laboratory methods are now available for detecting bacteriuria and identifying the organisms responsible for infection. These run in parallel with tests to determine the susceptibility of the uropathogens to antimicrobial agents. Commercial dipslides are agar-coated plastic slides which are dipped in urine and allowed to incubate in a bottle. Bacterial growth is compared with a visual standard to allow interpretation of colony density. This method correlates reasonable well with standard culture methods. The advantages of this method are that it allows immediate culture and obviates the need for transport or refrigeration.[86,87] Susceptibility test results are expressed either as susceptible, intermediate or resistant, or as the minimal inhibitory concentration in micrograms per ml.[88]

Dipstick urinalysis is too limited and inadequate as a screen for cystitis in young children, and urine culture should be performed. Hoberman and Wald[89] found that in children in a hospital setting, the positive predictive value of the combination of pyuria and bacteriuria (85%) allows prompt antimicrobial therapy before culture results are available. They recommended that the lower positive predictive value of the single finding of either pyuria or bacteriuria (40%) justifies delaying treatment until culture results are available.

LOCALIZATION OF INFECTION IN THE URINARY TRACT

Symptoms

The symptoms typically associated with cystitis in women are frequency of micturition and nocturia. Dysuria is also common and is often accompanied by suprapubic tenderness and pain. Recurrent painful macroscopic haematuria is also reported. Women may also complain that the urine is cloudy, malodorous or blood stained. Approximately one in three women presenting with symptoms of cystitis will also have an upper tract infection.[90] These infections are associated with loin pain and tenderness. Fever has long been accepted as the hallmark of pyelonephritis but in large studies both fever and loin pain have been present in subjects where the infection was localized to the bladder.[91] Only about half of patients in general practice with the typical symptoms of frequency, dysuria and suprapubic pain are found to have bacteriuria.[92] Cystitis may present with minimal or atypical symptoms of abdominal pain or discomfort, or painless haematuria. The diagnosis is particularly challenging in small children and the possibility should always be considered in the febrile sick child. Infections in older nursing-home residents may be difficult to detect as patients may present with atypical signs and symptoms, including the absence of pyrexia.[93] Hence, symptoms are often unreliable and when these are unclear, and in complicated cases or cases of recurrent cystitis, it may be necessary to perform tests to localize the site of infection in the urinary tract.[94]

Fairley washout test

By washing the bladder free of bacteria and collecting serial urine samples, Fairley proposed that these samples represent upper tract urine.[95] In this way Fairley was able to separate pyelonephritis from cystitis with some degree of confidence. However, the validity of the procedure in patients with spinal cord injury and reflux is doubtful.[96]

Catheterization

Urethral catheterization is useful to collect specimens for culture but may introduce urethral bacteria.

Marple[97] described the technique, which is still used today; small bacterial counts (100 cfu per ml) may indicate a UTI.[97] However, this is not recommended in routine cases because of the potential risks associated with urethral and bladder instrumentation.

Suprapubic aspiration of bladder urine is thought to provide the highest degree of reliability.[98] Indeed, it has been suggested that the presence of any bacteria in a bladder aspirate obtained by this technique will identify infection.[99]

It is possible to obtain a sample of renal urine by the technique of ureteral catheterization.[98] The problem with this is the risk of contamination by infected bladder urine following introduction of the cystoscope. Contamination is limited by employing rigorous bladder washout before catheterizing the ureters and obtaining serial cultures from each kidney. To improve the detection of pyelonephritis, the urine osmolality, specific gravity and creatinine concentration are also determined. Overall, although tedious and unpleasant for the patient, this is probably the best test to prove upper tract infection and disprove cystitis.[88]

Swabs

Direct culture of swabs from the urethra, vaginal vestibules and posterior fornix of the vagina are also used to localize infection in the lower genitourinary tract. In addition, this allows microscopic examination of wet preparations which can be diagnostic for pus cells, yeasts, fungi and *Trichomonas*.

Serum tests

When bacteria enter the body they elicit an antibody response. These antibodies react with the surface antigens of the bacteria. This antibody coating of the bacteria can be observed by mixing with fluorescence-conjugated globulin and viewing under a fluorescence microscope.[100] A positive test is a useful predictor of adult women who will require long-term therapy, but should not be used in children because of a high false-positive rate.[101,102] This is a valuable test in separating renal from bladder infections.[103] However, these tests are sometimes difficult to interpret.[104]

C-reactive protein (CRP) is a non-specific acute-phase reactant that appears in the serum in the presence of inflammation. Its value seems to be in the

assessment of febrile infants and children thought to have pyelonephritis. It is also useful as a measure of therapeutic response. In these studies, the level of CRP returned to normal within 7 days of onset of acute pyelonephritis.[103,105]

The measurement of serum antibody response to antigens on the urinary pathogens has also been used to localize the site of infection. Patients with acute pyelonephritis usually have a significant rise in serological titres, which correlate well with other tests of upper tract infection but are by no means diagnostic.[106] These elevated antibody titres reflect the severity of tissue invasion rather than site of infection, considerable overlap existing in the case of cystitis.[107]

RISK FACTORS

Host factors, more than bacterial virulence, are probably the most important contributors to infections.

Age

Most UTIs in healthy women in the sexually active age group present as bacterial cystitis.[108] The shorter urethra in women is the most likely explanation for the significant difference in the distribution of cystitis between men and women. The increasing prevalence of cystitis with increasing age is probably attributable to the presence of systemic disease, immobility, faecal and urinary dysfunction and urinary tract instrumentation. Yoshikawa *et al.*[93] noted that acute cystitis is one of the most common infections acquired in nursing homes and is among the most frequent reasons for transfer to an acute-care facility. In the elderly, virulence of the organisms and the host response to infection are similar to infections in younger patients.[109] Martinell *et al.*[110] followed women prospectively for a median of 23 years (range 13–88 years) from their first recognized symptomatic infection in childhood. The UTI attack rate (number of UTIs per individual per observation year) was highest during the first year of life (1.9), with a gradual decrease to the lowest rate (0.2) at 11–15 years of age. A moderate increase in attack rate (0.4) was seen in the late teens, extending through to the mid twenties.

In children, a strong correlation has been found between recurrent UTIs and non-neuropathic bladder dysfunction. Urodynamics studies have been found to be invaluable in the detection and treatment of such cases.[111] In another study of 41 children referred because of recurrent UTIs, 18 (44%) showed detrusor instability on cystometrogram.[112]

Obesity

Much information has been gained from a large study examining factors influencing the rate of first referral to hospital for urinary infection among 17 032 women. The risk of first referral declined with age, was higher in nulliparous women than in parous women, and was higher in non-obese than in obese women. The negative association between hospital referral for infection and obesity was unexpected and could not be explained in terms of age, parity or contraceptive diaphragm use.[113]

Sexual intercourse and behavioural patterns

Much has been written on women's health habits and behaviour such as voiding habits, diet, clothing and use of soaps as potential causes of cystitis. As individual factors they have only a small effect, but several of these together might substantially contribute to the risk of initial or recurrent cystitis.[114–116] The use of tampons is associated with a moderate risk of infection.[114]

Some behavioural factors have been shown to have a significant effect on the risk of initial and recurrent cystitis. There is a strong link with sexual intercourse, with 75–90% of women relating their infections to coitus.[117,118] There is also a 'dose–response' effect for increasing coital frequency.[119,120] Epidemiological and clinical evidence suggests that strains of *E. coli* which cause cystitis may be transmitted between sexual partners.[121]

The use of the contraceptive diaphragm and spermicide has also been implicated as a factor for recurrent UTIs.[116,122] This may be due to intermittent obstruction of the urethra as the rim presses on the urethra when left in for 6–8 hours after coitus, and to changes in the vaginal flora towards more enteric Gram-negative bacteria.[120] In one large study, the main increase in risk in current diaphragm users occurred during the first 24 months, when overall rates were 2–3 times higher in users than in non-users or ex-users of the diaphragm.[121]

Instrumentation of the urinary tract

Other important risk factors for cystitis include catheterization and instrumentation of the urethra and bladder. The incidence of UTI and cystitis following catheterization of a normal bladder is approximately 5%, despite a sterile technique. This is modified by the duration of catheterization, as well as the general well-being of the patient.[123] A patient has only a 50% probability of remaining free of infection for 4 days after catheterization.[124]

Efforts have been made to reduce infection associated with these invasive procedures. The antibacterial activity of silver-containing compounds has been employed in the manufacture of urinary catheters in an effort to reduce cystitis. However, a large randomized controlled trial using this type of catheter failed to demonstrate their efficacy in prevention of catheter-associated bacteriuria.[125]

Indwelling catheters are frequently used after vaginal hysterectomy but efforts have been made to avoid their use whenever possible. In a randomized controlled trial of catheterization vs no catheterization in women undergoing vaginal hysterectomy, there was a higher incidence of cystitis and more complications in the catheter group, and no incidence of urinary retention in the no-catheter group.[126] The rate of urinary infection following cystoscopy is approximately 7.5%.[127]

Residual urine

Deficient bladder emptying is an important factor predisposing to cystitis in adult women.[128] It has been suggested that residual urine is a facilitating host factor in the pathogenesis of symptomatic UTI in childhood. In one case–control study, residual urine was assessed by ultrasonography in children with a single attack of symptomatic lower urinary tract infection (LUTI) and in healthy controls. Residual urine was found significantly more often in 39 children during acute illness as well as during a follow-up of 6 months, compared with 55 control children.[129] Similar findings have been demonstrated in adults. In women with urinary retention, detrusor failure with low-pressure activity tends to be the prominent urodynamic abnormality as opposed to outlet obstruction. This occurs whether there is a neurological cause for retention or other non-neurological causes.[130]

Ageing women report similar symptoms of voiding difficulty as age-matched men. Madersbacher *et al.*[131] looked at age-related changes in urodynamic parameters and found a significant increase in post-void residual volume and a decrease in peak flow rate, average flow rate, voided volume and bladder capacity in both sexes with age. These data suggest a non-sex-specific ageing process of the lower urinary tract in the development, at least in part, of irritative urinary symptoms. Urinary retention can also develop due to a hypotonic bladder, increased sphincter tone, absent or decreased sensation of bladder fullness or urethral blockage. It may also occur as a result of bladder-neck surgery. Incomplete bladder emptying may lead to acute and recurrent cystitis and complicated infections.

Vesicoureteric reflux

At the time of micturition, the detrusor muscle contracts and VUR may occur. When the detrusor relaxes, urine then falls back into the bladder. This allows a stagnant pool of urine to be retained which will predispose to persistent cystitis. In this way, reflux may be involved in the pathogenesis of UTI. Alternatively, the presence of recurrent cystitis with inflammation around the ureteric orifice may make the physiological vesicoureteric valve mechanism incompetent and predispose to VUR. Baker and Barbaris[132] studied 200 girls with recurrent UTI and showed that 43% had VUR. Of 47 girls studied after only one episode of infection, 36% had VUR. They concluded that failure to investigate the child could mean that potentially severe urinary tract abnormalities could go undetected.[132]

Nosocomial urinary tract infections

UTIs represent approximately 40% of all nosocomial infections and urethral catheterization is the single most important predisposing factor. The National Survey of Infections in UK Hospitals reported that, of the total number of infections in hospital patients at any one time, urinary infection was second only to respiratory infection.[133] In addition to urethral catheterization, cystitis is usually secondary to urinary tract surgery or manipulation, and immobility, particularly in the elderly. The invading organism tends to be indigenous to the patient. Hospital infections may be prevented by careful catheter management while limiting the procedure to well-defined circumstances.

Environmental factors

It is possible that environmental factors have a part to play, placing some individuals at increased risk of infection. Sanderson and Alshafi demonstrated that it is possible to recover the causative organism from the bed sheets, floor and bedside chairs of patients with UTIs.[134]

Other factors

Blood-groups antigens are found on the surface of urothelial cells. These may affect bacterial adherence and increase the susceptibility to UTIs. Sheinfeld *et al.*[135] found an increased frequency of the Lewis blood-group phenotypes among women with recurrent UTIs.

Women with a history of previous febrile UTIs and renal scarring have a high risk for recurrent infections.[136]

Neurological disorders such as cerebrovascular accidents, Parkinson's disease, multiple sclerosis, spinal cord injury and peripheral neuropathy may result in loss of bladder reflex inhibition due to effects on the higher centres. The resultant functional urinary tract abnormalities may result in significant morbidity such as recurrent cystitis.[137]

RECURRENT INFECTION

Up to 26% of young women experience at least one culture-confirmed recurrence within 6 months of an initial infection.[138] Recurrent cystitis may be due to reinfection with different bacteria from outside the urinary tract as a new event. Re-infection accounts for 80% of recurrent UTIs and is not generally associated with physical abnormalities of the genitourinary tract.[139] The focus for these infections appears to be from the perineal flora.[140] Recurrent symptomatic UTIs in a given individual are usually due to reinfection with the same strain of organism rather than persistence of the pathogen within the urinary tract. The colonic flora is also a reservoir for these reinfecting strains.[141]

The other cause of recurrent UTI is reinfection due to the same organism which has persisted within the urinary tract. Several factors favour recurrent cystitis, and the source or focus of these persistent bacteria is usually a urological abnormality which is often correctable. Risk factors for the development of recurrent cystitis are given in Table 67.2. Other circumstances such as sexual relationships and sexual behaviour, excessive vaginal hygiene, vaginal tampons, the use of the contraceptive diaphragm, and clothing habits may play a role but this is controversial. The presence of haematuria as a symptom of initial infection is a strong predictor of recurrence. However, behavioural factors associated with the initial infection such as frequent sexual intercourse and diaphragm use are not such good predictors of recurrence.[142]

Relapse is diagnosed by recurrence of bacteriuria with the same organisms within 7 days of treatment and implies failure to eradicate the infection. In contrast, if bacteriuria is absent after treatment for 14 days or longer, and is then followed by recurrence of infection with the same or different organism, this is likely to be a reinfection.

The course of recurrent cystitis in adult women is rarely accompanied by upper tract dysfunction such as reflux, renal scarring or renal hypertension. In a prospective trial Ikaheimo *et al.*[142] followed-up 179 women (age range 17–82 years) for 12 months after an index episode of community-acquired acute cystitis caused by *E. coli*; 147 episodes of UTI were detected during follow-up, 131 of which were classified as recurrences occurring at least 1 month after the index episode. Forty-four per cent of women developed recurrent infections; *E. coli* caused 78% of the recurrent episodes. Virulence factors among the recurrence strains were identical to those among the index episode strains. The presence of these factors did not affect the risk of recurrence but did increase the likelihood that the index episode strain would persist and cause recurrent episodes of cystitis.[142]

Table 67.2. *Risk factors for recurrent urinary tract infection*

- Lower urinary tract obstruction and chronic retention of urine
- Stones and other foreign bodies in the bladder
- Trauma
- Enterovesical and vesicovaginal fistulae
- Urethral diverticula
- Malformations of the urinary tract
- Cystocoele
- Vesicoureteric reflux
- Infected periurethral glands
- Contraceptive-diaphragm use

PATHOLOGY AND MORPHOLOGY

Morphology of acute cystitis

In the early stages of inflammation the bladder mucosa becomes hyperaemic. As the inflammation becomes more severe, the walls may have focal or confluent haemorrhagic areas with grey–white or yellow exudate (suppurative cystitis). Ulceration may ensue as the granular mucosa becomes friable with deeper layers of inflammation and breaks down. With unchecked infection by a virulent organism in a bladder weakened by recurrent infection, deep ulceration and intramural abscess formation can occur. In severe cases with intense oedema and inflammation, ischaemia of the mucosa may occur, giving rise to areas of necrosis. In diabetic patients, gas-forming bacteria may cause bubbles in the submucosal connective tissue, called emphysematous cystitis.

Microscopic features of acute cystitis

Acute cystitis is characterized by an intense PMN-leucocyte infiltrate in the lamina propria and urothelium. In severe cases there may be sloughing of urothelial cells and fragmentation, with extensive mucosal denudation and exfoliation. There may also be evidence of increased vascularity, congestion and haemorrhage. Reactive changes may be present with urothelial hyperplasia and neutrophils migrating into the area of hyperplasia. Cytoplasmic vacuolizations, slight nuclear enlargement and enlarged nucleoli are common.

Morphology of chronic cystitis

The inflammation of chronic cystitis tends to be confluent, affecting most of the bladder wall and giving rise to a congested hyperaemic mucosa of varying degrees of severity. The trigone is sometimes more oedematous and infected than the rest of the bladder. Over time, with recurrent or persistent infection, chronic inflammatory changes may occur, with the mucosa becoming hyperaemic, granular and friable, with areas of petechial haemorrhage. Prominent folds of heaped-up mucosa are common, giving a papillary appearance. If associated with outlet obstruction, bladder trabeculation may occur. This is secondary to detrusor muscle hypertrophy and characteristically takes on the appearance of hypertrophied muscular bands with small sacular pouches in between.

Microscopic features of chronic cystitis

Chronic cystitis may have a variable appearance, but is often characterized by lymphocytes, monocytes and a dense plasma cell infiltrate in the lamina propria with histocytes and eosinophils. The lamina propria may be fibrotic, with persistent oedema and dilated congested vessels. The urothelial thickness may be variable depending on the degree of bladder contraction, distension and underlying pathology Normally there is a 5–7-cell layer thickness, but the urothelium may be thinned or hyperplastic. Consequent on inflammation there is healing and, after a repetitive insult, the process may result in proliferation of urothelium either downwards into the lamina propria, forming epithelial buds, or upwards, creating small villous surface projections. Clinical manifestation of chronic bacterial cystitis tends to be characterized by periods of exacerbation followed by remissions. Most cases tend not to be self-limiting and require specific therapy to bring about a resolution of the flare-up, and longer term treatment of the underlying pathology. Squamous metaplasia, where the urothelium is replaced by mature squamous epithelium, sometimes occurs as a consequence of chronic infection. Typically, keratinizing squamous metaplasia occurs and, if extensive, may lead to bladder dysfunction and reduced functional and structural capacity. Although it may have a greater malignant potential in men, it is generally accepted that squamous metaplasia is not a precursor of cancer in women.[143]

INVESTIGATIONS

Whom to investigate and when are often difficult decisions to make. In women who present with acute cystitis, opinions vary as to the extent of the investigation that is required, and which tests are appropriate. Table 67.3 lists patient groups in whom it would be prudent to evaluate further. Table 67.4 lists the methods of investigation. Invasive tests should probably be performed only when the acute attack has subsided so as to limit the associated morbidity.

Abnormalities of deficient bladder emptying that predispose to recurrent cystitis may be easily detected using non-invasive methods to determine urinary flow rates and residual urine.

Cystoscopy provides useful information and influences therapy in women with recurrent UTIs.[144] Cystoscopic findings in women with acute cystitis may be

Table 67.3. *Indications for further investigation of urinary symptoms*

- Children
- Proven recurrent infections
- Adults with childhood history of urinary tract infection
- Persistent haematuria
- Infection with an atypical or resistant organism
- Persistent infection
- Failure to respond to antimicrobial therapy

Table 67.4. *Types of investigation for cystitis*

Clinical indication	Test
Initial investigation	Dipstick Mid-stream urine sample – culture and sensitivity tests Full blood count, urea and electrolytes Urinary tract ultrasonography Postmicturition residual scan
Recurrent infections	Urine culture for fastidious organisms Cystourethroscopy Bladder wall biopsy
Scan suggests renal scarring	Renogram
Voiding difficulty Abnormal detrusor activity suspected	Uroflowmetry and urodynamics

misleading, however, because the acute inflammatory changes seen may be inconsistent with the degree of histological change.[145] Infection rates following flexible cystoscopy performed as an outpatient procedure are 2.2–7.5% and infection rates are similar in men and women. Infection rates are higher in patients with a history of cystitis or where an additional procedure is performed.[127,146]

Problems exist in the reporting of the histopathological findings from bladder biopsies showing chronic cystitis. Often there is too broad a spectrum of detail and terminology. By limiting these and using standardized criteria it is hoped that improvements will be made in the reporting of pathology to aid management of cystitis.[147]

It is generally accepted that ultrasonography and radiological investigations should not be undertaken on all women with cystitis or bacteriuria because they have a limited role in the evaluation of such cases in adults.[148,149] Most women will not have upper tract abnormalities and will have entirely normal urograms, so the risk and expense are not justified. These investigations should be reserved for women with other risk factors such as a history of unexplained haematuria, neurogenic bladder dysfunction or renal calculi.[144,148,150,151] However, this is not the case in children and will be addressed later in the chapter.

In a prospective study of women with recurrent UTI it was concluded that intravenous urography seldom reveals abnormalities that influence treatment in otherwise healthy women.[144] On the other hand, uroflowmetry and cystourethroscopy may yield helpful information. Also, urodynamics, including cystometry and videocystourethrography, may be of value in the assessment of patients with refractory recurrent cystitis. Koff *et al.*[152] performed a prospective uncontrolled study of children with recurrent UTIs and detrusor instability. Treatment of the uninhibited bladder contractions allowed 58% of patients to maintain sterile urine without subsequent antimicrobial therapy after cure of the initial infection. We have also found that women with recurrent cystitis have a significant incidence of abnormal detrusor activity on urodynamic testing compared with healthy controls. However, studies of the effect of treatment on the abnormal detrusor activity in women with recurrent cystitis have yet to be performed.

TREATMENT OF CYSTITIS

The objective of treatment is eradication of cystitis and prevention of recurrence. The aims of therapy are listed in Table 67.5. Host factors, clinical findings, and characteristics of the infection and the invading organism are all important in determining the appropriate agent for therapy. Therapeutic options include good general advice, adequate fluid intake, appropriate frequent voiding and post-coital micturition. The desired effect is to achieve a short voiding interval and a high flow rate while drinking a large amount of fluid to dilute the bacteria. This will dilute the inoculum and improve the washout mechanism. Spontaneous remission of infection occurs in up to 40% of adult women.[153] However, most patients will require antimicrobial therapy. Selection of the appropriate antimicrobial agent to achieve a high concentration of drug in the urine is vital to the success of therapy. Techniques to improve emptying of the bladder may be necessary, as well as other therapies or surgery to eliminate an underlying risk factor, particularly in difficult cases. In some cases of cystitis, the causative organisms are highly predictable and empirical therapy without pretreatment culture is recommended.[18] Spontaneous remission of cystitis for a 2-day period occurs in 5–7% of women;[154] it is no more likely in women with low urinary colony counts (100 to 10 000 cfu per ml) than in women with high colony counts (>10 000 cfu per ml).

There is a trend towards using clinical guidelines, coordinated primarily by nurses, to manage uncomplicated cystitis. Primary-care clinics which have implemented systems and tools to support nurse-coordinated care of such women have been very successful both in terms of cost of care and clinical outcome, and should be encouraged.[155] Situations that require particular attention include cystitis in pregnancy, children,

Table 67.5. *Aims of treatment*

- Clinical cure and relief of symptoms
- Microbiological cure
- Detection of predisposing factors
- Protection against upper tract involvement
- Selective approach to investigations
- Management of recurrence or persistence
- Explanation to the patient
- Prevention of recurrence

women with diabetes mellitus or neuropathic bladders, and catheterized subjects.

Choice of agent

The ideal drug is one that is specific for the bladder, achieves a high concentration in the urine and does not induce resistance in the organisms (Tables 67.6, 67.7). Drugs should be safe and efficacious, have a wide spectrum of activity and few side effects. Rapid and complete absorption from the gut is an advantage so that there is little residual drug to alter the normal bowel flora or induce resistance in the faecal reservoir. The antimicrobial agents usually selected attain high concentrations in the urine and the dilution resulting from a high fluid intake does not render them ineffective. Although the drug may be diluted and eliminated by voiding, there is evidence to suggest that dilution of the bacterial culture may increase drug efficacy.[156] Short duration of therapy of a drug that has

minimal side effects will help to ensure good patient compliance.

Duration and dosage of drug therapy

The duration and dosage of antimicrobial therapy varies widely. It is believed that the traditional dosage regimens for uncomplicated UTIs are excessive. Compliance is likely to be reduced with long duration of therapy, and there are increased chances of adverse reactions, the selection of resistant bowel organisms and *Candida* infections (both vaginal and oral). There is no convincing evidence that a long course of medication is more effective than a short one. Indeed, the use of single-dose therapy for uncomplicated UTIs is gaining support. Also, there is now increasing emphasis on reducing the cost of management of cystitis, by keeping the duration of treatment short and by being highly selective on diagnostic work-up and further investigations. It is not uncommon for women with a clinically obvious uncomplicated infection to receive a short course of empirical therapy.[157] In the past, courses of therapy usually lasted approximately 5 days. There is growing evidence in favour of shorter courses of therapy of 3 days, or even 24 hours, and single-dose regimens. Shorter courses are now recommended in uncomplicated infections where the urinary tract is normal and there is an effective washout mechanism (no voiding dysfunction). A single oral dose of an antimicrobial agent can be as effective as a conventional 3-day course for the treatment of uncomplicated cystitis.[158,159] Trimethoprim, co-trimoxazole (trimethoprim plus sul-

Table 67.6. *Profile of drugs used to treat cystitis*

- Specificity for the urinary tract
- High level of drug in urine
- Broad spectrum of activity
- Safe and efficacious
- Rapid and complete absorption
- Little alteration of normal bowel reservoir and vaginal flora
- Bactericidal for known uropathogens

Table 67.7. *Antimicrobials commonly used to treat cystitis*

Spectrum of activity	Drug
Gram-negative bacilli	Norfloxacin
Staphylococci	Ciprofloxacin
Most streptococci	Gentamicin Sulphonamides Co-trimoxazole (trimethoprim plus sulphamethoxazole) Trimethoprim Nitrofurantoin
Pseudomonas	Norfloxacin Ciprofloxacin Gentamicin

phamethoxazole), fostomycin trometamol and the 4-quinolones are the preferred agents for single-dose therapy.[158] Fostomycin tromethamine is the only antimicrobial approved by the Food and Drug Administration for single-dose therapy in women with acute cystitis. Stein[160] reviewed the clinical pharmacology of fostomycin in the treatment of uncomplicated cystitis. His study suggests that a single dose of this agent produces therapeutic concentrations in the urine for 2–4 days. It is active against common uropathogens, including organisms resistant to other antibiotics. Another advantage is that it appears to be safe during pregnancy.[161] However, there is still some contention – a review by Hooton and Stamm[57] suggests that a 3-day regimen is more effective treatment than a single-dose regimen for all antimicrobials tested.

Nitrofurantoin

Nitrofurantoin macrocrystals have the unique property of being specific to the urinary tract, limiting the potential effect of active drug on the faecal reservoir inducing resistance in the bowel flora. The drug is also bactericidal to common urinary pathogens.[161] These properties make it particularly useful for long-term low-dose prophylaxis. It is safe in pregnancy but is contraindicated in renal failure, even if renal function is only slightly impaired. It is bactericidal against Gram-negative bacilli except *Proteus* and *Pseudomonas*. Staphylococci, a common cause of catheter infection, are also sensitive.

Trimethoprim plus sulphamethoxazole

In a recent survey on the management of urinary infections in general practice, trimethoprim was the most popular antibiotic for treatment of acute cystitis and the most common duration of treatment was 5–7 days.[162]

Antimicrobial regimens with trimethoprim plus sulphamethoxazole seem to be more effective in the management of acute cystitis in women than those with beta lactam, regardless of duration.[57] These drugs are useful in clearing Gram-negative aerobic flora from the gut. Hence they are of value as a prophylactic treatment for the prevention of reinfection in women who possibly have a gut reservoir for organisms that may colonize the periurethral area. These drugs are usually used for a 6-month period and induce minimal faecal floral resistance.

Tetracyclines

Although tetracyclines induce little microbial resistance, this can occur and may be a factor in some treatment failures.[163]

Proteus mirabilis

Tawfik *et al.*[164] showed that amikacin significantly reduces the adhesion of proteus strains to the uroepithelial cells and that gentamicin exerts the same effect to a lesser extent. Both drugs inhibit swarming and motility of proteus strains, indicating their impact on the virulence factors of uropathogenic strains of proteus.[164]

Oestrogen therapy

Oestrogen deficiency in post-menopausal women is thought to be important in the genesis of lower urinary tract symptoms, in particular frequency, urgency and nocturia. The urethra and trigone of the bladder are rich in oestrogen receptors, so it is not surprising that oestrogen therapy has an effect on the lower urogenital tract.[165]

Systemic oestrogen replacement appears to alleviate the symptoms of urgency, frequency and dysuria in post-menopausal women. Furthermore, recurrent UTIs are a common finding in women who are oestrogen deficient, and there is good evidence to suggest that these can be prevented and even treated by the use of oestrogen therapy. This is probably achieved, in part, by modification of the vaginal flora.[166,167] Cardozo *et al.*[166] investigated the use of oestriol (3 mg orally daily for 3 months) in a double-blind, placebo-controlled trial. Although oestriol produced both subjective and objective improvement in lower urinary tract function, it was not significantly better than placebo.[168]

DIFFICULTIES IN MANAGEMENT

Unresolved bacteriuria

Refractory cases and resistance
Bacteriuria may prove to be refractory to treatment in a small number of women. This may be because of poor compliance leading to suboptimal incomplete

therapy; severe inflammation of the bladder wall with deep-seated forms of infection; or chronic urinary retention, usually associated with a neuropathic bladder. Antimicrobial therapy should be discontinued, the patient investigated, and management tailored to the patient.

Treatment may also be ineffective because the bacteria are resistant to the antimicrobial selected for treatment. This may follow empirical therapy in the absence of knowledge of the organism's sensitivity to antimicrobial agents. Alternatively, the infection may be due to previously susceptible bacteria that have subsequently developed resistance. Usually the patient has a history of recent antibiotic therapy, the treatment producing plasmid-mediated resistance transfer factors. This may also result in the development of resistance to other commonly used antimicrobial agents.

Mixed infection caused by organisms with different sensitivities is less common, but does occur. Laboratory culture may yield a pure growth of the predominant species and treatment in the clinical setting may result in continued growth and infection of the second organism, making therapy unsuccessful.

The emergence of resistant organisms has increased the importance of urine culture prior to therapy. Resistance to co-trimoxazole is an escalating problem; in situations where empirical therapy is used, alternative drugs should be considered. These alternatives include nitrofurantoin, a fluoroquinolone or a third-generation cephalosporin.[157]

Residual urine

Triple voiding at 1-minute intervals may reduce the quantity of residual urine. Another technique is to void at fixed regular intervals such as 3-hourly, to improve emptying and avoid overdistension of the bladder. Manual suprapubic pressure and different postures may also be used while voiding.[169] Chronic retention and subsequent recurrent cystitis are among the more frequent complications following spinal cord injuries.[165,170,171]

Urodynamic abnormalities

Lower urinary tract dysfunction may explain the marked tendency for recurrent infection despite treatment of bacteriuria. Wullt *et al.*[172] evaluated the influence of urodynamic factors on the establishment of bacteriuria after deliberate intravesical inoculations with *E. coli* in patients with recurrent UTIs. Successful

colonization could be established only in patients with defective bladder voiding. This suggests that urodynamic defects permit some non-virulent strains of microorganisms to establish in the bladder but that additional host factors determine if bacteriuria will persist. Conversely, bladder dysfunction may be the result of recurrent infection. It has been postulated that bladder dysfunction may result from generalized intravesical responses to injury mechanisms. To investigate this, Bagli *et al.*[173] measured the levels of basic fibroblast growth factor, a mediator of tissue response to injury, in children with voiding dysfunction and in healthy controls. The levels of this critical mediator of wound repair were significantly higher in the presence of voiding dysfunction, supporting the role of inflammation and repair in the genesis of urodynamic abnormalities in subjects with recurrent UTI.

Vesicoureteric reflux and pregnancy

It has been suggested that antireflux surgery in childhood would prevent significant upper tract infections in pregnancy. However, recent studies have suggested that this is not the case. Women who have undergone antireflux surgery are still at risk of UTIs and fetal morbidity. Those with renal scarring should, however, be considered for antireflux surgery before pregnancy to further reduce morbidity.[174]

PROPHYLAXIS

If the bacterial focus within the urinary tract cannot be removed, low-dose antimicrobial therapy should be considered to prevent the morbidity of recurrent infections.[175] Recurrent cystitis can be managed successfully by both short- and long-term low-dose prophylaxis, as well as self-start intermittent therapy or post-coital therapy.[176,177] The most effective drugs for this indication include norfloxacin, trimethoprim and nitrofurantoin, taken at night. It has also been demonstrated that a dose taken on alternate nights, 3 nights a week or after intercourse is just as effective. Post-coital administration of antibiotics such as cephalexin has been used as effective prophylaxis of recurrent UTIs in sexually active premenopausal women. In one study post-coital prophylaxis achieved identical results to daily administration but required only a third as many tablets.[178]

Short-term prophylaxis

Prophylactic antibiotics are often used at the time of surgery, during or after instrumentation or surgical procedures on the bladder, especially in a woman prone to cystitis. Antimicrobial prophylaxis does not reduce the incidence of transient perioperative bacteriuria and bacteraemia but certainly reduces the incidence of post-operative UTI. A short peroperative course of single or combination antibiotics represents sufficient prophylaxis.[179]

Long-term prophylaxis

The aims of long-term prophylaxis or suppression are to render the urine sterile, treat any persistent focus of infection and allow healing in the bladder wall, while reducing the likelihood of recurrent cystitis or relapse. Nitrofurantoin and co-trimoxazole have been used successfully and are recommended for this purpose.[180,181] If recurrence is prevented over the longer term, this will allow the local immune defences in the bladder wall to recover, particularly if they are badly damaged after a deep-seated infection. Medication should be taken at bedtime, after emptying the bladder for the last time. This will allow the drug to be retained in the bladder overnight and attain effective antimicrobial concentrations.

It has been proposed that vaginal application of *Lactobacillus lasei* may also reduce the reinfection rate in women with recurrent cystitis. This was examined by Baerheim *et al.*[182] in a randomized, double-blind, controlled trial of the vaginal application of *Lactobacillus* twice weekly in women with three or more episodes of cystitis during the previous 12 months. They found no difference in infection rate between the treatment and placebo groups.

Follow-up is important to check that the urine remains sterile, that symptoms improve and that side effects are monitored. An alternative treatment regimen may be required. Follow-up may be 3-monthly or at any time if symptoms recur. If symptomatic reinfection occurs during prophylaxis, urine samples should be obtained for culture and sensitivity tests. Treatment may be instituted at the full therapeutic dose and then continued at the prophylactic dose.

Prophylactic therapy has been shown to reduce recurrence by up to 95% compared with placebo; reinfection rates have been reduced from 2–3 per patient year to 0.1–0.4 per patient year.[139]

SPECIAL PROBLEMS

The elderly

The fall in circulating oestrogen after the menopause results in a decrease in lactobacilli colonization of the vagina, a lower vaginal pH and a subsequent increase in colonization with possible uropathogenic bacteria. This is thought to account partially for the higher incidence of bacteriuria in elderly women than elderly men.[183] Bacteriuria has a low predictive value for identifying febrile urinary infections in the elderly.[184] In the elderly, gross haematuria occurs more frequently in men than in women. Although bacteriuria is usually present, urinary infection alone is an infrequent cause of this condition. Indeed it has been shown that a febrile haematuria without irritative symptoms of cystitis probably does not require antimicrobial therapy.[185] Additionally, the prevalence in the elderly of Gram-positive organisms such as *Enterococcus faecalis*, coagulase-negative staphylococci and Group B streptococci is increasing.[186] UTIs in nursing-home residents are the most frequent source of bacteriuria in the elderly. Persistent bacteriuria is common in non-catheterized nursing-home residents, but there is little evidence that significant adverse outcomes result directly from this bacteriuric state.[187]

Overall it is evident that asymptomatic bacteriuria is frequent in elderly populations and it has a poor predictive value for identifying febrile urinary infection.[184] It has been estimated that, despite a high prevalence of bacteriuria, urinary infection contributes to less than 10% of episodes of clinically significant febrile morbidity. However there are few short- or long-term adverse outcomes attributable to this high prevalence and incidence of asymptomatic bacteriuria, and no evidence for an impact on survival. It is uncertain whether this contributes to the problem of antimicrobial resistance in these women.[188] Hence, it is suggested that asymptomatic bacteriuria, although quite common in the elderly, should rarely be treated.[189] Thus, currently there is no indication for the treatment of asymptomatic bacteriuria in the elderly except before invasive genitourinary procedures. The goal of treatment in symptomatic infection is relief of symptoms, not sterilization of the urine. The choice of antimicrobial agent for the treatment of symptomatic infections is similar to that for younger women, but it has been shown that the elderly are less likely to be cured by antibiotics, particularly short courses.[190]

Catheters

Indwelling catheters and their placement provide a microenvironment conducive to the growth of bacteria and infection. The frequency of catheter-acquired bacteriuria increases with the duration of catheterization, and failure to maintain a closed drainage system. The drainage bag often harbours polymicrobes, which enhances the transference of genetic information between strains of bacteria. Thus, it is not surprising that infections with multiple organisms tend to occur in women with long-term indwelling catheters.[191] In women catheterized for short periods of time (less than 2 weeks) after gynaecological or urological surgery, prophylaxis should be considered because acute cystitis is a risk. The incidence of catheter-associated infections has not been shown to decrease with interventions such as topical meatal antimicrobials, disinfectants added to the urinary drainage bag, antimicrobial coatings for catheters or antimicrobial irrigation.[192] Bacteriuria should be expected in women with long-term catheters; however, extended prophylaxis is not only expensive but is also likely to result in the selection of resistant organisms. Hence, antimicrobial treatment of asymptomatic bacteriuria is not justified in these women and should be reserved for those in whom it is clinically indicated.[193] When the catheter is removed, the urine should be cultured and any infection treated. Systemic antimicrobials given within 48 hours of catheter removal decrease the incidence of urinary infection but this is not currently recommended because of concerns about antimicrobial resistance.[192]

Suprapubic catheterization is recommended as an alternative to urethral catheterization because it is associated with a lower incidence of urinary infection and facilitates a controlled trial of micturition.[194]

Clean intermittent self-catheterization

Clean intermittent self-catheterization (CISC) is an excellent procedure for minimizing the risk of cystitis and urinary tract complications. Bacteriuria occurs in up to 61% of subjects performing long-term CISC but, despite this, the incidence of significant cystitis is approximately 6%. (The criteria for infection was greater than 100 cfu per ml.[195]) The reported incidence of cystitis in subjects performing CISC varies widely. In two good studies, the overall incidence of infection was 10.3 per 1000 patient days of CISC during early follow-up and 13.6 per 1000 patient days of CISC over an average of 22 months.[196,197] Pyuria is not a reliable indicator of infection in women performing CISC. Also, the leucocyte excretion rate overestimates terminal catheter urine and underestimates mid-stream catheter urine.[198]

The frequency of CISC is a good predictor for the risk of bacteriuria. Antibiotic use does not improve outcome greatly in these women and should be restricted. Catheterization should occur sufficiently often to ensure that the mean volume of each catheterization is kept to less than 400 ml.[199]

Diabetes mellitus

Bacteriuria and UTIs are more frequent in diabetic than non-diabetic women and the risk of complicated infections is higher. Also, infections tend to be more severe, particularly in patients with insulin-dependent diabetes. In one study, the point prevalence of UTIs at first screening was 3%, and over 18 months 12% of patients showed evidence of acute cystitis. Infection was also more frequent in women than in men (10% vs 5%; $p < 0.01$) and was significantly associated with the presence of peripheral neuropathy ($p < 0.05$).[200] The overall prevalence of significant asymptomatic bacteriuria in adult women with diabetes mellitus varies but is approximately 8% (85 cases per 1072 women).[201] In addition, women with bacteriuria are significantly more likely than non-bacteriuric women to have type 2 diabetes, longer duration of diabetes, peripheral neuropathy and heart disease.[202]

Diabetes mellitus has a number of long-term effects on the genitourinary system. The diabetic is a compromised host and at risk of bacterial cystitis. The increased susceptibility is due to the presence of microvascular disease which results in ischaemia of the bladder wall. This may also result in deficient mobilization of the mediators of the immune response, poor chemotaxis and defective phagocytosis. Diabetic neuropathy may involve the nerve supply to the bladder and result in an atonic detrusor with chronic retention of urine. Local hyperglycaemia, glycosuria and an impaired washout system create an environment within the bladder that is favourable for the growth of microorganisms. The severity and duration, as well as the type of diabetes mellitus, modify all these factors.[202] Because of a combination of these host and local risk factors, bacteriuria is more common in diabetic than non-diabetic women and predisposes them to bacterial cystitis. It is probable that is the increased susceptibility to infection, and not increased bacteriuria, that results in the increased incidence of cystitis in this group. Because infections tend to be more frequent and severe, they are more likely to result in secondary complications such as upper tract infections. Also rare complications are more likely to occur, such as emphysematous pyelonephritis and emphysematous pyelitis, so an early aggressive approach to treatment is recommended. Further investigations are also indicated more often to detect secondary complications and upper tract damage resulting from cystitis.[203]

Pregnancy

Asymptomatic bacteriuria occurs in 4–7% of pregnancies and is associated with the development of acute cystitis, pyelonephritis, preterm labour and low-birth-weight infants. The prevalence of bacteriuria in the first trimester of pregnancy is 5–6%, similar to that in non-pregnant women.[204] Asymptomatic bacteriuria plays an important role in the aetiology of urinary infection: if untreated, up to 30% of women will develop acute cystitis later in pregnancy. Treatment will reduce the infection rate to approximately 3%.[205]

The rate of urinary epithelial cell excretion is increased in pregnancy, and there is loss of the usual relationship between pyuria and urinary infection. Gallery et al. found that in early-morning urine samples, values of 2500 erythrocytes per ml or less and 30 hyaline or granular casts per ml or less can be accepted as normal.[206]

The susceptibility to cystitis in pregnancy may result from incomplete emptying and chronic residual urine due to the weight of the gravid uterus. Bacterial growth is also enhanced in pregnancy. It has been reported that the bacterial count of E. coli in the urine of pregnant women is twice that in non-pregnant women.[207] Women with cystitis and VUR as children have higher rates of cystitis with onset of sexual activity and during pregnancy than the general population.[208] Recurrent infections may also be a problem after delivery in women who have had bacteriuria in pregnancy, occurring in up to 25% of such cases.[209]

Serious infections, including acute cystitis, follow untreated silent bacteriuria in 25% of women.[210] Early detection and effective treatment of asymptomatic bacteriuria early in pregnancy can prevent the later occurrence of symptomatic infections.[211] Thus, information concerning bacteriuria in pregnancy is of particular interest to clinicians. If acute cystitis is not managed effectively, the subsequent risk of developing pyelonephritis is increased. Pyelonephritis is the most frequent severe bacterial infection complicating pregnancy, often with serious consequences. It is thought that up to 20% of women with severe pyelonephritis in pregnancy develop complications that include septic shock syndrome.[212] There have been reports that positive urine cultures for group B streptococci are associated with an increased risk of preterm delivery but this is controversial in the light of new studies. However, a clear association has been demonstrated between elevated levels of urinary antibodies to group B streptococci and E. coli antigens and preterm delivery. This is consistent with the possibility that a local inflammatory response to urogenital infection may be important in stimulating preterm labour.[213]

In a review of recent studies, particularly randomized controlled trials of maternal outcome, Villar and Bergsjø[214] found good evidence that urine culture and dipstick tests for leucocyte esterase and nitrite, with subsequent treatment of positive cases, reduced the risk of pyelonephritis and was cost-effective in pregnancy. This is the rationale for screening all pregnant women for bacteriuria and monitoring throughout pregnancy to identify recurrence after treatment with appropriate antibiotics. There is much criticism of antenatal care but one of the elements of these programmes which is of benefit is screening pregnant women using dipstick tests for leucocyte esterase and nitrite. Many maternity units practise a policy of screening for asymptomatic bacteriuria and treatment to prevent cystitis and pyelonephritis in pregnancy and there is good evidence to support this process. When compared with a policy of no screening, screening for and treatment of asymptomatic bacteriuria to prevent UTI in pregnancy is cost-beneficial whether based on the leucocyte esterase–nitrite dipstick or on urine culture. However, the culture strategy is not cost-beneficial when compared with the dipstick strategy.[215]

Many different screening techniques are used to detect asymptomatic bacteriuria in pregnancy as an alternative to standard urine culture. Bachman *et al.*[216] compared the results of three rapid screening tests with those of urine culture and found that urine dipstick testing for nitrites identified half of all patients with UTIs and was superior to urinalysis on follow-up visits. Although Gram staining is more expensive, it was more accurate for asymptomatic UTIs than urinalysis or urine dipstick testing.[216] Reagent strip testing (RST) such as Ames Multistix 8SG is another method to identify significant bacteriuria in pregnancy and provides a reliable and cheap alternative to microscopy and culture of all urine specimens. False negatives with RST screening are mainly with urine specimens containing low-grade urinary pathogens or genital tract contaminants.[217]

Uriscreen, a new rapid enzymatic screening test in the detection of significant bacteriuria, has been developed and tested in the USA and has been found to be a reliable alternative to culture screening of all pregnant women. It was estimated that a policy of performing urine culture during pregnancy only on women with a positive Uriscreen test would save as many as 80% of unnecessary cultures.[218] Invasive testing is probably best avoided in pregnancy because important correctable abnormalities occur infrequently.

Treatment in pregnancy

Treatment of positive cases will reduce the risk of cystitis and pyelonephritis and appears to be cost-effective.[214] Treatment of bacteriuria prevents up to 80% of cases of pyelonephritis and reduces the risk of preterm delivery.[219,220]

Certain antimicrobial agents should be avoided in pregnancy because of their adverse effects, but the same general principles of management apply as described earlier. Penicillins and cephalosporins are thought to be safe throughout pregnancy.[221] Nitrofurantoin and sulphonamides are safe in the first two trimesters; however, they should be avoided in the third trimester when nitrofurantoin may cause haemolytic anaemia in neonates, and sulphonamides may compete for fetal bilirubin-binding sites on albumin, causing neonatal hyperbilirubinaemia and kernicterus.[222,223] Tetracyclines, because of their chelating action, may cause hypoplasia

and staining of the child's teeth. They may also cause acute maternal liver decompensation and fetal malformations. The estolate salt of erythromycin should be avoided because it may cause cholestatic jaundice. Chloramphenicol may cause neonatal cardiovascular collapse. Fluoroquinolones may have an adverse effect on fetal cartilage formation. Trimethoprim is a folic acid antagonist and it would seem inherently sensible to avoid this drug preconceptually and in the first trimester if one wishes to avail of the benefits of folic acid supplements in preventing neural tube defects.[224]

Children

UTI is much more frequent in children than is widely believed. Greater awareness of the importance of investigation and management of cystitis in children is required because of the likelihood of complications. Low bacterial counts, the absence of pyuria or a finding of sterile pyuria are common in the course of acute or chronic cystitis and should not be disregarded as insignificant.[225] The relationship of acute cystitis and VUR with the potential for renal scarring and serious sequelae is well known.[226]

Jadresic *et al.* carried out a study of 57 432 children aged under 15 years, 7143 children aged under 2 years and their 195 general practitioners. They found that infection was underdiagnosed and, after a confirmed infection, only a minority of children received imaging for complications and microbiology follow-up to assess cure. The study also highlighted the practical difficulties faced by general practitioners as only a minority could obtain bacteriological confirmation of infection at weekends.[227] Voiding difficulties and constipation are also factors associated with UTIs in children.[228]

Asymptomatic bacteriuria is common in children practising clean intermittent catheterization but its significance is uncertain with regard to cystitis and renal scarring. Ottolini *et al.*[229] found that, in the absence of VUR, asymptomatic bacteriuria in these children was not a significant risk factor for renal scarring and does not require antibiotic therapy. UTIs are common in children and infective renal scarring, although rare, may be acquired following LUTI, especially in the presence of VUR, and has a risk of later hypertension and renal insufficiency.[230]

VUR is not usually diagnosed until it is complicated

by ascending UTI. The peak incidence for infection is in early infancy so it may be possible to prevent infections by screening newborn babies for familial ureteric reflux. Scott *et al.*[231] found that screening of pregnant women for VUR was worthwhile because the frequency of VUR among the newborn babies of women with such a history was significantly higher than in the general population (frequency of VUR 1–2%).

Investigation

It is not uncommon for cystitis to present without localizing signs or symptoms in young children, and urine culture maybe difficult to obtain reliably. Febrile infants with no apparent source of fever are twice as likely to have a UTI (7.5%) as those with a possible source of fever such as otitis media (3.5%). In infants with fever, one should consider UTI as a potential source and consider urine culture as part of the diagnostic evaluation.[232] Thus, many cases may go unrecognized and the condition is underdiagnosed in this group. It would therefore be unwise to consider the first diagnosed infection as the primary infection and children should be investigated further once an initial diagnosis is made, irrespective of sex. A delay in the diagnosis of upper tract damage may have profound effects on renal function. Whether a child should be investigated is an individual clinical decision; however, 70–80% of girls with bacteriuria have no radiological evidence of renal scarring when bacteriuria is first diagnosed.[233] Vernon *et al.*[234] found that children with a history of acute cystitis but unscarred kidneys on dimercaptosuccinic acid scans after the third birthday have about a 1 in 40 risk of developing a scar subsequently. After the fourth birthday, the risk is either very low or zero.[234]

With culture results as the validating standard, urinary Gram stain of urine is more reliable than urinalysis in detecting UTIs in young infants.[235] If a child is found to be febrile with pyuria and is suspected of having cystitis, it may be desirable to assess for complications or risk factors. Ultrasonography during bladder contractions is effective in detecting significant ureteric reflux in such cases.[236]

Management

Much of the risk of developing complications following LUTI in children is related to delay in diagnosis, appropriate imaging or in treating a confirmed infection. Efforts to reduce the incidence and severity of renal scarring following cystitis in infancy and childhood should be directed towards rapid diagnosis and early effective treatment.[237]

Treatment of UTIs in children ideally begins with culture-specific antimicrobial therapy, although treatment of a particularly sick child may be started before culture results are available. Treatment of asymptomatic bacteriuria in children is probably unnecessary if the renal tract is otherwise normal.[230]

The choice of antimicrobial agent is governed by the same principles as those employed in adults. In uncomplicated cystitis, short courses of 3–5 days duration is sufficient. If further investigations are required, the child should be maintained on low-dose antibiotic prophylaxis until work-up is complete.[228] Nitrofurantoin macrocrystals are an excellent choice in children and are well tolerated provided the dose does not exceed 3 mg/kg body weight/day. If VUR is diagnosed, effective management will often involve the use of antibiotics as prophylaxis against UTI. Intermittent, low-dose trimethoprim–sulphamethoxazole is effective for the prevention of recurrent UTI in children with VUR, even of higher grades.[238]

Compared with adults children rarely show serious adverse reactions to drugs. This is probably due to more cautious prescribing of the more toxic agents, the use of a limited number of drugs and attention to prescribing according to body weight.

Long-term suppressive therapy may be indicated in children with gross VUR or in cases of recurrent episodes of acute cystitis. The duration of suppressive therapy is judged by the results of subsequent investigations and may vary from 6 months to several years.

Renal transplant

Episodes of cystitis are frequent after renal transplant and may lead to upper tract infections. Muller *et al.*[239] have also shown that they are an important risk factor for the onset of chronic rejection, and that early and intense treatment is critical.[239] Goya *et al.* found that acute cystitis is common in the early period following renal transplantation, and administration of antimicrobial prophylaxis for approximately 4 months is recommended.[240]

The use of dipstick tests to exclude significant bacteriuria and reduce the necessity for routine microscopy and culture has been assessed in renal transplant patients. These tests appear to have a relatively low sensitivity and positive predictive value because of the underlying condition and therapies employed in these patients. Traditional microscopy and culture methods are more reliable and are recommended in these cases.[241]

Human immunodeficiency virus

Human immunodeficiency virus (HIV) infections can lead to UTIs and disturbances in micturition. However, urological disorders are usually due to complications of the infection involving higher centres of the brain, leading to voiding dysfunction.[242] HIV immunosuppression has been linked with an increased risk of developing urinary infections in men; however, this is not the case in women. Although high rates of significant bacteriuria can occur in women who are highly sexually active, this appears to be unrelated to HIV infection or the level of HIV-related immunosuppression and is generally asymptomatic or clinically indistinct.[243] If women do present with recurrent cystitis and have HIV infection, because of the complexity of urodynamic abnormalities in such subjects, urodynamic evaluation is essential for accurate diagnosis and treatment.[244]

Analgesia

Urinary discomfort is the second most common physical complaint affecting women and, in the case of cystitis, is a result of the inflammation that occurs with bacterial invasion of the bladder wall. In addition to antimicrobials, one should consider the use of urinary analgesics or antispasmodics for effective management.[245]

Antiseptics

There is some evidence that drinking cranberry juice can prevent recurrent cystitis. Cranberry juice is metabolized to hippuric acid, which probably has urinary antimicrobial activity by virtue of an acidifying effect on bladder urine.[246]

Post-therapy bacteriuria

The interpretation of bacteriologic outcome of antibiotic treatment for uncomplicated cystitis is often diffi-

cult and depends on the definition of significant bacteriuria used in the study or clinical setting. This was demonstrated in a large multicentre, randomized, double-blind, controlled trial of two antibiotics used to treat women with uncomplicated cystitis. Bacteriuria persisting for 5–9 days after the completion of therapy was documented in more women taking ritipenem acoxil than in those taking norfloxacin, but the two groups did not differ markedly with regard to bacteriological or clinical outcome 3–4 weeks after treatment.[247] Subanalyses of bacteriological outcome showed that failure rates varied between 6 and 67% for ritipenem and between 1 and 43% for norfloxacin, depending on management. It is still unclear how best to define significant post-therapy bacteriuria.

Prevention of cystitis

In a prospective randomized study of women undergoing caesarean section, Nagele *et al.*[248] analysed whether non-closure of the visceral peritoneum had advantages over suture peritonization with regard to postoperative morbidity. The incidence of febrile morbidity and cystitis and the need for antibiotics were all significantly greater when the peritoneum was closed. On this basis, they recommended that routine closure of the visceral peritoneum at caesarean delivery should be abandoned.[248]

Urethritis

Urethritis is defined as inflammation of the urethra. The clinical presentation is almost identical to that of acute cystitis, so there is considerable overlap in the assessment and investigation of both conditions. Significant urinary frequency due to urethritis in children is more common than is generally appreciated.[249]

The female urethral syndrome is a condition characterized by a lack of objective findings but with subjective complaints of retropubic pressure, dyspareunia, diurnal urinary frequency, dysuria and urethral irritation.[250] Sometimes sterile pyuria of unknown aetiology is also present. The pathogenesis of the urethral syndrome is not known and a specific secondary cause can be identified in only a minority of women.[251] There is no evidence of abnormal detrusor or urethral activity or any disease of the urinary tract. It is a condition of younger women, but can occur in any age group. In a study by Baldoni *et al.*,[252] women with a diagnosis of urethral syndrome found that their irritative symptoms were exacerbated in highly stressful situations.

PATHOGENESIS OF URETHRITIS

The urethral flora, like that of the vagina, is altered by age, local changes in pH, the use of antimicrobial drugs and reduced cellular glycogen. The microorganisms isolated from women with urethritis show the same virulence factors as the uropathogens causing acute cystitis. P-adhesion-expressing *E. coli* are commonly isolated from women with cystitis but the expression of these virulence factors on periurethral *E. coli* does not usually predict subsequent urethritis or periurethral infection.[17] Marrie *et al.*[253] showed that coliform organisms are only rarely isolated from the vaginal vestibule and external urethra of healthy premenopausal women and women of reproductive age. Inflammation is not always limited to the urethra but may also involve the bladder wall.[254]

There is now strong evidence that the microscopic para-urethral glands connected to the distal third of the urethra in the paravaginal space (homologous to the prostate) may become infected. This may be demonstrated clinically by palpating for localized tenderness and swelling through the anterior vaginal wall to one or both sides of the urethra.[250] However, because of their inaccessibility, the microbiology of the para-urethral glands and how they act as reservoirs for recurrent urethritis is incompletely understood.

It has been estimated that up to 50% of the US population will acquire a sexually transmitted disease by age 30–35 years.[255] *Chlamydia trachomatis* is the most common sexually transmitted bacteria in the industrialized world, with a prevalence of up to 20% in sexually active persons aged 25 years or less. Urethritis is one of the most common manifestations in women.[256] The most important and common causes of urethritis are infection with *C. trachomatis* and *Neisseria gonorrhoea*. Chlamydia infection of the urethra may occur concurrently in many cases of pelvic infection, and may be asymptomatic with no subjective signs of urinary frequency or dysuria.[257]

Gonococcal infection is often not confined to the urethra. On the basis of suprapubic aspiration, ascendant propagation of bacteria to the bladder was observed in 34.2% of women with gonococcal urethritis.[261]

Other infective causes of non-gonococcal urethritis include: *Ureaplasma urealyticum*, *Trichomonas vaginalis* and herpes simplex virus; rare causes include *Gardnerella vaginalis*, *S. saprophyticus*, *Candida albicans* and non-albicans.

Inflammatory reactions of the urethral wall are also known to occur by repeated introductions of a catheter into the urethra. The result may vary from minor degrees of inflammation to frank urethritis and postinflammatory urethral stricture formation.[259] With long-term follow-up, urethritis has been reported to occur in up to 19% of patients performing CISC.[260] Complications may be reduced by use of lubricants and smaller size catheters. Hydrophilic catheters, which bind water molecules to the catheter surface, are also recommended so that less trauma is induced. Indeed, urethral cytology has shown that women using such catheters have significantly less evidence of inflammation locally than women using conventional PVC catheters.[261]

INVESTIGATION OF URETHRITIS

Urethritis is a common cause of chronic pelvic pain in women and a careful history, with emphasis on urinary symptoms, may be the key to directing the investigations.[262] A thorough sexual history of the patient, including evaluation of sexual partners, is mandatory. Clinical evidence of infections, both locally and systematically, should be sought. This must be backed up by microbiological tests to document positive cultures.

The diagnosis may be made on the basis of the history, the clinical finding of a urethra that is tender to palpation, the presence of pus cells and culture of the same uropathogens as in cystitis but at much lower bacterial counts. Approximately 90% of women with 'low-count' bacteriuria will have pyuria that suggests urethritis.[71] It has been suggested that a differential in the urethrovesical urinary white cell count may distinguish urethritis from cystitis. The first 50 ml of voided urine probably contain the cells of the urethra. This count can be compared with another specimen passed at the end of micturition.[263]

Urethral swabs for culture and sensitivity may also be helpful in determining the presence and nature of urethritis. Swabs should be obtained at least 1 hour after the patient has urinated, to avoid contamination with bladder urine. The swab needs to be inserted approximately 3 cm into the urethra and rotated. Cotton swabs have a bactericidal effect and should be avoided.[264] Urethral smears are also useful in confirming evidence of inflammatory cells. Direct plating of specimens should be done for Gram staining as well as inoculation onto culture medium. In a Gram-stained urethral smear, more than four PMN leucocytes per hpf is strongly associated with urethritis. Alternatively, the presence of 15 or more PMN leucocytes in five random 400-power fields of the spun sediment of the first-void urine correlates with urethritis.[257,265]

C. trachomatis urethritis is often difficult to diagnose and needs expensive cell culture methods that are technically difficult. Horner *et al.*[257] demonstrated that, using a Gram-stained urethral smear, *C. trachomatis* infection of the urethra was strongly associated with five or more PMN leucocytes per hpf ($p < 0.0005$). Enzyme immunoassay (Chlamydiazyme) is used for the detection of chlamydial antigen. It is performed on the sediment of first-voided urine samples and is a reliable, rapid and non-invasive method of diagnosing chlamydia infection in men. However, it is not as specific and is considerably less sensitive in women.[266] Cystourethroscopy may be necessary and is also a useful means of differentiating cystitis from urethritis.

Ultrasonography has been used to investigate the urethrae of women who have frequency and urgency symptoms but is of somewhat limited value. Many have bladder-neck and sphincter incompetence, but these findings do not correlate well with clinical symptoms. In a study by Kuo,[267] transrectal ultrasonography was used to investigate the urethrae of women who had symptoms of frequency and urgency. Many had bladder-neck and sphincter incompetence but these findings did not correlate well with clinical symptoms. In addition, ultrasonography could not differentiate symptoms caused by the bladder from those caused by the urethra.[267]

High-resolution magnetic resonance imaging (MRI) with phased-array pelvic and endorectal coils has dramatically enhanced the ability to visualize abnormalities of the female urethra, including diverticulum, urethral trauma, fistula formation and periurethral abscesses.[268] Endovaginal MRI can be used to clearly demonstrate the anatomy of the urethra and also has a role in the evaluation of complex urethral and periurethral anomalies.[269,270]

TREATMENT OF URETHRITIS

Women presenting with symptoms suggestive of urethral syndrome are best assessed and managed using a multidisciplinary approach. Options should include local therapy, pain relief, possibly with the expertise of a pain-management team, and psychological support. Invasive and irreversible therapeutic or surgical procedures should be reserved as final options.

Single-dose antimicrobial regimens offer the advantage of reduced cost, good tolerability, minimal alteration of normal bacterial flora and the potential for good patient compliance. If empirical antimicrobial therapy is being considered for non-gonococcal urethritis, then tetracyclines such as doxycycline have an unusually broad spectrum of antimicrobial activity, are well tolerated and have a good safety profile.[271] Ofroxacin, 400 mg once daily for 7 days, is a safe and effective alternative to doxycycline in the treatment of non-gonococcal urethritis.[272] In a randomized, double-blind trial, minocycline, 100 mg nightly, was as effective as doxycycline, 200 mg nightly, (for 7 days) in the treatment of non-gonococcal urethritis, but was associated with less vomiting and gastrointestinal upset.[273]

Clinical cure rates for non-chlamydial, non-gonococcal urethritis are in excess of 85%, while eradication of *Chlamydia* occurs in almost 100% of cases. Azithromycin is an azalide antibiotic with substantial activity against *C. trachomatis*.[274,275] It is concentrated intracellularly and has a long half-life in serum and urethral tissues. A single 1 g dose of azithromycin was as effective for the treatment of uncomplicated chlamydial urethritis as a standard 7-day course of doxycycline and is proving to be an excellent alternative.[276]

Treatment of gonococcal urethritis is usually by a single intramuscular dose of ceftriaxone. Trovafloxacin is a new quinolone antibiotic with enhanced activity against *N. gonorrhoea*. Jones *et al.*[277] in the Trovafloxacin Gonorrhoea Study Group in the USA found that it compared favourably with ofloxacin as an excellent single-dose therapy for uncomplicated gonococcal urethritis.

Post-gonococcal urethritis due to concomitant *Chlamydia* infection has been found in 30.1% of patients. Because there is often this concomitant infection, a regimen of antimicrobials active against *Chlamydia* and non-gonococcal urethritis is recommended (for both patients and their partners) by the Centres for Disease Control.[278,279] This requires a 7-day treatment with a tetracycline. Alternatives include ofloxacin, 300 mg for 7 days, or azithromycin. Using these recommended regimens, microbiological cure rates are high in compliant women.[280]

Summary

As many as 50% of women report having at least one episode of cystitis in their lifetime. The normal urinary tract is sterile. Bacteria are flushed away periodically by urine and mucus flow, uroepithelial bactericidal activity and urinary secretory immunoglobulins. The prevalence of cystitis is modified by many factors. Those elements which contribute most are: lack of physical mobility and generalized ill-health in the patient, voiding difficulty with chronic residual urine, and urinary tract instrumentation. Organisms become pathogenic by virtue of their ability to survive and multiply in bladder urine. The presence of fimbriae or pili confers the ability to adhere to and colonize urothelial cells.

Acute cystitis may become a complicated UTI in the presence of structural abnormalities, metabolic abnormalities, abnormalities of the host response or uncommon, virulent and resistant uropathogens. We are gaining a better understanding of microbial virulence factors but much of the pathogenesis is unclear. In some cases the causative uropathogens are easily predictable and management strategies in uncomplicated cases depend on empirical therapy without urine culture. A more rigid approach with pretherapy culture, antimicrobial sensitivity tests and follow-up post-treatment cultures to demonstrate both clinical and microbiological cure should be mandatory in complicated cases. Provided the woman has a previously normal urinary tract, recurrent bacteriuria and cystitis is unlikely to cause upper tract complications. However, the need for investigation of the urinary tract, including more invasive testing, should also be considered for individual cases. Too often management strategies depend on clinical biases and trial and error, without any particular strategy. Primary-care clinics that have implemented systems and tools to support nurse-coordinated care of patients with cystitis have been very successful with respect to cost of care and clinical outcome. The use of clinical guidelines to manage uncomplicated cystitis coordinated primarily by the nurse practitioner should be encouraged.

Specialist care with the appropriate expertise, facilities for assessment and investigations, as well as a system of follow-up evaluation, must be available for the more difficult cases.

Future research is likely to focus on genetically determined cellular mechanisms that predispose individuals to isolated and recurrent UTIs.

REFERENCES

1. National Center for Health Statistics: 1985 Summary. National ambulatory medical care survey. *Adv Data* 1985; 128: 1–8

2. Asscher AW. Urinary tract infections. *J R Coll Physicians London* 1981; 15: 232–238

3. McLachlan M, Meller S, Jones E *et al*. Urinary tract in schoolgirls with covert bacteriuria. *Arch Dis Child* 1975; 50: 253–258

4. Yamamoto S, Tsukamoto T, Terai *et al*. Genetic evidence supporting the faecal–perineal–urethral hypothesis in cystitis caused by Escherichia coli. *J Urol* 1997; 157: 1127–1129

5. Johnson J, Brown J, Carlino U, Russo T. Colonisation with and acquisition of uropathogenic Escherichia coli as revealed by polymerase chain reaction-based detection. *J Infect Dis* 1998; 177: 1120–1124

6. Kallenius G, Svenson S, Hultberg H *et al*. P-fimbriae of pyelonephrogenic Escherichia coli: Significance for reflux and renal scarring – a hypothesis. *Infections* 1983: 11: 73–76

7. Kunin CM. *Detection, Prevention and Management of Urinary Tract Infection*. Philadelphia: Lea and Febiger, 1987; 57–124

8. Bollgren I, Winberg J. The periurethral aerobic flora in girls highly susceptible to urinary infections. *Acta Paediatr Scand* 1976; 65: 81–87

9. Stamey T, Sexton C. The role of vaginal colonisation. Enterobacteriaceae in recurrent urinary infections. *J Urol* 1975; 113: 214–217

10. Foxman B, Zhang L, Tallman P *et al*. Virulence characteristics of Escherichia coli causing first urinary tract infection predict risk of second infection. *J Infect Dis* 1995; 172: 1536–1541

11. Stamey TA. *Urinary Infections*. Baltimore: Williams & Wilkins, 1972

12. Lapides J. Pathophysiology of urinary tract infections. *Univ Michigan Medical Centre J* 1973; 39: 103–112

13. O' Grady F, Cattell WR. Kinetics of urinary tract infection II. The Bladder. *Br J Urol* 1966; 38: 156–162

14. O' Grady F, Richards B, McSherry M *et al.* Introital enter-obacteria, urinary infection and the urethral syndrome. *Lancet* 1970; 2: 1208–1210

15. Schlager TA, Whittam TS, Hendley JO *et al.* Comparison of expression of virulence factors by Escherichia coli causing cystitis and E. coli colonising the periurethra of healthy girls. *J Infect Dis* 1995; 172: 772–777

16. Wisinger DB. Urinary tract infection. Current management strategies. *Postgrad Med* 1996; 100: 229–236

17. Asscher A, Sussman M, Waters W *et al.* The clinical significance of asymptomatic bacteriuria in the non-pregnant woman. *J Infect Dis* 1969; 120: 17–21

18. Mabeck CE. Uncomplicated urinary tract infections in women. *Proc R Soc Med* 1971; 3: 31–35

19. Mannhardt W, Becker A, Putzer M *et al.* Host defence within the urinary tract. Bacterial adhesion initiates a uroepithelial defence mechanism. *Pediatr Nephrol* 1996; 10: 568–572

20. Schegel J, Cuellar J, O' Dell R. Bactericidal effect of urea. *J Urol* 1961; 86: 819–821

21. Culham D, Delgado C, Gyles C *et al.* Osmoregulatory transporter Prop influences colonisation of the urinary tract by Escherichia coli. *Microbiology* 1998; 144: 91–102

22. Norden C, Green G, Kass E. Antibacterial mechanisms of the urinary bladder. *J Clin Invest* 1968; 47: 2689–2700

23. Hicks R. The mammalian urinary bladder: an accommodating organ. *Biol Rev* 1975; 50: 215–246.

24. Lundberg JO, Ehren I, Jansson O *et al.* Elevated nitric oxide in the urinary bladder in infectious and non-infectious cystitis. *Urology* 1996; 48: 700–702

25. Natsis K, Toliou T, Stravoravdi P *et al.* Natural killer cell assay within bladder mucosa of patients bearing transitional cell carcinoma after interferon therapy: an immunohistochemical and ultrastructural study. *Int J Clin Pharm Res* 1997; 17: 31–36

26. Parsons C, Pollen J, Anwar H *et al.* Antibacterial activity of bladder surface mucin duplicated in the rabbit bladder by exogenous glycosaminoglcan (sodium pentosampolysulfate). *Infect Immun* 1980; 27: 876–881

27. Mulholland S, Qureshi S, Fritz R *et al.* Effect of hormonal deprivation on the bladder defence mechanism. *J Urol* 1982; 127: 1010–1013

28. Bartlett J, Onderdon A, Drude E *et al.* Quantitative bacteriology of the vaginal flora. *J Infect Dis* 1977; 136: 271–277

29. Burdon D. Immunoglobulins of the urinary tract, discussion on a possible role in urinary tract infection. In: Brumfitt W, Asscher A (eds) *Urinary Tract Infection.* London: Oxford University Press, 1973: 148–158

30. Tomasi TB. Mechanisms of immune regulation at mucosal surfaces. *Dev Infect Dis* 1983; 5: 5784–5792

31. Svanborg-Eden C, Svennerholm A. Secretory immunoglobulin A and G antibodies prevent adhesion of Escherichia to human urinary tract epithelial cells. *Infect Immun* 1978; 22: 790–797

32. Riedasch G, Heck P, Rauterberg E *et al.* Does low urinary IgA predispose to urinary tract infection? *Kidney Int* 1983; 23: 759–763

33. Jenkins MA. Clinical application of capillary electrophoresis to unconcentrated human urine proteins. *Electrophoresis* 1997; 18: 1842–1846

34. Tamm I, Horsfall F. Mucoprotein derived from human urine which reacts with influenza, mumps and Newcastle disease viruses. *J Exp Med* 1952; 95: 71–97

35. Kuriyama S, Silverblatt F. Effect of Tamm-Horsfall urinary glycoprotein on phagocytosis and killing of type I-fimbriated E. coli. *Infect Immun* 1986; 51: 193–198

36. Jelakovic B, Benkovic J, Cikes N *et al.* Antibodies to Tamm–Horsfall protein subunit prepared in vitro, in patients with acute pyelonephritis. *Eur J Clin Chem Clin Biochem* 1996: 34: 315–317

37. Hanson LA, Fasth A, Jodal U. Auto-antibodies to Tamm–Horsfall protein, a tool for diagnosing the level of urinary tract infection. *Lancet* 1976; 1: 226–228

38. Hopkins W, Heisey D, Lorentzen D, Venling D. A comparative study of major histocompatibility complex and red blood cell antigen phenotypes as risk factors for recurrent urinary tract infections in women. *J infect Dis* 1998; 177: 1296–1301

39. Yamamoto S, Wakata K, Yuri K *et al.* Assessment of the significance of virulence factors of uropathogenic Escherichia coli in experimental urinary tract infection in mice. *Microbiol Immunol* 1996; 40: 607–610

40. Fowler J, Stamey T. Studies of introital colonisation in women with recurrent urinary tract infections. VII. The role of bacterial adherence. *J Urol* 1977; 117: 472–476

41. Kozody, NL, Harding GK, Nicolle LE *et al.* Adherence of Escherichia coli to epithelial cells in the pathogenesis of urinary tract infection. *Clin Invest Med* 1985; 8: 121–125

42. Svanborg C, Hedlund M, Connell H *et al.* Bacterial adherence and mucosal cytokine responses. Receptors and transmembrane signaling. *Ann New York Acad Sci* 1996; 797: 177–190

43. Roberts JA. Factors predisposing to urinary tract infections in children. *Pediatr Nephrol* 1996; 10: 517–522

44. Svanborg-Eden C, Korhonen T, Lettler R Marild S. Pathogenic aspects of bacterial adherence in urinary tract infections. In: Losse H, Asscher A, Lison A (eds) *Pyelonephritis Vol IV, Urinary Tract Infection.* Stuttgart: Georg Thieme Verlag, 1980; 54–59

45. Domisgue G, Roberts H, Laucirica R *et al.* Pathogenic significance of P-fimbriated Escherichia Coli in urinary tract infections. *J Urol* 1985; 133: 983–989

46. Bullitt E, Makowski L. Bacterial adhesion pili are heterologous assemblies of similar subunits. *Biophys J* 1998; 74: 623–632

47. Blanco M, Blanco JE, Alonso MP, Blanco J. Virulence factors and O groups of Escherichia Coli isolates from patients with acute pyelonephritis, cystitis and asymptomatic bacteriuria. *Eur J Epidemiol* 1996; 12: 191–198

48. Ikaheimo P, Siitonen A, Karkkainen V *et al.* Characteristics of Escherichia coli in acute community-acquired cystitis of adult women. *Scand J Infect Dis* 1993; 25: 705–712

49. Funfstruck P, Smith J, Tschape H, Stein G. Pathogenic aspects of uncomplicated urinary tract infection: recent advances. *Clin Nephrol* 1997; 47: 13–18

50. Brooks H, O' Grady F, McSherry M, Cattell W. Uropathogenic properties of Escherichia coli in recurrent urinary tract infection. *J Med Microbiol* 1980; 13: 57–68

51. Finkelstein R, Scirotino C, McIntosh M. Role of iron in microbe–host interactions. *Rev Infect Dis* 1983; 5: 5759–5777

52. Hughes C, Hacker J, Roberts *et al.* Hemolysin production as a virulence maker in symptomatic and asymptomatic urinary tract infections caused by Escherichia coli. *Infect Immun* 1983; 39: 546–551

53. Connell R, de Man P, Jodal V *et al.* Lack of association between hemolysin production and acute inflammation in human urinary tract infection. *Microbiol Pathog* 1993; 14: 463–472

54. Montgomerie J, Bindereif A, Neilands J *et al.* Association of hydroxamate siderophore (aerobactin) with Escherichia coli isolated from patients with bacteremia. *Infect Immun* 1984; 46: 835–838

55. Hull P, Rudy D, Wieser I, Donovan W. Virulence factors of Escherichia coli isolates from patients with symptomatic and asymptomatic bacteriuria and neuropathic bladders due to spinal cord and brain injuries. *J Clin Microbiol* 1998; 36: 115–117

56. Stamey TA. Editorial: a clinical classification of urinary tract infections based upon origins. *South Med J* 1975; 68: 934

57. Hooton TM, Stamm WE. Diagnosis and treatment of uncomplicated urinary tract infection. *Infect Dis Clin North Am* 1997; 11: 551–581

58. Jarvis WR, Munn VP, Highsmith AK *et al.* The epidemiology of nosocomial infections. *Infect Control* 1985; 6: 68–74

59. Barnett BJ, Stephens DS. Urinary tract infection: an overview. *Am J Med Sci* 1997; 314: 245–249

60. Svanborg C, Godaly G. Bacterial virulence in urinary tract infection. *Infect Dis Clin North Am* 1997; 11: 513–529

61. Tolson P, Harrison B, Latta R *et al.* The expression of nonagglutinating fimbriae and its role in proteus mirabilis adherence to epithelial cells. *Can J Microbiol* 1997; 43: 709–717

62. Neu H. Urinary tract infections. *Am J Med* 1992, 92; 635–705

63. Kass EH. Asymptomatic infections of the urinary tract. *Trans Assoc Am Phys* 1956; 69: 56–64

64. Kass EH. The role of asymptomatic bacteriuria in the pathogenesis of pyelonephritis. In: Quinn EL, Kass EH (eds) *Biology of Pyelonephritis.* Boston: Little, Brown, 1960; 399–406

65. Stark R, Maki D. Bacteriuria in the catheterised patient. What quantitative level of bacteriuria is relevant? *N Engl J Med* 1984; 311: 560–564

66. Roberts AP, Robinson RE, Beard RW. Some factors affecting bacterial colony counts in urinary infection. *Br Med J* 1967; 1: 400–403

67. Kraft JK, Stamey TA. The natural history of symptomatic recurrent bacteriuria in women. *Medicine (Baltimore)* 1977; 56: 55–60

68. Mabeck CE. Studies in urinary tract infections: I The diagnosis of bacteriuria in women. *Acta Med Scand* 1969; 186: 1–2, 35–38

69. Kunin CM, White LV, Hua TH. A reassessment of the importance of the ìlow countî bacteriuria in young women with acute urinary symptoms. *Ann Int Med* 1993; 119: 454–460

70. Stamm WE. Quantitative urine cultures revisited. *Eur J Clin Microbiol* 1984; 3: 279–281

71. Stamm WE, Counts GW, Running KR *et al.* Diagnosis of coliform infection in acutely dysuric women. *N Engl J Med* 1982; 307: 463–468

72. Hindman R, Tronic B, Bartlett R. Effect of delay on culture of urine. *J Chem Microbiol* 1976; 4: 102–103

73. Beard RW, McCoy DR, Newton JR, Clayton SG. Diagnosis of urinary infections by suprapubic bladder puncture. *Lancet* 1965; 2: 610–611

74. Cohen HA, Woloch B, Linder N *et al.* Urine samples from disposable diapers: an accurate method for urine cultures. *J Fam Pract* 1997; 44: 209–212

75. Whitehall J, Shvartzman P, Muller MA. A novel method for isolating and quantifying urine pathogens collected from gel-based diapers. *J Fam Pract* 1995; 40: 476–479

76. Wagner MG, Smith FG, Tinglof BL *et al.* Epidemiology of proteinuria—a study of 4,807 school children. *J Paediatr* 1968; 73: 825–832

77. Morgan MG, McKenzie H. Controversies in the laboratory diagnosis of community-acquired urinary tract infection. *Eur J Clin Microbiol Infect Dis* 1993; 12: 491–504

78. Maskell R, Polak A. Bacteriological facilities for the diagnosis of urinary infection in general practice. In: Brumfitt W, Asscher A (eds) Urinary Tract Infections. Oxford: Oxford University Press; 3–10

79. Bailey RR, Blake E. A simple test for detecting pyuria. *NZ Med J* 1981; 682: 269–270

80. Perry JL, Wessner DE, Matthews JS, Wessner DE. Evaluation of leukocyte esterase activity as a rapid screening technique for bacteriuria. *J Clin Microbiol* 1982; 15: 852–854

81. Jou W, Powers R. Utility of dipstick urinalysis as a guide to management of adults with suspected infection or haematuria. *South Med J* 1998; 91: 266–269

82. Kopp J, Miller K, Mican J et al. Crystalluria and urinary tract abnormalities associated with indinavir. Ann Int Med 1997; 127: 119–125

83. Kunin CM, De Groot JE. Sensitivity of a nitrite indicator strip method in detecting bacteriuria in pre-school girls. *Paediatrics* 1977; 60: 244–245

84. Kunin CM. The quantitative significance of bacteria visualised in the unstained urinary sediment. *N Engl J Med* 1961; 265: 589–590

85. Robins DG, White RA, Rogers KB, Osman MS. Urine microscopy as an aid to detection of bacteriuria. *Lancet* 1975, 1: 476–478

86. Arneil GC, McAllister TA, Kay P. Measurement of bacteriuria by plain dipslide culture. *Lancet* 1973, 1: 94–95

87. Ellner PD, Papchristos T. Detection of bacteriuria by dipslide. *Am J Clin Pathol* 1975; 63: 516–521

88. Brumfitt W, Hamilton-Miller JMT. Urinary infection in the 1990s: the state of the art. *Infection* 1990; 18 (Suppl): 534–539

89. Hoberman A, Wald E. Urinary tract infections in young febrile children. *Pediatr Infect Dis J* 1997; 16: 11–17

90. Kurowski K. The women with dysuria. *Am Fam Phys* 1998; 57: 2155-2164; 2169–2170

91. Busch R, Huland H. Correlation of symptoms and results of direct bacterial localisation in patients with urinary tract infections. *J Urol* 1984; 132: 282–285

92. Mond NC, Percival A, Williams JD, Brumfitt W. Presentation, diagnosis and treatment of urinary tract infections in general practice. *Lancet* 1965, 1: 514–516

93. Yoshikawa TT, Norman DC. Approach to fever and infection in the nursing home. *J Am Geriat Soc* 1996; 44: 74–82

94. Pollock H. Laboratory techniques for detection of urinary tract infections and assessment of value. *Am J Med* 1983; 75: 79–84

95. Fairley KF, Carson NE, Gutch RC *et al.* Site of infection in acute urinary tract infection in general practice. *Lancet* 1971; 2: 615–618

96. Kuhlemeier KV, Lloyd LK, Storer SL. Failure of antibody-coated bacteria and bladder washout tests to localise infection in spinal cord injury patients. *J Urol* 1983; 130: 729–732

97. Marple CD. The frequency and character of urinary tract infections in an unselected group of women. *Ann Intern Med* 1941; 14: 2220

98. Stamey TA, Fair WR, Timothy M *et al.* Serum versus urinary antimicrobial concentrations in cure of urinary tract infections. *New Engl J Med* 1974; 291: 1159–1163

99. Monzon OT, Ory EM, Dobson HL. A comparison of bacterial counts of urine obtained by needle aspirations of the bladder catheterisation and mid-stream voided methods. *N Engl J Med* 1958; 259: 764–769

100. Thomas V, Shelokov A, Forland M. Antibody-coated bacteria in the urine and the site of urinary tract infection. *N Engl J Med* 1974; 290: 588–590

101. Rubin RR, Fang LT, Jones ST *et al.* Single dose amoxycillin therapy for urinary tract infection. *J Am Med Assoc* 1980; 244: 561–564

102. Forsum V, Hjelm E, Jonsell G. Antibody-coated bacteria in the urine of children with urinary tract infections. *Acta Paediatr Scand* 1976; 65: 639–642

103. Harding GK, Marrie TJ, Ronald AR *et al.* Urinary tract infection localization in women. *J Am Med Assoc* 1978; 240: 1147–1151

104. Mundt KA, Polk BF. Identification of site of urinary tract infections by antibody coated bacteria assay. *Lancet* 1979; 2: 1172–1175

105. Jodal U, Hanson LA. Sequential determination of C-reactive protein in acute childhood pyelonephritis. *Acta Paediatr Scand* 1976; 65: 319–322

106. Percival A, Brumfitt W, De Louvois J. Serum antibody levels as an indicator of clinically inapparent pyelonephritis. *Lancet* 1964; 2: 1027–1033

107. Ratner JJ, Thomas VA, Sandford BA, Forland M. Bacteria specific antibody in the urine of patients with acute pyelonephritis and cystitis. *J Infect Dis* 1981; 143: 404–412

108. Bailey RR. Management of lower urinary tract infections. *Drugs* 1993; 45 (Suppl 3): 139–144

109. Nicolle LE, Norris M, Finlayson M. Haemagglutination characteristics of Escherichia coli isolates from elderly women with asymptomatic bacteriuria. In: Kass EH, Svanborg-Eden C (eds) *Host-Parasite Interactions in Urinary Tract Infections.* Chicago: University of Chicago Press 1989; 62–65

110. Martinell J, Clarsson I, Lidin-Janson G, Jodal V. Urinary infection, reflux and renal scarring in females continuously followed for 13–38 years. *Pediatr Nephrol* 1995;9: 131–136

111. Van Gool JD, Kiyverberg MA, De Jong TP. Functional daytime incontinence: Clinical and urodynamic assessment. *Scand J Urol Nephrol Suppl* 1992; 141: 58–69

112. Qvist N, Nielsen KK, Kristensen ES *et al*. Detrusor instability in children with recurrent urinary tract infections and or enuresis. II. Treatment. *Urol Int* 1986; 41: 199–201

113. Vessey MP, Metcalfe M, McPherson K, Yeates D. Urinary tract infection in relation to diaphragm use and obesity. *Int J Epidemiol* 1987; 16: 441–444

114. Foxman B, Frerichs R. Epidemiology of urinary tract infection: II Diet, clothing and urination habits. *Am J Public Health* 1985; 75: 1314–1317

115. Elster A, Lach P, Roghmann K, McAnarney E. Relationship between frequency of sexual intercourse and urinary tract infections in young women. *South Med J* 1981; 74: 704–708

116. Foxman B, Chi J. Health behaviour and urinary tract infections in college-aged women. *J Clin Epidemiol* 1990; 43: 329–337

117. Nicolle LE, Harding GM, Preiksaitis J, Ronald AR. The association of urinary tract infection with sexual intercourse. *J Infect Dis* 1982; 146: 579–583

118. Leibovici L, Alpert G, Laor A *et al*. Urinary tract infections and sexual activity in young women. *Arch Int Med* 1987; 147: 345–347

119. Dennis R. Gurwith M, Gurwith D *et al*. Risk factors for urinary tract infection. *Am J Epidemiol* 1987; 126: 685–694

120. Hooton T, Scholes D, Hughes J. A prospective study of risk factors for symptomatic urinary tract infection in young women. *N Engl J Med* 1996; 335: 468-474

121. Foxman B, Zhang L, Tallman P *et al*. Transmission of uropathogens between sex partners. *J Infect Dis* 1997; 175: 989–992

122. Fihn SD, Johnson C, Roberts P *et al*. Associations between diaphragm use and urinary tract infection *J Am Med Assoc* 1985; 254: 240–245

123. Warren J, Platt R, Thomas R *et al*. Antibiotic irrigation and catheter-associated urinary tract infections. *N Engl J Med* 1978; 299: 570–573

124. Maizels M, Schaeffer A. Decreased incidence of bacteriuria associated with periodic installations of hydrogen peroxide into the urethral catheter drainage bag. *J Urol* 1980; 123: 841–845

125. Riley DK, Classen DC, Stevens LE, Burke JP. A large randomised clinical trial of a silver-impregnated urinary catheter: lack of efficacy and staphylococcal- superinfection. *Am J Med* 1995; 98: 349–356

126. Shmmit RL, Storal TG, Bran DF. Prospective comparisons of indwelling bladder catheter drainage versus no catheter after vaginal hysterectomy. *Am J Obstet Gynecol* 1994; 170: 1815–1818

127. Clark KR, Higgs MJ. Urinary infection following outpatient flexible cystoscopy. *Br J Urol* 1990; 66: 503–505

128. Hansoon S, Hyalmas K, Jodal V, Sixt R. Lower urinary tract dysfunction in girls with untreated asymptomatic or covert bacteriuria. *J Urol* 1990; 143: 313–315

129. Lidefelt K, Erasmie U, Bollgren I. Residual urine in children with acute cystitis and in healthy children: assessment by sonography. *J Urol* 1989; 141: 916–917

130. Wheeler J, Culkin D, Walter J, Flanigan R. Female urinary retention. *Urology* 1990; 35: 428–432

131. Madersbacher S, Pycha A, Schatzl G *et al*. The ageing lower urinary tract: a comparative urodynamic – study of men and women. *Urology* 1998; 51: 206–212

132. Baker R, Barbaris. HT. Comparative results of urological evaluation of children with initial and recurrent urinary tract infections. *J Urol* 1976; 116: 503–505

133. Meers PD. Infection in hospitals. *Br Med J* 1981; 282: 1246

134. Sanderson PJ, Alshafi KM. Environmental contamination by organisms causing urinary tract infection. *J Hosp Infect* 1995; 29: 301–303

135. Sheinfeld J, Schaeffer AJ, Cordon-Cardo C *et al*. Association of the Lewis blood group phenotype with recurrent urinary tract infections in women. *N Engl J Med* 1989; 320: 773–777.

136. Jacobson SH, Kallenius G, Luis LE, Svenson SB. Symptomatic recurrent urinary tract infections in patients with renal scarring in relation to fecal colonisation with P-fimbriated Escherichia coli. *J Urol* 1987; 137: 693–966

137. Kotkin L, Milam D. Evaluation and management of the urologic consequences of neurologic disease. *Techniq Urol* 1996; 2: 210–219

138. Foxman B. Recurring urinary tract infection: incidence and risk factors. *Am J Public Health* 1990; 80: 331–333

139. Nicolle LE, Ronald AR. Recurrent urinary tract infections in adult women: diagnosis and treatment. *Infect Dis Clin North Am* 1987; 1: 793–806

140. McGeachie J. Recurrent infection of the urinary tract: Re-infection or recrudescence? *Br Med J* 1966; 1: 952–954

141. Russo TA, Stapleton A, Menderoth S *et al.* Chromosomal restriction fragment length polymorphism analysis of Escherichia coli strains causing recurrent urinary tract infections in young women. *J Infect Dis* 1995 172: 440–445

142. Ikaheimo R, Siitomen A, Heiskanen T *et al.* Recurrence of urinary tract infections in a primary care setting: analysis of a 1 year follow-up of 179 women. *Clin Infect Dis* 1996; 22: 91–99

143. Midram J, Sanchez R, Gruhn J. Squamous metaplasia of the bladder: a study of 450 patients. *J Urol* 1974; 112: 479–482

144. Mogensen P, Hansen LK. Do intravenous urography and cystoscopy provide important information in otherwise healthy women with recurrent urinary tract infection? *Br J Urol* 1983; 55: 261–263

145. Marsh F, Banerjee R, Panchamia P. The relationship between urinary infection and cystoscopic appearance and pathology of the bladder in man. *J Clin Path* 1974; 27: 297–307

146. Manson AL. Is antibiotic administration indicated after outpatient cytoscopy? *J Urol* 1988; 140: 316–317

147. Thilagarajah Pt, Vale JA, Witherow RO, Walker MM. A clinicopathological approach to cystitis – recommendations for simplified pathology reporting. *Br J Urol* 1997; 79: 567–571

148. Engel G, Schaeffer A, Grayhack J, Mendel E. The role of excretory urography and cystoscopy in the evaluation and management of women with recurrent urinary tract infections. *J Urol* 1980; 123: 190–191

149. Fowler J, Pulaski E. Excretory urography cystography and cystoscopy in the evaluation of women with urinary tract infections. *N Engl J Med* 1981; 304: 462–465

150. Fairchild TN, Shuman W, Berger RE. Radiographic studies for women with recurrent urinary tract infections. *J Urol* 1982; 128: 344–345

151. Nickel JC, Wilson J, Morales A, Heaton J. Value of urologic investigations in a targeted group of women with recurrent urinary tract infections. *Can J Surg* 1991; 34: 591–594

152. Koff SA, Lapides J, Piazza DH. Association of urinary tract infections and reflux with uninhibited bladder contractions and involuntary sphincteric obstruction. *J Urol* 1979; 122: 373–376

153. Froom J. The spectrum of urinary tract infections in family practice. *J Fam Pract* 1980; 11: 385–391

154. Arav-Boger R, Leibovici L, Danon YL. Urinary tract infections with low and high colony counts in young women. Spontaneous remission and single-dose vs multiple-day treatment. *Arch Int Med* 1994; 154: 300–304

155. O'Connor PJ, Solberg LI, Christianson J *et al.* Mechanism of action and impact of a cystitis clinical practice guideline on outcomes and costs of care in an HMO. *Joint Commission J Quality Improvement* 1996; 22: 673–682

156. Garrod L, Lambert H, O'Grady F. *Antibiotic and Chemotherapy.* 4th edn Edinburgh: Churchill Livingstone, 1973; 403–405

157. Hooton TM. A simplified approach to urinary tract infection. *Hosp Pract* 1995; 30: 23–30

158. Bailey RR. Single oral dose treatment of uncomplicated urinary tract infections in women. *Chemotherapy* 1996; 42(suppl): 10–16

159. Delrio G, Dalet E, Aguilar L *et al.* Single dose rufloxacin versus 3 day norfloxacin treatment of uncomplicated cystitis. Clinical evaluation and pharmacodynamic considerations. *Antimicrob Agents Chemother* 1996; 40: 408–412

160. Stein GE. Single-dose treatment of acute cystitis with fostomycin tromethamine. *Ann Pharmacother* 1998; 32: 215–219

161. Stamey TA, Candy M, Mihara G. Prophylactic efficacy of nitrofurantoin macrocrystals and trimethoprim-sulphamethoxazole in urinary infections. *N Engl J Med* 1977; 296: 780–783

162. Brumfitt W, Hamilton-Miller JM. Consensus viewpoint on management of urinary infections. *J Antimicrob Chemother* 1994; 33(Suppl A): 147–153

163. Jones R, Vander Pol, B, Martin D, Shepard M. Partial characterisation of chlamydia trachomatis isolates resistant to multiple antibiotics. *J Infect Dis* 1990; 162: 1309–1315

164. Tawfik A, Ramadan M, Shibl, A. Inhibition of motility and adherence of proteus mirabilis to uroepithelial cells by subinhibitory concentrations of amikacin. *Chemotherapy* 1997; 43: 424–429

165. Iosif CS, Batra SC, Ek A *et al.* Estrogen receptors in the human female lower urinary tract. *Am J Obstet Gynecol* 1981; 141: 817–820.

166. Cardozo LD, Kelleher CL. Sex hormones, the menopause and urinary problems. *Gynecol Endocrinol* 1995; 9: 75–84

167. Raz R, Stamm WE. A controlled trial of intravaginal oestriol in post-menopausal women with recurrent urinary tract infections. *N Engl J Med* 1993; 329: 803–803

168. Cardozo L, Rekers H, Tapp A *et al.* Oestriol in the treatment of postmenopausal urgency: a multicentre study. *Maturitas* 1993; 18: 47–53

169. Adatto K, Doebele KG, Galland L, Granowetter L. Behavioural factors and urinary tract infections. *J Am Med Assoc* 1979; 241: 2525–2526

170. Ehren I, Alm P, Kinn AC. Renal and bladder functions in patients after spinal cord injuries. *Scand J Urol Nephrol* 1994; 28: 127–133

171. Chancellor MB, Riras W, Erhard MJ *et al*. Flexible cystoscopy during urodynamic evaluation of spinal cord injured patients. *J Endourol* 1993; 7: 531–535

172. Wullt B, Connell H, Rollano P, *et al*. Urodynamic factors influence the duration of Escherichia coli bacteriuria in deliberately colonised cases. *J Urol* 1998; 159: 2057–2062

173. Bagli D, Van Savage J, Khoury A *et al*. Basic fibroblast growth factor on the urine of children with voiding pathology. *J Urol* 1998; 158: 1123–1127

174. Bukowski T, Betrus G, Aquilina J, Permutter A. Urinary tract infections and pregnancy in women who underwent anti-reflux surgery in childhood. *J Urol* 1998; 159: 1286–1289

175. Pewitt EB, Schaeffer AJ. Urinary tract infection in urology, including acute and chronic prostatitis. *Infect Dis Clin North Am* 1997; 11: 623–646

176. Schaeffer AJ. Recurrent urinary tract infections in women. Pathogenesis and management. *Postgrad Med J* 1987; 81: 51–58

177. Brumfitt W, Hamilton-Miller JM. A comparative trial of low does cefaclor and macrocyrstaline nitrofurantoin in the prevention of recurrent urinary tract infection. *Infections* 1995; 23: 98–102

178. Ptan A, Sacks TG. Effective prophylaxis of recurrent urinary tract infections in premenopausal women by post coital administration of cephalexin. *J Urol* 1989; 142: 1276–1278

179. Larsen EH, Gasser TC, Madsen PO. Antimicrobial prophylaxis in urologic surgery. *Urol Clin North Am* 1986; 13: 591–604

180. Bailey R, Roberts A, Gower P, de Wardener H. Prevention of urinary tract infection with low-dose nitrofurantoin. *Lancet* 1971; 2: 1112–1114

181. Cattell W, Chamberlain D, Fry I *et al*. Long term control of bacteriuria with trimethoprim-sulphonamide. *Br Med J* 1971; 1: 377–379

182. Baerheim A, Larsen E, Digranes A. Vaginal applications of Lactobacilli in the prophylaxis of recurrent lower urinary tract infections in women. *Scand J Prim Health Care* 1994; 12: 239–243

183. Childs SJ, Egan RJ. Bacteriuria and urinary infections in the elderly. *Urol Clin North Am* 1996; 23: 43–54

184. Orr PH, Nicolle LE, Duckworth H *et al*. Febrile urinary infection in the institutionalised elderly. *Am J Med* 1996; 100: 71–77

185. Nicolle LE, Orr P, Duckworth H *et al*. Gross haematuria in residents of long term care facilities. *Am J Med* 1993; 94: 611–618

186. Nicolle LE. Topics in long term care: urinary tract infections in long term care facilities. *Infect Control Hosp Epidemiol* 1993; 14: 220–225

187. Eberle CM, Winsemius D, Garibaldi RA. Risk factors and consequences of bacteriuria in non-catheterised nursing home residents. *J Gerontol* 1993; 48: M266–271

188. Nicolle LE. Asymptomatic bacteriuria in the elderly. *Infect Dis Clin North Am* 1997 11: 647–662

189. Wood CA, Abrutyn E. Optimal treatment of urinary tract infections in elderly patients. *Drugs Ageing* 1996; 9: 352–362

190. Nicolle LE. Urinary tract infections in the elderly. *J Antimicrobial Chemotherapy* 1994; 33 (Suppl A): 99–109

191. Grahn D, Normal DC, White ML *et al*. Validity of urinary catheter specimen for diagnosis of urinary tract infection in the elderly. *Arch Intern Med* 1985; 145: 1858–1860

192. Nicolle LE. Prevention and treatment of urinary catheter related infections in older patients. *Drugs Ageing* 1994; 4: 379–391

193. Huth TS, Burke JP, Larson RA *et al*. Randomised trial of meatal care with silver sulfadiazine cream for the prevention of catheter associated bacteriuria. *J Infect Dis* 1992; 165: 14–18

194. Carty NJ, Yap J, Johnson CD. Prospective randomised trial of two devices for suprapubic catheterisation in general surgical patients. *Ann R Coll Soc Engl* 1994; 76: 194–196

195. National Institute on Disability and Rehabilitation Research Consensus Statement, Jan 27–29 1992. The prevention and management of urinary tract infections among people with spinal cord injuries. *J Am Paraplegia Soc* 1992; 15: 194–204

196. Rhame F, Perkash I. Urinary tract infections occurring in recent spinal cord injury patients on intermittent catheterisation. *J Urol* 1979; 122: 669–673

197. Perkash I, Giroux J. Clean intermittent catheterisation in spinal cord injury patients: a follow-up study. *J Urol* 1993; 149: 1068–1071

198. Gribble M, Puterman M, McCallum N. Pyuria: its relationship to bacteriuria in spinal cord injured patients on intermittent catheterisation. *Arch Phys Med Rehab* 1989; 70: 376–379

199. Bakke A, Pigrames A, Hoisaeter P. Physical predictors of infection in patients treated with clean intermittent catheterisation: a prospective 7 year study. *Br J Urol* 1997; 79: 85–90

200. Watts GF, O'Brien SF, Show KM. Urinary infection and albumen excretion in insulin-dependent diabetes mellitus: implications for the measurement of microalbumenuria. *Diabet Med* 1996; 13: 520–524

201. Zhassel GG, Nicolle LE, Harding GK. Prevalence of asymptomatic bacteriuria and associated host factors in women with diabetes mellitus. The Manitoba Diabetic Urinary infection Study Group. *Clin Infect Dis* 1995; 21: 316–322

202. Allen JC. The diabetic as a compromised host. In: Allen JC (ed) *Infection and the Compromised Host: Clinical Correlations and Therapeutic Approaches.* Baltimore: Williams & Wilkins, 1981; 229–270

203. Patterson JE, Andriole VT. Bacterial urinary tract infections in diabetes. *Infect Dis Clin North Am* 1997; 11: 735–750

204. Kass EH. Bacteriuria and pyelonephritis of pregnancy. *Arch Intern Med* 1960; 105: 194–198

205. Whalley PJ. Bacteriuria of pregnancy. *Am J Obstet Gynecol* 1967; 97: 723–738

206. Gallery ED, Ross M, Gyory AZ. Urinary red blood cell and cast excretion in normal and hypertensive human pregnancy. *Am J Obstet Gynecol* 1993; 168: 67–70

207. Roberts A, Beard R. Some factors affecting bacterial invasion of the bladder during pregnancy. *Lancet* 1965; 1: 1133–1136

208. Mansfield JT, Snow BW, Cartwright PC, Wadsworth K. Complications of pregnancy in women after childhood reimplantation for vesicoureteric reflux: an update with 25 years follow up. *J Urol* 1995; 154: 787–790

209. Gower P, Haswell B, Sidaway M *et al.* Follow up of 164 patients with bacteriuria of pregnancy. *Lancet* 1968; 1: 990–994

210. Cunningham FG, Lucas MJ. Urinary tract infections complicating pregnancy *Baillieres Clin Obstet Gynaecol* 1994: 8: 353–373

211. Kass EH. Prevention of apparently non-infectious disease by detection and treatment of infections of the urinary tract. *J Chronic Dis* 1962; 15: 665–673

212. Millar LK, Cox SM. Urinary tract infections complicating pregnancy. *Infect Dis Clin North Am* 1997; 11: 13–26

213. McKenzie H, Donnet ML, Howice PW *et al.* Risk of preterm delivery in pregnant women with group B streptococcal urinary infections or urinary antibodies to group B and E. coli antigens. *Br J Obstet Gynaecol* 1994; 101: 107–113

214. Villar J, Bergsjø P. Scientific basis for the content of routine antenatal care. I philosophy, recent studies and power to eliminate or alleviate adverse maternal outcomes. *Acta Obstet Gynecol Scand* 1997; 76: 1–14

215. Rouse DJ, Andrews WW, Goldenberg RL, Owen J. Screening and treatment of asymptomatic bacteriuria of pregnancy to prevent pyelonephritis: a cost-effectiveness and cost-benefit analysis. *Obstet Gynecol* 1995; 86: 119–123

216. Bachman JW, Heise RH, Balsseus JM, Timmerman MG. A study of various tests to detect asymptomatic urinary tract infections in an obstetric population. *J Am Med Assoc* 1993; 270: 1971–1974

217. Etherington IJ, James DK. Reagent strip testing of antenatal urine specimens for infection. *Br J Obstet Gynaecol* 1993; 100: 806–808

218. Hagay Z, Levy R, Miskin A *et al.* Uriscreen, a rapid enzymatic urine screening test: useful predictor of significant bacteriuria in pregnancy. *Obstet Gynecol* 1996: 87: 410–413

219. Kiningham RB. Asymptomatic bacteriuria in pregnancy. *Am Fam Phys* 1997 93; 47: 1232–1238

220. Lettieri L, Vintzileos AM, Rodis M *et al.* Does 'idiopathic' pre-term birth exist? *Am J Obstet Gynecol* 1993; 168: 1480–1485

221. Gerstner G, Müller G, Nahler G. Amoxicillin in the treatment of asymptomatic bacteriuria in pregnancy. A single dose of 3 g amoxicillin versus a 4 day course of 3 doses 750 mg amoxycillin. *Gynecol Obstet Invest* 1989; 27: 84-87

222. Harris RE. Antibiotic therapy of antepartum urinary tract infections. *J Int Med Res* 1980; 8(Suppl 1): 40–44

223. Schwarz RH. Considerations of antibiotic therapy during pregnancy. *Obstet Gynecol* 1981; 58: 95S–99S

224. Locksmith G, Duff P. Preventing neural tube defects: the importance of periconceptional folic acid supplements. *Obstet Gynecol* 1998; 91: 1027–1034

225. Pead L, Maskell R. Study of urinary tract infection in children in one health district. *Br Med J* 1994, 309: 631–634

226. Preston AA. Imaging strategies and discussion of vesicoureteric reflux as a risk factor in the evaluation of urinary tract infection in children. *Curr Opin Paediatr* 1994; 6: 178–182

227. Jadresic L, Cartwright K, Cowie N *et al.* Investigation of urinary tract infection in children. *Br Med J* 1993; 307: 761–764

228. Rushton HG. Urinary tract infections in children. Epidemiology, evaluation and management. *Pediatr Clin North Am* 1997; 44: 1133–1169

229. Ottolini MC, Shaer CM, Rushton FG *et al.* Relationship of asymptomatic bacteriuria and renal scarring in children with neuropathic bladders who are practising clean intermittent catheterisation. *J Paediatr* 1995: 127: 368–372

230. Clarke SE, Smellie JM, Prescod N *et al.* Technetium 99m-DMSA studies in pediatric urinary infection. *J Nucl Med* 1996; 35: 823–828

231. Scott JE, Swallow V, Coulthard MG *et al.* Screening of newborn babies for familial ureteric reflux. *Lancet* 1997; 350: 396–400

232. Hoberman A, Chao HP, Keller DM *et al.* Prevalence of urinary tract infection in febrile infants. *J Pediatr* 1993; 123: 17–23

233. Asscher A, McLachlan M, Jones R *et al.* Screening for asymptomatic urinary tract infection in schoolgirls. A two-centre feasibility study. *Lancet* 1973; 2: 1–4

234. Vernon SJ, Coulthard MG, Lambery HJ *et al.* New renal scarring in children who at age 3 and 4 years had had normal scans with dimercaptosuccinic acid: follow up study. *Br Med J* 1997; 315: 905–908

235. Lockhart GR, Lewander WJ, Cimini DM *et al.* Use of urinary Gram stain for detection of urinary tract infections in infants. *Ann Emerg Med* 1995; 25: 31–35

236. Hiraoka M, Hashimoto G, Hori C *et al.* Use of ultrasonography in the detection of ureteric reflux in children suspected of having urinary infection. *J Clin Ultrasound* 1997; 25: 195–199

237. Smellie JM, Poulton A, Prescod NP. Retrospective study of children with renal scarring associated with reflux and urinary infection. *Br Med J* 1994; 308: 1193–1196

238. Hori C, Hiraoka M, Tsukahara H *et al.* Intermittent trimethoprim-sulfamethoxazole in children with vesico ureteral reflux. *Paediatr Nephrol* 1997; 11: 328–330

239. Muller V, Becker G, Delfs M, Albrecht K *et al.* Do urinary tract infections trigger chronic kidney transplant rejection in man? *J Urol* 1998; 159: 1826–1829

240. Goya N, Tanabe K, Iguchi Y *et al.* Prevalence of urinary tract infection during outpatient follow-up after renal transplantation. *Infection* 1997; 25: 101–105

241. Hashnic P, Ho C, Morgan S, Stephenson JR. Routine urinalysis in renal transplant patients. *J Clin Pathol* 1995; 48: 383–384

242. Hermieu J, Delmas V, Boccon-Gibod L. Micturition disturbances and human immunodeficiency virus infection. *J Urol* 1996; 156: 157–159

243. Ojoo J, Paul J, Batchelor B *et al.* Bacteriuria in a cohort of predominantly HIV-1 seropositive female commercial sex workers in Nairobi, Kenya. *J Infect* 1996; 33: 33–37

244. Kance C, Bolton D, Connolly J, Tanagho E. Voiding dysfunction in human immunodeficiency virus infections. *J Urol* 1996; 155: 523–526

245. Hassay KA. Effective management of urinary discomfort. *Nurse Pract* 1995; 20(2): 36; 39–40; 42–44

246. Nazarko L. Infection control. The therapeutic uses of cranberry juice. *Nursing Standard* 1995; 9(34): 33–35

247. Interpretation of the bacteriologic outcome of antibiotic treatment for uncomplicated cystitis: impact of the definition of significant bacteriuria in a comparison of ritipenem acoxil with norfloxacin. Swedish Urinary Tract Infection Study Group. *Clin Infect Dis* 1995; 20: 507–513

248. Nagele F, Karas H, Spitzer D, Standach A *et al.* Closure or non closure of the visceral peritoneum at caesarean delivery. *Am J Obstet Gynecol* 1996; 174: 1366–1370

249. Robson W, Leung A. Extraordinary urinary frequency syndrome. *Urology* 1993; 42: 321–324

250. Gittes F, Nakamura R. Female urethral syndrome. A female prostatitis? *West J Med* 1996; 164: 435–438

251. Wesselmann U, Burnett A, Heinberg L. The urogenital and rectal pain syndromes. *Pain* 1997; 73: 269–294

252. Baldoni F, Ercolani M, Baldaro B, Trombini G. Stressful events and psychological symptoms in patients with functional urinary disorder. *Perceptual Motor Skills* 1995; 80: 605–606

253. Marrie T, Swantee C, Hartlen M. Aerobic and anaerobic urethral flora in healthy females in various physiological age groups and of females with urinary tract infections. *J Clin Microbiol* 1980; 11: 654–659

254. Tait J, Peddie B, Bailey R *et al.* Urethral syndrome (abacterial cystitis) – search for a pathogen. *Br J Urol* 1985; 57: 552–556

255. Handsfield H. Recent developments in STDs. II. Viral and other syndromes. *Hosp Pract (Off Ed)* 1992; 27: 175–182; 187; 191–192

256. Westrom L. Chlamydia trachomatis – clinical significance and strategies of intervention. *Sem Dermatol* 1990; 9: 117–125

257. Horner P, Hay P, Thomas B *et al.* The role of Chlamydia trachomatis in urethritis and urethral symptoms in women. *Int J STD AIDS* 1995; 6: 31–34

258. Pec J, Kliment J, Moravcik P *et al.* Isolation of Neisseria gonorrhoea and concomitant bacterial microflora from urine obtained by suprapubic bladder puncture in women with gonococcal urethritis. *Int Urol Nephrol* 1990; 22: 167–171

259. Sharfi A, Elarabi Y. The 'watering can' perineum: presentation and management. *Br J Urol* 1997; 80: 933–936

260. Wyndaele J, Maes D. Clean intermittent self-catheterisation: a 12 year follow-up. *J Urol* 1990; 143: 906–908

261. Vaidyanathan S, Soni B, Dundas S, Kirshnan KR. Urethral cytology in spinal cord injury patients performing intermittent catheterisation. *Paraplegia* 1994; 32: 493–500

262. Summitt RL. Urogynaecologic causes of chronic pelvic pains. *Obstet Gynecol Clin North Am* 1993; 20: 685–698

263 Moore T, Hira N, Stirland R. Differential urethrovesical urinary cell count. A method of accurate diagnosis of lower urinary tract infection in women. *Lancet* 1965; 1: 626–627

264. Kellogg D, Holmes K, Hill G. Cumitech 4: laboratory diagnosis of gonorrhoea. Washington DC: American Society for Microbiology, 1976

265. Bowie W. Urethritis and infections of the lower urogenital tract. *Urol Clin North Am* 1980; 7: 17–28

266. Adjei O, Lal V. Non invasive detection of Chlamydia trachomatis genital infection in asymptomatic males and females by enzyme immunoassay (Chlamydiazyme). *J Tropic Med Hygiene* 1994; 97: 51–54

267. Kuo HG. Trans-rectal sonography of the female urethra in incontinence and frequency-urgency syndrome. *J Ultrasound Med* 1996; 15: 363–370

268. Siegelman E, Banner M, Ramchandani P, Schnall M. Multicoil MR imaging of symptomatic female urethra and periurethral disease. *Radiographics* 1997; 17: 349–365

269. Tam I, Stoken J, Zwamborn A *et al.* Female pelvic floor: endovaginal MR imaging of normal anatomy. *Radiology* 1998; 206: 777–783

270. Nurenberg P, Zimmern P. Role of MR imaging with transrectal coil in the evaluation of complex urethral abnormalities. *Am J Roentgenol* 1997; 169: 1335–1338

271. Cunha B, Garabedian-Ruffalo S. Tetracyclines in urology: current concepts. *Urology* 1990; 36: 548–556

272. Kitchen V, Donegan C, Ward H *et al.* Comparison of ofloxacin with doxycycline in the treatment of non-gonococcal urethritis and cervical chlamydial infection. *J Antimicrob Chemother* 1990; 26(Suppl D): 99–105

273. Romanowski B, Talbot H, Stadnyk M *et al.* Minocycline compared with doxycycline in the treatment of non-gonococcal urethritis and mucopurulent cervicitis. *Ann Int Med* 1993; 119: 16–22

274. Thorpe E, Stamm W, Hook E *et al.* Chlamydial cervicitis and urethritis. Single dose treatment compared with doxycycline for seven days in community based practices. *Genitourin Med* 1996; 72: 93–97

275. Ridgeway G. Azithromycin in the management of chlamydia trachomatis infections. *Int J STD AIDS* 1996; 7(Suppl): 5–8

276. Martin D, Mroczkowski T, Dalu Z *et al.* A controlled trial of a single dose of azithromycin for the treatment of chlamydial urethritis and cervicitis. The Azithromycin for Chlamydial Infections Study Group. *N Engl J Med* 1992; 327: 921–925

277. Jones P, Schwebke J, Thorpe E *et al.* Randomised trial of trovafloxacin and ofloxacin for single-dose therapy of gonorrhoea. Trovafloxacin Gonorrhoea Study Group. *Am J Med* 1998; 104: 28–31

278. Anonymous. 1998 guidelines for treatment of sexually transmitted diseases. Centres for Disease Control and Prevention. *MMWR Morbid Mortal Wkly* 1998; 47: 1–11

279. Otubu J, Imade G, Sagay A, Tourobola O. Resistance of recent Neisseria gonorrhoea isolates in Nigeria and outcome of single dose treatment with ciprofloxacin. *Infection* 1992; 20: 339–341

280. Bowie WR. Effective treatment of urethritis. A practical guide. *Drugs* 1992; 44: 207–215

68

Frequency/urgency syndromes

B. Wise

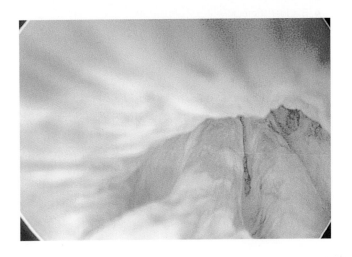

INTRODUCTION

Symptoms of urinary frequency and urgency are common and often coexist. Diurnal frequency is defined as the passage of urine more than seven times during waking hours (equivalent to every 2 hours). Nocturia is the interruption of sleep more than once a night specifically for micturition. Voiding patterns alter with age such that in elderly women, voiding two or more times at night may be considered normal. Those who void during the night due to insomnia or broken sleep do not have true nocturia. Urinary urgency is the sudden, strong desire to void. It may be followed immediately by involuntary loss of urine, constituting the symptom of urge incontinence. In a study by Bungay *et al.*[1] 20% of women were found to have urinary frequency and 15% complained of urgency. Each symptom may occur independently but often they present together in conjunction with other lower urinary tract symptoms. The causes of frequency and urgency are many and varied (Table 68.1); therefore, careful assessment of each patient is required to define the underlying pathology.

PATIENT ASSESSMENT

A detailed urological and gynaecological history should be obtained. Information about fluid intake, voiding habits and drug therapy should be collected. Abdominal and pelvic examinations will help to exclude pregnancy, a pelvic mass or a large urinary residual. A simple neurological examination of S2–4 will rule out major neurological impairment.

A urine specimen should be obtained for culture (including *Mycoplasma homonis* and *Ureaplasma urealyticum*) and cytological examination. High-vaginal, endocervical and urethral swabs may be taken to test for *Chlamydia* and other genitourinary pathogens. If tuberculous cystitis is suspected, three early-morning urine samples should be sent for acid-fast bacillus culture. Diabetes mellitus may be excluded by random blood glucose measurement or by glucose tolerance testing.

The patient should be asked to complete a voiding diary for at least 3 days to provide an objective assessment of fluid intake and voiding patterns. Excessive drinking may be identified and the patient should be encouraged to moderate fluid intake to approximately 1500 ml per day. Avoidance of caffeine-containing drinks and alcohol may relieve symptoms in some cases. Frequency and nocturia can be quantified from the diary and the number of episodes of urgency and incontinence can be recorded. The impact of treatment on symptomatology may also be assessed by this method.

If history and examination fail to reveal an obvious cause for the symptoms, further investigation by cysto-urethroscopy and cystometry may aid diagnosis. Cysto-urethroscopy can be performed under local or general anaesthesia and may reveal cystitis, a bladder tumour, bladder calculus, urethritis or a urethral diverticulum. Bladder biopsy in the presence of inflammation may lead to the diagnosis of interstitial cystitis. Subtracted cystometry may provide a diagnosis of detrusor instability (DI), a poorly compliant bladder or sensory urgency. Ultrasound assessment of a post-micturition residual will exclude chronic voiding difficulty due to outflow obstruction or detrusor failure.

Table 68.1. *The causes of urinary frequency and urgency*

- Excessive fluid intake
- Maladaptive learned behaviour (bad habits)
- Detrusor instability
- Sensory urgency
- Urinary tract infection
- Urethritis
- Bladder calculus
- Bladder tumour
- Diabetes mellitus
- Diabetes insipidus
- Pregnancy
- Pelvic mass
- Small capacity bladder
- Chronic urinary residual
- Cystocele
- Oestrogen deficiency
- Irradiation
- Diuretic therapy
- Congestive cardiac failure
- Renal impairment
- Urethral diverticulum
- Urethral syndrome
- Interstitial cystitis

DETRUSOR INSTABILITY

The normal bladder is a compliant reservoir which contracts only under voluntary control during micturition. An unstable bladder is one that contracts involuntarily, or can be provoked to do so.

The motor nerve supply to the detrusor is via the parasympathetic nervous system (S2–4), specifically to the pelvic nerve. Its effects are mediated by acetylcholine acting on muscarinic receptors.[2] There are predominantly two receptor types in the human bladder: M_2 (85%) and M_3 (10%).[3] Despite the dominance of the M_2 receptor, it appears that activation of the M_3 receptor is responsible for detrusor contraction. This is apparent from studies which show that 4-diphenylacetoxy-1,1-dimethylpiperidinium, a specific antagonist of the M_3 receptor subtype, blocks carbachol-induced bladder contractions *in vitro*. Antagonists of the M_1 and M_2 subtypes, however, have a more limited effect.[4] Sympathetic innervation is derived from the hypogastric nerve and acts predominantly on β-adrenoceptors to cause relaxation of the detrusor.

A detrusor contraction is initiated in the rostral pons. Efferent pathways emerge from the sacral spinal cord as the pelvic parasympathetic nerves and run forwards to the bladder. Acetylcholine is released at the neuromuscular junction, resulting in a coordinated contraction. A balance between parasympathetic and sympathetic stimulation is required for normal detrusor function.

DI is defined by the International Continence Society as a condition in which the detrusor is shown objectively to contract, either spontaneously or on provocation, during bladder filling, whilst the subject is attempting to inhibit micturition.[5] It is the second most common cause of urinary incontinence in women and is demonstrated in approximately 40% of referrals for urodynamic investigation. It has been estimated that the condition may occur to some degree in up to 10% of the population. The incidence of DI increases with age such that it is the most frequent cause of incontinence in the elderly.[6]

These uninhibited contractions may give rise to frequency, nocturia, urgency, urge incontinence and nocturnal enuresis, and it is usual for the patient to present with multiple symptoms.

Our understanding of the pathophysiology of DI is incomplete, and treatment of the condition is often ineffective. Few patients achieve a long-term cure of their symptoms, but the majority can derive some benefit from the treatment regimens currently available.

In a minority of women there is a detectable underlying neurological cause for their symptoms but this is not normally the case. DI may arise from poorly learnt bladder control as an infant, and indeed behavioural techniques such as bladder training can be effective for established DI. In a study of 46 children with urinary frequency, who had been previously toilet trained successfully, a psychological 'trigger' that preceded the onset of symptoms was identified in 40% of cases. The trigger often involved problems at school and, once resolved, led to a resolution in the urinary symptoms.[7] There is a strong association between childhood nocturnal enuresis and the development of DI in adult life.[8]

The psychoneurotic status of women with DI has been investigated by several authors, with conflicting results. Walters *et al.* evaluated 63 women with incontinence and 27 continent controls using formal psychometric testing.[9] They found no difference between the women with genuine stress incontinence (GSI) and those with DI. Women with DI scored significantly higher than controls on the scales for depression, hypochondriasis and hysteria. Norton *et al.* performed psychiatric assessments on 117 women attending the urodynamic clinic prior to investigation.[10] There was no increase in psychiatric morbidity in women with DI compared with those with GSI. Interestingly, women in whom no urodynamic abnormality could be found had the highest scores for anxiety and neuroticism. The measured levels were comparable with those of psychiatric outpatients. Moore and Sutherst evaluated treatment outcome in relation to psychoneurotic status.[11] Poor responders to oxybutynin therapy had a higher mean psychoneurotic score than responders, although one-third of poor responders had normal scores. Patients who responded well to therapy had scores similar to normal urban females.

Many women with DI show no evidence of an abnormal psychoneurotic state; this emphasizes the need for further research into the neurophysiology of lower urinary tract function to elucidate the physical cause of this condition.

In men there is an association between outflow obstruction due to benign prostatic hypertrophy and DI. In a large study by Webster, however, only one of 3000 women with DI had bladder-neck obstruction on meticulous urodynamic testing.[12] Following incontinence surgery, there is an increased incidence of DI.[13] This may arise from the development of relative outflow obstruction or, more likely, from the extensive bladder-neck dissection performed at operation. The prevalence of DI is correspondingly high in women who have undergone multiple bladder-neck procedures.

The pathophysiology of the unstable bladder is not

fully understood. Increased sensitivity of nerve endings in the bladder to local stimuli may result in abnormal reflex responses that result in frequency and urgency.[14] Low electrical sensitivity thresholds in the posterior urethrae of women with urgency syndromes have been demonstrated by Kieswetter.[15] Whether this is responsible for the generation of uninhibited detrusor motor activity has yet to be determined.

Relaxation of the urethral sphincter is known to precede contraction of the detrusor in a proportion of women with DI.[16] This may indicate a primary pathology of the urethra that triggers detrusor contraction, or merely represent part of a complex sequence of events that originate elsewhere. It has been suggested that incompetence of the bladder neck, allowing passage of urine into the proximal urethra, may result in an uninhibited contraction of the detrusor. However, in a study of 50 women, Sutherst and Brown were unable to provoke a detrusor contraction by rapidly infusing saline into the posterior urethra using modified urodynamic equipment.[17]

Brading and Turner suggest that the common feature in all cases of DI is a change in the properties of the smooth muscle of the detrusor which predisposes to unstable contractions. This change is caused by long-term reduction in the functional innervation of the bladder wall.[18] They dispute the concept of 'hyperreflexia' (i.e. increased motor activity to the detrusor) as the underlying mechanism of DI.

Clinical presentation

DI may present with any of the following symptoms:

- frequency,
- nocturia,
- urgency,
- urge incontinence,
- stress incontinence,
- nocturnal enuresis,
- coital incontinence.

The most frequent symptoms are urgency and frequency of micturition, which occur in approximately 80% of cases.[19] Nocturia occurs in almost 70% of patients. It should be remembered that nocturia is age-related such that over the age of 70 years it is normal to void twice during the night, increasing to three times over 80 years of age. Nocturnal enuresis is strongly correlated with DI.[8] Incontinence during sexual intercourse is a distressing symptom which may occur in women with DI or GSI. In the former, leakage usually occurs at orgasm whereas in the latter it occurs during penetration.[20]

A full clinical examination should be conducted as outlined above to exclude other causes of urinary symptoms; however, DI can only be diagnosed by subtracted cystometry. Figure 68.1 shows a cystometric trace from a patient with DI.

Treatment

Women with very mild or intermittent symptoms may require only reassurance and simple measures such as a reduction of excessive fluid intake, avoidance of caffeine and alcohol, or a change in voiding habits. Others with more incapacitating symptoms will require further treatment. The methods used attempt to improve central control of micturition, as in behavioural intervention, or to alter detrusor innervation using drugs, electrical stimulation or surgical techniques. If these measures fail, surgery to increase the size of the bladder 'reservoir', such as cystoplasty, may be undertaken. Conventional bladder-neck surgery rarely cures women with DI and may make the symptoms of frequency and urgency worse.

The main therapeutic options are shown below:

- drug therapy;
- behavioural therapy;
- maximal electrical stimulation;
- augmentation cystoplasty;
- urinary diversion.

Many other surgical techniques have been attempted in the past including: vaginal denervation,[21] selective sacral neurectomy,[22] cystodistension[23–26] and bladder transection.[27] All were reported as effective treatments initially but are not used routinely because of high complication rates or poor long-term efficacy. Transvesical blockade of nerve plexuses using phenol was introduced by Ewing in 1982,[28] with apparent efficacy in the treatment of the neuropathic bladder. Complications such as sciatic nerve palsy, ureteric sloughing and vesicovaginal fistulae have been reported. Subsequent studies failed to confirm the initial success of this technique,

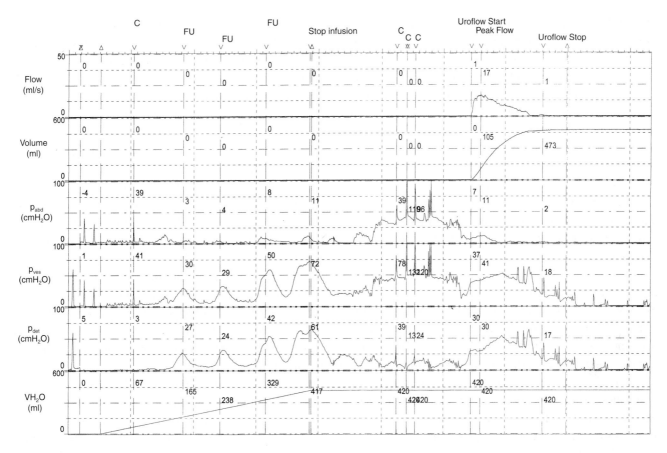

Figure 68.1. *A cystometrogram of a patient with idiopathic detrusor instability.* p_{abd}, *intra-abdominal pressure;* p_{ves}, *intravesical pressure;* p_{det}, *detrusor pressure;* VH_2O, *volume of water, C, cough; FU, First urge.*

with efficacy at about 50% for detrusor hyperreflexia and only 25% in cases of idiopathic DI.[29] The beneficial effect was usually temporary, lasting less than a year. Repeat injections were often unsuccessful and increased the risk of complications.[30]

Drug therapy

Drugs may be divided according to their pharmacological mode of action.

Antimuscarinic agents

The motor supply to the detrusor arises from S2–4 and is conveyed via the pelvic nerve. Acetylcholine is the neurotransmitter released from the nerve terminal and it acts at muscarinic receptors. Antimuscarinic agents would seem likely to be of benefit in the treatment of DI. Atropine is the classic antimuscarinic agent; however, its non-specific activity results in unacceptable side effects, limiting its clinical effectiveness. The side

effects include: dry mouth, blurred vision, tachycardia, drowsiness and constipation. Research into the pharmacokinetics and pharmacodynamics of atropine following intravesical instillation may allow this route of administration to be used, reducing systemic side effects.[31]

Propantheline is related to atropine but has fewer side effects. It is a quaternary ammonium analogue of atropine and has both antimuscarinic and antinicotinic properties, acting at both the ganglionic level and the neuromuscular junction. Intramuscular administration of propantheline was found to abolish involuntary detrusor contractions in 70% of patients but at the expense of urinary retention, requiring short-term self-catheterization in 50% of patients.[32] Efficacy data following oral administration are lacking, and the recommended dose of 15 mg four times a day may be too low. The dose may be increased to as much as 90 mg four times a day, but should be introduced slowly to minimize side effects. Gastrointestinal absorption is aided by taking the drug before meals.[33] Propantheline is a cheap drug with relatively few side effects and may be of particular use in the treatment of frequency.

Transdermal scopolamine was used in 10 patients with DI.[34] Only three patients reported symptomatic improvement; nine patients found that side effects were intolerable, requiring discontinuation of the drug in eight cases. Side effects included ataxia, blurred vision, dizziness and severe dry mouth.

Emepronium carrageenate is an anticholinergic agent derived from seaweed. It is used in Ireland and other parts of Europe but is not available in the United Kingdom.

Musculotropic relaxants

Oxybutynin is an antimuscarinic agent with an additional direct spasmolytic effect on the detrusor. It remains one of the most effective drugs available for the treatment of DI. In the first reported study in 1980, 30 patients were treated in a double-blind, placebo-controlled trial.[35] Of those treated with oxybutynin, 60% had improved symptoms compared with 8% of those receiving placebo. Seventeen patients experienced side effects, which caused nine patients to withdraw from the study.

Oxybutynin has been compared with propantheline in a variable-dose crossover trial.[36] It was found to be superior in terms of both symptomatic and cystometric improvement. In a large randomized, double-blind, multicentre study conducted by Thuroff *et al.*, the degree of symptomatic improvement and objective improvement in urodynamic variables were significantly greater for those treated with oxybutynin than for those receiving either propantheline or placebo.[37] Oxybutynin has been found to reduce the symptom of urgency in post-menopausal women with DI, but side effects were frequent.[38] In one study 76% of subjects experienced adverse effects while only 57% showed symptomatic improvement.[39]

Oxybutynin is an efficacious drug; however, the dose must be balanced with the patient's ability to tolerate the dry mouth and throat and lingering bad taste that accompany its use. Oxybutynin has a short half-life and is therefore effective soon after ingestion. A dose may be taken as prophylaxis to control symptoms for short periods, for example while shopping or at the cinema. The standard recommended dose is 5 mg twice daily,

and side effects are common at this dose. In practice, higher doses (up to 10 mg three times daily) may be tolerated by some women but compliance with treatment is improved by starting at 2.5 mg twice daily and slowly increasing the dose if required.

Low-dose oxybutynin (3 mg three times daily) was used by Moore *et al.* to treat 53 patients with DI.[40] Symptomatic cure or marked improvement was found in 60% of patients, and side effects resulted in discontinuation of therapy in only 7.5%.

Intravesical oxybutynin is useful for patients with detrusor hyperreflexia who need to self-catheterize or who have an indwelling catheter. Rectal oxybutynin produces higher steady-state plasma levels of the parent drug than oral administration, and these levels are maintained for more than 12 hours.[41] The levels of its *N*-desethyl metabolite, which is responsible for the side effects, are much lower following rectal administration and side effects are fewer compared with oral administration.

An oral controlled-release (CR) preparation has been developed to eliminate peak serum levels of oxybutynin and *N*-desethyloxybutynin. In a study of 128 patients randomized to receive either oxybutynin CR (10 mg once daily) or oxybutynin (5 mg twice daily) there was no difference in efficacy between the two treatment regimens; however, there was a 43% reduction in side effects in those treated with the CR preparation.[42]

Flavoxate is a tertiary amine with a paraverine-like effect on smooth muscle. It inhibits phosphodiesterase, increasing levels of cyclic AMP, which leads to muscle relaxation. Flavoxate also has analgesic and local anaesthetic properties. It is usually prescribed at a dose of 200 mg three times daily but is poorly absorbed from the gastrointestinal tract. Its true efficacy in the treatment of DI after either oral or parenteral administration is debatable, and its effects may be no better than placebo.[43,44] Terflavoxate is a related compound, the clinical efficacy of which has yet to be established.

Calcium channel blockers

Drugs that limit the availability of calcium ions may lead to smooth muscle relaxation. Until October 1991, terodiline was the most commonly prescribed drug for the treatment of DI in the United Kingdom. It is well absorbed from the gastrointestinal tract and reduces the frequency and the number of incontinence episodes in women with DI.[45] However, it was withdrawn voluntarily by the manufacturer following cardiac adverse events, mainly in elderly patients.

Verapamil has been administered alone or in combination with oxybutynin to 14 patients with DI.[46] Although verapamil alone had no clinical efficacy, 13 of the 14 patients experienced greater symptomatic benefit with combination therapy than with oxybutynin alone. In this way the dose of oxybutynin may be reduced and the incidence of side effects diminished.

Tolterodine

Tolterodine is a new molecule derived from terodiline specifically for the treatment of DI. As such it is the first drug in this field ever to be developed in this way. It is a non-selective antimuscarinic agent that acts on all muscarinic receptor subtypes. Tolterodine has greater affinity for bladder muscarinic receptors than salivary gland receptors; oxybutynin shows the opposite affinities.[47–52]

Tolterodine is rapidly and completely absorbed from the gastrointestinal tract, irrespective of food intake, and has a short plasma half-life (t_{max} = 1–3 hours; $t_{1/2}$ = 2–3 hours). It is metabolized in the liver and the active metabolite, DD01, has similar properties to the parent molecule (t_{max} = 1 hour; $t_{1/2}$ = 3–4 hours). The pharmacological effects result from the summed influence of parent drug and metabolite. Excretion of the drug and its metabolites is primarily through the kidneys (77%).

Seven per cent of Caucasians metabolize tolterodine slowly and metabolism is inhibited by fluoxetine. Patients over 80 years of age on concomitant medication may have 36% greater exposure to tolterodine; however, dose reduction is not required. Clinical trials have not shown any evidence of accumulation.[53]

Tolterodine is not associated with serious side effects. Detailed assessment of its effect on cardiac electrophysiology has shown that it has no clinically significant effects on the characteristics of the action potential and does not demonstrate properties conducive to Torsades de pointes. Safety data from clinical trials have demonstrated side effects consistent with an antimuscarinic agent.[47,53–56]

The clinical trials programme on tolterodine is the largest ever conducted on a drug of this class, involving 29 clinical trials on 2691 patients from 15 different countries. Data from these studies have shown that tolterodine is statistically and clinically superior to placebo in the treatment of the symptoms of DI. A dose of 2 mg twice daily is superior to 1 mg twice daily, although there is evidence of efficacy at the lower dose. Evidence of treatment efficacy is present after 4 weeks of therapy and is maximum after 5–8 weeks.[55–58]

Studies comparing tolterodine with oxybutynin (administered in doses ranging from 2.5 mg twice daily to 5 mg three times daily) have shown that the two drugs are equally efficacious. However, there were fewer side effects, especially dry mouth, reported by patients on tolterodine compared with those on oxybutynin. In addition, there were fewer dose reductions and treatment withdrawals in the tolterodine group.[54,59–60] Studies conducted in the elderly show tolterodine to be safe and effective in this group.[53,59]

Other drugs

Imipramine was initially tested as an antipsychotic agent, as it is an analogue of chlorpromazine, and was found to have antidepressant properties. It acts by inhibiting reuptake of noradrenaline and serotonin into the presynaptic membrane, thus potentiating their actions. This may result in bladder relaxation and increase outlet resistance. Imipramine also has antimuscarinic and local anaesthetic properties. It sometimes causes the common antimuscarinic side effects but, in addition, may cause tremor, sedation and even convulsions. Withdrawal reactions may occur if treatment is stopped abruptly; these include nausea, vomiting, malaise and depression. Electrocardiographic changes have been reported, including tachycardia, atrial flutter, atrial fibrillation, ventricular flutter and both atrioventricular and interventricular block. Imipramine is, however, a useful drug in the treatment of nocturia and nocturnal enuresis. In a study of 10 elderly patients with DI treated with imipramine, six became continent.[61] A dose of up to 150 mg may be taken safely, but the standard recommended dose is 50 mg twice daily. Other tricyclic antidepressants such as amitriptyline may be substituted for imipramine. Imipramine taken prophylactically prior to sexual intercourse may be of benefit to patients with coital incontinence at orgasm.[62]

1-Desamino-8-D vasopressin (DDAVP) is a long-acting, synthetic analogue of vasopressin, which is a peptide hormone consisting of eight amino acids. DDAVP may be administered intranasally or in tablet form and is effective for 12–24 hours, with a half-life of 75 minutes resulting from slow metabolic clearance.

Whilst it has full antidiuretic potency and increases permeability in the distal convoluted tubules and collecting ducts of the kidney, unlike vasopressin it has no significant effect on blood pressure. It has a lesser effect on smooth muscle contraction so pallor, bronchospasm, colic and coronary artery or uterine spasm do not occur. Studies have shown that a 50% reduction in urine production follows an intranasal dose of DDAVP of 20–40 µg.[63]

DDAVP is useful in the treatment of nocturia and nocturnal enuresis. Because the bladder fills more slowly and the total volume of urine is reduced, the number of uninhibited contractions is diminished. In a double-blind, placebo-controlled, crossover study of 12 patients, DDAVP significantly reduced the number of wet nights.[64] DDAVP also significantly reduced the number of night-time voids compared with placebo.[65] It is safe for long-term use;[66] however, caution must be exercised in patients with coronary artery disease, hypertension, heart failure or epilepsy.

Oral desmopressin has been investigated in a placebo-controlled trial of 25 adolescents with severe monosymptomatic nocturnal enuresis. At a dose of 400 µg there was a significant reduction in the number of wet nights compared with placebo. Over three months, approximately half of the patients on active therapy had one or no enuretic episodes per week. No serious adverse events were reported.[67]

There is an abundance of literature on oestrogens and the lower urinary tract; however, there have been few placebo-controlled trials using objective outcome measures. Oestrogen therapy does not improve incontinence due to DI; however, it may be of benefit in women with sensory urgency because it raises the sensory threshold of the bladder.[68] In a placebo-controlled trial, use of a daily low-dose intravaginal oestradiol tablet resulted in a significant reduction in the symptoms of urgency in a subgroup of post-menopausal women with urodynamically proven sensory urgency. No improvement in urinary symptoms was found for women with DI.[69]

Behavioural therapy

Bladder retraining or bladder drill was first described as 'bladder discipline' in 1966 by Jeffcoate and Francis.[70] They treated 246 women with urgency incontinence, a condition which we now know as DI, using a regimen of timed voiding. The interval between voids was gradually increased over a period of days to weeks. In 1978 Frewen reported a symptomatic cure rate of 82.5% in 40 patients treated with bladder drill for 3 months.[71] He believed that there was a psychogenic or emotive reason for the patients' symptoms. Further studies have produced similar success rates, with 86% of 150 patients with frequency and urgency becoming symptomatically cured after 3 months of bladder retraining.[72] This was irrespective of the presence or absence of DI. In 1981 Jarvis compared the efficacy of bladder drill and drug therapy and found the former to be more effective.[73] Bladder retraining may be the most effective therapy for DI; however, long-term studies show that relapse rates are high.[74]

Biofeedback

This involves the use of electronic equipment to monitor a normally subconscious physiological process and relay this information to the individual so that a change in a particular direction may be brought about. The information is fed back as an audible, tactile or visual signal. In a study of 27 patients with DI, 81% were improved following four to six 1-hour sessions of biofeedback using both audible and visual signals of detrusor overactivity.[75] Unfortunately, long-term results with such therapy are disappointing.

Other behavioural techniques such as hypnotherapy[76] have been used to treat DI, with some success. Such therapy is, however, complex and time-consuming and is often overlooked in favour of simpler drug treatments.

Acupuncture

Traditional Chinese acupuncture has been used by Philp *et al.*[77] to treat DI. Seventy per cent of 20 patients were improved, although only one converted to a stable bladder. Acupuncture is believed to work by increasing endogenous levels of endorphins and enkephalins in the cerebrospinal fluid. Enkephalins are known to inhibit detrusor contractility *in vitro*[78] and, conversely, naloxone, an opiate antagonist, decreases bladder capacity and increases detrusor pressure.[79] Pigne *et al.* found that 15 of 16 patients reported that urinary frequency and episodes of leakage were reduced following acupuncture treatment.[80] Gibson *et al.* treated 28 patients twice weekly for 5 weeks using infrared low-power laser on acupuncture points.[81] Following this, 50% of patients were initially cured of their symptoms and a further 25% improved; however, at 6 months 16 had relapsed.

Maximal electrical stimulation

In 1895 it was established that stimulation of the proximal end of a transected pudendal nerve resulted in detrusor relaxation.[82] Inhibition of detrusor contractility *in vivo* following vaginal or anal electrical stimulation using external electrodes is believed to occur via pudendal–pelvic and pudendal–hypogastric nerve reflexes. Long-term, low-amplitude stimulation of pudendal nerve afferents[83] and acute maximal electrical stimulation (MES) have proved to be effective in the treatment of DI.[84] Other studies have confirmed MES as a simple home treatment with efficacy equivalent to drug therapy and without significant side effects.[85-87]

Surgical techniques

Some patients fail to respond to drug therapy, or discontinue it due to side effects. They may then undergo MES or be treated with behavioural techniques. Those that remain symptomatic pose a difficult management problem. The only operation of proven benefit to patients with intractable DI is augmentation cystoplasty. It was first described by Bramble for the treatment of 15 patients with enuresis, of whom 87% were cured by the procedure.[88] The operation involves bisecting the bladder in the coronal plane anterior to the ureteric orifices to within 1 cm of the bladder neck. The distance is measured and a corresponding length of ileum is isolated, opened along its antimesenteric border and sutured as a patch into the defect. This segment acts by absorbing the effect of unstable contractions. Several studies have reported success rates of over 90%.[89,90] Voiding difficulty is common postoperatively, necessitating self-catheterization. The bowel segment produces mucus, which may be reduced by ingesting cranberry juice.[91] Adenocarcinoma arising in the bowel segment is a rare long-term complication.[92]

INTERSTITIAL CYSTITIS

This is an uncommon, disabling condition associated with chronic inflammation of the bladder. It was first described by Skene in 1887;[93] however, its aetiology remains obscure and its management difficult. Interstitial cystitis occurs much more frequently in women than in men with a 10 : 1 ratio of incidence.[94] The typical pre-sentation is with urinary frequency, urgency and bladder pain. The true prevalence of this condition is uncertain because of the subjective diagnostic criteria, and estimates vary between populations. Ten cases per 100 000 population has been reported in Finland, whereas a prevalence of 30–510 cases per 100 000 has been suggested in the US. It is unclear whether these estimates represent true differences in prevalence, or whether different criteria are used to define interstitial cystitis.

Interstitial cystitis is a serious, chronic condition which often results in significant disability. Many affected women are unable to work or cannot have sexual intercourse because of bladder pain. In some instances symptoms are so severe that the patient has considered suicide.

Aetiology

Possible causes of interstitial cystitis include: infection, lymphatic obstruction and endocrinological or psychosomatic disorders. No causative microorganism has been identified in affected patients although fastidious organisms play a role. Polymerase-chain-reaction amplification of DNA from cystoscopic bladder biopsies has failed to show evidence of infection with a specific organism in patients with interstitial cystitis compared with controls.[95-98] The prevalence of antibodies against *Helicobacter pylori* is similar in patients with interstitial cystitis compared with asymptomatic controls, suggesting that *H. pylori* is not a causative agent.[99]

Elbadawi has proposed a primary involvement of neurogenic inflammation in the pathogenesis of interstitial cystitis.[100,101] This in turn may trigger a sequence of events resulting in a leaky urothelium and mast cell activation.

An autoimmune disorder is also a possibility as there is an association between interstitial cystitis and systemic lupus erythematosus (SLE) and other collagen disorders.[102,103] Individuals with interstitial cystitis are 100 times more likely to have inflammatory bowel disease and 30 times more likely to have SLE.[104] Some patients have evidence of antinuclear antibodies[105] or antibladder antibodies.[106] A more recent study found autoantibodies in 50% of patients with interstitial cystitis.[107] Some of these autoantibodies were novel but others were shared with other diseases. It is not clear, however, whether this immune response is the primary cause of interstitial cystitis or a secondary response to bladder damage. Evidence against an immunological aetiology is the fact that symptoms may resolve completely following urinary diversion without cystectomy[108] and recurrence may occur in the bowel segment of a colocystoplasty.[109]

The glycosaminoglycan (GAG) layer of the transitional epithelium of the bladder is believed to have a protective function.[110] If it is deficient, microorganisms may penetrate the bladder wall, resulting in inflammation.[111] It has been suggested that similar deficiencies may allow urinary constituents to penetrate the detrusor muscle, resulting in the symptoms and histological features of interstitial cystitis.[112] However, evidence of a deficiency in the GAG layer in patients with histologically confirmed interstitial cystitis is lacking.[113]

Diagnosis

Patients usually present with frequency, nocturia, urgency, dysuria and suprapubic or perineal pain. Occasionally urge incontinence is also a feature. Symptoms are often relieved by micturition and exacerbated by caffeine and alcohol intake.[114] Symptoms are usually gradual in onset and progressive. Physical examination is often normal, although tenderness of the anterior vaginal wall may be present. Microscopic haematuria may occur with normal urine cytology. Cystometry usually reveals a reduced cystometric capacity, often with reduced bladder compliance.

Cystoscopy is the most useful diagnostic test and is best carried out under general anaesthesia to determine true bladder capacity. This is characteristically less than 400 ml. If the bladder is left distended for 1–2 minutes at bladder capacity and then drained, the terminal fluid is typically haematuric. Refilling the bladder may reveal the features of interstitial cystitis which include: subepithelial patechial haemorrhages (glomerulations), splotchy haemorrhages and linear cracking of the mucosa; ulcers and scarring may be features of late-stage disease.

Bladder-base biopsy is important to confirm the diagnosis and to exclude other inflammatory disorders such as tuberculosis, schistosomiasis or neoplastic change. The histological features of such biopsies are often non-specific. Chronic inflammation with submucosal oedema and vasodilatation is usually present. Fibrosis may be present, as may infiltration with round cells, plasma cells and eosinophils. Increased numbers of mast cells (more than 20 cells/mm^2 of detrusor muscle tissue)

are present in up to 50% of biopsies, although this finding may not be specific to interstitial cystitis.[115] A decrease in bladder perfusion in women with interstitial cystitis has been demonstrated by laser Doppler flowmetry.[116]

Treatment

Many therapeutic modalities have been tried in the treatment of interstitial cystitis, with varying degrees of success. Because the aetiology remains poorly understood, the treatment of this condition is largely empirical and there are few well-controlled, prospective studies from which to determine the most appropriate therapy. Suggested treatment regimens may be grouped as systemic, local or surgical.

Systemic treatment

Mast cells are present in increased numbers in the bladders of women with interstitial cystitis. The release of histamine from these cells may result in pain, inflammation and subsequent fibrosis. One study reported improvement in symptoms in a small group of patients treated with an antihistamine, and further assessment of this therapy would be worthwhile.[117]

Hydroxyzine has been evaluated in an open-label, non-consecutive case series of 150 patients with interstitial cystitis: a 40% reduction in symptom score was reported.[118]

Heparin may be administered subcutaneously or instilled into the bladder. It has an anti-inflammatory action and also mimics some of the characteristics of the GAG layer of the bladder. In an uncontrolled study, Parsons *et al.*[119] injected heparin subcutaneously for 1 week and this provided good symptomatic improvement. Alternatively, 10 000 IU heparin in 10 ml sterile water may be instilled into the bladder by the patient using a self-catheterization technique. This is performed several times each week and can be continued indefinitely.

Hyaluronic acid is an important GAG found in all connective tissue. When instilled into the bladder at a dose of 40 mg/week, the response rate was 30–70%.[120,121]

Pentosanpolysulphate is a synthetic analogue of sulphonated GAG. It augments the normal protective mucous layer of the bladder. Reports on efficacy are conflicting, although benefits in some placebo-controlled trials have been demonstrated.[119,122] Significant improvement can be expected in approximately 50% of patients with moderate disease. The activity was lower in those with severe disease. The usual dose is 100 mg three times daily and the incidence of side effects is low. In a longer term study, however, only 6.2–18.7% of patients benefited from this therapy,[123] and in another study 46% of patients discontinued therapy within the first 3 months.[124] A meta-analysis of four randomized controlled trials showed that pentosanpolysulphate is more efficacious than placebo in the treatment of pain, urgency and frequency associated with interstitial cystitis, but not nocturia.[125]

Amitriptyline has analgesic properties as well as anticholinergic and antihistaminic effects. Taken at doses of 25–75 mg at night, it improved pain and frequency in an uncontrolled study.[126] Tricyclic antidepressants may also help patients to cope with their symptoms by improving sleep and minimizing the depression that can accompany chronic disorders.

Anti-inflammatory and immunosuppresive agents would be expected to improve interstitial cystitis if it is an inflammatory disorder with an autoimmune basis. However, results are variable and unpredictable. There are no good studies on the use of steroids and the high doses used have resulted in frequent side effects. Badenoch[127] reported an improvement in 70% of patients but relapse rates were high and the duration of remission was unpredictable. Walsh[128] suggests that the response to steroids is unpredictable, while Messing and Stamey[108] report that improvement is likely only with high-dose regimens. Azathioprine, an immunosuppressant, has been reported to be efficacious in some studies.[129] Cyclosporin was been used to treat 11 patients with interstitial cystitis:[130] in 10 patients frequency of micturition decreased, voided volumes increased and bladder pain disappeared. After cessation of treatment, symptoms recurred in most patients. Benzydamine has analgesic and anti-inflammatory properties and has produced dramatic results in some patients.[131]

Hexamine hippurate, a urinary antiseptic, has been used with some success at a dose of 1 g twice daily (L. Cardozo; unpublished observations).

The true efficacy of many agents is uncertain because of the lack of good-quality prospective, randomized, placebo-controlled trials.

Local treatment

Many patients show a dramatic improvement in symptoms following cystodistension. Unfortunately, this is short-lived in most. The benefit is presumed to be secondary to ischaemic damage to afferent nerve plexuses or stretch receptors within the bladder wall. A number of different techniques are used. Dunn[132] reported symptomatic cure in over 60% of patients at a mean of 14 months after distension for 3 hours under anaesthesia. Bladder pressure was increased to the level of systolic blood pressure throughout this time. Other authors distend the bladder for different periods of time and at different pressures. Regional anaesthesia can be used for this procedure. Bladder rupture may occur in a small number of patients but can usually be managed conservatively.

Cystodistension has been carried out following electromotive drug administration (EMDA) of lignocaine and dexamethasone in 21 women with interstitial cystitis.[133] EMDA involves the active transport of ionized drugs by the application of an electric current to the bladder. Eighty-five per cent of patients had a good response, with a reduction in urinary frequency and pain scores. EMDA with lignocaine and adrenaline followed by cystodistension was efficacious in six patients with interstitial cystitis.[134]

Instillation therapy with dimethyl sulphoxide (DMSO), an industrial solvent, has been shown to be beneficial in the management of interstitial cystitis. The treatment regimen is easy to perform, inexpensive and can be performed as an outpatient procedure. DMSO has a number of pharmacological actions including local analgesia, anti-inflammatory activity and bacteriostasis. The patient is catheterized and 50 ml of a 50% solution of DMSO is instilled into the bladder. This is retained for 15–30 minutes; the bladder is then emptied by voiding. The treatment is performed every 1 or 2 weeks and four to six treatments may be required to achieve the maximum response. Patients who perform self-catheterization can administer DMSO themselves at home. Cataracts should be excluded prior to therapy. A significant improvement can be expected in 50–80% of patients with early interstitial cystitis.[135–137]

A prospective, randomized, controlled trial showed that intravesical *Bacille Calmette-Guérin* produced a 60% response rate compared with 27% in patients who received placebo.[138] In those patients who responded to treatment after 6 weeks, long-term follow-up ranging from 24 to 33 months showed that therapeutic benefit was maintained in 89% of patients.[139]

Surgical treatment

The surgical management of interstitial cystitis is frequently indicated and is reserved for those patients who have not responded to conservative management. The methods available can be grouped into either endoscopic or open procedures. Endoscopic surgery involves fulguration or resection of ulcers and is usually combined with other conservative therapies. Early reports of the use of the Nd:YAG laser are encouraging. Local injection of hydrocortisone or heparin around the ulcerated areas may be of benefit.

Open surgery is used as a last resort and the options available include partial cystectomy, augmentation cystoplasty, cystolysis and urinary diversion with or without cystectomy. Partial cystectomy is probably a poor option, because the disease may recur in the bladder remnant. Augmentation or substitution cystoplasty, where the supratrigonal portion of the bladder is removed, has been reported to be effective in cases of classic interstitial cystitis.[140] This procedure may be less successful in non-ulcer disease. Comparison of supratrigonal and subtrigonal cystectomy with orthotopic bladder substitution suggests that both are effective procedures for interstitial cystitis, with similar relief of symptoms. Supratrigonal cystectomy, however, is usually followed by normal voiding, whereas a significant proportion of patients undergoing subtrigonal cystectomy will require clean intermittent self-catheterization (41% in this study).[141]

Urinary diversion with total cystectomy/urethrectomy and the creation of a continent colonic reservoir was reported to have a success rate of 73% in a study of 22 patients with interstitial cystitis.[142] Diversion without cystectomy may be complicated by mucopurulent/bloody secretions from the defunctionalized bladder, pyocystis, urethral pain or sepsis.[143] Ultimately this may necessitate total cystectomy. The outcome of radical surgery may be improved by preoperative psychological evaluation and pain localization techniques using a multidisciplinary team approach.[142]

Cystolyses involves division of the sensory pathways to the upper part of the bladder and may be appropriate where the bladder is not contracted.

SENSORY URGENCY

Sensory urgency is a diagnosis made after urodynamic assessment. Affected patients have symptoms of frequency, urgency and sometimes urge incontinence and have no cystometric evidence of DI. Sensory urgency is thought to be due to a 'hypersensitive' bladder, although there are no generally agreed cystometric parameters that define this increased sensitivity. Some authors use the diagnostic criteria of the first sensation of filling to occur at less than 100 ml and the bladder capacity to be less than 400 ml. Because the diagnostic criteria are rather vague, the incidence of sensory urgency is unclear, but this diagnosis is made in approximately 10% of women investigated in our unit.[144] The aetiology of sensory urgency is poorly understood. However, psychological factors may be involved and affected women have been shown to be more anxious than those with GSI.[145] It is also probable that some do in fact have DI that was undetected at the time of laboratory urodynamics. Ambulatory testing may be appropriate further investigation in some patients.

Diagnosis requires a detailed history and examination, a urinary diary and cystometric examination. Once the diagnosis has been made on cystometry, cystoscopy and biopsy should be performed to exclude interstitial neoplastic conditions of the bladder wall, or other intravesical pathology. Most patients with sensory urgency respond to treatment with bladder retraining.[146] Anticholinergic therapy, for example propantheline, oxybutynin or tolterodine, can be used in addition to bladder retraining or in those for whom retraining is not effective. A combination of diazepam and anticholinergics has been reported to give reasonable results, either alone[147] or in combination with bladder retraining.[148]

REFERENCES

1. Bungay G, Vessey MP, McPherson CK. Study of symptoms in middle life with special reference to the menopause. *Br Med J* 1980; 281: 181–183

2. Kinder RB, Mundy AR. Atropine blockade of nerve-mediated stimulation of the human detrusor. *Br J Urol* 1985; 57: 418–421

3. Maeda A, Kubo T, Mishima M *et al.* Tissue distribution of mRNAs encoding muscarinic acetylcholine receptor subtypes. *FEBS Lett* 1988; 239: 339–342

4. Eglin RM, Whiting RL. Muscarinic receptor subtypes: a critique of the current classification and a proposal for a working nomenclature. *J Auton Pharmacol* 1986; 6: 323–346

5. The standardisation of terminology of lower urinary tract function. *Br J Obstet Gynaecol* 1990; Suppl 6: 1–6

6. Castleden CM, Duffin HM. Factors influencing outcome in elderly patients with urinary incontinence and detrusor instability. *Age Ageing* 1985; 14: 303–307

7. Zoubek J, Bloom D, Sedman AB. Extraordinary urinary frequency. *Pediatrics* 1990; 85: 1112–1114

8. Whiteside CG, Arnold GP. Persistent primary enuresis: a urodynamic assessment. *Br Med J* 1975; 1: 364–369

9. Walters MD, Taylor S, Schoenfeld LS. Psychosexual study of women with detrusor instability. *Obstet Gynecol* 1990; 75: 22–26

10. Norton KRW, Bhat AV, Stanton SL. Psychiatric aspects of urinary incontinence in women attending an outpatient clinic. *Br J Urol* 1990; 301: 271–272

11. Moore KH, Sutherst JR. Response to treatment of detrusor instability in relation to psychoneurotic status. *Br J Urol* 1990; 66: 486–490

12. Webster JR. Combined video/pressure/flow cystometography in female patients with voiding disturbances. *Urology* 1975; 5: 209–213

13. Cardozo LD, Stanton SL, Williams JE. Detrusor instability following surgery for genuine stress incontinence. *Br J Urol* 1979; 51: 204–207

14. Jeffcoate TNA, Francis WJA. Urgency incontinence in the female. *Am J Obstet Gynecol* 1966; 94: 604–609

15. Kieswetter J. Mucosal sensory threshold of urinary bladder and urethra measured electrically. *Urol Int* 1977; 32: 437–439

16. Wise BG, Cardozo LD, Cutner A *et al.* The prevalence and significance of urethral instability in women with detrusor instability. *Br J Urol* 1993; 72: 26–29

17. Sutherst JR, Brown M. The effect on the bladder pressure of sudden entry of fluid into the posterior urethra. *Br J Urol* 1978; 50: 406–409

18. Brading AF, Turner WH. The unstable bladder: towards a common mechanism. *Br J Urol* 1994; 73: 3–8

19. Cardozo LD, Stanton SL. Genuine stress incontinence and detrusor instability: a review of 200 cases. *Br J Obstet Gynaecol* 1980; 87: 184–190

20. Hilton P. Urinary incontinence during sexual intercourse: a common but rarely volunteered symptom. *Br J Obstet Gynaecol* 1988; 95: 377–381

21. Ingleman-Sundberg A. Partial denervation for detrusor dyssynergia. *Clin Obstet Gynecol* 1978; 21: 797–805

22. Mundy AR. Long term results of bladder transection for urge incontinence. *Br J Urol* 1983; 55: 642–644

23. Torrens MG, Griffith HB. The control of the uninhibited bladder by selective sacral neurectomy. *Br J Urol* 1974; 46: 639–644

24. Helmstein K. Treatment of bladder carcinoma by hydrostatic pressure technique. *Br J Urol* 1972; 44: 434–450

25. Dunn M, Smith JC, Ardan GM. Prolonged bladder distension as a treatment or urgency and urge incontinence of urine. *Br J Urol* 1974; 46: 645–652

26. Pengelly AW, Stephenson TP, Milroy ESG *et al.* Results of prolonged bladder distension as treatment for detrusor instability. *Br J Urol* 1978; 50: 243–245

27. Turner-Warwick RT, Ashken MH. The functional results of partial subtotal and total cystoplasty with special reference to ureterocaecoplasty, selective sphincterotomy and cystocystoplasty. *Br J Urol* 1976; 39: 3–12

28. Ewing R, Bultitude MI, Shuttleworth KED. Subtrigonal phenol injection for urge incontinence secondary to detrusor instability in females. *Br J Urol* 1982; 54: 689–692

29. Rosenbaum TP, Shah PJR, Worth PHL. Transtrigonal phenol: the end of an era? *Neurourol Urodyn* 1988; 7: 294–295

30. Wall LL, Stanton SL. Transvesical phenol injection of pelvic nerve plexuses in females with refractory urge incontinence. *Br J Urol* 1989; 63: 465–468

31. Enskat R, Deaney C, Charig C, Glickman S. Systemic absorption of atropine sulphate following intravesical instillation (abstract). International Continence Society (UK section) 5th Annual Meeting, University of Cambridge, April 1998; 16

32. Blaivas JG, Labib KB, Michalik SJ, Zayed AAH. Cystometric response to propantheline in detrusor hyperreflexia: therapeutic implications. *J Urol* 1980; 124: 259–262

33. Gibaldi M, Grundhofer G. Biopharmaceutic influences on the anticholinergic effect of propantheline. *Clin Pharmacol Ther* 1975; 18: 457–461

34. Cornella JL, Ostergard DR, Bent AE, Horbach NS. Prospective study using transdermal scopolamine in detrusor instability. *Urology* 1990; 25: 96–97

35. Moisey CU, Stephenson TP, Brendeler CB. The urodynamic and subjective results of treatment of detrusor instability with oxybutynin chloride. *Br J Urol* 1980; 52: 472–474

36. Holmes DM, Montz FJ, Stanton SL. Oxybutynin versus propantheline in the treatment of detrusor instability in the female: a patient regulated variable dose trial. *Proceedings of the Fifteenth Annual meeting of the International Continence Society*, London, 1985: 63–64

37. Thuroff JW, Bunke B, Ebner A *et al.* Randomised, double-blind multicentre trial on treatment of frequency, urgency and incontinence related to detrusor hyperactivity: oxybutynin versus propantheline versus placebo. *J Urol* 1991; 145: 813–816

38. Cardozo LD, Cooper D, Versi E. Oxybutynin chloride in the management of idiopathic detrusor instability. *Br Med J* 1987; 280: 281–282

39. Baigre RE, Kelleher JP, Fawcett DP, Pengelly AW. Oxybutynin, is it safe? *Br J Urol* 1988; 62: 319–322

40. Moore KH, Hay DM, Imrie AE *et al.* Oxybutynin hydrochloride (3 mg) in the treatment of women with idiopathic detrusor instability. *Br J Urol* 1990; 66: 479–485

41. Collas D, Malone-Lee JG. The pharmacokinetic properties of rectal oxybutynin – a possible alternative to intravesical administration. *Neurourol Urodyn* 1997; 16: 346–347

42. Birns J, Malone-Lee JG, and the Oxybutynin CR Study Group. Controlled-release oxybutynin maintains efficacy with a 43% reduction in side effects compared with conventional treatment. *Neurourol Urodyn* 1997; 16: 429–430

43. Brigg RS, Castleden CM, Asher MJ. The effect of flavoxate on uninhibited detrusor contractions and urinary incontinence in the elderly. *J Urol* 1980; 123: 665–666

44. Chapple CR, Parkhouse H, Gardener C, Milroy EJG. Double-blind, placebo-controlled, crossover study of flavoxate in the treatment of idiopathic detrusor instability. *Br J Urol* 1990; 66: 491–494

45. Tapp AJS, Fall M, Norgaard J *et al.* Terodiline: a dose titrated, multicenter study of the treatment of idiopathic detrusor instability in women. *J Urol* 1989; 142: 1027–1031

46. Bodner DR, Lindan R, Leffler E, Resnick MI. The effect of verapamil on the treatment of detrusor hyperreflexia in the spinal cord injured population. *Paraplegia* 1989; 27: 364–369

47. Nilvebrandt L, Hallen B, Larsson G. Tolterodine – a new bladder selective muscarinic receptor antagonist: preclinical pharmacological and clinical data. *Life Sci* 1997; 60: 1129–1136

48. Naerger, Fry CH, Nilvebrandt L. Effect of tolterodine on electrically induced contractions of isolated human detrusor muscle from stable and unstable bladders. *Neurourol Urodyn* 1995;14: 76–77

49. Nilvebrandt L, Stahl M, Andersson KE. Interaction of tolterodine with cholinergic muscarinic receptors in human detrusor. *Neurourol Urodyn* 1995; 14: 75–76

50. Nilvebrandt L, Sundquist S, Gillberg PG. Tolterodine is not subtype (M1–M5) selective but exhibits functional bladder selectivity *in vivo*. *Neurourol urodyn* 1196; 15: 310–311

51. Nilvebrandt L, Andersson KE, Gillberg PG *et al.* Tolterodine – a new bladder selective muscarinic receptor antagonist: preclinical pharmacological and clinical data. *Eur J Pharmacol* 1997; 327: 195–207

52. Nilvebrandt L, Gillberg PG, Sparf B. Antimuscarinic potency and bladder selectivity of PNU-200577, a major metabolite of tolterodine. *Pharmacol Toxicol* 1997; 81: 169–172

53. Malone-Lee JG, Walsh JB, Maugourd MF. Tolterodine in the Elderly Study Group. Safety and clinical efficacy of two dosages of tolterodine in comparison with placebo in the treatment of urinary urgency, frequency and urge incontinence in the elderly. Pharmacia & Upjohn, Data on file; 1988

54. Abrams P, Freeman RN, Anderstrom C, Mattiasson A. Efficacy and tolerability of tolterodine vs oxybutynin and placebo in patients with detrusor instability (abstract 402). *J Urol* 1997; 157; 103

55. Rentzhog L, Stanton SL, Cardozo LD *et al.* Efficacy and safety of tolterodine in patients with detrusor instability: a dose ranging study. *Br J Urol* 1998; 81: 42–48

56. Van Kerrebroeck PEVA, Amarenco G, Thuroff JW. Dose ranging study of tolterodine in patients with detrusor hyperreflexia. *Neurourol Urodyn* 1998; 17: 499–512

57. Millard R, Moore K, Dwyer P, Tuttle J. Clinical and urodynamic efficacy of tolterodine: a multicentre placebo-controlled trial. *Neurourol Urodyn* 1997; 16: 343–344

58. Appell RA. Clinical efficacy and safety of tolterodine in the treatment of overactive bladder: a pooled analysis. *Urology* 1997; 50(suppl 6A): 90–96

59. Malone-Lee JG, Eriksson M, Olofsson S, Lidberg M. Tolterodine vs oxybutynin study group. The comparative tolerability and efficacy of tolterodine 2 mg bid versus oxybutynin 2.5 to 5 mg bid in the treatment of the overactive bladder. Pharmacia & Upjohn, Data on file; 1998

60. Van Kerrebroeck PEVA, Serment G, Dreher E. Clinical efficacy and safety of tolterodine compared to oxybutynin in patients with overactive bladder. *Neurourol Urodyn* 1997; 16: 478–479

61. Castleden CM, George CF, Renwick AG, Asher MJ. Imipramine, a possible alternative to current therapy for urinary incontinence in the elderly. *J Urol* 1981; 125: 318–320

62. Cardozo LD. Sex and the bladder. *Br Med J* 1988; 296: 587–588

63. Monson JP, Richards P. Desmopressin urine concentration test. *Br Med J* 1979; 1: 2420–2423

64. Ramsden PD, Hindmarsh JR, Price DA *et al.* DDAVP for adult enuresis – a preliminary report. *Br J Urol* 1982; 54: 256–258

65. Hilton P, Stanton SL. The use of desmopressin (DDAVP) in nocturnal urinary frequency in the female. *Br J Urol* 1982; 54: 252–255

66. Knudsen UB, Rittig S, Pederen JB *et al.* Long term treatment of nocturnal enuresis with desmopressin – influence on urinary output and haematological parameters. *Neurourol Urodyn* 1989; 8: 348–349

67. Stenberg A, Lackgren G. Desmopressin tablets in the treatment of severe nocturnal enuresis in adolescents. *Pediatrics* 1994; 94: 841–846

68. Fantl JA, Wyman JF, Anderson RL *et al.* Postmenopausal urinary incontinence: comparison between non-oestrogen supplemented and oestrogen supplemented women. *Obstet Gynecol* 1988; 71: 823–828

69. Wise BG, Benness CJ, Cardozo LD, Cutner A. Vaginal oestradiol for lower urinary tract symptoms in post-menopausal women – a double-blind, placebo-controlled study. *Proceedings of the Seventh International Congress on the Menopause*, Stockholm, 1993: 15

70. Jeffcoate TNA, Francis WJA. Urgency incontinence in the female. *Am J Obstet Gynecol* 1966; 94: 604–618

71. Frewen WK. An objective assessment of the unstable bladder of psychological origin. *Br J Urol* 1978; 50: 246–249

72. Frewen WK. A reassessment of bladder training in detrusor dysfunction in the female. *Br J Urol* 1982; 54: 372–373

73. Jarvis GJ. A controlled trial of bladder drill and drug therapy in the management of detrusor instability. *Br J Urol* 1981; 53: 565–566

74. Holmes DM, Stone AR, Bary PR *et al.* Bladder training 3 years on. *Br J Urol* 1983; 55: 660–664

75. Cardozo LD, Abrams PH, Stanton SL, Feneley RCL. Idiopathic bladder instability treated by biofeedback. *Br J Urol* 1978; 50: 521–523

76. Freeman RM, Baxby K. Hypnotherapy for incontinence caused by the unstable bladder. *Br Med J* 1982; 284: 1831–1834

77. Philp T, Shah PJR, Worth PHL. Acupuncture in the treatment of bladder instability. *Br J Urol* 1988; 1: 490–493

78. Klarskov P. Enkephalin inhibits presynaptically the contractility of urinary tract smooth muscle. *Br J Urol* 1987; 59: 31–35

79. Murray KH, Feneley RCL. Endorphins – a role in lower urinary tract function? The effect of opioid blockade on the detrusor and urethral sphincter mechanisms. *Br J Urol* 1982; 54: 638–640

80. Pigne A, Degausac C, Nyssen C, Barrat J. Acupuncture and the unstable bladder. *Proceedings of the Fifteenth Annual Meeting of the International Continence Society*, London, 1985: 186–187

81. Gibson JS, Pardley J, Neville J. Infra-red low power laser therapy on acupuncture points for treatment of the unstable bladder. In: *Read by Titles. The Twentieth Meeting of the International Continence Society* 1990: 146–147

82. Griffiths J. Observations on the urinary bladder and urethra. Part 2. The nerves. Part 3. *Physiol J Anat Physiol* 1895; 29/61; 254

83. Fall M. Does electrostimulation cure urinary incontinence? *J Urol* 1984; 131: 664–667

84. Plevnik S, Janez J, Vrtacnik P *et al.* Short term electrical stimulation: home treatment for urinary incontinence. *World J Urol* 1986; 4: 24–26

85. Ohlsson BL, Fall M, Frankenberg-Sommar S. Effects of external and direct pudendal nerve maximal electrical stimulation in the treatment of the uninhibited overactive bladder. *Br J Urol* 1989; 64: 374–380

86. Jonasson A, Larsson B, Pschera H, Nyland L. Short term maximal electrical stimulation – a conservative treatment of urinary incontinence. *Gynecol Obstet Invest* 1990; 30: 120–123

87. Wise BG, Cardozo LD, Cutner A *et al.* Maximal electrical stimulation: an acceptable alternative to anticholinergic medication. *Int Urogynecol J* 1992; 3: 270–271

88. Bramble FJ. The treatment of adult enuresis and urge incontinence by enterocystoplasty. *Br J Urol* 1982; 54: 693–696

89. Mundy AR, Stephenson TP. 'Clam' ileocystoplasty for the treatment of refractory urge incontinence. *Br J Urol* 1985; 57: 641–646

90. McRae P, Murray KH, Nurse DE *et al.* Clam enterocystoplasty in the neuropathic bladder. *Br J Urol* 1987; 60: 523–535

91. Rosenbaum TP, Shah PJR, Rose GA, Lloyd-Davis RW. Cranberry juice helps the problem of mucus production in enterouroplastics. *Neurourol Urodyn* 1989; 8: 344–345

92. Stone AR, Davis N, Stephenson TP. Cancer associated with augmentation cystoplasty. *Br J Urol* 1987; 60: 236–238

93. Skene AJC. *Diseases of the Bladder and Urethra in Women.* New York: William Wood, 1887

94. Oravisto KJ. Epidemiology of interstitial cystitis. *Ann Chir Gynaecol* 1975; 64: 75–77

95. Keay S, Zhang CO, Baldwin BR *et al.* Polymerase chain reaction amplification of bacterial 16S rRNA genes in interstitial cystitis and control bladder biopsies. *J Urol* 1998; 159: 280–283

96. Hentz DM, Lacroix JM, Batra SD *et al.* Detection of eubacteria in interstitial cystitis by 16S rDNA amplification. *J Urol* 1997;158: 2291–2295

97. Duncan JL, Schaeffer AJ. Do infectious agents cause interstitial cystitis? *Urology* 1997; 49: 48–51

98. Haaraza M, Jalava J, Laato M *et al*. Absence of bacterial DNA in the bladder of patients with interstitial cystitis. *J Urol* 1996; 156: 1843–1845

99. English SF, Liebert M, Cross CA, McGuire EJ. The incidence of Helicobacter pylori in patients with interstitial cystitis. *J Urol* 1998; 159: 772–773

100. Elbadawi A. Interstitial cystitis: a critique of current concepts with a new proposal for pathologic diagnosis and pathogenesis. *Urology* 1997; 49: 14–40

101. Elbadawi AE, Light JK. Distinctive ultrastructural pathology of non-ulcerative cystitis: new observations and their potential significance in pathogenesis. *Urol Int* 1996; 56: 137–162

102. Fister GM. Similarity of interstitial cystitis (Hunner's ulcer) to lupus erythematosus. *J Urol* 1938; 40: 37–40

103. Manna L, Polito C, Papale MR *et al*. Chronic interstitial cystitis and systemic lupus erythematosus in an 8-year-old girl. *Pediatr Nephrol* 1998; 12: 139–140

104. Alagiri M, Chottiner S, Ratner V *et al*. Interstitial cystitis; unexplained associations with other chronic disease and pain syndromes. *Urology* 1997; 49: 52–57

105. Oravisto KJ. Interstitial cystitis as an autoimmune disease: a review. *Eur Urol* 1980; 6: 10–13

106. Jokinen EJ, Alfthan OS, Oravisto KJ. Antitissue antibodies of interstitial cystitis. *Clin Exp Immunol* 1972; 11: 333–337

107. Ochs RL. Autoantibodies and interstitial cystitis. *ClinLab Med* 1997; 17: 571–579

108. Messing EM, Stamey TA. Interstitial cystitis: early diagnosis, pathology and treatment. *Urology* 1978; 12: 381–385

109. McGuire ES, Lytton B, Carnog SL. Interstitial cystitis following colocystoplasty. *Urology* 1973; 2: 28–31

110. Parsons CL, Stauffer C, Schmidt JD. Bladder surface glycosaminoglycans: an efficient mechanism of environmental adaptation. *Science* 1980; 208: 605–608

111. Hanno PM, Parsons CL, Shrom SH. The protective effect of heparin on experimental bladder infection. *J Surg Res* 1978; 25: 324–327

112. Parsons CL, Schmidt JD, Pollen JY. Successful treatment of interstitial cystitis with sodium pentosan polysulfate. *J Urol* 1983; 130: 51–54

113. Collan Y, Alfthan O, Kivilaasko E, Oravisto KL. Electronic microscopic and histological findings in urinary bladder epithelium in interstitial cystitis. *Eur Urol* 1976; 2: 242–245

114. Koziol JA, Clark DC, Gittes RF, Tan EM. The natural history of interstitial cystitis: a survey of 374 patients. *J Urol* 1993; 149: 465–469

115. Dundore PA, Schwartz AM, Semerjian H. Mast cell counts are not useful in the diagnosis of nonulcerative interstitial cystitis. *J Urol* 1996; 156: 1445–1446

116. Irwin P, Galloway NT. Impaired bladder perfusion in interstitial cystitis: a study of blood supply using laser Doppler flowmetry. *J Urol* 1993; 149: 890–892

117. Simmons JL. Interstitial cystitis: an explanation for the beneficial effect of an antihistamine. *J Urol* 1961; 85: 149–152

118. Theoharides TC, Sant GR. Hydroxyzine therapy for interstitial cystitis. *Urology* 1997; 49: 108–110

119. Parsons CL, Benson G, Childs SJ. A quantitatively controlled method to study prospectively interstitial cystitis and demonstrate the efficacy of pentanopolysulfate. *J Urol* 1993; 159: 845–848

120. Porru D, Campus G, Tudino D *et al*. Results of treatment of refractory interstitial cystitis with intravesical hyaluronic acid. *Urol Int* 1997; 15: 26–29

121. Morales A, Emerson L, Nickel JC. Intravesical hyaluronic acid in the treatment of refractory interstitial cystitis. *Urology* 1997; 49: 111–113

122. Parsons CL, Mulholland SG. Successful therapy of interstitial cystitis with pentanopolysulfate. *J Urol* 1987; 138: 513–516

123. Jepsen JV, Sall M, Rhodes PR *et al*. Long-term experience with pentosanpolysulfate in interstitial cystitis. *Urology* 1998; 51: 381–387

124. Hanno PM. Analysis of long-term Elmiron therapy for interstitial cystitis. *Urology* 1997; 49: 93–99

125. Hwang P, Auclair B, Beechinor D *et al*. Efficacy of pentosanpolysulfate in the treatment of interstitial cystitis: a meta-analysis. *Urology* 1997; 50: 39–43

126. Hanno PM, Buehler J, Wein AJ. Use of amitriptyline in the treatment of interstitial cystitis. *J Urol* 1989; 141: 846–848

127. Badenoch AW. Chronic interstitial cystitis. *Br Med J* 1971; 43: 718–721

128. Walsh A. Interstitial cystitis. In: Harrison JH, Gittes RF, Perlmutter AD *et al*. (eds) *Campbell's Urology*, 4th edn. Philadelphia: WB Saunders, 1978: 693–707

129. Oravisto KJ, Alfthan OS. Treatment of interstitial cystitis with immunosuppression and chloroquine derivatives. *Eur Urol* 1976; 2: 82–84

130. Forsell T, Ruutu M, Isoniemi H *et al*. Cyclosporin in severe interstitial cystitis. *J Urol* 1996; 155: 1591–1593

131. Walsh A. Interstitial cystitis: observations on diagnosis and treatment with anti-inflammatory drugs, particularly benzydiamine. *Eur Urol* 1977; 3: 216–217

132. Dunn M. Interstitial cystitis: treated by prolonged bladder distension. *J Urol* 1977; 49: 641–645

133. Rosamilia A, Dwyer PL, Gibson J. Electromotive drug administration of lidocaine and dexamethasone followed by cystodistension in women with interstitial cystitis. *Int Urogynecol J* 1997; 8: 142–145

134. Gurpinar T, Wong HY, Griffith DP. Electromotive drug administration of intravesical lidocaine in patients with interstitial cystitis. *J Endourol* 1996; 10: 443–447

135. Sant GR. Intravesical 50% dimethyl sulfoxide in treatment of interstitial cystitis. *Urology* 1987; 29: 17–21

136. Mathews P, Barker S, Phillip PA. Prospective study of DMSO in treatment of chronic inflammatory bladder disease. *J Urol* 1986; 135: 187–189

137. Perez-Marrero R, Emerson LE, Feltis JT. A controlled study of dimethyl sulfoxide in interstitial cystitis. *J Urol* 1988; 140: 36–39

138. Peters K, Diokno A, Steinert B *et al.* The efficacy of Tice strain bacillus Calmette-Guerin in the treatment of interstitial cystitis: a double-blind, prospective, placebo-controlled trial. *J Urol* 1997; 157: 2090–2094

139. Peters KM, Diokno AC, Steinert BW, Gonzalez JA. The efficacy of intravesical bacillus Calmette-Guerin in the treatment of interstitial cystitis: long-term follow up. *J Urol* 1998; 159: 1483–1486

140. Peeker R, Aldenborg F, Fall M. The treatment of interstitial cystitis with supratrigonal cystectomy and ileocystoplasty: difference in outcome between classic and nonulcer disease. *J Urol* 1998; 159: 1479–1482

141. Linn JF, Hohenfellner M, Roth S *et al.* Treatment of interstitial cystitis: comparison of subtrigonal and supratrigonal cystectomy combined with orthotopic bladder substitution. *J Urol* 1998; 159: 774–778

142. Lotenfoe RR, Christie J, Parsons SA *et al.* Absence of neuropathic pelvic pain and favourable psychological profile in the surgical selection of patients with disabling interstitial cystitis. *J Urol* 1995; 154: 2039–2042

143. Grenados EA, Salvador J, Vicente J, Villvicencio H. Follow up of the remaining bladder after supravesical urinary diversion. *Eur Urol* 1996; 29: 308–311

144. Benness CJ, Barnick CG, Cardozo LD. Is there a place for videocystourethrography in the assessment of lower urinary tract dysfunction? *Neurourol Urodyn* 1989; 9: 299–300

145. Macaulay A, Stanton S, Holmes D. Micturition and the mind: psychological factors in the aetiology of urinary disorders in women. *Br Med J* 1987; 294: 540–543

146. Jarvis GJ. The management of urinary incontinence due to primary vesical sensory urgency by bladder drill. *Br J Urol* 1982; 54: 374–376

147. Frewen WK. Urgency incontinence. *J Obstet Gynaecol Br Commonw* 1972; 79: 77–79

148. Ferrie BG, Smith JS, Logan D. Experience with bladder training in 65 patients. *Br J Urol* 1984; 56: 482–484

69

Urethral syndrome

C. Benness

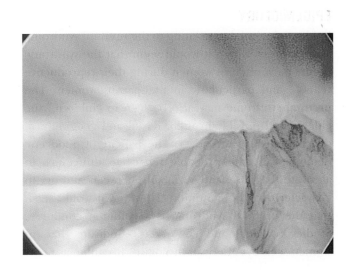

INTRODUCTION

The term 'urethral syndrome' was first used by Gallagher in 1932[1] and refers to a constellation of common lower urinary tract symptoms occurring in the absence of bacteriuria or other objective findings of urethral or bladder pathology. There is, however, no universally accepted definition of the urethral syndrome and it remains one of the most perplexing topics in urogynaecology. The symptoms vary greatly between affected individuals but the most common symptoms are urinary frequency, urgency and dysuria. Less common features include suprapubic and perineal discomfort, hesitancy and a sensation of incomplete bladder emptying. Urinary incontinence may occasionally be a feature.

The urethral syndrome is a significant clinical problem, giving rise to an estimated 5 million office visits per year in the US. The severity of the symptoms varies from very mild to severe and disabling. The urethral syndrome is essentially a diagnosis of exclusion, being made once urinary tract infection, detrusor instability, sensory urgency and local urethral pathology have been excluded. It is also a condition with multiple aetiologies. It is therefore not surprising that suggested treatment modalities range from local application of oestrogens or steroids, to surgery and even psychotherapy. Most, but not all, women with this syndrome can have their symptoms improved. However, patience is required by both physician and sufferer in the investigative work-up and implementation of a management plan. Unfortunately, a small group of patients have persistent chronic symptoms and remain a therapeutic dilemma.

EPIDEMIOLOGY

Epidemiological data relating to the urethral syndrome are scarce. However, it would seem that the syndrome occurs most often in women during their reproductive years,[2–5] and particularly in nulliparous women. The urethral syndrome may also be seen in children,[3] the elderly, and possibly in men. Racial and geographical distributions are unknown. The paucity of good epidemiological data probably relates to difficulties in accurate diagnosis and variability between authors in characterizing the condition. However, it would seem that the urethral syndrome is a common condition. Studies by Held and co-workers[6,7] indicate that, of women seen by American urologists, five times as many

have 'painful bladder syndrome' and sterile urine as have interstitial cystitis. Many of these women would be found to have the urethral syndrome following investigation. Scotti *et al.*[8] made the diagnosis of urethral syndrome in 20–30% of women with urinary complaints referred to their clinic.

DIFFERENTIAL DIAGNOSIS

Many lower urinary tract conditions can give rise to symptoms consistent with the urethral syndrome and need to be excluded. These include infection, urinary tract calculi, interstitial cystitis and urethral or bladder malignancy. Detrusor instability, urethral diverticulum, urethral caruncle, cystourethrocele and vaginitis should all be excluded.

PATHOGENESIS

The aetiology and pathogenesis of the urethral syndrome are still incompletely understood; however, it is certain that no single aetiological factor accounts for all cases. Popular theories as to the cause include infection, obstruction, spasm, oestrogen deficiency, and neurogenic and psychogenic mechanisms. One or more of these factors is likely to be present in the majority of women with the urethral syndrome. Other suggested aetiologies, with little supportive evidence, are reactions to environmental chemicals,[9] allergic conditions[10] and hormonal imbalance.[11]

Obstruction

Many investigators have proposed that the urethral syndrome could be caused by urethral stenosis and may thus be treated by surgery. Excellent results have been claimed for procedures that incise, dilate or resect the urethra. However, there is little evidence that many women with the urethral syndrome have objective urethral obstruction. Lyon and Smith[12] described a constrictive ring of fibrous tissue in the distal urethra of young girls. Urethral dilatation was associated with improvement in symptoms. It has been suggested that turbulent flow in the urethra secondary to stenosis may result in the backflow of bacteria into the proximal urethra.[13] However, Hole[14] did not find any difference in urethral calibre between women with frequency–dysuria syndrome and a control group.

Urethral stenosis has been described proximally as well as distally. Winsbury-White[15] and Young[16] both described vesical-neck obstruction and treatment by surgical resection. There is concern, however, that the procedures recommended to treat urethral obstruction may be of only temporary benefit, and by damaging the urethral sphincteric mechanism, may result in urinary incontinence.

Urethral spasm

Urethral spasm has been suggested as a cause of the urethral syndrome. Raz and Smith[17] demonstrated spasticity of the external urethral sphincter on urethral pressure profilometry in women with the urethral syndrome. They found that treatment with diazepam or α-blockers was more beneficial than urethral dilatation. Following the urodynamic investigation of 43 women with the urethral syndrome, Lipsky[18] found a group of younger women with incomplete relaxation or spasm of the external striated sphincter. Other researchers[19] found a high maximum urethral closure pressure in these women, associated with low flow rates and urethral instability. Multiple factors could be responsible for these findings, including a functional aetiology in some patients. It therefore remains unclear whether spasm, if it is a significant factor, is a primary or secondary phenomenon.

Infection

Infection is thought by some investigators to be an important cause of the urethral syndrome. Although there is no doubt that infection involving the urethra and bladder may result in lower urinary tract symptoms, bacteria are rarely retrieved from patients with the urethral syndrome. It has been suggested that fastidious organisms such as *Chlamydia trachomatis*, *Mycoplasma hominis* and *Ureaplasma urealyticum* may give rise to symptoms in women with the urethral syndrome, but these organisms are difficult to culture and identify.[20,21] Against this theory is the general agreement that the majority of women with symptoms and colonization of the lower urinary tract with such organisms will have pyuria; the diagnosis of the urethral syndrome is therefore excluded. Furthermore, some authors have found that there is no difference in the ratios of positive cultures of implicated organisms from women with the urethral syndrome or from controls.[22,23]

Endoscopy of the lower urinary tract may indicate erythema, inflammatory polyps, urethritis and cobblestoning of the trigone, suggestive of an infectious or inflammatory aetiology. However, most of these findings can also be caused by other mechanisms such as trauma or hormonal changes.[24] It is therefore unlikely that infection is a factor in the aetiology of the urethral syndrome in many women.

Hypo-oestrogenism

The female genital and urinary tracts are intimately associated. They share a common embryology, both arising from the primitive urogenital sinus. High-affinity oestrogen receptors have been identified in the bladder, trigone and urethra in both animal and human studies.[25] It is therefore not surprising that changes in oestrogen levels influence the lower urinary tract as well as the genital tract in women. Symptomatic, clinical and urodynamic changes of the lower urinary tract occur with fluctuation of the female sex steroids. This occurs during pregnancy, the menstrual cycle and at the menopause. The urethra is therefore an oestrogen-sensitive tissue. Post-menopausal oestrogen deficiency results in atrophic changes in the bladder and urethra and may give rise to irritative bladder and urethral symptoms. Endoscopy in post-menopausal women often indicates a pale, stenotic and friable urethra. Youngblood *et al.*[26] demonstrated that oestrogen therapy (diethylstilboestrol) produced considerable improvement in post-menopausal urethral syndrome. Hypo-oestrogenism should therefore be considered seriously as a possible aetiological factor in post-menopausal women with symptoms suggestive of the urethral syndrome.

Psychogenic factors

The urethral syndrome may have a psychogenic aetiology in some women. Carson *et al.*[27] found higher scores of hysteria and hypochondriasis in 160 women with the urethral syndrome, tested using the Minnesota Multiphasic Personality Inventory. In a subgroup referred for psychiatric counselling, 13 out of 15 achieved total resolution of symptoms following therapy. However, more recent studies[28,29] have not found a significant association between the urethral syndrome and psychiatric morbidity. It is also possible that psychological problems in women with the urethral syndrome may be more a consequence of organic disease than a significant pathogenic factor in the condition.

DIAGNOSIS

Because the diagnosis of the urethral syndrome is essentially one of exclusion, a fairly extensive investigative work-up is often required to make the diagnosis and to avoid overlooking organic pathology. A thorough history is important, including questions about the onset and duration of symptoms, any exacerbating factors such as sexual intercourse, and previous history of sexually transmitted disease.

A general physical and neurological examination should be performed, including documentation that the sacral segments S2–4 are intact. Pelvic assessment should include checking for evidence of pelvic relaxation, urethral–hymenal fusion, a pelvic mass or urethral caruncle. A catheter specimen of urine for microscopy and culture should be obtained. Urethral and cervical cultures for *Chlamydia* should be obtained in sexually active women. There is generally a low yield from radiological studies in women with symptoms suggestive of the urethral syndrome. However, an intravenous urogram may be necessary to exclude other rare causes of similar symptoms (e.g. urethral diverticulum).

Cystourethroscopy

Women with the urethral syndrome do not usually show significant abnormality of the urethra or bladder on endoscopic assessment. However, atrophic changes suggestive of hypo-oestrogenism may be apparent in post-menopausal women. The main indication for cystourethroscopy is to rule out conditions with similar symptomatology. These include urethritis, trigonitis, urethral and bladder diverticula, interstitial cystitis and premalignant and malignant conditions of the bladder. Following inspection of the urethra and bladder, the urethra should be massaged by a finger in the vagina as the endoscope is being withdrawn. During this process, a careful search is made for exudate from glandular orifices or diverticula.

Urodynamic studies

Urodynamic investigations are not necessary in all women in whom the diagnosis of the urethral syndrome is suspected. However, they are useful in those with significant urinary frequency and urgency. Urodynamic testing is also indicated in those women with urinary incontinence or a history suggestive of neurological disease. If the patient's bladder can be comfortably filled to normal capacity and the patient has normal bladder compliance, then the conditions of detrusor instability, interstitial cystitis and sensory urgency are largely excluded. During cystometry, provocative measures such as changing position, hand-washing in cold water, and heel-bouncing increase the sensitivity for diagnosing detrusor instability.

Uroflowmetry is a simple non-invasive test which can assess voiding function objectively and should be performed if urodynamic testing is undertaken in these women. Some authors suggest that this is potentially the most diagnostic of the urodynamic investigations.[30]

TREATMENT

A wide range of treatment options have been advocated for the management of women with the urethral syndrome. Because this condition may be caused by a number of different aetiologic factors, no one therapy is effective for all women. Therefore, the guiding principle in the management of the urethral syndrome is to treat the most probable cause after a thorough diagnostic work-up has been performed. Supportive therapy is required for all women with the urethral syndrome, regardless of the underlying aetiology. Patience and understanding are of the utmost importance in the management of patients with chronic and recurring lower urinary tract symptoms.

Women whose symptoms are thought to be due to an infection should be treated with antibiotics. These are patients who, from urine culture, have an infection with less than 10 colony-forming units per ml or who have sterile pyuria. However, some authors would exclude this latter group from the diagnosis of urethral syndrome. Antibiotic therapy based on culture and sensitivities from urethral swabs should be used when available. If chlamydial infection is suspected, a 10-day course of a tetracycline should be given. Stamm *et al.*[31] found that doxycycline was significantly more effective than placebo in a double-blind randomized trial. Erythromycin can also be used if pyuria persists. It is effective against *Chlamydia* and many of the anaerobes that have been implicated in the urethral syndrome.

There are some data to support the use of long-term low-dose antibiotic prophylaxis in women with symptoms consistent with the urethral syndrome and a past history of recurrent urinary tract infections. Kraft and Stamey[32] showed that some patients with recurrent bacteriuria may experience irritable voiding symptoms when their urine is uninfected and then develop documented bacteriuria within several months.

Noxious agents, bubble baths, tampons and chemical substances such as deodorant soaps should be avoided if these are suspected as a possible cause for the patient's symptoms.

All post-menopausal women, whether or not they have objective evidence of oestrogen deficiency, should try local oestrogen therapy,[33] as creams, ovules or tablets. Initially this should be on a daily basis for 4–8 weeks and can then be used less frequently. Local effects on the vagina and lower urinary tract are more prominent with local oestrogen therapy than with systemic oestrogen therapy. Patients should be warned that the clinical benefits of local oestrogen therapy may take 1–3 months to become fully apparent.

If no improvement is found after antimicrobial therapy, treatment with oestrogens or both of these, then urethral dilatation may be considered. This time-honoured technique is combined with anterior vaginal wall massage (Fig. 69.1). The rationale is that obstructed, inflamed or infected urethral glands will be massaged against the rigid dilator. Bergman *et al.*[34] reported a trial in 60 women with the urethral syndrome, comparing this technique with placebo or treatment with tetracycline for 10 days. A 75% subjective improvement was noted in the urethral dilatation group, which was significantly better than either the placebo or tetracycline treatment.

Numerous other treatment modalities have been recommended. These include non-surgical therapies such as psychotherapy, biofeedback, anti-inflammatory agents and bladder instillations, including dimethyl-sulphoxide and silver nitrate. More invasive therapeutic options include urethral resection, fulguration and treatment with cryosurgery. Most of the studies of these techniques have significant methodological problems, making interpretation difficult. There is also the constant problem in studies of the urethral syndrome of non-rigid criteria to determine the diagnosis. It is important to bear in mind the findings of Carson *et al.*[27] and Zufall,[35] who demonstrated excellent results with

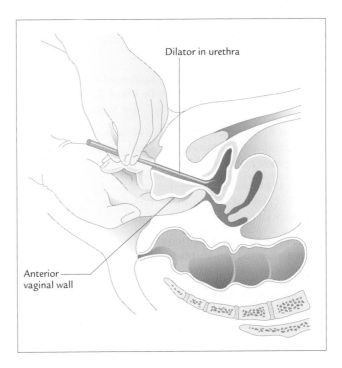

Figure 69.1. *Technique of urethral dilatation and massage through the anterior vaginal wall.*

observation alone in over 85% of women. In general, treatment for the urethral syndrome should initially take a conservative approach, as this is usually as effective as surgery, is less expensive and is associated with less morbidity.

REFERENCES

1. Gallagher D, Montgomerie J, North J. Acute infections of the urinary tract and the urethral syndrome in general practice. *Br Med J* 1965; 543: 622–624

2. Carson CC, Osborne D, Segura JW. Psychologic characteristics of patients with urethral syndrome. *J Clin Psychol* 1979; 35: 312–316

3. Kaplan WE, Firlit CF, Schoenberg HW. The female urethral syndrome; external sphincter spasm as etiology. *J Urol* 1980; 124: 48–50

4. Mabry EW, Carson CC, Older RA. Evaluation of women with chronic voiding discomfort. *Urology* 1981; 18: 244–247

5. Smith P. The management of the urethral syndrome. *Br J Hosp Med* 1979; 22: 578–580

6. Held P, Hanno P, Wein A, Pauly M. Epidemiology of interstitial cystitis: Incidence of interstitial cystitis from a

natural sample of urologists. Presented at the NIH-NIDDK workshop on interstitial cystitis, Bethesda USA, August 1997.

7. Held P, Hanno P, Wein A *et al*. Epidemiology of interstitial cystitis. In: Hanno P, Staskin D, Krane R, Wein A (eds) *Interstitial Cystitis*. New York: Springer-Verlag, 1990; 29–48

8. Scotti R, Ostergard DR. Predictive value of urethroscopy in genuine stress incontinence and vesical instability. *Int Urogynecol J* 1993; 4: 255–258

9. Bell I. The kinin system theory of mechanism for food and chemical sensitivities. Presented at the Ninth Advanced Seminar in Clinical Ecology, Toronto, 1975

10. Gilmore N, Vane J. Hormones released into the circulation when the urinary bladder of the anaesthetised dog is distended. *Clin Sci* 1971; 41: 69–72

11. Zondek B, Bromberg Y. Endocrine allergy: clinical reactions of allergy to endogenous hormones and their treatment. *J Obstet Gynaecol Br Emp* 1947; 54: 1–4

12. Lyon R, Smith D. Distal urethral stenosis. *J Urol* 1963; 89: 414–416

13. Corriere J. McClure J, Lipschultz L. Contamination of bladder urine by urethral particles during voiding: urethrovesical reflux. *J Urol* 1972; 107: 399–401

14. Hole R. The calibre of the adult female urethra. *Br J Urol* 1972; 44: 68–71

15. Winsbury-White H. Two cases of retention of urine in women. *Lancet* 1936; 2: 1008–1009

16. Young H. The pathology and treatment of obstructions at the vesical neck in women. *J Am Med Assoc* 1940; 115: 2133–2138

17. Raz S, Smith R. External sphincter spasticity syndrome in female patients. *J Urol* 1976; 115: 443–447

18. Lipsky H. Urodynamic assessment of women with the urethral syndrome. *Urologe A* 1976; 15: 207–212

19. Barbalias G, Meares E. Female urethral syndrome: clinical and urodynamic perspectives. *Urology* 1984; 23: 208–215

20. Bruce A, Chadwick P, Hassen A, Van Cott GF. Recurrent urethritis in women. *Can Med Assoc J* 1973; 108: 973–979

21. Stamm W, Wagner K, Amsel R *et al*. Causes of the acute urethral syndrome in women. *N Engl J Med* 1980; 303: 409–411

22. Gillespie W, Henderson E, Linton K, Smith P. Microbiology of the urethral (frequency and dysuria) syndrome. A controlled study with 5-year review. *Br J Urol* 1989; 64: 270–274

23. Tait J, Peddie B, Bailey R *et al*. Urethral syndrome – search for a pathogen. *Br J Urol* 1985; 57: 522–526

24. Messing EM. Interstitial cystitis and related syndromes. In: Walsh PC, Gittes RF, Perlmutter AD, Stamey TA (eds) *Campbell's Urology*, 5th edn. Philadelphia: WB Saunders, 1985; 1070–1092

25. Ingelman-Sundberg A, Rosen J, Gustafson SA, Carlstrom K. Cytosol estrogen receptors in the urogenital tissues in stress incontinent women. *Acta Obstet Gynecol Scand* 1981; 60: 585–588

26. Youngblood VH, Tomlin EM, Davis JB. Senile urethritis in women. *J Urol* 1957; 78: 150–153

27. Carson CC, Segura JW, Osborne DM. Evaluation and treatment of the female urethral syndrome. *J Urol* 1980; 124: 609–615

28. Sumners D, Kelsey M, Chait I. Psychological aspects of lower urinary tract infections in women. *Br Med J* 1992; 304: 17–19

29. Nazaret I, King MB. The urethral syndrome: a controlled evaluation. *J Psychosom Res* 1993; 37: 737–743

30. Schmidt RA, Tanagho EA. Urethral syndrome or urinary tract infection? *Urology* 1981; 18: 454–458

31. Stamm WE, Running K, McKevitt M *et al*. Treatment of the acute urethral syndrome. *N Engl J Med* 1981; 304: 956–960

32. Kraft JK, Stamey TA. The natural history of symptomatic recurrent bacteriuria in women. *Medicine (Baltimore)* 1977; 56: 55–61

33. Benness C, Wise B, Cutner A, Cardozo L. Does low-dose vaginal estradiol improve frequency and urgency in postmenopausal women? *Int Urogynecol J* 1992; 3: 281–282

34. Bergman A, Karram M, Bhattia N. Urethral syndrome. A comparison of different treatment modalities. *J Reprod Med* 1989; 34: 157–162

35. Zufall R. Infectiveness of treatment of urethral syndrome in women. *Urology* 1978; 12: 337–339

70

Vaginitis

K. Boos

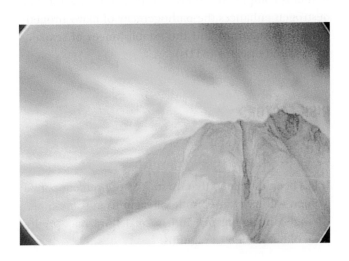

INTRODUCTION

Vulvovaginal pain, itching and burning, often accompanied by vaginal discharge, are the classic symptoms of vaginitis. These symptoms account for as many as 5 million primary-care visits per year in the USA.[1] The common infectious conditions include candidiasis, trichomoniasis, bacterial vaginosis (BV) and group B streptococcal vaginitis.

AETIOLOGY

There is certainly some doubt about what should be regarded as normal vaginal flora.[2] In general terms, the flora of the vagina consists of aerobic, facultative and obligate anaerobic bacteria. These exist together and interact with each other and with host factors to maintain a healthy equilibrium. Both endogenous and exogenous mechanisms may disrupt this equilibrium and give rise to an inflammatory response within the vagina.

PATHOGENESIS

The vagina has certain defences that must be overcome by pathogenic organisms before infection can be established. Studies have shown that it is local epithelial, and not systemic, immunization that provides a high and long-lasting level of immunity from infection, particularly from sexually transmitted viral infections.[3] Numerous studies have examined the influence of the female sex hormones – oestrogen and progesterone – on urogenital infections.[4] The interaction between these hormones in the adult female and the immune system is complex but there is evidence to suggest that oestrogen enhances the pathogenicity of many urogenital microorganisms and the establishment of sexually transmitted diseases (STDs).

RISK FACTORS

Age

It has been estimated that up to 75% of premenopausal women will have an episode of vaginitis at some time.[5] Changes in vaginal pH and normal flora may predispose older women to vaginitis.

Sexual activity

It is debatable whether sexual activity contributes to recurrent vaginitis, in particular vulvovaginal candidiasis. Both partners should receive treatment and should possibly refrain from intercourse to give the best chance of healing and to break the cycle of vaginal infection. However, it has been suggested that certain sexual activities are associated with repeated episodes of vulvovaginal candidiasis. Hellberg and co-workers found that significant sexual variables included early age at first intercourse, casual sex partners in the previous month, sex during menstruation and regular oral sex. Recurrent infection was not, however, associated with multiple sexual partners.[6]

Diabetes mellitus

Vaginal symptoms attributable to vaginal candidiasis are common in young women with type I diabetes. However, the relationship between these symptoms and glycated haemoglobin is weak, and the symptoms are not confined to women with poor diabetic control.[7]

Human immunodeficiency virus infection

Women constitute the fastest growing segment of adults with acquired immune deficiency syndrome (AIDS), representing 18% of all cases in the USA in 1994. Heterosexual transmission is now the dominant route by which women are infected. Vaginitis due to *Candida*, *Trichomonas* and BV are common findings among women who are seropositive for human immunodeficiency virus (HIV).[8] Frankel *et al.*[9] investigated the presence of gynaecological disease in women infected with HIV: the prevalence of vaginitis was 51%. For predicting gynaecological disease, gynaecological symptoms had a sensitivity of 76% and a positive predictive value of 95% but a negative predictive value of only 41%. Frankel *et al.* also found a high prevalence of co-morbid gynaecological disease among women infected with HIV. Only 9% of the women were admitted to hospital for primary gynaecological or genitourinary problems but, after evaluation, 83% of them were found to have gynaecological disease, including genital condylomata, genital herpes and pelvic inflammatory disease.[9]

PRINCIPLES OF DIAGNOSIS

In general practice, it may be quite difficult to establish the exact cause of vaginal symptoms. It is common to attribute symptoms to a candidal infection and to institute empirical therapy without prior microscopy or culture of vaginal fluid. This practice has led to much misdiagnosis and inadequate therapy. Berg *et al.*[10] reported that when comparing clinical findings and comprehensive microbiology, up to 50% of women diagnosed with vulvovaginal candidiasis had other conditions.

In very young girls, pelvic examination may be difficult; vaginal secretion may be collected using vaginal washes. In cases of alleged sexual abuse in girls prior to the menarche, vaginal-wash techniques have been shown to be useful and show promise as a diagnostic procedure for STDs.[11]

Vaginal pH may be a useful, effective and inexpensive marker for the presence of bacterial pathogens within the vagina and as a marker for the menopausal status of women. A vaginal pH of 4.5 is consistent with a premenopausal serum oestradiol level and the absence of bacterial pathogens. An elevated vaginal pH – in the range 5.0–6.5 – suggests a diagnosis of either bacterial pathogens or decreased serum oestradiol. In women with an elevated pH, vaginal culture should establish the diagnosis. In the absence of bacterial pathogens, a vaginal pH of 6.0–7.5 is strongly suggestive of the menopause.[12]

Screening tests

Rapid antigen tests for *Neisseria gonorrhoea* and *Chlamydia trachomatis* have been shown to be inaccurate for screening women with disturbed vaginal lactobacilli flora. Donders *et al.*[13] found that detectors of endocervical antigens of *C. trachomatis* and *N. gonorrhoea* lacked sensitivity in pregnant and infertile women living in an area with a high prevalence of chlamydia cervicitis, gonorrhoea and trachomatis vaginitis.

Chacko *et al.*[14] assessed the ability of the leucocyte esterase (LE) dipstick of vaginal secretions to detect *Trichomonas*, *Candida* and BV and the LE dipstick of both vaginal and cervical secretions to detect gonococcal and chlamydia infection and polymorphonuclear (PMN) cells. The LE dipstick was only a moderately good screening test for vaginal infection but was a good screening test for cervical infection.[14]

PRINCIPLES OF TREATMENT

Over-the-counter medication

Many women who experience what they believe to be a vaginal yeast infection use over-the-counter (OTC) antifungal agents, which they perceive to be safe, efficacious, convenient and cost-effective.[15] Nyirjesy *et al.*[16] investigated the use of OTC and alternative medicines in the treatment of women with chronic vaginal symptoms. The median duration of symptoms was 2 years and 73.3% of women had self-treated with OTC medicines such as miconazole (74% of OTC users), clotrimazole (38.2%) or providone-iodine (13.2%). Alternative treatments were used by 41.9% of women: most frequently used were: acidophilus pills, orally (50%) or vaginally (11.4%); yogurt, orally (20.5%) or vaginally (18.2%); vinegar douches (13.6%) and boric acid (13.6%). Although most women thought that vulvovaginal candidiasis was the cause of their symptoms, the most common diagnoses at initial presentation were candidiasis in 27.6%, vulvovestibulitis in 17.1%, irritant dermatitis in 15.2% and BV in 10.5%. Women who actually had candidiasis were more likely to have used alternative medicines that were unlikely to be of benefit.

The ingestion of yogurt has traditionally been advocated as prophylaxis for both recurrent candidal vaginitis and BV. Shaler *et al.*[17] compared the ingestion of yogurt that contained live *Lactobacillus acidophilus* with pasteurized yogurt for these conditions. They found that daily ingestion of 150 ml of yogurt enriched with *L. acidophilus* was associated with an increased prevalence of colonization of the rectum and vagina by the bacteria and may have reduced the episodes of BV.[17]

CANDIDAL VAGINITIS

Candida infections account for 20–25% of cases of infectious vaginitis; 80–92% of cases of vulvovaginal candidiasis are attributed to *Candida albicans*.[18] However, the incidence of non-albicans vaginal infection is increasing. Spinillo *et al.* evaluated the prevalence of, and risk factors for, fungal vaginitis caused by non-albicans species in a vaginitis clinic setting.[19] The prevalence had increased sharply from 9.9% in 1988 to 17.2% in 1995. Those at increased risk of non-albicans vaginitis include patients with HIV or recurrent vaginal candidiasis.

Risk factors for vulvovaginal candidiasis include diabetes mellitus, and the use of antibiotics and the oestrogen-containing contraceptive pill. Candida infection is also more common in women using intra-uterine devices and vaginal sponges for contraception.[20]

Diagnosis

One of the most characteristic features of candida vaginitis is intense pruritis associated with a creamy discharge. Kurowski[21] has suggested that urinary symptoms such as dysuria may be the principal complaint of women with vaginitis infections (atrophic or chemical).

In the presence of candida infection the vaginal pH remains unchanged (4–4.5) and the amine sniff test is negative. Polarizing saline microscopy reveals the presence of budding yeast and pseudohyphae in up to 40% of samples. Examination with the addition of 10% potassium hydroxide shows a positive result with the presence of pseudohyphae in 70% of samples. Microscopy may also show the presence of a large number of PMN leucocytes. In the case of women with negative microscopy in whom there is a strong clinical suspicion of candidiasis, one should perform a culture of vaginal secretions.

Because *Candida* are normal commensals in the vaginal flora, treatment is only recommended in symptomatic women with clinical disease. In the past it was thought unnecessary to treat the male sexual partner. However, it would seem prudent to do so because, even though candidiasis is not an STD, infection has been associated with sexual intercourse. Treatment of the male partner may help to break the cycle of recurrent infection possibly associated with sexual intercourse.[22]

Reef *et al.*[23] have suggested that topical antimycotic drugs can achieve cure rates for vulvovaginal candidiasis in excess of 80%. However, it is generally accepted that, in uncomplicated cases, there is little difference in efficacy between various formulations or routes of administration.[24]

Duration of treatment

In uncomplicated cases of candidal vaginitis, single-dose regimens are highly effective and are recommended. In complicated cases one should consider underlying predisposing factors which, if treated, will optimize cure rates. Culture may also reveal unexpected or atypical pathogens such as *C. glabrata* which are less susceptible to the usual antimicrobials and require more specific therapy.[25] Therapy for up to 14 days is recommended to achieve best results in complicated cases.[25]

Suppressive therapy

Treatment of recurrent vaginitis can be difficult and challenging because the patient's morale falls with each recurrence of vaginitis. Long-term suppressive therapy is recommended in these cases. Azole resistance is rare but problems may occur. Regimens include ketoconazole or itraconazole daily, fluconazole once weekly or clotrimazole vaginal suppositories once weekly. Suppressive therapy for at least 6 months achieves best results and is recommended.[23]

BACTERIAL VAGINOSIS

BV is the most common cause of vaginal discharge in women of childbearing age.[26] It is a clinical syndrome defined microbiologically where lactobacilli-dominated vaginal flora is replaced by an abundant complex flora dominated by strict and facultative anaerobic bacteria constituted by *Gardnerella*, micrococci, streptococci and staphylococci.[27] Thorsen *et al.* demonstrated that this may be due to an intermicrobial interaction in which the microorganisms *G. vaginalis*, anaerobic bacteria and *Mycoplasma hominis* constitute the pathological core of BV.[28] BV characteristically shows a relapsing and remitting course with apparently spontaneous cure or resolution.

Virulence of BV

Sialidases are enzymes produced by microorganisms present in the microflora of patients with BV. They confer virulence not only by destroying the mucins and enhancing adherence of bacteria, but also by impairing a specific IgA-mediated immune response in the host against other virulence factors such as cytotoxin and haemolysin from *G. vaginalis*.[29]

Risk factors

BV may be found in up to 68% of all women without evidence of vaginal disease.[30] Additionally, BV will be detected in the vaginal secretions of almost all women with non-specific vaginitis.[31–34] Some risk factors have been implicated in the pathogenesis of this condition. BV arises most often in the first 7 days of the menstrual cycle and resolves spontaneously in mid-cycle.[26] In a study by Priestley *et al.*[35] BV seemed to be related to frequent use of scented soap and there was an additive effect of clothing and hygiene factors.

Among post-menopausal women attending a vaginitis clinic, a diagnosis of BV, candidal vaginitis or trichomonas vaginitis was made in approximately one-third of symptomatic patients. In the remaining women, in whom there was no microbiological evidence of such infections, symptoms were mostly due to atrophic vaginitis, non-anaerobic bacterial infections, local irritants or allergens, or dermatological conditions.[36] BV is also found more often in black than in non-black women.[37] Also, recurrence of BV often follows an episode of candidiasis.[26]

Diagnosis

BV is usually considered to be present if the following are detected:[38]

- grey–white vaginal discharge;
- vaginal pH > 4.5;
- positive 'whiff' test;
- presence of epithelial cells classified as clue cells.

Because BV is not caused by any single agent, the current diagnostic approach is to provide as much evidence as possible on the basis of some characteristic findings. The Amsel criteria are often used and define BV as being present if three of the four following criteria are found:[33]

- homogeneous vaginal discharge;
- vaginal pH > 4.3;
- positive whiff test;
- presence of clue cells on wet microscopy of the vaginal fluid.

As a refinement, it is recommended that at least 20% of the epithelial cells present be defined as clue cells.[34]

Gram stain of vaginal fluid is another method used reliably as a diagnostic standard to detect BV.[39,40] The Gram stain provides a direct view of the bacteriological

morphotypes and is unaffected by factors such as menses or recent sexual intercourse, which may alter vaginal pH, and by technical variables such as observer interpretation of clue cells.[34] It has excellent inter and intra-observer reproducibility and correlates well with the clinical signs of BV, including pH, positive whiff test and clue cells.[41] The sensitivity and specificity of the Gram stain are 89% and 83%, respectively.[42]

Another technique is to examine cervical cytology smears for evidence of BV. Cervical cytological tests have a sensitivity of 55% and specificity of 98%. They have an excellent positive predictive value (96%) in diagnosing BV.[43]

Complications

On the basis of histological, microbiological or laparoscopic evidence, BV is associated with an increased risk of upper genital tract infections (adjusted odds ratio: 3.0; 95% confidence intervals: 1.2–7.6). BV-associated (anaerobic Gram-negative) bacteria also play a role in the aetiology of endometritis in women with clinically suspected pelvic inflammatory disease.[44] However, it is not yet clear whether treatment of BV can reduce the risk of this ascending infection.[38] Research has also suggested that BV may increase the survival of HIV-1 infection in the genital tract, and that loss of lactobacilli or the presence of BV may increase susceptibility to HIV-1.[45]

BV may be important in the development of cervical intra-epithelial neoplasia (CIN) because the abnormal microflora can produce carcinogenic nitrosamines; however, Frega *et al.*,[27] in a study of over 1000 women, found no significant correlation between CIN and BV.

Oral contraceptive and condom use seem to exert protective effects against the development of BV. The use of intra-uterine devices shows no association with subsequent BV.[46]

Treatment

Clindamycin, metronidazole, cefmetazole, amoxycillin and amoxycillin clavulanate are highly active against BV-associated anaerobic isolates, except mobiluncus species, which are resistant to metronidazole. Ceftazidime and ofloxacin are variably effective, while cefaclor was shown to be the least effective agent.[47]

Vaginal clindamycin (2% vaginal cream once daily for 7 days) is effective and safe in the treatment of BV compared with placebo. Treatment of the male partner of women with BV does not significantly reduce the woman's risk of recurrence of the condition.[48]

Treatment in pregnancy with topical clindamycin or metronidazole is also effective in returning the vaginal flora to normal but may be less effective in preventing the increased incidence of adverse pregnancy outcomes.[49]

SEXUALLY TRANSMITTED DISEASES

The problems caused by STDs such as vaginitis have continued to increase over the last decade. These conditions are recognized as major causes of morbidity and may cause serious illness and psychological distress. There is no room for the previous complacent opinion that STDs are of little importance, and the clinician must strive not only for effective treatment but also to develop wide-ranging preventative measures. STDs are the most common communicable diseases found in the world today and the number of patients treated each year continues to rise. This increase in incidence has occurred despite rapid advances in diagnostic facilities and the ready availability of the drugs that cure each condition. Table 70.1 lists the most frequent infecting organisms.

Edwards and Carne[50] have reviewed the literature on the role of oral sex in the transmission of STDs that can cause vaginitis. They found that oral sex was a common sexual practice among both heterosexual and homosexual couples and that orogenital sex can transmit HIV from penis or vagina to mouth. Receptive orogenital sex carries a small risk of human papillomavirus infection and possibly hepatitis C, while insertive orogenital contact is an important risk factor for acquisition of herpes simplex virus 1. The relative importance of oral sex as a route for transmission of viruses is likely to increase as other high-risk sexual practices are avoided for fear of acquiring HIV infection.[51]

The three most frequent presenting symptoms of STD are urethral discharge, genital ulceration and vaginal discharge, with or without vulval irritation. It may be quite obvious that symptoms have developed after a recent sexual contact or a change of partner. Also, the partner may have symptoms of an STD. However, it is often the case that these classical clues to the diagnosis are lacking and one must add to the evidence by an extensive sexual history, physical examination and include microbiological, and possibly serological, tests. This requires time and skill. It is recommended that the woman attend a genitourinary medicine clinic where these facilities are readily available. These clinics have considerable expertise, given their large throughput of patients, and the capability for follow-up to prove both clinical and microbiological cure. They also offer contact-tracing to ensure effective treatment and to prevent spread of disease. Table 70.2 shows the plan of investigation of an STD.

Trichomonas spp. are usually best isolated from the posterior fornix; *N. gonorrhoeae* and *Chlamydia* are best isolated from swabs of the endocervix and urethra. A Cusco speculum should be used to visualize the lower genital tract and allow appropriate swabs to be taken. Table 70.3 shows the basic principles to be considered when investigating a patient with an STD. Table 70.4 shows possible reasons for treatment failure.

Table 70.1. *Sexually transmitted pathogenic microorganisms*

Bacteria	Viruses
Chlamydia trachomatis	herpes simplex types 1 and 2
Neisseria gonorrhoea	papillomavirus
Treponema pallidum	hepatitis A and B
Haemophilus ducrey	HIV
	cytomegalovirus
Mycoplasmas	**Protozoa**
Ureaplasma urealyticum	*Trichomonas vaginalis*
Mycoplasma hominis	

Table 70.2. *Investigations required for accurate diagnosis of sexually transmitted disease*

Detailed sexual history	Type of sexual contact
	Number of partners
	Symptoms in contacts
	Sexual habits
	Sites of sexual contact
Clinical signs and symptoms	
Recurrent symptoms	
General symptoms (complications)	
Microbiological tests	
Serological tests	

Vaccines against STDs

Many viral and bacterial pathogens enter the body through the epithelium of the genital tract. One of the major goals of a vaccine against STDs is to induce in the genital epithelium an immune response capable of controlling the entry of the pathogen.[51]

Medaglini *et al.*[51] developed vaccines against STDs based on the use of non-pathogenic Gram-positive bacteria as live vaccine vectors. They developed genetic systems for the expression of antigens on the surface of the human commensals *Streptococcus gordonii* and *Lactobacillus*. Vaginal colonization of women expressing human papillomavirus and HIV antigens induced antigen-specific vaginal IgA and serum IgG. Local and systemic immune responses were also detected in monkeys immunized intravaginally with recombinant *S. gordonii*. These results show great promise for the development of vaccines against STDs by using colonization Gram-positive bacteria as live vectors to induce immunity.

Table 70.3. *Management plan for sexually transmitted disease*
Health education
General hygiene
Chemotherapy
Investigation and treatment of contacts
Follow-up
Assess clinical and microbiological cure or improvement
Need for further therapy
Manage treatment failures

Table 70.4. *Possible reasons for treatment failure in women with sexually transmitted disease*
Reinfection
Multiple infecting organisms
Poor or non-compliance with therapy (patient or contact)
Problems with chemotherapy
Wrong drug
Drug resistance
Inadequate dose of drug
Inadequate duration of therapy

TRICHOMONIASIS

Trichomonas is a pear-shaped parasitic protozoon which is highly pathogenic to the vagina and responsible for trichomoniasis, the most common non-viral STD.[52] This organism is frequently present together with other infectious agents. It is associated with male and female genitourinary infections, perinatal complications and an increased risk of HIV transmission.

Parasitic infection with *Trichomonas* affects approximately 180 million people annually worldwide.[53] Trichomoniasis accounts for 15–20% of cases of infectious vaginitis, but is important because it is associated with a high prevalence of co-infection with *C. albicans* and other STDs.[54] Laga *et al.*[55] showed that it is also a significant risk factor for HIV-1 transmission in women.

Pathogenicity

The pathogenesis of *Trichomonas vaginalis* is complex and poorly understood but involves adhesion to the vaginal epithelium, haemolysis and the action of soluble factors such as cysteine proteinases and cell-detaching factors. The proteinases are capable of degrading human IgG and secretory IgA, thereby avoiding an immune reaction.[56] Cysteine proteinases interact with the resident vaginal flora and can survive in a hostile environment. To be functional they must be activated by disulphide-reducing agents. The human vagina has a reducing environment adequate for the action of trichomonal proteinases, which helps to explain the host susceptibility to these pathogens.[57]

Diagnosis

The most common clinical findings in trichomoniasis include a malodorous, purulent, grey, possibly frothy, discharge, with dyspareunia and pruritis. Vulvovaginal reddening is commonly present. In some cases, urinary symptoms of frequency and dysuria are also present, suggesting bladder and urethral inflammation. The pH of the vaginal secretion is 5–6 and the amine test is often positive. On a saline-net mount, microscopy demonstrates abundant PMN leucocytes, but studies suggest that motile trichomonads are seen in only 50–70% of culture-confirmed cases.[58,59] Diagnosis can be difficult because the symptoms of trichomoniasis mimic those of other sexually transmitted vaginal infections and detection methods lack precision.

The vaginal introitus is a novel, highly effective site for collection of samples of *C. trachomatis* for testing by the polymerase chain reaction. The sensitivity of vaginal introital swabs for the detection of *C. trachomatis* vaginal infection was 92% (95% confidence intervals: 83–100). This is higher than with culture or enzyme immunoassay of the cervix or urethra.[60]

Treatment of trichomoniasis

The mainstay of treatment for trichomoniasis is oral metronidazole. The sexual partners of women with infection must also be treated, *T. vaginalis* being detected in up to 40% of these men.[55] Treatment options include oral metronidazole for 7 days or a single 2 g oral dose. Cure rates are said to exceed 90% when both sexual partners are treated.[55] In the USA, oral metronidazole is practically the only treatment option for *T. vaginalis*. DuBouchet *et al.*[61] compared the safety and efficacy of 0.75% metronidazole vaginal gel (twice daily for 7 days) and oral metronidazole (250 mg three times daily for 7 days): the gel preparation was not as effective as oral metronidazole. Spence *et al.*[62] found that the minimum effective single oral dose of metronidazole for trichomoniasis is 1.5 g.

ATROPHIC VAGINITIS

There are approximately 10 million climacteric and post-menopausal women in England and Wales and therefore 1 in 5 of the population is potentially at risk of the symptoms of urogenital oestrogen deficiency.[63]

At approximately 40 years of age the frequency of ovulation declines, initiating a period of waning ovarian function – the climacteric. This results in menstrual irregularities, the menopause and, finally, generalized atrophy of all oestrogen-sensitive tissues.

The female genital and urinary tracts develop in close proximity, both arising from the embryological urogenital sinus. Human and animal studies have shown that the adult female urogenital tissues are oestrogen sensitive, and oestrogen and progesterone receptors have been identified in the human urethra, bladder, vagina and pelvic floor, irrespective of hormonal status.[64–67] Fluctuations in sex steroids, in particular oestrogens, result in symptomatic and cytological changes. This has been demonstrated during the menstrual cycle, in pregnancy and following the menopause.[68–70] Circulating oestrogen levels fall at the time of the menopause, and there is urogenital atrophy, which causes symptoms of dryness, itching, burning, dyspareunia and discharge, and an increased incidence of urinary symptoms, including dysuria, frequency, nocturia, urgency and incontinence.

The epithelium, connective tissue, vascular tissue and muscle layers of the vagina are affected by oestrogen status. Urogenital atrophy and, in particular, atrophic vaginitis are manifestations of oestrogen deficiency after the menopause. Symptoms usually present 10 years or more after the last menstrual period.[71] Because urogenital atrophy presents so long after the symptoms usually associated with the climacteric and menopause, it is often underdiagnosed and inadequately or inappropriately treated. Women will often present not only with vaginal symptoms but, because the atrophic process also affects the lower urinary tract, she may have irritative urinary symptoms. These symptoms are listed in Table 70.5.

Oestrogen therapy

Oestrogen therapy increases the number of intermediate and superficial cells in the vaginas of post-menopausal women and similar changes have been demonstrated in the urethra and bladder.[72]

Vaginal oestradiol is useful in the management of atrophic vaginitis. In a placebo-controlled study of 164 women, 78.8% of women who received vaginal oestradiol and 81.9% of those who received placebo had moderate-to-severe vaginal atrophy before treatment, decreasing to only 10.7% and 29.9%, respectively, after 12 weeks' therapy.[73]

Table 70.5. *Symptoms of urogenital atrophy*

Vaginal	Urinary
Dryness	Frequency
Burning	Urgency
Discharge	Nocturia
Dyspareunia	Dysuria
Soreness	Recurrent urinary tract infections

Low-dose local therapy appears to be most beneficial in the management of symptoms due to vaginal atrophy. A silicone vaginal ring that releases 5–10 μg oestradiol every 24 hours for a minimum of 90 days has been evaluated[74]. Its efficacy, safety and acceptability were assessed in 222 post-menopausal women with symptoms and signs of vaginal atrophy. Maturation of the vaginal epithelium, measured cytologically, was significantly improved during treatment, as were symptoms of vaginal dryness, pruritis vulvae, dyspareunia and urinary urgency. Cure or improvement of atrophic vaginitis was recorded in more than 90% of women and most of the women found this form of treatment acceptable, even during sexual intercourse. There was, however, no placebo group in this study.

Cardozo *et al.*[75] performed a meta-analysis to evaluate the efficacy of oestrogen therapy in the management of symptoms and signs associated with urogenital atrophy in post-menopausal women. Peer-reviewed original publications in English were included, and urogenital atrophy had to have been assessed by at least one of the following outcomes: patient symptoms, physician's report, pH, or cytological change. In addition, the data had to allow comparison between treated and control groups in controlled trials or an estimated change in uncontrolled series. Methods of meta-analysis were applied to controlled clinical trials and uncontrolled studies. The meta-analysis revealed a statistically significant benefit of oestrogen therapy for all outcomes studied. The addition of data from 54 uncontrolled case series yielded information on patient symptoms in 24 treatment groups. All routes of administration appeared to be effective, and maximum benefit was obtained 1–3 months after the start of treatment. As expected, the lowest systemic absorption of oestrogen was seen with oestriol. The authors concluded that oestrogen is efficacious in the treatment of vaginal atrophy and that low-dose oestradiol preparations are as effective as systemic oestrogen therapy in the management of symptoms and signs of urogenital atrophy in post-menopausal women.[75]

This meta-analysis clearly demonstrated that oestrogen therapy is beneficial for the treatment of the symptoms and signs associated with urogenital atrophy in post-menopausal women. It also demonstrated that oestrogen taken orally or vaginally and in all dosage regimens was effective. Local low-dose oestradiol or oestriol was as effective as systemic oestrogen therapy but did not cause the same increase in serum oestrone or oestradiol levels. The study could not, however, make recommendations regarding the most effective type of oestrogen, route of administration or duration of therapy.

It is estimated that 10–25% of women receiving systemic hormone-replacement therapy still experience vaginal symptoms, so it may be desirable to add low-dose preparations as an adjunct to improve symptom relief.[76]

Adverse events

Local low-dose oestrogen therapy is virtually free from side effects. There have been occasional reports of vaginal bleeding in women with a uterus but usually the endometrium remains atrophic despite prolonged treatment in some cases.[77] Reported side effects and complications of oestrogen therapy in the management of post-menopausal urinary incontinence have also been few. Breast tenderness, heavy irregular withdrawal bleeding and palpitations have been reported, and there have been isolated cases of myocardial infarction, which were probably unrelated to therapy.

The following conclusions can be drawn from the published data relating to the use of oestrogen therapy in the treatment of post-menopausal urogenital problems:

- There have been very few appropriate placebo-controlled studies using subjective and objective parameters for assessment – so more are urgently needed.
- Local low-dose oestrogen therapy is effective in the management of atrophic vaginitis.
- Systemic oestrogen therapy apparently alleviates the symptoms of urgency, urge incontinence, frequency, nocturia and dysuria.
- As yet there are inadequate data available to identify the best treatment in terms of dose, route of administration or type of oestrogen.

Oestrogen supplementation definitely improves quality of life for many post-menopausal women and therefore makes them better able to cope with other disabilities. Perhaps the role of oestrogen in the management of post-menopausal urinary disorders is as an adjunct to other methods of treatment such as surgery, physiotherapy or drugs; this is certainly a hypothesis that should be tested.

RECURRENT VAGINITIS

Recurrent vaginitis is defined as four or more infections per year. Sobel[78] estimated that recurrent vulvovaginitis occurs in less than 5% of healthy women and, in the majority, no apparent cause can be found. A minority of cases are associated with diabetes mellitus or immunosuppressed states such as the result of chemotherapy or infection with HIV.[78] In cases where an infectious aetiology can be found, recurrent vaginitis is caused primarily by *C. albicans*, and there are no known exogenous predisposing factors to explain the incidence of symptomatic infection in most women. The incidence of vaginal candidiasis is increased in women with depressed cell-mediated immunity; however, studies suggest that cell-mediated immunity may not be the predominant host defence mechanism against *C. albicans* vaginal infections. Instead, locally acquired mucosal immunity, distinct from that in the peripheral circulation, is considered to be an important host defence.[79]

Hilton *et al.*[80] found an association between recurrent candidal vaginitis and inheritance of the Lewis blood group antigens, giving rise to an increased susceptibility in the host.

EFFECT OF TREATMENT

The effect of treatment regimens for vaginitis and cervicitis on vaginal colonization by lactobacilli was investigated by Agnew and Hillier.[81] They evaluated women receiving therapy for *C. trachomatis*, BV, vaginal candidiasis or mucopurulent cervicitis. Doxycycline, azithromycin, clotrimazole and fluconazole had little effect on vaginal colonization by lactobacilli. Metronidazole and ampicillin caused a modest increase in lactobacilli levels.

VAGINITIS IN PREGNANCY

BV is associated with complications of pregnancy, accounting for 40% of the attributable risk for spontaneous birth at less than 32 weeks of gestation.[37] Maffei *et al.*[84] investigated women who presented with recurrent vaginal candidiasis in pregnancy. The strain of *C. albicans* isolated was analysed by morphotyping, antifungal typing and genotyping. The changes observed were the emergence of strains resistant to miconazole, which was the drug used for the treatment of the first episode of vaginitis. There was good evidence to suggest that, in pregnant women, recurrent vaginal candidiasis was caused by the persistence of a single yeast genotype that had undergone morphological and behavioural changes in the presence of antifungal agents.[82]

BV tends not to occur in the presence of hydrogen-peroxide-producing strains of lactobacilli in the vaginal flora. However, it has been shown that in some pregnant women, hydrogen-peroxide-producing lactobacilli had not protected them from developing BV. It is possible that in these women a change to an abnormal bacterial flora, with progression to vaginosis, can occur before the complete disappearance of lactobacilli, and that other, as yet unidentified, factors contribute to this progression.[83]

Screening in pregnancy

Despite spontaneous recovery of BV during pregnancy, there is still no change in poor perinatal outcome from preterm birth.[84] It is beneficial and cost-effective to screen for BV to prevent preterm birth only in obstetric populations where both the prevalence of BV and the incidence of preterm delivery are high.[85] In the USA, this can best be done with screening and treatment for BV at the initial antenatal examination (9 weeks of pregnancy).[86]

Treatment in pregnancy

Metronidazole is the drug of choice for pregnant women, but should be avoided in the first trimester because of the potential for teratogenicity. McDonald *et al.*[87] performed a randomized placebo-controlled trial to assess whether metronidazole treatment of women with a heavy growth of *G. vaginalis* in mid-pregnancy would reduce the risk of spontaneous preterm birth. Intent-to-treat analysis showed no difference between metronidazole and placebo groups in overall preterm or spontaneous preterm birth. Interestingly, however, among women with a history of previous preterm birth, metronidazole reduced the subsequent risk of spontaneous preterm delivery.[87]

SUMMARY

Vaginitis is a common condition among women of all ages. Vaginal irritation associated with a discharge is a common symptom of an infectious cause. Identifying the underlying aetiology may be difficult because of the large number of pathogens that can cause vaginitis, This is made even more challenging because several host factors that make the individual susceptible to recurrent infections by more than one organism may coexist. The history and clinical findings may help to make a pre-emptive diagnosis but it is prudent to perform tests to make an accurate diagnosis.

In addition to an infectious cause, non-bacterial infections and non-infectious causes such as allergic and post-menopausal vaginitis with epithelial atrophy should be considered in the differential diagnosis.

Diagnostic tests include: cytological examination of the vaginal discharge; bacterial and fungal cultures and microscopic examination of Gram-stained vaginal smears; the amine whiff test; pH assessment and wet-mount examinations. Venous-blood specimens may be considered to test for antibodies to syphilis and HIV. Once the source and type of infection have been determined, treatment options usually involve oral antibiotics or antifungals or topical vaginal preparations.

REFERENCES

1. Freeman S. Common genitourinary infections. *J Obstet Gynecol Neonatal Nurs* 1995; 24: 735–742

2. Stephenson J. Studies suggest a 'darker' side of benign microbes. *J Am Med Assoc* 1997; 278: 2051–2052

3. Gallichau W, Rosenthal K. Long-term immunity and protection against herpes simplex virus type 2 in the murine female genital tract after mucosal but not systemic immunisation. *J Infect Dis* 1998; 177: 1155–1161

4. Sonnex C. Influence of ovarian hormones on urogenital infections. *Sex Trans Infect* 1998; 74: 11–19

5. Hurley P, DeLouvois J. Candida vaginitis. *Postgrad Med J* 1979; 55: 645–647

6. Hellberg D, Zdolsek B, Nilsson S, Mardh P. Sexual behaviour of women with repeated episodes of vulvovaginal candidiasis. *Eur J Epidemiol* 1995; 11: 575–579

7. Gibb D, Hockey S, Brown L, Hunt H. Vaginal symptoms and insulin dependent diabetes mellitus. *New Engl Med J* 1995; 108: 252–253

8. Cu-Uvin S, Flanigan T, Rich J *et al.* Human immunodeficiency virus infection and acquired immunodeficiency syndrome among North American women. *Am J Med* 1996; 101: 316–322

9. Frankel R, Selwyn P, Mezger J, Andrews S. High prevalence of gynecologic disease among hospitalised women with human immunodeficiency virus infection. *Clin Infect Dis* 1997; 25: 706–712

10. Berg A, Heidrich F, Fihns *et al.* Establishing the cause of genitourinary symptoms in women in a family practice: comparison of clinical examinations and comprehensive microbiology. *J Am Med Assoc* 1984; 251: 620–651

11. Embree J, Lindsay P, Williams T *et al.* Acceptability and usefulness of vaginal washes in premenarcheal girls as a diagnostic procedure for sexually transmitted diseases. The Child Protection Centre at the Winnipeg Children's Hospital. *Pediatr Infect Dis J* 1996; 15: 662–667

12. Caillouette J, Sharp C, Zimmerman G, Roy S. Vaginal pH as a marker for bacterial pathogens and menopausal status. *Am J Obstet Gynecol* 1997; 176: 1270–1275

13. Donders G, van Gerven V, de Wet H *et al.* Rapid antigen tests for Neisseria gonorrhoea and Chlamydia trachomatis are not accurate for screening women with disturbed vaginal lactobacillary flora. *Scand J Infect Dis* 1996; 28: 559–562

14. Chacko M, Kozinetz C, Hill R *et al.* Leukocyte esterase dipstick in a rapid screening test for vaginitis and cervicitis. *J Pediatr Adolesc Gynecol* 1996; 9: 185–189

15. Lipsky M, Taylor C. The use of over-the-counter antifungal vaginitis preparations by college students. *Fam Med* 1996; 28: 493–495

16. Nyirjesy P, Weitz M, Grody M, Lorber B. Over-the-counter and alternative medicines in the treatment of chronic vaginal symptoms. *Obstet Gynecol* 1997; 90: 50–53

17. Shaler E, Battino S, Weiner E *et al.* Ingestion of yoghurt containing lactobacillus acidophilus compared with pasteurized yoghurt as prophylaxis for recurrent candidal vaginitis and bacterial vaginosis. *Arch Fam Med* 1996; 5: 593–596

18. Odds F. Candidosis of the genitalia. *Candida and Candidosis: a Review and Bibliography*, 2nd Edn. London: Balliere Tindall, 1988; 124–135

19. Spinillo A, Capuzzo E, Gulminetti P *et al.* Prevalence of and risk factors for fungal vaginitis caused by non-albicans species. *Am J Obstet Gynecol* 1997; 176: 138–141

20. Foxman B. The epidemiology of vulvovaginal candidiasis: risk factors. *Am J Pub Health* 1990; 80: 329–331

21. Kurowski K. The women with dysuria. *Am Fam Physician* 1998; 57: 2155–2164, 2169–2170

22. Geiger A, Foxman B. Risk factors in vulvovaginal candidiasis: a case control study among university students. *Epidemiology* 1996; 7: 182–187

23. Reef S, Levine W, McNeil M *et al.* Treatment options for vulvovaginal candidiasis. *Clin Infect Dis* 1995; 20: S80–S90

24. Sobel J, Brooker D, Stein G *et al.* Single oral dose fluconazole compared with conventional clotrimazole topical therapy of candida vaginitis. *Am J Obstet Gynecol* 1995; 172: 1263–1268

25. Sobel J, Chaim W. Treatment of Torulopsis glabrata vaginitis: a retrospective review of boric acid therapy. *Clin Infect Dis* 1997; 24: 649–652

26. Hay P, Ugwumada A, Chowns J. Sex, thrush and bacterial vaginosis. *Int J STD AIDS* 1997; 8: 603–608

27. Frega A, Stentella P, Spera G *et al.* Cervical intraepithelial neoplasia and bacterial vaginosis: correlation or risk factor? *Eur J Gynaecol Oncol* 1997; 18: 76–77

28. Thorsen P, Jensen F, Jeune B *et al.* Few micro-organisms, associated with bacterial vaginosis may constitute the pathologic core: a population-based microbiologic, study among 3596 pregnant women. *Am J Obstet Gynecol* 1998; 178: 580–587

29. Cauci S, Priussi S, Moute R *et al.* Immunoglobulin A response against Gardnerella vaginalis hemolysin and sialidase activity in bacterial vaginosis. *Am J Obstet Gynecol* 1998; 178: 511–515

30. Totten P, Amsel R, Hale J *et al.* Selective differential human blood bilayer media for isolation of Gardnerella (Haemophilus) vaginalis. *J Clin Microbiol* 1982; 15: 141–147

31. Holmes K, Spiegel C, Amsel *et al.* Non-specific vaginosis. *Scand J Infect Dis Suppl* 1981; 26: 110–114

32. Hill GB. The microbiology of BV. *Am J Obstet Gynecol* 1993; 169: 450–454

33. Amsel R, Totten P, Spiegll C *et al.* Non-specific vaginitis: diagnostic criteria and microbial and epidemiological associations. *Am J Med* 1983; 74: 14–22

34. Eschenbach D, Hillier S, Critchlow C *et al.* Diagnostic and clinical manifestations of bacterial vaginosis. *Am J Obstet Gynecol* 1988; 158: 819–28.

35. Priestley C, Jones B, Dhar J, Goodwin L. What is normal vaginal flora? *Genitourin Med* 1997; 73: 23–28

36. Spinillo A, Bernuzzi A, Cerini C *et al.* The relationship of bacterial vaginosis, candida and trichomonas infection to symptomatic vaginitis in post-menopausal women attending a vaginitis clinic. *Maturitas* 1997; 27: 253–260

37. Goldenberg R, Iamis J, Mercer B *et al.* The pre-term prediction study: the value of new vs standard risk factors in predicting early and all spontaneous pre-term births. NICHD MFMM Network. *Am J Pub Health* 1998; 88: 233–238

38. Peipert J, Montagno, A, Cooper A, Sing C. Bacterial vaginosis as a risk factor for upper genital tract infections. *Am J Obstet Gynecol* 1997; 177: 1184–1187

39. Nugent R, Krohn M, Hillier S. Reliability of diagnosing bacterial vaginosis is improved by a standardised method of gram stain interpretation. *J Clin Microbiol* 1991; 29: 297–301

40. Spiegel C, Amsel R, Holmes K. Diagnosis of bacterial vaginosis by direct gram stain of vaginal fluid. *J Clin Microbiol* 1983; 18: 170–177

41. Hillier S, Krohn M, Nugent R, for the Vaginal Infections and Prematurity Study Group. Characteristics of three vaginal flora patterns assessed by grain stain among pregnant women. *Am J Obstet Gynecol* 1992; 166: 938–944

42. Schwebke J, Hillier S, Sobel J *et al.* Validity of the vaginal grain stain for the diagnosis of bacterial vaginosis. *Obstet Gynecol* 1996; 88: 573–576

43. Davis J, Connor E, Clarke P *et al.* Correlation between cervical cytologic results and Gram stain as diagnostic tests for bacterial vaginosis. *Am J Obstet Gynecol* 1997; 177: 532–535

44. Hillier S, Kiviat N, Hawes S *et al.* Role of bacterial vaginosis-associated microorganisms in endometritis. *Am J Obstet Gynecol* 1996; 175: 435–441

45. Sewankambo N, Gray R, Waiver M *et al.* HIV-1 infections associated with abnormal vaginal flora morphology and bacterial vaginosis. *Lancet* 1997; 350: 546–550

46. Shoubnikova M, Hellberg D, Nilsson S, Mardh P. Contraceptive use in women with bacterial vaginosis. *Contraception* 1997; 55: 355–358

47. Puapermpoonsiri S, Watanabe K, Kato N, Veno K. In vitro activities of 10 antimicrobial agents against bacterial vaginosis-associated anaerobic isolates from pregnant Japanese and Thai women. *Antimicrob Agents Chemother* 1997; 41: 2297–2299

48. Colli E, Landoni M, Pavazzini F. Treatment of male partners and recurrence of bacterial vaginosis: a randomised trial. *Genitour Med* 1997; 73: 267–270

49. Majeroni B. Bacterial vaginosis: an update. *Am Fam Physician* 1998; 57: 1285–1289

50. Edwards S, Carne C. Oral sex and the transmission of viral STDs. *Sex Transm Infect* 1998; 74: 6–10

51. Medaglini P, Oggloni M, Pozzi G. Vaginal immunisation with recombinant gram positive bacteria. *Am J Reprod Immun* 1998; 39: 199–208

52. Petrin D, Delgaty K, Bhatt P, Garber G. Clinical and microbiological aspects of Trichomonas vaginalis. *Clin Microbiol Rev* 1998; 11: 300–317

53. Lossick J. Epidemiology of urogenital trichomoniasis. In: Homigberg BM (ed) *Trichomonads Parasitic Infections in Humans*. New York: Springer-Verlag, 1990; 311–323

54. Wolner-Hanssen P, Krieger J, Stevens C *et al*. Clinical manifestations of vaginal trichomoniasis. *J Am Med Assoc* 1989; 261: 571–576

55. Laga M, Manoka A, Kivuvu M *et al*. Non-ulcerative sexually transmitted diseases as risk factors for MV-1 transmission in women: result from a cohort study. *AIDS* 1993; 7: 95–102

56. Provenzano D, Alderete J. Analysis of human immunoglobulin-degrading cysteine proteinases of trichomonas vaginalis. *Infect Immun* 1995; 63: 3388–3395

57. Alderete J, Provanzano D. The vagina has reducing environment sufficient for activation of Trichomonas vaginalis cysteine proteinases. *Genitourin Med* 1997; 73: 291–296

58. Krieger J, Tam M, Stevens C *et al*. Diagnosis of trichomoniasis: comparison of conventional wet-mount examinations with cytogenic studies, cultures and monoclonal antibody staining of direct specimens. *J Am Med Assoc* 1988; 259: 1223–1227

59. Fouts A, Kraus S. Trichomonas vaginalis: reevaluation of its clinical presentation and laboratory diagnosis. *J Infect Dis* 1980; 141: 137–143

60. Urieseufelt H, Heine R, Rideout A *et al*. The vaginal introitus: a novel site for Chlamydia trachomatis testing in women. *Am J Obstet Gynecol* 1996; 174: 1542–1546

61. DuBouchet L, McGregor J, Ismail M, McCormack W. A pilot study of metronidazole vaginal gel versus oral metronidazole for the treatment of trichomonas vaginalis vaginitis. *Sex Trans Dis* 1998; 25: 176–179

62. Spence M, Harwell T, Davies M, Smith J. The minimum single oral metronidazole dose for treating trichomoniasis: a randomised blinded study. *Obstet Gynecol* 1997; 89: 699–703

63. Central Statistics Office. *Annual Abstract of Statistics*, no 127. London: HMSO, 1991

64. Cardozo LD. Role of oestrogens in the treatment of female urinary incontinence. *J Am Geriatr Soc* 1990; 38: 326–328

65. Batra SC, Iosif LS. Female urethra: a target for oestrogen action. *J Urol* 1983; 129: 418–420

66. Batra SC, Iosif LS. Progesterone receptors in the female lower urinary tract. *J Urol* 1987; 138: 1301–1304

67. Blakeman P, Hilton P, Bulmer J. Mapping oestrogen and progesterone receptors throughout the female lower urinary tract. *Neurourol Urodyn* 1996; 15: 324–325

68. Van Geelen JM, Desburg WH, Thomas CMG, Martin CB. Urodynamic studies in the normal menstrual cycle: the relationship between hormonal changes in the menstrual cycle and urethral pressure profiles. *Am J Obstet Gynecol* 1981; 141: 384–392

69. Tapp AJS, Cardozo LD. The postmenopausal bladder. *Br J Hosp Med* 1986; 35: 20–23

70. McCallin PE, Stewart-Taylor E, Whitehead RW. A study of the changes in cytology of the urinary sediment during the menstrual cycle and pregnancy. *Am J Obstet Gynecol* 1950; 60: 64–74

71. Iosif C. Effects of protracted administration of oestriol on the lower genitourinary tract in postmenopausal women. *Acta Obstet Gynecol Scand* 1992; 251: 115–120

72. Samsioe G, Jansson I, Mellstrom D, Svandborg A. Occurrence, nature and treatment of urinary incontinence in a 70-year-old female population. *Maturitas* 1985; 7: 335–342

73. Eriksen PS, Rasmussen H. Low-dose 17 beta estradiol vaginal tablets in the treatment of atrophic vaginitis: a double-blind placebo controlled study. *Eur J Obstet Gynae Reprod Biol* 1992; 44: 137–144

74. Smith P, Heimer G, Lindskog M, Ulmsten U. Oestradiol-releasing vaginal ring for treatment of post menopausal urogenital atrophy. *Maturitas* 1993; 16: 145–154

75. Cardozo L, Bachmann G, Mc Clish D *et al*. Meta-analysis of estrogen therapy in the management of urogenital atrophy in postmenopausal women: second report of the Hormones and Urogenital Therapy Committee. *Obstet Gynecol* 1998; 92: 722–727

76. Smith R, Studd J. Recent advances in hormone replacement therapy. *Br J Hosp Med* 1993; 49: 799–809

77. Samsioe G. The menopause revisited. *Int J Obstet Gynecol* 1995; 51: 1–13

78. Sobel J. Epidemiology and pathogenesis of recurrent vulvovaginal candidiasis. *Am J Obstet Gynecol* 1985; 152: 924–935

79. Fidel P, Sobel J. Immunopathogenesis of recurrent vulvovaginal candidiasis. *Clin Microbiol Rev* 1996; 9: 335–348

80. Hilton E, Chandrasekavan V, Rindos P, Isenberg H. Association of recurrent candidal vaginitis with inheritance of Lewis blood group antigens. *J Infect Dis* 1995; 172: 1616–1619

81. Agnew K, Hillier S. The effect of treatment regimens for vaginitis and cervicitis on vaginal colonisation by lactobacilli. *Sex Transm Dis* 1995; 22: 269–273

82. Maffei C, Paula C, Mazzocato T, Francheschini S. Phenotype and genotype of candida albicans strains isolated from pregnant women with recurrent vaginitis. *Mycopath* 1997; 137: 87–94

83. Rosenstein I, Fontaine E, Morgan D *et al*. Relationship between hydrogen peroxide-producing strains of lactobacilli and vaginosis-associated bacterial species in pregnant women. *Eur J Clin Microbiol Infect Dis* 1997; 16: 517–522

84. Gratacos E, Figueras F, Barranco M *et al.* Spontaneous recovery of bacterial vaginosis during pregnancy is not associated with an improved perinatal outcome. *Acta Obstet Gynecol Scand* 1998; 77: 37–40

85. Glantz J. Screening and treatment of bacterial vaginosis during pregnancy: a model for determining benefit. *Am J Perinatol* 1997; 14: 487–490

86. McGregor J, Roberts A. First antenatal visits and metronidazole. *Am J Obstet Gynecol* 1997; 176: 887–888

87. McDonald H, O'Loughlin J, Vigneswaran R *et al.* Impact of metronidazole therapy on pre-term birth in women with bacterial vaginosis flora (Gardnerella vaginalis) – a randomised, placebo controlled trial. *Br J Obstet Gynaecol* 1997; 104: 1391–1397

71

Laparoscopic treatment of pelvic pain

R. W. Dover, C. J. G. Sutton

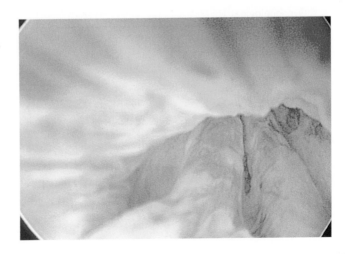

INTRODUCTION

Pelvic pain is a common symptom amongst women of reproductive age, and its diagnosis and management constitute a considerable part of a gynaecologist's workload. Women with acute pain usually present via the emergency department. The pain is usually severe and of recent onset and requires skilled assessment in order to distinguish gynaecological causes from diseases of adjacent organs or structures (Table 71.1).

Pelvic pain of more than 6 months' duration is usually labelled as chronic pelvic pain, and the differential diagnosis is usually more complex and requires careful evaluation of the physical, psychological and emotional state of the patient[1] (Table 71.2).

If one overlooks the difficulties of defining the condition, and focuses on the patients themselves, the magnitude and importance of the problem become obvious. One author comments that chronic pelvic pain is responsible for approximately 5% of new gynaecological referrals at his hospital,[2] but unfortunately there is no community-based study from the UK that allows us to estimate the prevalence of chronic pelvic pain within the whole population. Such a study in the United States has been published, quoting a prevalence rate of 15%.[3] The study also made an economic assessment of the problem: in addition to the medical costs associated with hospital attendance and treatments, 15% of the employed women reported time lost from work and

Table 71.1. *Causes of acute pelvic pain*

Gynaecological	Non-gynaecological
Uterus	Gastrointestinal
miscarriage	appendicitis
acute degeneration of a fibroid	diverticulitis
endometritis	obstruction (adhesions/volvulus)
perforation (after insertion of IUCD/surgery)	constipation
Fallopian tubes	ischaemia
ectopic pregnancy	gastroenteritis
acute salpingitis	Urological
torsion (e.g. hydrosalpinx)	cystitis/pyelonephritis
Ovary	renal/ureteric colic
cyst accident/ovulation	retention
torsion	Other
tubo-ovarian abscess	musculoskeletal
metabolic	
idiopathic	

IUCD, intra-uterine contraceptive device

Table 71.2. *Causes of chronic pelvic pain*

Gynaecological	Non-gynaecological
Uterus	Gastrointestinal
primary dysmenorrhoea	adhesions
adenomyosis	constipation
fibroids	diverticular disease
Fallopian tube	irritable bowel syndrome
chronic salpingitis	Urological
Ovary	retention
benign and malignant cysts	urethral syndrome
endometriotic cysts	interstitial cystitis
entrapment by adhesions	Other
remnant syndrome	musculoskeletal
General	nerve entrapment
endometriosis	idiopathic
venous congestion	

45% reported reduced productivity. Although there is no population-based UK study, a recent paper[4] has reviewed all published work and quotes prevalence rates for dysmenorrhoea of 45–97% and for abdominal pain of 23–29%. The authors make the valid point that the definitions used vary widely, and that the selection criteria in some cases may not have been truly representative of the population as a whole.

The next step, once these patients have been identified, is to attempt to reach a diagnosis. The literature is replete with the potential difficulties of assessment in these women, and stresses the importance of the medical history as potentially the most important part of the process.[2,5] The other issue that is constantly highlighted is the possibility of previous sexual abuse, which is more prevalent in women with chronic pelvic pain. This issue in the UK setting has been reviewed by Collett *et al.*[6] Some clinicians have a special interest in this area and will take the time to explore all areas of the history. However, it is most likely that the patient will undergo a diagnostic laparoscopy. Because of the number of patients who may suffer from pelvic pain it is not surprising that their investigation may account for more than 40% of all laparoscopic procedures in some units.[7]

The next area of interest is to consider the pathology encountered at the time of the diagnostic laparoscopy. In view of the confusion surrounding the definition of the condition under investigation, it should come as no surprise that the reported findings vary considerably from one unit to the next. It must be remembered, however, that these differences could also be explained in terms of different local referral practices, and the special interest and reputation of the clinician involved. With these reservations in mind, a superficial review of the published literature reveals that, at the time of diagnostic laparoscopy for chronic pelvic pain, the incidence of endometriosis is 16–33.3%, and the incidence of adhesions is 23.1–40%; negative findings may be encountered in 14.8–30% of cases.[8–11] There appears to be considerable variation in these figures, and other papers quoting negative laparoscopy rates of 65%[1] or 10–90%[12] do little to clarify the issue.

It is possible to discern some common themes from these confusing statements. While the exact proportions may vary considerably, it does appear that endometriosis and pelvic adhesions will be diagnosed in a large subgroup; however, the fact that pathology is demonstrable does not imply that the relationship between it and the symptoms is a causal one. There is also the indisputable fact that diagnostic laparoscopy will be negative in a percentage of patients.

The rest of this chapter focuses on the various laparoscopic techniques that are available to treat endometriosis and pelvic adhesions and gives some measure of their success. The treatment of other pathologies such as chronic infection will not be covered, but options for laparoscopic treatment in cases where no pathology has been demonstrated is discussed briefly in the section on denervation.

LAPAROSCOPIC TREATMENT OF ENDOMETRIOSIS

Endometriosis may be present in the pelvis in three main areas: peritoneal deposits, ovarian endometriomas and rectovaginal septum deposits, and it has been suggested that these are in fact three separate conditions.[13] The treatment of disease in each of these sites will be considered separately.

Peritoneal disease

Endometriosis of the pelvic peritoneum may be superficial or deep. Indeed it has been suggested that deep deposits (>3mm) may be present in up to 60% of patients with this condition.[14] The identification of deep disease is essential, since treatment – either vaporization or excision – needs to extend down to the level of normal tissue. Failure to appreciate the depth of a lesion may therefore lead to inadequate treatment and incomplete relief of symptoms. This is particularly true for deposits infiltrating deeply into the bladder, which may penetrate through the mucosa and give rise to cyclical haematuria. If this is the case, cure can be achieved only by complete excision of the lesion and laparoscopic suturing of the defect in the bladder, followed by catheter drainage for a 'urological week'.

Most lesions do not penetrate the full thickness of the bladder wall, but it is important to remove all of the endometriotic implants and the vessels arising from angioneogenesis that are supplying them. The choice between laser ablation or electrosurgical resection of focal disease is usually a matter of individual preference, but may be influenced by the range of equipment available and the location of the deposits concerned. The relative merits of these two techniques have been covered elsewhere.[15] In our centre we tend to use carbon dioxide laser vaporization with a rotating mirror delivery system, employing the laser in super-pulse or ultra-pulse mode for more effective cutting. An electrosurgical needle is the dominant method of treatment for peritoneal disease, but on occasions we use excision, especially if the uterosacral ligaments are involved.

Whilst most clinicians are familiar with the use of lasers in the operating theatre, and will have read papers describing the technique of laser ablation of endometriotic deposits, most would probably be surprised to learn that the first study subjecting this therapy to the rigours of a prospective, randomized, double-blind study was not published until 1994.[16] An earlier report regarding the use of laser ablation in the treatment of pelvic pain secondary to endometriosis was produced by this unit:[17] of 228 consecutive patients treated for endometriosis, pelvic pain was improved in 126 of 181 women (69.6%) who suffered with it. The authors had some reservations about the design of this study and consequently embarked on a prospective, randomized trial. Although the findings of this study have been well publicized, there are several interesting aspects that bear closer inspection.

The study examined patients with symptoms suggestive of endometriosis who were recruited and then randomized to receive either a diagnostic laparoscopy only, or laparoscopy combined with laser ablation of all visible deposits of endometriosis and uterine nerve transection. Of the patients eligible for analysis, 62.5% of those who received laser therapy reported that symptoms were better or improved. This finding was statistically different from the 22.6% who had improved in the group that received laparoscopy alone.

When the results were analysed stage by stage, it was discovered that response rates were lowest amongst those with stage I disease; if these patients were excluded from the final analysis, then 73.7% of patients with mild or moderate disease obtained benefit. The authors suggested that endometriosis was in fact a chance finding in this group with minimal disease, and was not responsible for their symptoms. Some credence is given to this suggestion by the finding that three of the five women who did not derive benefit from laser ablation had no residual disease when they underwent a second laparoscopy. This obviously raises doubts about the pathology responsible for their symptoms. It

is suggested that, in cases of minimal disease, the diagnosis of endometriosis, which was invariably based on the interpretation of vascular patterns, may have been incorrect. It was suggested that the affected areas should be biopsed at the time of treatment so that a histological diagnosis is available to help further treatment planning, should the response to laser ablation be suboptimal. This is of more than just academic interest because a diagnosis of endometriosis can have far-reaching consequences for a woman.

The other aspect of the study that needs to be considered is that in the two other patients who showed no improvement after laser laparoscopy, endometriosis had recurred but was not present at the site of previous laser treatment. This reminds us that endometriosis can be an aggressive and progressive condition, and that on some occasions laser surgery may need adjuvant medical therapy.

The patients were followed-up for 1 year after surgery and it is of some significance that, of those who responded initially, symptom relief was maintained in 90%.[18]

The main criticism directed at this study was that patients in the treatment arm received both laser ablation and uterine nerve transection, and it was therefore unclear which was responsible for the symptomatic benefit.[19] To clarify this issue, a second prospective, double-blind study was undertaken, in which patients were randomized to receive laser ablation either alone or in addition to uterine nerve transection. Although this study is not yet finished, recruitment is complete, and interim analysis appears to suggest that there is no difference in the degree of symptomatic relief between the two groups.[20] If this finding is confirmed in the final analysis, then not only will it validate the earlier study, but it will also demonstrate that, where pathology is encountered, the addition of a denervation procedure does not provide additional symptomatic relief.

Ovarian endometriomas

These lesions are readily treated using laparoscopic methods, which are as effective as treatment by laparotomy, but have the benefit of the shorter recovery time associated with endoscopic surgery.[21] Therapeutic options are based on either vaporization of the lining of the structure, or stripping of the capsule.[22] Whichever method is adopted, it is paramount that the whole of the internal aspect of the capsule is closely inspected before treatment in order to exclude the presence of an underlying malignancy. The use of multiple biopsies to allow subsequent histological assessment is encouraged. In our department we aim to completely vaporize the cyst lining using a potassium titanyl phosphate (KTP/532) laser at the time of laparoscopy. Other centres use a carbon dioxide laser and adopt a three-stage approach.[23] A retrospective review of all patients treated in this unit over a 10-year period[24] revealed that 74% of patients reported improvement or resolution of their pain. Whilst this finding is encouraging, it is tempered by the fact that the recurrence rate was 19% during the study period and subsequent 2-year follow-up.[25] Several facts need emphasising, however. First, not all the endometriomas occurred in the same site, nor indeed the same ovary; secondly, this recurrence rate is in broad agreement with that of 11% quoted by others.[21] Lower rates of recurrence have also been quoted – 3.2% (1/31) – but follow-up extended to only 6 months in this study.[26]

The evidence therefore suggests that although laparoscopic treatment of ovarian endometriomas is possible, in common with peritoneal disease, there is a problem with recurrent disease. The incidence and delayed nature of recurrent disease should always be borne in mind when counselling patients prior to surgery, and also those with a resurgence of symptoms.

Rectovaginal septum endometriosis

The presence of endometriosis in the rectovaginal septum can be particularly painful, but is also difficult to treat. In some cases a retroperitoneal nodule will be seen at the time of laparoscopy, lying in the posterior fornix of the vagina and extending down into the septum. Unfortunately, in many cases a deeply infiltrating septal lesion is almost impossible to see at the time of laparoscopic assessment and may be missed. These nodules are, however, palpable on combined rectovaginal examination, particularly at the time of menstruation. Although these patients will constitute a minority of those presenting to a gynaecological clinic with chronic pelvic pain, there are some important points to raise.

- Most of these lesions are amenable to endoscopic laser surgery, as demonstrated in a series reported by

Donnez *et al.*[27] The number of women with each of the presenting symptoms was not clearly defined, but it appears that most patients suffered from severe pelvic pain, severe dysmenorrhoea and severe dyspareunia. Of the 242 patients followed-up for more than 2 years, only 3.7% experienced recurrent severe dysmenorrhoea, and 1.2% dyspareunia. Whilst the figures are not readily available, the impression is one of major symptomatic benefit.

- The second issue arising from this study is that, although the surgeons were amongst the most experienced in the world, four patients out of 497 who were treated by laparoscopy suffered a rectal perforation. It is therefore only too clear that any woman suffering from this condition should be referred to a suitably qualified surgeon.

PELVIC DENERVATION PROCEDURES

As well as treating visible organic pathology at the time of laparoscopic assessment, the ability to interrupt several of the neural pathways responsible for the transmission of pain has also been used. Indeed there are many who advocate the use of these methods when no pathology is demonstrable. There are two commonly used techniques: uterine nerve transection and presacral neurectomy (PSN).

Uterine nerve transection

The idea is to disrupt the course of pain fibres as they leave the uterus, in an effort to decrease dysmenorrhoea; this is not a new idea, having previously been described over 40 years ago.[28] The original paper reported that, by transecting the uterosacral ligaments close to their point of origin on the cervix (a technique that could be performed either abdominally or vaginally) it was possible to achieve complete pain relief in 86% of women with primary dysmenorrhoea and 86.8% of women with secondary dysmenorrhoea.

The advent of the non-steroidal anti-inflammatory agents and combined contraceptive pill tended to focus attention on the medical management of these conditions, rather than the surgical, and the technique became almost forgotten. The emergence of laparoscopic surgery and the ability to divide these nerves without the need for open surgery generated much interest in resurrecting this technique, which had produced such good results. The technique is now a common procedure in ours and many other units around the world. Two recent review articles have described the history, anatomical rationale and the various methods of dividing the nerves that are currently employed in this technique.[29,30]

It is of considerable relevance that in these times of evidence-based medicine, laparoscopic uterine nerve ablation (LUNA) has been subjected to the rigors of a prospective, randomized, double-blind study.[31] Although the numbers in this report were small, and the surgeons used electrosurgery rather than laser, the results still warrant mention. In women with severe dysmenorrhoea but no obvious pathology, 81% of those undergoing LUNA reported almost complete relief of pain at 3 months, although this fell to 45% at 12 months. None of those in the control group reported any benefit. A different study looked at the outcome of patients with primary dysmenorrhoea and an improvement rate of 73% was reported.[29] Other reported rates of improvement for primary dysmenorrhoea range from 50 to 73%.[11,32–34] These differences may be due to differing patient subgroups, and perhaps the degree of demarcation of the uterosacral ligaments, since if they are poorly developed an incomplete procedure is often performed.[29]

The group of patients who find that their dysmenorrhoea worsens after this operation is of particular interest. Daniell[33] reported that 10% of his patients with primary dysmenorrhoea experienced deterioration in symptoms after surgery. Because preoperative counselling includes an explanation of this potential development to the patient, it has been suggested that this may be a self-fulfilling prophecy, whereas it does not occur if you do not inform your patient of the possibility, as is the policy in other units.[29]

One publication[35] has provided evidence suggesting that the benefits of a LUNA procedure could be due to an entirely different mechanism. Nisolle *et al.*[35] demonstrated that, in patients with an apparently normal pelvis at the time of laparoscopy, histological evidence of endometriosis may be found in biopsy samples of the uterosacral ligaments in 6% of cases. There is obviously considerable debate about the significance of this finding. If it transpires that these deposits are located laterally to the usual site of a LUNA procedure, this may help to explain why not all patients derive the same degree of benefit from this operation.

The last area to be considered is that of safety. Although widely performed, LUNA is not without risks since the rectum, ureter and uterine artery are all within the immediate vicinity. Two deaths due to postoperative haemorrhage,[33] and two cases of severe uterine prolapse[36] have been reported.

Presacral neurectomy

Interruption of the hypogastric plexus at the sacral promontory has been used for more than 60 years to provide relief from pelvic pain and dysmenorrhoea. An early review of this topic showed that significant relief could be obtained from these symptoms in 80% of patients.[37] This procedure has been well described in three recent reviews.[30,38,39]

Rather than performing a traditional excisional neurectomy, some workers recommend a divisional neurotomy, which is far quicker and, in the short term at least, appears to be just as effective.[40]

While there have been several publications considering the role of LUNA in patients with pelvic pain and a negative laparoscopy, most of the literature relating to PSN combines it with other therapeutic procedures. However, Candiani *et al.*[41] have found that the addition of PSN made no difference to patient outcome. Seventy-one patients with stage III or IV endometriosis and pelvic pain were assigned to conservative surgery alone, or with the addition of PSN. Postoperatively there was no significant difference in the reduction of dysmenorrhoea, dyspareunia and intermenstrual pain between the two study groups. The findings of this paper are contradicted by those of Tjaden *et al.*[42] which showed such overwhelming benefit from the addition of PSN that the trial was halted on the grounds that it would be unethical to continue because the response rate was so good.

Perry and Perez[43] have raised the important issue of the reasons for failure of PSN. Although they reported a successful outcome in most of 103 women treated for pelvic pain or dysmenorrhoea, the interest lies within a small subgroup. Of the patients in the study, 11 had previously undergone LUNA, without symptomatic benefit, yet all experienced alleviation of midline pain following PSN. The authors noted that the most common reason for PSN failing to improve midline pain was incomplete division of the presacral nerve. This is a reflection of operator experience and confidence, and is reflected in our own practice where we see patients referred for assessment of their pelvic pain, having previously undergone a LUNA procedure, only to find little evidence of this at the time of surgery. We would suggest that the above observation could also be applied to LUNA.

Several themes run through the literature on PSN, one being that patient assessment is paramount, especially with regard to the location of the pain. Reports have suggested that PSN is useful in the treatment of midline pain, but of no benefit when the pain is more lateral.[44] This is supported by a report revealing that out of 27 women undergoing PSN, midline pain was relieved in 22 and reduced in a further four; however, lateral pain remained in three of 12 cases.[45]

Another theme common to most of these publications is that PSN should be reserved for patients with midline pain in whom previous attempts at medical therapy have failed. It should also be remembered that there are many potential complications associated with this procedure. Immediate complications include damage to major vessels,[30,45] and long-term problems such as constipation are common.

In view of the above evidence it seems prudent that patients are carefully assessed and counselled prior to this procedure, and that it is performed by a competent and experienced endoscopic surgeon. Since transection of the uterosacral ligaments is easier to perform and less dangerous than division of the presacral nerve, the suggestion that PSN should be reserved for patients who have undergone an adequate transection of the uterosacral ligaments but still have persistent pelvic pain and dysmenorrhoea seems wise.[30]

ADHESIOLYSIS

Laparoscopic adhesiolysis crosses the boundary of gynaecological and general surgery. Adhesiolysis usually involves enterolysis – the release of adhesions involving the bowel – and a high degree of experience is required because of the risk of causing an intestinal perforation. Introduction of the trocar can be hazardous, and surgeons should be aware of the different methods by which this can be achieved and the various techniques available for enterolysis. These have been reviewed recently.[30,46]

As with the other causes of chronic pelvic pain, the relationship between adhesions and chronic pelvic pain

is unclear, with several workers describing the presence of adhesions in 23–25% of patients with chronic pain, but also in 14–17% of women without pain.[7,47] Coupled with this are the observations that, of women with adhesions, 50% have no risk factors for their development,[30] and 66% have a completely normal abdominopelvic examination.[48] Whilst there appears to be little correlation between the degree of the adhesions and the severity of the symptoms,[49] the pain does seem to be located at the site of the adhesions in most cases.[49,50] If adhesions are relatively common in the asymptomatic population, what is it that makes certain adhesions painful, and does dividing them make any difference?

Laparoscopic laser adhesiolysis was reported to produce pain relief in 76% of women;[51] the authors noted that success was usual in patients who had a thick adhesive band limiting the mobility of the small intestine. This finding is corroborated by an important randomized trial in which 48 patients with stage II–IV adhesions either underwent adhesiolysis via a midline laparotomy, or were merely clinically observed.[52] At 9–12 months follow-up there was no significant difference between the groups with regard to pelvic pain. More importantly, the improvement rate in the control group was 50%. A small subgroup of patients with severe, dense, vascular lesions involving the bowel did, however, show a significant improvement (89%) compared with the control group (17%).

A review of the efficacy of adhesiolysis quotes improvement rates that vary between 63 and 89%.[30] The design of these studies varied widely, however, and the period of review was only 1 month in some cases. Of interest is the fact that 4.7–23% of patients derive some initial benefit but then develop a recurrence of their symptoms; it has been suggested that this is due to reformation of adhesions.[53] This makes it mandatory to scrutinize the length of follow-up, since good results at 1 month may have deteriorated dramatically by 12 months. The improvement rates should also be interpreted in light of the 50% response rate in the control group described above.

Fayez and Clark[50] appear to report much better results than other studies. In this study 156 patients with chronic pelvic pain associated with postoperative adhesions were treated with laser adhesiolysis. Complete relief, defined as disappearance of symptoms and an ability to carry on with normal daily activity during the 12-month follow-up period, was reported in 137 (88%)

patients. The remaining 19 (12%) improved, but to a lesser degree. However, five of these 19 (3% overall), in all of whom severe, dense adhesions had been divided, presented with a recurrence of their symptoms after only 4–6 months. These women underwent repeat surgery, which confirmed the presence of adhesions at the site of pain, and subsequently rendered them pain free. It is not clear why the results should be so much better in this study than others. However, the prevention of *de-novo* adhesions at the time of initial surgery and of redevelopment after adhesiolysis are areas that are attracting considerable interest.

It is difficult to decide what recommendations can be made from the above data. However confusing the results may be, it seems sensible to attempt to prevent the initial formation of adhesions at the time of surgery. To this end, the use of laparoscopy for the initial surgery, which causes fewer postoperative adhesions than laparotomy, seems sensible.[54]

The main issue is the treatment that should be offered to patients with pelvic pain and adhesions. One study showed that adhesiolysis, combined with a second procedure in poor responders, gave excellent results,[50] whereas others have shown that improvement can be achieved in the majority, but that this is often little better than can be achieved by a conservative approach. Taking an evidence-based approach, it could be argued that adhesiolysis should be offered only to women with stage IV adhesions involving the bowel, and should not be offered to those with lesser pathology. This approach may need to be modified in light of the development of conscious pain mapping (discussed below); however, if it can be demonstrated unequivocally that the adhesion is the source of the pain, rather than an incidental finding, then adhesiolysis becomes a far more attractive option.

CONSCIOUS PAIN MAPPING

Laparoscopy under general anaesthesia allows a thorough evaluation of a patient's pelvis but does not permit the surgeon to assess the significance of these findings. The concept of performing an interactive procedure where the surgeon is able to probe a lesion to see if it is responsible for the symptoms is obviously an attractive one. However, equipment manufacturers have only recently produced small-diameter laparoscopes with high-quality resolution that have made the widescale use of microlaparoscopy a feasible prospect. For this procedure a laparoscopy is performed with a 2 mm laparoscope under local anaesthesia and intravenous sedation. The lack of general anaesthesia allows a degree of surgeon–patient interaction, and means the surgeon can gently probe all the pelvic organs or demonstrable pathology to see if any significant discomfort is produced. In theory this should enable the surgeon to differentiate between symptomatic and asymptomatic incidental findings and, therefore, to tailor patient care more appropriately.

It should be remembered that performance of laparoscopy under local anaesthetic has long been established, and that no increase in either the morbidity or mortality rate amongst 250 000 patients has been reported.[55]

An early study on this subject compared the performance of office microlaparoscopy under local anaesthetic (OLULA) in a group of patients with chronic pelvic pain, and a second group undergoing assessment for infertility.[56] The operation was well tolerated by 20 of the 22 patients; two procedures were terminated, one because of benzodiazepine-induced disorientation in a non-English-speaking patient, and one because of an intra-operative anxiety attack in a patient with a history of severe anxiety disorders. These two cases obviously give some useful information as to the future selection criteria for this technique.

This study produced two areas of interest in addition to the profound reduction in the cost of the procedure by avoiding expensive hospital charges, First, in three patients with chronic pelvic pain, an area of marked pain sensitivity was diagnosed. Two of these related to deposits of endometriosis but, importantly, both patients had other areas of endometriosis within the pelvis that did not produce increased pain sensitivity. In the third patient, the area of increased sensitivity related to a loop of bowel adherent to the anterior abdominal wall. This is of considerable interest because, as mentioned earlier, whilst adhesions are found in many patients with chronic pelvic pain, they are also found in 14–17% of asymptomatic patients. The use of OLULA could therefore potentially allow surgeons to discriminate between symptomatic and asymptomatic adhesions in a patient with chronic pelvic pain, so that adhesiolysis, a potentially dangerous procedure, can be restricted to the areas where it would be expected to be of some benefit.

The second interesting finding was that 10 of the 11 patients with chronic pelvic pain had a generalized visceral hypersensitivity to pain; this was not found in any of the patients being investigated for underlying infertility. The authors proposed several explanations for this finding and also suggest that, in the future, this may act as a marker for a certain subgroup of patients and may be of some prognostic significance.

A second paper on this topic[57] also demonstrated that this technique was highly acceptable to the patients, and reviewed the findings of 50 consecutive patients undergoing microlaparoscopy for chronic pelvic pain. Operative as well as diagnostic procedures were performed, and 14 of the 48 women who needed therapeutic procedures had these performed under local anaesthesia. The incidence of significant adhesions was 62%, and all of these were lysed, irrespective of whether they were tender at the time of probing. Twenty-five of these 31 women had pain on manipulation of their adhesions, but it is not clear whether their outcome was any better than that of the six women who had lysis of non-tender, perhaps asymptomatic, adhesions. This is obviously an important area of interest worthy of further work, a point noted by the authors. Thirteen of these women had a markedly tender appendix during their pain mapping, and all underwent appendicectomy, with subsequent symptomatic relief. Abnormal histological findings were present in nine women, and seven women, including all those with normal histology, had severe periappendiceal adhesions. The authors made the critical point that although two of these appendices appeared distorted secondary to the presence of faecaliths, the others appeared macroscopically normal and would have been missed by performing a traditional laparoscopy on an unconscious patient; conscious pain mapping was the only technique capable of demonstrating this pathology

SUMMARY

At present it is not entirely clear what clinical features are required to make a diagnosis of chronic pelvic pain. Until that definitive statement is published and adhered to throughout the scientific and medical communities, it will continue to be difficult to compare one putative treatment with another. However, for the time-being, there are several aspects of this condition that can be critically reviewed.

- The investment of time with the patient during the initial consultation may well pay dividends. A thorough history may suggest other pathology such as irritable bowel syndrome, or an underlying unrelated anxiety disorder that may manifest as pelvic pain, and needs addressing before more invasive investigation of the pelvis. This degree of assessment may well prevent many patients undergoing unnecessary laparoscopy.

- Diagnostic laparoscopy will reveal pathology in a variable percentage of cases, and the rationale for treating these findings laparoscopically has been discussed above. It should be remembered that this treatment can often be performed at the same time as the initial diagnostic laparoscopy, but also that other treatments are available for conditions such as endometriosis, notably medical management, hysterectomy and bilateral oophorectomy.

- That pathology can be demonstrated and treated does not necessarily imply that symptomatic relief will follow. Indeed, it should not be forgotten that these lesions may not be causal or may return rapidly following treatment, especially when dealing with endometriosis and adhesions.

- In cases where pain persists, there is the option of performing one of the pelvic denervation procedures. It cannot be stressed too firmly, however, that these techniques have their limitations and, if they have any role at all, it is in patients with midline, not lateral, pain. One should not forget that procedures such as PSN can be highly dangerous and should only be performed in adequately investigated and counselled patients, and by suitably experienced surgeons.

- Finally, a negative laparoscopy does not imply that there is no organic cause for the pain. The widespread use of OLULA and conscious pain mapping in this subgroup of patients may lead to the demarcation of sensitive foci within the pelvis that may be of prognostic importance and amenable to treatment. Alternatively, it may indicate which areas of pathology are responsible for the symptoms when faced with multiple possibly non-significant lesions. The possible benefits of this technique in assessing patients with chronic pelvic pain should not be underestimated, and it may be that this development is entirely responsible for a marked improvement in our comprehension of the pathophysiology of this poorly understood condition.

REFERENCES

1. Beard RW. Chronic pelvic pain. *Br J Obstet Gynaecol* 1998; 105: 8–10

2. Stones RW. Chronic pelvic pain. Review 97/01. Personal Assessment in Continuing Education. London: Royal College of Obstetricians and Gynaecologists, 1997

3. Mathias SD, Kupperman M, Liberman RF *et al.* Chronic pelvic pain: prevalence, health related quality of life and economic correlates. *Obstet Gynecol* 1996; 87: 321–327

4. Zondervan KT, Yudkin PL, Vessey MP *et al.* The prevalence of chronic pelvic pain in women in the United Kingdom: a systematic review. *Br J Obstet Gynaecol* 1998; 105: 93–99

5. Porpora MG, Gomel V. The role of laparoscopy in the management of pelvic pain in women of reproductive age. *Fertil Steril* 1997; 68: 765–779

6. Collett BJ, Cordle CJ, Stewart CR. A comparative study of women with chronic pelvic pain, chronic nonpelvic pain and those with no history of pain attending general practitioners. *Br J Obstet Gynaecol* 1998; 105: 87–92

7. Howard FM. The role of laparoscopy in the evaluation of chronic pelvic pain. Promises and pitfalls. *Obstet Gynecol Surv* 1993; 48: 117–118

8. Kontoravdis A, Chryssikopoulos A, Hassiakos D *et al.* The diagnostic value of laparoscopy in 2365 patients with acute and chronic pelvic pain. *Int J Gynaecol Obstet* 1996; 52: 243–248

9. Howard FM. Laparoscopic evaluation and treatment of women with chronic pelvic pain. *J Am Assoc Gynecol Laparosc* 1994; 1: 325–331

10. Newham AP, van der Spuy ZM, Nugent F. Laparoscopic findings in women with chronic pelvic pain. *S Afr Med J* 1996; 86: 1200–1203

11. Wiborny R, Pichler B. Endoscopic dissection of the uterosacral ligaments for the treatment of chronic pelvic pain. *Gyne Endosc* 1998; 7: 33–35

12. Howard FM. The role of laparoscopy in the evaluation of chronic pelvic pain: pitfalls with a negative laparoscopy. *J Am Assoc Gynecol Laparosc* 1996; 4: 85–94

13. Donnez J, Nisolle M, Casanas-Roux F. Three-dimensional architectures of peritoneal endometriosis. *Fertil Steril* 1992; 57: 980–983

14. Martin DC, Hubert GD, Levy BS. Depth of infiltration of endometriosis. *J Gynecol Surg* 1989; 5: 55–60

15. Redwine D. Non-laser resection of endometriosis. In: Sutton C, Diamond M (eds) *Endoscopic Surgery for Gynaecologists*. London: WB Saunders, 1993; 220–228

16. Sutton CJG, Ewen SP, Whitelaw N, Haines P. Prospective, randomised, double-blind, controlled trial of laser laparoscopy in the treatment of pelvic pain associated with minimal, mild, and moderate endometriosis. *Fertil Steril* 1994; 62: 696–700

17. Sutton CJG, Hill D. Laser laparoscopy in the treatment of endometriosis. A 5-year study. *Br J Obstet Gynaecol* 1990; 97: 181–185

18. Sutton CJG, Pooley AP, Ewen SP *et al.* Follow-up report on a randomised controlled trial of laser laparoscopy in the treatment of pelvic pain associated with minimal to moderate endometriosis. *Fertil Steril* 1997; 68: 1070–1074

19. Reiter RC. Letter to the editor. *Fertil Steril* 1995; 63: 1355–1356

20. Dover RW, Pooley AP, Sutton CJG. Prospective, randomised, double-blind trial of laparoscopic laser uterine nerve ablation in the treatment of pelvic pain associated with endometriosis. *Br J Obstet Gynecol* 1997; 105(Suppl. 17): 52

21. Bateman BG, Kolp LA, Mills S. Endoscopic versus laparotomy management of endometriomas. *Fertil Steril* 1994; 62: 690–695

22. Semm K, Freidrich ER. *Operative Manual for Endoscopic Abdominal Surgery*. Chicago: Year Book, 1987

23. Donnez J, Nisolle M, Wayembergh M *et al.* CO_2 laser laparoscopy in peritoneal endometriosis and in ovarian endometrial cysts. In: Donnez J (ed) *Laser Operative Laparoscopy and Hysteroscopy*. Louvain, Belgium: Nauwelaerts, 1989, 53–78

24. Sutton CJ, Ewen SP, Jacobs SA *et al.* Laser laparoscopic surgery in the treatment of ovarian endometriomas. *J Am Assoc Gynecol Laparosc* 1997; 4: 319–323

25. Sutton CJ. Endometriosis. *Infertil Reprod Med Clin North Am* 1995; 6: 591–613

26. Marrs RP. The use of potassium-titanyl-phosphate laser for laparoscopic removal of ovarian endometrioma. *Am J Obstet Gynecol* 1991; 164: 1622–1628

27. Donnez J, Nisolle M, Gillerot S *et al.* Rectovaginal septum adenomyotic nodules: a series of 500 cases. *Br J Obstet Gynaecol* 1997; 104: 1014–1018

28. Doyle JB. Paracervical uterine denervation by transection of the cervical plexus for the relief of dysmenorrhoea. *Am J Obstet Gynecol* 1955; 70: 1–16

29. Sutton C, Whitelaw N. Laparoscopic uterine nerve ablation for intractable dysmenorrhoea. In: Sutton C, Diamond M (eds) *Endoscopic Surgery For Gynaecologists*. London: WB Saunders, 1993; 159–168

30. Daniell JF, Lalonde CJ. Advanced laparoscopic procedures for pelvic pain and dysmenorrhoea. In: Sutton C

(ed) *Advanced Laparoscopic Surgery.* London: Balliere Tindall, 1995; 795–808

31. Lichten EM, Bombard J. Surgical treatment of dysmenorrhoea with laparoscopic uterine ablation. *J Reprod Med* 1987; 32: 37–42

32. Daniell JF, Feste J. Laser laparoscopy. In: Keye WR (ed) *Laser Surgery in Gynaecology and Obstetrics.* Boston: GK Hall, 1985; 147–165

33. Daniell JF. Fibreoptic laser laparoscopy. *Ballieres Clin Obstetr Gynecol Laparoscopic Surgery.* 1989; 3: 545–562

34. Daniell JF, Feste JR. Laser laparoscopy. In: Keye WR (ed) *Laser Surgery in Gynecology and Obstetrics.* Boston: GK Hall, 1985; 147–165

35. Nisolle M, Paindevine B, Bourdon A *et al.* Histologic study of peritoneal endometriosis in infertile women. *Fertil Steril* 1990; 53: 984–988

36. Good MC, Copas PR, Doody MC. Uterine prolapse after laparoscopic uterosacral transection. A case report. *J Reprod Med* 1992; 37: 995–996

37. Black WT. Use of presacral sympathectomy in the treatment of dysmenorrhoea: A second look after 25 years. *Am J Obstet Gynecol* 1964; 89: 16–32

38. Daniell E, Dover RW. Laparoscopic use of the argon beam coagulator. In: Sutton C (ed) *Endoscopic Surgery for Gynaecologists,* 2nd edn. London: WB Saunders, 1998; 105–110

39. Biggerstaff ED, Foster SN. Laparoscopic surgery for dysmenorrhoea: uterine nerve ablation and presacral neurectomy. In: Sutton C (ed) *Gynecological Endoscopic Surgery.* London: Chapman & Hall, 1997; 63–83

40. Daniell W, Kurtz BR, Gurley LD *et al.* Laparoscopic presacral neurectomy vs neurotomy: use of the argon beam coagulator compared to conventional technique. *J Gynecol Surg* 1993; 9: 169–173

41. Candiani G, Fedele L, Vercellini P *et al.* Presacral neurectomy for the treatment of pelvic pain associated with endometriosis: a controlled study. *Am J Obstet Gynecol* 1992; 167: 100–103

42. Tjaden B, Schlaff WD, Kimball A *et al.* The efficacy of presacral neurectomy for the relief of midline dysmenorrhoea. *Obstet Gynecol* 1990; 76: 89–91

43. Perry CP, Perez J. The role for laparoscopic presacral neurectomy. *J Gynecol Surg* 1993; 9: 165–168

44. Nezhat C, Nezhat F. A simplified method of laparoscopic presacral neurectomy for the treatment of central pelvic pain due to endometriosis. *Br J Obstet Gynaecol* 1992; 99: 659–663

45. Biggerstaff ED, Foster S. Presacral neurectomy for treatment of midline pelvic pain: laparoscopic approach with laparoscopic treatment of a single major complication. *J Am Assoc Gynecol Laparos* 1994; 1: S4: 17

46. Daniell JF, Dover RW. Laparoscopic enterolysis. In: Sutton C (ed) *Endoscopic Surgery for Gynaecologists,* 2nd edn. London: WB Saunders, 1998; 390–397

47. Trimbos JB, Trimbos-Kemper GCM, Peters AAW *et al.* Findings in 200 consecutive asymptomatic women having a laparoscopic sterilisation. *Arch Gynecol Obstet* 1990; 247: 121–124.

48. Cunanan RG, Courey NG, Lippes J. Laparoscopic findings in patients with pelvic pain. *Am J Obstet Gynecol* 1983; 146: 589–591

49. Stout AL, Steege JF, Dodson WC *et al.* Relationship of laparoscopic findings to self-report of pelvic pain. *Am J Obstet Gynecol* 1991; 164: 73–79

50. Fayez JA, Clark RR. Operative laparoscopy for the treatment of localised chronic pelvic-abdominal pain caused by postoperative adhesions. *J Gynecol Surg* 1994; 10: 79–83

51. MacDonald R, Sutton CJG. Adhesions and laser laparoscopic adhesiolysis. In: Sutton CM (ed) *Lasers in Gynaecology.* London: Chapman & Hall, 1992; 95–113

52. Peters AAW, Trimbos-Kemper GCM, Admiraal C *et al.* A randomised clinical trial on the benefit of adhesiolysis in patients with intraperitoneal adhesions and chronic pelvic pain. *Br J Obstet Gynaecol* 1992; 99: 59–62

53. Steege JF, Stout AL. Resolution of chronic pelvic pain after laparoscopic lysis of adhesions. *Am J Obstet Gynecol* 1991; 165: 278–283

54. Lundorff P, Hahlin M, Kallfelt B *et al.* Adhesion formation after laparoscopic surgery in tubal pregnancy: A randomised study versus laparotomy. *Fertil Steril* 1991; 55: 911–915

55. Metha PV. A total of 250,136 laparoscopic sterilisations by a single operator. *Br J Obstet Gynaecol* 1989; 96: 1024–1034

56. Palter SF, Olive DL. Office microlaparoscopy under local anaesthesia for chronic pelvic pain. *J Am Assoc Gynecol Laparos* 1996; 3: 359–364

57. Almeida OD, Val-Gallas M. Conscious pain mapping. *J Am Assoc Gynecol Laparos* 1997; 4: 587–590

72

Sports and fitness activities

K. Bø

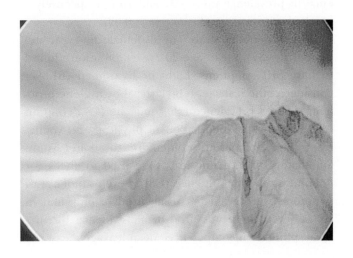

INTRODUCTION

Urinary incontinence is usually regarded as a problem affecting older, post-menopausal, multiparous women.[1] However, several epidemiological studies have demonstrated that symptoms of stress urinary incontinence (SUI) are also frequent in populations of young nulliparous women.[1–9] Prevalence rates vary between 12 and 52% and may be explained by differences in definition, study design and populations. Prevalence rates are usually lower when the International Continence Society (ICS) definition of the symptoms causing social and hygiene problems is introduced.[6,10]

SUI is the most common type of urinary incontinence in women.[11] Urodynamic assessment is needed to distinguish between different subtypes of urinary incontinence.[12,13] Since the literature on urine loss associated with sport and fitness is based mostly on epidemiological studies, the term SUI will be used. SUI implies that urine loss occurs during an increase in intra-abdominal pressure. Therefore, one may expect that women with this condition are likely to experience urine loss during participation in most forms of physical activity. Leakage is less likely to occur in sedentary women who are less exposed to physical exertions, although the underlying condition may be present.

Studies have shown that SUI is common among physical-education/sport students, women who exercise for fitness and female elite athletes. Bø et al.[7] found that 26% of young physical-education students had urinary leakage during different forms of physical activity (questionnaire response rate 84%). A group of women exercising three times a week in addition to daytime physical activities at the university was compared with a group of sedentary nutrition students; the difference in prevalence rates – 31 and 10%, respectively – reached statistical significance ($p = 0.02$).

In a subsequent study[14] of all female first-year students (n = 37), mean age 20.2 years, 38% were found to have SUI symptoms. Eight of 13 women (61.5%) considered the leakage to be a social or hygiene problem, giving a prevalence rate using the ICS definition of 21.6% for this population of physically fit, young, exercising, nulliparous women. In this latter study, ambulatory urodynamic tests were used to check for genuine stress incontinence (GSI). Seven women with symptoms were evaluated using urodynamics, and in six of seven there was urodynamic evidence for urethral sphincter incompetence. Mean leakage measured

by pad test with standardized bladder volume was 12 g (range 0–46).

Nygaard et al.[9] studied incontinence and exercise in a group of 326 women presenting to private gynaecology offices (questionnaire response rate 50%). Eighty-nine per cent exercised at least once a week; the average was three times per week for 30–60 minutes per session. Forty-seven per cent reported some degree of incontinence.

Knowledge about incontinence in female elite athletes is sparse. Nygaard et al.[1] surveyed all 156 women participating in varsity athletics at a large state university. The questionnaire response rate was 92%. The mean age was 19.9 ± 3.3 years and all the women were nulliparous. The women were asked whether they had ever experienced urinary leakage during participation in sports or during coughing, sneezing, heavy lifting, walking to the bathroom, sleeping or on hearing the sound of running water. They rated the frequency of leakage on a five-point scale. Twenty-eight per cent reported urine loss while participating in their sport. Two-thirds of the women who leaked during athletics were incontinent 'more often' than 'rarely'. The proportions in different sports were: gymnastics 67%, basketball 66%, tennis 50%, field hockey 42%, track events 29%, swimming 10%, volleyball 9%, softball 6% and golf 0%. Sixteen per cent were incontinent during practice sessions and 14% during competition. Forty-two per cent reported urine loss during at least one of the activities of daily life, 18% 'more often' than 'rarely'. Twenty-one per cent reported urine loss only during daily life and not during sports, and 7% noted incontinence only during sports.

To find out whether high-impact activity contributes to later urinary incontinence, Nygaard[15] compared former female Olympians who had competed in swimming (low impact) and gymnastics or track and field (high impact). One hundred and four women participated (response rate 51%). When doing their sport as Olympians, high-impact athletes had a higher prevalence of incontinence (36%) than low-impact athletes (4.5%). However, when studied more than 20 years after the end of their sporting career, there was no significant difference in prevalence of incontinence between the groups. It was concluded that participation in regular, strenuous, high-impact activity when young does not predispose a woman to significant urinary leakage later in life.

CONSEQUENCES OF STRESS URINARY INCONTINENCE DURING PHYSICAL ACTIVITY

Urinary incontinence may lead to withdrawal from social activities and reduction of well-being.[16] Norton *et al.*[17] reported that urinary leakage frequently interfered with daily life in more than 50% of their study group. Fall *et al.*[11] reported that 42% of women with incontinence had problems during sport and physical activities.

Bø *et al.*[18] found that two-thirds of sedentary women with GSI reported that urinary leakage was a cause of inactivity. Of 52 women, 27 had tried to participate in specific sport and fitness activities but had withdrawn from one or more activities because of leakage; 19 of these 27 women had withdrawn from aerobics or dance activities, showing that this is one of the most popular fitness activities among women. They all reported that the major leakage occurred during high-impact activities during aerobics session, and especially when performing 'jumping jacks'/'star jumps' (jumping with legs in subsequent abduction and adduction; see Figure 72.1a), which is one of the most frequently used high-impact exercises in aerobics, dance and general fitness programmes.

This is consistent with the study of Nygaard *et al.*[9] in which women reported that running and high-impact aerobics were the activities that resulted in urinary leakage. Thirty per cent of the exercisers noted incontinence during at least one type of exercise, and 20% of the women who were incontinent during a specific activity stopped the activity solely because of incontinence. Eighteen per cent changed the way they performed an exercise because of leakage, and 55% wore a pad during exercise. Frequency, time spent per session, and duration of a particular exercise had no significant impact on the prevalence of incontinence.[9]

Regular participation in sports and fitness activities is an important factor for women's health at all ages. Moderate physical activity can be an important factor in prevention of coronary heart disease, high blood pressure, osteoporosis, musculoskeletal diseases, obesity, breast and colon cancer and anxiety and depression.[19] If a consequence of incontinence is withdrawal from physical activity, the impact on women's health may be enormous.

CAN PHYSICAL ACTIVITY CAUSE URINARY INCONTINENCE?

Several risk factors have been suggested for the development of female urinary incontinence: hereditary weak connective tissue, weak or non-functional pelvic floor muscles, hormonal factors, dyssynergia between detrusor and urethral smooth and striated muscle activity, pregnancy and vaginal delivery, heavy physical exertion, inactivity, obesity, cigarette smoking, menopause and old age have all been suggested as aetiological factors.[20,21] Until now there has been little evidence supporting a strong causal effect of any of these factors. Urinary incontinence in women probably has a multifactorial aetiology, or may be due to failure of one or more factors to compensate for any other weak factor. The speed and strength of contraction of the pelvic floor muscles may be one such important factor.[22]

Optimal pelvic floor muscle function implies that the pelvic floor is positioned in an adequate anatomical position, and with sufficient cross-sectional area, to give structural support for the vagina, bladder and the urethra in order to prevent descent during increases in intra-abdominal pressure. The muscles must be in a neurological state of 'readiness for action', allowing a quick and strong response, or must be part of a 'feed-forward' loop, automatically contracting simultaneously with, or before, increases in intra-abdominal pressure.

Pelvic floor muscles in female athletes

Typically there are two contradicting myths about female athletes and the strength of their pelvic floor muscles. Myth number one is that general physical activity strengthens the pelvic floor, thus making the pelvic floor muscles strong in female athletes. So far, no research has verified this hypothesis. The fact that so many female athletes report SUI[1,7] contradicts the view that general physical activity may strengthen the pelvic floor and thereby prevent leakage.

No studies have yet focused on measuring pelvic floor muscle strength in female elite athletes and age-matched controls. However, Bø *et al.*[14] did not find any significant difference between a group of incontinent female sport students compared with a comparable group of continent women. However, the sample was small, and other studies have found significantly stronger pelvic floor muscles in continent women than in women with GSI.[22,23] Further studies are needed to answer this question.

Myth number two is that heavy exercise (e.g. marathon running), with repetitive bouncing towards the pelvic floor, or weight lifting may overload the pelvic floor and weaken the muscles over time. Nichols and Milley[24] suggested that the cardinal and uterosacral ligaments, pelvic floor muscles and the connective tissue of the perineum may be damaged permanently because of repeated increases in intra-abdominal pressure arising from manual work or chronic cough. According to this theory, strenuous exercise raises the intra-abdominal pressure and may contribute to the development of GSI in some women.

Davis and Goodman[25] studied 512 of 2651 female soldiers who entered the airborne infantry and found that nine developed urinary incontinence during the training period. Urodynamic investigation demonstrated detrusor instability in three and GSI in six of the women. At the end of the training period all six women with GSI had a definite cystourethrocele, a hypermobile vesical neck with loss of the posterior ureterovesical angle and visible urine loss on Valsalva manoeuvre. Four of the women reported feeling a tearing pain in their lower quadrant on impact during a parachute jump, and one woman related a similar event during heavy lifting and when performing sit-ups. Parachute jumping is an extremely high-impact activity; however, from the data available to date it is not possible to conclude whether moderately high-impact activities can cause damage to connective tissue or pelvic floor muscles. It is probable that a considerable proportion of women are able to perform high-impact activities without experiencing incontinence.

Another factor that may contribute to GSI in female elite athletes is hypothalamic amenorrhoea due to intensive exercise, eating disorders or a combination of both, resulting in low levels of oestrogen.[1] However, the association between low oestrogen levels and prevalence of GSI is not clear.[26] Most of the women with GSI in the studies of Bø et al.[14] and Nygaard et al.[1] had regular menstrual cycles.

Nygaard et al.[1] suggest that gymnasts, for example, may have chosen their sport because of hypermobility, and that changes in collagen concentration may be one factor in the higher prevalence of incontinence in gymnasts. However, although some studies have shown reduction in collagen tissue in women with incontinence compared with continent women,[27] the link between collagen, hypermobility and GSI is not clear. There are no studies comparing the collagen structure in gymnasts or other athletes with or without GSI with matched controls.

ASSESSMENT OF INCONTINENCE DURING PHYSICAL ACTIVITY

Usually the diagnosis of GSI is made during assessment in a half-sitting, lithotomy position. The validity of this evaluation can be questioned, however, because most women leak only in a standing position. The original ICS pad test did not involve physical activity at all. However, a test developed later included activities such as stair-climbing and jumping.[12] Hennalla et al.[28] and Hagen et al.[29] have designed tests based on physical activities. The latter's test involved running, jumping jacks, standing up and laying down, and abdominal curls, and was found to be nine times as provocative as the ICS test involving physical activity. The authors concluded that assessment of the degree of SUI has to be physically provocative to detect GSI. Nygaard et al. reported that 7% of women admitted to urine loss during sports only, and that 40% and 17% first noted urinary incontinence during sport while in high school or junior high school, respectively.[1]

Because of methodological problems, there is a lack of studies describing bladder and urethral function during physical activity. James[30] argued that assessment of SUI should be performed in standing and working positions and during physical activity. Applying ambulatory bladder pressure measurements, he demonstrated that peaks in bladder pressure, which rises during running and jumping, occurred when the feet touched the ground. Although the pressure was higher during coughing, some women leaked only during exercise.

Kulseng-Hanssen and Klevmark[31] improved the methodology by placing bladder and urethral transducer catheters in a silicon cuff, which was then sutured to the external urethral opening to keep it stable during activity. Figure 72.1b shows measurements during jumping and coughing in a woman with GSI. In 16 of the patients, 115 leakage episodes were seen in 45 minutes. In 92 of these episodes the decrease in maximum urethral pressure was greater than the increase in detrusor pressure. Some patients complained of urinary leakage during strenuous exercise (running and

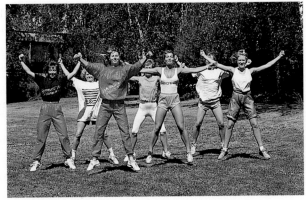

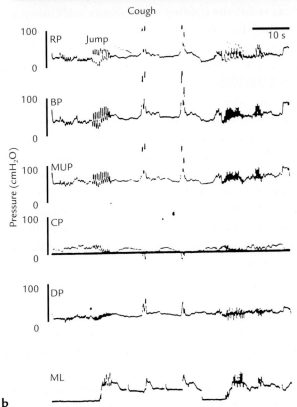

Figure 72.1. *a) 'Jumping jacks' make most women with genuine stress incontinence leak. b) Trace from a stress incontinent patient during jumping and coughing. RP, rectal pressure; BP, blood pressure; MUP, maximum urethral pressure; CP, closure pressure; DP, detrusor pressure; ML; leakage. (From ref. 31, with permission; photo courtesy of Ronny Kristensen, AFJ-Foto.)*

muscles, some women may need even more vigorous and continuous activities to provoke the leakage that they experience outside the laboratory.

Nygaard *et al.*[32] comparing the flexibility of the foot arches in 47 continent and incontinent varsity athletes and found that it was significantly lower in the incontinent women ($p < 0.03$). They suggested that the way in which impact forces are absorbed may be an aetiological factor for stress incontinence, and that more research is required to understand how impact forces are transmitted to the pelvic floor. The high prevalence of urine loss in gymnasts may be explained by the extremely high impact during landing and take-off and the transmission of this pressure to the pelvic floor.

TREATMENT

Prevention during exercise

Because of the health benefits of regular moderate exercise, it is important to emphasize that women should be advised not to stop exercising because of urinary leakage. However, the woman can be advised to choose low-impact activities such as walking, dancing, low-impact aerobics, step training, cycling, swimming or cross-country skiing.

If an incontinent woman wants to participate in high-impact aerobics classes, she may use low-impact alternatives, for example walking while others are running, and doing 'step touch' while others are doing jumping jacks, etc. In addition, if she leaks or feels downward pressure during sit-ups she should be advised to try to contract the pelvic floor muscles before doing abdominal curls or sit-ups.

A good alternative is to exercise the transverse abdominal muscle, an important abdominal muscle to train. This internal abdominal muscle can be easily contracted in a crawling position with one hand on the lower abdominal wall (Fig 72.2). The exercise is performed by lifting the abdominal wall away from the hand and holding the contraction for 6–8 seconds. This contraction puts very little, if any, pressure on the pelvic floor, and can be done in prone, supine, sitting and standing positions.

The woman should be encouraged to use specially designed protection during exercise. Fortunately some

jumping for longer periods of time), although leakage was undetected even in this test. Similar results were seen in the study of Bø *et al.*[14] where the test did not detect leakage in four subjects with a convincing history of urinary leakage. Because GSI may occur due to fatigue of the striated urethral wall and pelvic floor

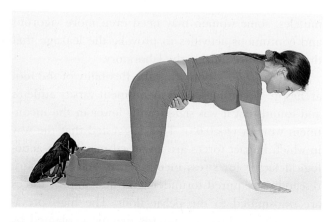

Figure 72.2. *Exercise for the transverse abdominal muscle. (Photo courtesy of Ronny Kristensen, AFJ-Foto.)*

of the best protecting pads are now manufactured in small sizes, making them more comfortable for active women to wear while exercising. In addition, women may use urethral or vaginal devices to prevent leakage during physical activity.[33,34] In a study by Glavind,[35] six women with stress incontinence demonstrated total dryness when using a vaginal device during 30 minutes of aerobic exercise.

Pelvic floor muscle training

Several randomized controlled trials have demonstrated a positive effect of pelvic floor muscle training on GSI.[36,37] Bø *et al.*[18] found that after specific strength training of the pelvic floor muscles, 17 of 23 women had improved symptoms (i.e. less incontinence) during jumping and running, and 15 during lifting. In addition, significant improvement was obtained while dancing, hiking, during general exercise, and in an overall score of ability to participate in different activities.[18] Urine loss was measured using a pad test with standardized bladder volume during exercise comprising running, jumping jacks and sit-ups.[38] There was a significant reduction in urine loss from a mean of 27 g (95% confidence intervals [CI]: 8.8–45.1; range 0–168) to 7.1 g (95% CI: 0.8–13.4; range 0–58.3) ($p < 0.01$) after pelvic floor muscle training.

There seem to be no published data on the effect of pelvic floor muscle training in female elite athletes. However, as these women are used to regular training and are highly motivated to exercise, one would expect the effect to at least as effective, if not more effective, in this specific group of women.

Pelvic floor muscle training should be the first choice of treatment for several reasons:

- It has proved to be effective when conducted intensively with a close follow-up.
- It is a functional, physiological and non-invasive treatment with no known side effects.
- It can be very cost-effective when compared with other treatment modalities.
- The women is given the opportunity to take control of her own health. She learns body awareness and, if successful, the training may enhance self-esteem and coping strategies.

CONCLUSIONS

SUI is prevalent in women exercising at all levels. It is not yet possible to conclude whether strenuous physical activity may cause GSI or genital prolapse. More research is needed to understand how impact from different exercises affects pelvic organs, connective tissue and pelvic floor muscles. The effect of pelvic floor muscle training in elite athletes has not yet been evaluated. However, from the current knowledge of the effect of pelvic floor muscle training, it is suggested as the first choice of treatment.

REFERENCES

1. Nygaard I, Thompson F, Svengalis S, Albright J. Urinary incontinence in elite nulliparous athletes. *Obstet Gynecol* 1994; 84: 183–187

2. Nemir A, Middleton R. Stress incontinence in young nulliparous women. *Am J Obstet Gynecol* 1954; 68: 1166–1168

3. Wolin L. Stress incontinence in young, healthy nulliparous female subjects. *J Urol* 1969; 101: 545–549

4. Hørding U, Pedersen K, Sidenius K, Hedegaard L. Urinary incontinence in 45-year-old women. *Scand J Urol Nephrol* 1986; 20: 183–186

5. Jolleys J. Reported prevalence of urinary incontinence in women in a general practice. *Br Med J* 1988; 296: 1300–1302

6. Sommer P, Bauer T, Nielsen K *et al.* Voiding patterns and prevalence of incontinence in women: a questionnaire survey. *Br J Urol* 1990; 66: 12–15

7. Bø K, Mæhlum S, Oseid S, Larsen S. Prevalence of stress urinary incontinence among physically active and

sedentary female students. *Scand J Sports Sci* 1989; 11: 113–116

8. Simeonova Z, Bengtsson C. Prevalence of urinary incontinence among women at a Swedish primary health care centre. *Scand J Prim Health Care* 1990; 8: 203–206

9. Nygaard I, DeLancey JOL, Arnsdorf L, Murphy E. Exercise and incontinence. *Obstet Gynecol* 1990; 75: 848–851

10. Elving L, Foldsprang A, Lam G, Mommsen S. Descriptive epidemiology of urinary incontinence in 3,100 women age 30–59. *Scand J Urol Nephrol Suppl* 1989; 125: 37–43

11. Fall M, Frankenberg S, Frisen M *et al.* 456 000 svenskar kan ha urininkontinens. Endast var fjærde søker hjelp før besværen. *Laekartidningen* 1985; 82: 2054–2056

12. Abrams P, Blaivas JG, Stanton SL, Andersen JT. The standardisation of terminology of the lower urinary tract function. *Scand J Urol Nephrol Suppl* 1988; 114: 5–19

13. Cundiff G, Harris R, Coates K, Bump R. Clinical predictors of urinary incontinence in women. *Am J Obstet Gynecol* 1997; 177: 262–267

14. Bø K, Stien R, Kulseng-Hanssen S, Kristoffersen M. Clinical and urodynamic assessment of nulliparous young women with and without stress incontinence symptoms: a case control study. *Obstet Gynecol* 1994; 84: 1028–1032

15. Nygaard I. Does prolonged high-impact activity contribute to later urinary incontinence? A retrospective cohort study of female olympians. *Obstet Gynecol* 1997; 90: 718–722

16. Hunskaar S, Vinsnes A. The quality of life in women with urinary incontinence as measured by the sickness impact profile. *J Am Geriatr Soc* 1991; 39: 378–382

17. Norton P, MacDonald LD, Sedgwick PM, Stanton SL. Distress and delay associated with urinary incontinence, frequency, and urgency in women. *Br Med J* 1988; 297: 1187–1189

18. Bø K, Hagen R, Kvarstein B, Larsen S. Female stress urinary incontinence and participation in different sport and social activities. *Scand J Sports Sci* 1989; 11: 117–121

19. Bouchard C, Shephard R, Stephens T *et al* (eds) *Physical Activity, Fitness, and Health. Consensus Statement.* Champaign, IL: Human Kinetics; 1993

20. Bø K. Physical activity, fitness and bladder control. In: Bouchard C, Shephard RJ, Stephens T (eds) *Physical Activity, Fitness, and Health.* Champaign, IL: Human Kinetics; 1994; 774–795

21. Bø K. Risk factors for development and recurrence of urinary incontinence. *Curr Opin Urol* 1997; 7: 193–196

22. Lose G. Simultaneous recording of pressure and cross-sectional area in the female urethra: a study of urethral closure function in healthy and stress incontinent women. *Neurourol Urodyn* 1992; 11: 54–89

23. Hahn I. *Pelvic Floor Training for Genuine Stress Urinary Incontinence.* PhD thesis, University of Gothenberg; 1993

24. Nichols D, Milley P. Functional pelvic anatomy: the soft tissue supports and spaces of the female pelvic organs. *The Human Vagina.* Amsterdam: Elsevier/North-Holland Biomedical Press, 1978; 21–37

25. Davis G, Goodman M. Stress urinary incontinence in nulliparous female soldiers in airborne infantry training. *J Pelvic Surg* 1996; 2: 68–71

26. Fantl J, Cardozo L, McClish D. Estrogen therapy in the management of urinary incontinence in postmenopausal women; a meta-analysis. First report of the hormones and urogenital therapy committee. *Obstet Gynecol* 1994; 83: 12–18

27. Ulmsten U, Ekman G, Giertz G, Malmstrøm A. Different biochemical composition of connective tissue in continent and stress incontinent women. *Acta Obstet Gynecol Scand* 1987; 66: 455–457

28. Hennalla SM, Kirwan P, Castleden DM *et al.* The effect of pelvic floor muscle exercises in the treatment of genuine stress incontinence in women at two hospitals. *Br J Obstet Gynecol* 1988; 95: 81–92

29. Hagen R, Kvarstein B, Bø K *et al.* A simple pad test with fixed bladder volume to measure urine loss during physical activity (Abstract). *Proceedings of the International Continence Society Annual Meeting.* Oslo: International Continence Society, 1988; 88–89

30. James E. The behaviour of the bladder during physical activity. *Br J Urol* 1978; 50: 387–394

31. Kulseng-Hanssen S, Klevmark B. Ambulatory urethrocystorectometry: A new technique. *Neurourol Urodyn* 1988; 7: 119–130

32. Nygaard I, Glowacki C, Saltzman L. Relationship between foot flexibility and urinary incontinence in nulliparous varsity athletes. *Obstet Gynecol* 1996; 87: 1049–1051

33. Thyssen H, Lose G. Long-term efficacy and safety of a disposable vaginal device (Continence Guard) in the treatment of female stress incontinence. *Int Urogynecol J* 1997; 8: 130–133

34. Staskin D, Bavendam T, Miller J. Effectiveness of a urinary control insert in the management of stress urinary incontinence; results of a multicenter study. *Urology* 1996; 47: 629–636

35. Glavind K. Use of a vaginal sponge during aerobic exercises in patients with stress urinary incontinence. *Int Urogynecol J* 1997; 83: 51–53

36. Bø K. Physiotherapy to treat genuine stress incontinence. *Int Cont Surv* 1996; 6: 2–8

37. Wilson D, Bø K, Bourcier A *et al.* Conservative management in women. Committee 14. In: Abrams P, Khoury S, Wein A (eds) *Incontinence.* Plymouth: Health Publication Ltd, 1999; 579–636

38. Bø K, Hagen RH, Kvarstein B *et al.* Pelvic floor muscle exercise for the treatment of female stress urinary incontinence: III. Effects of two different degrees of pelvic floor muscle exercise. *Neurourol Urodyn* 1990; 9: 489–502

73

Problems associated with sexual activity

A. Hextall, L. Cardozo

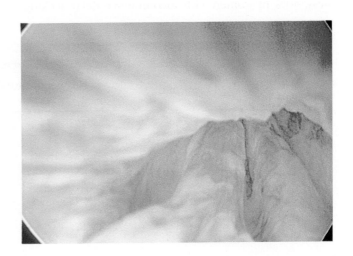

INTRODUCTION

Urinary incontinence may have an adverse effect on almost every aspect of a woman's life, including sexual relations with her partner.[1] A woman's sexuality is concerned not only with her sexual activity, but also with the perception of her own image and the formation of relationships with others.[2] Nearly 50% of women presenting with incontinence, frequency or urgency report feeling odd or different from other people because of their bladder problems and 40% feel less attractive.[3] Poor self-esteem is a frequent problem and difficulties with personal relationships may contribute to the depression and social isolation often felt by women with bladder dysfunction.[4,5]

Sexual intercourse may have an impact on the bladder in several important ways:

- Coital incontinence may give rise to sexual problems for the woman, her partner or both where none had previously existed.
- Incontinence during intercourse may be blamed for problems within a relationship, although a degree of sexual dysfunction may have already existed.
- Sexual activity can give rise to urogenital problems, for example dysuria and urinary tract infection (UTI).

In this chapter we review the impact of urinary incontinence in the sexually active woman and examine the role of sexual intercourse in the pathophysiology of UTI.

PREVALENCE OF COITAL INCONTINENCE

Despite increasing media attention and public awareness, 40% of women with incontinence delay seeking treatment because of embarrassment about their condition.[3] Discussing their urinary problem with a doctor or nurse is very difficult for many women and this may explain why symptoms of coital incontinence are not always volunteered immediately. For example, in a survey of 400 incontinent women, of whom 324 were sexually active, only two women mentioned the problem except in response to direct enquiry.[6] Clinicians may also feel uncomfortable or concerned about their ability to take an adequate history regarding what may be considered a private problem. Some hospitals use a pre-consultation questionnaire and while this may be time saving and give valuable information, further enquiry is often necessary. As with other history taking, it is important to put the patient at ease,[7] perhaps asking about other urinary symptoms or medical complaints first. Open questions such as 'Is there anything else you would like to discuss?' or 'Many women with incontinence leak during sex. Is this problem for you?' are then a good way forward. It may also be appropriate to ascertain if the coital incontinence has had any impact on the patient's relationship with her partner, although it should be noted that for some couples leakage during intercourse may not necessarily give rise to any sexual dysfunction.

The exact prevalence of coital incontinence in the community is not known. However, several studies have attempted to determine frequency of coital incontinence among women presenting with a variety of urinary complaints (Table 73.1). The retrospective nature of some of the studies, variations in questionnaire design and sensitivity, and type of study population may account for some of the observed differences. The four largest reports suggest a prevalence of between 24 and 34%;[6,8–10] the 62% reported by Walters *et al.*[11] requires

Table 73.1. *The prevalence of coital incontinence among women presenting with lower urinary tract symptoms*

Reference	Number of sexually active women	Sexually active women with coital incontinence (%)
Hilton[6]	324	24
Korda *et al.*[8]	839	23
Thiede and Thiede[9]	235	27
Vierhout and Gianotten[10]	254	34
Walters *et al.*[11]	42	62

cautious interpretation because of the small number of patients studied. It is clear that coital incontinence may occur in women with many types of lower urinary tract dysfunction. Most studies do not show any significant differences in the overall prevalence of coital incontinence between women with genuine stress incontinence (GSI) or detrusor instability (DI). In addition, urodynamic studies usually fail to discriminate between those women likely to leak during sexual activity and those who do not.

Some reports have attempted to assess if the timing of the incontinence occurring during sexual activity differed in women with GSI or DI. Hilton[6] found that in two-thirds of affected women the incontinence occurred during penile penetration whereas in the remaining third it was restricted to orgasm. In the group who experienced leakage on penetration, 70% had GSI and only 4% had DI, whereas in the group that experienced leakage during orgasm 42% had GSI and 35% had DI. It was concluded that incontinence occurring during penetration was frequently associated with GSI, and women who experienced leakage during orgasm alone were more likely to have DI. However, others have found that 77% of women with GSI and coital incontinence experience urine loss at orgasm.[10]

PATHOPHYSIOLOGY OF COITAL INCONTINENCE

There are a number of theoretical reasons why women may develop coital incontinence but practical difficulties have limited attempts at clarification. Riley and co-workers[12] used ultrasonography to show that penetrative intercourse in humans is associated with considerable displacement of the female pelvic anatomy. A high degree of indentation and stretching of the anterior vaginal wall and bladder base occurs in both the missionary and female-superior positions, and illustrates how the lower urinary tract may become traumatized during intercourse and give rise to post-coital urinary symptoms.[13] The presence of the erect penis in the vagina may therefore displace the bladder neck and disturb the continence mechanism.[10] Women with a degree of urethral sphincteric incompetence may be expected to be at particular risk of coital incontinence. However, urodynamic studies have failed to show that women who leak during penetration have lower urethral pressures than continent controls.[6]

Penile stimulation of the trigone and bladder base

may provoke abnormal detrusor contractions during intercourse, resulting in raised intravesical pressures and incontinence. A similar effect may also occur at orgasm,[14] particularly given the increased prevalence of DI in women who leak only at climax. However, cystometry has not been performed in asymptomatic women during sexual intercourse to confirm or refute this hypothesis.

The phenomenon of female ejaculation has a long and often disputed history, with considerable debate still occurring between gynaecologists and sex therapists as to its existence and possible origin. Grafenberg[15] reported the expulsion of large quantities of clear fluid at the peak of orgasmic response, which was thought to originate from the urethral glands. However, other authors have suggested that urinary leakage is a more likely, but less socially acceptable, explanation.[16] It does seem clear, however, that many women report having fluid release at the time of orgasm. Anderson Darling and co-workers[17] performed an anonymous survey of 2350 professional women in the United States and Canada. Of the 1172 (50%) of women whose responses were used in the analysis, 40% reported having experienced ejaculation at the moment of orgasm, with almost 10% admitting that they 'frequently' urinated at climax.

INCONTINENCE AND SEXUAL DYSFUNCTION

Several studies have examined the prevalence of sexual dysfunction among middle-aged women, the group most likely to be affected by coital incontinence. Osborn and co-workers[18] interviewed 436 women aged 35–59 years, with a male partner, who were identified from a general practitioner database. One-third of women had at least one operationally defined sexual problem (impaired interest 17%; vaginal dryness 17%; infrequent orgasm 16%; dyspareunia 8%), but only 10% of women regarded themselves as having sexual dysfunction. Sexual difficulties were also found in 45% of 40-year-old Danish women surveyed by Garde and Lunde[19] and 63% of non-randomly selected American women using a broad definition of sexual dysfunction.[20]

In the study by Osborn and co-workers,[18] the only gynaecological factor that was associated with sexual dysfunction was the presence of stress incontinence occurring once or more a week, regardless of age.

Sexual problems are certainly more frequent amongst women with incontinence than the background community rates; this may be explained in part by the presence of a number of physical and psychological factors (Table 73.2). Sutherst[21] reported that 46% of incontinent patients felt that their sex life had been adversely affected by their bladder problem; 35% said that intercourse took place less frequently; 12% had ceased to have any sexual activity. It is possible that psychosexual abnormalities may be related to urinary symptoms in general, rather than specific diseases of the lower urinary tract.[11,22] However, Field and Hilton[23] found that significantly more women with DI had sexual dysfunction (71%) than had those with GSI (29%). An interesting finding was that in women in whom no urodynamic abnormality was detected 54% reported sexual problems. This may be related to the fact that women in this group tend to have higher anxiety and neuroticism scores than do women with DI or GSI.[24]

Urinary incontinence and urogenital prolapse have similar aetiologies and the two conditions frequently coexist.[25] Weber and co-workers[26] compared the sexual function of 80 women complaining of prolapse, with or without incontinence, with 30 continent controls. Only 45 (56%) of the women with prolapse and 17 (57%) of the women without prolapse were currently sexually active. Of the sexually active women with prolapse, 70%

Table 73.2. *Reasons why incontinence may lead to sexual dysfunction*
Reduced sexuality
• Poor self-esteem
• Depression
• Decreased libido
• Presence of pads/pants
• Reduced spontaneity
Performance anxiety
• Concerns about odour
• Fear of leakage occurring during penetration or at orgasm
Pain
• Urinary dermatitis
• Dyspareunia from previous prolapse or continence surgery
Adverse reaction from partner
• Reduced attraction
• Erectile dysfunction

said that their prolapse or incontinence had not led to a change in interest in sexual activity or intercourse. Indeed, anecdotal evidence suggests that many women with severe prolapse, and even those with a pessary *in situ*, can continue having relatively normal intercourse. One of the main findings of this study and others[18,23] is that in women with urinary symptoms, sexual dysfunction and inactivity become increasingly common with age.

Several epidemiological studies have reported a tendency towards a gradual decline in sexual activity in both men and women with ageing.[27,28] Impaired mobility, psychological disturbance, chronic illness and the use of medication, particularly sedatives, are also important factors associated with a decline in sexual activity[29,30] and each becomes more prevalent with advancing age. Most population studies also show that sexual difficulty is related to continence status. Reduced sexual function has also been reported in over 50% of women with multiple sclerosis.[31] This is a particular problem for women over the age of 50 years, and is strongly correlated with bladder and bowel dysfunction.

In some women the onset of incontinence may coincide with the menopause,[32] which is itself a significant risk factor for sexual problems. During the climacteric, many women and their partners experience a decline in sexual interest, activity and responsiveness.[33] The problem is not restricted to women. Approximately one in five women attending a menopause clinic had a partner suffering from medical, psychiatric or sexual problems that contributed to the deterioration in the couple's sex life.[34] In a recent study of 2465 community-dwelling Swedish women aged over 55 years, the most frequent reason for cessation of sexual activity was lack of a partner.[35] The prevalence of male sexual dysfunction among the partners of women having treatment for urogynaecological problems is unknown.

Hysterectomy is the most frequently performed major gynaecological operation but whether the procedure has a major impact on urinary or sexual function remains a controversial issue.[36] A number of physical and psychological factors, including cultural beliefs, preconceived views on the role of the uterus and knowledge of reproductive anatomy, are important but are difficult to quantify. In general, gynaecologists tend to reassure women that hysterectomy is unlikely to have a significant effect on their sex life and may even enhance it, particularly if concerns about troublesome vaginal bleeding and pelvic pain are eradicated. There is some evidence to support this view. Virtanen and co-workers[37] studied 102 women undergoing abdominal hysterectomy for benign disease and found a significant decrease in the number of women with dyspareunia 12 months after surgery. The current debate is whether subtotal hysterectomy, where the cervix is preserved, offers any psychosexual benefits over total hysterectomy; the results of prospective randomized, double-blind studies are awaited with interest. Perhaps not surprisingly, however, it is clear that women undergoing hysterectomy and radiotherapy for gynaecological malignancy experience more sexual dysfunction than those undergoing hysterectomy for benign disease.[38]

A number of factors may therefore contribute to the sexual dysfunction in women with urinary incontinence. The psychological consequences of this distressing condition, once established, can become incorporated into an individual's lifestyle and personality. Sexual dysfunction often becomes worse over time because of the development of performance anxiety, where the goal of sexuality is no longer enjoyment, but 'getting it right'. Such factors, described by Masters and Johnson as 'spectating', are important in perpetuating sexual difficulties.[39] This may have major implications for the treatment of these women, as the successful management of lower urinary tract symptoms may not necessarily improve their sexual dysfunction.

TREATMENT OF INCONTINENCE AND SEXUAL DYSFUNCTION

Treatments for urinary incontinence are almost always assessed in terms of objective changes in urodynamic results and subjective improvement in urinary symptoms. More recently this limited approach has been extended and now quality-of-life measures are becoming much more important, particularly in the evaluation of new techniques. Conservative therapies such as pelvic floor exercises or electrical stimulation carry virtually no long-term sequelae. However, for women with incontinence or prolapse opting for surgical treatment, the type of operation and subsequent risks of dyspareunia are important considerations.

For some patients simple measures such as emptying the bladder before sex or a change of position are effective in reducing the risk of coital leakage. However, few studies have assessed the effect of treatment on coital incontinence, despite the fact that urinary incontinence and sexual dysfunction are so closely related; most have considered it only as a secondary outcome measure after results of therapy for stress or urge incontinence have been presented. Hilton[40] reported that the cure rate for coital incontinence may be lower than that of other symptoms of stress incontinence, with only 66% of women reporting a cure compared with 88% in other circumstances. There is a paucity of information about the benefits of non-surgical treatments on sexual activity in women with urinary symptoms, and there are no randomized trials comparing surgical and non-surgical treatments.

Haase and Skibsted[41] performed a prospective study of 55 women undergoing a primary surgical procedure for stress incontinence or prolapse. Postoperatively 13 women experienced an improvement in their sex life, 35 no change and five a deterioration. Improvement resulted from a cure of coital incontinence; deterioration resulted from dyspareunia secondary to a posterior vaginal wall repair. Although colposuspension alters the vaginal axis, none of the 14 patients who underwent this procedure alone, or the six women who underwent this procedure in combination with a vaginal repair, reported any dyspareunia. Two other studies have addressed the same issue and found that 8% (three out of 36)[42] and 18% (seven out of 39)[43] of women complained of postoperative dyspareunia, although in the latter series no attempt was made to exclude the effects of previous surgery. Pain on intercourse following vaginal surgery has been known to be a problem for many years[44,45] and remains a significant cause of sexual morbidity.[46]

It is unusual for women with DI to present only with the symptom of urinary leakage during intercourse. Bladder retraining and anticholinergic therapy are the treatments of choice but their cure rate in this situation remains unclear. Imipramine has been advocated as a particularly useful treatment.[16]

Women who have a urinary diversion for intractable incontinence may find an improvement in their sex life following surgery. Nordstrom and Nyman[47] investigated the effect of ileal-conduit urinary diversion on the sexual function of 15 women who were undergoing the procedure for incontinence mainly because of spinal cord injury or radiotherapy for gynaecological malignancy. Seven women (47%), four of whom were sexually inactive before surgery, reported increased sexual desire and activity and found their overall sex life to be more satisfying following surgery. In a larger series of 126 men and 46 women, 56% of patients had reduced sexual desire following ileal loop urostomy.[48] Schover and von Eschenbach[49] interviewed nine sexually active women before and after radical cystectomy. (Six of the women also received preoperative irradiation.) All seven of the women who resumed sexual activity experienced initial dyspareunia but this eventually improved.

Catheterization may be indicated for women with acute or chronic urinary retention or a neuropathic bladder or sometimes for incontinence. Clean intermittent self-catheterization is of particular benefit to women who remain sexually active.[50] Long-term urethral catheterization has the drawback of discomfort, urethral trauma and a high incidence of contamination from perineal flora which may lead to symptomatic infection. Suprapubic catheterization is often more comfortable, and should always be considered if the patient wants to continue with sexual relations.

Even when the physical aspects of coital incontinence have been treated there may well be psychological sequelae. Thus, overall management must take account of both aspects.[51] A sympathetic approach is required, with the aim of helping the couple come to terms with their disability, which will hopefully allow them to have a mutually enjoyable sex life despite their problem.[40]

URINARY TRACT INFECTION AND SEXUAL INTERCOURSE

Generations of women have recognized the association between sexual intercourse and the development of urinary symptoms. Nulliparity and a rigid perineum contribute to the development of post-coital dysuria, also known as 'honeymoon cystitis'. Kunin and McCormack[52] showed that nuns have a lower prevalence of bacteriuria than other populations of women in early adult life. Organisms are massaged into the urethra and bladder during intercourse and, if they are not voided soon after, they multiply and cause infection. Buckley *et al.*[53] found an increase in the urinary bacterial count after coitus in 30% of women, and Nicolle[54] reported that both symptomatic and asymptomatic bacteriuria was more frequent the day after intercourse.

Several behavioural factors have been shown to enhance the risk of UTI following sexual intercourse. These include: deferred voiding after intercourse,[55] frequency of intercourse,[56] low fluid intake[57] and deferred voiding after the initial urge to micturate.[58]

A large prospective study by Hooton and co-workers examined the risk factors for UTI in young women.[59] A total of 796 healthy, sexually active women were included on the basis that they were starting a new contraceptive method and were willing to participate in the study. Two cohorts of women were investigated for a total of 323 person-years of follow-up. The annual incidence of acute cystitis was 0.7 episodes per person-year among university students (90% were confirmed infections on culture) and 0.5 per person-year among women enrolled in a health maintenance programme. Using multivariate analysis, the authors were able to identify contraceptive diaphragm and spermicide use, recent sexual intercourse and a history of recurrent UTI as independent risk factors for UTI among women at each study site. The relative risk of UTI increased from 1.0 for unmarried women who had not been sexually active in the previous week to 9.0 for women who had had intercourse seven times during that period.

Some women are particularly sensitive to post-coital urinary tract dysfunction due to the development of a relatively high urethral pressure following intercourse. Contraceptive diaphragms may also reduce urinary flow, and research has shown that the risk of referral to hospital for UTI is two to three times higher amongst diaphragm users than among well-matched controls.[60] Spermicidal cream and the use of spermicidal-lubricated condoms can sometimes result in vaginal and urethral irritation.

Several simple measures may be effective in reducing the risk of post-coital UTI. Close attention to perineal hygiene, change of coital technique, use of a vaginal lubricant and avoidance of the contraceptive diaphragm may all be successful first-line measures. Women should be encouraged to drink fluid before anticipated sex to facilitate post-coital voiding. Other unproven interventions include the ingestion of cranberry or blueberry juice.[61] These juices contain a substance that reduces bacterial adhesion to uroepithelial cells.[62,63] While they may have a place in reducing the risk of bacteriuria and pyuria in elderly women,[64] their role in prophylaxis against infection following intercourse has yet to be established.

For women who do not respond to simple measures, regular or intermittent antibiotic prophylaxis is usually effective.[65,66] We have found norfloxacin (400 mg taken around the time of intercourse) to be effective. The role of oestrogen therapy for post-menopausal women with recurrent UTIs is controversial and is discussed further in Chapter 66. Those women who continue to have post-coital symptoms should undergo further investigation. Mid-stream urine analysis is mandatory and culture for fastidious organisms, including *Mycoplasma hominis* and *Ureaplasma urealyticum*, is often worthwhile. Acute urethritis may also be caused by *Chlamydia* which, although difficult to isolate, responds well to a 14–21-day course of doxycycline. Underlying abnormalities such as voiding difficulties and vesicoureteric reflux should always be considered, and imaging of the renal tract with ultrasonography, intravenous pyelography or videocystourethrography may be necessary. It is also sometimes appropriate to perform a cystourethroscopy to exclude a urethral diverticulum or an intravesical foreign body such as a calculus. Our policy is also to take a bladder biopsy, even if the cystoscopic appearance is normal, because 50% of women will have histological evidence of underlying chronic cystitis in this situation.[67]

CONCLUSIONS

Urinary symptoms may have a profound effect on the sexual health of women. Coital incontinence is a relatively frequent problem encountered in the urogynaecology clinic but few women admit to this symptom unless asked directly. The pathogenesis is not entirely understood but it is clear that urinary leakage during intercourse can occur on penetration, orgasm, or both, in women with a variety of different urinary problems. Sexual dysfunction may continue even when other urinary symptoms have been treated successfully and objective urodynamic evaluation fails to detect any residual abnormality. Sexual intercourse is a risk factor for the development of post-coital urinary symptoms and UTI. For many women simple measures such as maintaining good perineal hygiene, passing urine after sex and avoiding the contraceptive diaphragm are all that is necessary. Prophylactic antibiotics, taken either after intercourse or on a regular basis, are effective second-line measures. However, some women with persistent problems require investigation to exclude an underlying urogenital abnormality.

REFERENCES

1. Kelleher CJ, Cardozo LD, Wise BG *et al.* The impact of urinary incontinence on sexual function. *Neurourol Urodyn* 1992; 11: 359–360

2. Wheeler V. A new kind of loving? The effect of continence problems on sexuality. *Professional Nurse* 1990; June: 492–496

3. Norton PA, MacDonald LD, Sedgwick PM *et al.* Distress and delay associated with urinary incontinence, frequency, and urgency in women. *Br Med J* 1988; 297: 1187–1189

4. Stone CB, Judd GE. Psychogenic aspects of urinary incontinence in women. *Clin Obstet Gynecol* 1978; 21: 807–815

5. Macauley AJ, Stern RS, Holmes DM *et al.* Micturition and the mind: psychological factors in the aetiology and treatment of urinary symptoms in women. *Br Med J* 1987; 294: 540–543

6. Hilton P. Urinary incontinence during sexual intercourse: a common, but rarely volunteered, symptom. *Br J Obstet Gynaecol* 1988; 95: 377–381

7. Tomlinson J. ABC of sexual health. Taking a sexual history. *Br Med J* 1998; 317: 1573–1576

8. Korda A, Cooper M, Hunter P. Coital incontinence in an Australian Population. *Asia Oceania J Obstet Gynaecol* 1989; 15: 313–315

9. Thiede HA, Thiede FK. A glance at the urodynamic database. *J Reprod Med* 1990; 35: 925–931

10. Vierhout ME, Gianotten WL. Mechanisms of urine loss during sexual activity. *Eur J Obstet Gynecol Reprod Biol* 1993; 52: 45–47

11. Walters MD, Taylor S, Schoenfeld LS. Psychosexual study of women with detrusor instability. *Obstet Gynecol* 1990; 75: 22–26

12. Riley AJ, Lees WR, Riley EJ. An ultrasound study of human coitus. In: Bezemer W (ed) *Sex Matters.* Amsterdam: Elsevier Science, 1992; 29–32

13. Kelleher CJ, Cardozo LD. Sex and the bladder. *Sexual Marital Ther* 1993; 8: 231–241

14. Khan Z, Bhola A, Starer P. Urinary incontinence during orgasm. *Urology* 1988; 31: 279–282

15. Grafenberg E. The role of the urethra in female orgasm. *Int J Sexol* 1950; 3: 145–148

16. Cardozo LD. Sex and the bladder. *Br Med J (Clin Res Ed)* 1988; 296; 587–588

17. Anderson Darling C, Davidson JK, Conway-Welch C. Female ejaculation: perceived origins, the Grafenberg spot/area and sexual responsiveness. *Arch Sex Behav* 1990; 19: 29–47

18. Osborn M, Hawton K, Gath D. Sexual dysfunction among middle aged women in the community. *Br Med J* 1988; 296: 959–962

19. Garde K, Lunde I. Female sexual behaviour: a study in a random sample of 40-year-old Danish women. *Maturitas* 1980; 2: 225–240

20. Franke E, Anderson C, Rubenstein D. Frequency of sexual dysfunction in normal couples. *New Engl J Med* 1978; 299: 111–115

21. Sutherst JR. Sexual dysfunction and urinary incontinence. *Br J Obstet Gynaecol* 1979; 86: 387–388

22. Clark A, Romm J. Effect of urinary incontinence on sexual activity in women. *J Reprod Med* 1993; 38: 679–683

23. Field SM, Hilton P. The prevalence of sexual problems in women attending for urodynamic investigation. *Int Urogynecol J* 1993; 4: 212–215

24. Norton KRW, Bhat AV, Stanton SL. Psychiatric aspects of urinary incontinence in women attending an outpatient urodynamic clinic. *Br Med J* 1990; 301: 271–272

25. Stanton SL. Vaginal prolapse. In: Shaw R, Soutter P, Stanton SL (eds) *Gynaecology*. Edinburgh: Churchill Livingstone, 1992; 437–447

26. Weber AM, Walters MD, Schover LR *et al.* Sexual function in women with uterovaginal prolapse and urinary incontinence. *Obstet Gynecol* 1996; 85: 483–487

27. Verwoert A, Pfeiffer E, Wang H. Sexual behaviour in senescence: changes in sexual activity and interest in aging men and women. *J Geriatr Psychiatry* 1969; 2: 163–180

28. Diokno AC, Brown MB, Herzog R. Sexual function in the elderly. *Arch Intern Med* 1990; 150: 197–200

29. Nilsson L. Sexuality in the elderly. *Acta Obstet Gynecol Scand* 1987; 140: 52–58

30. Mooradian AD, Greiff V. Sexuality in older women. *Arch Intern Med* 1990; 150: 1033–1038

31. Bakke A, Myhr KM, Gronning M *et al.* Bladder, bowel and sexual dysfunction in patients with multiple sclerosis – a cohort study. *Scand J Urol Nephrol Suppl* 1996; 179: 61–66

32. Hextall A, Cardozo LD. The menopause and lower urinary tract dysfunction. *Urogynaecologia Int J* 1997; 11: 103–107

33. Graziottin A. Sexuality and the menopause. In: Studd JW (ed) *The Modern Management of the Menopause. Annual review 1998*. Carnforth, Lancashire: Parthenon, 1998; 49–58

34. Sarrel PM, Whitehead MI. Sex and menopause: defining the issues. *Maturitas* 1985; 7: 217–224

35. Lindgren R, Berg G, Hammar M *et al.* Hormone replacement therapy and sexuality in a population of Swedish postmenopausal women. *Acta Obstet Gynecol Scand* 1993; 72: 292–297

36. Thakar R, Mayonda I, Stanton SL *et al.* Bladder, bowel and sexual function after hysterectomy for benign conditions. *Br J Obstet Gynaecol* 1997; 104: 983–987

37. Virtanen H, Makinen J, Tenho T *et al.* Effects of abdominal hysterectomy on urinary and sexual symptoms. *Br J Urol* 1993; 72: 868–872

38. Lalos O, Lalos A. Urinary, climacteric and sexual symptoms one year after treatment of endometrial and cervical cancer. *Eur J Gynaecol Oncol* 1996; 17: 128–136

39. Masters WH, Johnson VE. *Human Sexual Inadequacy*. London: Churchill Livingstone, 1970

40. Hilton P. Sexuality and urinary incontinence. *Br J Sex Med* 1989; 6: 230–233

41. Haase P, Skibsted L. Influence of operations for stress incontinence and/or genital descensus on sexual life. *Acta Obstet Gynecol Scand* 1988; 67: 659–661

42. Walter S, Olsen KP, Frimodt-Moller C *et al.* [Urinary incontinence in women treated with colposuspension. Clinical urodynamic and radiological assessment.] *Ugeskr Laeger* 1975; 137: 2979–2981

43. Kampar AL, Tikjob G, Bay-Nielsen A. Kolposuspension a. M. Burch. *Ugeskr Laeger* 1982; 144: 1921

44. Jeffcoate TNA. Posterior colpoperineorrhaphy. *Am J Obstet Gynecol* 1959; 77: 490–502

45. Francis WJA, Jeffcoate TNA. Dyspareunia following vaginal operations. *J Obstet Gynaecol Br Commonw* 1961; 1–10

46. Kahn M, Stanton SL. Posterior colporrhaphy: its effects on bowel and sexual function. *Br J Obstet Gynaecol* 1997; 104: 82–86

47. Nordstrom GM, Nyman CR. Male and female sexual function and activity following ileal conduit urinary diversion. *Br J Urol* 1992; 70: 33–39

48. Boyd SD, Feinberg SM, Skinner DG *et al.* Quality of life survey of urinary diversion patients: comparison of ileal conduits versus continent Kock ileal reservoirs. *J Urol* 1987; 138: 1387–1389

49. Schover LR, von Eschenbach AC. Sexual function and female radical cystectomy: a case series. *J Urol* 1985; 134: 465–468

50. Roe BH, Brocklehurst JC. Study of patients with indwelling catheters. *J Adv Nurs* 1987; 12: 713–719

51. Ramage M. ABC of sexual health. Management of sexual problems. *Br Med J* 1998; 317: 1509–1512

52. Kunin CM, McCormack RC. An epidemiology study of

bacteriuria and blood pressure among nuns and working women, *New Engl J Med* 1968; 278: 635–642

53. Buckley RM, McGuckin M, MacGregor RR. Urine bacterial counts after sexual intercourse. *New Engl J Med* 1978; 298: 321–324

54. Nicolle LE, Harding GK, Preiksaitis J *et al.* The association of urinary tract infection with sexual intercourse. *J Infect Dis* 1982; 146: 579–583

55. Strom BL, Collins M, West SL. Sexual activity, contraception use, and other risk factors for symptomatic and asymptomatic bacteriuria. *Ann Int Med* 1987; 107: 816–823

56. Foxman B, Frerichs RR. Epidemiology of urinary tract infection 1. Diaphragm use and sexual intercourse. *Am J Pub Health* 1985; 75: 1308–1313

57. Ervine C, Komaroff AL, Pass TM. Behavioural factors and urinary incontinence. *J Am Med Assoc* 1980; 243: 330–331

58. Adatto K, Doebele KG, Galland L, Granowetter L. Behavioural factors and urinary tract infection. *J Am Med Assoc* 1979; 241: 2525–2526

59. Hooton TM, Scholes D, Hughes JP *et al.* A prospective study of risk factors for symptomatic urinary tract infection in young women. *New Engl J Med* 1996; 335: 468–474

60. Gillespie L. The diaphragm, an accomplice in recurrent urinary tract infections. *Urology* 1984; 254: 240–245

61. Ronald AR. Sex and urinary tract infections (Editorial). *New Engl J Med* 1996; 335: 511–512

62. Sobota AE. Inhibition of bacterial adherence by cranberry juice: potential use for the treatment of urinary tract infection. *J Urol* 1984; 131: 1013–1016

63. Ofek I, Goldhar J, Zafriri D *et al.* Anti-*Escherichia coli* adhesion activity of cranberry and blueberry juices. *New Engl J Med* 1991; 324: 1599

64. Avorn J, Monane M, Gurwitz J *et al.* Cranberry juice's effects on urinary tract infection. *J Am Med Assoc* 1994; 271: 751–754

65. Pfau A, Sacks T, Engelstein D. Recurrent urinary tract infections in premenopausal women: prophylaxis based on an understanding of the pathogenesis. *J Urol* 1983; 129: 1153–1157

66. Stapleton A, Latham RH, Johnson C *et al.* Postcoital antimicrobial prophylaxis for recurrent urinary tract infection. *J Am Med Assoc* 1990; 264: 703–706

67. Hextall A, Boos K, Aslam N *et al.* The value of a cystoscopy for diagnosing chronic cystitis in women with irritative urinary symptoms or recurrent urinary tract infections. *Int Urogynecol J* 1997; 8: 62

74

Nulliparous women

A. Bourcier

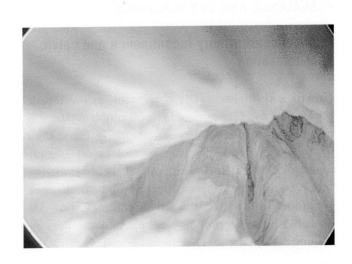

INTRODUCTION

Over the last few decades, urinary and faecal incontinence, as well as vaginal prolapse, have been thought to be related to the weakening of the striated muscles with age and to the overstretching of the pelvic muscles during childbirth, leading to damage of the pelvic floor muscles and/or sphincters.

Although there has been very little research on identification of patients at risk for pelvic disorder, I believe that there are 'intrinsic' and 'extrinsic' factors which are associated with pelvic floor dysfunction. It is generally accepted that female pelvic floor disorders occur widely and that this is a frequent problem relating to parity, menopause and age, but specialists in this field are less aware of the prevalence in younger women, particularly nulliparous women.

A number of features of modern living result in urological symptoms that represent a high risk to the pelvic floor musculature: the greater proportion of women in the work force, the tendency to become pregnant after the age of 40 years, and the desire to keep in shape through fitness programmes. This type of dysfunction relates to 'mechanical' defects. Overall health, environment, social contacts and internal psychological processes are possible contributors to a 'psychogenic' disturbance. In urodynamic laboratories it is not uncommon to encounter nulliparous women complaining of leakage during running or complaining of frequency/urgency symptoms. However, the number of younger women reporting symptoms of urinary stress incontinence (USI) or voiding difficulties and seeking treatment is surprisingly high.

PREVALENCE AND DEMOGRAPHICS

Prevalence of urinary incontinence and pelvic floor relaxation

Urinary incontinence (UI) is common in the female population and is considered to be a problem affecting mostly multiparous women or the elderly. Pelvic floor dysfunction, specifically urinary and faecal incontinence, is thought to be widespread. Pelvic floor disorder is a general term that is used to describe conditions which affect the female continence mechanisms and genital prolapse. Sexual and psychogenic voiding dysfunction has been investigated less, and data

on these conditions affecting nulliparous women are limited or even absent. The prevalence of pelvic floor disorders in the general population, of any age, ranges from 26 to 57%,[1–4] with only 4% of subjects designated incontinent by all definitions. Incontinence was considered bothersome by 21–64% of subjects. Predisposing factors have not been clearly identified. Although most of the studies support increasing age and parity as risk factors, other studies have shown only a minimal increase in prevalence with age or a higher prevalence in younger age groups.

Reports of the prevalence of USI in nulliparous[5,6] or young women after childbirth vary considerably. Nulliparous women are thought to complain less of the symptoms of USI than parous women. The prevalence rates, as discussed previously, bring into question age as a true risk factor. Although Brocklehurst[2] and Molander[7] support increasing age as a risk factor, earlier studies have shown only a minimal increase in prevalence with age or a higher prevalence in younger groups (between 4 and 25% at age 18–24 years).[1–4] Holst and Wilson[8] reported that nulliparous women reported incontinence less often than primiparous women, but that incontinence changed insignificantly with increasing parity (3% in 18–24 year olds). Bø et al.[9] reported that 38% of 37 physical-education students had symptoms of UI. Harris et al.[10] examined differences between parous and nulliparous women presenting with UI and pelvic organ prolapse (POP). A total of 722 consecutive referrals with UI or POP were evaluated, 62 of whom were nulliparous; 70% had UI (66% genuine stress incontinence [GSI], 19% detrusor instability [DI], and 15% GSI and DI); 30% had at least stage III POP. There were significant differences in the distribution of diagnoses according to parity, with the nulliparous group much less likely to have POP (11 vs 32%). Nulliparous women were younger, had less anterior vaginal descent, less bladder-neck mobility and narrower genital hiatus and perineal body measurements. The authors concluded that nulliparous women are less likely to present with POP, and those with GSI tend to be older, have less bladder-neck mobility and lower maximal urethral closure pressures than parous women. Janssen et al.[11] asked a series of 310 healthy nulliparous women, aged 12–18 years, to complete a questionnaire, with an 82% response rate. Altogether 29% of the 265 nulliparous women were incontinent; 11% had USI, 13% had urge incontinence and 5% had mixed symptoms. In addition, 28% had giggle incontinence, 11% reported that they had regular urinary leakage (more than once a week) and the majority of the women with USI used pads. Only 33% of these nulliparous women considered their symptoms to be a real handicap.

Prevalence of USI in physically active women and sportswomen

Despite the lack of reliable studies, the prevalence of incontinence is significantly higher in physically active women than in sedentary women. The prevalence of USI in young female athletes and women who exercise ranges from 8 to 40%. In one series of studies,[12,13] approximately 30% of young, healthy, nulliparous women who practised sports on a regular basis experienced problems of incontinence. There have been few studies on the problems of USI related to sports.

Nygaard[14] studied the relationship between exercise and incontinence using a self-administered questionnaire assessing the prevalence of both exercise and incontinence in 326 women with a mean age of 38.5 years, who exercised regularly and who were attending private gynaecology offices: 47% of regularly exercising women reported some degree of incontinence. In another study, Nygaard *et al.*[15] determined the prevalence of UI symptoms during endeavours among a group of nulliparous elite college varsity female athletes by asking them to fill in a questionnaire about the occurrence of UI while participating in their sport and during activities of daily life. A total of 156 women participated, with a mean age of 19.9 years; all the women were nulliparous. Overall, 40 athletes (28%) reported urine loss while participating in their sport. The proportions in different sports were: gymnastics 67%, basketball 66%, tennis 50%, field hockey 42%, track 29%, swimming 10%, volleyball 9% and golf 0%. The authors concluded that physical stress is common in young, fit, nulliparous women. In another study, Nygaard *et al.*[16] surveyed 144 nulliparous varsity athletes at a state university, with a mean age of 19.9 years. Overall, 28% noted urine loss while participating in their sport. Bø *et al.*[17,18] have shown a prevalence of USI in physical-education students of 26% and showed that the prevalence of USI in physically active students is significantly higher than in sedentary women. Bourcier and Juras[19] investigated USI during sports and fitness activities in 59 women divided into two groups. Group I (n = 28)

represented female athletes; their mean age was 25.5 years (range 21–29) and mean parity 0.5 (range 0–1). Group II (n = 31) represented women practising sports on a regular basis; their mean age was 28 years (range 23–32) and mean parity 1 (range 0–2). The degree of USI was defined as severe (dripping incontinence on exercising), moderate (incontinence with heavy lifting or running) or mild (incontinence on jumping). The prevalence of USI symptoms in group I was: 7% severe, 24% moderate and 33% mild; prevalence rates in group II were 5%, 20% and 28%, respectively. Fall *et al.*[20] reported that 42% of women with incontinence had problems relating to sport and fitness activities.

Bourcier *et al.*[21] also studied the relationship between physical activities and incontinence. A self-administered questionnaire was used to assess the prevalence of exercise and incontinence in two groups of women: 480 women with a mean age of 48.5 years and no regular practice of sports (group I), and 120 women with a mean age of 28 years, practising sports on a regular basis (group II). They found that the urine loss was related to sneezing or coughing in 87% of group I, and to running or tennis in 38%, and to aerobics in 35% of group II.

Jacquetin *et al.*[22] surveyed 155 healthy nulliparous students, mean age 20 years, using a questionnaire on USI related to practice of sports. All the subjects were involved in sports and had begun their physical activities at the age of 6 years. The activities included gymnastics, basketball and volleyball. Of the 155 students studied, 22% had some degree of USI and 9.7% reported leakage at least weekly. More than 24% of the women complained of embarrassment; 6.5% used an absorbent pad during practice and 44% wanted medical information on their problem and to seek medical care.

Prevalence of other dysfunctions

Interstital cystitis, frequency–urgency syndrome, nocturnal enuresis, giggle incontinence, vulvodynia, vaginismus and other sexual and psychogenic disturbances are common in nulliparous women but information regarding the prevalence is missing. An extensive review of the literature failed to identify specific data on the prevalence or incidence of these psychogenic dysfunctions, or of pelvic relaxation with or without vaginal prolapse.

AETIOLOGIC FACTORS AND PATHOPHYSIOLOGY

Contrary to commonly held assumptions, pelvic floor dysfunction in nulliparous women appears to be due to a combination of different factors which can be classified into two main categories: 'intrinsic' or underlying factors and 'extrinsic' or environmental factors.

UI can be caused by anatomical, pathological or physiological factors affecting the urinary tract. The most common type of USI results from loss of support by the pelvic floor musculature and loss of suspension by the connective tissue in the ligaments fascia. Another cause is intrinsic urethral sphincter deficiency which arises from loss of urethral connective elements and urethral vasculature. Wilson[23] has described general principles associated with the development of UI:

- the genotype of the individual and the way in which that genotype interacts with the environment;
- structural and functional abnormalities which may lead to conditions including genital prolapse, incontinence and anorectal dysfunction;
- adverse environmental factors (work, physical activities).

Intrinsic factors

Heredity

It has been suggested that a genetic defect in the connective tissue may be a major factor in the aetiology of USI. Langer et al.,[24] in a study of 259 women suffering from USI, concluded that this condition is about three times more prevalent in first-degree female family members of women who suffer from this disorder, in comparison with the relatives of continent women. This familial tendency does not relate to age, parity or maximum birth weight. Hence, it might reflect an inherited factor that predisposes to the development of USI.

Race

USI seems to have a high prevalence in the white population. Zaccharin[25] measured anatomical differences (pubouerthral attachments) in Asians and whites in an attempt to explain differences in the prevalence of USI. He reported that the fascia of the pelvic structures in cadavers of Chinese women was dense and thick compared with that observed in cadavers of white women.

Anatomical abnormalities

Defects or damage to the upper suspensory ligaments cause a different type of prolapse.[26] It is also possible that a congenital defect of the puborectalis fibres and/or a widened levator ani hiatus may impede pelvic floor closure during times of increased intra-abdominal pressure.

Connective tissue

Makinen et al.[27] studied the perivaginal fascia, demonstrating fewer fibroblasts and an alteration in the orientation of collagen fibrils in women with prolapse compared with normal women. Norton et al.[28,29] showed generalized joint laxity in women with prolapse, and suggested that genital prolapse is part of a more generalized connective tissue disorder. The incidence of pelvic relaxation was significantly higher in women with hypermobile joints than in a control group with no clinical joint laxity. Connective tissue defects have also been suggested as a cause of, or at least to have a relationship with, joint hypermobility and POP. Sayer et al.[30] studied biopsies of pubocervical fascia from women who had USI with or without bladder-neck prolapse. The women who had bladder-neck prolapse appeared to have an alteration in the collagen component of the fascia. Keane et al.[31,32] reported that nulliparous women who developed USI have evidence of a change in the proportion of type I to type III collagen in the endopelvic fascia. These studies demonstrate that deficiencies in collagen may be responsible for GSI in nulliparous women.

Neurological abnormalities

There may be intrinsic conditions that lead to neurological disorders of the pelvic floor or bladder, for example spina bifida occulta. A woman with this neurological defect may be asymptomatic for most or all of her life. Therefore, the sacral nerve roots may not be sufficiently compromised to affect the pelvic floor and the bladder. USI in these patients is related to weakness of the external sphincter mechanism. Certainly, co-ordinated behaviour is often lost in abnormal conditions, as has been shown for the levator ani,[33] and the urethral and anal sphincters.[34]

Lower motor neuron disorders such as lumbar disc disease in nulliparous women could be associated with a spectrum of detrusor and outlet dysfunctions. Lumbar disc disease typically affects the L4–L5 and L5–S1 interstices. When a disc compresses the nerve roots, signs and symptoms may include pain and numbness, muscle wasting and occasionally bowel and/or bladder incontinence.

Extrinsic factors

Different extrinsic (environmental) factors in individuals who are at risk for developing USI or POP may interfere with or enhance the intrinsic factors in the onset of USI described above. These extrinsic factors include pregnancy and childbirth, hormonal modification and conditions of increased intra-abdominal pressure.

Pregnancy and childbirth

Pregnancy may promote USI in several ways: progesterone-mediated relaxation of smooth muscle, changes in connective tissue, pressure of the uterus, and inherent previous anatomical defects. Different findings support the following hypotheses:

- USI is a common complaint during pregnancy, 31–46% of women reporting symptoms in one study,[35] and 60% in another study.[36]
- In women who had USI before pregnancy, symptoms are invariably worse during pregnancy.

Hormonal effects

Many women complain of an exacerbation of their UI and pelvic floor relaxation just before menses, which may reflect the smooth muscle relaxant property of progesterone. Loss of oestrogen may affect mucosal coaptation of the urethra through decreased vascularity and thinning of the urethral lining.

Conditions of increased intra-abdominal pressure

The following conditions may promote the development of USI or POP:

- chronic pulmonary disease such as bronchitis and asthma;
- smoking is known to be associated with USI;[37]
- chronic straining at bowel movements;
- lifting may alter pelvic floor function, particularly lifting of excessively heavy loads.

BASIC INVESTIGATIONS

Snooks *et al.*[38] investigated 29 nulliparous women using transvaginal ultrasonography to assess whether their bladder necks were open or closed at rest. Overall, a 21% incidence of an open bladder neck was recorded. It is likely that the true incidence of an open bladder neck in young nulliparous women is higher than this, since none of these patients had troublesome stress incontinence. Since women with an open bladder neck are more likely to develop stress incontinence if the integrity of the distal sphincter mechanism is compromised by neural damage, antenatal recognition of this problem should contraindicate traumatic vaginal delivery. Sampselle[39] studied pelvic muscle strength and USI in 20 nulliparous women at 32–36 weeks *ante partum* and 6 weeks *post partum*. Measurements included a digital muscle strength score, observed incontinence and urine flow interruption. Pelvic muscle strength decreased from the ante-partum to the post-partum periods in women who had vaginal deliveries.

FUNCTIONAL ASSESSMENT OF THE PELVIC FLOOR MUSCLES

Functional assessment of the pelvic floor muscles in nulliparous women is similar to that for pelvic floor dysfunction, and includes digital testing, functional stop test, vaginal cones, perineometry and surface electromyography (EMG) studies.

Vaginal cones were designed as a biofeedback method for testing and exercising the pelvic floor muscles. They may also be used as a method of evaluation, being a measure of the weight a subject can hold in the vagina and the time while exercising. Different protocols of assessment have been proposed; as the muscle strength increases, heavier cones can be retained.

The EMG (computerized EMG biofeedback) response to pelvic floor contraction is an alternative method of monitoring baseline/resting tone, strength, endurance and other activity patterns. Different surface EMGs provide information about muscle events and assess the magnitude and timing of overall muscle contraction and relaxation, with the objective of obtaining data on normal and abnormal physical function of the pelvic floor muscle. We provide different techniques which will ensure accuracy in recording the details of pelvic floor muscle function and, depending on the data, specific pelvic muscle training programmes.

RE-EDUCATION AND PREVENTION

Many women complaining of lower urinary tract dysfunction could benefit from different techniques of re-education. The problem of UI in women is now discussed widely in newspapers, women's magazines and on television. Re-education techniques must be selected rationally and each caregiver should adapt the treatment according to the patient's pathology. Treating and managing urogynaecological disorders requires different stages for the treatment to be successful.

It is thought that every woman should benefit from muscular training to develop contraction of the levator ani before any increase in intra-abdominal pressure, particularly with strenuous effort during physical activities. During the first interview the therapeutic plan must be explained and the need to persevere with the exercises emphasized.

If nulliparous women were better informed of the fact that many problems are caused by pelvic floor weakness, many of them would implement conservative treatment, such as physiotherapy. In fact, everyone should know that any damage in this area may lead to disturbance in family and professional life. Pelvic floor disorders disrupt family life in young women. Urinary problems may interfere with sexual activity in a number of ways and all of these social consequences cause embarrassment and can lead to depression.

Lack of knowledge about the structure and function of the pelvic floor muscles makes it difficult to perceive the sensation of contracting or relaxing these muscles. Videos can help the patient to gain a better understanding of the anatomy and function of the pelvic floor muscles and the role of pelvic muscle training. In physiotherapy, we were surprised to find a difference in the voluntary perineal command according to the patient's sex. Whereas men control their pelvic floor muscles properly and are able to stop their urine flow, some women have a real problem controlling this musculature. More than 22% of young nulliparous women cannot correctly contract their pelvic floor muscles and achieve a contraction that increases the intra-abdominal pressure. This incorrect manoeuvre has been called the 'reversed perineal command'[40] and is now called 'paradoxical puborectalis contraction'. From a practical standpoint it is possible to make this paradoxical perineal command disappear after a few practice sessions; 'active pushing' and 'holding in' are performed in these women in order to learn the resulting consequences.

In normal healthy nulliparous women the pelvic floor muscles show a reflex increase in activity during increases in intra-abdominal pressure: during this event, the activity of the sphincter increases, reflecting an increase in efferent firing in the pudendal nerve and an increase in outlet resistance, which contributes to the maintenance of urinary continence. One of the aims of rehabilitation is to re-establish this reflex. It is important at this stage to know if the patient can contract against gravity (sitting and standing) in order to propose a training programme in a gravity-resisted position. Functional neuromuscular electrostimulation has been used in medical practice for many years, the basis of which is restoration of normal physiological reflex mechanisms in abnormal nerves and muscles. Electrical stimulation has become popular for the treatment of GSI by enhancing the periurethral sphincter, and urge incontinence, by inhibiting the overactive detrusor. We have never used such a therapy for nulliparous women. Extracorporeal magnetic stimulation is a safe and effective technique for rebuilding strength and endurance in the muscles of the pelvic floor and continence system, and could be used as first-line treatment for nulliparous women. This stimulation does not involve a probe and is therefore non-invasive, making it an appropriate treatment for pelvic floor dysfunction in nulliparous women.[41]

Behavioural modification includes the analysis and alteration of the possible interactions between the patient's symptoms and the environment. This method aims to identify the micturition complaint and the factors that may influence the development or maintenance of presenting symptoms. There are various techniques, such as bladder training, habit training and prompted voiding. Different types of bladder training may be used, including bladder drill, bladder habit retraining and bladder retraining. Techniques of urgency control include a variety of distraction and relaxation techniques, and use of pelvic floor muscle contractions to control a specific urge. The efficacy rate of bladder drill alone ranges from 12 to 90%.[42]

CONCLUSIONS

Pelvic floor dysfunction, specifically that resulting in UI, occurs widely, even in nulliparous women, but with varying reported prevalence rates. Protective and predisposing factors have not been clearly identified. In addition, there is a need for examination of the prevalence, incidence and risk factors for pelvic relaxation and faecal incontinence.

The data from these studies demonstrate perfectly well that UI is not rare and we think that young incontinent women need an appropriate treatment to prevent possible aggravation of the symptom; it seems logical to develop strategies to screen those with high risk factors. Pelvic floor re-education seems to be a promising prophylactic option. It may be possible that ante-partum pelvic floor training, using similar techniques but without electrical stimulation, could limit the degree of muscle overdistension or stretch injury to the pudendal nerves during parturition. Should all nulliparous women at risk for pelvic floor dysfunction have pelvic floor re-education before pregnancy and what type? Which women should be selected for this therapy? These are certainly questions that could be answered from a prospective study.

REFERENCES

1. Diokno AC, Brock BM, Brown MB, Herzog R. Prevalence of urinary incontinence and other urological symptoms in the non-institutionalized elderly. *J Urol* 1986; 135: 1022–1025

2. Brocklehurst JC. Urinary incontinence in the community: analysis of a Mori poll. *Br Med J* 1993; 306: 832–834

3. Thomas TM, Plymat KR, Blannin J, Meade TW. Prevalence of urinary incontinence. *Br J Urol* 1980; 281: 1243–1245

4. Burgio KL, Matthews KA, Engel BT. Prevalence, incidence and correlates of urinary incontinence in healthy, middle-aged women. *J Urol* 1991; 146: 1255–1259

5. Nemir A, Midleton R. Stress incontinence in young nulliparous women. *Am J Obstet Gynecol* 1954; 68: 1166–1168

6. Wolin JH. Stress incontinence in young healthy nulliparous female subjects. *J Urol* 1969; 101: 545–549

7. Molander U, Milsom I, Ekelund P, Mellstrom D. An epidemiological study of urinary incontinence and related urogenital symptoms in elderly women. *Maturitas* 1990; 12: 51–60

8. Holst K, Wilson PD. The prevalence of female urinary incontinence and reason for seeking treatment. *N Z Med J* 1988; 101: 756–758

9. Bø K, Kristofferson M, Kulseng-Hanssen S, Stien R. Clinical and urodynamic assessment of nulliparous young women with and without stress incontinence symptoms: a case-control study. *Obstet Gynecol* 1994; 84: 1028–1032

10. Harris RL, Cundiff GW, Coates KW, Bump RC. Urinary incontinence (UI) and pelvic organ prolapse (POP) in nulliparous women. Proceedings of the International Continence Society 26th Annual Meeting. Athens: International Continence Society, 1996; 384

11. Janssen T, Crick D, Scroeder C, Schulman CC. Prevalence of urinary incontinence in nulliparous women aged 12–18: data suggesting the need for a screening program. Proceedings of the International Continence Society 26th Annual Meeting. Athens: International Continence Society, 1996; 385

12. Rekers H, Drogendjik AC, Valkenberg H, Riphagen F. Urinary incontinence in women from 35 to 79 years of age: prevalence and consequences. *Eur J Obstet Gynecol Reprod Biol* 1992; 43: 229–234

13. Jolleys JV. Reported prevalence of urinary incontinence in a general practice. *Br Med J* 1998; 296: 1300–1302

14. Nygaard I. Exercise and incontinence. *Obstet Gynecol* 1990; 75: 848–850

15. Nygaard IE, Albright JP, Svengalis SL, Thompson FL. Urinary incontinence in elite nulliparous athletes. *Obstet Gynecol* 1994; 84: 183–187

16. Nygaard I, Thompson FL. Prevalence of urinary incontinence in college varsity athletes. *Proceedings of the American UroGynecological Society*. San Antonio: AUGS, 1993; 89–91

17. Bø K, Mæhlum S, Oseid S, Larsen S. Prevalence of stress urinary incontinence amongst physically active and sedentary female students. *Scand J Sports Sci* 1989; 11: 113–116

18. Bø K, Hagen R, Kvarstein B, Larsen S. Female stress urinary incontinence and participation in different sports and social activities. *Scand J Sports Sci* 1989; 11: 117–121

19. Bourcier AP, Juras JC. Urinary incontinence in sports and fitness activities (abstract). *Med Sci Sports Exerc* 1994; 26 (Suppl): 5

20. Fall M, Frankenberg S, Frisen M *et al.* 456,000 svenskar kan ha urininkontinens. Endast var fjarde soker hjalp for besvaren. *Laeakrtidningen* 1995; 82: 2054–2056

21. Bourcier AP, Dentz JP, Juras CJ. Le plancher pelvien et le sport; le sport aprés 40 ans. Proceedings of Troisième Rencontre Sport-Santé-Médecine, Angers: Troisième Rencontre Sport-Santé-Médecine, November 1997; 24–26

22. Jacquetin B, Lambert T, Grunberg P, Descamps C. Incontinence urinaire de la femme sportive. In: *Le Pelvis Féminin, Statique et Dynamique*. Paris: Masson 1993; 142–144

23. Wilson J. Current status of teratology – general principles and mechanisms derived from animal studies. In: Wilson J, Fraser F (eds) *Handbook of Teratology*. New York: Plenum, 1997

24. Langer R, Mushkat Y, Bubosky I. Is urinary stress incontinence hereditary? Proceedings of the International Continence Society 24th Annual Meeting, Prague. *Neurourol Urodyn* 1994; 13: 96

25. Zaccharin RF. A 'Chinese anatomy': the pelvic supporting tissue of the Chinese and Occidental female compared and contrasted. *Aust N Z Obstet Gynaecol* 1977; 17: 1–5

26. DeLancey JOL. Functional anatomy of the pelvic floor and urinary continence mechanism. In: Schûssler B, Laycock J, Norton P, Stanton S (eds) *Pelvic Floor Re-education*. London: Springer Verlag, 1994; 9–21

27. Makinen J, Sonderstrom KO, Kuhoma P, Hirvonen T. Histological changes in the vaginal connective tissue of patients with and without uterine prolapse. *Arch Gynecol* 1986; 239: 17–20

28. Norton P, Baker J, Sharp H, Warenski J. Genitourinary prolapse. Relationship with joint mobility. *Neurourol Urodyn* 1990; 9: 321–322

29. Norton P, Boyd C, Deak S. Collagen synthesis in women with genital prolapse of stress incontinence. *Neurourol Urodyn* 1992; 11: 300–301

30. Sayer T, Hosker GL, Dixon JS, Warrell DW. A study of paraurethral connective tissue in women with stress incontinence. *Neurourol Urodyn* 1990; 9: 319–320

31. Keane DP, Sims TJ, Bailey AJ, Abrams P. Analysis of pelvic floor electromyography and collagen status in premenopausal nulliparous females with genuine stress incontinence. *Neurourol Urodyn* 1992; 11: 40–46

32. Keane DP, Bailey AJ, Abrams P, Sims TJ. Analysis of collagen status in premenopausal nulliparous women with genuine stress incontinence. *Br J Obstet Gynaecol* 1997; 104: 994–998

33. Bourcier A. Final general discussion. In: Bock G, Whelan J (eds) *Neurobiology of Incontinence*. Amsterdam: *Ciba Found Symp* 1990: 318; 151

34. Vereechen RL, Verduyn H. The electrical activity of the paraurethral and perineal muscles in normal pathological conditions. *Br J Urol* 1970; 42: 457–463

35. Burgio KL, Locher JL, Zyczynski H *et al.* Urinary incontinence during pregnancy in a racially mixed sample. Characteristics and predisposing factors. *Int Urogynecol J Pelvic Floor Dysfunct* 1996; 7: 67–71

36. Mellier G, Delille MA. Urinary disorders during pregnancy and post partum. *Rev Fr Gynecol Obstet Reprod* 1990; 85: 525–527

37. Bump R, McClish D. Cigarette smoking and pure genuine stress incontinence of urine: a comparison risk factors and determinants between smokers and non-smokers. *Am J Obstet Gynecol* 1994; 170: 579–582

38. Snooks SJ, Setchell M, Henry MM, Swash M. Risk factors in childbirth causing damage to the pelvic floor innervation. *Br J Urol* 1989; 64: 357–359

39. Sampselle CM. Changes in pelvic muscle strength and USI associated with childbirth. *J Obstet Gynecol Nurs* 1990; 19: 371–377

40. Bourcier A. Pelvic floor rehabilitation. In: Raz S (ed) *Female Urology*, 2nd edn. Philadelphia: WB Saunders, 1996; 263–283

41. Galloway NTM, Appell RA. Extracorporeal magnetic stimulation therapy for urinary incontinence. In: Appell RA, Bourcier, La Torre F (eds) *Pelvic Floor Dysfunction, Investigation and Conservative Treatment*. Rome: C.E.S.J.; 1999: 291–294

42. Jarvis GJ, Millard R. Controlled trial of bladder drill for detrusor instability. *Br Med J* 1980; 281: 1322–1323

75

Pregnancy and childbirth

P. Toozs-Hobson, A. Cutner

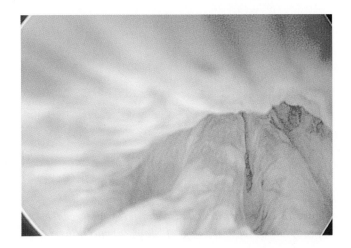

INTRODUCTION

Pregnancy is a time when the body undergoes many physiological and anatomical alterations. This adaptation during confinement and delivery affects all body systems. Examples include increased cardiac and renal output, increased gas exchange across the lung alveoli and changes to the body metabolism and the immune system.

The pelvis and lower genitourinary tract differ from the other systems in that they undergo profound changes that may not completely revert to the pre-pregnancy state. This occurs for a variety of reasons including the effects of hormones, pressure from the gravid uterus and circumstances surrounding the delivery. Anatomical alterations in the connective tissue lead to a decrease in the tensile qualities of the pelvic connective tissue. Together these changes commonly result in urinary symptoms (Fig. 75.1).

This chapter will concentrate on relating the development of symptoms to urodynamic diagnoses and to changes that have occurred to produce these symptoms. We have subdivided the chapter into the following sections:

1. Voiding patterns
2. Urgency and urge incontinence
3. Stress incontinence
4. Voiding difficulties
5. Faecal incontinence
6. Vaginal prolapse

VOIDING PATTERNS

In the non-pregnant female, sex-steroid receptors are found throughout the trigone, urethra and vagina. They are also found in transitional epithelium that has undergone squamous metaplasia in the bladder.[2] During pregnancy, the level of oestrogen increases to over 100 times that in the non-pregnant state.[3] The exact effect of this hormonal flux on the lower urinary tract has yet to be fully established.

Urine production and bladder storage

Urine production rises in pregnancy as a result of a 25% increase in renal perfusion and glomerular filtration rate. In addition there is a decrease in production of antidiuretic hormone.[4] Two studies[5,6] have looked at urine production and quantified the increase (Table 75.1). Together these effects give rise to changes in the pattern of voiding. Other factors such as increased fluid intake[3,6,7] affect voiding patterns but whether increased urine output follows increased fluid intake or *vice versa* is unknown.

Early animal studies[8] examining the effect of pregnancy on bladder muscle suggest that pregnancy reduces vesical tone and increases bladder capacity. The results of studies in human pregnancy performed using simple cystometry have been conflicting, with some authors[9,10] finding evidence of bladder atony in the third trimester and reduced intravesical pressure for any given bladder volume. By 6 weeks *post partum* there was a return to normal bladder tone. Francis,[11]

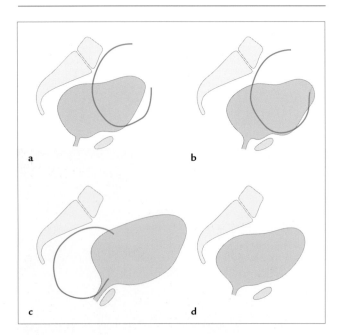

Figure 75.1. *Movements of the bladder in (a) late pregnancy, (b) early labour, (c) second stage of labour, (d) after delivery.*

Table 75.1. *Urine output (litres) in pregnancy*

	Trimester			Non-pregnant
	First	Second	Third	
Francis *et al.*[5]	1.9	2.0	1.8	1.5
Parboosingh and Doig[6]	1.3	1.3	1.3	1.1

however, found the reverse, with decreasing bladder capacity towards term and evidence of increased bladder tone.

Frequency and nocturia

Urinary frequency is one of the earliest symptoms of pregnancy – it may be noticed even before the first missed period. There have been several reports[5,6,12–14] on the prevalence of frequency and nocturia but different authors have used varying definitions and this may reflect the differences in findings.

The first large-scale study of bladder function in pregnancy assessed 400 women and defined frequency as at least seven daytime voids and one night-time void.[5] In this study 59.5% experienced frequency in early pregnancy, 61% in mid pregnancy and 81% in late pregnancy. Once frequency occurred it tended not to resolve but, rather, got worse. Parboosingh and Doig[6] defined nocturia as night-time voiding on three nights in a week. In their cross-sectional study of 100 patients, the prevalence of nocturia was 58% in the first trimester, 57% in the second trimester and 66% in the third trimester. They also found that most of their patients accepted nocturia as a normal feature of pregnancy, it causing distress in less than 4% of women.

Stanton *et al.*[13] defined frequency as seven or more daytime voids and nocturia as two or more night-time voids. They found that frequency was more common in nulliparous than multiparous women, but this difference was statistically significant only at 38 weeks and 40 weeks' gestation. Cutner[14,15] found that although 43% of women complained of diurnal frequency and 34% of nocturia in early pregnancy, 91% overall complained of an increased voiding pattern. Thus, an increased voiding pattern appears to be almost universal and explains why frequency is considered to be a symptom of pregnancy. In addition, Cutner[7] looked at the effects of parity and race on voiding patterns in early pregnancy. The prevalence of frequency was higher in black, nulliparous women compared with white, nulliparous women and the prevalence of nocturia was higher in black parous women compared with white parous women.

Cutner[7] demonstrated a correlation between the maximum volumes voided and the first sensation and bladder capacity on urodynamic testing. In early pregnancy those women with nocturia had reduced bladder

capacities. However, there was little difference in bladder capacity between those women with and without diurnal frequency; this is in agreement with the findings of Francis[1,5] (Fig. 75.2).

Factors affecting symptoms

Two studies[7,13] have examined the relationship between fetal head position in the last 4 weeks of pregnancy and urinary frequency. There was no change in frequency with the engagement of the head. These studies also

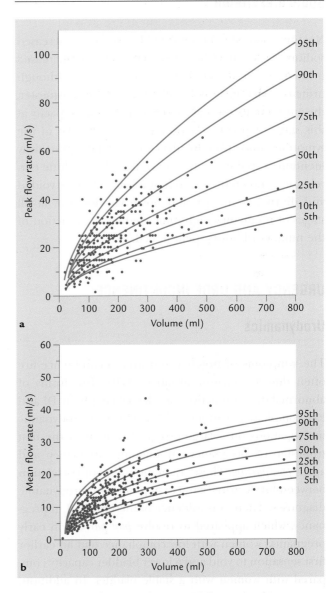

Figure 75.2. *Nomograms for (a) peak and (b) mean urinary flow rate during pregnancy. Curves indicate centiles.*

showed that frequency generally resolves *post partum*. Women with a greater increase in the number of voids in pregnancy are more likely to continue to suffer from these symptoms *post partum*.[7]

If the number of voids is related to the first sensation and bladder capacity, which in turn is related to the presence of low compliance, one might expect that this effect would be more marked in the day than at night when the uterus would no longer exert such a marked pressure on the bladder. Thus whether pressure from an enlarged uterus results in frequency remains controversial.[16–20]

Sodium excretion

Nocturia may also be explained in part by increased sodium excretion at night, which results in increased urine production and, therefore, nocturia.[6,12] Although urine production at night falls off in the third trimester, the authors suggest that a decreased bladder capacity at this stage of pregnancy prevents improvement in the symptom of nocturia. In addition, two of the previously mentioned studies[5,7] have shown that there is little correlation between the maximum volume of urine voided and diurnal frequency and nocturia. However, at all stages of pregnancy night-time voiding is a function of the number of hours spent in bed.[7,14]

URGENCY AND URGE INCONTINENCE

Urodynamics

The symptoms of urgency and urge incontinence are often due to detrusor instability (DI). Two forms of abnormal detrusor activity are described: phasic DI and low compliance. Cutner[7,14,21–23] performed urodynamic investigations on a large group of women in the first trimester of pregnancy, in ongoing pregnancy and again *post partum*. These studies found poor correlation between lower urinary tract symptoms and urodynamic diagnoses. There was evidence of increased DI in pregnancy, which appeared to resolve *post partum*. In early pregnancy, women with low compliance had an earlier first sensation to void and a lower bladder capacity compared with women with a stable bladder. In addition, women with phasic DI had an increased prevalence of urethral instability in pregnancy. These findings suggest

that the two conditions (low compliance and phasic DI) may well have different aetiologies in pregnancy although in the non-pregnant state they may lead to similar symptomatology.

Animal work

Further work aimed at determining the cause of irritative bladder symptoms in pregnancy has entailed the use of animal models. Lee *et al.*[24] demonstrated an increased compliance in the bladder of New Zealand White rabbits. They also showed changes in the sensory thresholds which may be responsible for urgency. These changes were thought to occur as a result of changes in the levels of sex steroids in pregnancy.

Symptoms

Stanton *et al.*[13] showed an increased incidence of urgency and urge incontinence in pregnancy. Urge incontinence had a peak incidence of 19% in multiparous women. They suggested that the symptoms were produced by the changes due to pregnancy and the pressure effects of the gravid uterus.

Cutner[7] found the prevalence of urgency and urge incontinence to be 60% and 10%, respectively. Seventy-five women with these symptoms agreed to undergo urodynamics: 55% had abnormal detrusor activity. The finding of abnormal detrusor activity did not correlate individually with symptoms of urgency; this is not surprising as the symptoms are known to correlate poorly with diagnosis.[25–27] In addition, there was a significant correlation between severe antenatal symptoms and the persistence of symptoms postnatally.

STRESS INCONTINENCE

Incidence of symptoms

Stress incontinence is known to result from increased parity (Table 75.2) but whether pregnancy itself or childbirth is the primary cause remains in doubt. Thomas *et al.*[28] undertook a large epidemiology study, showing that stress incontinence is related to parity. These results were supported by Foldspang *et al.*[29] in their cross-sectional study of 3114 women.

Iosif[30] and Ingermarsson,[31] in two retrospective

Table 75.2. *Incidence of stress incontinence relating to pregnancy*

Time of onset	% of symptoms[30]	% of population	
		Iosif and Ingermarsson[31]	Viktrup and Lose[33]
Before pregnancy	8.5	2	4
Permanent from pregnancy	23	5	NR
Temporary in pregnancy	50	11	32
Postnatally	19	4	7

NR; not reported

studies involving over 1400 women, found an overall incidence of stress incontinence of 22%. Half the symptoms were temporary, but in women with ongoing complaints most symptoms started antenatally. The authors found no significant difference between women who developed symptoms postnatally and continent controls with respect to the duration of labour, mode of delivery or infant weight. Interestingly, the incidence of stress incontinence in the mothers of patients with stress incontinence was also five times greater than in the control group, suggesting hereditary factors.

Beck and Hsu[32] retrospectively investigated 1000 women who were attending their gynaecological outpatient clinic. Thirty-one per cent of the women admitted to the symptom of stress incontinence, of whom 246 (79%) said the stress incontinence was associated with a previous pregnancy and 82% said it first occurred antenatally.

Four studies have examined the incidence of stress incontinence prospectively in pregnancy. Francis[11] found that, overall, 53% of nulliparous women and 84% of multiparous women admitted to stress incontinence antenatally, showing that it rarely occurred for the first time *post partum*. These findings have been confirmed by three other studies.[7,13,33]

Causes of stress incontinence

Problematic stress incontinence prior to pregnancy has been reported to be associated with a decrease in mature collagen.[34] This results in less cross linking of the collagen strands, the effect of which is to reduce the tensile strength of connective tissue. These findings have also been reported in parous women who have developed genitourinary prolapse in later life.[35]

Peptide hormones such as relaxin may also play a role in connective tissue metabolism during pregnancy.[36] This hormone, produced mainly by the placenta, reaches highest plasma levels during pregnancy and has been shown to induce collagen remodelling and consequent softening of the tissues of the birth canal.[37]

Landon *et al.*[38] demonstrated that the rectus sheath of women undergoing caesarean section was significantly weaker than that of non-pregnant women. This has subsequently been shown to be due to increases in glycosaminoglycans in the connective tissue and a reduction in total collagen.[39] These results suggest overstretching and tissue remodelling consistent with both the mechanical and endocrine effects of pregnancy. The extent to which these changes are reversed *post partum* has not been investigated.

Urodynamics

Continence is maintained by a combination of factors including the intrinsic urethral pressure and extrinsic compression of the urethra. Several authors have used urethral pressure profilometry to look at the effect of pregnancy on the intrinsic urethral pressure. Iosif and Ulmston[40] followed-up 26 women, 12 of whom developed stress incontinence in pregnancy (Fig. 75.3). They found that continent women had gradual increases in functional urethral length (FUL) and maximal urethral closure pressure (MUCP) during pregnancy. After delivery these measurements reverted to those found early in pregnancy. By contrast, in women who developed stress incontinence, FUL and MUCP did not increase during pregnancy. Women with temporary or no symptoms had a positive pressure profile, whereas

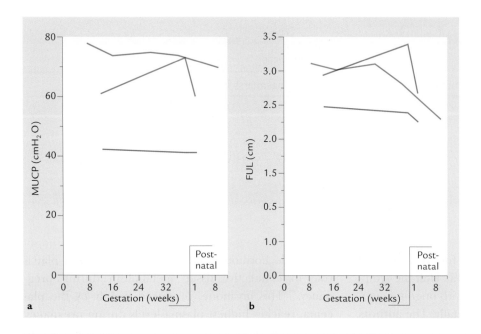

a

b

Figure 75.3. *Changes in (a) maximal urethral closure pressure (MUCP) and (b) functional urethral length (FUL) during pregnancy. (Data are from ref. 30 [— continent, — incontinent] and — ref. 41.)*

those with persistent problems had a negative pressure profile, a shorter FUL and a lower MUCP. Van Geelen *et al.*[41] examined mode of delivery and found that vaginal delivery was associated with a decrease in MUCP and FUL relative to the measurements early in pregnancy. The post-partum changes observed after vaginal delivery were not influenced by the duration of the second stage of labour, the presence of episiotomy or the weight of the infant. Caesarean section preserved MUCP and FUL. They also noted that the women who complained of symptoms had a negative pressure profile on coughing.

Imaging of the bladder neck and urethra

Recent advances in ultrasonography have facilitated measurement of the urethral sphincter volume[42] (Fig. 75.4). A reduction in urethral sphincter volume has been shown to be associated with the development of stress incontinence.[43] Recent studies[44,45] have also shown that a decrease in MUCP correlates with a decrease in volume and maximal cross-sectional area of the urethra in women who develop stress incontinence after delivery. Vaginal delivery is also associated with a decrease in the sphincter volume compared with caesarean section.

Perineal ultrasonography has been used to investigate bladder-neck position and the proximal urethra. Transperineal ultrasonography was chosen because the distortion of the anatomy by the probe is less than with a vaginal probe.[46]

Meyer *et al.*[47] investigated 214 women, 74 of whom were nulliparous, 29 had had one delivery, 64 had had two or more vaginal deliveries and 16 had had forceps deliveries. They also examined 32 women who complained of stress incontinence. There was a significant increase in bladder-neck movement on Valsalva manoeuvre in both the incontinent women and those who had undergone forceps delivery. The possibility of hypermobility predisposing to stress incontinence has been substantiated by King and Freeman.[48] In this

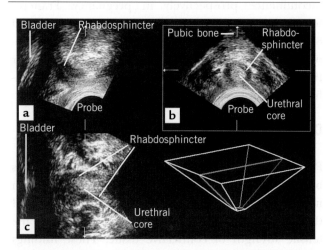

Figure 75.4. *Ultrasonography of the urethral spincter: (a) coronal section; (b) transversion section; (c) sagittal section.*

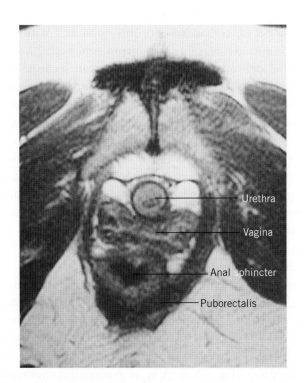

Figure 75.5. *Magnetic resonance imaging of the pelvic floor.*

Urethra
Vagina
Anal sphincter
Puborectalis

Table 75.3. *Effect of infant weight on incidence (%) of symptoms of stress incontinence*		
	Infant weight	
Symptoms of stress incontinence	Over 4 kg	Under 4 kg
Antenatal	10	6.9
Postnatal	34	30.6

Data from ref. 51.

preliminary study they found a significant antenatal increase in bladder-neck mobility in those women who subsequently experienced post-partum stress incontinence compared with the continent post-partum group.

Recently, the use of magnetic resonance imaging (MRI) has led to increased interest in anatomy. To date only one study using MRI has looked longitudinally at changes in the pelvis due to childbirth,[49] and did not find any significant changes (Fig. 75.5). This is almost certainly due to current limitations in investigating functional anatomy. The development of faster MRI will allow the dynamic assessment of the pelvic floor[50] and may yet supersede ultrasonography.

Factors affecting the development of stress incontinence

Maternal and infant weight

Krue *et al.*[51] investigated infant birth weight in 194 women who delivered vaginally and found an increased incidence of both antenatal and postnatal symptoms in women having a baby weighing more than 4 kg (Table 75.3).

The same group also reported an increased incidence of stress incontinence in women with a body mass index above 30 kg/m^2.[52]

Duration of labour

Cutner[7] has shown a correlation between the duration of the first stage of labour and the degree of postnatal symptoms of stress incontinence. Viktrup *et al.*[33] correlated the development of postnatal urinary symptoms with infant weight, episiotomy and duration of the second stage of labour. They also found that caesarean section conferred some protection against the development of incontinence. At 3 months *post partum* all obstetric correlations had disappeared in the women who remained symptomatic. At 1 year *post partum* only 3% of women admitted to urinary stress incontinence.

Mode of delivery and use of epidural anaesthesia

Both the development of incontinence and vaginal delivery are associated with a reduction in the rhabdosphincter volume.[44,45] These studies suggest that the symptom of stress incontinence may be physiological in pregnancy and occurs when urethral parameters cannot increase. It may be that susceptible women are those who will sustain sphincter damage as a result of childbirth. However, should delivery occur without trauma to the pelvic floor and urethral sphincter mechanism, continence will be regained.

Instrumental delivery (ventouse extraction or forceps delivery) is often cited as a factor in the development of urinary symptoms. In England the assisted-delivery rate among primiparous women varies from 10% to 24%. In 1993 the rates in the UK for forceps delivery and ventouse extraction were 6.6% and 3.5%, respectively.[54] Given the relatively frequent use of these instruments, there is a paucity of objective evidence to support the claim of their involvement in the aetiology of stress incontinence. One postal study did, however, demonstrate a tenfold increase in stress incontinence (68 vs 6.8%) with instrumental delivery.[55] This publication stands virtually alone in suggesting an increase in the incidence of incontinence after instrumental delivery. Dimpfl *et al.*[56] showed that vaginal delivery and maternal age over 30 years increased stress incontinence. They found associations with the use of ventouse and forceps, but these findings were not statistically significant.

Wilson *et al.*[57] performed an epidemiological study of 1800 women 3 months after delivery; they found no difference in the incidence of incontinence between women who had had a forceps delivery and those who had had a normal vaginal delivery. Jackson *et al.*[58] also showed little difference in the incidence of incontinence regardless of the use of epidural anaesthesia or instrumental delivery. This study did report an increase in stress incontinence in women with a short second stage of labour (less than 20 minutes in primiparous women without epidural anaesthesia and less than 45 minutes in women with epidural anaesthesia).

Viktrup and Lose[33] also analysed the use of epidural anaesthesia and found a higher incidence of stress incontinence in women who received epidural pain relief during labour (Table 75.4).

In contrast to Jackson *et al.*,[58] Viktrup and Lose[33] reported a correlation between incontinence and increased duration of the second stage of labour in those who received epidural anaesthesia. At 1 year, 7% of those who received epidural anaesthesia were symptomatic, compared with 3% of controls. These figures were not significantly different, however, reflecting the small numbers in the groups.

Caesarean section is thought to protect against pelvic floor damage and dysfunction. In one survey,[59] 31% of female obstetricians described caesarean section as their personal preferred method of delivery, with 80% citing fear of pelvic floor damage as the reason.

It has been proposed that caesarean section may reduce the incidence of incontinence after delivery.

Skoner *et al.* concurred with this opinion.[60] Wilson *et al.*[57] reported rates of urinary incontinence of 27% after vaginal delivery and 5% after caesarean section. The protective effect seemed to lessen with subsequent instrumental deliveries, and three caesarean sections conferred no advantage over vaginal births. Conversely, Iosif and Ingermarsson[31] found significant differences in symptoms when they retrospectively analysed results from 204 women undergoing elective caesarean section. They concluded that stress incontinence results from a combination of hereditary disposition, changes during pregnancy and damage during delivery.

Pelvic floor and nerve damage

The birth canal undergoes considerable distortion during parturition. The pudendal nerve, which supplies the pelvic floor, is vulnerable to damage because it runs around the edge of the birth canal. The pelvic floor itself may be damaged by tearing during birth or by an episiotomy (Fig. 75.6). Use of forceps increases the diameter of the head during delivery,[61] potentially increasing trauma to the birth canal.

Sampselle[62] showed that pelvic floor contractility and strength correlate inversely with the development of symptoms after childbirth, suggesting that antenatal pelvic floor exercises may protect against the develop-

Table 75.4. Incidence of incontinence associated with epidural anaesthesia during childbirth		
	Epidural (n = 45)	No epidural (n = 163)
Incontinent	12 (27)	21 (13)
No incontinence	33 (73)	142 (87)

Data are number (percentage) of women affected.
Data from ref. 33.

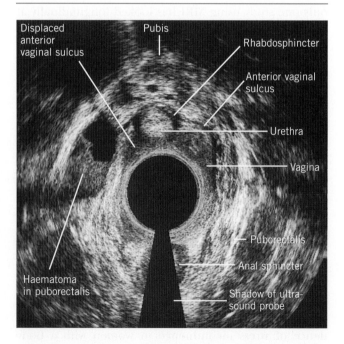

Figure 75.6. *Ultrasonography of pelvic floor damage.*

ment of stress incontinence. Marshall *et al.*[63] reported a significant decrease in pelvic floor contractility in multiparous physiotherapists compared with their nulliparous counterparts. Changes in the electromyograph (EMG) readings of the levator ani muscle were less significant. These changes can be explained in part by increases in the contractility of the levator hiatus that result from delivery.[64]

Allen *et al.*[65] recruited 129 women and examined changes in the EMG and pudendal nerve terminal latency due to childbirth. The results suggest that pudendal nerve damage may play an important part in the development of prolapse and incontinence. This study demonstrated that damage to the pudendal nerve was relatively common, occurring in up to 85% of women. They suggested that failure of normal reinnervation resulted in loss of normal function.

Further evidence supporting this theory was provided by a small comparative study[56] which showed characteristic changes in the muscle EMG in women with stress incontinence compared with nulliparous continent women. Similar findings by Gilpin *et al.*[66] showed an alteration of muscle fibre type, consistent with denervation, after vaginal delivery. However, Helt *et al.*[67] were unable to find muscle changes consistent with denervation injuries. The differences between these two groups may be explained by the fact that different areas of the levator ani muscle were biopsied in the two studies.

Tetzchner *et al.*[68] provided further evidence that women with stress incontinence had a significant increase in the motor latency of the pudendal nerve. The development of a pudendal neuropathy was associated with the use of ventouse extraction to deliver the baby. These findings are in agreement with earlier studies.[69] The same group had reported earlier[70] that multiparity, forceps delivery, prolonged second-stage labour, third-degree tear and high infant birth weight were important factors in the development of pudendal nerve injury, but not incontinence. Other studies[71,72] have demonstrated a relationship between perineal descent and prolongation of the pudendal nerve motor latency.

Perineal descent commonly occurs with distortion of the birth canal during the active second stage of labour. It can also occur with chronic constipation as a sequel to childbirth. It is important to remember that the pudendal nerve supplies the urethra and pelvic floor.

Thus, neuropathy of the pudendal nerve may reflect events in the urethra rather than the pelvic floor. Both vaginal delivery and the development of incontinence are associated with a reduction in the volume of the rhabdosphincter.[43,44] This hypothesis was not substantiated by the only study to date to investigate urethral sphincter innervation.[73] In this study, 33 women with urodynamically proven stress incontinence were compared with 35 controls. There was no statistical difference in the duration of the motor unit potential between these two groups. This study was cross-sectional and therefore did not allow comparison of the changes that occurred as a result of childbirth.

Episiotomy may protect against perineal descent and could be expected to protect the pudendal nerve and help to prevent stress incontinence. One study[74] followed-up 190 women for 4 years and found no difference in the incontinence rate between women who had undergone episiotomy and those who had not. In the largest prospective trial comparing liberal and restricted use of episiotomy[75] no difference was found in incontinence rates between the two treatment groups.

Ethnic variations

The reported ethnic differences in non-pregnant populations have also been described relating to pregnancy and childbirth. Burgio *et al.*[76] studied 523 women and found an incidence of stress incontinence of 62.5% in white women and 46.4% in black women. Cutner[7] found that black women had greater MUCP, maximum urethral pressure, FUL and anatomical urethral length in pregnancy compared with white women.

VOIDING DIFFICULTIES

Antenatal voiding difficulties

Uroflowmetry

Two studies on uroflowmetry in pregnancy have been published.[7,77] Fischer and Kittel[77] measured the peak flow rate and volume voided at different stages of pregnancy in 290 women; 128 of their pregnancies were normal; 103 received treatment with salbutamol for premature labour. The study also included 46 postpartum women and 19 normal non-pregnant controls. This study concluded that there was a significant increase in the peak urine flow rate in the second trimester of pregnancy compared with normal controls and women in the first or third trimester of pregnancy. These differences could, however, be explained in part by different volumes of urine passed. Not surprisingly, tocolytics were associated with reduced flow rates.

Cutner[7] assessed symptoms of voiding difficulties and peak flow rates and volumes voided in 400 women at different stages of pregnancy. He found that there was no difference in the symptoms of slow stream or incomplete bladder emptying with regard to the peak flow rate once the volume voided was taken into account. Indeed, symptoms of voiding difficulties appear to be a function of increasing voiding frequency. He constructed nomograms for the peak flow rate and average flow rate, taking the volume voided into account, and generated equations demonstrating their relationship.

Urinary retention

The classic cause of urinary retention in early pregnancy is incarceration of the retroverted uterus at 14–16 weeks' gestation. This has been attributed to mechanical pressure on the neck of the bladder with elongation of the urethra. However, there is little difficulty in passing a catheter in the initial stages of retention in these cases. Francis[5] has shown that the theory of urethral elongation is not valid. She examined the radiographs of six women who had urethrocystography carried out at the time of retention and did not find elongation of the urethra or elevation of the urethrovesical junction in these patients. She suggested that retention is caused by the retroverted uterus interfering with the normal opening mechanism of the internal urethral meatus. When retention has been present for some time, oedema of the bladder neck may make it difficult to pass a catheter as a secondary effect.

Post-partum voiding difficulties

Although the modern management of labour may have decreased the incidence of post-partum urinary retention, it is still the most common time for retention to occur in relation to pregnancy. Unfortunately, this is frequently overlooked and may lead to long-term sequelae.[79] Possible predisposing factors for post-partum retention are trauma, analgesia and prolonged labour. Spasm of the external urethral sphincter caused by pain was thought by Francis to contribute to retention following vaginal delivery.[5]

Epidural analgesia

Epidural anaesthesia has a number of effects on bladder function. It can take up to 8 hours for normal sensation to return,[80] and it is common for a diuresis to occur during this time, which can further increase the risk of bladder distension. Sacral root blockade preferentially paralyses the parasympathetic supply to the bladder over the sympathetic supply to the urethral sphincter.[81] It has been shown that urinary residuals are increased 2–5 days after delivery with an epidural during labour.[82] This suggests that other effects associated with regional blockade may delay the return to normal function after delivery. One factor that often affects the bladder is overdistension during labour when an indwelling urinary catheter has not been used.

Epidural analgesia was not initially considered to cause an increase in urinary retention.[83–85] The authors of these studies considered instrumental delivery to be the primary cause of post-partum lower urinary tract dysfunction. A more recent report[86] concluded that patients who give birth vaginally with an epidural block may be at increased risk of developing asymptomatic urinary retention.

The effect of epidural analgesia on bladder function following caesarean section has been assessed by Kerr-Wilson and McNally.[87] They concluded that epidural analgesia may predispose to urinary retention following caesarean section, and advocated the use of an indwelling catheter at the time of surgery.

Post-partum urinary retention is undoubtedly distressing at the time but there may also be long-term sequelae. Tapp *et al.*[88] described six women who developed acute retention *post partum*. Two patients had permanent voiding difficulties, two required self-catheterization 6 months *post partum* and two had altered bladder sensation although were voiding normally. Five of the six patients had had epidural analgesia, and four had had an instrumental delivery. Four had residual urine volumes in excess of 1 litre when catheterized. However, this small retrospective study does not preclude the possibility that these patients may have had an underlying neuropathy that resulted in their voiding difficulties, rather than retention secondary to labour.

Management after retention

Overdistension injury can potentially lead to permanent bladder dysfunction but is entirely avoidable by careful vigilance and proper management. Attention should be paid to those patients at risk of developing retention, including those who have had a traumatic delivery, prolonged labour, epidural analgesia or caesarean section. Voiding alone is not an adequate assessment of bladder function because it may be incomplete, leading to increasingly large urinary residuals. Input–output charts are generally inadequate following delivery because diuresis may occur and women are encouraged to increase their fluid intake to promote breastfeeding. The minimum requirement is that women at risk should complete an output chart to check that they are voiding at least 200 ml urine at intervals of more than 2 hours. Frequent small volumes of urine indicate incomplete voiding. If necessary, a disposable catheter can be passed to ensure the bladder is empty. If a woman is unable to void after delivery, a catheter should be passed within 6–8 hours to avoid overdistension of the bladder. If a second catheterization is required then it is advisable to leave an indwelling catheter in position for 48 hours. If voiding is still unsatisfactory then a suprapubic catheter is recommended, together with investigations for possible underlying causes (e.g. neurological or pharmacological). A suprapubic catheter will also allow the mother to leave hospital with her baby after being given instructions on how to manage the catheter. Arrangements should be made for its removal when her urinary residuals are satisfactory.

FAECAL INCONTINENCE

Long-term incontinence of flatus or faeces occurs in about 5% of women after childbirth;[89,90] faecal urgency without incontinence occurs in a further 2%.[89] Two types of damage have been proposed as mechanisms for the development of incontinence: pudendal nerve damage and direct trauma. Neither, however, is found universally and this tends to suggest that faecal incontinence after childbirth has a multifactorial origin.

Damage to the pudendal nerve has been comprehensively investigated using pudendal nerve terminal latency measurements and EMG studies[65,67–68] and has been associated with the development of faecal symptoms. Additional evidence for transient alteration in pudendal nerve function has been found by studying anal canal sensation after delivery.[91] Vaginal delivery was associated with decreased anal sensation whereas no change in sensation was found in women undergoing caesarean section. In an early paper, Parks et al.[92] showed that denervation was most prominent in the external anal sphincter (which is also more likely to be disrupted during childbirth).

The presence of a neuropathy has also been correlated with the length of the second stage of labour, size of the infant and instrumental delivery.[69] MacAuthur et al.[89] also found that the use of forceps and ventouse were independent risk factors for developing faecal incontinence. (Thirty-three per cent of women who had instrumental deliveries and 14% of women who had spontaneous vaginal deliveries complaining of symptoms.) These results demonstrated that emergency caesarean section in labour conferred no protection over the development of symptoms. Constipation after delivery may be one factor that prolongs damage to the pudendal nerve, straining at stool increasing perineal descent.

Direct trauma to the anal sphincter mechanism has also been proposed as a factor in the development of symptoms. This has been investigated using endo-anal ultrasonography to image the internal and external anal sphincters. Sultan et al.[93] found previously unrecognized anatomical defects in the anal sphincter after vaginal delivery in 35% of primiparous women. This study also correlated the presence of a defect with a decrease in the pressures measured on anal manometry. Sultan et al.[93] also investigated multiparous women and found only a further 4% increase in the incidence of damage over primiparous women. This suggests that the first delivery is the most important for causing damage to the anal sphincter. These findings are supported by an ultrasonography study[94] which demonstrated scarring in the anal sphincter in 19 of 57 parous women attending the gynaecology outpatient department for reasons other than faecal incontinence. Other studies have aimed to define the part of the sphincter that is most important in the development of symptoms. Burnett et al.[95] found that damage to the external anal sphincter was common in women with faecal incontinence symptoms. This observation was confirmed by Sorensen et al.[96] who compared symptoms with reported trauma to the anal sphincter at the time of delivery.

The use of perineal ultrasonography has also been reported. Ultrasound evidence correlated with the finding of an anal spincter defect at surgery in symptomatic women.[97] These studies have shown that damage to the anal sphincter is relatively common, but occurs as an occult finding in between three and seven times as many women as have symptoms.

The incidence of symptomatic incontinence after a primary repair is 37–49%.[96,98] It may be that the risk of developing symptoms is proportional to the amount of the sphincter disrupted and that many of the asymptomatic disruptions are of a small degree. This question may be answered with three-dimensional ultrasonography or MRI, which now allow more extensive investigation of the anal sphincter (Fig. 75.7).

Fornell *et al.*[99] prospectively followed-up 51 women who had sustained a rupture to their anal sphincter and 31 women who had not, as determined using ultrasonography. They reported that the incidence of recognized sphincter rupture was 2.4%. The women with a rupture had reduced anal manometry scores compared with those without a rupture. The incidence of symptoms of faecal incontinence was 40% in both groups but symptoms were more severe in the women who had sustained a rupture. Snooks *et al.*[100] looked at the incidence of both sphincter and nerve damage. Their study showed that 60% of women who have anal sphincter defects also have prolonged pudendal terminal latencies, suggesting that the two injuries may be related in the development of faecal symptoms. Felt-Bersma and Cuesta[101] suggested that the mechanisms of the injuries may be different, labour being associated with damage to the pudendal nerve and vaginal delivery with sphincter damage (Table 75.5).

The only long-term follow-up study to date has shown that the incidence of faecal symptoms remains high.[102] In contrast to most studies, this study suggests that long-term symptoms are not related to delivery type. However, this study was retrospective and may not solely reflect the contribution of the index delivery (i.e. the delivery that symptoms are related to) to the development of faecal incontinence.

Repair of anal sphincter damage

Consensus on repair of anal sphincter disruption now seems to be in favour of an overlap repair,[103] although this is not advocated universally.[104] Fang *et al.*[105] proposed that good results were achieved using an overlap repair, providing there was an intact neuromuscular bundle. They also stipulated that extensive dissection to remove scar tissue, or division between internal and external sphincters should be avoided.

VAGINAL PROLAPSE

Childbirth is often cited as one of the principal causes of vaginal prolapse and it is estimated that 50% of

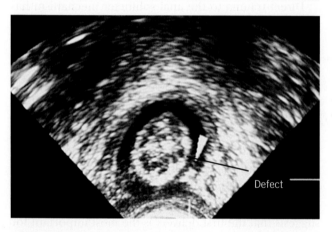

Figure 75.7. *Anal sphincter damage.*

Table 75.5. *The long-term incidence (%) of post-partum faecal symptoms*				
	Type of incontinence			
	Flatus	Bothersome flatus	Frequent faecal	Bothersome faecal
Sphincter rupture	30	58	6.9	27
Episiotomy	42	30	18	25
Caesarean section	36	15	0	15

Data from ref. 101.

parous women have some degree of prolapse.[106] In a recent epidemiological study of more than 17 000 women, age, weight and parity were found to correlate independently with inpatient admission for prolapse.[107] Vaginal delivery causes damage to the endopelvic fascia[108] and levator hiatus.[109] Such studies suggest that alterations in the pelvic floor lead to a gradual weakening of the support for the pelvic organs. This results in a gradual increase in displacement over time, which is increased as the tissues naturally weaken; prolapse may then gradually occur universally.

CONCLUSIONS

Urinary symptoms are frequently associated with pregnancy in both the antenatal and postnatal periods. Many large-scale symptomatic studies have demonstrated the prevalence of the different symptoms. Smaller studies involving urodynamic investigations, imaging techniques and electrophysiological investigations have started to elucidate the underlying causes for these symptoms.

Urinary frequency is the most frequent symptom and occurs as a function of increased urine output. Whereas nocturia is due to a combination of increased urine output, reduced bladder capacity and increased time spent in bed, urgency may be associated with temporary changes in the sensory threshold of the bladder. There also appears to be an increase in detrusor activity in pregnancy. Whether this increase is a manifestation of pregnancy has never been investigated prospectively. There is no evidence to support the suggestion that DI occurs as a result of childbirth.

Symptoms of stress incontinence are frequent during pregnancy, but most are temporary during confinement and resolve postnatally. In addition, *de-novo* leakage appears to be uncommon after delivery. Studies to date suggest that pregnancy and hereditary factors are also influential in the genesis of permanent stress incontinence. Loss of urethral sphincter volume may occur during pregnancy, labour or delivery. There is evidence overall to support the suggestion that the first caesarean section is at least partially protective against the development of stress incontinence; however, the effect on the bladder of repeated pelvic surgery has yet to be evaluated.

Voiding difficulties are a concern mainly in the postnatal period, and long-term problems arise if a woman is left in urinary retention. All women with epidural anaesthesia, extensive trauma or difficulties passing urine during the perinatal period should be catheterized with an indwelling catheter.

Faecal incontinence appears to be related to disruption of the neuromuscular function of the anal sphincter. Nerve damage and sphincter damage are both independent factors associated with the development of faecal symptoms. Careful attention to the repair of anal sphincter damage is probably the single most important factor in reducing these symptoms.

REFERENCES

1. Cardozo L, Cutner A. Lower urinary tract symptoms in pregnancy. *Br J Urol* 1997; 80(Suppl 1): 14–23

2. Blakeman P, Hilton P, Bulmer JN. Mapping oestrogen and progesterone receptors throughout the female lower urinary tract. *Neurourol Urodyn* 1996; 15: 324–325

3. Chard T, Lilford R. Cell biology, embryology and the placenta. *Basic Sciences for Obstetrics and Gynaecology*, 3rd edn. London: Springer Verlag, 1989; 1–38

4. Dewhurst J, DeSwiet M, Chamberlain G (eds) Physiology. *Basic Sciences in Obstetrics and Gynaecology*. London: Churchill Livingstone, 1986; 128–206

5. Francis WJA. Disturbances of bladder function in relation to pregnancy. *J Obstet Gynecol Br Empire* 1960; 67: 353–366

6. Parboosingh J, Doig A. Studies of nocturia in normal pregnancy. *Obstet Gynecol Br Commonw* 1973; 80: 888–895

7. Cutner A. *The Lower Urinary Tract in Pregnancy*. MD thesis, University of London, 1993

8. Langworthy OR, Brack CB. The effect of pregnancy and the corpus luteum upon the vesical muscle. *Am J Obstet Gynecol* 1939; 37: 121–125

9. Youssef AF. Cystometric studies in gynecology and obstetrics. *Obstet Gynecol* 1956; 8: 181–188

10. Muellner SR. Physiological bladder changes during pregnancy and the puerperium. *J Urol* 1939; 41: 691–695

11. Francis WJA. The onset of stress incontinence. *J Obstet Gynaecol Br Empire* 1960; 67: 899–903

12. Parboosingh J, Doig A. Renal nyctohemeral excretory patterns of water and solutes in normal human pregnancy. *Am J Obstet Gynecol* 1973; 116: 609–615

13. Stanton SL, Kerr-Wilson R, Harris GV. The incidence of urological symptoms in normal pregnancy. *Br J Obstet Gynaecol* 1980; 87: 897–900

14. Cutner A, Cardozo LD, Benness CJ *et al.* Detrusor instability in early pregnancy. *Neurourol Urodyn* 1990; 9: 328–329

15. Cutner A, Carey A, Cardozo LD. Lower urinary tract symptoms in early pregnancy. *J Obstet Gynaecol* 1992; 12: 75–78

16. Shutter HW. Care of the bladder in pregnancy, labor, and the puerperium. *J Am Med Assoc* 1992; 79: 449–453

17. Hundley Jr JM, Siegel IA, Hachtel FW, Dumler JC. Some physiological and pathological observations on the urinary tract during pregnancy. *Surg Gynecol Obstet* 1938; 66: 360–379

18. Malpas P, Jeffcoate TNA, Lister UM. The displacement of the bladder and urethra during labour. *J Obstet Gynaecol Br Empire* 1949; 56: 949–960

19. Marchant DJ. The urinary tract in pregnancy. *Clin Obstet Gynaecol* 1978; 21: 817–914

20. Langer R, Golan A, Neuman M *et al.* The effect of large uterine fibroids on urinary bladder function and symptoms. *Am J Obstet Gynecol* 1990; 163: 1139–1141

21. Cutner A, Cardozo LD, Benness CJ. Assessment of urinary symptoms in early pregnancy. *Br J Obstet Gynaecol* 1991; 98: 1283–1286

22. Cutner A, Cardozo LD, Benness CJ. Assessment of urinary symptoms in the second half of pregnancy. *Int Urogynecol J* 1992; 3: 30–32

23. Cutner A, Cardozo LD. The association between pregnancy and abnormal detrusor activity. *J Obstet Gynaecol* 1996;16: 143–145

24. Lee JG, Wein AJ, Levin RM. Effects of pregnancy on urethral and bladder neck function. *Urology* 1993; 42: 747–752

25. Cardozo LD, Stanton SL. Genuine stress incontinence and detrusor instability: a review of 200 patients. *Br J Obstet Gynaecol* 1980; 87: 184–190

26. Cantor TJ, Bates CP. A comparative study of symptoms and objective urodynamic findings in 214 incontinent women *Br J Obstet Gynaecol* 1980; 87: 889–892

27. Jarvis GJ, Hall S, Stamp S *et al.* An assessment of urdynamic examination in incontinent women. *Br J Obstet Gynaecol* 1980; 87: 893–896

28. Thomas TM, Plymat KR, Blannin J, Meade TW. Prevalence of urinary incontinence. *Br Med J* 1980; 8: 1243–1245

29. Foldspang A, Mommsen S, Lam GW, Elving L. Parity as a correlate of adult urinary incontinence prevalence. *J Epidemiol Social Med* 1992; 46: 595–600

30. Iosif S. Stress incontinence during pregnancy and in puerperium. *Int J Gynaecol Obstet* 1981; 19: 13–20

31. Iosif CS, Ingermarsson I. Prevalence of stress incontinence among women delivered by elective caesarean section. *Int J Gynaecol Obstet* 1982; 20: 87–89

32. Beck RP, Hsu N. Pregnancy, childbirth and the menopause related to the development of stress incontinence. *Am J Obstet Gynecol* 1965; 91: 820–823

33. Viktrup L, Lose G. Epidural anaesthetic during labour and stress incontinence after delivery. *Obstet Gynaecol* 1993; 82: 87–89

34. Keane DP, Sims TJ, Abrams P, Bailey AJ. Analysis of collagen status in premenopausal nulliparous women with genuine stress incontinence. *Br J Obstet Gynaecol* 1997; 104: 994–998

35. Jackson S, Avery N, Eckford S *et al.* Connective tissue analysis in genitourinary prolapse. *Neurourol Urodyn* 1995; 14: 412–414

36. Bell RJ, Eddie LW, Lester AR *et al.* Relaxin in human pregnancy serum measured with an homologous radioimmunoassay. *Obstet Gynecol* 1987; 69: 585–589

37. Bani D. Relaxin: a pleiotropic hormone. *Gen Pharmacol* 1997; 28: 13–22

38. Landon CR, Crofts CE, Smith ARB, Trowbridge EA. Mechanical properties of fascia during pregnancy: a possible factor for the development of stress incontinence of urine. *Contemp Rev Obstet Gynecol* 1990; 2: 40–46

39. Lavin JM, Smith ARB, Anderson J *et al.* The effect of the first pregnancy on the connective tissue of the rectus sheath. *Neurourol Urodyn* 1997; 16: 381–382

40. Iosif S, Ulmston U. Comparative urodynamic studies of continent and stress incontinent women in pregnancy and in the puerperium. *Am J Obstet Gynecol* 1981; 140: 645–650

41. Van Geelen JM, Lemmens WA, Eskes TK, Martin CB. The urethral pressure profile in pregnancy and after delivery in healthy nulliparous women. *Am J Obstet Gynecol* 1982; 144: 636–649

42. Noble JG, Dixon PJ, Rickards D, Fowler CJ. Urethral sphincter volumes in women with obstructed voiding and abnormal sphincter electromyographic activity. *Br J Urol* 1995; 76: 741–746

43. Athanasiou S, Boos K, Khullar V *et al.* Pathogenesis of genuine stress incontinence and urogenital prolapse. *Neurourol Urodyn* 1996; 15: 339–340

44. Toozs-Hobson P, Athanasiou SA, Khullar V *et al.* Why do women develop incontinence after childbirth? *Neurourol Urodyn* 1997; 16: 384–385

45. Toozs-Hobson P, Athanasiou S, Anders K *et al.* Changes in the urethral sphincter in relationship to childbirth and the development of stress incontinence. *Int Urogynaecol J Pelvic Floor Dysfunct* 1997; 8: 59

46. Wise BG, Burton G, Cutner A, Cardozo LD. Effect of vaginal ultrasound probe on lower urinary tract function. *Br J Urol* 1992; 70: 12–16

47. Meyer S, De Grandi P, Schreyer A, Caccia G. The assessment of bladder neck position and mobility in continent women using perineal ultrasound: a future office procedure. *Int Urogynecol J Pelvic Floor Dysfunct* 1996; 7: 138–146

48. King J, Freeman R. Can we predict antenatally those patients at risk of postpartum stress incontinence? *Neurourol Urodyn* 1996; 15: 330–331

49. Hayat SK, Thorp JM, Kullar JA *et al.* Magnetic resonance imaging of the pelvic floor in the postpartum patient. *Int Urogynecol J Pelvic floor Dysfunct* 1996; 7: 321–324

50. Bø K, Lilleas F, Talseth T. Dynamic MRI of the pelvic floor and coccygeal movement during pelvic floor contraction and straining. *Neurourol Urodyn* 1997; 16: 409–410

51. Krue S, Jensen H, Aggar AO, Rasmussen KL. The influence of infant birth weight on post partum stress incontinence in obese women. *Arch Gynecol Obstet* 1997; 259: 143–145

52. Rasmussen KL, Krue S, Johansson LE *et al.* Obesity as a predictor of postpartum urinary symptoms. *Acta Obstet Gynecol Scand* 1997; 76: 359–362

53. Drife JO. Choice and instrumental delivery. *Br J Obstet Gynaecol* 1996; 103: 608–611

54. Meinru GI. An analysis of recent trends in vacuum extraction and forceps delivery in the United Kingdom. *Br J Obstet Gynaecol* 1996; 103: 168–170

55. Chiarelli P, Campbell E. Incontinence during pregnancy. Prevalence and opportunities for continence promotion. *Aust N Z J Obstet Gynaecol* 1997; 37: 66–73

56. Dimpfl T, Hesses U, Schussler B. Incidence and cause of postpartum stress incontinence. *Eur J Obstet Gynecol Reprod Biol* 1992; 43: 29–33

57. Wilson PD, Herbison RM, Herbison GP. Obstetric practice and the prevalence of urinary incontinence three months after delivery. *Br J Obstet Gynaecol* 1996; 103: 154–161

58. Jackson S, Barry C, Shepherd A, Abrams P. Management of delivery in primiparous women: effect on subsequent urinary incontinence. *Neurourol Urodyn* 1997; 16: 387–388

59. Al-Mufti R, McCarthy A, Fisk NN. Obstetricians personal choice and mode of delivery [letter]. *Lancet* 1996; 347: 544

60. Skoner MM, Thompson WD, Caron VA. Factors associated with risk of stress urinary incontinence in women. *Nurs Res* 1994; 43: 301–306

61. Hibbard BM, McKenna DM. The obstetric forceps. Are we using the appropriate tools? *Br J Obstet Gynaecol* 1990; 97: 963

62. Sampselle CM. Changes in pelvic muscle strength and stress urinary incontinence associated with childbirth. *J Obstet Gynecol Neonatal Nurs* 1990; 19: 371–377

63. Marshall K, Walsh DM, Baxter GD. The effect of a first delivery on the integrity of the pelvic floor musculature. *Neurourol Urodyn* 1996; 15: 436–437

64. Toozs-Hobson P, Athanasiou S, Khullar V *et al.* Does vaginal delivery damage the pelvic floor? *Neurourol Urodyn* 1997; 16: 384–385

65. Allen RE, Hosker GL, Smith AR, Warrell DW. Pelvic floor damage and childbirth: a neurophysiological study. *Br J Obstet Gynaecol* 1990; 97: 770–779

66. Gilpin SA, Gosling JA, Smith AR, Warrell DW. The pathogenesis of genitourinary prolapse and stress incontinence of urine. A histopathological and histochemical study. *Br J Obstet Gynaecol* 1989; 96: 15–23

67. Helt M, Benson JT, Russell B, Brubaker L. Levator ani muscle in women with genitourinary prolapse: indirect assessment by muscle histopathology. *Neurourol Urodyn* 1996; 15: 17–29

68. Tetzchner T, Sorenson M, Jonsson L *et al.* Delivery and pudendal nerve function. *Acta Obstet Gynecol Scand* 1997; 76: 324–331

69. Snooks SJ, Swash M, Mathers SE, Henry MM. Effect of vaginal delivery on the pelvic floor; 5 year follow up. *Br J Surg* 1990; 77: 1358–1360

70. Snooks SJ, Swash M, Henry MM, Setchell M. Risk factors in childbirth causing damage to the pelvic floor innervation. *Int J Colorectal Dis* 1986; 1: 20–24

71. Ho YH, Goh HS. The neurophysiological significance of perineal descent. *Int J Colorectal Surg* 1995; 10: 107–111

72. Jorge JM, Wexner SD, Ehrenpresis ED *et al.* Does perineal descent correlate with pudendal neuropathy? *Dis Colon Rectum* 1993; 36: 475–483

73. Barnick CG, Cardozo LD. Denervation and re-innervation of the urethral sphincter in the urethral sphincter in the aetiology of genuine stress incontinence: an electromyography study. *Br J Obstet Gynaecol* 1994; 101: 559–560

74. Rockner G. Urinary incontinence after perineal trauma at childbirth. *Scand J Caring Sci* 1990; 4: 169–172

75. Sleep J, Grant A. West Berkshire perineal management trial. Three year follow up. *Br Med J Clin Res Ed* 1987; 295: 749–751

76. Burgio KL, Locher JL, Zyczynski H *et al.* Urinary incontinence during pregnancy in a racially mixed group: characteristics and predisposing factors. *Int Urogynecol J Pelvic floor Dysfunct* 1996; 7: 69–73

77. Fischer W, Kittel K. Harnflußmessungen in der Schwangerschaft und im Wochenbett (Urine flow studies

in pregnancy and puerperium). *Zent bl Gynakol* 1990; 112: 593–600

78. Haylen BT, Ashby D, Sutherst JR *et al.* Maximum and average flow rates in normal male and female populations – the Liverpool nomograms. *Br J Urol* 1989; 64: 30–38

79. Dolman M. Midwives recording of urinary output. *Nurs Stand* 1992; 6: 26–27

80. Khullar V, Cardozo LD. Bladder sensation after epidural analgesia. *Neurourol Urodyn* 1993; 12: 424–425

81. Torrens MJ. Urodynamic analysis of differential sacral nerve blocks and sacral neurectomy. *Urol Int* 1975; 30: 85–91

82. Tapp AJS, Meir H, Cardozo LD. The effect of epidural analgesia on post-partum voiding. *Neurourol Urodyn* 1987; 6: 235–237

83. Grove LH. Backache, headache and bladder dysfunction after delivery. *Br J Anaesth* 1973; 45: 1147–1149

84. Crawford JS. Lumber epidural block in labour: a clinical analysis. *Br J Anaesth* 1972; 44: 66–74

85. Kranz MI, Edwards WI. Anaesthesia and urinary retention in obstetrics. *J Indian State Med Assoc* 1974; 76: 329–330

86. Weil A, Reyes H, Rottenberg RD *et al.* Effect of lumber epidural analgesia on lower urinary tract function in the immediate postpartum period. *Br J Obstet Gynaecol* 1983; 90: 428–432

87. Kerr-Wilson RHJ, McNally S. Bladder drainage for caesarean section under epidural analgesia. *Br J Obstet Gynaecol* 1986; 93: 23–30

88. Tapp AJS, Meir H, Cardozo LD. The effect of epidural analgesia on post-partum voiding. *Neurourol Urodyn* 1987; 6: 235–237

89. MacAurthur C, Bick DE, Keighley MRB. Faecal incontinence after childbirth. *Br J Obstet Gynaecol* 1997; 104: 45–60

90. Ryhammer AM, Beck KM, Laurberg S. Multiple vaginal deliveries increase the risk of permanent incontinence of flatus and urine in normal premenopausal women. *Dis Colon Rectum* 1995; 38: 1206–1209

91. Cornes H, Bartolo D, Stirrat GM. Changes in anal canal sensation after childbirth. *Br J Surg* 1991; 78: 74–77

92. Parks AG, Swash M, Urich H. Sphincter denervation in anorectal incontinence and rectal prolapse. *Gut* 1977; 18: 656–665

93. Sultan AH, Kamm MA, Hudson CN *et al.* Anal sphincter disruption during vaginal delivery. *N Engl J Med* 1993; 329: 1905–1911

94. Frudinger A, Bartram CI, Spencer JA, Kamm MA. Perineal examination as a predictor of underlying anal sphincter damage. *Br J Obstet Gynaecol* 1997; 104: 1009–1013

95. Burnett SJ, Spence-Jones C, Speakman CT *et al.* Unsuspected sphincter damage following childbirth revealed by anal endosonography. *Br J Radiol* 1991; 64: 225–227

96. Sorensen M, Tetzscner T, Rasmussen OO *et al.* Sphincter rupture in childbirth. *Br J Surg* 1993; 80: 392–394

97. Peschers UM, DeLancey JO, Schaer GN. Exoanal ultrasound of the anal sphincter: normal anatomy and sphincter defects. *Br J Obstet Gynaecol* 1997; 104: 999–1003

98. Sultan AH, Kamm MA, Bartram CI, Hudson CN. Third degree obstetric anal sphincter tears: risk factors and outcome of primary repair. *Br Med J* 1994; 308: 887–891

99. Fornell EK, Berg G, Hallbook O *et al.* Clinical consequences of anal sphincter rupture during vaginal delivery. *J Am Coll Surg* 1996; 183: 553–558

100. Snooks SJ, Henry MM, Swash M. Faecal incontinence due to external anal sphincter division in childbirth is associated with damage to the innervation of the pelvic floor musculature: a double pathology. *Br J Obstet Gynaecol* 1985; 92: 824–828

101. Felt-Bersma RJ, Cuesta MA. Faecal incontinence: which test which treatment? *Neth J Med* 1994; 44: 182–188

102. Nygaard IE, Rao SS, Dawson JD. Anal incontinence after anal sphincter disruption: a 30 year retrospective cohort study. *Obstet Gynecol* 1997; 89: 896–901

103. Gibbs DH, Hooks VH. Overlapping sphincteroplasty for acquired anal incontinence. *South Med J* 1993; 86: 1376–1380

104. Arnaud A, Sarles JC, Sielezneff I *et al.* Sphincter repair without overlapping for faecal incontinence. *Dis Colon Rectum* 1991; 34: 744–747

105. Fang DT, Nivatvongs S, Vermeulen FD *et al.* Overlapping sphincteroplasty for acquired anal incontinence. *Dis Colon Rectum* 1984; 27: 720–722

106. Beck RP, Nordstrom L. A 25 year experience with 519 anterior colporrhaphy prcedures. *Obstet Gynecol* 1991; 78: 1011–1018

107. Mant J, Painter R, Vessey M. Epidemiology of genital prolapse: observations from the Oxford Family Planning Association Study. *Br J Obstet Gynecol* 1997; 104: 579–585

108. Monga A. Fascia-defects and repair. *Curr Opin Obstet Gynecol* 1996; 8: 366–371

109. Athanasiou S, Boos K, Khullar V *et al.* Pathogenesis of genuine stress incontinence and urogenital prolapse. *Neurourol Urodyn* 1996; 15: 339–340

76

Menopause

A. Hextall, L. Cardozo

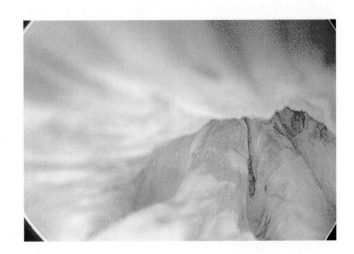

INTRODUCTION

Ovarian function starts to decline from as early as the 20th week of embryological life, and oestrogen production falls to a critical level during a period known as the climacteric. De Gardanne coined the term 'la menespausie' from the Greek *men* (month) and *pausis* (cessation).[1] The menopause is diagnosed when a woman has not had a period for 12 months. Aristotle (384–322 BC)[2] recognized that menstruation normally stopped at about the age of 40 years but that some women continued to have periods until their 50th year. In the 17th century less than a third of women lived to experience the menopause. However, increased life expectancy during the last century means that many women will spend a significant part of their life in the post-menopausal years and will therefore be at risk of the effects of oestrogen deficiency.

The average age at the menopause is now generally accepted to be 50 years, but some variation is thought to exist between different countries and geographical regions.[3] In 1990 there were approximately 467 million women aged 50 years and above in the World; this number is expected to have increased to 1200 million by the year 2030[4] (Fig. 76.1). Post-menopausal women make up over 15% of the population in industrialized countries, with a growth rate of 1.5% predicted until the 2020s.

Hormonal changes occurring at the time of the menopause have an impact on all oestrogen-sensitive tissues, and the female urogenital tract is no exception. Oestrogen deficiency, particularly when prolonged, is associated with a wide range of urinary symptoms including frequency, nocturia, incontinence, urinary tract infections (UTIs) and the 'urge syndrome'. These may coexist with vaginal symptoms of dryness, itching, burning and dyspareunia.

HORMONAL INFLUENCES ON THE FEMALE LOWER URINARY TRACT

The female lower urinary and genital tracts both arise from the primitive urogenital sinus and develop in close anatomical proximity from early in the first trimester of pregnancy (Fig. 76.2). Oestrogen receptors are consistently expressed in the squamous epithelium of the proximal and distal urethra and vagina, and in areas of the trigone of the bladder that have undergone squamous metaplasia[5,6] (Fig. 76.3). However, they are not present in the transitional epithelium of the bladder dome, reflecting the different embryological origin of this tissue. The pubococcygeus muscle of the pelvic floor is also oestrogen sensitive.[7,8] Oestrogen increases cell cycle activity in the female lower urinary tract,[9] demonstrated by an increase in the number of intermediate

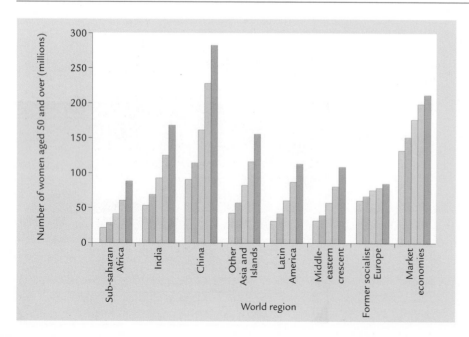

Figure 76.1. *Summary statistics for number of menopausal women by World region, 1990–2030:* ▪ *1990;* ▪ *2000;* ▪ *2010;* ▪ *2020;* ▪ *2030.*

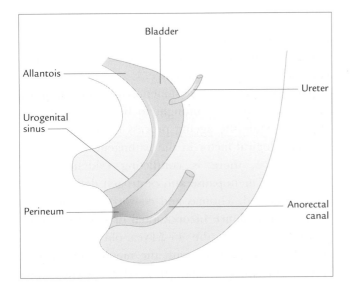

Figure 76.2. *Embryology of the female lower urinary tract.*

and superficial cells in the urethra and bladder,[10] with similar changes occurring in the vagina, in post-menopausal women.[11] Alterations in urinary cytology during the menstrual cycle are comparable with those seen in vaginal cytology,[12] changes that also occur in the urinary sediment following treatment with oestrogens.[13]

Progesterone receptors are expressed inconsistently in the lower urinary tract and may be dependent on the oestrogen status of the woman.[7,14] Androgen receptors are found in the female bladder and urethra, but their role is at present unclear.[15]

Cyclical variations in the levels of sex steroids during the menstrual cycle may lead to both symptomatic and urodynamic changes. Van Geelen[16] measured the urethral pressure profiles of 27 nulliparous women with normal ovulatory cycles and found an increase in the functional urethral length mid-cycle and early in the luteal phase. The data suggested a causal relationship between changes in serum oestradiol and alterations in urethral length. During pregnancy many women complain of urinary symptoms that are due only in part to an increase in urine output and pressure effects from the gravid uterus.[17–19] However, the prevalence of detrusor instability is significantly greater antenatally than postnatally,[20] suggesting a hormonal effect, thought to be mediated through progesterone.

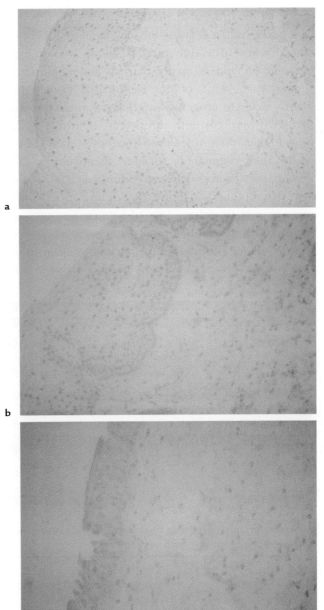

Figure 76.3. *Oestrogen receptors are expressed in the squamous epithelium of the vagina (a) and urethra (b) but not in the transitional epithelium of the bladder dome (c). Oestrogen receptor-positive cell nuclei appear brown; oestrogen receptor-negative nuclei appear blue. (Provided by Blakeman et al. based on the data in ref. 6.)*

PREVALENCE OF POST-MENOPAUSAL URINARY SYMPTOMS

Urinary symptoms secondary to oestrogen deficiency may develop many years after the menopause and may, therefore, be under-reported by both patient and doctor. Epidemiological studies have shown that the incidence of urogenital problems increases with age, with many women delaying the seeking of treatment for several years. In a study of 2045 British women aged between 55 and 85 years, Barlow and co-workers[22] showed that 48.5% of post-menopausal women had been affected by urogenital symptoms at some time and that 11% were currently affected by individual symptoms (Table 76.1). At least two-thirds of women did not relate their vaginal or urinary complaint to the menopause. Iosif and Bekassy[22] studied 2200 women aged 61 years and also found a high prevalence of lower urinary tract disorders, 49% of women having some symptoms. In addition, 70% of the women with incontinence related the onset of their urinary leakage to the time of their final menstrual period. Urinary tract

symptoms are certainly frequent following the menopause: of women who attend a menopause clinic, one in five complain of severe urgency and nearly half complain of stress incontinence.[24]

The prevalence of post-menopausal incontinence in the community is thought to be between 16 and 29%.[24–26] While the ageing process is clearly a significant aetiological factor in the pathogenesis of urinary incontinence, there is conflicting evidence as to whether the menopause and oestrogen deficiency are also implicated. Thomas and co-workers[27] found that the peak prevalence of occasional or regular incontinence occurred in the 45–54-year-old age group, a period which coincides with the menopause in most women (Fig.76.4). Jolleys[24] surveyed 937 women regis-

Table 76.1. *Prevalence of urogenital symptoms by age in the preceding two years*

Age group (years)	All	55–64	65–74	75–84	> 85
TOTAL	2011 [2011]	662 [706]	697 [678]	539 [517]	113 [109]
Urgency, dysuria, frequency	312 (16)	101 (14)	96 (14)	95 (18)	19 (18)
Urinary incontinence	172 (9)	46 (7)	45 (7)	65 (13)	16 (14)
Vaginal itching	217 (11)	68 (10)	72 (11)	65 (12)	15 (13)
Vaginal dryness	156 (8)	75 (11)	4 (7)	34 (7)	3 (2)
Painful intercourse	33 (2)	23 (3)	8 (1)	2 (0–4)	0

Values are given as n with weighted totals in brackets or percentages in parentheses.
Reproduced from ref. 21 with permission.

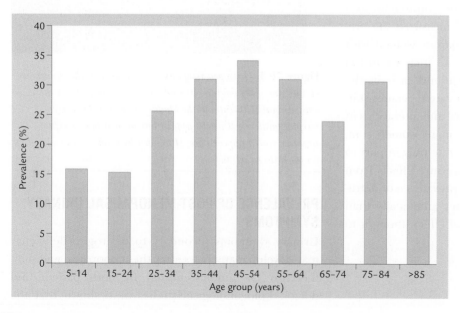

Figure 76.4. *Prevalence of occasional or regular incontinence in women. (Data from ref 27.)*

tered with a rural general practice and detected similar changes in the prevalence of incontinence with age (Fig. 76.5). A similar pattern appears to occur in hospital practice: Hilton[29] reported that the mean age of women referred to a urogynaecology unit was almost identical to the age of the natural menopause. Urge incontinence in particular occurs more frequently after the menopause[30] (Fig. 76.6). Most studies, however, show that many women develop incontinence at least 10 years before the menopause; Jolleys[24] found

that significantly more premenopausal women than post-menopausal women were affected. In addition, the prevalence of stress incontinence in the community actually starts to fall after the menopause, particularly in age groups that are most likely to be affected by relative oestrogen deficiency. These data probably simply confirm that the development of urinary incontinence is a multifactorial process, and that the menopause is just one of a number of aetiological factors.

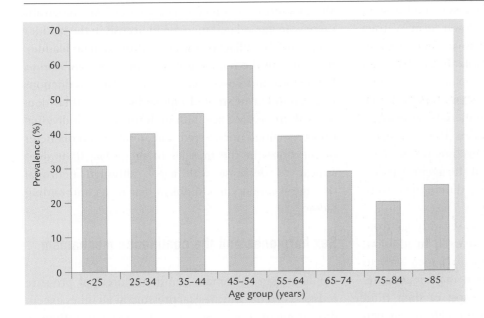

Figure 76.5. *Prevalence of stress urinary incontinence with increasing age. (Data from ref. 24.)*

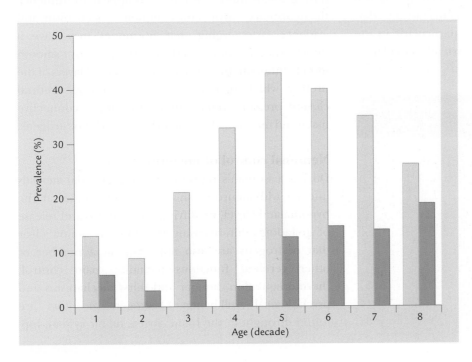

Figure 76.6. *Changes in prevalence of symptoms of stress incontinence ( ) and urge incontinence ( ) with increasing age. (Data from ref. 29.)*

MENOPAUSE AND THE CONTINENCE MECHANISM

Effects of ageing

Many women consider the development of urinary symptoms as they get older to be a normal phenomenon rather than the manifestation of a disease.[30] In a study by Gjorup and co-workers,[31] over 50% of women aged more than 75 years thought that their symptoms were normal for elderly people. The ageing population is at risk for a number of systemic illnesses and transient problems that may present with lower urinary tract symptoms, including diabetes mellitus, congestive cardiac failure and renal disease (Table 76.2). A patient with impaired mobility may develop urinary incontinence if suitable access to a toilet is not available, a situation which may be exacerbated if medications such as diuretics or hypnotics are being taken. However, symptomatic and functional changes certainly do occur in the lower urinary tract as a result of the ageing process itself; these changes are difficult to differentiate from those due to oestrogen deficiency.

The prevalence of nocturia increases with age from 10.5% (50–59 years) to 50% (> 80 years).[32] In addition, the proportion of women with nocturia secondary to nocturnal polyuria also rises after the menopause. Younger women tend to excrete most of their fluid intake during the day, whereas in the elderly this pattern may be reversed. Postural effects may lead to daytime pooling of extracellular fluid, particularly in the ankles. This fluid returns to the systemic circulation during the night, leading to an increase in urine output. This combined with abnormal sleep patterns may lead to nocturia. Impaired secretion of antidiuretic hormone may also be a factor in some women.

Urodynamic studies have shown that the bladder becomes less efficient with age.[33–35] Elderly women have a reduced urine flow rate, increased urinary residual, higher first sensation to void and increased bladder capacity, although bladder capacity may decrease in the eighth and ninth decades. Detrusor pressures at urethral opening and closure during voiding decrease in absolute terms as women become older.[36] Histologically there is an age-related increase in fibrosis in the bladder neck[37] and in collagen content[38] of the female bladder. In a study of the female urethral sphincter *post mortem*, Perucchini and co-workers[39] demonstrated reductions in the number of striated muscle fibres and their density with increasing age, although the size of individual fibres remained unchanged. The number and diameter of the fibres in the muscles of the pelvic floor does appear to decrease with age,[40] although neuronal damage secondary to childbirth may be a confounding factor.[41,42]

Sex hormones and the continence mechanism

For a woman to remain continent, urethral pressure must exceed the intravesical pressure at all times except during micturition.[43] Sex steroids appear to influence the neuronal control of the continence mechanism, and evidence is emerging that hormones may have a direct (non-genomic) effect on detrusor smooth muscle function. In addition, the functional layers of the urethra which help to maintain a positive urethral closure pressure (epithelium, vasculature, connective tissue and muscle) all appear to be targets for oestrogens.

Neuronal control of micturition

During a woman's reproductive life, gonadal steroids interact with neurotransmitters/neuropeptides at the hypothalamic level, modifying the synthesis and release of gonadotrophin-releasing hormone. It is now clear that oestrogens are also important in a number of other cerebral functions including pain control, thermoregulation, hunger and thirst mechanisms and psychological well-being. Oestrogen receptors are found throughout the brain cortex, limbic system, hip-

Table 76.2. *Transitional causes of urinary incontinence in the elderly*

- Urinary tract infection
- Faecal impaction
- Oestrogen deficiency
- Restricted mobility
- Drug therapy
- Depression
- Confusional state

pocampus and cerebellum.[44,45] In these regions oestrogens can alter the synthesis, release and metabolism of neurotransmitters such as dopamine, acetylcholine, serotonin and melatonin. This may explain why oestrogen supplementation can improve cognitive function and enhance mood and psychological well-being in the perimenopausal and post-menopausal periods.[46–49]

Recent animal studies have shown that androgen receptors are present in the pontine micturition centre.[50] They are also present in the preoptic area of the hypothalamus, an area of the forebrain which may play an important role in the initiation of micturition. Further work is required to establish the exact type and distribution of sex-steroid receptors in the human micturition pathways and their importance in the control of the continence mechanism.

Detrusor function

Oestrogen appears to have a direct effect on detrusor function by modifying muscarinic receptors[51,52] and inhibiting the influx of extracellular calcium ions into muscle cells.[53] Studies of female rats have shown that oophorectomy alters the pressure–flow characteristics of micturition.[54] This effect may be only partly reversed by oestrogen supplementation and is possibly age dependent. It is not clear if similar effects occur in humans. Oestrogen may theoretically play a role in the treatment of sensory and motor urge incontinence. Oestradiol reduces the amplitude and frequency of spontaneous rhythmic contractions, which has been associated with detrusor instability.[55] In addition, pretreatment of rats with oestrogen *in vivo* reduces the contractile response of isolated detrusor muscle.[56] There is also evidence to suggest that the sensory threshold of the bladder may be raised by oestrogen supplementation.[57]

In general, progestogens have an adverse effect on the continence mechanism. Elliot and Castleden[58] have shown that progesterone blocks the inhibitory effect of oestradiol on detrusor muscle contractions in the rat. The effect of oestrogen on the responsiveness of muscarinic receptors therefore appears to be modified by progesterone. Clinically, progestogens are associated with an increase in irritative bladder symptoms[59,60] and urinary leakage in those women with incontinence taking hormone-replacement therapy (HRT).[61] However, progestogens do not appear to alter significantly the urethral pressure profile of continent women.[62]

Urethral function

Oestrogen improves the 'maturation index' of urethral squamous epithelium,[63] increases urethral closure pressure and improves pressure transmission to the proximal urethra.[64–66] There is evidence to suggest that the vasodilatory effects of oestrogens that occur in the systemic and cerebral circulations[67–69] may also occur in the urogenital tract. Using urethral pressure profilometry, Versi and Cardozo[70] showed that vascular pulsations seen secondary to blood flow in the urethral submucosa and urethral sphincter increase in size in response to oestrogen. Attempts have been made to quantify changes in urethral blood flow in response to oestrogen therapy using Doppler ultrasonography.[71] Unfortunately, the reproducibility of this technique is limited by difficulties in imaging the same vessel repeatedly and natural variation in the blood flow through pelvic vessels.

Alpha-adrenoceptors in the urethral sphincter are sensitized by oestrogens, helping to maintain muscular tone.[72] Finally, connective tissue metabolism is stimulated by oestrogens, increasing production of collagen in periurethral tissues and, therefore, possibly reversing the changes that occur as result of ageing.[73]

The oestrogen status of the patient can therefore have a significant effect on urethral pressure,[74] and this may be particularly important when there is already some impairment of urethral function.

OESTROGEN TREATMENT FOR INCONTINENCE

Oestrogens may be useful for the treatment of urinary incontinence for a number of reasons (Table 76.3). Salmon[75] first reported the successful use of oestrogens to treat urinary incontinence over 50 years ago. It is now well recognized that there is a poor correlation between a woman's symptoms and the diagnosis made following appropriate investigation.[76] Unfortunately, early trials took place before the widespread introduction of urodynamic studies and, therefore, almost certainly included a heterogeneous group of individuals with a number of different pathologies. Lack of objective outcome measures also limits interpretation of these studies.

Table 76.3. *Mechanisms by which oestrogens may improve female urinary incontinence*

- Increased urethral closure pressure
  - Increased urethral cell maturation
  - Increased urethral blood flow
  - Increased α-adrenergic receptor sensitivity in urethral smooth muscle
- Improved abdominal pressure transmission to proximal urethra
- Stimulation of periurethral collagen production
- Improved neuronal control of micturition
- Increased sensory threshold of the bladder
- Improved mood and quality of life
- Reduced incidence of urinary tract infection

Oestrogen treatment for stress incontinence

The role of oestrogen in the treatment of stress incontinence is controversial, even though a number of studies have been reported. Some studies gave promising results but this may be because they were observational, and were not randomized, blinded or controlled. The situation is further complicated by the fact that a number of different types of oestrogen have been used, with various doses, routes of administration and durations of treatment. The concurrent use of progestogens in women with a uterus to prevent endometrial hyperplasia may also be a confounding factor. A meta-analysis from the Hormones and Urogenital Therapy (HUT) Committee helped to clarify the situation.[78] Of 166 articles published in English between 1969 and 1992, only six reported controlled trials; 17 reported uncontrolled series. The results showed that there was a significant subjective improvement for all patients, including those with genuine stress incontinence (GSI), possibly because oestrogens improve feelings of well-being and quality of life. However, assessment of the objective parameters revealed that there was no change in the volume of urine lost. Maximum urethral closure pressure did increase significantly, but this result was influenced by only one study showing a large effect. In a further review, Sultana and Walters[78] examined eight controlled and 14 uncontrolled prospective trials and included all types of oestrogen treatment. They also found that oestrogen therapy was not an efficacious treatment for stress incontinence but might be useful for associated symptoms of urgency and frequency.

Two studies using oral oestrogen were reported after the HUT Committee meta-analyses. Fantl *et al.*[79] studied 83 hypo-oestrogenic women with urodynamic evidence of GSI and/or detrusor instability; they were treated with conjugated equine oestrogens (0.625 mg) and medroxyprogesterone (10 mg cyclically) for 3 months or received placebo tablets. At the end of the study period the clinical and quality-of-life variables had not changed significantly in either group. Jackson *et al.*[80,81] treated 68 post-menopausal women with GSI or mixed incontinence with oestradiol valerate (2 mg) or placebo, daily for 6 months. Again, there were no significant changes in subjective or objective outcome measures between the two groups.

Oestrogen does not appear to be an effective treatment for stress incontinence when taken alone. However, several studies have shown that it may have a role in combination with other therapies. Beisland and co-workers[82] treated 24 women with GSI using phenylpropanolamine (50 mg twice daily) and oestriol (1 mg per day vaginally), separately or in combination. Symptoms were cured in eight women receiving the combination treatment and were improved in a further nine women; the combination was more effective than either drug alone. Hilton and co-workers[83] used oestrogen (vaginal or oral) alone or in combination with phenylpropanolamine to treat 60 post-menopausal women with GSI in a double-blind, placebo-controlled study. The symptoms of stress incontinence improved subjectively in all groups but objectively only in the women taking the combination therapy. This type of treatment may be particularly useful for women with mild stress incontinence or for whom surgery is not appropriate.

It is unclear if oestrogen supplementation can be used as prophylaxis against the development of urinary incontinence in perimenopausal women.

Oestrogen treatment for urge incontinence

Oestrogen has been used for many years to treat post-menopausal urgency and urge incontinence but few controlled trials have been performed to confirm that it is of benefit. Walter[84] found that a daily combination of oestradiol (2 mg) and oestriol (1 mg) cured the symptom of urge incontinence in seven of 11 women, whereas a placebo cured symptoms in only one of 10 women. Samsioe[10] treated 34 women aged 75 years with oral oestriol (3 mg daily) in a double-blind, placebo-controlled, crossover study. Overall, a substantial subjective improvement was found in the 12 women with urge incontinence and eight women with mixed incontinence. The results of these two studies should be interpreted with caution because of the small patient numbers and lack of objective outcome measures, despite the known large placebo effect that occurs in the treatment of this condition.

A double-blind multicentre study of 64 post-menopausal women with the 'urge syndrome' did not confirm these results.[85] Before treatment all women underwent urodynamic investigation to establish that they had either sensory urgency or detrusor instability. They were then randomized to receive either oral oestriol (3 mg) or placebo daily for 3 months. Compliance was confirmed by a significant improvement in the maturation index of vaginal epithelial cells in the treatment group but not in the placebo group. Oestriol produced subjective and objective improvements in urinary symptoms but was not significantly better than placebo. In a further study, sustained-release vaginal tablets containing 25 mg 17β-oestradiol or placebo were used to treat 110 post-menopausal women.[87] Urodynamic investigations confirmed that the women had sensory urgency, detrusor instability or a normal study. At the end of the 6-month treatment period the only significant difference between the treatment and placebo groups was an improvement in the symptom of urgency in the women who had a diagnosis of sensory urgency. It is possible that this low dose of local oestrogen reversed atrophic changes in the lower urinary/genital tract rather than treating the underlying pathology.

These studies may not have shown any benefit because the wrong type of oestrogen was used for too short a period of time or the oestrogen may have been given via the wrong route. Oestriol is a naturally occurring oestrogen but has little effect on the endometrium and does not prevent osteoporosis. It is therefore questionable whether the low dose used in these studies is sufficient to treat urinary symptoms. 17β-oestradiol is absorbed well from sustained-release vaginal tablets and this has been shown to induce maturation of the vaginal epithelium within 14 days;[87] however, higher systemic levels may be needed for therapy to be effective.

OESTROGEN DEFICIENCY AND RECURRENT URINARY TRACT INFECTION

UTIs occur in women of all ages. They are a particular problem in the elderly, with a reported incidence of 20% in community-dwelling women and sometimes over 50% in institutionalized patients.[88,89] Pathophysiological changes that may account for this increase in risk include impairment of bladder emptying, poor perineal hygiene and both faecal and urinary incontinence. At present there is no conclusive evidence that impairment of immune function as a result of ageing *per se* is an independent risk factor for the development of UTI.[90] However, once an infection is acquired, the elderly are usually sicker and at considerably greater risk of dying than the young.

Alterations in the vaginal flora after the menopause are also thought to place women at an increased risk of UTI, particularly if they are sexually active. There is an increase in the vaginal pH and a decrease in the number of lactobacilli, allowing colonization with Gram-negative bacteria which act as uropathogens. However, the exact role of the menopause as an aetiological factor in the development of UTI may have been overstated. Analysis of mid-stream urine (MSU) specimens sent to our hospital from the community indicate that the proportion of positive results increases with age in both men and women, with no specific changes in the rate of infection occurring at or after the menopause[91] (Fig 76.7).

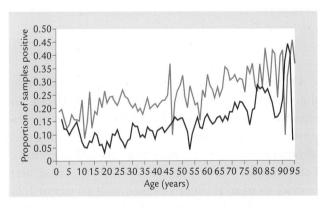

Figure 76.7. *Proportion of mid-stream urine (MSU) samples that were positive, by subject's age. Analysis of all MSU samples sent to the Department of Microbiology at King's College Hospital, London, from the community in 1997. The proportions for females (—) are calculated and plotted at each year of age. For males (—), from whom there were fewer samples, the proportion plotted at a given age is calculated over a 3-year age interval around that age.*

Table 76.4. *Summary of randomized controlled trials of oestrogen for UTI*

Study	Study group	Type of oestrogen	Route of delivery	Duration of therapy	Results
Kjaergaard *et al.* (1990)[95]	21 post-menopausal women with recurrent cystitis; 10 active treatment 11 placebo	Oestradiol	Vaginal tablets	5 months	• No statistical difference in number of positive cultures between the two groups
Kirkengen *et al.* (1992)[96]	40 post-menopausal women with recurrent UTIs; 20 active treatment 20 placebo	Oestriol	Oral	12 weeks	• Both oestriol and placebo significantly reduced the incidence of UTIs ($p < 0.05$) • Oestriol was significantly more effective than placebo after 12 weeks ($p < 0.05$)
Raz and Stamm (1993)[97]	93 post-menopausal women with recurrent UTIs; 50 active treatment 43 placebo	Oestriol	Vaginal cream	8 months	• Significant reduction in the incidence of UTIs in treatment group compared with placebo group ($p < 0.001$)
Cardozo *et al.* (1998)[98]	72 post-menopausal women with recurrent UTIs; 36 active treatment 36 placebo	Oestriol	Oral	6 months' treatment; further 6 months' follow-up	• Urinary symptoms and incidence of UTIs reduced in both groups; oestriol no better than placebo
Eriksen 1999[99]	108 women with recurrent UTIs 53 active group 55 no treatment	Oestradiol	Estring (vaginal ring)	36 weeks for the active group; 36 weeks or until first recurrence for the controls	• Cumulative likelihood of remaining free of infection was 45% in active treatment group and 20% in control group ($p = 0.008$)

UTI, urinary tract infection

Oestrogen reverses the microbiological changes in the vaginal flora that occur after the menopause, an effect which enables it to be used for treatment or prophylaxis. Early small uncontrolled studies[92,93] using oral or vaginal oestrogen appeared to give promising results. For example, Brandberg and co-workers[94] used oral oestriol to treat 41 elderly women with recurrent UTI and showed that their vaginal flora was restored to the premenopausal type and they required fewer antibiotics. Subsequent randomized trials have shown rather mixed and largely disappointing benefits[95–98] (Table 76.4). Kirkengen and co-workers[96] randomized 40 elderly women with recurrent UTIs to receive either oral oestriol (3 mg per day for 4 weeks followed by 1 mg per day for 8 weeks) or matching placebo. There was no difference between oestriol and placebo after the first treatment period; however, after the second treatment period, oestriol was significantly better than placebo in reducing the incidence of UTIs.

A randomized, double-blind, placebo-controlled study of 93 post-menopausal women also showed that *intravaginal* oestriol cream prevented recurrent UTIs in women presenting with this problem.[97] MSU cultures were obtained at enrolment, monthly for 8 months and whenever urinary symptoms occurred. Changes in the vaginal pH and colonization with lactobacilli occurred within 1 month of the start of treatment in the oestriol group only, and the incidence of UTI in this group was significantly reduced compared with that in the placebo group (0.5 vs 5.9 episodes per patient per year). Unfortunately we were unable to repeat these results in a double-blind, placebo-controlled, study of *oral* oestriol in the prevention of recurrent UTI in elderly women.[98] Although both oestriol and placebo improved urinary symptoms during the trial, the incidence of UTI did not differ significantly between the two groups.

In the largest report to date, Eriksen[99] conducted a multicentre, randomized, open, parallel-group trial of 108 post-menopausal women with recurrent, symptomatic, bacteriologically confirmed UTIs. The women were randomly assigned to receive either Estring (7.5 μg oestradiol/24 hours)(Pharmacia & Upjohn) or no oestrogen treatment. After 36 weeks of study the cumulative likelihood of remaining free of infection was 45% in the women with the vaginal oestrogen is also supported by the HUT committee who concluded in their third report that it seemed to be of benefit when used in women with this problem[100].

CONCLUSIONS

Oestrogen has important physiological effects on the female lower urinary tract throughout adult life; fluctuations in its level produce symptomatic, histological and functional changes. The menopause and subsequent oestrogen deficiency have been implicated in the pathogenesis of a number of urogenital problems including incontinence, the urge syndrome and recurrent UTIs. Oestrogens do objectively improve urinary leakage when used alone to treat urinary incontinence but are more effective when given in combination with α-adrenergics. HRT does appear to improve irritative urinary symptoms of frequency and urgency, possibly by reversing urogenital atrophy. Treatment for several weeks or even months may be needed for maximum efficacy but the optimal route of delivery and duration of therapy remain to be determined. There is conflicting evidence regarding the benefits of oestrogen for prophylaxis against recurrent UTIs. Further studies are required before conclusions can be made about the role of oestrogen for this indication.

REFERENCES

1. Wilbush J. La Menespausie – the birth of a syndrome. *Maturitas* 1979; 1: 145–151

2. Aristotle. *Historia Animalium,* book VII c.350 BC. Creswell R (translator), London: George Bell and Sons, 1897

3. Research on the menopause in the 1990s. Report of a WHO Scientific Group. In: WHO Technical Report Series 866. Geneva, Switzerland: WHO, 1994

4. Hill K. The demography of the menopause. *Maturitas* 1996; 23: 113–127

5. Iosif CS, Batra S, Ek A. Estrogen receptors in the human female lower urinary tract. *Am J Obstet Gynecol* 1981; 141: 817–820

6. Blakeman PJ, Hilton P, Bulmer JN. Mapping oestrogen and progesterone receptors throughout the female lower urinary tract. *Neurourol Urodyn* 1996; 15: 324–325

7. Ingelman-Sundberg A, Rosen J, Gustafsson SA. Cytosol oestrogen receptors in urogenital tissues in stress incontinent women. *Acta Obstet Gynecol Scand* 1981; 60: 585–586

8. Smith P. Estrogens and the urogenital tract. *Acta Obstet Gynecol Scand* 1993; 72(Suppl): 1–26

9. Blakeman PJ, Hilton P, Bulmer JN. Oestrogen status and cell cycle activity in the female lower urinary tract. *Neurourol Urodyn* 1996; 15: 325–326

10. Samsioe G, Jansson I, Meelstrom D *et al.* Occurrence, nature and treatment of urinary incontinence in a 70 year old female population. *Maturitas* 1985; 7: 335–342

11. Smith PJB. The effect of oestrogens on bladder function. In: Campbell S (ed) *Management of the Menopause and Post-menopausal Years.* Lancaster: MTP, 1976; 291–298

12. McCallin PF, Taylor ES, Whitehead RW. A study of the changes in the urinary sediment during the menstrual cycle. *Am J Obstet Gynecol* 1950; 60: 64–74

13. Soloman C, Panagotopoulos P, Oppenheim A. The use of urinary sediment as an aid in endocrinological disorders in the female. *Am J Obstet Gynecol* 1958; 76: 56–60

14. Batra SC, Iosif CS. Progesterone receptors in the female lower urinary tract. *J Urol* 1987; 138: 1301–1304

15. Blakeman PJ, Hilton P, Bulmer JN. Androgen receptors in the female lower urinary tract. *Int Urogynecol J* 1997; 8: S54

16. Van Geelen JM, Doesburg WH, Thomas CMG. Urodynamic studies in the normal menstrual cycle: the relationship between hormonal changes during the menstrual cycle and the urethral pressure profile. *Am J Obstet Gynecol* 1981; 141: 384–392

17. Stanton SL, Kerr-Wilson R, Harris VG. The incidence of urological symptoms in normal pregnancy. *Br J Obstet Gynaecol* 1980; 87: 897–900

18. Cutner A, Carey A, Cardozo LD. Lower urinary tract symptoms in early pregnancy. *J Obstet Gynaecol* 1992; 12: 75–78

19. Chaliha C, Kalia V, Stanton SL *et al.* What does pregnancy and delivery do to bladder function? A urodynamic viewpoint. *Neurourol Urodyn* 1998; 17: 415–416

20. Cutner A. *The Lower Urinary Tract in Pregnancy.* MD thesis, University of London, 1993

21. Barlow DH, Cardozo LD, Francis RM *et al.* Urogenital ageing and its effect on sexual health in older British women. *Br J Obstet Gynaecol* 1997; 104: 87–91

22. Iosif CS, Bekassey Z. Prevalence of genito-urinary symptoms in the late menopause. *Acta Obstet Gynecol Scand* 1984; 63: 257–260

23. Cardozo LD, Tapp A, Versi E. The lower urinary tract in peri- and post-menopausal women. In: Samsioe G, Bonne Erickson P (eds) *The Urogenital Oestrogen Deficiency Syndrome.* Bagsverd, Denmark: Novo Industri AS, 1987; 10–17

24. Jolleys JV. Reported prevalence of urinary incontinence in a general practice. *Br Med J* 1988; 296: 1300–1302

25. Rekers H, Drogendijk AC, Valkenburg H *et al.* Urinary incontinence in women from 35 to 79 years of age: prevalence and consequences. *Eur J Obstet Gynecol Reprod Biol* 1992; 43: 229–234

26. Vetter NJ, Jones DA, Victor CR. Urinary incontinence in the elderly at home. *Lancet* 1981; 2: 1275–1277

27. Thomas TM, Plymat KR, Blannin J *et al.* Prevalence of urinary incontinence. *Br Med J* 1980; 281: 1243–1245

28. Hilton P. *Urethral Pressure Measurement by Micro Transducer: Observations on the Methodology, the Pathophysiology of Stress Incontinence and the Effects of Treatment in the Female.* MD thesis, University of Newcastle upon Tyne, UK, 1981

29. Kondo A, Kato K, Saito M *et al.* Prevalence of hand washing incontinence in females in comparison with stress and urge incontinence. *Neurourol Urodyn* 1990; 9: 330–331

30. Svanberg A. The gerontological and geriatric study in Göteborg, Sweden. *Acta Med Scand* 1977; 611: 1–37

31. Gjorup T, Hendriksen C, Lund E *et al.* Is growing old a disease? A study of the attitudes of elderly people to physical symptoms. *J Chron Dis* 1987; 40: 1095–1098

32. Swithinbank LV, Vestey S, Abrams P. Nocturnal polyuria in community dwelling women. *Neurourol Urodyn* 1998; 17: 314–315

33. Rud T, Anderson KE, Asmussen M *et al.* Factors maintaining the urethral pressure in women. *Invest Urol* 1980; 17: 343–347

34. Malone Lee J, Waheda I. The characterisation of detrusor contractile function in relation to old age. *Br J Urol* 1993; 72: 873–880

35. Collas DM, Malone Lee J. Age-associated changes in detrusor sensory function in women with lower urinary tract symptoms. *Int Urogynecol J* 1996; 7: 24–29

36. Wagg AS, Lieu PK, Ding YY. A urodynamic evaluation of age associated changes in urethral function in women with lower urinary tract symptoms. *J Urol* 1996; 156: 1984–1988

37. Brocklehurst JC. Ageing of the human bladder. *Geriatrics* 1972; 27: 154

38. Susset JG, Servot-Viguier D, Lamy F *et al.* Collagen in 155 human bladders. *Invest Urol* 1978; 16: 204–206

39. Perucchini D, DeLancey JOL, Patane L *et al.* The number and diameter of striated muscle fibres in the female urethra. *Neurourol Urodyn* 1997; 16: 405–406

40. Kolbl H, Strassegger H, Riis PA. Morphological and functional aspects of pelvic floor muscles in patients with pelvic relaxation and genuine stress incontinence. *Obstet Gynecol* 1989; 74: 789–795

41. Smith ARB, Hosker GL, Warrell DW. The role of partial denervation of the pelvic floor in the etiology of genito-urinary prolapse and stress incontinence of urine. *Br J Obstet Gynaecol* 1989; 96: 24–28

42. Allen RE, Warrell DW. The role of pregnancy and childbirth in the partial denervation of the pelvic floor. *Neurourol Urodyn* 1992; 6: 183–184

43. Abrams P, Blaivas JG, Stanton SL *et al.* The standardisation of terminology of lower urinary tract dysfunction. *Br J Obstet Gynaecol* 1990; 97: 1–16

44. Maggi A, Perez J. Role of female gonadal hormones in the CNS. *Life Sci* 1985; 37: 893–906

45. Smith SS. Hormones, mood and neurobiology – a summary. In: Berg G, Hammar M (eds) *The Modern Management of the Menopause.* Carnforth: Parthenon, 1993; 204

46. Schneider MA, Brotherton PL, Hailes J. The effect of exogenous oestrogens on depression in menopausal women. *Med J Aust* 1977; 2: 162–163

47. Sherwin BB. Affective changes with estrogen and androgen replacement therapy in surgically menopausal women. *J Affect Disord* 1988; 14: 177–187

48. Ditkoff EC, Crary WG, Cristo M. Estrogen improves psychological function in asymptomatic post-menopausal women. *Obstet Gynecol* 1991; 78: 991–995

49. Best NR, Rees MP, Barlow DH *et al.* Effect of estradiol implant on noradrenergic function and mood in menopausal subjects. *Psychoneuroendocrinology* 1992; 17: 87–93

50. Blok BFM, Holstege G. Androgen receptor immunoreactive neurons in the hypothalamic preoptic area project to the pontine micturition center in the male cat. *Neurourol Urodyn* 1998; 17: 404–405

51. Shapiro E. Effect of oestrogens on the weight and muscarinic receptor density of the rabbit bladder and urethra. *J Urol* 1986; 135: 1084–1087

52. Batra S, Anderson KE. Oestrogen-induced changes in muscarinic receptor density and contractile responses in the female rat urinary bladder. *Acta Physiol Scand* 1989; 137: 135–141

53. Elliott RA, Castleden CM, Miodrag A *et al.* The direct effects of diethylstilboestrol and nifedipine on the contractile responses of isolated human and rat detrusor muscles. *Eur J Clin Pharmacol* 1992; 43: 149–155

54. Diep N, Yokota T, Soo Choo M *et al.* Effect of estrogen supplementation of ovariectomized rats on micturition. *Neurourol Urodyn* 1998; 17: 405–406

55. Shenfield OZ, Blackmore PF, Morgan CW *et al.* Rapid effects of estradiol and progesterone on tone and spontaneous rhythmic contractions of the rabbit bladder. *Neurourol Urodyn* 1998; 17: 408–409

56. Elliott RA, Castleden CM, Miodrag A. The effect of *in vivo* oestrogen pretreatment on the contractile response of rat isolated detrusor muscle. *Br J Pharmacol* 1992; 107: 766–770

57. Fantl JA, Wyman JF, Anderson RL *et al.* Post-menopausal urinary incontinence: comparison between non-estrogen and estrogen supplemented women. *Obstet Gynecol* 1988; 71: 823–828

58. Elliott RA, Castleden CM. Effect of progestogens and oestrogens on the contractile response of rat detrusor muscle to electrical field stimulation. *Clin Sci* 1994; 87: 337–342

59. Burton G, Cardozo LD, Abdalla H *et al.* The hormonal effects on the lower urinary tract in 282 women with premature ovarian failure. *Neurourol Urodyn* 1992; 10: 318–319

60. Cutner A, Burton G, Cardozo LD *et al.* Does progesterone cause an irritable bladder? *Int Urogynecol J* 1993; 4: 261

61. Benness C, Gangar K, Cardozo LD *et al.* Do progestogens exacerbate urinary incontinence in women on HRT? *Neurourol Urodyn* 1991; 10: 316–318

62. Raz S, Ziegler M, Laine M. The effect of progesterone on the adrenergic receptors of the urethra. *Br J Urol* 1973; 45: 131–135

63. Bergman A, Karram MM, Bhatia NN. Changes in urethral cytology following estrogen administration. *Gynecol Obstet Invest* 1990; 29: 211–213

64. Hilton P, Stanton SL. The use of intravaginal oestrogen cream in genuine stress incontinence. *Br J Obstet Gynaecol* 1983; 90: 940–944

65. Bhatia NN, Bergman A, Karram MM *et al.* Effects of oestrogen on urethral function in women with urinary incontinence. *Am J Obstet Gynecol* 1989; 160: 176–181

66. Karram MM, Yeko TR, Sauer MV *et al.* Urodynamic changes following hormone replacement therapy in women with premature ovarian failure. *Obstet Gynecol* 1989; 74: 208–211

67. Ganger KF, Vyas S, Whitehead RW *et al.* Pulsatility index in the internal carotid artery in relation to transdermal oestradiol and time since the menopause. *Lancet* 1991; 338: 839–842

68. Jackson S, Vyas S. A double-blind, placebo controlled study of post-menopausal oestrogen replacement therapy and carotid artery pulsatility index. *Br J Obstet Gynaecol* 1998; 105: 408–412

69. Penotti M, Farina M, Sironi L *et al.* Long term effects of post-menopausal hormone replacement therapy on pulsatility index of internal carotid and middle cerebral arteries. *Menopause* 1997; 4: 101–104

70. Versi E, Cardozo LD. Urethral instability: diagnosis based on variations in the maximum urethral pressure in normal climacteric women. *Neurourol Urodyn* 1986; 5: 535–541

71. Jackson S, McDonnell C, James M *et al.* Is post-menopausal urethral blood flow affected by hormone replacement therapy? A placebo controlled pilot study. *Neurourol Urodyn* 1997; 16: 352–353

72. Screiter F, Fuchs P, Stockamp K. Estrogenic sensitivity of alpha receptors in the urethral musculature. *Urol Int* 1976; 31: 13–19

73. Jackson S, Avery N, Shepherd A *et al.* The effect of oestradiol on vaginal collagen in post-menopausal women with stress urinary incontinence. *Neurourol Urodyn* 1996; 15: 327–328

74. Rud T. The effects of estrogens and gestogens on the urethral pressure profile in urinary continent and stress incontinent women. *Acta Obstet Gynecol Scand* 1980; 59: 265–270

75. Salmon UL, Walter RI, Gast SH. The use of estrogen in the treatment of dysuria and incontinence in post-menopausal women. *Am J Obstet Gynecol* 1941; 14: 23–31

76. Jarvis GJ, Hall S, Stamp S *et al.* An assessment of urodynamic investigation in incontinent women. *Br J Obstet Gynaecol* 1980; 87: 184–190

77. Fantl JA, Cardozo LD, McClish DK *et al.* Estrogen therapy in the management of urinary incontinence in post-menopausal women: a meta-analysis. *Obstet Gynecol* 1994; 83: 12–18

78. Sultana CJ, Walters MD. Estrogen and urinary incontinence in women. *Maturitas* 1995; 20: 129–138

79. Fantl JA, Bump RC, Robinson D *et al.* Efficacy of estrogen supplementation in the treatment of urinary incontinence. *Obstet Gynecol* 1996; 88: 745–749

80. Jackson S, Shepherd A, Abrams P. The effect of oestradiol on objective urinary leakage in post-menopausal stress

incontinence; a double blind placebo controlled trial. *Neurourol Urodyn* 1996; 15: 322–323

81. Jackson S, Shepherd A, Abrams P. Does oestrogen supplementation improve the symptoms of post-menopausal urinary stress incontinence? A double blind placebo controlled trial. *Neurourol Urodyn* 1997; 16: 350–351

82. Beisland HO, Fossberg E, Moer A *et al.* Urethral insufficiency in post-menopausal females: treatment with phenylpropanolamine and estriol separately and in combination. *Urol Int* 1984; 39: 211–216

83. Hilton P, Tweddel AL, Mayne C. Oral and intravaginal estrogens alone and in combination with alpha adrenergic stimulation in genuine stress incontinence. *Int Urogynecol J* 1990; 12: 80–86

84. Walter S, Wolf H, Barlebo H *et al.* Urinary incontinence in post-menopausal women treated with oestrogen. *Urol Int* 1978; 33: 135–143

85. Cardozo LD, Rekers H, Tapp A *et al.* Oestriol in the treatment of post-menopausal urgency: a multicentre study. *Maturitas* 1993; 18: 47–53

86. Benness C, Wise BG, Cutner A *et al.* Does low dose vaginal estradiol improve frequency and urgency in post-menopausal women? *Int Urogynecol J* 1992; 3: 281

87. Nilsson K, Heimer G. Low dose oestradiol in the treatment of urogenital oestrogen deficiency – a pharmacokinetic and pharmacodynamic study. *Maturitas* 1992; 15: 121–127

88. Sandford JP. Urinary tract symptoms and infection. *Ann Rev Med* 1975; 26: 485–905

89. Boscia JA, Kaye D. Asymptomatic bacteria in the elderly. *Infect Dis Clin North Am* 1987; 1: 893–903

90. Horan MA, Parker SG. Infections, aging and host response. In: Horan MA, Little RA (eds) *Injury in the Aging.* Cambridge: Cambridge University Press, 1998; 126–146

91. Hextall A, Hooper R, Cardozo LD *et al.* Does the menopause influence the risk of bacteriuria? *Int J Urogynecol* 2001 (in press)

92. Parsons CL, Schmidt JD. Control of recurrent lower urinary tract infections in post-menopausal women. *J Urol* 1982; 128: 1224–1226

93. Privette M, Cade R, Peterson J *et al.* Prevention of recurrent urinary tract infections in post-menopausal women. *Nephron* 1988; 50: 24–27

94. Brandberg A, Mellstrom D, Samsioe G. Low dose oral oestriol treatment in elderly women with urogenital infections. *Acta Obstet Gynecol Scand* 1987; 140: 33–38

95. Kjaergaard B, Walter S, Knudsen A *et al.* Treatment with low dose vaginal estradiol in post-menopausal women. A double blind controlled trial. *Ugeskr Laeger* 1990; 152: 658–659

96. Kirkengen AL, Anderson P, Gjersoe E *et al.* Oestriol in the prophylactic treatment of recurrent urinary tract infections in post-menopausal women. *Scand J Prim Health Care* 1992; 10: 139–142

97. Raz R, Stamm WE. A controlled trial of intravaginal estriol in post-menopausal women with recurrent urinary tract infections. *New Engl J Med* 1993; 329: 753–756

98. Cardozo LD, Benness C, Abbott D. Low dose oestrogen prophylaxis for recurrent urinary tract infections in elderly women. *Br J Obstet Gynaecol* 1998; 105: 403–407

99. Eriksen B. A randomized, open, parallel group-study on the preventive effect of an estradiol-releasing vaginal ring (Estring) on recurrent urinary tract infections in postmenopausal women. *Am J Obstet Gynecol* 1999; 180: 1072–1079

100. Cardozo L, Lose G, McClish D *et al.* A systematic review of oestrogens for recurrent urinary tract infections. *Int Urogynecol J* 2001 (in press)

77

Anal incontinence

L. Brubaker

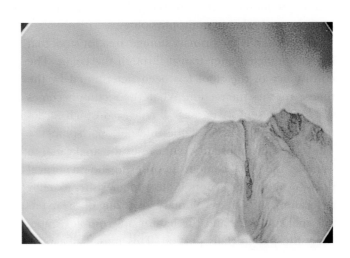

INTRODUCTION

Many challenges face the woman who suffers from anal incontinence. A major barrier to treatment is the embarrassing nature of the disorder itself, which causes most patients and their physicians to avoid discussion. Physicians may have expertise in other areas of the pelvis, but may have limited knowledge or ability in solving symptoms of anal incontinence. The symptoms of anal incontinence can include involuntary loss of gas, liquid or solid stool. Obviously, a high frequency of symptoms is particularly disturbing, but less frequent loss of solid stool can also be devastating. Understandably, the loss of anal contents during intimate times can adversely affect a woman's quality of life.

Physicians, nurse midwives and other pelvic health providers have an important opportunity to minimize anal sphincter disruption during vaginal delivery. In addition, the healthcare team can facilitate early recognition and treatment for symptomatic patients by routinely enquiring about pelvic symptoms. Although some health providers may not feel trained to provide care for anal incontinence, appropriate referral to a colleague with interest and expertise in this area can aid the patient and provide prompt resolution of her symptoms. This chapter will focus on the prevention, diagnosis and clinically relevant treatment of anal incontinence.

CLINICALLY RELEVANT ANATOMY AND NEUROPHYSIOLOGY

There are fascinating chapters and even whole textbooks on the anatomy and physiology of the lower gastrointestinal tract. Fortunately, general clinical care can be rendered with a working knowledge of the anatomy and relevant neurophysiology.

The rectum is the primary storage area for stool that has accumulated after transit through the colon. The consistency of the stool has been determined by the time is reaches the rectum. When the rectum becomes distended, a sensory message is conveyed which causes momentary relaxation of the internal anal sphincter. This critically important event causes the anal canal to 'sample' the rectal contents in order to allow a cortical decision about defecation. If the woman wishes to defer defecation, she causes voluntary squeezing of the external anal sphincter and the levator ani complex, especially the puborectalis portion. This muscular activity

relocates the sampled rectal bolus up and out of the anal canal, returning it to the rectum for storage until further peristalsis occurs. When it is the right time and place for defecation, these voluntary muscles cease firing, relaxing completely, and a brief initial Valsalva manoeuvre causes movement of the rectal bolus into the anal canal for expulsion.

This skill of deferred defecation, so essential to our modern way of living, depends on many important features:

- The continence mechanism works best when the stool transit time is within a normal range – even otherwise continent women may experience anal incontinence during severe diarrhoea which simply overwhelms the continence system.
- The storage area in the rectum requires the rectal wall to be distensible, compliant and capable of sending a sensory message.
- The voluntary muscles should be contracting during faecal storage and must be in the anatomically correct position to allow an acute anorectal angle, so that the faecal bolus is supported over the levator plate, and not directly over the anal canal.
- The external anal sphincter should be circumferentially intact throughout its length.
- The neuromuscular integrity of the smooth and skeletal muscles is essential for optimal function.
- The integrity of the outflow system itself needs to be intact (e.g. devoid of fistula, etc.).

These simple concepts can be points of controversy for scholars in this area. The origins and current knowledge of pelvic muscles are areas of considerable debate; similarly, there is some indecision about the innervation of the levator ani. Although these are fascinating areas for scholars of anatomy and neuroanatomy, the woman who suffers from a symptom such as faecal soiling is more concerned with resolution of symptoms. Thus, these scholarly debates will be put aside for this chapter, and clinical terms, albeit arbitrary, will be used to convey concepts important for patient care.

AETIOLOGY OF COMMON CAUSES FOR ANAL INCONTINENCE

The aetiology of symptoms can be clarified using questions designed to assess the common causes for anal incontinence. When a woman is unable to sense a faecal bolus and experiences insensible passage of gas or stool, disorders such as sensory abnormality of the rectal wall or more global neural problems become likely. When a woman senses an urge to defecate but is unable to defer passage of gas or stool, the voluntary muscle systems, including the external anal sphincter, become suspect. Symptoms that are present only during bouts of diarrhoea suggest an underlying transit disorder which may be amenable to treatment. Thus, the circumstances of anal loss, the consistency of the lost material (gas, liquid or solid) and the presence or absence of sensation are important first-line questions. Many clinical algorithms for treatment of faecal incontinence suggest early, empirical treatment with bulking agents, predominately dietary fibre. Fibre promotes a bulkier stool, which may enhance rectal sensation. Additionally, increased fibre content may cause liquid stool to adhere together, occasionally slowing abnormally fast colonic transit. Unfortunately, many patients and providers have a poor understanding of normal fibre requirements. Typically, intake of dietary fibre should be 25–30 g per day; however, this intake may be difficult to achieve given the calorie-restricted diets that many women follow. Although rigorous attention to dietary sources is possible, it is frequently necessary to use some form of fibre supplement. Many formulations are available, including tablets, wafers, bars, and powder that dissolves in juice.

In the more acute post-partum setting, anatomical anal sphincter disruption should be considered. In a landmark study using anal ultrasonography before and after delivery, Sultan[1] demonstrated an extraordinarily high rate of undetected sphincter rupture in primiparas. In addition, other investigators have documented abnormalities in anal pressure[2,3] and electrodiagnostic parameters. These studies cause concern and may leave the obstetric provider wondering about prevention, natural history and intervention for such damage. These topics will be discussed later in this chapter.

EVALUATION TECHNIQUES

As with virtually every clinical problem, a systematic framework for evaluation facilitates appropriate diagnosis and logical treatment. Age-appropriate gastrointestinal cancer testing should be up to date. The history should include onset, circumstances and contents of anal loss. Prior treatment efforts, both non-surgical and surgical, should be reviewed. Other associated pelvic symptoms should be assessed as anal incontinence frequently coexists with other pelvic abnormalities of support and/or function. The general urogynaecological history is reviewed elsewhere.[4] On the basis of the history, the physician should formulate a mental list of likely diagnoses. For ambulatory women with a normal bowel this usually includes anatomical anal sphincter disruption, anatomical outflow disruption (fistulae), abnormal anorectal sensation, abnormal rectal compliance or abnormal transit. Table 77.1 lists the symptoms frequently reported for these diagnoses.

Physical examination

The physical examination includes the entire pelvic floor. The integrity of the sacral innervation should be ascertained by testing the voluntary and reflex motor

Table 77.1. *Symptoms for common causes of anal incontinence in ambulatory women*

Differential diagnosis	Symptoms	
	Able to feel urge to defecate?	Able to defer voluntary defecation?
Anal sphincter disruption	Typically, yes	May be impaired, depending on utility of levator muscles
Fistula	Typically, yes	Yes, but soils between voluntary defecation
Sensation	No, or poorly	No; unable to sense process until anal contents outside body
Compliance	Variable	Variable, typically yes
Transit	Typically, yes	Variable; diarrhoea difficult to defer; constipation easy to defer

activity, as well as sensation in the sacral dermatomes. Screening that reveals abnormalities may be followed by more accurate diagnostic testing. The anatomical integrity of the external anal sphincter can be assessed grossly by palpation. Sphincter disruption is frequently associated with a loss of radial skin folds over the areas of muscle loss. This physical sign is extremely helpful when prior sphincter and/or perineal surgery has been minimal. With multiple previous attempts at repair, this physical finding may become more difficult to interpret and alternative diagnostic techniques are required.

In addition to the routine parts of a gynaecological examination, the speculum part of the examination should look specifically for traces of stool in the vaginal vault, which would raise suspicion of a fistula. In the post-partum woman the likely sites of fistulae are along the line of the prior episiotomy. Fistulae at other sites may be present in women with an abnormal bowel (e.g. Crohn's disease, prior pelvic radiation treatment). Occasionally, this examination for occult fistulae must be performed under anaesthesia.

The bimanual examination should search for standard causes of pelvic pathology. Beyond visceral abnormalities, it is important to determine the symmetry and status of the levator muscle as well as the baseline tone and voluntary squeeze activity of the anal sphincter itself. Clinical evaluation by digital examination is generally the first approach, whereas quantitative assessments may be required for complex patients or in research settings. Following the history and physical examination, a single likely diagnosis should be formulated. Table 77.2 lists the techniques for screening examinations and 'gold-standard' diagnostic tests.

Anal ultrasonography

Anal ultrasonography is a valuable tool for determining the anatomical integrity of the anal sphincter. Before the advent of this technique, anal sphincter mapping was widely performed using electromyography (EMG) to localize the limits of the 'healthy' muscle and map areas of scarring. Although this technique is effective, it is understandably painful for the patient. Concentric anal ultrasonography probes allow full visualization of the anal sphincter and can facilitate an understanding of the anatomical extent of sphincter disruption. Additional information regarding the smooth muscle portions of the sphincter can be obtained. This information is not obtained by needle mapping because smooth muscle is not studied during clinical EMG examinations. Knowledge of the ultrasound appearance of the normal sphincter is a prerequisite for interpreting images that may show abnormalities. As with all imaging procedures, the patient's orientation in the specific image must be known. There are variations across specialties and geographical regions, with some investigators using a side-lying position (defects on the image typically appear at the 3:00 position) and others using the dorsolithotomy position (defects on the image typically appear at the 12:00 position). It is well documented that anal sphincter ultrasonography is superior to clinical examination for detection of anal sphincter disruption in the post-partum setting. However, there is no evidence supporting the routine use of this modality in other settings when anal sphincter disruption is historically consistent and clinically apparent.

Anal manometry was used widely for many years but has become less popular of late; some investigators still

	Screening technique	Gold-standard diagnostic test
Anatomical sphincter disruption	Physical examination	Anal ultrasonography
Fistula	Office examination	Examination under anaesthesia; possibly imaging
Anal sensation	Questions about faecal urge	Manometry
Sacral innervation	Clinical sacral reflexes	Electrodiagnostic: quantitative sacral reflexes, EMG
Pudendal nerve integrity	None	Electrodiagnosis: needle EMG and latency studies

Table 77.2. *Screening examinations and 'gold-standard' diagnostic tests*

EMG, electromyography

strongly advocate the routine use of this modality, however.[5,6] Manometry is essential in determining whether the normal anorectal inhibitory reflex is present. This reflex occurs when there is sufficient rectal distension and the anal sphincter relaxes to allow sampling of the rectal contents. Although this reflex is typically absent in Hirschsprung's disease, the absence of this reflex would be an unusual abnormality in ambulatory women with anal incontinence. Manometry can provide additional information about the appropriateness of rectal sensation and compliance, as well as the power of the sphincter at rest and with voluntary activation (squeeze pressures). Voluntary sphincter activity can usually be estimated by digital examination.

Electrodiagnostic tests

Electrodiagnostic techniques are being described more frequently in articles on anal incontinence, particularly with regard to outcomes of sphincteroplasty. The pudendal nerve terminal motor latency (PNTML) test is a variant of a nerve conduction time test. The correct performance and interpretation of the test requires basic knowledge of the principles of electrodiagnostic medicine.[7] Standard values for PNTML have not been clearly established across the clinically relevant age span; because of the difficulty in obtaining standard data, most investigators extrapolate from a small data pool obtained from middle-aged women. This issue is critical for the correct interpretation of individual test results, as well as larger data sets reported in research publications. The most problematic portion of the PNTML test is that a normal value does not necessarily indicate a lack of neuropathy, since the test measures only the fastest conducting nerve fibre. Although a decrease in the amplitude of the motor response may be used as a clue to abnormality, variations in recording technique may affect the reproducibility of the amplitude. In addition, there are many statistical concerns in analysing and reporting these measures.

Many investigators augment the PNTML studies with motor unit potential morphology, typically obtained with a concentric EMG needle. These studies provide more direct evidence of neuropathy or, rarely, myopathy. For neurophysiological testing, a composite of multiple tests provides the most reasonable clinical interpretation. Rarely should a single value be interpreted as abnormal without reproduction and corroboration by ancillary tests. These tests have not gained widespread clinical use and there is an unmet demand for equipment and expertise in this rapidly evolving field.

CLINICAL APPROACH FOR COMMON CAUSES

Acute obstetric management

Obstetricians must meet the daunting task of balancing the needs of the unborn fetus with the maternal concerns, including immediate and long-term pelvic floor damage. There are many perspectives in the literature on the best way to accomplish this task. Maternal–fetal specialists have an understandable bias toward fetal well-being, with a lesser appreciation of the health of the maternal pelvic floor. Urogynaecology, colorectal and urology specialists frequently see the most symptomatic post-partum women and may therefore overinterpret the risks of vaginal delivery by focusing on the numerator, but not the denominator, of the problem. Retrospective epidemiological studies are plagued with problems of patient recall, lack of charted information and poor characterization of the problem under study. Thus, recommendations in this realm await large clinical trials with well-studied outcome measures that are recorded over many years.

An obstetrician is often the first physician to diagnose anatomical anal sphincter disruption following vaginal delivery. The literature has many reports of deteriorating anal sphincter function following vaginal delivery. These examples demonstrate that even when the gross anatomical components of the sphincter remain intact, damage to the neural elements may cause symptoms such as faecal urgency and flatal incontinence to occur. Although there are no recommendations for avoidance of these types of symptoms *post partum*, expert opinion is virtually unanimous that avoidance of sphincter rupture is preferable to rupture with any form of repair.[8–11] Techniques to minimize the risk of anal sphincter rupture include avoidance of midline episiotomy, substituting a mediolateral incision, or keeping the perineum intact. Most obstetricians use some form of perineal incision for instrumented deliveries, although Klein *et al.* proffer data with short-term follow-up that question this dogma.[12]

Repair of sphincter and lacerations

The optimal repair for a torn anal sphincter is debatable. However, there is general agreement on several basic tenets:

- The repair should provide adequate length and approximation of the full-length of the sphincteric complex, including internal and external anal sphincters. Some investigators have demonstrated that symptomatic patients may have ultrasound evidence of persistent disruption following acute sphincter repair.[13–15] The recommendation for a complete repair is in keeping with the anatomy of the torn muscle and its underlying connective tissue and mucosal structures.
- Experts agree that infection is a chief threat to the long-term health of the anatomical repair. Thus, antibiotics are frequently used, although there is no controlled clinical trial supporting this recommendation.
- Finally, experts recognize that an intact anatomical repair does not necessarily equate with absence of symptoms, probably because of concomitant neural insult.[16–18]

The end-to-end repair technique has been the standard for many decades. Some investigators feel that this simple technique does not hold up well under the known tension of the repair and have recommended an alternative, overlapping technique.[11,15,19,20] However, there is scant data available to document the effectiveness of any technique as a first-line choice for repair. Strict adherence to surgical techniques of careful tissue handling and haemostasis are essential. It is prudent to use antibiotics and to avoid post-repair constipation or impaction.

On occasion, despite optimal care, a delivery-induced sphincter rupture will break down following repair. This generally occurs within days to weeks of the initial repair. Anecdotal reports suggest that patients with impending breakdown report more episiotomy-site drainage and pain. It may be difficult for a new mother to know what to expect and what is normal following episiotomy repair with sphincteroplasty. It is therefore prudent to perform timely physical examinations on any patient who initiates contact regarding unusual perineal symptoms in this setting.

If there is suspicion that the repair site is infected, treatment with antibiotics and local hygiene measures should be initiated immediately and the patient closely followed-up. When breakdown occurs despite attempts at early recognition and intervention, the physician will be faced with the prospect of a discouraged patient who must face repeat repair at some point. The timing of this repair is debated, but experts agree on several key concepts. Prior to repeat repair, the tissue should be non-friable and free of infection, and patient support and care of the newborn baby should be assessed. Success with early repair has been reported[21–23] with an acceptably low risk of fistula complications.

Repairs of third-degree and fourth-degree lacerations may heal incompletely, leaving a symptomatic fistulous tract. While upsetting to the patient, repair of these fistulae should be delayed until there is no infection or inflammation. The repair of fistulae is discussed later in this chapter. However, in the post-partum setting, assurance of anal sphincteric integrity should be part of the routine preoperative evaluation in order to avoid the unhappy result of an excellent fistula repair that unmasks an inadequate anal sphincter repair.

CHRONIC ANAL INCONTINENCE

Although post-partum sphincter disruption is a frequent cause of anal incontinence in women, there are other causes. Some patients may be at increased risk for clinical symptoms later in life based on occult post-partum damage or they may have no such predisposing factors.

Medically, disorders that alter stool consistency and/or transit may cause a woman with an otherwise intact anal sphincteric mechanism to develop symptoms of anal incontinence. Anecdotally it appears that all but the most extreme of these stool alterations can be tolerated by patients without occult damage. However, in the presence of previous damage, symptoms may occur following procedures such as cholecystectomy, which frequently causes loose stool, or medications that have diarrhoea-like side effects. The temporal onset of the symptoms is an important clue to these medically predisposing situations. Often medications can be altered to avoid these troublsome side effects.

When a woman reports diarrhoea-like stool, an appropriate medical work-up for bowel pathogens and neoplasms should be considered. The diagnosis of irritable bowel syndrome is one of exclusion that should be made in consultation with a primary or specialty bowel physician. These patients may respond to oral agents that mechanically slow transit. Over-the-counter medications are frequently used.

The power of the anal sphincter and levator ani muscle is essential for deferring stool leakage. When this muscle has adequate innervation, muscle strength can be augmented with a progressive exercise programme. It is often helpful to have a physiotherapist as a dedicated member of the pelvic floor team. While 'adequate innervation' is an interesting research topic, this can be determined clinically by asking the patient to demonstrate voluntary muscle contraction. Progressive exercise programmes should enhance strength, endurance and timing of muscle use.

Surgery may be considered for women with anatomical distortions and for those with severe symptoms who require various forms of faecal diversion. Anal sphincteroplasty is frequently considered for a woman who reports symptoms remote from any form of pelvic trauma yet is found to have sphincter disruption on physical examination. Of course, the interesting question is what mechanism has kept them continent all the time that the anal sphincter was not intact. Despite the anatomical abnormality, it is prudent to review thoroughly the history and physical examination for other aetiologies that may be treated non-surgically. Similarly, the neuromuscular status of the sphincter should be clarified before repair in these settings, given the inexorable neuromuscular decline with ageing.

The role of faecal diversion to protect a fresh repair is evolving. While diverting colostomy was frequently performed before or during sphincteroplasty by some investigators[14,24-25] others do not use this except for complicated, repeat repairs.[26,27] Sphincteroplasty in this setting must follow several surgical principles. The edges of the sphincter must be identified and mobilized, taking care to avoid further injury to the inferior haemorrhoidal nerve, which approaches the muscle laterally. Any rectal mucosal defects should be repaired. The overlapping technique, usually without excision of intervening scarring, is currently favoured by surgeons[14,26,28,29] (Fig. 77.1). Rarely, a patient may present many years after vaginal delivery with a cloacal-like distortion. The Noble–Mengert–Fish procedure[31] and the Warren flap[32] are traditional layered approaches for these repairs.

Rectovaginal fistulae can complicate episiotomy repair, gynaecological or anorectal surgery, or may

occur in an abnormal bowel. When the fistula involves the abnormal bowel (e.g. radiation damage or neoplasm) or the upper half of the rectovaginal septum, colostomy and transabdominal repair should be seriously considered.[33,34] Transabdominal repairs are beyond the scope of this chapter.

The approach to the fistulous tract may be transvaginal, transperineal or transanal. These approaches share the need for preoperative bowel preparation, which includes a clear liquid diet for 48 hours, mechanical cleansing and antibiotics. The common rectovaginal fistula is simple, low and small (< 2.5 cm in diameter). Key surgical principles for repair include isolation of the fistulous tract with wide mobilization of the surrounding viscera and closure in anatomical layers. Additional tissues (e.g. labial fat pads) can be mobilized to provide layers, although this is rarely necessary in a primary repair of a simple fistula. By providing a minimum of 2 cm of free tissue adjacent to the fistula margins, the surgeon optimizes the chance of a successful tension-free closure.

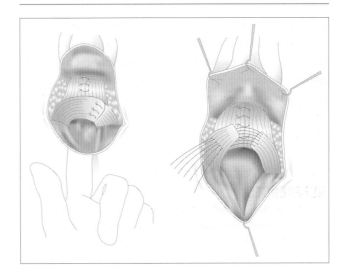

Figure 77.1. *Overlapping sphincteroplasty. Six mattress sutures of 2/0 polyglycolic acid are placed to bring each fibrous end as far as possible to the opposite side. Three sutures are placed in each end of the sphincter. The sutures should be placed so that the sphincter can be tightened to allow the entrance of just the tip of the index finger into the anal canal. The sutures are then tied, completing the wrap. At this time, any tears that have occurred in either the vaginal or the rectal mucosa should be meticulously repaired with fine chromic catgut sutures.*

An alternative to a simple layered closure is a group of anterior rectal wall advancement procedures. These procedures involve mobilizing the anterior wall from the perineum to well above the fistulous site, pulling the rectal wall down below the perineal skin and excising the excess wall.[35] Modifications of the original approach have included mobilizing only a trapezoidal portion of the anterior rectal wall.

SUMMARY

Anal incontinence may present as an acute or long-term consequence of vaginal delivery. Occult injury to the gross anatomical integrity and the delicate neuromuscular control of the sphincter appear frequently. Other less frequent aetiologies include infection, neoplasm and an intrinsically abnormal bowel. Careful assessment of the interactions of stool consistency and transit and anatomical integrity of the sphincteric mechanism typically provide a working diagnosis. Further tests to clarify the diagnosis may be considered, depending on the risk–benefit ratio for the individual patient and the proposed therapy. Simple, non-surgical interventions such as dietary modification and muscle rehabilitation may be initiated in appropriate patients without extensive evaluation. Risks and complications understandably increase with surgical intervention and additional testing is often warranted. Consultation with an interested specialist may be helpful for women with refractory symptoms or complex or recurrent disorders.

REFERENCES

1. Sultan AH, Kamm MA, Hudson CN *et al.* Anal-sphincter disruption during vaginal delivery. *N Engl J Med* 1993; 329: 1905–1911

2. Tetzschner T, Sorensen M, Lose G *et al.* Anal and urinary incontinence in women with obstetric sphincter rupture. *Br J Obstet Gynaecol* 1996; 103: 1034–1040

3. Uustal Fornell EK, Berg G, Hallbook O *et al.* Clinical consequences of anal sphincter rupture during vaginal delivery. *J Am Coll Surg* 1996; 183: 553–558

4. Brubaker L. Initial assessment: the history in women with pelvic floor problems. *Clin Obstet Gynecol* 1998; 41: 657–662

5. Rao SS, Patel RS. How useful are manometric tests of anorectal function in the management of defecation disorders? *Am J Gastroenterol* 1997; 92: 469–475

6. Falk PM, Blatchford GJ, Cali RL *et al.* Transanal ultrasound and manometry in the evaluation of faecal incontinence. *Dis Colon Rectum* 1994; 37: 468–472

7. Brubaker L, Saclarides TJ (eds) *The Female Pelvic Floor: Disorders of Function and Support.* Philadelphia: F. A. Davis, 1996

8. DeLancey JOL, Toglia MR, Perucchini D. Internal and external anal sphincter anatomy as it relates to midline obstetric lacerations. *Obstet Gynecol* 1997; 90: 924–927

9. Engel AF, Kamm MA, Sultan AH *et al.* Anterior anal sphincter repair in patients with obstetric trauma. *Br J Surg* 1994; 81: 1231–1234

10. Kamm MA. Obstetric damage and faecal incontinence. *Lancet* 1994; 344: 730–733

11. Sultan AH. Anal incontinence after childbirth. *Curr Opin Obstet Gynecol* 1997; 9: 320–324

12. Klein MC, Janssen PA, MacWilliam L *et al.* Determinants of vaginal-perineal integrity and pelvic floor functioning in childbirth. *Am J Obstet Gynecol* 1997; 176: 403–410

13. Nielsen MB, Dammegaard L, Pedersen JF. Endosonographic assessment of the anal sphincter after surgical reconstruction. *Dis Colon Rectum* 1994; 37: 434–438

14. Sitzler PJ, Thomson JP. Overlap repair of damaged anal sphincter. A single surgeon's series. *Dis Colon Rectum* 1996; 39: 1356–1360

15. Ternent CA, Shashidharan M, Blatchford GJ *et al.* Transanal ultrasound and anorectal physiology findings affecting continence after sphincteroplasty. *Dis Colon Rectum* 1997; 40: 462–467

16. Jacobs PPM, Scheuer M, Kuijpers JHC *et al.* Obstetrical faecal incontinence. Role of pelvic floor denervation and results of delayed sphincter repair. *Dis Colon Rectum* 1990; 33: 494–497

17. Simmang C, Birnbaum EH, Kodner IJ *et al.* Anal sphincter reconstruction in the elderly: does advancing age affect outcome? *Dis Colon Rectum* 1994; 37: 1065–1069

18. Sangwan YP, Coller JA, Barrett RC *et al.* Unilateral pudendal neuropathy. Impact on outcome of anal sphincter repair. *Dis Colon Rectum* 1996; 39: 686–689

19. Wexner SD, Gonzalez-Padron A, Rius J *et al.* Stimulated gracilis neosphincter operation. Initial experience, pitfalls and complications. *Dis Colon Rectum* 1996; 39: 957–964

20. Nielsen MB, Hauge C, Rasmussen OO *et al.* Anal endosonographic findings in the follow up of primarily sutured sphincteric ruptures. *Br J Surg* 1992; 79: 104–106

21. Hauth JC, Gilstrap LC 3rd, Ward SC *et al.* Early repair of an external sphincter ani muscle and rectal mucosal dehiscence. *Obstet Gynecol* 1986; 67: 806–809

22. Hankins GD, Hauth JC, Gilstrap LC 3rd *et al.* Early repair of episiotomy dehiscence. *Obstet Gynecol* 1990; 75: 48–51

23. Arona AJ, al-Marayati L, Grime DA *et al.* Early secondary repair of third- and fourth-degree perineal lacerations after outpatient wound preparation. *Obstet Gynecol* 1995; 86: 294–296

24. Parks AG, McPartlin JF. Late repair of injuries of the anal sphincter. *Proc Roy Soc Med* 1971; 64: 1187–1189

25. Yoshioka K, Keighley MRB. Critical assessment of the quality of continence after postanal repair for faecal incontinence. *Br J Surg* 1989; 76: 1054–1057

26. Fleshman JW, Peters WR, Shemesh EI *et al.* Anal sphincter reconstruction: anterior overlapping muscle repair. *Dis Colon Rectum* 1991; 34: 739–743

27. Fleshman JW, Kodner IJ, Fry RD *et al.* Anal incontinence. In: Zuidema GD, Condon RE (eds) *Shackleford's Surgery of the Alimentary Tract, Volume IV: Colon.* Philadelphia: W. B. Saunders, 1996; 386–401

28. Beart RW, Block GE. Anal incontinence. In: Block GE, Mossa AR (eds) *Operative Colorectal Surgery.* Philadelphia: W.B. Saunders, 1994; 417–427

29. Corman ML. Anal incontinence. *Colon and Rectal Surgery,* 3rd edn. Philadelphia: J. B. Lippincott, 1993; 188–261

30. Thorson AG. Surgical repair of anal sphincters following injury. In: Fielding LP, Goldberg SM (eds) *Rob and Smith's Operative Surgery, Surgery of the Colon, Rectum and Anus.* Oxford: Butterworth–Heinemann, 1993; 747

31. Noble GH. A new operation for complete laceration of the perineum designed for the purpose of eliminating danger of infection from the rectum. *Trans Am Gynecol Soc* 1902; 27: 357–363

32. Warren JC. A new method of operation for the relief of rupture of the perineum through the sphincter and rectum. *Trans Am Gynecol Soc* 1882; 7: 322–330

33. Schrock TR. Rectovaginal fistula. In: Block GE, Mossa AR (eds) *Operative Colorectal Surgery.* Philadelphia: W. B. Saunders, 1994; 429–443

34. Tsang CBS, Rothenberger DA. Rectovaginal fistulas: therapeutic options. *Surg Clin N Am* 1997; 77: 95–114

35. Mengert WG, Fish SA. Anterior rectal wall advancement. Technic [sic] for repair of complete perineal laceration and rectovaginal fistula. *Obstet Gynecol* 1955; 5: 262–267

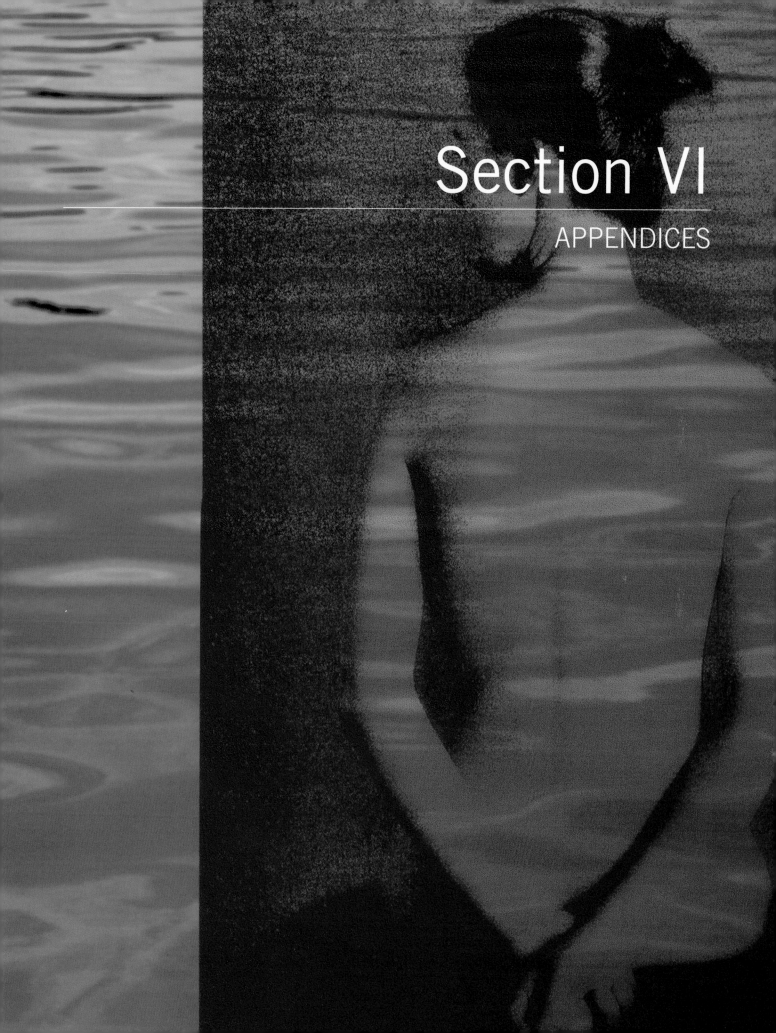

Section VI

APPENDICES

78

Outcome measures in women with lower urinary tract symptoms

G. Lose

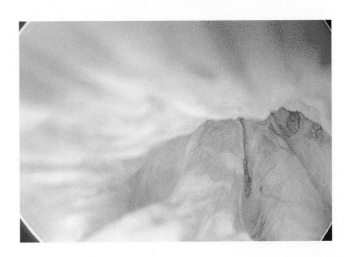

INTRODUCTION

Assessment of the clinical outcome of intervention in women with lower urinary tract symptoms (LUTS) is impaired by the lack of standardization and unclear reliability of many outcome measures. Generally there is a need to improve the methodological quality of outcome studies.[1,2] Consequently, at the moment it is very difficult to assess the effects of various types of intervention and to compare the results of studies.

MULTIDIMENSIONAL PHENOMENA

Disorders or health conditions such as LUTS represent multidimensional phenomena with far-reaching effects that may be quantified within various areas or domains. The complex interaction between different domains can be described by the World Health Organization (WHO) International Classification of Impairments, Disabilities and Handicaps (ICIDH)-2 disease model, which offers a coherent view of different dimensions of health at biological and social levels[3] (Fig. 78.1).

Disablement is seen as an interaction/complex relationship between the health condition and contextual factors (i.e. environmental and personal factors). The interaction works in both directions, and even the presence of the consequences may modify the health condition itself. One may experience impairment without activity or participation being limited.

The ICIDH-2 classification provides a common framework for understanding and communicating the different dimensions of disablement and health, and permits evaluation of outcomes in different cultures.

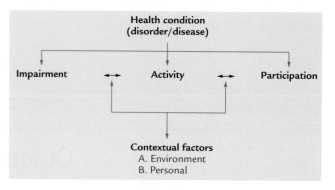

Figure 78.1. *Current understanding of interactions within the WHO ICIDH-2 model. Definitions:* **Health condition** *– an alteration or attribute of the health status of an individual that may lead to distress, interference with daily activities, or contact with health services; it may be a disease (acute or chronic), disorder, injury or trauma, or reflect other health-related states such as pregnancy, ageing, stress, congenital abnormality or genetic predisposition.* **Impairment** *– a loss or abnormality of a body structure or of a physiological or psychological function.* **Activity** *– the nature and extent of functioning at the whole-person level. Activities may be limited in nature, duration and quality.* **Participation** *– the nature and extent of a person's involvement in life situations in relationship to impairments, activities, health conditions and contextual factors. Participation may be restricted in nature, duration and quality.* **Contextual factors** *– the complete background to a person's life and living, in terms of external environmental factors and internal personal factors. (Arrows mean 'may lead to'). (From ref. 3.)*

Table 78.1. *Outcome measures within different domains according to the ICS recommendations*	
I The patient's observations (symptoms)	• General or condition-specific
II Quantification of symptoms (e.g. urine loss)	• Diary (frequency/volume chart) • Pad-weighing tests
III Clinician's observations	• Pelvic muscle activity • Uroflowmetry • Pressure–flow study • Electromyography • Nerve stimulation • Urethral pressure measurement • Imaging
IV Quality of life	• Generic and condition-specific
V Socioeconomic costs	

From ref. 4.

MULTIDIMENSIONAL APPROACH TO LUTS

The International Continence Society (ICS) has recently recommended a multidimensional approach to the evaluation of the outcome of therapeutic interventions in women with LUTS;[4] the domains described are listed in Table 78.1.

The 'patient's observation', 'quantification of symptoms' and 'clinician's observation' quantify measures within the ICIDH-2 levels of 'health condition' (pathological changes) and 'impairment' (signs are exteriorized), while 'quality-of-life' and 'socioeconomic' measures quantify qualities within the levels of 'activity' and 'participation' in the ICIDH-2 model.

There is dynamic interaction between the factors in the ICIDH-2 model and *intervention* at one level has the potential to modify other related elements. *The interactions are not always in a predictable one-to-one relationship to each other.*

Table 78.2. *Checklist for outcome studies in women with LUTS*

I	The purpose of the study	• What are the reasons for this particular study? • What do the investigators want to show?
II	Patient groups	• Definition of patient groups • Inclusion/exclusion criteria
III	Disease/disorder	• Causal or symptomatic treatment? • Arrest of a process? • Reversible changes?
IV	Intervention	• Description of the intervention • Intervention-related complications, morbidity and mortality
V	Study design and controls	• Ideally intervention studies should have a control group and should be randomized • Define endpoints • Define response criteria • Nature of trial e.g. double blind, placebo controlled, crossover • Adverse events, dropouts
VI	Methods of measurement	• Characterization of methods, test–retest data in the hands of the investigators • Change in circumstances or procedures prior to and after intervention • Interindividual variation (plus differences between centres in multicentre trials) • Normal values
VII	Statistics	• Power of the study • Reason for choise of statistical method • Compliance • Statistician involved?
VIII	Timescale	• Why was outcome evaluated at a particular time in relation to the intervention? • Long-term outcome?
IX	Expected outcome	• Degree of improvement • Risk–benefit analysis • Patient expectations • Effects on quality of life • Socioeconomic factors
X	Interpretation of data	• Comparison with outcome in other studies • Unexpected/adverse findings • Limitations • Clinical significance • Theoretical importance • Possible ways of improving the study • Conclusions for future investigations

Outcome measures should be selected within the context of a specific study and the researchers should choose reliable methods or describe their methodology and provide reproducibility data or indicate its absence.[4]

The time frame for evaluation of intervention is also an important factor that needs to be standardized to allow for understanding and comparison between studies. The time frame of the intervention and its expected outcome should be considered when designing a study. Long-term outcome should be measured whenever possible. Statistical expertise is vital and should be applied from the beginning of the study.

CHECKLIST FOR OUTCOME STUDIES IN WOMEN WITH LUTS

Whenever an outcome study on LUTS is planned, series of questions should be considered and addressed appropriately. Table 78.2 serves as a checklist.[5]

It is important to improve the quality of outcome studies. This requires a rigorous pragmatic methodology and a multidimensional approach.

REFERENCES

1. Black NA, Downs SH. The effectiveness of surgery for stress incontinence in women: A systematic review. *Br J Urol* 1996; 78: 497–510

2. Urinary incontinence in adults: acute and chronic management. AHCPR publ. no. 96-0682. Rockville, MD: Agency for Health Care Policy and Research, Public Health Service. US Department of Health and Human Services, March 1996

3. *International Classification of Impairment Activities and Participation: A Manual of Dimensions of Disablement and Health (ICIDH-2)*. Geneva: WHO, August 1997

4. Lose G, Fantl SA, Victor A *et al.* Outcome measures for research in adult women with symptoms of lower urinary tract dysfunction. *Neurourol Urodyn* 1998; 17: 255–562

5. Mattiasson A, Djurhuus JC, Fonda D *et al.* Standardization of outcome studies in patients with lower urinary tract dysfunction: a report on general principles from the Standardisation Committee of the International Continence Society. *Neurourol Urodyn* 1998; 17: 249–253

79

The purpose of standardization of terminology and methods in patients with lower urinary tract dysfunction

A. Mattiasson
(Coordinating Chairman of the Standardization Committee of the ICS)

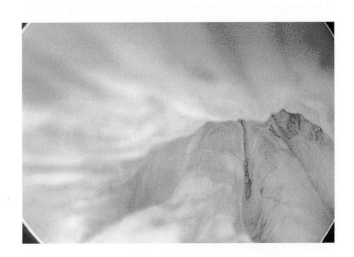

INTRODUCTION

The standardization of terminology and methods used to characterize the lower urinary tract (LUT) is motivated first and foremost by the need for communication and documentation. As in other contexts, to achieve satisfactory communication it is vital that people speak the same language and that the terms used have the same meaning for everyone who uses them. This is not simply a matter of characterizing and classifying different types of dysfunction, but also of applying methods and quantifying different findings in terms of measurements. We also need to ensure that the methods we use are well defined and characterized with regard to suitability, sensitivity and reproducibility. In short, we need a common language with definitions of what is normal and what is abnormal. In the case of abnormalities, it is assumed that we can measure how large the abnormality is in relation to what is normal, to an earlier situation or to another chosen definition of the desirable state. The measurements and the measures we choose also need to be standardized so that we know that our measurements and investigations are comparable over time and between different places.

WHAT IS A STANDARD?

Standardization is a tool for quality assurance, and the production of standards is itself a part of such work. Standards are needed in all three principal sections of quality-assurance work:

- in the structure,
- in the process,
- for describing the result.

The procedure of standardization is one of writing down terms, descriptions of methods and measures which, at present and for the foreseeable future, are judged to best reflect the pathological condition/function/dysfunction in both qualitative and quantitative terms. It is, therefore, an intraprofessional agreement, which sometimes has to be a compromise since practicability is important – the methods and terms must be perceived as being adequate and reflecting everyday reality. Sometimes the demand for precision has to be combined with demands for practicability. A standard – whether it concerns a term or a measure – must be practical, simple and perceived as meaningful to use; it must have a high degree of acceptance.

Describing and measuring the functions of the LUT is not as easy as one might think. In biological systems with superimposed functional disorders it is difficult to capture the overall picture purely statistically using simple means. Standardization is based on what is common to patients with a certain type of complaint, even if there are significant differences in other respects when the pathological picture is described more precisely at an individual level. We often know more about the manifestations of a disease than about its true intrinsic nature. Standardization will therefore be designed primarily to describe secondary manifestations – the consequences (e.g. a detrusor contraction) instead of the primary cause (e.g. a lesion in the nervous system).

One problem with standardization of the LUT is that often the symptoms do not go hand in hand with urodynamic findings, which is what we usually measure. There is, therefore, a lack of correlation between subjective and objective measurements. It is clear from the above argument that a standard in itself does not have to express what is true. Standards can be said to express what we believe to be correct, but are not, therefore, necessarily synonymous with what is correct. We endeavour to bridge this discrepancy so that the standard we agree to use is as true as possible.

For whom?

Standardization is just as important for day-to-day practice as for scientific studies. Ideally this should be common ground for researchers, clinicians and others, that is, all those who need to communicate within the subject area.

Information and knowledge are vital tools if agreed standards are to be used by everyone. Quick, effective dissemination guaranteed by established scientific journals with a wide circulation in the target group is one of the prerequisites. Another is that each and every one of us must take standards on board and adjust our terminology and shape our work to correspond with what has been agreed. A very important link, and one which must not be neglected, is to create understanding through education and training of colleagues in different areas and the staff with whom one is working in this context. It may seem obvious to use (correspondingly) accepted designations for conditions and methods in one's own laboratory, and to be familiar with, for example, the test–retest variations in one's analyses for different sexes of different ages. However, most of us need to take a very large step in this direction before we can be sure that this really is the case.

Current standards must be accepted and used if it is to be possible to compare data from different researchers both within and between studies. Because this is so often not the case, the conclusions from meta-analyses, for example, are often regarded with a touch of scepticism.

What should be done?

First, it is important to create standards around the most frequent diseases/disorders and examination methods. That is why the Standardization Committee of the International Continence Society (ICS) has chosen to work with the major diagnosis groups of: women, men, children, the old and frail, and patients with neurogenic functional disorders of the LUT. The most significant methods for diagnosis and follow-up, both in quantitative and qualitative terms, are, of course, the first to be considered for standardization. Traditional urodynamic investigations can be mentioned in this context, but newer examination methods such as ambulatory urodynamics, imaging, etc. are also relevant. General recommendations under the heading 'good urodynamic practice' and signal processing are also important.

If the recommendations or, in some cases, guidelines produced are to be received with respect and used, those doing the work must be experts who are well grounded in their respective fields.

How often?

There are no set rules or recommendations stating how long a standard should be regarded as valid. Some well-established standards are impossible to question (e.g. the length of a metre). In dynamic areas that develop quickly (e.g. computer technology) increased understanding may mean that previously agreed standards need to be replaced relatively often with new ones that are up to date. The demand for change must always be weighed against the need for continuity. To some extent one is, of course, dependent on respecting traditions that have become established within certain fields over a number of years. This has turned out to be

particularly true of our terminology. It also has to be remembered that the introduction of a new standard may make it impossible to make comparisons with historical data. At the same time it is important that current standards are not perceived as either an expression of rules that are too rigid or a desperate insistence on the old for its own sake.

When it comes to setting a standard for the first time, one has greater freedom than when an existing standard needs updating. It is also important that standardization is kept up to date and is considering when new fields are developed, when new technology becomes available and as the understanding of the causes and manifestations of diseases increases. Renewal always means a simultaneous and recurrent rejuvenation process in the groups working on these questions. Many more people than those who currently take an active interest in standardization will have to do so in the future if we are to have the best possible tools to work with. Involving both young people, who we already know will be responsible for formulating the problems of the future, and more experienced colleagues in this work is the best we can do.

Methods, measurements and terms

Ideally the methods we use should reflect pathological activity and degree of damage etc., and the findings should agree with the patient's perception of the whole thing (i.e. symptomatology, level of discomfort and quality-of-life factors). There is often a discrepancy between these measurements, which is why each observation we make must be considered on its own merits, and why we should be careful with regard to making assumptions about correlations that are not proven. A good example here is the lack of correlation between the symptoms and the degree of obstruction in benign prostatic hypertrophy.

If it is impossible to reflect all pathological activity with one method, which is usually the case, it is reasonable to demand that what is examined is representative of the disease/disorder or, from the point of view of the method used, really hits the target picture. Regardless of which perspective is preferred, that of the examined or the examiner, the next major problem is whether the methods used block the view between the examiner and the object. We often ascribe a greater degree of sensitivity and specificity to methods than we have reason to.

In reality, however, we often do not know the reproducibility of a method at our own clinic, in our own laboratory or in our own hands. Since we cannot readily establish whether there is a significant change over time unless the observed difference lies outside the test–retest interval, most of us have no way of establishing whether there is a small difference between two instances of measurement.

As well as making intra-individual comparisons, inter-individual comparisons are also needed, usually with reference to what is normal for the age and sex in question. Unfortunately, there is a lack of normative data and, with a few exceptions, we have no validated nomograms for urodynamic investigations.

Normality

We know all too little about what is normal when it comes to the LUT. This may seem strange; however, consider the bladder and urethra as an example. We would like to know what is normal from both a quantitative and a qualitative point of view. However, normality can only be described almost solely in qualitative terms such as 'not leaking', and 'emptying completely without difficulty'. As soon as we come to individual measurements in the normal population of both sexes and for different ages we have very few studies to use as a basis. This makes it difficult to draw a boundary between normal and abnormal; the problem becomes particularly difficult when it comes to differentiating between the results of ageing and the consequences of disease.

OUTCOME RESEARCH

Outcome refers to the result of intervention in a patient or group of patients. Usually the same type of measurement is performed before and after a particular period of a particular treatment; the treatment outcome is compared with the accepted standard treatment for the disease in question and, if possible, a placebo as well. There are variations on this theme. It is now recommended that when performing outcome research on patients with LUT dysfunction, measurements from as many as possible of the following five domains are considered:

- the patient's medical history;
- quantification of symptoms (e.g. urine loss);
- anatomical and functional data;
- quality of life;
- socioeconomic factors.

Well-developed measurements are not available for all these areas; intensive work is being done to produce good measurements of quality of life for different groups and of the social and economic consequences of LUT dysfunction. The patient's medical history and experience of the situation have come to control treatment more and more, and our previously rather one-sided focus on anatomical and functional measurements is now being supplemented by consideration of the patient's symptoms and level of discomfort, as well as quality-of-life and socioeconomic factors. Our ability to describe what we can offer patients and society in such terms will be vital in determining how well we succeed in maintaining awareness of these disease groups in comparison with other types of disease and dysfunction.

In the first three areas listed above there ought to be plenty of good appropriate measurements which could be recommended and, where appropriate, combined in different indices to capture a pathological picture. A comprehensive examination of work in the area of incontinence research on men, women, children, the old and frail, and patients with neurogenic disorders has instead revealed an apparent large-scale lack of knowledge in this field. There is a particular lack of knowledge in the pathophysiological area, that is, the actual reasons for LUT dysfunction. We also have difficulty differentiating between dysfunction that is due to disease and that which is a consequence of the ageing process. In some cases we may come to the conclusion that they are the same and that our present approach is in need of adjustment.

We should also acknowledge that we are never, or rarely, able to reverse the course of a disease with our interventions, but are able merely to slow down and, at best, stop its development. Some consequences, such as thickening of the bladder wall if outflow is obstructed, are reversible in many cases, but we never achieve an entirely normal situation. We can provide a partial or complete symptomatic recovery and a partial but incomplete pathophysiological recovery. We really need to establish a new balance between the organs involved and their control systems, that is, balance at a point that is different from that if the individual were counted as normal. This approach makes it much easier to see the outcome of treatment in relation to what is possible and reasonable. One should also ask oneself, perhaps first and foremost, what the patient wishes to achieve.

For the reasons given above, cure and normalization are not realistic goals for treatment whereas improvement towards a situation that is perceived as normal by the patient is more achieveable. At best this will be a large improvement, but in other cases we are looking at small steps forward.

CLINICAL RESEARCH ASSESSMENT GROUPS

On the basis of the arguments above with regard to outcome, it is easy to conclude that we have large gaps in our knowledge. Once we have agreed on how best to conduct outcome research in principle, we need to formulate a plan as to how the missing knowledge is best acquired. This task has been assigned within the ICS to the Clinical Research Assessment groups; these groups correspond to the structure of the outcome groups: one each for women, men, children, the old and frail, and patients with neurogenic LUT dysfunction. There are great opportunities to make an international, multidisciplinary contribution to this area in a logical, structured and meaningful way.

We seem to have had a tendency over the years to contribute pieces to a jigsaw, each of which is nicely shaped and coloured, but where the different pieces do not fit together to provide a single, coherent picture. It is for this reason that we should now work together to plan the future picture and the size and shape of the pieces of the LUT puzzle.

Specific questions for each diagnosis group

Current recommendations and guidelines are best read in the relevant reports from the Standardization Committee of the ICS, listed at the end of the chapter. The following describes some of the questions with which the Standardization Committee is currently grappling, illustrating some of the issues already raised about drawing boundaries and replacing standards.

It is of central importance to characterization of a dysfunctional state in the LUT that both the internal and external characteristics of the disorder/disease are encompassed in the terms we decide to use, and that the methods applied to measurement reflect the same things. Precision requires complete understanding of the nature of the disease in terms of both its pathophysiology and how advanced the disease is. However we do not have complete information for any of the major diagnosis groups – incontinence, obstruction and neurogenic disorders – so we cannot be certain that we have used terms which exactly describe the internal and external characteristics of these disorders. In order to throw light on our difficulties and sometimes, failures, I will give examples from each of the three main areas. These should not be interpreted as proposals for immediate changes to current standards, but rather serve the purpose of providing food for thought.

Incontinence

Incontinence as a symptom, a sign and a condition

As well as defining urinary incontinence as a social and hygienic problem, we are in the habit of defining incontinence as a symptom, a sign and a condition. The first two definitions do not in themselves present a problem but we need to discuss what is meant by incontinence as a condition. Hitherto we meant the underlying pathological condition or disorder. This way of looking at it is probably incorrect since, from a medical point of view, incontinence is a consequence and not a cause. The condition in itself means, of course, the involuntary passing of urine through the urethra – such a definition by no means refers to the pathological condition. This means that we need to redefine the condition of incontinence.

Motor and sensory urge incontinence

According to the current definition, motor urge incontinence exists when we can detect motor activity urodynamically, usually in the bladder in the form of hyperactivity, combined with the patient's experiences of the urge to pass urine and urine leakage. If such hyperactivity cannot be detected, we talk about sensory urge incontinence. This is an inappropriate term, however, since urine cannot reasonably pass through the urethra unless motor activity – an increase in pressure in the bladder and/or a decrease in pressure in the urethra – occur. Logically speaking, urge incontinence should therefore be regarded as motor incontinence in all cases. There are several explanations for this, including the fact that hyperactivity in the bladder does not always occur during cystometric examination, and that we usually measure the pressure ratios in the urethra.

A reduction in pressure in the urethra can, of course, be combined with a feeling of the urge to pass urine, but also with incontinence.

Obstruction

We have adopted a definition of obstruction in pressure–flow terms, the recommended nomogram being based on the original diagram of Abrams–Griffiths.[1] There are other similar classifications that are essentially the same, for example Schäfer's nomogram.[2] These nomograms are probably a simplification of a more complex reality; none of them takes into account the significance of the temporal component, for example. If a patient with symptoms has two consecutive measurements approaching the obstructed range, and we assume that these two observations in the form of plots on the pressure–flow nomogram are significantly different but still within the normal range, this might very well be an indication of an obstruction. The obstruction may not yet be particularly pronounced or developed, but an obstructive process is nevertheless involved. This patient still ends up inside the so-called normal range in the current nomogram. This is, of course, because our present definition does not take into account a temporal component in the *dynamic* process of obstruction. What we have at the moment is a static, physical classification of obstruction and non-obstruction. What we need is a biological and dynamic definition, that is, a *biodynamic* definition.

Neurogenic dysfunction

We now know that primarily non-neurogenic pathological conditions in experimental models give rise to neurogenic changes, and neural plasticity is thought to be an important factor in coping with the situation that arises in the case of infravesical obstruction. We suspect that these secondary neurogenic changes are important in terms of pathological development, but are not sure what role they play. It may be appropriate to consider both primary and secondary neurogenic disorders, primary disorders being diseases of the nervous system that affect the functioning of the LUT, and secondary disorders being those that begin in other organs (e.g. the bladder, urethra or prostate). It also follows that LUT disorders might be regarded as primary or secondary in nature. Future research may provide answers to these questions.

THE FUTURE

The importance of broad-based commitment and the pursuit of standardization as a continuous process, with repeated questioning of the terminology used and the methods available, cannot be stressed enough. The more people who contribute to the work on standardization, the better it will be. It does, after all, concern our common use of language and our common methods, that is, our ability to communicate with each other. What can be more important to us than keeping that ability alive?

REFERENCES

1. Abrams P, Griffiths DJ. The assessment of prostatic obstruction from urodynamic measurements and from residual urine. *Br J Urol* 1979; 51: 129–134

2. Schäfer W. The contribution of the bladder outlet to the relation between pressure and flow rate during micturition. In: Hinman F Jr (ed) *Benign Prostatic Hypertrophy*. New York: Springer Verlag, 1983; 470–496

BIBLIOGRAPHY: REPORTS FROM THE STANDARDIZATION COMMITTEE OF THE ICS

1. Bates P, Bradley WE, Glen E *et al*. First report on the standardisation of terminology of lower urinary tract function. Urinary incontinence. Procedures related to the evaluation of urine storage: cystometry, urethral closure pressure profile, units of measurements. *Br J Urol* 1976; 48: 39–42; *Eur Urol* 1976; 2: 274–276; *Scand J Urol Nephrol* 1976; 11: 193–196; *Urol Int* 1976; 32: 81–87

2. Bates P, Glen E, Griffiths D *et al*. Second report on the standardisation of terminology of lower urinary tract function. Procedures related to the evaluation of micturition: Flow rate, pressure measurement, symbols. *Acta Urol Jpn* 1977; 27: 1563–1566; *Br J Urol* 1977; 49: 207–210; *Eur Urol* 1977; 3: 168–170; *Scand J Urol Nephrol* 1977; 11: 197–199

3. Bates P, Bradley WE, Glen E *et al*. Third report on the standardisation of terminology of lower urinary tract function. Procedures related to the evaluation of micturition: pressure flow relationships, residual urine. *Br J Urol* 1980; 52: 348–359; *Eur Urol* 1980; 6: 170–171; *Acta Urol Jpn* 1980; 27: 1566–1568; *Scand J Urol Nephrol* 1980; 12: 191–193

4. Bates P, Bradley WE, Glen E *et al*. Fourth report on the standardisation of terminology of lower urinary tract function. Terminology related to neuromuscular dysfunction of lower urinary tract. *Br J Urol* 1981; 52: 333–335;

Urology 1981; 17: 618–620; *Scand J Urol Nephrol* 1981; 15: 169–171; *Acta Urol Jpn* 1981; 27: 1568–1571

5. Abrams P, Blaivas JG, Stanton SL *et al.* Sixth report on the standardisation of terminology of lower urinary tract function. Procedures related to neurophysiological investigations: electromyography, nerve conduction studies, reflex latencies, evoked potentials and sensory testing. *World J Urol* 1986; 4: 2–5; *Scand J Urol Nephrol* 1986; 20: 161–164

6. Rowan D, James ED, Kramer AEJL *et al.* (ICS working party on urodynamic equipment) Urodynamic equipment: technical aspects. *J Med Eng Technol* 1987; 11; 57–64

7.* Abrams P, Blaivas JG, Stanton SL, Andersen JT. The standardisation of terminology of lower urinary tract function. *Scand J Urol Nephrol Suppl* 1988; 114; 5–19

8. Andersen JT, Blaivas JG, Cardozo L, Thüroff J. Lower urinary tract rehabilitation techniques: seventh report on the standardization of terminology of lower urinary tract function. *Int Urogynecol J* 1992; 3: 75–80

9.* Bump RC, Mattiasson A, Bø K *et al.* The standardization of terminology of female pelvic organ prolapse and pelvic floor dysfunction. *Am J Obstet Gynecol* 1996; 175: 10–17

10. Thüroff J, Mattiasson A, Andersen JT *et al.* Standardization of terminology and assessment of functional characteristics of intestinal urinary reservoirs. *Neurourol Urodyn* 1996; 15: 499–511; *Br J Urol* 1996; 78: 516–523; *Scand J Urol Nephrol* 1996; 30: 349–356

11. Griffiths D, Höfner K, van Mastrigt R *et al.* Standardization of terminology of lower urinary tract function: pressure-flow studies of voiding, urethral resistance, and urethral obstruction. *Neurourol Urodyn* 1997; 16: 1–18

12. Fonda D, Resnick NM, Colling J *et al.* Outcome measures for research of lower urinary tract dysfunction in frail older people. *Neurourol Urodyn* 1998; 17: 273–381

13. Lose G, Fantl SA, Victor A *et al.* Outcome measures for research in adult women with symptoms of lower urinary tract dysfunction. *Neurourol Urodyn* 1998; 17: 255–562

14. Mattiasson A, Djurhuus JC, Fonda D *et al.* Standardization of outcome studies in patients with lower urinary tract dysfunction: a report on general principles from the Standardisation Committee of the International Continence Society. *Neurourol Urodyn* 1998; 17: 249–253

15. Nordling J, Abrams P, Ameda K *et al.* Outcome measures for research in treatment of adult males with symptoms of lower urinary tract dysfunction. *Neurourol Urodyn* 1998, 17: 263–371

* Reports 7 and 9 are reproduced in Chapters 80 and 81, respectively, of this volume.

The standardization of terminology of lower urinary tract function recommended by the International Continence Society

P. Abrams, J. G. Blaivas, S. L. Stanton, J. T. Andersen (Chairman)
ICS Committee on Standardization of Terminology

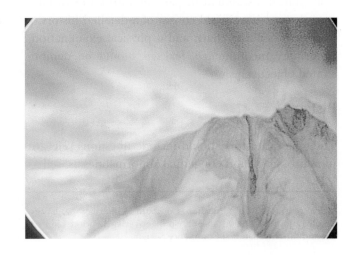

INTRODUCTION

The International Continence Society (ICS) established a committee for the standardization of terminology of lower urinary tract function in 1973. Five of the six reports from this committee, approved by the Society, have been published.[1-5] The fifth report, on quantification of urine loss, was an internal ICS document but appears, in part, in this document.

These reports are revised, extended and collated in this monograph. The standards are recommended to facilitate comparison of results by investigators who use urodynamic methods. These standards are recommended not only for urodynamic investigations carried out on human patients but also during animal studies. When using urodynamic studies in animals the type of any anesthesia used should be stated. It is suggested that acknowledgement of these standards in written publications be indicated by a footnote to the section 'Methods and Materials' or its equivalent, to read as follows: 'Methods, definitions and units conform to the standards recommended by the International Continence Society, except where specifically noted.'

Urodynamic studies involve the assessment of the function and dysfunction of the urinary tract by any appropriate method. Aspects of urinary tract morphology, physiology, biochemistry, and hydrodynamics affect urine transport and storage. Other methods of investigation such as the radiographic visualization of the lower urinary tract is a useful adjunct to conventional urodynamics.

This monograph concerns the urodynamics of the lower urinary tract.

CLINICAL ASSESSMENT

The clinical assessment of patients with lower urinary tract dysfunction should consist of a detailed history, a frequency/volume chart, and a physical examination. In urinary incontinence, leakage should be demonstrated objectively.

History

The general history should include questions relevant to neurological and congenital abnormalities as well as information on previous urinary infections and relevant surgery. Information must be obtained on medication with known or possible effects on the lower urinary tract. The general history should also include assessment of menstrual, sexual and bowel function, and obstetric history.

The urinary history must consist of symptoms related to both the storage and the evacuation functions of the lower urinary tract.

Frequency/volume chart

The frequency/volume chart is a specific urodynamic investigation recording fluid intake and urine output per 24-hour period. The chart gives objective information on the number of voidings, the distribution of voidings between daytime and nighttime and each voided volume. The chart can also be used to record episodes of urgency and leakage and the number of incontinence pads used. The frequency/volume chart is very useful in the assessment of voiding disorders, and in the follow-up of treatment.

Physical examination

Besides a general urologic and, when appropriate, gynecologic examination, the physical examination should include the assessment of perineal sensation, the perineal reflexes supplied by the sacral segments S2–S4, and anal sphincter tone and control.

PROCEDURES RELATED TO THE EVALUATION OF URINE STORAGE

Cystometry

Cystometry is the method by which the pressure/volume relationship of the bladder is measured. All systems are zeroed at atmospheric pressure. For external transducers the reference point is the level of the superior edge of the symphysis pubis. For catheter-mounted transducers the reference point is the transducer itself.

Cystometry is used to assess detrusor activity, sensation, capacity, and compliance.

Before starting to fill the bladder the residual urine may be measured. However, the removal of a large volume of residual urine may alter detrusor function, especially in neuropathic disorders. Certain cystometric parameters may be significantly altered by the speed of bladder filling (see *Compliance*, page 1044).

During cystometry it is taken for granted that the patient is awake, unanesthetized and neither sedated nor taking drugs that affect bladder function. Any variations should be specified.

General information

The following details should be given:

1. Access (transurethral or percutaneous);
2. Fluid medium (liquid or gas);
3. Temperature of fluid (state in degrees Celsius);
4. Position of patient (e.g., supine, sitting, or standing);
5. Filling method – may be by diuresis or catheter. Filling by catheter may be continuous or incremental; the precise filling rate should be stated. When the incremental method is used the volume increment should be stated. For general discussion, the following terms for the range of filling rate may be used:
   a. Up to 10 ml/min is *slow fill cystometry* ('physiological' filling).
   b. 10–100 ml/min is *medium fill cystometry*.
   c. Over 100 ml/min is *rapid fill cystometry*.

Technical information

The following details should be given:

1. Fluid-filled catheter – specify number of catheters, single or multiple lumens, type of catheter (manufacturer), size of catheter.
2. Catheter tip transducer – list specifications.
3. Other catheters – list specifications.
4. Measuring equipment.

Definitions

Cystometric terminology is defined as follows:

- *Intravesical pressure* is the pressure within the bladder.
- *Abdominal pressure* is taken to be the pressure surrounding the bladder. In current practice it is estimated from rectal or, less commonly, extraperitoneal pressure.
- *Detrusor pressure* is that component of intravesical pressure that is created by forces in the bladder wall (passive and active). It is estimated by subtracting abdominal pressure from intravesical pressure. The

simultaneous measurement of abdominal pressure is essential for interpretation of the intravesical pressure trace. However, artifacts on the detrusor pressure trace may be produced by intrinsic rectal contractions.

- *Bladder sensation.* Sensation is difficult to evaluate because of its subjective nature. It is usually assessed by questioning the patient in relation to the fullness of the bladder during cystometry.

Commonly used descriptive terms include:

- *First desire to void.*
- *Normal desire to void,* – defined as the feeling that leads the patient to pass urine at the next convenient moment, but voiding can be delayed if necessary.
- *Strong desire to void* – defined as persistent desire to void without the fear of leakage.
- *Urgency* – defined as a strong desire to void accompanied by fear of leakage or fear of pain.
- *Pain.* The site and character of pain should be specified. Pain during bladder filling or micturition is abnormal.

The use of objective or semi-objective tests for sensory function, such as electrical threshold studies (sensory testing), is discussed in detail under *Sensory testing* (see page 1042).

The term 'Capacity' must be qualified as follows:

Maximum cystometric capacity, in patients with normal sensation, is the volume at which the patient feels he/she can no longer delay micturition. In the absence of sensation the maximum cystometric capacity cannot be defined in the same terms and is the volume at which the clinician decides to terminate filling. In the presence of sphincter incompetence the maximum cystometric capacity may be significantly increased by occlusion of the urethra, e.g., by Foley catheter.

The *functional bladder capacity*, or voided volume, is more relevant and is assessed from a frequency/volume chart (urinary diary).

The *maximum (anesthetic) bladder capacity* is the volume measured after filling during a deep general or spinal / epidural anesthetic, specifying fluid temperature, filling pressure, and filling time.

Compliance indicates the change in volume for a change in pressure. Compliance is calculated by dividing the volume change (ΔV) by the change in detrusor pressure (Δp_{det}) during that change in bladder volume ($\Delta V / \Delta p_{det}$). Compliance is expressed as milliliters per centimeters of water pressure. (See also *Compliance*, page 1044.)

Urethral presssure measurement

It should be noted that the urethral pressure and the urethral closure pressure are idealized concepts which represent the ability of the urethra to prevent leakage (see *Urinary incontinence*, page 1045). In current urodynamic practice the urethral pressure is measured by a number of different techniques which do not always yield consistent values. Not only do the values differ with the method of measurement, but there is often lack of consistency for a single method; for example, the effect of catheter rotation when urethral pressure is measured by a catheter-mounted transducer.

Intraluminal urethral pressure may be measured:

- At rest, with the bladder at any given volume;
- During coughing or straining;
- During the process of voiding (see *Urethral pressure profile during voiding*, page 1039).

Measurements may be made at one point in the urethra over a period of time, or at several points along the urethra consecutively forming a *urethral pressure profile* (UPP).

Two types of UPP may be measured in the *storage phase*:

1. Resting urethral pressure profile – with the bladder and subject at rest;
2. Stress urethral pressure profile – with a defined applied stress (e.g., cough, strain, Valsalva).

In the storage phase the *urethral pressure profile* denotes the intraluminal pressure along the length of the urethra. All systems are zeroed at atmospheric pressure. For external transducers the reference point is the superior edge of the symphysis pubis. For catheter-mounted transducers the reference point is the transducer itself. Intravesical pressure should be measured to exclude a simultaneous detrusor contraction. The subtraction of intravesical pressure from urethral pressure produces the *urethral closure pressure profile*.

It is essential to record both intravesical and intraurethral pressures simultaneously during stress urethral profilometry.

General information
The following details should be given:

1. Infusion medium (liquid or gas);
2. Rate of infusion;
3. Stationary, continuous, or intermittent withdrawal;
4. Rate of withdrawal;
5. Bladder volume;
6. Position of patient (supine, sitting, or standing).

Technical information
The following details should be given:

1. Open catheter: specify type (manufacturer), size, number, position, and orientation of side or end hole.
2. Catheter-mounted transducers: specify manufacturer; number of transducers; spacing of transducers along the catheter; orientation with respect to one another; transducer design, e.g., transducer face depressed or flush with catheter surface; catheter diameter; and material. The orientation of the transducer(s) in the urethra should be stated.
3. Other catheters, e.g., membrane, fiberoptic: specify type (manufacturer), size, and number of channels as for microtransducer catheter.
4. Measurement technique: for stress profiles the particular stress employed should be stated, e.g., cough or Valsalva.
5. Recording apparatus: describe type of recording apparatus. The frequency response of the total system should be stated. The frequency response of the catheter in the perfusion method can be assessed by blocking the eyeholes and recording the consequent rate of change of pressure.

Definitions
Terminology referring to profiles measured in storage phase (see Fig. 80.1) is defined as follows:

Maximum urethral pressure is the maximum pressure of the measured profile.

Maximum urethral closure pressure is the maximum difference between the urethral pressure and the intravesical pressure.

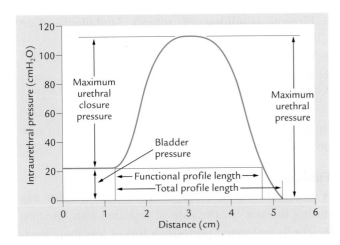

Figure 80.1. *Diagram of a female urethral pressure profile (static) with ICS recommended nomenclature.*

Functional profile length is the length of the urethra along which the urethral pressure exceeds intravesical pressure.

Functional profile length (on stress) is the length over which the urethral pressure exceeds the intravesical pressure on stress.

Pressure 'transmission' ratio is the increment in urethral pressure on stress as a percentage of the simultaneously recorded increment in intravesical pressure. For stress profiles obtained during coughing, pressure transmission ratios can be obtained at any point along the urethra. If single values are given, the position in the urethra should be stated. If several pressure transmission ratios are defined at different points along the urethra, a pressure 'transmission' profile is obtained. During 'cough profiles' the amplitude of the cough should be stated if possible. *Note:* The term 'transmission' is in common usage and cannot be changed. However, 'transmission' implies a completely passive process. Such an assumption is not yet justified by scientific evidence. A role for muscular activity cannot be excluded.

Total profile length is not generally regarded as a useful parameter.

The information gained from urethral pressure measurements in the storage phase is of limited value in the assessment of voiding disorders.

Quantification of urine loss

Subjective grading of incontinence may not indicate reliably the degree of abnormality. However, it is important to relate the management of the individual patients to their complaints and personal circumstances, as well as to objective measurements.

In order to assess and compare the results of the treatment of different types of incontinence in different centers, a simple standard test can be used to measure urine loss objectively in any subject. In order to obtain a representative result, especially in subjects with variable or intermittent urinary incontinence, the test should occupy as long a period as possible; yet it must be practical. The circumstances should approximate to those of everyday life, yet be similar for all subjects to allow meaningful comparison. On the basis of pilot studies performed in various centers, an internal report of the ICS[6] recommended a test occupying a 1-hour period during which a series of standard activities was carried out. This test *can* be extended by further 1-hour periods if the result of the first 1-hour test were not considered representative by either the patient or the investigator. Alternatively, the test can be repeated, after filling the bladder to a defined volume.

The total amount of urine lost during the test period is determined by weighing a collecting device such as a nappy, absorbent pad, or condom appliance. A nappy or pad should be worn inside waterproof underpants or should have a waterproof backing. Care should be taken to use a collecting device of adequate capacity. Immediately before the test begins the collecting device is weighed to the nearest gram.

Typical test schedule

1. Test is started without the patient voiding.
2. Preweighed collecting device is put on and first 1-hour test period begins.
3. Subject drinks 500 ml sodium-free liquid within a short period (max. 15 min), then sits or rests.
4. Half-hour period: subject walks, including stair climbing equivalent to one flight up and down.
5. During the remaining period the subject performs the following activities:
   a. Standing up from sitting, 10 times;
   b. Coughing vigorously, 10 times;
   c. Running on the spot for 1 min;
   d. Bending to pick up small object from floor, 5 times;
   e. Washing hands in running water for 1 min.
6. At the end of the 1-hour test the collecting device is removed and weighed.

7. If the test is regarded as representative, the subject voids and the volume is recorded.

8. Otherwise the test is repeated, preferably without voiding.

If the collecting device becomes saturated or filled during the test it should be removed and weighed, and replaced by a fresh device. The total weight of urine lost during the test period is taken to be equal to the gain in weight of the collecting device(s). In interpreting the results of the test it should be borne in mind that a weight gain of up to 1 g may be due to weighing errors, sweating, or vaginal discharge.

The activity program may be modified according to the subject's physical ability. If substantial variations from the usual test schedule occur, these should be recorded so that the same schedule can be used on subsequent occasions.

In principle the subject should not void during the test period. If the patient experiences urgency, then he/she should be persuaded to postpone voiding and to perform as many of the activities in the section on *Procedures related to neurophysiological evaluation of the urinary tract during filling and voiding* (page 1039) as possible in order to detect leakage. Before voiding the collection device is removed for weighing. If voiding cannot be postponed, then the test is terminated. The voided volume and the duration of the test should be recorded. For subjects not completing the full test the results may require separate analysis, or the test may be repeated after rehydration.

The test result is given in grams urine lost in the 1-hour test period in which the greatest urine loss is recorded.

Additional procedures

Provided that there is no interference with the basic test, additional procedures intended to give information of diagnostic value are permissible. For example, additional changes and weighing of the collecting device can give information about the timing of urine loss; the absorbent nappy may be an electronic recording nappy so that the timing is recorded directly.

Presentation of results

The following details should be given:

1. Collecting device;

2. Physical condition of subject (ambulant, chair-bound, bedridden);
3. Relevant medical condition of subject;
4. Relevant drug treatments;
5. Test schedule.

In some situations the timing of the test (e.g., in relation to the menstrual cycle) may be relevant.

Findings

A record should be made of the weight of urine lost during the test (in the case of repeated tests, greatest weight in any stated period). A loss of less than 1 g is within experimental error and the patient should be regarded as essentially dry. Urine loss should be measured and recorded in grams.

Statistics

When performing statistical analysis or urine loss in a group of subjects, nonparametric statistics should be employed, since the values are not normally distributed.

PROCEDURES RELATED TO THE EVALUATION OF MICTURITION

Measurement of urinary flow

Urinary flow may be described in terms of *rate* and *pattern* and may be *continuous* or *intermittent*. *Flow rate* is defined as the volume of fluid expelled via the urethra per unit time. It is expressed in milliliters per second.

General information

The following details should be given:

1. Voided volume;
2. Patient environment and position (supine, sitting, or standing);
3. Filling:
   a) By diuresis (spontaneous or forced: specify regimen);
   b) By catheter (transurethral or suprapubic);
4. Type of fluid.

Technical information

The following details should be given:

1. Measuring equipment;

2. Solitary procedure or combined with other measurements.

Definitions

The terminology referring to urinary flow is defined as follows:

1. *Continuous flow* (Fig. 80.2):
   Voided volume is the total volume expelled via the urethra.
   Maximum flow rate is the maximum measured value of the flow rate.
   Average flow rate is voided volume divided by flow time. The calculation of average flow rate is only meaningful if flow is continuous and without terminal dribbling.
   Flow time is the time over which measurable flow actually occurs.

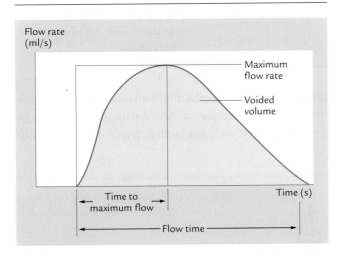

Figure 80.2. *Diagram of a continuous urine flow recording with ICS recommended nomenclature.*

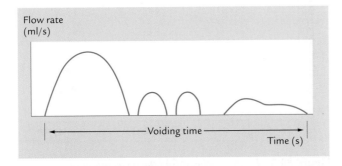

Figure 80.3. *Diagram of an interrupted urine flow recording with ICS recommended nomenclature.*

Time to maximum flow is the elapsed time from onset of flow to maximum flow.
The flow pattern must be described when flow time and average flow rate are measured.

2. *Intermittent flow* (Fig. 80.3):
   The same parameters used to characterize continuous flow may be applicable, if care is exercised, in patients with intermittent flow. In measuring flow time the time intervals between flow episodes are disregarded.
   Voiding time is total duration of micturition, i.e., includes interruptions. When voiding is completed without interruption, voiding time is equal to flow time.

Bladder pressure measurements during micturition

The specification of patient position, access for pressure measurement, catheter type, and measuring equipment are as for cystometry (see *Cystometry*, page 1032).

Definitions

The terminology referring to bladder pressure during micturition is defined as follows (Fig. 80.4):

Opening time is the elapsed time from initial rise in detrusor pressure to onset of flow. This is the initial isovolumetric contraction period of micturition. Time lags should be taken into account. In most urodynamic systems a time lag occurs equal to the time taken for the urine to pass from the point of pressure measurement to the uroflow transducer.

The following parameters are applicable to measurements of each of the pressure curves – intravesical, abdominal, and detrusor pressure:

Premicturition pressure is the pressure recorded immediately before the initial isovolumetric contraction.

Opening pressure is the pressure recorded at the onset of measured flow.

Maximum pressure is the maximum value of the measured pressure.

Pressure at maximum flow is the pressure recorded at maximum measured flow rate.

Contraction pressure at maximum flow is the difference between pressure at maximum flow and premicturition pressure.

Postmicturition events (e.g., after contraction) are not well understood and so cannot be defined as yet.

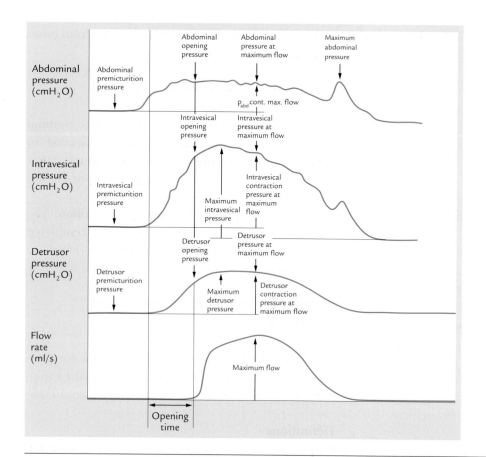

Figure 80.4. *Diagram of a pressure–flow recording of micturition with ICS recommended nomenclature.*

Pressure flow relationships

In the early days of urodynamics the flow rate and voiding pressure were related as a 'urethral resistance factor.' The concept of a resistance factor originates from rigid tube hydrodynamics. The urethra does not generally behave as a rigid tube; it is an irregular and distensible conduit and its walls and surroundings have active and passive elements which influence the flow through it. Therefore a resistance factor cannot provide a valid comparison between patients.

There are many ways of displaying the relationships between flow and pressure during micturition. An example is suggested in the third ICS report[3] (Fig. 80.5). As yet, available data do not permit a standard presentation of pressure/flow parameters.

When data from a group of patients are presented, pressure flow relationships may be shown on a graph, as illustrated in Figure 80.5. This form of presentation allows lines of demarcation to be drawn on the graph to separate the results according to the problem being studied. The points shown in Figure 80.5 are purely illustrative to indicate how the data might fall into groups. The group of equivocal results might include either an unrepresentative micturition in an obstructed or an unobstructed patient, or underactive detrusor function with

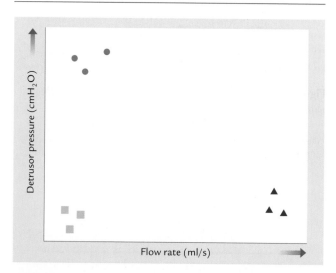

Figure 80.5. *Diagram illustrating the presentation of pressure–flow data on individual patients in three groups of three patients (● obstructed; ▲ unobstructed; ▣ equivocal).*

or without obstruction. This is the group which invalidates the use of the term 'urethral resistance factors.'

Urethral pressure measurements during voiding

The voiding urethral pressure profile (VUPP) is used to determine the pressure and site of urethral obstruction. Pressure is recorded in the urethra during voiding. The technique is similar to that used in the UPP measured during storage (the resting and stress profiles; see *Urethral pressure measurement*, page 1034).

General and technical information should be recorded as for UPP during storage (see *Urethral pressure measurement*, page 1034).

Accurate interpretation of the VUPP depends on the simultaneous measurement of intravesical pressure and the measurement of pressure at a precisely localized point in the urethra. Localization may be achieved by radiopaque marker on the catheter, which allows the pressure measurements to be related to a visualized point in the urethra.

This technique is not fully developed, and a number of technical as well as clinical problems need to be solved before the VUPP is widely used.

Residual urine

Residual urine is defined as the volume of fluid remaining in the bladder immediately following the completion of micturition. The measurement of residual urine forms an integral part of the study of micturition. However, voiding in unfamiliar surroundings may lead to unrepresentative results, as may voiding on command with a partially filled or overfilled bladder. Residual urine is commonly estimated by the following methods:

1. Catheter or cystoscope (transurethral, suprapubic);
2. Radiography (excretion urography, micturition cystography);
3. Ultrasonics;
4. Radioisotopes (clearance, gamma camera).

When estimating residual urine the measurement of voided volume and the time interval between voiding and residual urine estimation should be recorded. This is particularly important if the patient is in a diuretic phase. In the condition of vesicoureteric reflux, urine may re-enter the bladder after micturition and may falsely be interpreted as residual urine. The presence of urine in bladder diverticula following micturition presents special problems of interpretation, since a diverticulum may be regarded either as part of the bladder cavity or as outside the functioning bladder.

The various methods of measurement each have limitations as to their applicability and accuracy in the various conditions associated with residual urine. Therefore it is necessary to choose a method appropriate to the clinical problems. The absence of residual urine is usually an observation of clinical value, but does not exclude infravesical obstruction or bladder dysfunction. An isolated finding of residual urine requires confirmation before being considered significant.

PROCEDURES RELATED TO NEUROPHYSIOLOGICAL EVALUATION OF THE URINARY TRACT DURING FILLING AND VOIDING

Electromyography

Electromyography (EMG) is the study of electrical potentials generated by the depolarization of muscle. The following refers to striated muscle EMG. The functional unit in EMG is the motor unit. This comprises a single motor neuron and the muscle fibers it innervates. A motor unit action potential is the recorded depolarization of muscle fibers which results from activation of a single anterior horn cell. Muscle action potentials may be detected either by needle electrodes or by surface electrodes.

Needle electrodes are placed directly into the muscle mass and permit visualization of the individual motor unit action potentials. Surface electrodes are applied to an epithelial surface as close to the muscle under study as possible. Surface electrodes detect the action potentials from groups of adjacent motor units underlying the recording surface.

EMG potentials may be displayed on an oscilloscope screen or played through audio amplifiers. A permanent record of EMG potentials can only be made using a chart recorder with a high-frequency response (in the range of 10 KHz).

EMG should be interpreted in the light of the patient's symptoms, physical findings, and urologic and urodynamic investigations.

General information

The following details should be given:

1. EMG (solitary procedure, part of urodynamic or other electro-physiological investigation).
2. Patient position (supine, standing, sitting, or other).
3. Electrode placement:
   a. Sampling site – intrinsic striated muscle of the urethra, periurethral striated muscle, bulbocavernosus muscle, external anal sphincter, pubococcygeus, or other. State whether sites are single or multiple, unilateral or bilateral. Also state number of samples per site.
   b. Recording electrode – define the precise anatomical location of the electrode. For needle electrodes, include site of needle entry, angle of entry, and needle depth. For vaginal or urethral surface electrodes, state method of determining position of electrode.
   c. Reference electrode position.

Note: ensure that there is no electrical interference with any other machines, e.g., x-ray apparatus.

Technical information

The following details should be given:

1. Electrodes:
   a. Needle electrodes – design (concentric, bipolar, monopolar, single fiber, other); dimensions (length, diameter, recording area); electrode material (e.g., platinum).
   b. Surface electrodes – type (skin, plug, catheter, other); size and shape; electrode material; mode of fixation to recording surface; conducting medium (e.g., saline, jelly).
2. Amplifier (make and specifications).
3. Signal processing (data: raw, averaged, integrated, or other).
4. Display equipment (make and specifications to include method of calibration, time base, full scale deflection in microvolts and polarity):
   a. Oscilloscope;
   b. Chart recorder;
   c. Loudspeaker;
   d. Other.
5. Storage (make and specifications):
   a. Paper;
   b. Magnetic tape recorder;
   c. Microprocessor;
   d. Other.
6. Hard copy production (make and specifications):
   a. Chart recorder;
   b. Photographic/video reproduction of oscilloscope screen;
   c. Other.

EMG findings

Individual motor unit action potentials

Normal motor unit potentials have a characteristic configuration, amplitude and duration. Abnormalities of the motor unit may include an increase in the amplitude, duration, and complexity of waveform (polyphasicity) of the potentials. A polyphasic potential is defined as one having more than five deflections. The EMG findings of fibrillations, positive sharp waves, and bizarre high-frequency potentials are thought to be abnormal.

Recruitment patterns

In normal subjects there is a gradual increase in 'pelvic floor' and 'sphincter' EMG activity during bladder filling. At the onset of micturition there is complete absence of activity. Any sphincter EMG activity during voiding is abnormal unless the patient is attempting to inhibit micturition. The finding of increased sphincter EMG activity during voiding, accompanied by characteristic simultaneous detrusor pressure and flow changes is described by the term 'detrusor-sphincter-dyssynergia.' In this condition a detrusor contraction occurs concurrently with an inappropriate contraction of the urethral and/or periurethral striated muscle.

Nerve conduction studies

Nerve conduction studies involve stimulation of a peripheral nerve and recording the time taken for a response to occur in muscle innervated by the nerve under study. The time taken from stimulation of the nerve to the response in the muscle is called the 'latency'. Motor latency is the time taken by the fastest motor fibers in the nerve to conduct impulses to the muscle and it depends on conduction distance and the conduction velocity of the fastest fibers.

General information

Also applicable to reflex latencies and evoked potentials (see page 1042). The following details should be given:

1. Type of investigation:
   a. Nerve conduction study (e.g., pudendal nerve);
   b. Reflex latency determination (e.g., bulbocavernosus);
   c. Spinal evoked potential;
   d. Cortical evoked potential;
   e. Other.
2. Is the study a solitary procedure or part of urodynamic or neurophysiological investigations?
3. Patient position and environmental temperature, noise level, and illumination.
4. Electrode placement. Define electrode placement in precise anatomical terms. The exact interelectrode distance is required for nerve conduction velocity calculations.
   a. Stimulation site (penis, clitoris, urethra, bladder neck, bladder, or other).
   b. Recording sites (external and sphincter, periurethral striated muscle, bulbocavernosus muscle, spinal cord, cerebral cortex or other). When recording spinal evoked responses, the sites of the recording electrodes should be specified according to the bony landmarks (e.g., L4). In cortical evoked responses the sites of the recording electrodes should be specified as in the international 10–20 system.[6] The sampling techniques should be specified (single or multiple, unilateral or bilateral, ipsilateral or contralateral, or other).
   c. Reference electrode position.
   d. Grounding electrode site. Ideally this should be between the stimulation and recording sites to reduce stimulus artifact.

Technical information

Also applicable to reflex latencies and evoked potentials (see Reflex latencies, page 1042). The following details should be given:

1. Electrodes (make and specifications). Describe separately stimulus and recording electrodes as below:
   a. Design (e.g., needle, plate, ring, and configuration of anode and cathode where applicable);
   b. Dimensions;
   c. Electrode material (e.g., platinum);
   d. Contact medium.
2. Stimulator (make and specifications):
   a. Stimulus parameters (pulse width, frequency, pattern, current density, electrode impedance in Kohms). Also define in terms of threshold (e.g., in case of supramaximal stimulation).
3. Amplifier (make and specifications):
   a. Sensitivity (mV–µV);
   b. Filters – low pass (Hz) or high pass (kHz);
   c. Sampling time (ms).
4. Averager – make and specifications:
   a. Number of stimuli sampled.
5. Display equipment (make and specifications to include method of calibration, time base, full scale deflection in microvolts, and polarity):
   a. Oscilloscope.
6. Storage (make and specifications):
   a. Paper;
   b. Magnetic tape recorder;
   c. Microprocessor;
   d. Other.
7. Hard copy production (make and specification):
   a. Chart recorder;
   b. Photographic/video reproduction of oscilloscope screen;
   c. XY recorder;
   d. Other.

Description of nerve conduction studies

Recordings are made from muscle, and the latency of response of the muscle is measured. The latency is taken as the time to onset of the earliest response.

To ensure that response time can be precisely measured, the gain should be increased to give a clearly defined take-off point (gain setting at least 100 µV/div and using a short time base, e.g., 1–2 ms/div).

Additional information may be obtained from nerve conduction studies, if, when using surface electrodes to record a compound muscle action potential, the amplitude is measured. The gain setting must be reduced so that the whole response is displayed and a longer time base is recommended (e.g., 1 mV/div and 5 ms/div). Since the amplitude is proportional to the number of motor unit potentials within the vicinity of the recording electrodes, a reduction in amplitude indicates loss of motor units and therefore denervation. (*Note:* A prolongation of latency is not necessarily indicative of denervation.)

Reflex latencies

Reflex latencies require stimulation of sensory fields and recordings from the muscle which contracts reflexly in response to the stimulation. Such responses are a test of reflex arcs, which comprise both afferent and efferent limbs and a synaptic region within the central nervous system. The reflex latency expresses the nerve conduction velocity in both limbs of the arc and the integrity of the central nervous system at the level of the synapse(s). Increased reflex latency may occur as a result of slowed afferent or efferent nerve conduction or due to central nervous system conduction delays.

General and technical information

The same technical and general details apply as discussed above under *Nerve conduction studies* (page 1040).

Description of reflex latency measurements

Recordings are made from muscle, and the latency of response of the muscle is measured. The latency is taken as the time to onset of the earliest response.

To ensure that response time can be precisely measured, the gain should be increased to give a clearly defined take-off point (gain setting at least 100 µV/div and using a short time base, e.g., 1–2 ms/div).

Evoked responses

Evoked responses are potential changes in central nervous system neurons resulting from distant stimulation, usually electrical. They are recorded using averaging techniques. Evoked responses may be used to test the integrity of peripheral, spinal, and central nervous pathways. As with nerve conduction studies, the conduction time (latency) may be measured. In addition, information may be gained from the amplitude and configuration of these responses.

General and technical information

See *Nerve conduction studies* (page 1040).

Description of evoked responses

When describing the presence or absence of stimulus evoked responses and their configuration the following details should be given:

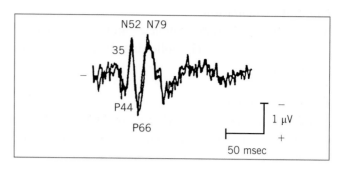

Figure 80.6. *Multiphasic evoked response recorded from the cerebral cortex after stimulation of the dorsal aspect of the penis. The recording shows the conventional labelling of negative (N) and positive (P) deflections, with the latency of each deflection from the point of stimulation in milliseconds.*

1. Single or multiphasic response.
2. Onset of response – defined as the start of the first reproducible potential. Since the onset of the response may be difficult to ascertain precisely, the criteria used should be stated.
3. Latency to onset – defined as the time (in milliseconds) from the onset of stimulus to the onset of response. The central conduction time relates to cortical evoked potentials and is defined as the difference between the latencies of the cortical and the spinal evoked potentials. This parameter may be used to test the integrity of the corticospinal neuraxis.
4. Latencies to peaks of positive and negative deflections in multiphasic response (Fig. 80.6). P denotes positive deflections. N denotes negative deflections. In multiphasic responses, the peaks are numbered consecutively (e.g., P1, N1, P2, N2 ...) or according to the latencies to peaks in milliseconds (e.g., P44, N52, P66 ...).
5. The amplitude of the responses is measured in microvolts.

Sensory testing

Limited information, of a subjective nature, may be obtained during cystometry by recording such parameters as the first desire to micturate, urgency, or pain. However, sensory function in the lower urinary tract can be assessed by semi-objective tests by the measurement of urethral and/or vesical sensory thresholds to a standard applied stimulus such as a known electrical current.

General information

The following details should be given:

1. Patient's position (supine, sitting, standing, other);
2. Bladder volume at time of testing;
3. Site of applied stimulus (intravesical, intraurethral);
4. Number of times the stimulus was applied and the response, e.g., the first sensation or the sensation of pulsing;
5. Type of applied stimulus:
   a. Electrical current – it is usual to use a constant current stimulator in urethral sensory measurement. State electrode characteristics and placement as in section on EMG (page 1039); electrode contact area and distance between electrodes if applicable; impedance characteristics of the system; type of conductive medium used for electrode/epithelial contact. *Note: Topical anaesthetic agents should not be used.* Also state stimulator make and specifications; and stimulation parameters (pulse width, frequency, pattern, duration, current density).
   b. Other (e.g., mechanical, chemical).

Definition of sensory thresholds

The vesical/urethral sensory threshold is defined as the least current which consistently produces a sensation perceived by the subject during stimulation at the site under investigation. However, the absolute values will vary in relation to the site of the stimulus, the characteristics of the equipment, and the stimulation parameters. Normal values should be established for each system.

CLASSIFICATION OF LOWER URINARY TRACT DYSFUNCTION

The lower urinary tract is composed of the *bladder* and *urethra*. They form a functional unit and their interaction cannot be ignored. Each has two functions, the bladder to store and void, the urethra to control and convey. When a reference is made to the hydrodynamic function or to the whole anatomical unit as a storage organ – the vesica urinaria – the correct term is the *bladder*. When the smooth muscle structure known as the m.detrusor urinae is being discussed, then the correct term is *detrusor*. For simplicity the bladder/detrusor and the urethra will be considered separately so that a classification based on a combination of functional anomalies can be reached. Sensation cannot be precisely evaluated but must be assessed. This classification depends on the results of various objective urodynamic investigations. A complete urodynamic assessment is not necessary in all patients. However, studies of the filling and voiding phases are essential for each patient. As the bladder and urethra may behave differently during the storage and micturition phases of bladder function it is most useful to examine bladder and urethral activity separately in each phase.

Terms used should be objective and definable, and ideally should be applicable to the whole range of abnormality. When authors disagree with the classification presented below, or use terms which have not been defined here, they should ensure that the meaning of their terminology is made clear.

Assuming the absence of inflammation, infection, and neoplasm, *lower urinary tract dysfunction* may be caused by:

1. Disturbance of the pertinent nervous or psychological control system;
2. Disorders of muscle function;
3. Structural abnormalities.

Urodynamic diagnoses based on this classification should correlate with the patient's symptoms and signs. For example, the presence of an unstable contraction in an asymptomatic continent patient does not warrant a diagnosis of detrusor overactivity during storage.

The storage phase

Bladder function during storage

This may be described according to:

- Detrusor activity
- Bladder sensation
- Bladder capacity
- Compliance

Detrusor activity

In this context detrusor activity is interpreted from the measurement of detrusor pressure (p_{det}). Detrusor activity may be:

- Normal
- Overactive

In *normal detrusor function* the bladder volume increases during the filling phase without a significant rise in pressure (accommodation). No involuntary contractions occur despite provocation. A normal detrusor so defined may be described as 'stable'.

Overactive detrusor function is characterized by involuntary detrusor contractions during the filling phase, which may be spontaneous or provoked and which the patient cannot completely suppress. Involuntary detrusor contractions may be provoked by rapid filling, alterations of posture, coughing, walking, jumping, and other triggering procedures. Various terms have been used to describe these features and they are defined as follows:

The *unstable detrusor* is one that is shown objectively to contract, spontaneously or on provocation, during the filling phase while the patient is attempting to inhibit

micturition. Unstable detrusor contractions may be asymptomatic or may be interpreted as a normal desire to void. The presence of these contractions does not necessarily imply a neurologic disorder. Unstable contractions are usually phasic in type (Fig. 80.7a). A gradual increase in detrusor pressure without subsequent decrease is best regarded as a change of compliance (Fig. 80.7b).

Detrusor hyperreflexia is defined as overactivity due to disturbance of the nervous control mechanisms. The term 'detrusor hyperreflexia' should only be used when there is objective evidence of a relevant neurologic disorder. The use of conceptual and undefined terms such as 'hypertonic,' 'systolic,' 'uninhibited,' 'spastic,' and 'automatic' should be avoided.

Bladder sensation

During filling, bladder sensation can be classified in qualitative terms (see *Cystometry*, page 1032) and by objective measurement (see *Sensory testing*, page 1042). Sensation can be classified broadly as follows:

- Normal
- Increased (hypersensitive)
- Reduced (hyposensitive)
- Absent.

Bladder capacity

(See *Cystometry*, page 1032)

Compliance

This is defined as: $\Delta V/\Delta p$ (see *Cystometry*, page 1032). Compliance may change during the cystometric examination and is variably dependent upon a number of factors including:

1. Rate of filling;
2. The part of the cystometrogram curve used for compliance calculation;
3. The volume interval over which compliance is calculated;
4. The geometry (shape) of the bladder;
5. The thickness of the bladder wall;
6. The mechanical properties of the bladder wall;
7. The contractile/relaxant properties of the detrusor.

During normal bladder filling little or no pressure change occurs and this is termed 'normal compliance'.

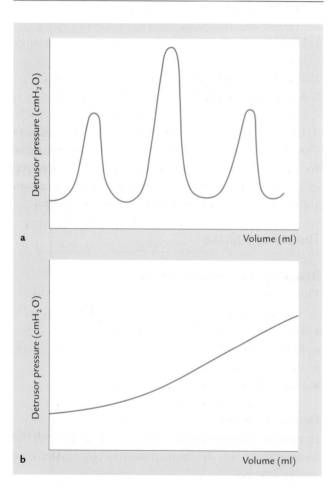

Figure 80.7. *Diagrams of filling cystometry: (a) typical phasic unstable detrusor contraction; (b) gradual increase of detrusor pressure with filling characteristic of reduced bladded compliance.*

However, at present there is insufficient data to define normal, high and low compliance.

When reporting compliance, specify:

1. The rate of bladder filling;
2. The bladder volume at which compliance is calculated;
3. The volume increment over which compliance is calculated;
4. The part of the cystometrogram curve used for the calculation of compliance.

Urethral function during storage

The urethral closure mechanism during storage may be:

- Normal
- Incompetent.

The *normal urethral closure mechanism* maintains a positive urethral closure pressure during filling even in the presence of increased abdominal pressure. Immediately prior to micturition the normal closure pressure decreases to allow flow.

An *incompetent urethral closure mechanism* is defined as one which allows leakage or urine in the absence of a detrusor contraction. Leakage may occur whenever intravesical pressure exceeds intraurethral pressure (genuine stress incontinence) or when there is an involuntary fall in urethral pressure. Terms such as 'the unstable urethra' await further data and precise definition.

Urinary incontinence

This is defined as involuntary loss of urine which is objectively demonstrable and a social or hygienic problem. Loss of urine through channels other than the urethra is extraurethral incontinence.

Urinary incontinence denotes:

1. A symptom;
2. A sign;
3. A condition.

The symptom indicates the patient's statement of involuntary urine loss, the sign is the objective demonstration of urine loss, and the condition is the urodynamic demonstration of urine loss.

Symptoms

These can be defined as follows:

- *Urge incontinence* – the involuntary loss of urine associated with a strong desire to void (urgency). *Urgency* may be associated with two types of dysfunction:
  - Overactive detrusor function (*motor urgency*)
  - Hypersensitivity (*sensory urgency*).
- *Stress incontinence* – the symptom indicates the patient's statement of involuntary loss of urine during physical exertion.
- *'Unconscious' incontinence* – incontinence may occur in the absence of urge and without conscious recognition of the urinary loss.
- *Enuresis* – any involuntary loss of urine. If the term is used to denote incontinence during sleep, it should always be qualified with the adjective 'nocturnal'.
- *Post-micturition dribble* and *continuous leakage* – denote other symptomatic forms of incontinence.

Signs

The sign stress incontinence denotes the observation of loss of urine from the urethra synchronous with physical exertion (e.g., coughing). Incontinence may also be observed without physical exercise. Post-micturition dribble and continuous leakage denote other signs of incontinence. Symptoms and signs alone may not disclose the cause of urinary incontinence. Accurate diagnosis often requires urodynamic investigation in addition to careful history and physical examination.

Conditions

These can be defined as follows:

- *Genuine stress incontinence* – the involuntary loss of urine occurring when, in the absence of a detrusor contraction, the intravesical pressure exceeds the maximum urethral pressure.
- *Reflex incontinence* – loss of urine due to detrusor hyperreflexia and/or involuntary urethral relaxation in the absence of the sensation usually associated with the desire to micturate. This condition is only seen in patients with neuropathic bladder/urethral disorders.
- *Overflow incontinence* – any involuntary loss of urine associated with overdistension of the bladder.

The voiding phase

The detrusor during voiding
During micturition the detrusor may be:

- Acontractile
- Underactive
- Normal.

The *acontractile detrusor* is one that cannot be demonstrated to contract during urodynamic studies. *Detrusor areflexia* is defined as acontractility due to an abnormality of nervous control and denotes the complete absence of centrally coordinated contraction. In detrusor areflexia due to a lesion of the conus medullaris or sacral nerve outflow, the detrusor should be described as *decentralized* – not denervated, since the peripheral neurons remain. In such bladders pressure fluctuations of low amplitude, sometimes known as 'autonomous' waves, may occasionally occur. The use of terms such as 'atonic,' 'hypotonic,' 'autonomic,' and 'flaccid' should be avoided.

Detrusor underactivity is defined as a detrusor contraction of inadequate magnitude and/or duration to effect bladder emptying with a normal time span. The term should be reserved as an expression describing detrusor activity during micturition. Patients may have underactivity during micturition and detrusor overactivity during filling.

Normal detrusor contractility. Normal voiding is achieved by a voluntarily initiated detrusor contraction that is sustained and can usually be suppressed voluntarily. A normal detrusor contraction will effect complete bladder emptying in the absence of obstruction. For a given detrusor contraction, the magnitude of the recorded pressure rise will depend on the degree of outlet resistance.

Urethral function during micturition
During voiding urethral function may be:

- Normal
- Obstructive
  - overactivity
  - mechanical.

Normal – the normal urethra opens to allow the bladder to be emptied.

Obstruction – this occurs when the urethral closure mechanism contracts against a detrusor contraction or fails to open at attempted micturition. Synchronous detrusor and urethral contraction is *detrusor/urethral dyssynergia*. This diagnosis should be qualified by stating the location and type of the urethral muscles (striated or smooth) which are involved. Despite the confusion surrounding 'sphincter' terminology, the use of certain terms is so widespread that they are retained and defined here. The term *detrusor/external sphincter dyssynergia* or *detrusor-sphincter-dyssynergia (DSD)* describes a detrusor contraction concurrent with an involuntary contraction of the urethral and/or periurethral striated muscle. In the adult, detrusor sphincter dyssynergia is a feature of neurologic voiding disorders. In the absence of neurologic features the validity of this diagnosis should be questioned. The term *detrusor/bladder neck dyssynergia* is used to denote a detrusor contraction concurrent with an objectively demonstrated failure of bladder neck opening. No parallel term has been elaborated for possible detrusor/distal urethral (smooth muscle) dyssynergia.

Overactivity of the striated urethral sphincter may occur in the absence of detrusor contraction, and may prevent voiding. This is not detrusor/sphincter dyssynergia.

Overactivity of the urethral sphincter may occur during voiding in the absence of neurologic disease and is termed *dysfunctional voiding*. The use of terms such as 'non-neurogenic' and 'occult neuropathic' should be avoided.

Mechanical obstruction – this is most commonly anatomical, e.g., caused by urethral stricture.

Summary
Using the characteristics of detrusor and urethral function during storage and micturition an accurate definition of lower urinary tract behaviour in each patient becomes possible.

UNITS OF MEASUREMENT
In the urodynamic literature pressure is measured in centimeters of water and *not* in millimeters of mercury. When Laplace's law is used to calculate tension in the bladder wall, it is often found that pressure is then measured in dyne/cm^2. This lack of uniformity in the systems used leads to confusion when other parameters,

Table 80.1. *Recommended units of measurement*

Quantity	Acceptable unit	Symbol
Volume	milliliter	ml
Time	second	s
Flow rate	milliliters/second	ml/s
Pressure	centimeters of water[a]	cmH$_2$O
Length	meters or submultiples	m, cm, mm
Velocity	meters/second or submultiples	m/s, cm/s
Temperature	degrees Celsius	°C

[a]The SI unit is the pascal (Pa), but it is only practical at present to calibrate our instruments in cmH$_2$O. One centimetre of water pressure is approximately equal to 100 pascals (1 cmH$_2$O = 98.07 Pa = 0.098 kPa).

which are a function of pressure, are computed – for instance, 'compliance', contraction force, velocity, etc. From these few examples it is evident that standardization is essential for meaningful communication. Many journals now require that the results be given in SI units. This section is designed to give guidance in the application of the SI system to urodynamics and defines the units involved. The principal units to be used are listed in Table 80.1.

SYMBOLS

It is often helpful to use symbols in a communication. The system in Table 80.2 has been devised to standardize a code of symbols for use in urodynamics. The rationale of the system is to have a basic symbol representing the physical quantity with qualifying subscripts. The list of basic symbols largely conforms to

Table 80.2. *List of symbols*

Basic symbols		Urologic qualifiers		Value	
Pressure	p	Bladder	ves	Maximum	max
Volume	V	Urethra	ura	Minimum	min
Flow rate	Q	Ureter	ure	Average	ave
Velocity	v	Detrusor	det	Isovolumetric	isv
Time	t	Abdomen	abd	Isotonic	ist
Temperature	T	External stream	ext	Isobaric	isb
Length	l			Isometric	ism
Area	A				
Diameter	d				
Force	F				
Energy	E				
Power	P				
Compliance	C				
Work	W				
Energy per unit volume	e				

$p_{det/max}$ = maximum detrusor pressure
e_{ext} = kinetic energy per unit volume in the external stream

international usage. The qualifying subscripts relate to the basic symbols for commonly used urodynamic parameters.

REFERENCES

1. Bates P, Bradley WE, Glen E *et al.* First report on the standardisation of terminology of lower urinary tract function. Urinary incontinence. Procedures related to the evaluation of urine storage – cystometry, urethral closure pressure profile, units of measurement. *Br J Urol* 1976; 48: 39–42; *Eur Urol* 1976; 2: 274–276; *Scand J Urol Nephrol* 1976; 11: 193–196; *Urol Int* 1976; 2: 81–87

2. Bates P, Glen E, Griffiths D *et al.* Second report on the standardisation of terminology of lower urinary tract function. Procedures related to the evaluation of micturition – flow rate, pressure measurement, symbols. *Acta Urol Jpn* 1977; 27: 1563–1566; *Br J Urol* 1977; 49: 207–210; *Eur Urol* 1977; 3: 168–170; *Scand J Urol Nephrol* 1977; 11: 197–199

3. Bates P, Bradley WE, Glen E *et al.* Third report on the standardization of terminology of lower urinary tract function. Procedures related to the evaluation of micturition: pressure flow relationships, residual urine. *Br J Urol* 1980; 52: 348–350; *Eur Urol* 1980; 6: 170–171; *Acta Urol Jpn* 1980; 27: 1566–1568; *Scand J Urol Nephrol* 1980; 12: 191–193

4. Bates P, Bradley WE, Glen E *et al.* Fourth report on the standardization of terminology of lower urinary tract function. Terminology related to neuromuscular dysfunction of lower urinary tract. *Br J Urol* 1981; 53: 333–335; *Urology* 1981; 17: 618–620; *Scand J Urol Nephrol* 1981; 15: 169–171; *Acta Urol Jpn* 1981; 27: 1568–1571

5. Abrams P, Blaivas JG, Stanton SL *et al.* Sixth report on the standardization of terminology of lower urinary tract function. Procedures related to neurophysiological investigations. Electromyography, nerve conduction studies, reflex latencies, evoked potentials and sensory testing. *World J Urol* 1986; 4: 2–5; *Scand J Urol Nephrol* 1986; 20: 161–164; *Br J Urol* 1986; 59: 300–307

6. Jasper HH. Report to the committee on the methods of clinical examination in electroencephalography. *Electroencephalogr Clin Neurophysiol* 1958; 10: 370–375

The standardization of terminology of female pelvic organ prolapse and pelvic floor dysfunction

R. C. Bump, A. Mattiasson, K. Bø, L. P. Brubaker, J. O. L. DeLancey,
P. Klarskov, B. L. Shull, A. R. B. Smith

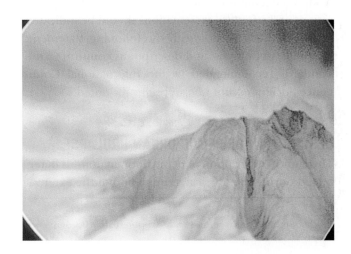

INTRODUCTION

The International Continence Society (ICS) has been at the forefront in the standardization of terminology of lower urinary tract function since the establishment of the Committee on Standardization of Terminology in 1973. This committee's efforts over the past two decades have resulted in the world-wide acceptance of terminology standards that allow clinicians and researchers interested in the lower urinary tract to communicate efficiently and precisely. While female pelvic organ prolapse and pelvic floor dysfunction are intimately related to lower urinary tract function, such accurate communication using standard terminology has not been possible for these conditions.

There is no universally accepted system for describing the anatomic position of the pelvic organs. Many reports use terms for the description of pelvic organ prolapse which are undefined; none of the many aspiring grading systems has been adequately validated with respect either to reproducibility or to the clinical significance of different grades. The absence of standard, validated definitions prevents comparisons of published series from different institutions and longitudinal evaluation of an individual patient. A primary goal of this report is to introduce a system that will allow the accurate, quantitative description of pelvic support findings in individual patients.

This document is a first effort toward the establishment of standard, reliable, and validated descriptions of female pelvic anatomy and function. The subcommittee acknowledges a need for well designed reliability studies to evaluate and validate various descriptions and definitions. We have tried to develop guidelines that will promote new insights rather than existing biases. Acknowledgement of these standards in written publications and scientific presentations should be indicated in the Methods Section with the following statement: 'Methods, definitions, and descriptions conform to the standards recommended by the International Continence Society, except where specifically noted'.

DESCRIPTION OF PELVIC ORGAN PROLAPSE

The clinical description of pelvic floor anatomy is determined during the physical examination of the external

genitalia and vaginal canal. The specifics of the examination technique are not dictated by this document, however authors should precisely describe their specific technique. Segments of the lower reproductive tract will replace such terms as 'cystocele, rectocele, enterocele, or urethrovesical junction' because these terms may imply an unrealistic certainty as to the structures on the other side of the reproductive tract bulge, particularly in women who have had previous prolapse surgery.

Conditions of the examination

Many variables of examination technique may influence findings in patients with pelvic organ prolapse. It is critical that the examiner sees and describes the maximum protrusion noted by the individual subject during her daily activities. Therefore the criteria for the end point of the examination and the full development of the prolapse must be specified in any report.

Suggested criteria for demonstration of maximum prolapse should include one or all of the following:

a. Any protrusion of the vaginal wall has become tight during straining by the patient.
b. Traction on the prolapse causes no further descent.
c. The subject confirms that the size of the prolapse and extent of the protrusion seen by the examiner is as extensive as the most severe protrusion which she has experienced. The means of this confirmation should be specified. For example, the subject may use a small handheld mirror to visualize the protrusion.
d. A standing, straining examination confirms that the full extent of the prolapse was observed in other positions used.

Other variables of technique that should be specified during the quantitative description (page 1051) and the ordinal staging (page 1054) of pelvic organ prolapse include the following:

a. the position of the subject (e.g., supine lithotomy, lateral Sims' position, specified degrees of upright, erect sitting, standing, etc);
b. the type of examination table or chair used;
c. the type of standard vaginal specula, retractors, or tractors used;

Article reprinted with permission of the International Continence Society.

d. diagrams of any customized retraction, traction, or measuring devices used;

e. the type (e.g., Valsalva maneuver, cough) and, if measured, intensity (e.g., vesical or rectal pressure rise) of straining used to develop the prolapse maximally;

f. fullness of bladder, and, if the bladder was empty, whether this was by spontaneous voiding or by catheterization;

g. content or rectum;

h. the method by which any quantitative measurements were made (e.g., estimation by visualization or palpation, direct measurement with a calibrated device, etc).

There is a critical need to define the importance of all variables of technique as they relate to the ease of assessment and reproducibility of measurements. Researchers should determine the inter-observer and intra-observer reliability of measurements made with their assessment techniques before utilizing them as baseline and outcome variables. Manuscript descriptions of assessment techniques should include sufficient detail to ensure that other researchers can precisely replicate them.

Quantitative description of pelvic organ position

This description system is a tandem profile in that it contains a series of component measurements grouped together in combination, but listed separately in tandem, without being fused into a distinctive new expression or 'grade'. It allows for the precise description of an individual woman's pelvic support without assigning a 'severity value'. Second, it allows accurate site-specific observations of the stability or progression of prolapse over time by the same or different observers. Finally, it allows similar judgements as to the outcome of surgical repair of prolapse. For example, noting that a surgical procedure moved the vaginal apex from 0.5 cm beyond the hymeneal ring to 0.5 cm above the hymeneal ring denotes more meager improvement than stating that the prolapse was reduced from Grade 3 to Grade 1 as would be the case using some current grading systems.

Definition of anatomic landmarks

Prolapse should be evaluated by a standard system relative to clearly defined anatomic points of reference.

These are of two types, fixed reference points and defined points for measurement.

Fixed point of reference

Prolapse should be evaluated relative to a fixed anatomic landmark which can be consistently and precisely identified. The hymen will be the fixed point of reference used throughout this system of quantitative prolapse description.

Visually, the hymen provides a precisely identifiable landmark for reference. Although it is recognized that the plane of the hymen is somewhat variable depending upon the degree of levator ani dysfunction, it remains the best landmark available. 'Hymen' is preferable to the ill-defined and imprecise term 'introitus'. The anatomic position of the six defined points for measurement (see *Defined points for measurement* below) should be centimeters above or proximal to the hymen (negative number) or centimeters below or distal to the hymen (positive number) with the plane of the hymen being defined as zero (0). For example, a cervix that protruded 3 cm distal to the hymen would be +3 cm.

Palpably, the ischial spines provide precisely identifiable landmarks. In the sitting or standing position or in situations with limited viability due to obesity or limited ability for hip abduction, the position of the cervix or the leading point of the prolapse relative to the ischial spines may be measured by palpation. Measurements so obtained should be normalized to the level of the hymen by noting the distance between the ischial spines and the plane of the hymen. For example, a cervix that is 3 cm distal to the ischial spines would be at −2 cm if the spines were 5 cm above the plane of the hymen.

Defined points for measurement

Anterior Vaginal Wall   Because the only structure directly visible to the examiner is the surface of the vagina, anterior prolapse should be discussed in terms of a segment of the vaginal wall rather than the organs which lie behind it. Thus, the term 'anterior vaginal wall prolapse' is preferable to 'cystocele' or 'anterior enterocele' unless the organs involved are identified by ancillary tests.

Point Aa   A point located in the midline of the anterior vaginal wall 3 cm proximal to the external urethral meatus. This corresponds to the approximate location of the 'urethrovesical crease', a visible landmark of variable prominence that is obliterated in many patients. By definition, the range of position of Point Aa relative to the hymen is −3 to +3 cm.

Point Ba   A point that represents the **most distal (i.e., most dependent)** position of the upper portion of the anterior vaginal wall from the vaginal cuff or anterior vaginal fornix to Point Aa. By definition, Point Ba is at −3 cm in the absence of prolapse and would have a positive value equal to the position of the cuff in women with total post-hysterectomy vaginal eversion.

Vaginal Apex   These points represent the most proximal locations of the normally positioned lower reproductive tract.

Point C   A point that represents either the most distal (i.e., most dependent) edge of the cervix or the leading edge of the vaginal cuff scar in a woman who has undergone total hysterectomy.

Point D   A point that represents the location of the posterior fornix (or pouch of Douglas) in a woman who still has a cervix. It represents the level of uterosacral ligament attachment to the proximal posterior cervix. It is included as a point of measurement to differentiate suspensory failure of the uterosacral-cardinal ligament complex from cervical elongation. When the location of Point C is significantly more positive than the location of Point D, this is indicative of cervical elongation which may be symmetrical or eccentric (e.g., involving only the anterior lip of the cervix due to a prior laceration). Point D is omitted as a point for measurement in the absence of the cervix.

Posterior Vaginal Wall   Analogous to anterior prolapse, posterior prolapse should be discussed in terms of segments of the vaginal wall rather than the organs which lie behind it. Thus, the term 'posterior vaginal wall prolapse' is preferable to 'rectocele' or 'enterocele' unless the organs involved are identified by ancillary tests. If small bowel appears to be present in the recto-vaginal space, the examiner should comment on this fact and should clearly describe the basis for this clinical impression (e.g., by observation of peristaltic activity in the distended posterior vagina, by palpation of loops of small bowel between an examining finger in the rectum and one in the vagina, etc). In such cases, a 'pulsion' addendum to the point Bp position should be noted (e.g., Bp = +5[pulsion]). See *Supplementary physical examination techniques* points a and b, page 1056.

Point Bp   A point that represents the **most distal (i.e., most dependent)** position of the upper portion of the posterior vaginal wall from the vaginal cuff or posterior vaginal fornix to Point Ap. By definition, Point Bp is at −3 cm in the absence of prolapse and would have a positive value equal to the position of the cuff in a woman with total post-hysterectomy vaginal eversion.

Point Ap   A point located in the midline of the posterior vaginal wall 3 cm proximal to the hymen. By definition, the range of position of Point Ap relative to the hymen is −3 to +3 cm.

Other landmarks and measurements

The *genital hiatus* is measured from the middle of the external urethral meatus to the posterior midline hymen. If the location of the hymen is distorted by a loose band of skin without underlying muscle or connective tissue, the firm palpable tissue of the perineal body should be substituted as the posterior margin for this measurement.

The *perineal body* is measured from the posterior margin of the genital hiatus (as just described) to the mid-anal opening. Measurement of the genital hiatus and perineal body are expressed in centimeters.

The total *vaginal length* is the greatest depth of the vagina in cm when Point C or D is reduced to its full normal position. Note: Eccentric elongation of a prolapsed anterior or posterior vaginal wall should not be included in the measurement of total vaginal length. (See Fig. 81.4a and accompanying discussion). The points and measurements discussed in this section are presented in Figure 81.1.

Making and recording measurements

The position of Points Aa, Ba, Ap, Bp, C, and (if applicable) D with reference to the hymen should be measured and recorded. Positions are expressed as centimeters above or proximal to the hymen (negative number) or centimeters below or distal to the hymen (positive number) with the plane of the hymen being defined as zero (0). While an examiner may be able to make measurements to the nearest half (0.5) cm, it is doubtful that further precision is possible. All reports should clearly specify how measurements were derived. For example, were direct measurements made using a probe, ruler, glove, speculum or other device marked in centimeters, were indirect measurements made with the examiner's fingers and then measured off a centimeter tape, were measurements estimated by the examiner without using a graduated device, or were combinations of techniques used? If customized measuring devices were used, diagrams of such should be included in any manuscript or presentation.

Measurements may be recorded as a simple line of numbers (e.g., −3, −3, −7, −9, −3, −3, 9, 2, 2 for Points Aa, Ba, C, D, Bp, Ap, total vaginal length, genital hiatus, and perineal body respectively). Note that the last three numbers have no sign (i.e., − or +) attached to them because they denote lengths and not positions relative to the hymen. Alternatively, a three-by-three 'tic-tac-toe' grid can be used to organize concisely the measurements as noted in Figure 81.2. If point D is not

applicable due to a prior hysterectomy, this should be noted as such with 'NA' or '—' in either the line of numbers or in the grid.

Figure 81.3 is a line diagram contrasting measurements indicating normal support to those of post hysterectomy vaginal eversion.

In the example of normal support (Fig. 81.3A), Points Aa and Ba and Points Ap and Bp are all −3 since there is no anterior or posterior wall descent. The lowest point of the cervix is 8 cm above the hymen (−8) and the posterior fornix is 2 cm above this (−10). The vaginal length is 10 cm and the genital hiatus and perineal body measure 2 and 3 cm respectively.

Point Aa anterior wall	Point Ba anterior wall	Point C cervix or cuff
Genital hiatus	Perineal body	Total vaginal length
Point Ap posterior wall	Point Bp posterior wall	Point D posterior fornix

Figure 81.2. *A three-by-three grid for recording the quantitative description of pelvic organ prolapse.*

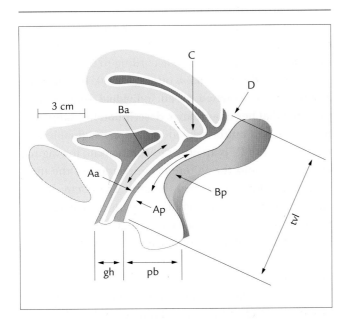

Figure 81.1. *Six points, genital hiatus (gh), perineal body (pb) and total vaginal length (tvl) used for prolapse quantitation.*

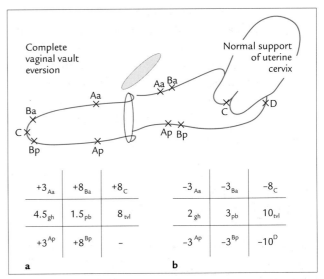

Figure 81.3. *(a) Complete eversion; (b) normal support.*

In the example of complete eversion (Figure 81.3b), the most distal point of the anterior wall (Point Ba), the vaginal cuff scar (Point C), and the most distal point of the posterior wall (Point Bp) are all at the same position (+8) and Points Aa and Ap are maximally distal (both at +3). The fact that the total vaginal length equals the maximum protrusion reflects the fact that the eversion is total.

Figure 81.4 is a line diagram representing predominant anterior and posterior vaginal wall prolapse with partial vault descent.

In the example of a predominant anterior support defect (Fig. 81.4a), the leading point of the prolapse is the upper anterior vaginal wall, Point Ba (+6). Note that there is significant elongation of the bulging anterior wall. Point Aa is maximally distal (+3) and the vaginal cuff scar is 2 cm above the hymen (C = −2). The cuff scar has undergone 4 cm of descent since it would be at −6 (the total vaginal length) if it were perfectly supported. In this example, the total vaginal length is not the maximum depth of the vagina with the elongated anterior vaginal wall maximally reduced, but rather the depth of the vagina at the cuff with Point C reduced to its normal full extent as specified in *Other landmarks and measurements* on page 1052.

In the example of the predominant posterior support defect (Fig. 81.4b), the leading point of the prolapse is the upper posterior vaginal wall, Point Bp (+5). Point Ap is 2 cm distal to the hymen (+2) and the vaginal cuff

scar is 6 cm above the hymen (−6). The cuff has undergone only 2 cm of descent since it would be at −8 (the total vaginal length) if it were perfectly supported.

Ordinal staging of pelvic organ prolapse

The tandem profile for quantifying prolapse just described provides a precise description of anatomy for individual patients. However, because of the many possible combinations, such profiles cannot be directly ranked; the many variations are too numerous to permit useful analysis and comparisons when populations are studied. Consequently they are analogous to other tandem profiles such as the TNM Index for various cancers. For the TNM description of individual patient's cancers to be useful in population studies evaluating prognosis or response to therapy, they are clustered into an ordinal set of stages. Ordinal stages represent adjacent categories that can be ranked in an ascending sequence of magnitude, but the categories are assigned arbitrarily and the intervals between them cannot be actually measured.

While the committee is aware of the arbitrary nature of an ordinal staging system and the possible biases that it introduces, we conclude such a system is necessary if populations are to be described and compared, if symptoms putatively related to prolapse are to be evaluated, and if the results of various treatment options are to be assessed and compared.

Stages are assigned according to the most severe portion of the prolapse when the full extent of the protrusion has been demonstrated according to the criteria in *Conditions of the examination* on page 1050. **In order for a stage to be assigned to an individual subject, it is essential that her quantitative description be completed first.** The 2 cm buffer related to the total vaginal length in Stages 0 and IV is an effort to compensate for vaginal distensibility and the inherent imprecision of the measurement of total vaginal length. The 2 cm buffer around the hymen in Stage II is an effort to avoid confusing a stage to a single plane and to acknowledge practical limits of precision in this assessment.

Stage 0

No prolapse is demonstrated. Points Aa, Ap, Ba, and Bp are all at −3 cm and either Point C or D is between −X cm and −(X − 2) cm, where X = the total vaginal length in cm [i.e., the quantitation value of point C or

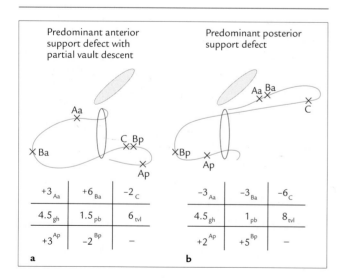

Figure 81.4. *(a) predominant anterior prolapse; (b) predominant posterior prolapse.*

D is $\leq -(X - 2)$ cm]. Figure 81.3a represents Stage 0 pelvic organ prolapse.

Stage I

The criteria for Stage 0 are not met but the most distal portion of the prolapse is more than 1 cm above the level of the hymen (i.e., its quantitation value is < -1 cm). Stage I can be subgrouped according to which portion of the lower reproductive tract is the *most distal* part of the prolapse using the following letter qualifiers: a = anterior vaginal wall, p = posterior vaginal wall, C = vaginal cuff, Cx = cervix, and Aa, Ap, Ba, Bp, and D for the Points of measurement already defined. (e.g., I-Cx if the cervix is the most distal, I-Bp if the upper posterior wall is most distal, or I- if the junction of the distal and proximal anterior wall is the most distal part of the prolapse.

Stage II

The most distal portion of the prolapse is 1 cm or less proximal to or distal to the plane of the hymen (i.e., its quantitation value is ≥ -1 cm but $\leq +1$ cm). Stage II can be subgrouped according to the scheme described under Stage I (e.g., II-a, II-C, or II-Bp).

Stage III

The most distal portion of the prolapse is more than 1 cm below the plane of the hymen but protrudes no further than 2 cm less than the total vaginal length in cm [i.e., its quantitation value is $> +1$ cm but $< +(X - 2)$ cm where X = total vaginal length]. Stage III can be subgrouped according to the scheme described under Stage I. For example, Fig. 81.4a represents State III-Ba and Fig. 81.4b represents Stage III-Bp prolapse.

Stage IV

Essentially complete eversion of the total length of the lower genital tract is demonstrated. The distal portion of the prolapse protrudes to at least $(X - 2)$ cm where X = the total vaginal length in cm [i.e., its quantitation value is $\geq + (X - 2)$ cm]. In most instances, the leading edge of Stage IV prolapse will be the cervix or vaginal cuff scar. Rare exceptions to this can be noted according to the subgrouping scheme described under Stage I. Figure 81.3b represents Stage IV-C prolapse. Table 81.1 summarizes the staging system.

Table 81.1. *ICS pelvic organ prolapse ordinal staging system*

Stage 0	Points Aa, Ap, Ba, & Bp are all at −3 cm *and* Either Point C or D is at $\leq - (X - 2)$ cm
Stage I	The criteria for Stage 0 are not met *and* The leading edge of prolapse is < −1 cm
Stage II	Leading edge of prolapse is ≥ −1 cm but ≤ +1 cm
Stage III	Leading edge of prolapse is > +1 cm but < + (X − 2) cm
Stage IV	Leading edge of prolapse is ≥ + (X − 2) cm

X = Total Vaginal Length in centimeters in Stages 0, III, and IV

Stages I through IV can be subgrouped according to which portion of the lower reproductive tract is the leading edge of the prolapse using the following qualifiers: a = anterior vaginal wall, p = posterior vaginal wall, C = vaginal cuff, Cx = cervix, and Aa, Ba, Ap, Bp, and D for the defined points of measurement. (e.g., IV-Cx, II-a, or III-Bp)

ANCILLARY TECHNIQUES FOR DESCRIBING PELVIC ORGAN PROLAPSE

This series of procedures may help to further characterize pelvic organ prolapse in an individual patient. They are considered ancillary either because they are not yet standardized or validated or because they are not universally available to all patients.

Authors utilizing these procedures should include the following information in their manuscripts.

a. Describe the objective information they intended to generate and how it enhanced their ability to evaluate or treat prolapse.
b. Describe precisely how the test was performed, any instruments that were used, and the specific testing conditions (see *Conditions of the examination*, page 1050) so that other authors can reproduce the study.
c. Document the reliability of the measurement obtained with the technique.

Supplementary physical examination techniques

Many of these techniques are essential to the adequate pre-operative evaluation of a patient with pelvic organ prolapse. While they do not directly affect either the tandem profile or the ordinal stage, they are important for the selection and performance of an effective surgical repair. These techniques include, but are not necessarily limited to, the following:

a. performance of a digital rectal-vaginal examination while the patient is straining and the prolapse is maximally developed to differentiate between a high rectocele and an enterocele;
b. digital assessment of the contents of the rectal-vaginal septum during the examination noted in a. above to differentiate between a 'traction' enterocele (the posterior cul-de-sac is pulled down with the prolapsing cervix or vaginal cuff but is not distended by intestines) and a 'pulsion' enterocele (the intestinal contents of the enterocele distend the rectal-vaginal septum and produce a protruding mass);
c. Q-tip testing for the measurement of urethral axial mobility;
d. measurements of perineal descent;
e. measurements of the transverse diameter of the genital hiatus or of the protruding prolapse;
f. measurements of vaginal volume;
g. description and measurement of rectal prolapse;
h. examination techniques for differentiating between various types of defects (e.g., central versus paravaginal defects of the anterior vaginal wall).

Endoscopy

Cystoscopic visualization of bowel peristalsis under the bladder base or trigone may identify an anterior enterocele in some patients. The endoscopic visualization of the bladder base and rectum and observation of the voluntary constriction and dilation of the urethra, vagina, and rectum has, to date, played a minor role in the evaluation of pelvic floor anatomy and function. When such techniques are described, authors should include the type, size, and lens angle of the endoscope used, the doses of any analgesic, sedative, or anesthetic agents used, and a statement of the level of consciousness of the subject in addition to a description of the other conditions of the examination.

Photography

Still photographic documentation of prolapse beyond Stage II may utilized both to document serial changes in individual patients and to illustrate findings for manuscripts and presentations. Photographs should contain an internal frame of reference such as a centimeter ruler or tape.

Imaging procedures

Different imaging techniques have been used to visualize pelvic floor anatomy, support defects, and relationships among adjacent organs.

These techniques may be more accurate than physical examination in determining which organs are involved in pelvic organ prolapse. However, they share the limitations of the other techniques in this section, i.e., a lack of standardization, validation, and/or availability. For this reason, no specific technique can be recommended but guidelines for reporting various techniques will be considered.

General guidelines for imaging procedures

Landmarks should be defined to allow comparisons with other imaging studies and the physical examination. The lower edge of the symphysis pubis should be given high priority as a landmark. Other examples of bony landmarks include the superior edge of the pubic symphysis, the ischial spine, the obturator foramen, and the promontory of the sacrum.

All reports on imaging techniques should specify the following:

a. position of the patient including the position of her legs. (Images in manuscripts should be oriented to reflect the patient's position when the study was performed and should not be oriented to suggest an erect position unless the patient was erect.);
b. specific verbal instructions given to the patient;
c. bladder volume and content and bowel content, including any pre-study preparations;
d. the performance and display of simultaneous monitoring such as pressure measurements that might be used to document that exposures were made at the most appropriate moment.

Ultrasonography

Continuous visualization of dynamic events is possible. All reports using ultrasound should include the following information:

a. transducer type and manufacturer (e.g., sector, linear, MHz);
b. transducer size;
c. transducer orientation;
d. route of scanning (e.g., abdominal, perineal, vaginal, rectal, urethral).

Contrast radiography

Contrast radiography may be static or dynamic and may include voiding colpo-cysto-urethrography, defecography, peritoneography, and pelvic fluoroscopy among others. All reports of contrast radiography should include the following information:

a. projection (e.g., lateral, frontal, horizontal, oblique);
b. type and amount of contrast media used and sequence of opacification of the bladder, vagina, rectum and colon, small bowel, and peritoneal cavity;
c. any urethral or vaginal appliance used (e.g., tampon, catheter, bead-chain);
d. type of exposures (e.g., single exposure, video);
e. magnification – an internal reference scale should be included.

Computed tomography and magnetic resonance imaging

These techniques do not allow for continuous imaging under dynamic conditions. Currently available equipment usually dictates supine scanning. Specifics of the technique should be specified including:

a. the specific equipment used, including the manufacturer;
b. the plane of imaging (e.g., axial, sagittal, coronal, oblique);
c. the field of view;
d. the thickness of sections and the number of slices;
e. the scan time;
f. the use and type of contrast;
g. the type of image analysis.

Surgical assessment

Intra-operative evaluation of pelvic support defects is intuitively attractive but as yet of unproven value. The effects of anesthesia, diminished muscle tone, and loss of consciousness are of unknown magnitude and direction. Limitations due to the position of the patient must also be evaluated.

PELVIC FLOOR MUSCLE TESTING

Pelvic floor muscles are voluntarily controlled, but selective contraction and relaxation necessitates muscle awareness. Optimal squeezing technique involves contraction of the pelvic floor muscles without contraction of the abdominal wall muscles and without a Valsalva maneuver. Squeezing synergists are the intraurethral and anal sphincteric muscles. In normal voiding, defecation, and optimal abdominal-strain voiding, the pelvic floor is relaxed, while the abdominal wall and the diaphragm may contract. With coughs and sneezes and often when other stresses are applied, the pelvic floor and abdominal wall are contracted simultaneously.

Evaluation and measurement of pelvic floor muscle function includes 1) an assessment of the patient's ability to contract and relax the pelvic muscles selectively (i.e., squeezing without abdominal straining and vice versa) and 2) measurement of the force (strength) of contraction.

There are pitfalls in the measurement of pelvic floor muscle function because the muscles are invisible to the investigator and because patients often simultaneously and erroneously activate other muscles. Contraction of the abdominal, gluteal, and hip adductor muscles, Valsalva maneuver, straining, breath holding, and forced inspirations are typically seen. These factors affect the reliability of available testing modalities and have to be taken into consideration in the interpretation of these tests.

The individual types of tests cited in this report are based both on the scientific literature and current clinical practice. It is the intent of the committee neither to endorse specific tests or techniques nor to restrict evaluations to the examples given. The standards recommended are intended to facilitate comparison of results obtained by different investigators and to allow investigators to replicate studies precisely.

For all types of measuring techniques the following should be specified:

a. patient position, including the position of the legs;
b. specific instructions given to the patient;
c. the status of bladder and bowel fullness;
d. techniques of quantification or qualification (estimated, calculated, directly measured);
e. the reliability of the technique.

Inspection

A visual assessment of muscle integrity, including a description of scarring and symmetry, should be performed. Pelvic floor contraction causes inward movement of the perineum and straining causes the opposite movement. Perineal movements can be observed directly or assessed indirectly by movement of an externally visible device placed into the vagina or urethra. The abdominal wall and other specified regions might be watched simultaneously. The type, size and placement of any device used should be specified as should the state of undress of the patient.

Palpation

Palpation may include digital examination of the pelvic floor muscles through the vagina or rectum as well as assessment of the perineum, abdominal wall, and/or other specified regions. The number of fingers and their position should be specified. Scales for the description of the strength of voluntary and reflex (e.g., with coughing) contractions and of the degree of voluntary relaxation should be clearly described and intra- and inter-observer reliability documented. Standardized palpation techniques could also be developed for the semiquantitative estimation of the bulk or thickness of pelvic floor musculature around the circumference of the genital hiatus. These techniques could allow for the localization of any atrophic or asymmetric segments.

Electromyography

Electromyography from the pelvic floor muscles can be recorded alone or in combination with other measurements. Needle electrodes permit visualization of individual motor unit action potentials, while surface or wire electrodes detect action potentials from groups of adjacent motor units underlying or surrounding the electrodes. Interpretation of signals from these latter electrodes must take into consideration that signals from erroneously contracted adjacent muscles may interfere with signals from the muscles of interest. Reports of electromyographic recordings should specify the following:

a. type of electrode;
b. placement of electrodes;
c. placement of reference electrode;
d. specifications of signal processing equipment;
e. type and specifications of display equipment;
f. muscle in which needle electrode is placed;
g. description of decision algorithms used by the analytic software.

Pressure recording

Measurements of urethral, vaginal, and anal pressures may be used to assess pelvic floor muscle control and strength. However, interpretations based on these pressure measurements must be made with a knowledge of their potential for artifact and their unproven or limited reproducibility. Anal sphincter contractions, rectal peristalsis, detrusor contractions, and abdominal straining can affect pressure measurements. Pressures recorded from the proximal vagina accurately mimic fluctuations in abdominal pressure. Therefore it may be important to compare vaginal pressures to simultaneously measured vesical or rectal pressures. Reports using pressure measurements should specify the following:

a. the type and size of the measuring device at the recording site (e.g., balloon, open catheter, etc);
b. the exact placement of the measuring device;
c. the type of pressure transducer;
d. the type of display system;
e. the display of simultaneous control pressures.

As noted in the section on *Inspection* (above), observation of the perineum is an easy and reliable way to assess for abnormal straining during an attempt at a pelvic muscle contraction. Significant straining or a Valsalva maneuver causes downward/caudal movement of the perineum; a correctly performed pelvic muscle contraction causes inward/cephalad movement of the perineum. Observation for perineal movement should be considered as an additional validation procedure whenever pressure measurements are recorded.

DESCRIPTION OF FUNCTIONAL SYMPTOMS

Functional deficits caused by pelvic organ prolapse and pelvic floor dysfunction are not well characterized or absolutely established. There is an ongoing need to develop, standardize, and validate various clinimetric scales such as condition-specific quality-of-life questionnaires for each of the four functional symptom groups (described below) thought to be related to pelvic organ prolapse.

Researchers in this area should try to use standardized and validated symptom scales whenever possible. **They must always ask precisely the same questions regarding functional symptoms before and after therapeutic intervention.** The description of functional symptoms should be directed toward four primary areas: 1) lower urinary tract, 2) bowel, 3) sexual, and 4) other local symptoms.

Urinary symptoms

This report does not supplant any currently approved ICS terminology related to lower urinary tract function.[1] However, some important prolapse related symptoms are not included in the current standards (e.g., the need to manually reduce the prolapse or assume an unusual position to initiate or complete micturition). Urinary symptoms that should be considered for dichotomous, ordinal, or visual analog scaling include, but are not limited to, the following:

a. stress incontinence
b. frequency (diurnal and nocturnal)
c. urgency
d. urge incontinence
e. hesitancy
f. weak or prolonged urinary stream
g. feeling of incomplete emptying
h. manual reduction of the prolapse to start or complete voiding
i. positional changes to start or complete voiding.

Bowel symptoms

Bowel symptoms that should be considered for dichotomous, ordinal, or visual analog scaling include, but are not limited to, the following:

a. difficulty with defecation
b. incontinence of flatus
c. incontinence of liquid stool
d. incontinence of solid stool
e. fecal staining of underwear
f. urgency of defecation
g. discomfort with defecation
h. digital manipulation of vagina or perineum to complete defecation
i. feeling of incomplete evacuation.

Sexual symptoms

Research is needed to attempt to differentiate the complex and multifactorial aspects of 'satisfactory sexual function' as it relates to pelvic organ prolapse and pelvic floor dysfunction. It may be difficult to distinguish between the ability to have vaginal intercourse and normal sexual function. The development of satisfactory tools will require multidisciplinary collaboration. Sexual function symptoms that should be considered for dichotomous, ordinal, or visual analog scaling include, but are not limited to, the following:

a. Is the patient sexually active?
b. If she is not sexually active, why?
c. Does sexual activity include vaginal coitus?
d. What is the frequency of vaginal intercourse?
e. Does the patient experience pain with coitus?
f. Is the patient satisfied with her sexual activity?
g. Has there been any change in orgasmic response?

Other local symptoms

We currently lack knowledge regarding the precise nature of symptoms that may be caused by the presence of a protrusion or bulge. Possible anatomically based symptoms that should be considered for dichotomous, ordinal, or visual analog scaling include, but are not limited to:

a. vaginal pressure or heaviness;

b. vaginal or perineal pain;

c. sensation or awareness of tissue protrusion from the vagina;

d. low back pain;

e. abdominal pressure or pain;

f. observation or palpation of a mass.

REFERENCE

1. Abrams P, Blaivas JG, Stanton SL, Andersen JT. The International Continence Society Committee on Standardization of Terminology. The standardization of terminology of lower urinary tract function. *Scand J Urol Nephrol* 1988; 114S: 5–19 [Also see Chapter 80.]

ACKNOWLEDGEMENTS

The subcommittee would like to acknowledge the contributions of the following consultants who contributed to the development and revision of this document:

W. Glenn Hurt, M.D., Richmond, VA, U.S.
Bernhard Schüssler, M.D., Luzern, Switzerland
L. Lewis Wall, M.D.D.Phil., New Orleans, LA, U.S.

Index